Ketogenic

The Science of Therapeutic Carbohydrate Restriction in Human Health

Ketogenic

The Science of Therapeutic Carbohydrate Restriction in Human Health

Edited by

Timothy David Noakes
Department of Health and Wellness Sciences, Cape Peninsula University of Technology, Cape Town, South Africa; Nutrition Network, Cape Town, South Africa

Tamzyn Murphy
Nutrition Network, Cape Town, South Africa

Neville Wellington
Nutrition Network, Cape Town, South Africa

Hassina Kajee
Nutrition Network, Cape Town, South Africa

Sarah M. Rice
Nutrition Network, Cape Town, South Africa

Managing Editors

Jayne Bullen
Nutrition Network, Cape Town, South Africa

Candice Egnos
Nutrition Network, Cape Town, South Africa

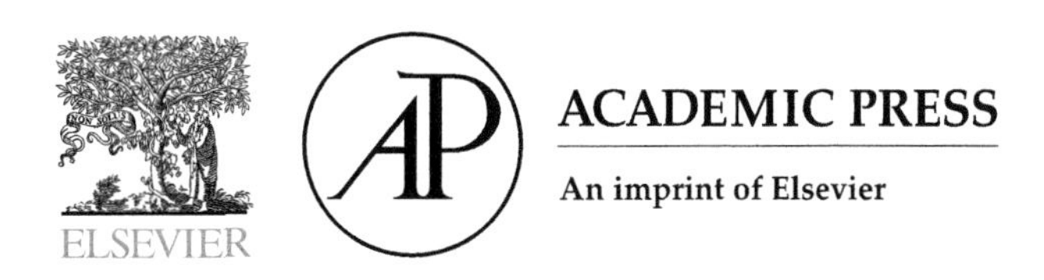

Academic Press is an imprint of Elsevier
125 London Wall, London EC2Y 5AS, United Kingdom
525 B Street, Suite 1650, San Diego, CA 92101, United States
50 Hampshire Street, 5th Floor, Cambridge, MA 02139, United States
The Boulevard, Langford Lane, Kidlington, Oxford OX5 1GB, United Kingdom

ISBN: 978-0-12-821617-0

For Information on all Academic Press publications
visit our website at https://www.elsevier.com/books-and-journals

Publisher: Nikki P. Levy
Acquisitions Editor: Nicole Denis
Editorial Project Manager: Lena Sparks
Production Project Manager: Bharatwaj Varatharajan
Cover Designer: Christian J. Bilbow

Typeset by MPS Limited, Chennai, India

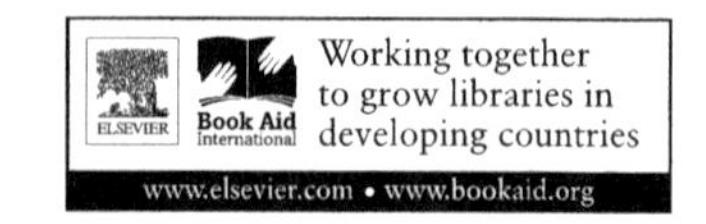

Contents

Part 4
Managing the patient

List of contributors

Joan Adams HPCSA Professional Conduct Commitee, Arcadia, Pretoria, South Africa

Ali Irshad Al Lawati Diwan of Royal Court, Muscat, Oman

Nadir Ali Webster, TX, United States

Gabriel Arismendi-Morillo Instituto de Investigaciones Biológicas, Facultad de Medicina, Universidad del Zulia, Maracaibo, Venezuela

Shawn Baker Revero, San Francisco, CA, United States

Miki Ben-Dor Department of Archaeology, Tel Aviv University, Tel Aviv, Israel

Miriam Berchuk Alberta Health Services, Calgary, Alberta, Canada

Amy Berger Nutritionist in Private Practice

Anne-Sophie Brazeau McGill University, Montreal, Canada

Natasha Campbell-McBride GAPS Science Foundation, Cambridge, United Kingdom

David Cavan Independent consultant, London, United Kingdom

Ann M. Childers Oregon City, OR, United States

Christos Chinopoulos Department of Medical Biochemistry, Semmelweis University, Budapest, Hungary

Catherine Crofts School of Interprofessional Health, Auckland University of Technology, Auckland, New Zealand

Mark Cucuzzella West Virginia University School of Medicine, Morgantown, WV, United States

Robert Cywes JSAPA Metabolic Centre, Jupiter, FL, United States

Trudi Deakin X-PERT Health, Hebden Bridge, West Yorkshire, United Kingdom

David M. Diamond University of South Florida, Tampa, FL, United States

Dominic P. D'Agostino Department of Molecular Pharmacology and Physiology, University of South Florida, Tampa, FL, United States

Georgia Edes Psychiatrist in Private Practice

Julienne Fenwick Best of both Wellness, Hermanus, Western Cape, South Africa

Gary Fettke Launceston, Tasmania, Australia

Mark I. Friedman Nutrition Science Initiative, San Diego, CA, United States

Jason Fung Scarborough Hospital Network, Scarborough, Ontario, Canada

Elizabeth Gonzalez UCF Medical School, Orlando, FL, United States

Cliff Harvey Holistic Performance Institute, Auckland, New Zealand

Michael Hoffmann University of Central Florida, Orlando, FL, United States; Orlando VA Medical Center, Orlando, FL, United States

Joan Ifland Food Addiction Reset LLC, Vashon, WA, United States

Diana Isaacs Cleveland Clinic, Cleveland, OH, United States

Hassina Kajee Nutrition Network, Cape Town, South Africa

Miriam Kalamian Dietary Therapies LLC, Hamilton, MT, United States

Bob Kaplan Independent researcher, Wayland, MA, United States

Daniel Katambo Afyaplanet, Dagoretti Corner, Nairobi, Kenya

Eric H. Kossoff Departments of Neurology and Paediatrics, Johns Hopkins Hospital, Baltimore, MD, United States

Meredith M. Kossoff Cornell University, Ithaca, NY, United States

Ian Lake Aspen Medical Practice, Gloucester, United Kingdom; Everyone Health, Cambridge, United Kingdom; The Fasting Method, New York City, NY, United States

Brian Lenzkes Internal Medicine, San Diego, CA, United States

Sean McKelvey Institute for Personalized Nutrition Therapy, Vancouver, Canada

Nafeeza Hj Mohd Ismail School of Medicine, International Medical University, Kuala Lumpur, Federal Territory of Kuala Lumpur, Malaysia

Purna Mukherjee Biology Department, Boston College, Boston, MA, United States

Campbell Murdoch Millbrook Surgery, Somerset, United Kingdom

Tamzyn Murphy Nutrition Network, Cape Town, South Africa

Timothy David Noakes Department of Health and Wellness Sciences, Cape Peninsula University of Technology, Cape Town, South Africa; Nutrition Network, Cape Town, South Africa

Connor Ostoich Scarborough Hospital Network, Scarborough, Ontario, Canada

Amber O'Hearn Independent Researcher, Toronto, Canada

Nadia Pataguana Public Health Collaboration, United Kingdom

David Perlmutter American Nutrition Association, Hinsdale, IL, United States; University of Miami Miller School of Medicine, Miami, FL, United States

Graham Phillips iHeart Pharmacy Group, Hertfordshire, United Kingdom

Mathew C.L. Phillips Waikato Hospital, Hamilton, New Zealand

Laurie Rauch Physiological Sciences, Faculty of Health Sciences, University of Cape Town, Cape Town, South Africa

Sarah M. Rice Nutrition Network, Cape Town, South Africa

Karen Riley Institute for Personalized Nutrition Therapy, Vancouver, Canada

Caroline Roberts Virta Health, Denver, CO, United States

Elisa Marie Rossi UCF Medical School, Orlando, FL, United States

Fabian Rossi UCF Medical School, Orlando, FL, United States; Clinical Neurophysiology Lab, Orlando VA Medical Center, Orlando, FL, United States

Joshua Rossi UCF Medical School, Orlando, FL, United States

Catherine Saenz Exercise Science, Ohio State University, Columbus, OH, United States

Thomas N. Seyfried Biology Department, Boston College, Boston, MA, United States

James Smith Division of Exercise Science and Sports Medicine, University of Cape Town, Cape Town, South Africa

Angela A. Stanton Stanton Migraine Protocol, Anaheim, CA, United States

Mateja Stephanovic Scarborough Hospital Network, Scarborough, Ontario, Canada

Martha Tettenborn Kemble, Ontario, Canada

David Unwin Norwood Surgery, Southport, United Kingdom

Jen Unwin Norwood Surgery, Southport, United Kingdom

Christopher Webster Division of Exercise Science and Sports Medicine, University of Cape Town, Cape Town, South Africa

Neville Wellington Private Practice, Cape Town, South Africa; Kenilworth Diabetes Medical Centre, Cape Town, South Africa; Nutrition Network, Cape Town, Western Cape, South Africa

Eric C. Westman Division of General Internal Medicine, Department of Medicine, Duke University Medical Centre, Durham, NC, United States

Nasha Winters Metabolic Terrain Institute of Health, Wilmington, DE, United States

Susan Wolver VCU Medical Weight Loss Program, Richmond, VA, United States

William S. Yancy, Jr. Division of General Internal Medicine, Department of Medicine, Duke University Medical Centre, Durham, NC, United States; Center of Innovation to Accelerate Discovery and Practice Transformation, Durham Veterans Affairs Medical Centre, Durham, NC, United States; Duke Diet and Fitness Centre, Duke University Health System, Durham, NC, United States

Caryn Zinn Auckland University of Technology, Auckland, New Zealand

Preface

(Robert) Atkins reinvented the nineteenth century Banting diet in 1963, although it took another 30 years to reach prime time in the public consciousness. His regimen closely resembled the 'Eskimo diet' that Joslin had inflicted upon his mother in 1898 [1], the actual Inuit diet advocated for health reasons by the explorer Vilhjalmur Stefansson [2] and the diet tested upon overweight DuPont executives by Alfred Pennington in the 1930s. It should by now come as no surprise to the reader that the new diet worked (for some), generated passion, was condemned, vindicated, grudgingly accepted and finally forgotten.

L. Sawyer and A.M. Gale. Diet, delusion and diabetes. *Diabetologia* 2009, 52, 4.

My dietary Damascene moment occurred on a Saturday morning in December 2010. Probably not by chance, perhaps by divine intervention, I was introduced to the book – The New Atkins for a New You [3] – written by Drs Eric Westman, Steve Phinney and Jeff Volek. At first I was mortified. How, I wondered, could these three associate with the man whose promotion of a diet loaded with 'artery-clogging' saturated fats would send all its followers to an early grave?

My instant of doubt occurred as I read the foreword to their book:

In more than 150 articles these three international experts on the use of the low-carbohydrate diets to combat obesity, high cholesterol and Type-2 diabetes mellitus have led the way in repeatedly proving how a low-carbohydrate approach is superior to a low-fat one.

How could this possibly be credible, I wondered. Not once in my academic training had I been introduced to any of these concealed studies. But who was I to believe? These three dissidents? Or my heavily credential academic mentors, all of whom had taught me their shared version of what constitutes a healthy diet during my medical training in Cape Town? And all of whom had convinced me to eat and promote their 'heart-healthy', prudent, low-fat, 1977 US Dietary Guidelines diet pyramid, 'in moderation', which I did, dutifully, for the next 34 years.

But within 2 hours of opening the three dissidents' book, the scales of those lost years fell from my eyes. The secreted scientific evidence that they presented appeared overwhelming. Like Saul, I was now on the road to a transformation of holy proportions. That same day I began my personal experiment with the low-carbohydrate high-(healthy) fat (LCHF) diet, also known as therapeutic carbohydrate restriction (TCR). And the rest, as they say, is now history.

Why was this personal experience which I suspect is shared by the majority of, if not all, the authors of this magnum opus, so necessary for us to arrive at a carefully concealed truth?

The likely explanation is that all of us share a common metabolism, present also in most of those now living in the developed and developing world. Our metabolism is simply not designed to cope with foods that raise our blood glucose and insulin concentrations every few hours, daily, 350 days a year for decades; a diet high in carbohydrates that in our ignorance, most of us have promoted since at least 1977. The diet that, we eventually realized, had made us sick and unhealthy and, in my case, caused me also to develop type 2 diabetes (T2D).

But the only way our programmed stupidities would ever admit that revelation was when we finally summoned the courage to ignore everything our education had taught us about 'healthy' diets, and, instead, to do the exact opposite. After which we experienced the full range of dramatic health transformations that are described in these pages and which in my case, included putting my T2D into a medically impossible remission.

Without that common experience, there would not have been authors to explain these truths.

The idea of compiling this textbook with the goal of educating healthcare providers of these realities and how best they might assist the world's neglected metabolic majority was not mine. It came from the team at The Noakes Foundation, most especially Drs Hassina Kajee and Neville Wellington, and our CEO, Jayne Bullen, together with Candice Egnos. They argued that a novel medical discipline often requires the compilation of a textbook to show sceptical healthcare providers that, yes, there is indeed a large body of published scientific evidence backed up by extensive clinical experience, examining TCR. What is more, this published evidence establishes that TCR is entirely safe and highly effective in the management of a wide range of chronic medical conditions.

But without the support of our 62 expert contributors, each of whom provided their expertise without any thoughts of personal remuneration, we could not have amassed this information.

Ultimately, this work reflects the combined contribution of those selfless individuals. But that is just the nature of the professionals involved in promoting TCR and the LCHF lifestyle. The message, not the individual, is what is ultimately important. Thank you all for your generosity, your courage, and your determination to change the future course of healthcare across the globe.

For what their contributions establish once and for all is that the popular opinion that TCR has no evidence-based support is nonsensical. Instead, this textbook definitively establishes that TCR is perhaps the most studied and definitely the most effective dietary intervention known to modern medicine. In these pages, you will find the hardcore scientific evidence to support that judgement.

We invite you to test that opinion by examining what we have jointly contributed.

Perhaps, like us, in these pages you will discover your own Damascene revelation.

Timothy David Noakes
Department of Health and Wellness Sciences, Cape Peninsula University of Technology, Cape Town, South Africa
Emeritus Professor, Division of Exercise Science and Sports Medicine, University of Cape Town, Cape Town, South Africa
Sports Science Institute of South Africa, Cape Town, South Africa
Nutrition Network, Cape Town, South Africa
The Noakes Foundation, Cape Town, South Africa
Eat Better South Africa, Cape Town, South Africa

References

[1] Joslin EP. Treatment of Diabetes Mellitus. 2nd ed. Philadelphia: Lea and Ferbiger; 1917.

[2] Lieb CW. The effect of an exclusive, long-continued meat diet. Based on the history, experiences and clinical survey of Vilhjalmur Stefansson, Arctic explorer. J Am Med Assoc 1926;87:25–6.

[3] Westman EC, Phinney SD, Volek JS. The New Atkins for the New You. *The Ultimate Diet for Shedding Weight and Feeling Great.* New York, NY.: Atria Books; 2010.

Introduction

At the time the low carbohydrate movement exploded into mainstream science, there was a disjointed scientific community of practitioner pioneers dotted around the globe.

Reducing carbohydrate intake a decade ago was considered a fad diet, something that will pass like many other things that have contested the incorrect dietary guidelines. The same guidelines have contributed to an epidemic of diabetes, obesity and most other chronic and metabolic diseases [1,2]. There were a few strong global voices and pillared efforts to do something in the area, flying flags and sharing good research, but it seemed that no one in policy and dietary guidance was listening. As the new science emerged, it was clear that we had to move forward in a more cohesive and evidence-based way.

Industry was running rife with diabetes and obesity, along with the many other syndromes that we now know are connected to the broader, complex condition known as insulin resistance; they were slowly building momentum and becoming the dire health tsunami we now face and are stuck with as a planet. Healthcare is now doing the tireless, unrewarding work of mopping them up, with little success.

Healthcare workers at the time were getting their continued professional development notches from fancy pharmaceuticals-funded events that came with sweet treats and sweet handshakes [3]. These meetings between doctors and big pharma led, and sadly still lead today, to the branded prescription book for patients [3].

One could call it industry-driven science and learning. We were in a situation where a patient would go to a doctor for medical advice for a chronic condition that was just rearing its head and leave with advice and/or medication that would be guaranteed, for the most part, to make them ill and possibly do more harm than good over time.

When we look back on the past 50 years of global treatment of disease, we see a scary evolving picture. The food industry, and big food in particular, influences consumer choice and shapes demand. Highly processed, addictive foods influence consumer taste and choices [4]. Along with processing and flavour additives, the demand for sugar has escalated at an unimaginable rate, which has fueled the demand for more [4]! Sugar addiction and the addiction to highly processed, often high fat carbohydrate laden foods, fueled by the low fat generation, lay the foundations for a silent health tsunami on a scale no one in the 60s could ever have foreseen or predicted. But here we are today, dealing with a massively obese, diabetic, hypertensive population. Children are having early onset diabetes and fatty liver disease [5] and paediatric bariatric surgery presents ethical dilemmas [6,7] such that alternative approaches demand consideration [8,9].

The simple truth is that we need a full societal change in the way that diet and lifestyle are treated. They need to be brought back into the core principles and ethical tenets of medicine. Doctors and healthcare have to start refocussing on the somehow forgotten link between a patient's landscape, what they eat and their health. By landscape, I mean the trauma they may face, their stress levels, sleep, exercise patterns and the quality of their lives. We need a full change in the way that we eat and understand diet and its role in our health.

Unable to find answers from their doctors, patients would write to us at The Noakes Foundation, asking Prof Noakes why their doctors would not support their successes on the then called Banting diet.

"I have lost 32 kgs, am off all my medications and my diabetes/hypertension have reversed, but my doctor will not agree that I am on the right path" was the kind of email we were getting regularly, far too often to ignore.

We started to look for doctors who understood how to help these patients, for referral reasons, and apart from those who are now our medical directors, they were few and far between.

We knew that we had to build a practising community of some kind to support patients, via their doctors, to make them better and improve their lives. And clearly, we had no time to waste!

Fast track several years and we have now taken over 20 trainings to the medical community and trained thousands of medical professionals around the world in how to apply this simple dietary advice to patient care responsibly, meaningfully, robustly and confidently. We have a huge and growing body of evidence alongside global partners and hubs of excellence in all areas of life.

This textbook was developed as a reference guide to support our medical community adjacent to their training. This essential approach to the treatment of the plethora of medical conditions with metabolic underpinnings (not least among these, type 2 diabetes, hypertension and obesity) has to be clearly included in medicine in the future, in significant mainstream ways.

What we know now is the following:

- Changing the way dietary medicine is approached will require a huge, systemic societal shift
- This implies that all areas of society are impacted: what we eat, how we eat and how we get food to people around the world is a multifactorial and complex story that is associated with our climate, ecology, community, history, beliefs, ancestry and also our genetics and beliefs.

When looking at the physiological impact of insulin resistance and its ability to affect most or all systems of the body, the complexity of this particular project is immense. It requires a massive scope of specialisations, broad and different areas of medicine and pathophysiology and a deep, complex understanding of disease pathways and progression. I would like to thank and take a deep bow to the extraordinary professionals from so many fields and places in the world who agreed to write, contribute, edit and co-create this essential piece of literature.

We are honoured to have been able to publish this volume of knowledge in this way and with this degree of expertise, knowledge, care, precision, depth and, also, love and are deeply grateful to our incredible, committed team of researchers, editors, scientists and doctors who hold this space and know beyond any doubt that:

Integratively applied, this knowledge is already changing and will change the face of health for our planet.

The science is now overwhelming, and it is essential to put this evidence in the public domain in a way that can make a real difference to people's lives, alongside old medical textbooks. It can no longer be ignored or set aside or passed off for a medication manual. Diabetes, alongside its related metabolic diseases, can and will no longer be considered a terminal disease because in light of the evidence presented in this textbook, its patients and treating practitioners will no longer accept or allow that to happen, when appropriate dietary intervention can change lives.

Our immense gratitude goes to Prof Tim Noakes for his tireless work in Challenging Beliefs and uncovering the errors in science, to Elsevier for taking on this big idea with and for us, and then to each of our 62 contributors, 7 editors and 5 reviewers for their tireless hard work in taking this book to print. Huge congratulations to the team at Nutrition Network for the years of tirelessly working on this book and its content and in particular to Tamzyn Murphy for her exceptional editing.

Really, when it comes to this body of work, manifest into this profound and important book, only two words apply:

Sorry to the millions that have succumbed to diseases that they should not have due to false dietary information and incorrect nutritional science that they listened to, and

Thank you to the thousands who are part of this massive change that is manifesting, helping to secure future healthy outcomes for humanity.

We have a lot of work to do.

Jayne Bullen
Nutrition Network, Cape Town, South Africa
The Noakes Foundation, Cape Town, South Africa
Eat Better South Africa, Cape Town, South Africa

References

[1] Harcombe Z, Baker JS, Cooper SM, Davies B, Sculthorpe N, DiNicolantonio JJ, et al. Evidence from randomised controlled trials did not support the introduction of dietary fat guidelines in 1977 and 1983: a systematic review and meta-analysis. Open Heart 2015;2(1):e000196.
[2] O'Keefe J. Problems with the 2015 Dietary Guidelines for Americans: an alternative. Missouri medicine 2016;113:74–8.
[3] Amazon.com: Bad Pharma: How Drug Companies Mislead Doctors and Harm Patients. Goldacre, Ben: Books [Internet]. [cited 2022 Aug 15]. 9780865478008. Available from: https://www.amazon.com/Bad-Pharma-Companies-Mislead-Patients/dp/0865478007.
[4] Schiestl ET, Rios JM, Parnarouskis L, Cummings JR, Gearhardt AN. A narrative review of highly processed food addiction across the lifespan. Prog Neuropsychopharmacol Biol Psychiatry 2021;106:110152.
[5] Schwarz JM, Noworolski SM, Erkin-Cakmak A, Korn NJ, Wen MJ, Tai VW, et al. Effects of dietary fructose restriction on liver fat, de novo lipogenesis, and insulin kinetics in children with obesity. Gastroenterology. 2017;153(3):743–52.
[6] Hofmann B. Bariatric surgery for obese children and adolescents: a review of the moral challenges. BMC Med Ethics 2013;14:18.
[7] Moreira LAC. Ética e aspectos psicossociais em crianças e adolescentes candidatos a cirurgia bariátrica. Rev Bioét 2017;25(1):101–10.
[8] Cakmak HM, Ilknur Arslanoglu, Sungur MA, Bolu S. Clinical picture at attendance and response to flexible family based low-carb life style change in children with obesity. Int J Child Health Nutr 2021;10(1):9–16.
[9] Zinn C, Lenferna De La Motte KA, Rush A, Johnson R. Assessing the nutrient status of low carbohydrate, high-fat (LCHF) meal plans in children: a hypothetical case study design. Nutrients. 2022;14(8):1598.

Part 1

Nutritional fundamentals

Chapter 1

Understanding human diet, disease, and insulin resistance: scientific and evolutionary perspectives

Timothy David Noakes[1,2], Catherine Crofts[3] and Miki Ben-Dor[4]

[1]*Department of Health and Wellness Sciences, Cape Peninsula University of Technology, Cape Town, South Africa,* [2]*Nutrition Network, Cape Town, South Africa,* [3]*School of Interprofessional Health, Auckland University of Technology, Auckland, New Zealand,* [4]*Department of Archaeology, Tel Aviv University, Tel Aviv, Israel*

1.1 Understanding human diet and disease – the scientific and evolutionary evidence

1.1.1 Evolutionary evidence: the species-specific natural human diet

1.1.1.1 Defining a species specific diet

The success of a species is determined by its ability to survive and to procreate. The primary condition for survival is the ability to acquire and assimilate a sufficient quantity of appropriate food, daily. This food must be secured in competition with other animals and then eaten, digested, and absorbed to serve either as energy or as nutrients for other bioprocesses.

Thus, in competition with other species, all living creatures are under constant evolutionary pressure to optimise their bodily structures efficiently to acquire, eat, digest, and metabolise specific foods in an environment that is as favourable to those needs as is possible. But no animal can adapt to eating all the foods that are available in any particular environment.

Evolution is a process of selection between alternative solutions to these challenges, under the constant pressure of trade-offs. 'The concept of trade-offs underpins much of the research in evolutionary organismal biology, physiology, behavioural ecology, and functional morphology' [1].

With regard to food choices, this means that every adaptation to the consumption of one type of food may make an animal less able to obtain, digest, or metabolise another type of food. When hominins descended from the trees, some six million years ago, and began to exploit more terrestrial resources, the shape of their bodies changed to favour bipedal locomotion. This in turn allowed hominins to cover long distances on land and to view the landscape from a greater height.

However, bipedal locomotion meant hominins became less effective than other competing primates at acquiring high-hanging fruits [2]. Having their noses at a higher level, far from the ground, also impaired their ability to track other animals by smell and to locate underground food sources. But by developing a larger brain, they were better able to obtain meat without the need for speed or other key physical features of other predators with whom they were in competition [3]. However, to offset the greatly increased energy demand of the larger brain, hominins had to reduce the size of their energetically expensive gut by as much as 40% [4]. This decrease in gut size caused a substantial reduction in the ability to ferment highly fibrous plant-based food sources in a much shortened large bowel (colon).

Thus, this newly acquired ability to obtain meat from animal sources came with a significant trade-off – a diminished capacity to extract nutrients from lower quality, fibrous plants and fruits. The internal structure of the gut also had to change substantially, further limiting humans' future food choices.

In summary, evolution is very much a process of trade-offs, surrendering one ability in order to obtain another. In nutritional terms, evolution leads to optimal but different diets for all the different species on the planet. We now refer to each of these different diets as the natural (species-specific) diet for that species.

Ketogenic. DOI: https://doi.org/10.1016/B978-0-12-821617-0.00011-5

1.1.1.2 The herbivorous gut

With the adoption of agriculture approximately 11,500 years ago, humans, specifically adapted for animal food consumption, needed to bypass some of these physiological evolutionary constraints by adopting plant-sourced foods as a primary food type. This involved a critical switch from what is the species-specific natural human diet. As will be shown later in the chapter, the more recent introduction of novel industrially produced, highly addictive foods made predominantly from grains, seed oils, and sugar or high fructose corn syrup has been associated with profoundly deleterious physiological consequences for all humans.

We begin by reconstructing how humans' species-specific natural diet came about. Although humans are the descendants of primates, we evolved to eat differently.

Chimpanzees, our closest phylogenetic relatives, have eaten the same diet for the past six million years comprising, for the most part, fibre-laden fruits, plant stems, and leaves, with a small additional contribution from meat [5].

The challenge posed for all mammals eating a plant-based diet is that none has the capacity to digest the cellulose (fibre) that forms the cell lining of all plants. To overcome this deficiency, mammals eating plant materials have developed a symbiotic relationship with anaerobic gut bacteria. Billions of anaerobic bacteria are given safe residence in specially adapted intestinal organs, where they busily ferment ingested cellulose into usable mammalian food. In chimpanzees, this special organ is a voluminous large bowel (colon), making chimpanzees 'hindgut fermenters' [6], a feature they share with horses, pigs, zebras, elephants, warthogs, rhinoceroses, rabbits and other rodents. In other grass-eating ruminants, including cattle, sheep, antelope, and gazelles, the special fermenting organ is a four-chambered stomach in the foregut. Hence they are referred to as 'foregut fermenters'.

The basis for this mammal-bacteria symbiosis is that, in exchange for an environment where they can safely reproduce, the bacteria convert the cellulose into a form of saturated fat called volatile short-chain fatty acids, on which the host mammal bases its existence [7]. The important point is this: grass-eating ruminants convert 100% nutrient-poor carbohydrate food (grass) into the energy-dense saturated fatty acids that are essential for mammalian survival. When humans eat those ruminants, that process also ensures our survival.

To summarise, the specifically adapted fore- and hind- guts of herbivores can rightly be labelled super-specialised organs for manufacturing saturated fats from cellulose. All plant-eating mammals use that cellulose as the growth medium for the bacteria in their intestines. These bacteria then produce the fatty acids that are missing in the nutrient-poor grass, roots, fruits, and shoots on which these mammals must survive. What is more, when absorbed by the herbivores' intestines, the cell bodies of these dead bacteria provide the protein needed for their own tissue growth.

1.1.1.3 Specialised omnivores

In the pre-agricultural era, humans were the only primates able to source and to survive on a completely carnivorous diet. Omnivory is defined as the ability to obtain energy from two or more trophic levels of food sources, in the case of humans, from both animals and plants. A common belief is that humans are omnivores and thus have substantial flexibility in their food choices. However, this human *potential* for omnivory means that humans can, at least acutely, replace animal-based foods with plant-sourced foods should that choice be imposed by constraints in their natural environment. It does not indicate that omnivory is the sole dietary choice for humans.

When living in their natural environments, omnivorous species are seldom fully adapted to obtain their nutrition equally from more than one trophic level of food. Chimpanzees, for example, are omnivores since they consume meat on occasion. However chimpanzees are unable to compensate for the dietary deficiencies caused by a lack of fruit, by simply switching to eating more meat as the dominant component of their diet. Chimpanzees simply do not have the biological capabilities to obtain enough meat to avoid starvation if fruits and plants suddenly became unavailable. Designed by a specific evolutionary history, their morphology and physiology have adapted chimpanzees to live in trees where they are best able to obtain and digest fruits and shoots. Alternatively, wolves can gorge on berries during the summer and autumn. But they are far better equipped to hunt animals; making them specialised carnivores but, at the same time, facultative omnivores.

The energetic returns for modern hunter-gatherers from hunting animals are tens of times greater than the returns from gathering plants (tables 3 and 4 in Ref. [8]). In the past, this difference would have been even greater due to the relatively greater abundance of large animals compared to edible plants [9]. To obtain the equivalent amount of energy from the environment, a human who had to 'shop in nature's supermarket' in the pre-agricultural era, would have had to 'pay' tenfold more in energetic terms to gather and consume plants than to hunt animals.

This means that early humans could not easily have switched from animals to plants as a food source. Thus it is perhaps not surprising that among mammals, most omnivores are specialised, consuming over 70% of their food from either plant or animal sources.

1.1.1.4 Did all early humans eating their species-specific natural diet have a shortened life-expectancy?

A common misconception is that all humans eating the pre-industrial species-specific human diet died at a young age. This would indicate that modern humans would be ill-advised to adopt that specific diet.

This misconception is based on the finding that modern human life expectancy at birth is twice that of humans living in the pre-industrial era. However, this is potentially misleading because the rate of death at birth or shortly thereafter was 100 times greater in the past than it is today (fig. 7 in Ref. [10]). So to compensate for the large number of infants dying before the age of one in the pre-industrial era, an equal number of adults would have had to live to age 70 to produce an overall average life expectancy of 35 years.

Moreover, recent studies of modern hunter-gatherers find that most adult hunter-gatherers who reach maturity survive to become grandparents, despite an absence of protection from predators and without access to the medical and sanitary services that modern societies provide [10].

We can now turn to a more complete reconstruction of the natural, species-specific evolutionary human diet.

1.1.1.5 Reconstructing the natural, species-specific, evolutionary human diet

The natural diets of most living species can be determined by observing what those species eat in their natural environments. However, humans have progressed far from the state in which they and their ancestors lived for millions of years; first by domesticating their food sources during the last 10,000 years, and more recently by industrialising the production of the foods we now eat.

In an attempt to reconstruct our ancestors' diet, intuitively we turn to archaeologists who dig *Homo*'s base camps that are millions of years old. But if we rely only on the pre-historical archaeological record, with its thousands of sites containing fossilised animal bones including just a few sites with plant residues, we might conclude that humans are specialised hypercarnivores. However this archaeological view of the natural human diet is biased by the different preservation potentials of plant and animal remains over millions of years. Therefore, while archaeology can reveal a great deal about what animal foods we ate, it tells us very little about the relative contribution of animals or plants to the diet eaten by early hominins.

Consequently, most scientists attempting to reconstruct the natural human diet have focused on the food choices of modern hunter-gatherer groups in remote corners of the world [11–18]. But more recent research shows that modern ecological conditions are so different from those that prevailed during the long history of human evolution that this information does not provide a valid measure of the natural species-specific human diet [9,19–21].

So, if we cannot rely on the archaeological record and recent ethnographic observations, where do we find the best evidence for what constitutes the natural, species-specific human diet?

The growth of paleobiology as a vibrant scientific discipline provides the basis for a different approach to rediscover the natural human diet [22]. This approach assumes that the shape of the human body, the structure of our organs, our genetic composition, and our metabolism are largely the result of adaptations to our species-specific diet during our evolution as the genus *Homo*. Paleobiology enables a review of unique features in human morphology and physiology which can only have developed in humans that eat a species-specific diet [20,21].

Table 1.1. lists 14 biological human features which indicate that a specialised carnivorous diet drove human evolution, with plants as a fall-back food. Additional evidence from archaeology, palaeontology, and zoology support the conclusion that humans evolved as hypercarnivores, obtaining at least 70% of their calories from animal-sourced foods [19,21]. Increased consumption of plant-sourced foods becomes evident only toward the end of the Pleistocene, 80,000–15,000 years ago. By which time *Homo sapiens* had been established as a distinct species for more than 200,000 years.

1.1.1.6 The critical role of animal fat in human evolution

The evidence that humans were carnivorous during the Palaeolithic period has important implications for our understanding of the biology of fat and protein consumption and metabolism in humans. Carnivores have a large capacity to consume protein for energy. Cats, for example, can obtain over 70% of their energy from the metabolism of protein [55]. Consumption of protein for energy requires the removal of the toxic nitrogen element from the protein molecule.

TABLE 1.1 Biological features and other evidence for the evolution of humans as specialised carnivores (Extended explanations can be found in Ben-Dor et al. [21]).

Biological feature	Explanation
High energy requirements	Humans have high energetic requirements for a given body mass. Hunting provides tenfold higher energetic return than does the consumption of plants (tables 3 and 4 in Ref. [8]) [23].
Large brain	In primates, a larger brain is associated with the consumption of high-quality, high-energy, and nutrient-dense foods. Having the largest brain among primates, humans targeted the highest energy and nutrient-dense foods, specifically animal fats and proteins [24,25] (brain size declined at an exponentially increasing rate during the terminal Pleistocene and subsequent Holocene (40,000 years ago to recent time)). Over this period, diet quality declined as humans increased their consumption of plants [26].
Higher fat reserves	With much larger body fat reserves than primates, humans are uniquely adapted to survive prolonged periods without eating [27]. This adaptation allowed survival during those frequent periods when contact with large hunted prey was erratic.
Fat metabolism	There is evidence for substantial genetic changes that allow for greater fat metabolism in *Homo*. Genetic changes in the FADS (fatty acid desaturase) gene in African humans 85,000 years ago allowed for a slight increase in the conversion of linolenic acid (the plant docosahexaenoic acid (DHA) precursor) to DHA [28,29].
Adaptation to higher fat consumption	The study of Swain-Lenz et al. [30] 'suggests that humans shutdown regions of the genome to accommodate a high-fat diet while chimpanzees open regions of the genome to accommodate a high sugar diet'.
Late adaptations to consumption of tubers	Groups that consume high quantities of tubers have specific genetic adaptations to deal with the toxins and antinutrients present in tubers. Other humans are not well adapted to consume large quantities of tubers [31].
Stomach acidity	Higher stomach acidity is found in carnivores. Higher stomach acidity inactivates meat-borne pathogens. Stomach acidity in humans is even higher than in carnivores, probably to deal with higher pathogen load, due to the continuous consumption of carcasses of large prey over days and weeks [32].
Insulin resistance (IR)	Carnivores have a natural state of IR. This reduces their reliance on smaller carbohydrate (glucose/glycogen) reserves. Humans may develop IR when eating a carbohydrate-rich diet. Herders have higher IR than farmers [33,34].
Gut morphology	Human's gut morphology and relative size are fundamentally different from those of chimpanzees. Longer small intestine and a shorter large intestine, as found in humans, are the typical morphological features of the carnivore's gut [35].
Mastication	Humans show a reduced size of the masticatory system, already present in *H. erectus*, compared to early hominins, who relied on terrestrial vegetation as a primary food source. This is compatible with meat and fat consumption [4,36].
Postcranial morphology	Unique postcranial morphological features of *Homo* include the following: (1) increased body size in *H. erectus*; (2) set of adaptations to endurance running in *H. erectus*, useful in hunting, especially in the heat; (3) shoulders adapted to spear-throwing in *H. erectus* [37–39].
Adipocyte morphology	Similar to the adipocyte morphology in carnivores: '...the energy metabolism of humans is adapted to a diet in which lipids and proteins rather than carbohydrates, make a major contribution to the energy supply' [40].
Age at weaning	Carnivores wean at a younger age, as do humans. Early weaning 'highlight(s) the emergence of carnivory as a process fundamentally determining human evolution' [41].
Longevity	Kaplan et al. [42] hypothesised that due to a prolonged childhood, the survival of a large fraction of each group of humans depended on the presence of experienced hunters. Extended longevity in humans may have evolved to allow the survival of these hunters, whose hunting proficiency peaks by age 40.

(Continued)

TABLE 1.1 (Continued)

Biological feature	Explanation
Archaeology	
Stone tools	Stone tools that are specific to plant food utilisation only appeared around 40,000 years ago. Their prevalence increases just before the appearance of agriculture [43].
Zooarchaeology	Evidence of access to large prey first appears in *H. erectus* archaeological sites 1.5 million years ago. Humans even hunted large carnivores [44,45].
Targeting fat	At substantial energetic costs, humans concentrated on hunting the fattest animals; they preferentially carried fatty animal parts back to base camps and exploited bone fat [46,47].
Stable Isotopes	Nitrogen isotope measurements of human fossil collagen residues are the most extensively used method for determining what humans ate in the last 50,000 years. All studies show that humans were highly carnivorous until very late, ending just before the appearance of modern agriculture (Table in Ref. [21]); [48].
Dental pathology	Dental caries, evidence of substantial consumption of carbohydrates, appeared only some 15,000 years ago in groups with evidence of plant food consumption [49].
Behavioural adaptations	A comparison of human behaviour patterns with those of chimpanzees and social carnivores shows that humans have carnivore-like behaviour patterns. Food sharing, alloparenting, labour division, and social flexibility are among the typical behaviours of carnivores [50].
Palaeontology	Evidence that hunting by *H. erectus* 1.5 million years ago was associated with the extinction of several large, but not smaller, carnivores. This suggests that *H. erectus* became a member of the large carnivores' guild [51]. Extinctions of large herbivores were associated with the arrival of humans on continents and islands, for example, in Australia and the Americas [52].
Zoology	Amongst the carnivores, predation on large prey is exclusively associated with hypercarnivory. Humans were predators of large prey [19–21,53,54].

However, humans have a limited capacity to perform this removal. It is estimated that nitrogen removal becomes limiting when protein intake exceeds 35%–45% of the total caloric intake [56]. This limitation means that 55%–65% of calories in the human diet must come from animal fat or from fat and carbohydrates in plant materials. Since humans were hunters of large animals and large animals store over 50% of their calories as fat [19], it may be deduced that fat provided a very high percentage of the ingested calories of early humans.

A comprehensive review led Jochim [57] to formulate the Fat Hypothesis, which proposes that a hunted prey's fat content was an essential criterion that directed early humans' hunting decisions. He writes [[57], p. 87]: 'The most efficient procurement of fatty meat is given priority over that of lean meat in the decision-making process, as is that of big meat package over small'. At times, the hunted prey was abandoned once it was deemed fatless [58,59]. Humans preferentially hunted large animals as they contained a higher body fat content [19,47,60]. They specifically exploited those animal body parts that contain greater amounts of fat [61,62]. They also selectively hunted adult prey in their physical prime because this group of animals contains more fat than do the easier-to-catch younger and older animals [19,63]. Finally, at great energetic expense, they extracted fat by boiling bones [46,64].

In summary, the physiological and archaeological evidence supports the conclusion that the natural species-specific human diet involved the daily consumption of significant amounts of animal fat and protein.

1.1.1.7 Summary of evidence for the species-specific natural human diet

The evidence presented here and elsewhere [20,21] strongly supports the hypothesis that humans evolved to become specialised carnivores. This dietary pattern lasted until very late into the Pleistocene period, approximately 15,000 years ago. A slight modification towards a greater inclusion of plants may have started in Africa some 85,000 years ago. This is suggested by changes in the FADS group of genes. That trend has increased in intensity towards the arrival of the Neolithic culture and the beginning of agriculture, starting between 11,000 and 5000 years ago, depending on the geographic region.

It is clear from the evidence presented in Table 1.1 that the evolutionary adaptations to the consumption of large quantities of meat and fat remain deeply embedded in human biology.

1.1.1.8 The appearance of agriculture causes the first changes to the species-specific natural human diet

The next stage in the evolution of the human diet began with the domestication of plants, starting about 10,000 years ago in The Fertile Crescent in Asia [65].

The addition of cereals and grains to the human diet reduced human reliance on hunting, fishing, and gathering. A secure source of storable, year-round food allowed the growth of stable communities living together in towns and villages. Jared Diamond suggests that, for the future of the earth and the human species, agriculture was 'the worst mistake in the history of the human race' [66]. According to Diamond, the adoption of farming produced a number of serious disadvantages, including starvation, epidemic diseases and malnutrition. By 3000 BC humans living on cereals and grains had lost at least 13 cm in height.

Since then, agriculture has coexisted in different communities with either hunting and gathering or exclusively with the herding of domesticated and semi-domesticated animals.

Never in our pre-history has there been a group of humans that existed solely on the exclusive cultivation or gathering of plants or on a purely vegetarian/vegan diet.

1.1.1.8.1 The health and diets of farmers compared to hunter-gatherers

During most of the Holocene, the period of improved (warmer) climate that started approximately 11,650 years ago, the human diet became more varied than it had ever been. We find societies living side by side but eating diets that range from almost exclusively animal-based to predominantly agricultural- and plant-based. But it is clear that the health of those societies that continued to eat an animal-based diet was superior.

In 1877, Lieutenant Scott, a US cavalry scout, wrote about the Cheyenne scouts, whose actions led to the defeat of General Custer at the Battle of the Little Bighorn in 1876 [67]: '... they were all keen, athletic young men, tall and lean and brave, and I admired them as real specimens of manhood more than anybody of men I have ever seen before or since. They were perfectly adapted to their environment, and knew just what to do in every emergency and when to do it, without any confusion or lost motion. Their poise and dignity were superb; no royal person ever had more assured manners. I watched their every movement and learned lessons from them that later saved my life many times on the prairie'. Scott also noted that the Crow, the enemies of the Cheyenne, hunted bison once a week from large herds and that their camp, 'was full of meat drying everywhere. Everybody was carefree and joyous'.

Others reported that the American Plains Indians were free of the diseases that afflicted European settlers, including diabetes, cancer, heart disease, and most infectious diseases: 'It is rare to see a sick body amongst them' and that they are 'unacquainted with a great many diseases that afflict the Europeans such as gout, gravel and dropsy, etc'. [68]. Plains Indians were also amongst the tallest peoples then living on earth [69]. Today type 2 diabetes mellitus (T2D) and obesity are rampant among their descendants [70].

Another group of hunter-gatherers, the Inuit of the Arctic, consumed diets based on meat and animal fat, as did the Masai herders living close to the Equator, as well as the herders of the high plateau of Central Asia. Other hunter-gatherers living in warmer climates subsisted on a diet with a higher component of plants [18], whereas coastal societies lived on fish and other aquatic foods.

In the same historical period, peoples who lived close to the large rivers - such as the Nile, the Euphrates, the Indus and the Yangtze - relied on an agricultural diet high in plant-based foods, supplemented with dairy and meat from domesticated animals. Besides the change in food acquisition methods, the post-Palaeolithic period is also characterised by the more intensive use of food processing methods [71].

However this change to the agricultural diet was clearly associated with worsening human health.

In their seminal book, *Paleopathology at the Origins of Agriculture*, Cohen et al. [72] show that the transition to agriculture was forced rather than voluntary; a change born of a shortage of natural foods and not the result of sudden, marvellous inventions in plant and animal domestication. Based mainly on studies of bone pathology, these authors show that humans suffered many novel chronic diseases after switching from a diet based on hunting to one grounded on the consumption of domesticated foods. North America, where agricultural groups lived side by side with hunter-gatherers, provides pathological evidence that the hunter-gatherers were healthier than the agriculturalists. Steckel et al. [73] have written: 'Diet was also closely related to change in the health index, with performance being nearly 12 points lower under the triad of corn, beans, and squash than with the more diverse diet of hunter-gatherer groups'.

Africa also includes ethnic groupings that chose to eat different diets either predominantly carnivorous or mainly plant-based. In 1931, Orr and Gilks [74] compared the health and physical attributes of the Kikuyu, a 'vegetarian tribe' eating predominantly cereals supplemented with roots and fruits, with the 'largely carnivorous' Masai, whose diet comprised milk, meat and raw blood. Compared to adult Kikuyu, adult Masai were about 5 inches (13 cm) taller, 23 pounds (10 kg) heavier, and 50% stronger when tested with a hand dynamometer. In addition, bony deformities, dental caries, anaemia, pulmonary conditions, and tropical ulcers were more prevalent in the Kikuyu, whereas rheumatoid arthritis and 'intestinal stasis' were more common in the Masai [74].

The effects on human health of the transition to farming are also revealed in the mummified bodies in South America and Egypt. The mummies from groups eating the agricultural diet exhibit a wide range of diseases, including tuberculosis and cancer [75–80].

It seems that, with time, humans learned how to overcome some but perhaps not all of the unhealthy effects of eating the agricultural diet.

1.1.2 Food as a source of health and disease: the evidence

1.1.2.1 The health-promoting diet of the Mid-Victorians (1850–80)

Victorian England, between 1850 and 1880, provides an excellent example of the state of health before the change to the human diet caused by the introduction of industrially mass-produced food. This mid-Victorian period is now recognised as the golden era of British health. It is explained by the high quality of the mid-Victorians' diet [81–84].

Farm-produced real foods were available in such abundance that even the working-class poor ate highly nutritious foods. As a result, life expectancy in Britain in 1875 was equal to, or even surpassed that of modern Britons. This was especially true for men (whose life expectancy was higher by about three years). In addition, the profile of diseases was quite different from those prevalent in Britain today. The authors concluded:

> *[This] shows that medical advances allied to the pharmaceutical industry's output have done little more than change the manner of our dying. The Victorians died rapidly of infection and/or trauma, whereas we die slowly of degenerative disease. It reveals that with the exception of family planning, the vast edifice of twentieth century healthcare has not enabled us to live longer but has in the main merely supplied methods of suppressing the symptoms of degenerative disease which have emerged due to our failure to maintain mid-Victorian nutritional standards [84].*

This mid-Victorians' healthy diet included freely available and cheap vegetables such as onions, carrots, turnips, cabbage, broccoli, peas, and beans; fresh and dried fruit, including apples; legumes and nuts, especially chestnuts, walnuts, and hazelnuts; fish, including herring, haddock, and John Dory; other seafood, including oysters, mussels and whelks; meat, which was considered 'a mark of a good diet', so much so that 'its complete absence was rare', was sourced from free-range animals, especially pork, and also included offal such as brain, heart, pancreas (sweetbreads), liver, kidneys, lungs, and intestine; eggs from hens that were kept by most urban households; and hard cheeses [84].

Their healthy diet was therefore low in cereals, grains, sugar, trans-fats, and refined flour, and high in fibre, phytonutrients, and omega-3 polyunsaturated fatty acids, entirely compatible with the modern Paleo or low-carbohydrate high-fat (LCHF) diets [84].

But this period of nutritional 'paradise' changed drastically after 1875, when cheap imports of white flour, tinned meat, sugar, canned fruits and condensed milk became more readily available [84]. The result was immediately noticeable. By 1883, the British infantry was forced to lower by three inches, its minimum height for recruits; by 1900, 50% of British volunteers for the Anglo-Boer War were rejected because of undernutrition [82]. The changes were associated with an alteration in disease patterns in these populations, as clearly described by Yellowlees [85] (see later) in the patients in his rural medical practice in the Scottish Highlands.

The remarkable health of other pre-industrial societies eating their traditional diets and conversely its immediate destruction with the adoption of the industrial (colonial) diet, has been captured in the unique and remarkable writings of Dr. Weston Price.

1.1.2.2 Weston Price investigates the health and diet of traditional societies

In the 1930s, Weston Price, a dentist in Cleveland, Ohio, USA, noticed that dental caries were becoming more prevalent in his young patients. At the time he had observed that the teeth of children with type I diabetes prescribed high-fat diet in the pre-insulin era, were free of caries [86]. The diet comprised milk, cream, butter, eggs, meat, cod liver oil, bulky vegetables, and fruit. His own experiments had also shown that one meal a day high in fat-soluble vitamins could prevent the progression of dental decay in children with active dental caries [87]. He also knew that the teeth of ancient South African fossils did not have dental caries [88]. He wondered whether perhaps a recent dietary change could explain the increase in dental caries among the children in his dental practice. He knew that to answer that question, he would need to travel the world in search of peoples who were still eating the 'control' diet that they had eaten before the spread of the modern industrial diet. If they were healthy, he would know that the adoption of that novel diet is a key driver of the ill-health of modern humans.

1.1.2.2.1 The healthy populations

With his wife in support, over the next decade, Price examined the teeth and general health of the Swiss inhabitants of the Lötschental Valley; of Scottish families living on the Outer and Inner Hebrides; of the Inuit (Eskimos) of Alaska; of the Indians of north, west and central Canada, the western United States and Florida; of the Melanesians and Polynesians inhabiting eight archipelagos of the Southern Pacific; of six tribes in eastern and central Africa, including the Masai; of the Aborigines of Australia; of Malay tribes living on islands north of Australia; of the Maori of New Zealand; and of South Americans in Peru and the Amazon Basin. Wherever possible, the health of those continuing to eat traditional foods was compared with that of others in the area who had begun to eat imported diet of processed foods. Prices travelled with a mobile laboratory as well as photographic equipment to collect food samples and to photograph the teeth and faces of the people they examined, as well as recording their general state of health. They also analysed these traditional foods for the presence of vitamins and minerals. The results of this six-year project are described in the remarkable book 'Nutrition and Physical Degeneration' [89].

The Prices discovered that those farmers and herders who adhered to their traditional diets were, in general, very healthy. Specifically, those who continued to eat the foods of their ancestors showed:

- an almost total absence of tooth decay;
- broad faces, wide nostrils and perfect dental arches;
- superior immunity, demonstrated by an absence of tuberculosis in some communities (such as the Swiss of the Lötschental Valley); and
- an absence of most of the modern 'chronic diseases of lifestyle', including cancer, rheumatic diseases, and other autoimmune diseases.

For example, they described the Inuit of Alaska as 'an example of physical excellence and dental perfection such as has seldom been excelled by any race in the past or present' and as 'robust, muscular and active, inclining rather to sparseness than corpulence, presenting a markedly healthy appearance. The expression of the countenance is one of habitual good humor. The physical constitution of both sexes is strong'.

His findings of the generally good health of the Inuit matched those of Harvard biologist Vilhjalmur Stefansson who wrote several books describing his multi-year experience of living with the Inuit and eating their very low carbohydrate animal-based diet [90]. Stefansson also observed that the Innuit appeared to be free of cancer [91].

In Australia, Weston Price reserved special praise for the health and physical abilities of those Aborigines who continued to live in accordance with their traditional ways. However, he also observed that, like the Inuit and the American Plains Indians, Aboriginal health deteriorated catastrophically once their diet began to include wheat flour and sugar: 'While these evidences of superior physical development demand our most profound admiration, their ability to build superb bodies and maintain them in excellent condition in so difficult an environment commands our genuine respect. It is a supreme test of human efficiency. It is doubtful if many places in the world can demonstrate so great a contrast in physical development and perfection of body as that which exists between the primitive Aborigines of Australia who have been the sole arbiters of their fate, and those Aborigines who have been under the influence of the white man. The white man has deprived them of their original habitats and is now feeding them in reservations while using them as laborers in modern industrial pursuits' ([89], p. 152).

In many cases, he documented the unique nutritional solutions that a group would adopt to ensure their health. For example, those living in the secluded Loetschental Valley of Switzerland, paid special attention to the cheese made from the milk of cows, fed on the new grasses of summer. It was stored and used throughout the year to feed the young. Those young people were so physically perfect that they provided the pool for the Pontifical Swiss Guard in the Vatican.

In Africa, he noticed that, 'The natives of Africa know that certain insects are very rich in special food values at certain seasons, also that their eggs are valuable foods'. From another African tribe with exceptional health and remarkable physiques, the herding Neurs of Sudan, he learned that 'they have a belief which to them is their religion, namely, that every man and woman has a soul which resides in the liver and that a man's character and physical growth depend upon how well he feeds that soul by eating the livers of animals'. The liver is so sacred that it may not be touched by human hands. It is accordingly always handled with their spear or saber, or with specially prepared forked sticks. It is eaten both raw and cooked.

In many places, the Prices found that certain foods such as fish and fish eggs, were traded over long distances with other groups that had no access to aquatic resources. On the island of Viti Levu in Fiji, trade continued between the shore and the interior tribes even during periods of bitter warfare. The interior group would leave mountain plant foods in known caches at night; in return, the shore groups would leave seafoods. In many of these groups, a special diet was prescribed to newly married couples and to pregnant women.

In the Peruvian Andes, the Prices found young children with pouches filled with fish eggs that they had collected hundreds of miles away on the Pacific coast. Analysing these fish eggs, Price found that they contained a high level of what he termed 'Factor X', which he deemed essential for healthy growth. He identified Factor X in different foods of many societies, including in the special cheese of the Swiss Loetschental Valley. Factor X was later identified as vitamin K2, which is responsible, among other effects, for the orderly distribution of calcium to various bodily organs.

Comparing the vitamin content of traditional and modern foods, Price concluded that the most crucial difference between the two can be found in the higher content of fat-soluble vitamins like A, D, and Factor X (vitamin K2). He wrote: 'I have shown that the primitive races studied were dependent upon one of three sources for some of these fat-soluble factors, namely, sea foods, organs of animals or dairy products. These are all of animal origin'.

This remarkable book provides an image of traditional societies with astonishing practical knowledge on how to prepare foods optimally for the promotion of health. Their knowledge had been accumulated over countless generations, largely via anecdotes and without the use of the scientific method. Today we would not consider that this method of knowledge accumulation – anecdote versus randomised controlled trial – is scientifically acceptable.

1.1.2.2.2 The first appearance of specific diseases in these populations

Already at the time of the Prices' travels, those traditional peoples who lived closer to the sea ports or the trading posts that followed the spread of colonialism, had begun to replace their traditional diets with the industrially-prepared foods that include white flour and sugar. This development allowed Price to compare the health of individuals in the same ethnic groups and living in the same regions who subsisted either on their traditional diets or on the modern industrial diet. He noted an obvious trend: as soon as communities began to eat the 'modern foods of commerce' - the name he gave to foods containing white flour and sugar – their health declined dramatically and predictably. Not only did the rate of dental caries increase substantially in both the young and old but the facial structures of the children were dramatically changed with dire consequences for their health: 'It is remarkable that regardless of colour the new generations born after the adoption by primitives of deficient foods develop in general the facial and dental arch deformities and skeletal defects' [89].

Significantly, the shape of the nose did not allow for optimal nose breathing, and the crania narrowed, with flat cheeks compared to the broad facial form of those who continued to consume their traditional diets (Fig. 1.1).

1.1.2.2.3 The contribution of Weston Price to modern nutrition science

The first scientific contribution made by the Prices was a renewed appreciation of the nutritional importance of vitamins and minerals. Not that the Prices knew which specific vitamins or minerals were involved. But they did realise that something special was present in the specific cheese, fish eggs, liver, or a myriad of other vitamin-containing foods that were unique to the diets of the different healthy populations that they studied.

Secondly, they learned how these traditional societies prepared each food source to remove specific deleterious effects. Many foods, mostly plants, have chemicals that are toxic to humans. Plants invest heavily in defending themselves from consumption. They do this by producing toxins and anti-nutrients especially in their seeds, which are the energy-dense parts that mammals prefer. This explains why humans cannot safely eat raw wheat, rice, or beans. The harmful chemical compounds in most plants include rapidly-acting toxins, as well as toxins that produce more subtle effects with prolonged consumption [92,93]. They also contain compounds that reduce the digestibility of the plant macronutrients and interfere with mineral absorption [16].

Humans have developed a number of methods of food preparation or preservation that neutralise, partly or wholly, these deleterious chemical compounds in plants (see reviews in Refs [94,95]).

The best known and arguably the oldest preparation method is 'thermal processing', be it roasting, cooking, or baking. The cooking of plants has been practiced since at least the Palaeolithic era [95–97]. Fermentation, which is the

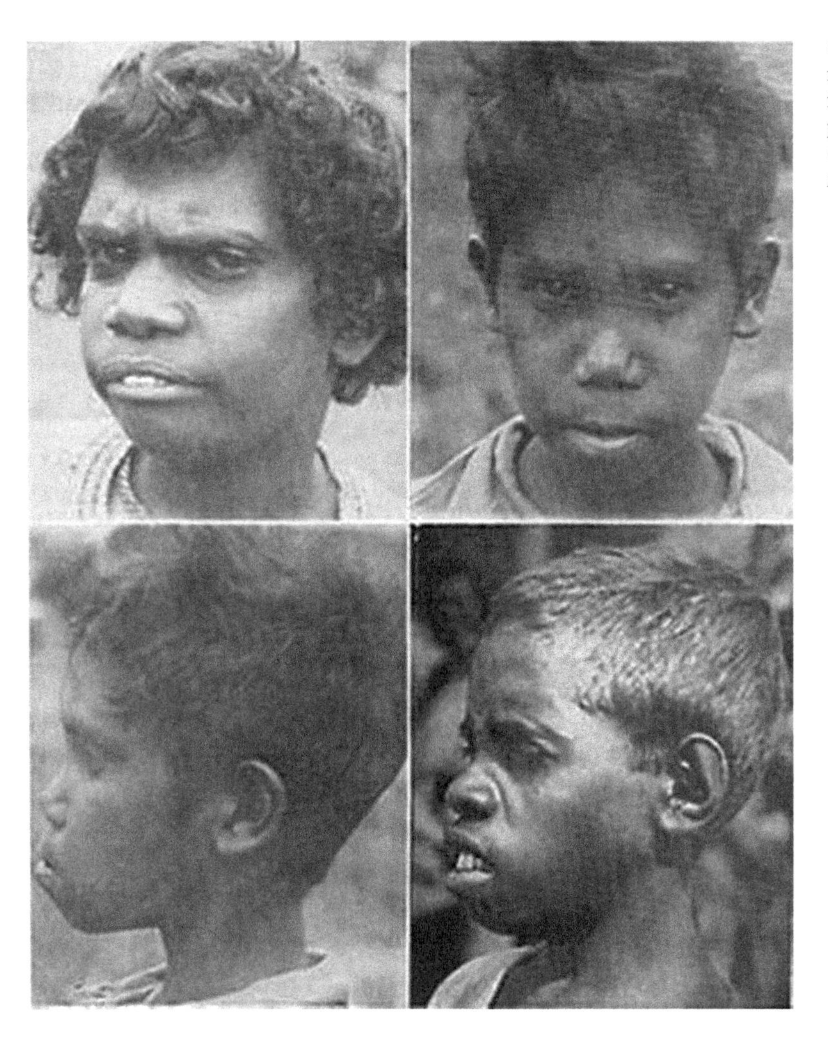

FIGURE 1.1 Deformity patterns produced in the modernised Aborigines of Australia by white men's food. Note the undershot mandible, upper left, the pinched nostrils and facial deformity in all four [89].

external pre-digestion of food by bacteria, also dates back to the Palaeolithic era [98]. Fermentation is widely used to prepare plants, as well as dairy products, and sometimes meat.

For example, the rising of dough is a form of fermentation. Thus the preparation of bread combines two food preparation methods: fermentation and heat processing (baking). In societies in South America and Africa whose staple food is maize, the maize is fermented and cooked with lime, in a process named nixtamalisation, which removes the antinutrients that interfere with plant nutrient digestion and absorption [99]. Sprouting and soaking are also effective in neutralising plant toxins and are used to prepare legumes and cereals, amongst other foods.

1.1.2.2.4 Summary

To summarise, the study of traditional, healthy societies teaches us that humans built countless food systems by trial and error, each unique to a particular environment. These systems included a unique set of essential foods that originated within those environments, as well as methods for removing toxins from plants to increase the absorbability of their contained nutrients. Most importantly, being relatively small and stable, these traditional societies could ensure that this knowledge was passed down from generation to generation.

In overview, we can see that an originally meat-dominated diet, during the first 2.5 million years of human evolution, transformed a few thousand years ago into thousands of locally adapted diets, each forming a complete nutritional system aligned with a specific local agricultural system that provided healthy nutrition for all members of these local communities.

However, as the very reason for the Prices' travels shows, signs of deterioration, both in dental and general health, appeared in the first half of the 20th century in America and other non-secluded parts of the world. Industrialisation and the global trend of urbanisation seem to have broken the transference of communal nutritional knowledge.

Urbanisation also eliminated easy access to foods that had secured the health of traditional societies over hundreds of generations.

But the Prices were not alone in alerting the world to the critical importance of diet and dietary changes in determining human health.

1.1.2.3 Major General Professor Sir Robert McCarrison studies the different diets of Indian peoples living on the Asian subcontinent

The quest for proper nutrition for the masses became a subject of public concern in the British Empire at the beginning of the 20th century. This situation called for a more systematic scientific approach to find proper nutritional solutions to health which could be applied to large industrialised societies. One of the original pioneers of this research was Major General Professor Sir Robert McCarrison [100].

McCarrison was the first scientist to study the effects of nutritionally deficient diets, establishing how particular nutritional deficiencies caused specific medical conditions, including goitre, cretinism, and beriberi. On the advice of 1932 Nobel laureate Sir Charles Sherrington, McCarrison accepted the position of Director of Nutritional Research at Coonoor in Tamil Nadu, India. There, as Sherrington had suggested, he set about investigating the dietary patterns of the different Indian communities across the Asian sub-continent. Subsequently in the prestigious Cantor Lectures [101], McCarrison reviewed the findings from his early work.

His methods were simple – a large number of albino rats were fed either 'good' or 'faulty' diets, modelled on the diets of the 'healthy' Sikhs from the Punjab in the North and the 'less healthy' Madrassas from the South. During this research none of the thousands of stock (control) albino rats fed the 'good' Sikhs' diet ever became ill.

From these experiments 'on several thousand deficiently-fed rats', McCarrison provided a detailed list of some 80 ailments, all recognised in humans (Table 1.2), that were found at autopsy in animals eating the deficient diet. The ailments affected most bodily organs, namely, skin, eye, ear, nose, lungs, alimentary tract, urinary tract, reproductive system, blood, lymph, endocrine glands, heart, and the nervous system.

McCarrison also identified a deleterious influence of a faulty diet on mental function. In one experiment, he tested the diet of 'the poorer classes in England' that consumed mainly white bread, margarine, over-sweetened tea with a little milk, cabbage, and tinned meat and tinned jam. The experimental rats, he wrote 'were nervous and apt to bite the attendants; they lived unhappily together and by the sixtieth day of the experiment they began to kill and eat the weaker ones amongst them. When they had disposed of three in this way, I was compelled to segregate the remainder ...'.

McCarrison's wished to determine if these different dietary patterns might explain the different body shapes, physical abilities and disease patterns in the different ethnic groupings in India: 'Indeed, nothing could be more striking than the contrast between the manly, stalwart and resolute races of the north – the Pathans, Baluchis, Sikhs, Punjabis, Rajputs, and Maharattas – and the poorly developed, toneless and supine people of the east and south: Bengalis, Madrassas, Kanarese and Travancorians', he wrote (p. 268 in Ref. [100]). McCarrison noted that the Pathans are meat-eaters whereas the Bengalis, Madrassas and Kanarese are, for the most part, vegetarian.

He found that in humans, as in the rats, there was a strong correlation between diet and health. He found that the Madrassas, who lived mainly on plant foods, were between two and ten times 'sicker' in a range of illnesses than were the Punjabis [101].

His explanation was: 'As we pass from the north to the east, south-east, south-west and south of India, there is thus a gradual fall in the nutritive value of cereal grains forming the staples of the national diet, this fall reaching the lowest limit amongst the rice-eaters of the east and south. There is also a gradual fall in the amount of animal protein, animal fats and vitamins entering into these diets' (p. 267 in Ref. [100]).

He concluded that protein was an essential component of a healthy diet: 'It will be obvious from these considerations that the insufficient ingestion, absorption or assimilation of proteins, or of proteins of the right kind, will tend to degradation of vital processes; a degradation manifested in stunting of growth, poor physique, lack of energy, resource and initiative, digestive disturbances and impaired action of glandular organs' [101]. While he understood that proteins from plants were labelled 'second-class' proteins, he recognised their value to the peoples he was studying: 'the use of milk and cheese should be greatly extended. Much greater use should also be made of the better class vegetable proteins, such as those of soya bean, legumes and nuts, and much less use of the flesh of animals. Apart from every other consideration the use of meat as the main source of proteins is as uneconomical as it is unnecessary...' [101].

Yet he argued: 'The poorer classes, according to the degree of their poverty, drop out, in part or in whole, the more expensive or less easily obtainable items: milk, milk products, animal fats, legumes, fruit and vegetables. So that as the

TABLE 1.2 Diseases detected at autopsy in rats and other animals fed the faulty Indian diet [101].

System	Disease description
Skin	Loss of hair, gangrene of the feet and tail, dermatitis, ulcers, abscesses, oedema
Eye	Conjunctivitis, corneal ulceration, xerophthalmia, panophthalmitis, cataract
Ear	Otitis media, pus in the middle ear
Nose	Rhinitis, sinusitis
Lungs and respiratory system	Adenoids, pneumonia, broncho-pneumonia, bronchiectasis, pleurisy, pyothorax, haemothorax
Gastrointestinal tract	Dental disease, dilatation of the stomach, gastric ulcer, epithelial new growths in the stomach (two cases of cancer), duodenal ulcer, duodenitis, enteritis, colitis, stasis, intussusception and a condition of the lower bowel suggestive of a pre-cancerous state
Urinary tract	Pyonephrosis, hydronephrosis, pyelitis, renal calculus, nephritis, urethral calculus, dilated ureters, vesical calculus, cystitis, encrusted cystitis
Reproductive system	Endometritis, ovaritis, death of the foetus in utero, premature birth, uterine haemorrhage, testicular disease
Blood	Anaemia, a pernicious type of anaemia, Bartonella muris anaemia
Lymph	Cysts, abscesses, enlarged glands
Endocrine glands	Goitre, lymph-adenoid goitre, adrenal hypertrophy, atrophy of the thymus, haemorrhagic pancreatitis (very occasionally)
Heart	Cardiac atrophy, cardiac hypertrophy, myocarditis, pericarditis, hydropericardium
Nervous system	Polyneuritis, beri-beri, degenerative lesions
Bone	Crooked spine, distorted vertebrae (no work was done on rickets – a known 'deficiency disease')
General	Malnutritional oedema, scurvy, pre-scorbutic states

people are poorer and poorer their diets are more and more cereal in nature, more and more imbalanced, more and more depleted of animal protein, animal fats, vitamins and essential nutrients' (p. 270 in Ref. [100]).

A key weakness of this poor diet, he observed, 'takes the form of an excessive richness of the food in carbohydrates' (p. 271 in Ref. [100]).

Ultimately McCarrison contributed this wisdom that continues to be largely ignored by the medical and dietetics professions: 'The newer knowledge of nutrition has revealed, and reveals the more with every addition to it, that a chief cause of the physiological decay of organs and tissues of the body is faulty food, wherein deficiencies of some essentials are often combined with excess of others. It is reasonable, then, to assume that dietetic malnutrition is a chief cause of many degenerative diseases of mankind. However, this may be, it seems clear that the habitual use of a diet made up of natural foodstuffs, in proper proportions one to another, and produced on soils that are not impoverished is an essential condition for the efficient exercise of the function of nutrition on which the maintenance of health depends. This, combined with the proper exercise of the body and of its adaptive functions, is mankind's main defence against degenerative diseases: a bulwark, too, against those of infectious origin. Such, at least, is the conclusion to which my own studies in deficiency disease have led me' (p. 305–306 in Ref. [100]).

And: 'I know of nothing so potent in maintaining good health in laboratory animals as perfectly constituted food; I know of nothing so potent in producing ill health as improperly constituted food. This, too, is the experience of stock-breeders. Is man an exception to a rule so universally applied to the higher animals?' [100].

His key message summarises so much of what is the goal of all the authors contributing to this textbook: 'Some years ago I made the statement that the 'newer knowledge of nutrition is the greatest advance in medical science since the days of Lister. When physicians, medical officers of health and the lay public learn to apply the principles which this new knowledge has to impart ... then will it do for medicine what asepsis has done for surgery'. I see no reason, in the later days, to detract from this view; on the contrary, there is every reason to emphasise it the more, particularly in regard to preventive medicine' [101].

1.1.2.4 Drs. Cleave, Campbell and Yudkin describe the dangers of sugar and the saccharine diseases

In the course of his career as a naval surgeon sailing around the world, Captain T.L. Cleave [102] in collaboration with South African physician G.D. Campbell [103], formulated the hypothesis that a variety of medical conditions – including dental caries and associated periodontal disease, peptic ulcers, obesity, diabetes, colonic stasis 'and its complications of varicose veins and haemorrhoids', heart attack (coronary thrombosis) and certain gut infections – are caused by diets high in sugar and refined carbohydrates, and should therefore be termed the 'saccharine diseases'. As a result, 'in any disease in man due to alterations in his food from the natural state, the refined carbohydrates, both on account of the magnitude and the recentness of the alterations, are always the foods most likely to be at fault; **and not the fats**' (p. 9 in Ref. [103]).

Cleave and Campbell built their hypothesis on evidence that global sugar consumption began to increase exponentially after 1850, increasing fivefold within the next century, reaching 110 pounds per individual per year in the United Kingdom by 1950. They next compared the health and diets of Indians living in India with those in South Africa. Despite eating less carbohydrate and more protein and fat, South African Indians had much higher rates of T2D, which Cleave and Campbell concluded must be due to the roughly 10-times greater consumption of sugar (110 vs 12 pounds) by Indians living in South Africa [103].

Next they showed that urbanised Zulu-speaking South Africans in Durban, who also ate more sugar than their rural compatriots, developed high rates of T2D after living in the city for 20 or more years. This became known as the Rule of Twenty Years, as it takes 20 years of exposure to a high-sugar diet before T2D develops (pp. 46–49 in Ref. [103]).

Cleave and Campbell also noted that 'until the disastrous rinderpest of 70 years ago the Zulus (of South Africa) have been predominantly meat-eaters', so that they wondered if 'the more carnivorous peoples of the world are more vulnerable to the diabetogenic effects of the consumption of refined carbohydrates than are the more vegetarian peoples, or are they less vulnerable?' (p. 50 in Ref. [103]).

The studies of O'Dea and her colleagues [104–106] support this interpretation as they clearly establish that Australian Aborigines are insulin resistant even when eating their traditionally very low-carbohydrate diet. Perhaps this can be generalised to all populations that traditionally ate carnivorous diets?

Cleave and Campbell next presented evidence that T2D is more common in countries that eat more sugar. Like Weston Price, they argued that the rising incidence of T2D in American Indians, the Inuit, the Icelanders, the 'Black Jews' who moved to Israel from Yemen, and the Pacific Islanders coincided with the adoption of the high-sugar Western diet. Interestingly, Cleave and Campbell understood that 'obesity is not due to diabetes, nor diabetes to obesity, but both arise from a common cause' (p. 59 in Ref. [103]).

The evidence is now clear that they are correct: IR is the underlying condition that is present before the development of either obesity or T2D [107].

Cleave and Campbell's description of the Saccharine Diseases received strong support from Professor John Yudkin during his career as Professor of nutrition and dietetics at the University of London from 1954 to 1971. Yudkin also argued that: 'The diet of early man contained little carbohydrate. With the discovery of agriculture, the amount of carbohydrate increased, and the amounts of protein and fat decreased ... Increasing prosperity, both between countries and within a country, leads to an increasing proportion of sugar being bought in manufactured foods, rather than as household sugar. It is suggested that the effect of this is that wealthier countries, and the wealthier section of a national population, tend to have a higher intake of calories from the accompanying flour, chocolate, fat and other ingredients of these manufactured foods ... one of the effects of this contribution of calories from sugar-containing foods is to reduce the consumption of nutritionally desirable foods, such as fruit and meat ... In the wealthier countries, there is evidence that sugar and sugar-containing foods contribute to several diseases, including obesity, dental caries, diabetes mellitus and myocardial infarction ... the known association of the prevalence of diabetes and of myocardial infarction with the level of fat intake is fortuitous and secondary. It is more likely that the primary association is with levels of sugar intake, which I have shown are, in turn, closely related to levels of fat intake' [108].

For suggesting this hypothesis and for devoting the latter part of his scientific career to the study of the medical consequences of this increased sugar consumption, Yudkin was demonised and ultimately excommunicated from the research community, losing his academic position and his status as a researcher, including all his funding. He was never under any doubt that the sugar industry directed his ex-communication: 'It is difficult to avoid the conclusion that this is the result of the vigorous, continuing and expanding activities of the sugar industry' (p. 188 in Ref. [109]).

1.1.2.5 *Dr. Walter Yellowlees describes the changes in the health of a rural Scottish farming community in less than 40 years between 1948 and 1981*

Dr. Walter Yellowlees graduated in medicine from Edinburgh University in 1941. He served with the Royal Army Medical Corps during the latter years of the World War II, winning the Military Cross for outstanding bravery 'for tending the wounded under heavy fire ... and for being the last to leave the battlefield'. For 33 years after the war he worked as a medical practitioner in a traditional, rural Scottish farming community, retiring in 1981.

In 1993, he wrote his autobiography to record the precipitous deterioration in the health of the community he had served and observed. He wanted to explain what he considered to be the real causes of this rapid health decline and to express his frustration that no one in his profession seemed particularly concerned to expose them: 'If a GP (general practitioner) lives up to the traditions of his calling, he must forever seek to understand why this particular patient is suffering from this particular complaint' (p. 14 in Ref. [85]).

That tradition of his calling meant that in Yellowlees's world, the archetypical GP is honour bound to take a 'much wider view which encompasses not only the patient's disease but, also, his way of life, food, relationships, and environment. The latter attitude, in the Hippocratic tradition, assumes that health is the normal inheritance of mankind and seeks to know what has gone wrong to disturb that inheritance'. Or the doctor can view the patient's illness as 'an unfortunate happening, a haphazard quirk of fate' (p. 14 in Ref. [85]).

In choosing the first option, Yellowlees discovered a perplexing paradox. He struggled to understand why, during the 20th century, 'thanks to better sanitation, clean water, preventive inoculation and improved housing, the incidence of infective diseases caused by bacteria or viruses has greatly diminished', yet, in his own medical lifetime, he had personally observed a dramatic increase in the incidence of degenerative diseases, the so-called diseases of lifestyle, which he concluded could not be conveniently rationalised by 'better methods of diagnosis or the ageing of the population' (p. 14 in Ref. [85]).

His conclusion was exactly the same as those of Price, Cleave, Campbell and Yudkin. It was that this alarming deterioration was the result of a change in diet, as sugar, refined flour and processed foods had replaced the traditional foods on which his people had lived for centuries: 'Food and drink, highly processed and degraded by a multitude of additives, consumed by an ever expanding urban-based population inevitably brings a heavy load of degenerative disease. In Scotland, especially, refined sugar and constipating white flour are still consumed in huge quantities. Obesity and diabetes are rife; the overall incidence of cancer increases' (p. 17 in Ref. [85]).

Yellowlees, like probably all the authors of this textbook, could not understand why something so obvious to him was apparently beyond the understanding of almost all of his medical colleagues.

But he suggested that there were probably three reasons for the 'wilderness of confusion' about the true causes of the rapidly increasing ill health he encountered in rural Scotland.

The first, he suggested, was 'the frailty of human nature on the part of scientists, engaged in nutrition research, who get hold of an idea and refuse to accept any evidence, however compelling, which casts doubt on its veracity' (p. 195 in Ref. [85]).

The second was 'the dominant role of commercial interests in determining the dietary habits of consumers, as well as in shaping developments in agriculture and in medical practice' (p. 195 in Ref. [85]).

'Food manufacturers', he argued, 'equipped with their immensely powerful weapons of mass advertising, join the fray; they do so either openly to the consumer or through a more subtle approach to doctors and dieticians by financing research, publications or conferences' (p. 15 in Ref. [85]).

As to the third reason, Yellowlees suggested that the medical profession had capitulated in the face of these commercial forces. Doctors, he argued, 'are meant to be scientists and science is supposed to reveal the truths of the material world'. Instead, they had forsaken Christian values and become too scared to be deemed either 'judgmental' or 'moralising'.

The result he considered was this: 'The third and daunting part of my wilderness is the spiritual darkness which, in the second half of this century, has cast a deepening shadow over all our affairs. By darkness I mean the loss of loyalty, honesty, integrity, and decency without which human transactions revert to the violence and inhumanity of the beast. These sad trends follow the retreat of Christianity and the rise of humanist false prophets who preach the supremacy not of God, but of human reason; they seek to rule the world, not by God-given wisdom, but by the power of money' (pp. 15–16 in Ref. [85]).

Finally, he asked: 'Are doctors to remain silent when they believe the truth is being perverted?' (p. 195 in Ref. [85]).

His final conclusion sounds as if it came directly from Sir Robert McCarrison: 'Human health depends above all on sound nutrition; sound nutrition means growing food and using it in accordance with nature's laws; of all foods made 'unnatural' by industrial processing the commonest are refined sugar, refined flour and certain processed vegetable oils. I know of no research that refutes this simple concept'. (p. 14 in Ref. [85]).

1.1.2.6 Summary

Is it really surprising that there is such a strong relationship between food and health, as McCarrison, Price, Cleave, Campbell, and Yellowlees have described? Obtaining and digesting food is a significant part of humans' daily activities, one that involves the closest exposure of the body to its environment. We import relatively large chunks of the external environment deep into our bodies, where they are processed before providing the building blocks for all our cells. The food materials we allow to enter our bodies can either provide the healthy nutrients that allow us to survive and thrive, or they can cause harm.

Considering all the evidence presented in this chapter, it is difficult to avoid the conclusion that many, if not most of the modern humans' ailments are the direct result of a 'faulty' diet.

But instead of embracing this clear evidence and consuming a diet to which our bodies are evolutionarily adapted, humans spend billions of dollars researching specific chemical treatments (patented pharmaceutical drugs) for each of these hundreds of different ailments, all of which are most probably caused by eating highly processed, unnatural foods.

For we have waived responsibility for our food preparation to commercial entities, whose highest priority is to lessen production costs, while attempting to minimise and sometimes cleverly bypass governmental regulations.

All in the pursuit of maximum profits, not optimum human health.

Some 70% of the foods in the modern American diet including wheat, corn (maize), seed oils, and sugars, were not consumed during the 2.5 million years in which our species evolved. These foodstuffs can therefore be defined as *non-species-specific*; that is, they are unnatural for consumption by our species. Moreover the seed oils (soy, corn, and canola), which now provide 21% of the calories in the modern American diet, did not exist as food even 100 years ago.

Sugar, which provides some 15% of calories in the current diet, became a commodity only at the beginning of the slave trade in the 1500 s [102,103,108–110] with consumption already increasing eightfold from 1840 to 1895 [111]. Cleave [111] makes the compelling point that since there is a latency period of perhaps 20–50 years before a dietary change can explain the subsequent epidemic of coronary heart disease beginning after the 1920s, any dietary change considered causal of that epidemic must have begun by the 1870s. The increased global consumption of sugar neatly fulfils that requirement.

1.1.3 The pitfalls of modern industrial food preparation

The modern health crisis is caused by the ultra-processed industrial diet and dietary changes following the introduction of mass food manufacturing.

The modern, ultra-processed industrial diet that is now consumed by most populations around the world, deviates profoundly from the diet of traditional agricultural societies that was common less than a 100 years ago.

Traditional food preparation methods are not used in modern industrial food preparation.

The change in the primary food sources eaten by humans may form only a part of the difference between what we eat and what our ancestors ate. As we have described, traditional food preparation techniques such as fermentation, soaking, sprouting, and nixtamalisation, were practised in preindustrial and even early industrial societies to remove plant toxins and increase the absorption of energy, vitamins, and minerals from grains, vegetables, and milk, respectively. But these methods are no longer commonly followed.

Ultra-processed foods (UPFs) [112,113] now dominate the global food system [114], providing up to 58% of the energy consumption and 90% of calories from added sugars in the US diet [115]. UPFs include breakfast cereals, savoury snacks, reconstituted meat products, frankfurters, pre-packaged frozen dishes, soft and/or sweetened drinks, distilled alcoholic beverages, and supplements. Most of the methods used to mass-produce these industrial foods do not fully utilise the anti-nutrient removal methods developed by traditional societies. Thus the nutritional value of these industrially produced 'foods' is further compromised.

Observational studies confirm the association between the consumption of ultra-processed foods and a range of non-communicable diseases [116] including T2D [117], all-cause and cardiovascular mortality [118,119] and obesity [120], including visceral obesity [121]. UPFs also impair skeletal maturation in rats [122], a finding McCarrison would have predicted. As yet no randomised controlled trials have been conducted to test these relationships.

1.1.3.1 The prescription of polyunsaturated fatty acids in seed oils to replace saturated fats

Most explanations of why the current dietary guidelines have failed to prevent obesity and related chronic diseases typically ignore the obvious evolutionary mismatch between this novel diet and the natural species-specific diet on which humans evolved. A good example is the recommendation to limit the consumption of saturated fat. But animal fat, the primary source of saturated fats in the diet, has been an essential component of the humans' natural diet for millions of years and has always been cherished by traditional societies [123].

Although some studies using surrogate markers have concluded that the replacement of saturated fats with seed oils should improve future health [124,125], controlled long-term clinical trials measuring hard clinical endpoints have failed not only to support this conclusion but also, in fact, have identified seed oils as the probable cause of increased risk of mortality [126,127]. Industrially-produced seed oils were first offered less than a century ago, much later than even grains and sugar.

Thus the Recovered Minnesota Coronary Experiment (RMCE) [127] found that persons randomised to the intervention diet which replaced saturated fat with the polyunsaturated fatty acid (PUFA), linoleic acid, were at an 22% higher risk of death for each 0.78 mmol/L (30 mg/dL) reduction in blood cholesterol concentrations. This adverse effect was especially apparent in those over 65 years of age. The Recovered Sydney Diet Heart Study (RSDHS) [126] also found that the replacement of dietary saturated fat with linoleic acid was associated with increased all-cause mortality and with increased death from both cardiovascular disease and coronary heart disease.

Another recently published study found that those with the highest intakes of hydrogenated seed oils had a 68% increased risk for myocardial infarction [128]. No other dietary fat source was associated with increased mortality from ischaemic heart disease, cardiovascular disease, stroke, or all-causes.

Reviewing the additional evidence provided by the two recovered studies, Ramsden et al. (p. 13 in Ref. [127]) emphasise that: 'Increasing dietary linoleic acid has been shown to increase oxidised linoleic acid derivatives in a dose-dependent manner in many tissues. These oxidised derivatives, along with other non-cholesterol lipid mediators, have been implicated in the pathogenesis of many diseases including coronary heart disease, chronic pain, and steatohepatitis'.

In fact, the explosive growth in the consumption of industrially-produced polyunsaturated fats from seed oils, mainly soy oil containing a high level of linoleic acid, is another obvious dietary candidate for the increasing ill-health of modern humans.

The relative chemical instability of seed oils and their tendency to oxidise in the body and turn into potentially deleterious compounds, ceramide 1 phosphate and 4-hydroxynonenal, [129,130], emphasises their potential role in the promotion of insulin resistance, obesity, cardiovascular and autoimmune diseases, cancer, and diabetes [131–136]. More long-term clinical studies are needed to establish any role of seed oils in the growth of all these now common diseases.

In reviewing all the current evidence, Lawrence concludes that 'PUFAs are unstable to chemical oxidation and their oxidation products are harmful in a variety of ways. PUFAs also form powerful signalling agents that can initiate inflammation which can have dire health consequences...If saturated fats are replaced by carbohydrates in the diet, there would be no significant improvement in serum cholesterol and it can result in a more atherogenic lipoprotein profile. When looking at much of the data in the context of known biochemical and physiological mechanisms, it appears that saturated fats are less harmful than the common alternatives' (pp. 7–8 in Ref. [137]).

1.1.3.2 The increased consumption of grains

The second-largest dietary change since 1970 has been the increased consumption of grains. Two features of modern bread production stand out: a significant recent genetic change in grain species combined with a dramatic shift in processing techniques due to the industrialisation of bread production [138].

The original wheat genus, einkorn (*T. monococcum*), differs significantly from modern wheat (*T. aestivum*) in the number of harmful chemical constituents it contains, something that the germination and fermentation methods used by the historic agriculturists would have either reduced or removed [139]. Although germination is still used in the preparation of modern mass-produced bread, fermentation time has been reduced from the ideal of 6–12 h to less than 1 h. Additionally, industrially ground flour is devoid of those enzymes that are usually active in antinutrient removal. The result is that the prevalence of various wheat-associated harmful conditions continues to increase [140] and, perhaps as a consequence, the consumption of gluten-free foods has become increasingly popular [140–142].

1.1.3.3 The increased consumption of sugar and high fructose corn syrup

Sugar is the third food that is unnatural and whose consumption has increased since 1970. Global sugar consumption increased by 30% between 1970 and 2017. There is now a general consensus that Cleave, Campbell and Yudkin were correct and that high consumption of sugar produces many harmful effects [110,143]. This increased consumption has been associated with a partial replacement of cane sugar in some countries with high-fructose corn syrup that contains 55% fructose compared to 50% fructose in sugar. Excessive consumption of fructose (as opposed to glucose) can lead to non-alcoholic fatty liver disease (NAFLD), inflammation, oxidative stress, overweight, and other pathologic conditions [144].

The addictive nature of the modern highly processed industrial diet.

Increasing attention is now being placed on the addictive nature [145] of modern ultra-processed foods [146,147] and their contribution to overeating [148] and the development of obesity (perhaps also related to a lower protein content) [149].

1.1.4 Summary

The first section of this chapter shows how humans and their ancestors have maintained their health and thrived on a wide range of different diets. During the first 2.5 million years of our evolution, humans consumed an animal-based, fat-rich diet to which their physiology and metabolism became very well adapted. With the establishment of agriculture about 10,000 years ago, more plant-sourced foods entered the human diet.

After a bumpy start and with time, humans developed food systems that allowed them to stay almost as healthy on an agricultural diet as they had been for more than 2 million years on the natural species-specific diet. But the modern industrial diet that has become ever more prevalent since World War II has been associated with a progressive impairment in human health across the globe.

The cause appears to be that more than 50% of the calories consumed in the modern industrial (American) diet come in the form of seed oils, grains and sugar; often in a diet comprising ultra-processed foods. While grains ($\sim$18,000 years) and sugar ($\sim$400 years) have been in the human diet for some time, industrially-produced seed oils have been eaten by humans for little more than a century.

It is clear that the replacement of animal-based foods with industrially-produced food has led to the dramatic worsening of human health described by, amongst others, Weston Price, Cleave, Campbell, Yudkin and Yellowlees.

The increased consumption of grains and especially industrially-extracted seed oils has led to a reduction in the consumption of saturated fat compared to consumption patterns 2–3 million years ago. Yet according to the popular current dietary dogma, it is an increased consumption of saturated fat that is the main dietary cause of worsening human health.

Conversely the key evidence shows that as humans have reduced their consumption of saturated fat, rates of ill-health have increased. This might suggest that saturated fat makes a positive rather than a negative contribution to human health. The evolutionary perspective we present in this chapter, supports this interpretation.

Appearing before the 1980 US House of Representatives Agricultural Committee, to comment on the formation of the (still) current dietary guidelines, Dr. Philip Handler, then president of the National Academy of Science, asked: 'What right has the federal government to propose that the American people conduct a vast nutritional experiment, with themselves as subjects, on the strength of so very little evidence that it will do them any good?' (p. 51 in Ref. [150]).

In retrospect, the experiment has been a catastrophic failure. Could it be that in the modern era of mass manufacturing of ultra-processed foods, we find ourselves in a similar situation to that which humans faced at the beginning of the agricultural era? Do we lack the necessary knowledge of how to be healthy in this radically changed dietary environment? Could it be that, like McCarrison's rats, humans have developed scores of novel diet-induced illnesses specifically because our nutrition is now dependent on mass produced ultra-processed foods that are so far removed from the species-specific diet that kept humans healthy for millions of years?

The respected biologist Theodosius Dobzhansky wrote: 'Nothing in biology makes sense, except in the light of evolution' [151]. He suggests that the ultimate test of any explanation in biology is that it must make evolutionary sense.

Let us hope that the light of human evolution that we have presented here, will guide future research into the relationship between food and health and, in particular, the formulation of future dietary guidelines that will restore human health.

1.2 Insulin resistance: a unifying feature of chronic disease

Catherine Crofts

Before the discovery of insulin, diagnosis of diabetes was akin to death sentence. The question became, 'for how long could death be delayed?' With the discovery of insulin in 1920, the use of the life-saving medicine has become widespread. However, for a variety of reasons, insulin could not be quantified until the 1960s. This meant that what we understand about insulin was based on its actions; especially glucose as this could be quantified. Many of the assumptions we make today about insulin are due to the delays in understanding insulin and its overarching role in controlling metabolism and health.

1.2.1 History

During the 1920–30s there was a general belief that all causes of diabetes mellitus could be explained by a deficiency of insulin. This theory was challenged separately by Harris and Himsworth. Harris [152] theorised via case studies that pancreatic dysfunctions would likely result in insulin's under- (hypo) or over- (hyper) secretion (insulinism). Himsworth, through a series of experiments in the 1930s, recognised that there were groups of patients who were 'insulin sensitive' and those who were 'insulin resistant'. He proposed that a state of diabetes might result from 'inefficient action of insulin as well as a lack of insulin' [153]. Unfortunately, both Harris' and Himsworth's work suffered by a lack of bioassay to accurately quantify blood insulin concentration and was also interrupted by World War II. It would not be until the 1970s and the work of Reaven before the belief that all diabetes mellitus was caused by a deficiency of insulin would be successfully challenged [154].

Although insulin bioassays were pioneered in the 1950s, it took the development of the insulin radioimmunoassay in the 1960s, by Yalow and Berson, to confirm that plasma insulin concentration in people with IR diabetes were much higher compared to people with normoglycaemia [153]. Kraft recognised that the aetiology of T2D likely stemmed from hyperinsulinaemia that occurred while the patient was still normoglycaemic. A subsequent collaboration with Crofts and colleagues [155] showed that, according the World Health Organization criteria [156], at least 85% of people with an impaired glycaemic response (impaired fasting glucose, impaired glucose tolerance or diabetes mellitus, n = 3750, 46% of sample) also had elevated insulin concentration; with 2-h postprandial concentration proving more diagnostic of hyperinsulinaemia than fasting concentration [157]. Although Kraft did not collect longitudinal data, Hayashi and colleagues conducted a longitudinal study in 400 Japanese American men living in Seattle [158]. They collected insulin and glucose samples every 30 min during a 2-h 75 g oral glucose tolerance test and also analysed their results based on the insulin response pattern. They found that people with a time to maximum insulin concentration of 60 min or greater had at least a 15% chance of developing T2D over the following 10 years, while those who took 120 min or greater to reach maximal insulin concentration had a 35%–50% chance of developing T2D over the same time period.

Due to the difficulties with assaying insulin, researchers tended to infer IR using insulin-mediated glucose disposal techniques in either the basal or postprandial state [159]. It became apparent that people with T2D (known then as maturity or late onset diabetes) had higher insulin concentrations and a diminished insulin response [154]. It was concluded that hyperglycaemia developed when the pancreas was no longer capable of maintaining the compensatory hyperglycaemia needed to overcome the 'defect' in insulin's action [154].

Unfortunately for medical science, the fundamental challenge with these theories stemmed from the belief that it was the hyperglycaemia causing the complications arising from diabetes mellitus. However, this is not the case for the many people with T2D. The Action to Control Cardiovascular Risk in Diabetes Study group [160] (ACCORD study) concluded that intensive glucose lowering increased mortality risks, did not lower cardiovascular risks and caused significant weight gain.

This suggests that insulin itself may be one of the drivers of cardiovascular disease. Reaven continued to champion this belief especially after linking glucose intolerance, hyperinsulinaemia, and carbohydrate-induced hypertriglyceridaemia with cardiovascular disease. With the later addition of essential hypertension, Reaven coined the term 'Syndrome X' for people who had 'insulin resistance, compensatory hyperinsulinaemia, varying degrees of glucose tolerance, hypertriglyceridaemia and suppressed HDL cholesterol concentrations' [153]. As hyperinsulinaemia/IR became associated with more metabolic abnormalities and clinical manifestations, such as endothelial dysfunction or central obesity, the term 'Syndrome X' was retired in favour of the term Metabolic Syndrome' (MetS). Yet, as became later known, many of the sequelae of IR would also directly, or indirectly, result in increased IR (Fig. 1.2), which confounds understanding the underlying pathologies [161].

With different clinical diagnostic definitions (Table 1.3) the link to IR or hyperinsulinaemia has been somewhat lost. As will be discussed in this section, most of the diagnostic criteria can manifest as a result of IR and/or hyperinsulinaemia, thus limiting the clinical utility for understanding the syndrome [164].

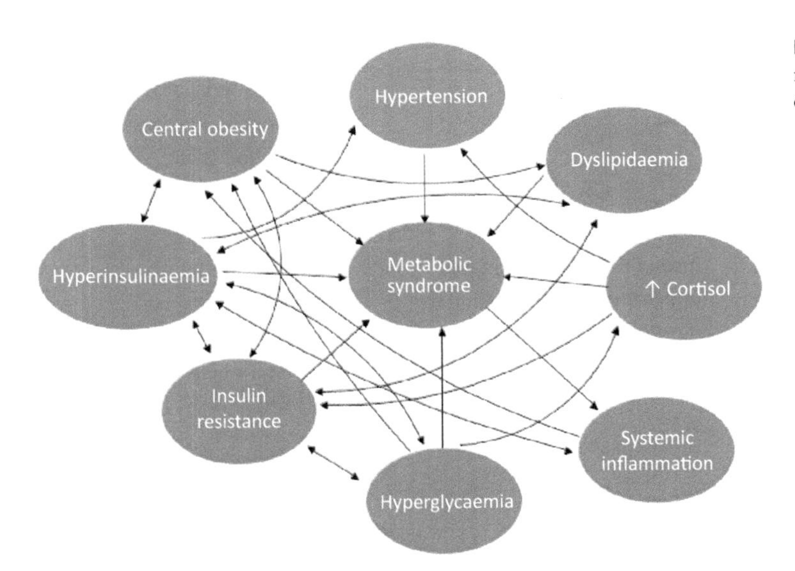

FIGURE 1.2 Interconnected nature of the symptoms of metabolic syndrome. Arrows indicate the best-known evidence of directionality.

1.2.2 Insulin

Insulin, produced by the β-cells of the pancreas, is the body's only hormone to lower blood glucose concentration. With autocrine, paracrine, and endocrine characteristics [165], in combination with adequate substrate supply and under the influence of other hormones, insulin orchestrates an integrated anabolic response to nutrient availability. Yet insulin is also a pleiotropic hormone as it can simultaneously influence multiple phenotypic traits across most body systems.

1.2.2.1 Insulin: synthesis and release

Insulin is a dipeptide formed from A and B peptide chains connected by disulphide bonds. Initially synthesised as the polypeptide preproinsulin, a signal peptide is rapidly cleaved to form proinsulin, which is the A and B chains connected by C (connecting) peptide. Proinsulin is stored in readily-releasable or reserve-pool vesicles [166] in a calcium- and zinc-rich environment [159]. It is estimated that a very small fraction (1%–5%) of insulin is in the readily-releasable vesicles with the remainder (95%–99%) in the reserve pool [167]. After maturation, vesicle exocytosis releases an equimolar ratio of c-peptide and insulin into the portal vein in response to a variety of stimuli: predominantly elevated glucose concentration, fuel secretagogues, such as arginine, hormones, including osteocalcin, glucagon-like peptide-1 (GLP-1), and gastric inhibitory peptide (GIP), or via s vagal nerve stimulation [168] as shown in Table 1.4. Glucose-stimulated insulin secretion can be further augmented by various stimuli including incretins, β-cell to β-cell interaction [166], and acute elevations of non-esterified fatty acids, or β-hydroxybutyrate [159].

1.2.2.1.1 Basal insulin release

Insulin is typically described as being released from the pancreas in both a basal and bolus response to maintain homoeostasis [159], although this model is likely an oversimplification of a complex process. The mechanism by which basal (fasting) insulin is secreted is not fully elucidated but theorised to involve both serotonin and osteocalcin and/or the incretins [171,177]. It is estimated that the basal rate of insulin secretion is 0.25–1.5 units of insulin per hour and that basal secretion accounts for approximately 50% of total daily insulin [159]. Basal insulin is released from the pancreas in a rhythmic and pulsatile manner with circadian and ultradian periodicities [178] as depicted in Fig. 1.3. Although the ultradian periodicity ranges from 40 to 180 min [166,178,179], this is further modulated by fast oscillations that vary between 5 and 15 min. These latter oscillations are believed to be influenced by the individual's personal degree of IR [180]. Finally, insulin is secreted in pulses from the pancreas approximately every 4 min [178]. Calcium and/or cAMP oscillations are hypothesised to be the direct cause of the insulin oscillations [166].

TABLE 1.3 Definitions of metabolic syndrome.

	The National Cholesterol Education Program Adult Treatment Panel III (NCEP ATP III)	**WHO**	**International Diabetes Federation (IDF)**
	Three or more variables	**Insulin resistance/glucose impairment disorder plus two or more variables**	**Central obesity plus two or more variables**
Central obesity	Waist circumference 102 cm (male) > 88 cm (female)	Body mass index 30 kg/m^2 *or* Waist-to-hip ratio 0.9 (male) > 0.85 (female)	Body mass index 30 kg/m^2 *or* Waist circumference ≥ 90–94 cm (male; ethnicity dependent) ≥ 80 cm (female)
Dyslipidaemia	HDL cholesterol < 1.0 mmol/L (male) (39 mg/dl) (male) < 1.3 mmol/L (female) (50 mg/dl) (female) Triglycerides 1.7 mmol/L (150 mg/dl) *and/or* dyslipidaemic medication	HDL cholesterol < 0.9 mmol/L (male) (35 mg/dl) (male) < .0 mmol/L (female) (39 mg/dl) (female) Triglycerides 1.7 mmol/L (150 mg/dl) *and/or* dyslipidaemic medication	HDL cholesterol < 1.03 mmol/L (male) (40 mg/dl) (male) < 1.29 mmol/L (female) (50 mg/dl) (female) Triglycerides 1.7 mmol/L (150 mg/dl) *and/or* dyslipidaemic medication
Glycaemic profile	Confirmed glucose impairment disorder	Confirmed glucose impairment disorder as per Table 1.2 *or* Normoglycaemia *and* glucose uptake below the lowest quartile for background population under hyperinsulinaemic, euglycaemic conditions	Fasting glucose ≥ 5.6 mmol/L (100.8 mg/dl) *or* Confirmed T2D
Hypertension	Blood pressure > 135/85 mm Hg *and/or* antihypertensive medication	Blood pressure > 140/90 mmHg *and/or* antihypertensive medication	Blood pressure > 135/85 mm Hg *and/or* antihypertensive medication
Microalbuminuria	N/A	Albumin excretion > 20 μg/min	N/A

Data taken from: Cleeman J. National Cholesterol Education Program ATP III Guidelines At-A-Glance Quick Desk Reference: 6. https://www.nhlbi.nih.gov/files/docs/guidelines/atglance.pdf; [162] Consensus statements [International Diabetes Federation (IDF) [163]]. [cited 2022 Jun 14]. Available from: https://www.idf.org/e-library/consensus-statements/60-idfconsensus-worldwide-definitionof-the-metabolic-syndrome.html; World Health Organization. Definition, diagnosis and classification of diabetes mellitus and its complications. Retrieved from Geneva: http://whqlibdoc.who.int/hq/1999/WHO_NCD_NCS_99.2.pdf.

1.2.2.1.2 Bolus insulin release

The biphasic mechanism by which bolus insulin is released following glucose stimulation is well established (Fig. 1.4). Briefly, glucose enters the β-cell via glucose transporters (GLUT), stimulating mitochondrial oxidative ATP synthesis. (Although traditionally believed to be GLUT (type) 2) [159], accumulating evidence suggests that GLUT1 and GLUT3 are predominant in human pancreatic β- cells [177,181]. An adequate amount of ATP closes the K_{ATP} channel, leading to depolarisation of the cell membrane, which triggers an influx of Ca^{2+}, resulting in exocytosis of insulin stored in the readily-releasable vesicles [159,166]. In a healthy person, this first-phase insulin release should occur over approximately 15–30 min (depending on administration route), and leads to the 30 min insulin peaks seen on oral glucose tolerance tests [155,158]. The second phase of insulin secretion likely represents both readily-releasable and reserve-pool vesicles[159,166] and is induced by fuel secretagogues. The second phase is characterised by a nadir following the first phase and has a lower amplitude and longer duration and lasts as long as the stimulus on the β-cells [178].

The rationale for the pulsatility is that it is more effective at reducing blood glucose concentration [166] and is hypothesised to reduce the risk of downregulating the insulin receptor (INSR) through overstimulation. The ultradian

TABLE 1.4 Substances affecting insulin release from β-cells.

Substance	Action on β-cells	Mechanism
Glucose[a]	Stimulant	Increased glycolysis and increased ATP production [169]
Glucagon	Stimulant	Directly and via GLP-1 receptors on the β-cell [170]
Osteocalcin	Stimulant	Both direct and by increasing GLP-1 [171]
GLP-1	Stimulant	Via GLP-1 receptors on the β-cell in the presence of elevated glucose concentrations [167]
GIP	Stimulant	Via GIP receptors on the β-cell in the presence of elevated glucose concentrations [172]
Acetylcholine	Regulatory	Directly via muscarinic receptors on β-cell (stimulant) and indirectly via muscarinic receptors on δ-cells which stimulate somatostatin secretion (suppression) [173]
Arginine	Augments insulin release	Membrane depolarisation [174]
Adrenaline	Suppressant	Via α-2 adrenoreceptors on the β-cell [175]
Somatostatin	Suppression	Directly via paracrine processes [176]

[a]*Most important secretagogue.*

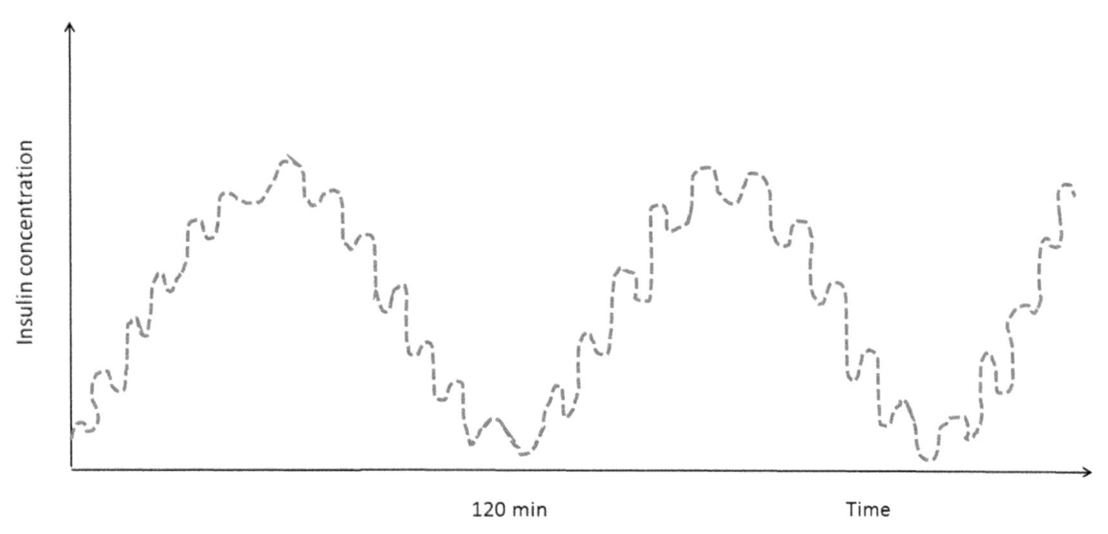

FIGURE 1.3 A conceptual model of the oscillatory nature of insulin secretion in the fasted state.

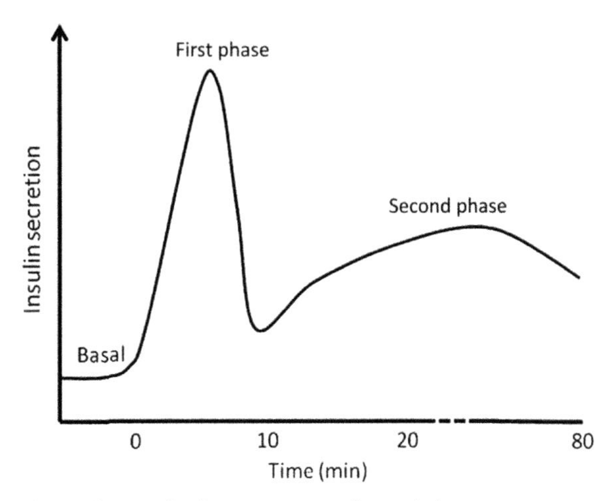

FIGURE 1.4 Conceptual model of biphasic insulin secretion in response to a glucose bolus.

periodicity is tightly coupled with the ultradian rhythms of the neuroendocrine, cardiovascular, and autonomic nervous systems and contributes to sympathovagal balance [182].

Suppression of insulin secretion is mediated via a variety of hormones, including the somatostatin, corticosteroids, and catecholamines, especially α2-adrenoreceptors, with the latter two typically during stress or exercise [159] (Table 1.4).

1.2.2.2 Insulin: mechanism of action

All of insulin's physiological effects occur following binding to the INSR, which is on the plasma membrane of many different somatic cell types. It is suggested that lower insulin doses invoke metabolic effects while larger amounts invoke mitogenic effects, with the latter predominantly via the mitogen-activated protein kinase (MAPK) pathways [169].

1.2.2.2.1 Main effects of insulin

Insulin principally acts on three main body tissues (skeletal muscle, white adipose tissue (WAT), and hepatocytes) through both direct and indirect effects with both metabolic and mitogenic actions (Table 1.5). Insulin's effects via acting on the central and peripheral nervous systems, vascular or endocrine systems can have systemic consequences.

Nutrient metabolism Insulin orchestrates fuel flux and metabolism through direct and indirect mechanisms with major pathways including gluconeogenesis, glycogen synthesis, and suppression of proteolysis or lipolysis.

Hepatic glucose flux (gluconeogenesis, glycogen synthesis) is regulated through insulin, fuels and glucagon working in concert [169]. Insulin suppresses gluconeogenesis directly via gene transcription and indirectly via suppressing lipolysis (reduction in substrate availability) [169]. It also suppresses glucagon release by the reduction of enzymatic expression and/or activity [183]. Insulin is well recognised to have anabolic effects in human skeletal muscle predominantly through suppressing proteolysis [184].

Electrolyte homoeostasis Insulin lowers serum concentration of phosphate, potassium, and magnesium by promoting cellular uptake [185]. Within the renal system, insulin promotes sodium reabsorption in the distal nephron and may promote calcium excretion [186].

TABLE 1.5 Direct and indirect actions of insulin in metabolically healthy systems.

Tissue	Effect
Hepatocyte	• Stimulates glycogen synthase and glycogen production • Inhibits glycogen phosphorylase and glycogenolysis • Stimulates de novo lipogenesis • Stimulates protein anabolism • Transcriptionally inhibits gluconeogenesis, • Inhibits ketogenesis via inhibiting β-oxidation • Indirectly inhibits gluconeogenesis by inhibiting lipolysis and releasing fatty acid and glycerol substrates • Indirectly inhibits gluconeogenesis via suppressing the release of glucagon
Skeletal muscle	• Upregulate GLUT4 translocation for glucose absorption • Stimulates glycogen synthase and glycogen production
White adipose tissue	• Stimulates lipogenesis • Suppresses lipolysis
Nervous system	• Neuronal growth stimulant
Vascular system	• Activates eNOS thus maintaining endothelial health
Electrolyte balance	• Increases cellular uptake of phosphate, potassium, and magnesium • Promotes renal absorption of sodium • Promotes renal excretion of calcium

Nervous system Insulin's pleiotropic effects are well demonstrated in the nervous system where its effects on glucose and energy homoeostasis are more indirect, via insulin's essential roles on neuronal health and development. While insulin is essential for both central and peripheral neuronal growth via activation of the Akt pathways [187], due to the predominant expression of GLUT1 and GLUT 3, neurons are considered 'insulin-responsive' rather than 'insulin-dependent'[188].

In the central nervous system, insulin is transcytosed across the blood brain barrier [169] where INSRs are widely expressed, especially in the hypothalamus, hippocampus and cerebral cortex all of which are involved in regulating metabolic homoeostasis [189,190]. Brain insulin signalling is pivotal for regulating the hypothalamic-pituitary-adrenal axis, promotes synaptic plasticity, influences proliferation of glial cells, and has a central role for glycaemic control with mechanisms yet to be fully determined; thus highlighting insulin's significant role within the brain [169,191].

Vascular system Within the vascular system, insulin has a number of vital roles, especially in vasoconstriction and coagulation. INSRs are widely expressed on both vascular endothelium and platelets. When insulin binds to the endothelial receptors, it activates endothelial nitric oxide (NO) synthase (eNOS). The subsequent production of NO prevents vasoconstriction, inflammatory cell adhesion, and platelet aggregation to the endothelial wall [192]. With respect to coagulation, insulin modulates platelet aggregation, preventing over-activation [193] while it also modulates fibrinolysis [194], thus impacting many aspects of vascular health.

1.2.2.3 Insulin resistance and hyperinsulinaemia

1.2.2.3.1 Insulin resistance: important for human survival?

IR is a poorly defined concept that aims to explain the pathophysiology of T2D. The term itself can be traced to the observations of Himsworth in the 1930s where people who required larger doses of insulin to maintain euglycaemia were termed 'insulin resistant'. Historically, IR has a glucocentric focus, which has resulted in increased attention to myocytes, hepatocytes, and WAT as these tissues can manage significant glucose flux and disposal.

What has been overlooked is that IR *per se* is an important physiological state that is evolutionarily important for human survival. Biochemically, mitochondria use fuels from a variety of sources (e.g. glucose, pyruvate, lactate, acetoacetate, and fatty acids) to generate ATP, preferentially from oxidative phosphorylation as this generates the maximal amount of ATP and other products (e.g. proteins, hormones, and enzymes) with a minimal amount of reactive oxidative species (ROS) and other undesirable by-products. Certain cells have a higher glucose demand including: retinal cells, renal medulla cells, red blood cells, and the central nervous system, whereas other cells can use fatty acids and ketone bodies (e.g. skeletal muscle). During times of food shortages, especially of carbohydrate-rich foods (e.g. during winter), IR is physiologically important to ensure that cells with a higher reliance on glucose receive sufficient amounts, whereas cells with lower glucose requirements do not use the scarce resource. Furthermore, it is well recognised that different life-stages, especially pregnancy [195] and puberty [169], are associated with transient IR in healthy individuals. In these instances, IR is of physiological benefit and necessary for development and growth.

This means that IR can be divided into acute (IR_A) and chronic (IR_C) subtypes with IR_A being the physiologically important and *reversible* subtype for evolutionary survival. Conversely, IR_C is associated with the pathogenesis of metabolic diseases, especially T2D. Although, as to be discussed in later chapters, IRC can be improved, whether IR_C can be improved, placed into remission, or reversed, but cure remains uncertain.

1.2.2.3.2 Physiology and pathophysiology of insulin resistance

Traditionally, the biochemical principles behind IR_C and IR_A are similar and revolve around glucose disposal in the skeletal muscle, which is a major site of insulin-mediated glucose disposal. Most glucose taken into skeletal muscle is converted to glycogen to be used as a local energy source and cannot be re-released back into the bloodstream for other tissues [196]. Therefore, inducing IR in skeletal muscle was vital for survival in evolutionary terms. In times of poor food availability, adequate glycogen could be 'locked' away in skeletal muscles for 'flight-fight' emergencies, while fat was used for basal energy expenditure and the body's glucose, primarily from hepatic gluconeogenesis, used for the other tissues that had a higher physiological need for glucose. IR_A can develop within hours, with triggers such as short-term stressors (i.e. pain, fasting/starvation, acute stress, or impaired sleep) and are believed to impart increased rates of survival. By contrast IR_C is believed to develop over years if not decades [197].

Acute insulin resistance This means that the mechanism for IR_A is predominantly the inhibition of GLUT4, especially in skeletal muscle. Although insulin, or muscle contractions, induce the translocation of GLUT4 to the cell surface

[169], a variety of processes can impede GLUT4 translocation including acute pain/injury [198], corticosteroids, sympathetic activity [199], and pregnancy [169]. The precise mechanism by which fasting induces IR in humans has not yet been resolved, however, elevated concentration of glycogen and increased lipid accumulation have both been observed after a 72-h fast and both mechanisms decrease GLUT4 translocation [200]. In hepatocytes IR_A results in increased gluconeogenesis [169]. Key features of IR_A are timeline and reversibility. IR_A is generally associated with a clear timeline and/or endpoint (e.g. pregnancy or winter) or a short-term challenge (e.g. injury) where the person would either survive or die. It can also be swiftly reversed with the removal of the challenge (e.g. childbirth, increased food availability).

Chronic insulin resistance By contrast, IR_C is due to a combination of decreased insulin receptor (INSR) expression at cell surface (receptor defects) and impaired signal transduction (post-receptor defects) [169]. However, it is likely that a combination of IR_C and hyperinsulinaemia is required to develop the pathologies associated with IR_C. A decrease in INSR numbers means that a higher insulin concentration (compensatory hyperinsulinaemia) is needed to achieve the same biological result, while impaired signal transduction means a decreased biological response no matter the insulin concentration [169].

Within skeletal muscle, IR_C is a combination of INSR and post-receptor defects resulting in a blunting of insulin's ability to both translocate GLUT4 to the cell surface and stimulate glycogen synthesis [169]. This leads to impaired uptake of glucose from the bloodstream, which leads to glycaemic stress on other tissues, including the pancreas, which results in compensatory hyperinsulinaemia. Interestingly, insulin's mitogenic effects on skeletal muscle are not impaired and may even be enhanced due to the compensatory hyperinsulinaemia [169].

In hepatocytes, through a variety of complex biochemical mechanisms [169], both increased IR (resulting in increased hepatic gluconeogenesis) and increased insulin action (increased lipogenic flux) are observed. This paradox is believed to result from a combination of hepatic IR and insulin-independent pathways. IR results in inadequate suppression of gluconeogenesis and a decrease in hepatic glycogen synthesis while insulin-independent nutrient-sensitive pathways drive the re-esterification of circulating fatty acids and de novo lipogenesis to increase hepatic triglyceride concentration [169].

WAT is both a nutrient sink and an endocrine organ. Although not a significant site of insulin mediated glucose disposal ($<5\%$), this process is necessary to generate the glycerol-3-phosphate needed for fatty acid esterification and correct lipid storage. Therefore, IR in WAT results in incomplete suppression of lipolysis and improper lipid storage thus facilitating lipid storage in non-adipose tissues [169]. The aetiology of IR in WAT remains the subject of debate. However, what is recognised is that hypertrophy of WAT induces low levels of chronic and systemic inflammation with an increased release of cytokines, especially from visceral fat deposits. Despite insulin per se being anti-inflammatory [201], the net effect of hyperinsulinaemia is increased systemic inflammation due to increased visceral obesity, and so it will be described accordingly [202].

1.2.2.3.3 Aetiology of insulin resistance

The aetiology of IR and/or hyperinsulinemia is complex and likely to have multiple pathways/triggers as shown in Fig. 1.5.

Different ethnic populations have different prevalence rates of IR_C, that cannot be completely explained by rates of obesity, fat distribution, glucose concentration, or socioeconomic status [203–206]. The *thrifty-gene* hypothesis suggests that ease of fat accumulation and or IR_A, aided survival for certain populations, especially hunter-gatherer. However, no specific gene, polymorphism or mitochondrial mutation has yet been identified to confirm the theory ([207]).

The most significant contributor to IR_C is believed to be overnutrition. Modern processed foods are often considered to be energy dense but nutrient poor and contribute to an increased risk of obesity, dyslipidaemia, and hypertension – all markers of hyperinsulinaemia [208,209]. Nutrient deficiencies, especially vitamins D or B12, magnesium, and folate, are also associated with increased IR as well as being independently associated with other metabolic disorders such as nitric oxide (NO) synthase dysfunction [210,211]. Obesity and/or hyperplasia disorders may further aggravate these nutrient deficiencies by increasing the effective volume of distribution (i.e. vitamins may be stored or sequestered in adipose tissue).

Although obesity is a significant contributor to the aetiology of IR and hyperinsulinaemia, it is argued that it is not obesity *per se* that is the causative factor. People with simple obesity (absence of other symptoms of MetS) maintain first-phase insulin secretion. Furthermore, although the prevalence of a population with a BMI > 30 kg/m^2 is greater in USA compared to Japan, the prevalence of T2D is similar ([166]).

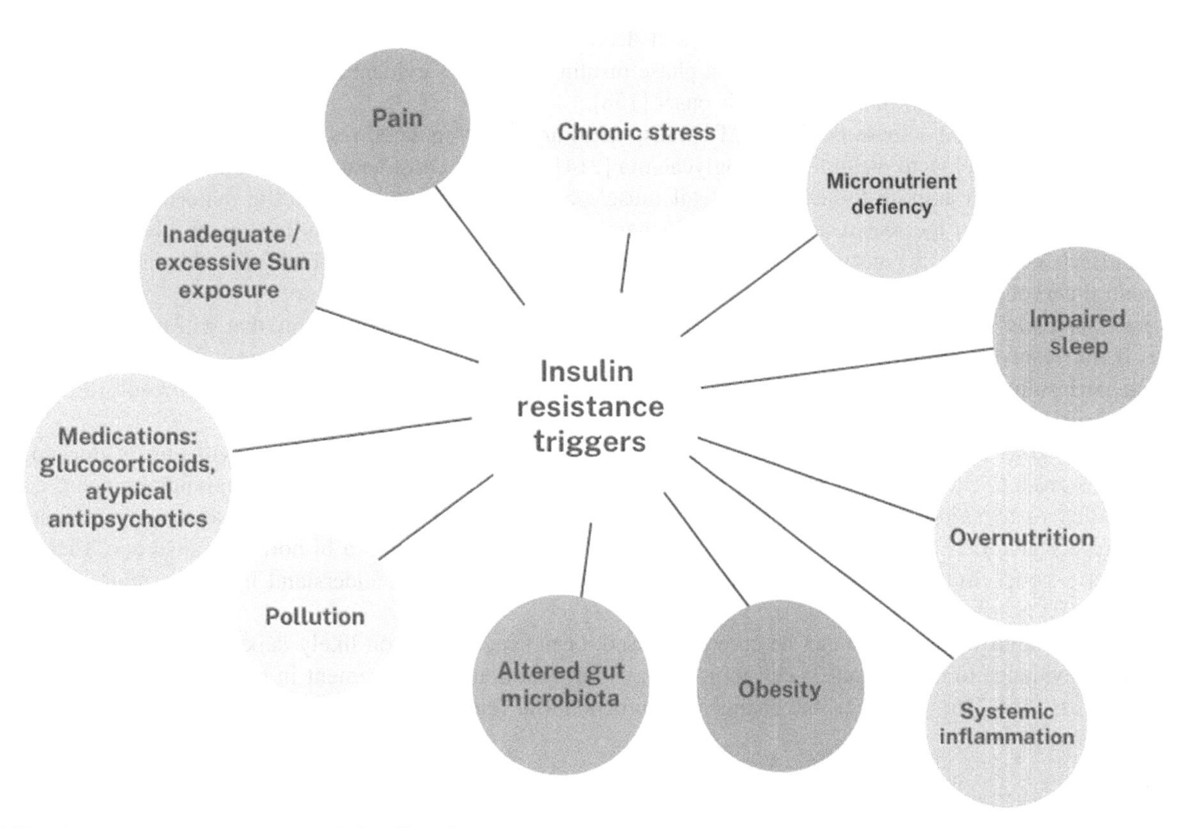

FIGURE 1.5 Aetiologic pathways of chronic insulin resistance.

Other aspects of modern living are also significant contributors to hyperinsulinaemia, especially anything that disturbs autonomic (sympathovagal) balance. Evolutionarily, humans were not designed to function under allostatic or sympathetic overload (chronic stress) [212]. Excessive and continuous release of glucocorticoids, catecholamines, and other mediators, will suppress immune function, increase appetite, and aggravate hypertension and IR. However, this allostatic overload can also cause insomnia and other sleep disturbances. Disturbed sleep often results in increased stress and other psychological pressures the following day, which may further impact allostatic load and appetite and continue the destructive cycle.

Poor sleep quality is indisputably associated with IR/hyperinsulinaemia and with many of its sequelae. Poor sleep is clearly related to modern living (e.g. excessive light (especially in the blue-spectrum), noise, bedroom temperature and/or humidity, shift-work and excessive mental stimulation too close to bedtime). Sleep deprivation disturbs insulin secretion oscillations through a variety of mechanisms. It also increases cortisol secretion (impairing GLUT4 translocation) and catecholamine release. Furthermore, sleep deprivation increases ghrelin and decreases leptin, thus affecting appetite control [182]. Sleep quality is also crucial to good metabolic health. A decreased quantity of deep non-REM sleep (also referred to as stages 3 and 4 slow wave sleep) can impair the central glymphatic drainage system, which may impact cognition, centrally mediated IR, and neuronal health and activity [213].

1.2.2.3.4 Shift from normoglycaemia-hyperinsulinaemia to hyperglycaemia-hyperinsulinaemia

The metabolically healthy are initially normoglycaemic-normoinsulinaemic. Repeated exposure to one or more insulin resistance triggers, especially overnutrition, causes a slight elevation in plasma glucose – still well within the normal reference range of 3.5–5.3 mmol/L (63–95 mg/dL) – but enough to cause glycaemic stress on mitochondria. This glycaemic stress causes an increase in systemic mitochondrial respiration, a decrease in oxidative phosphorylation reactions and overall production of ATP, as well as concurrent increases in glycolytic reactions and production of reactive oxidative species (ROS). This process reduces effective cellular communication and protein/other substrate production and increases the cell's need for antioxidants. This drives a number of different processes including a loss of the first phase insulin release for reasons not fully elucidated but hypothesised to involve a less hyperpolarisable inner mitochondrial membrane [177]. Observations show a decrease in quantity and/or impaired exocytosis of the readily releasable insulin vesicles [166]. This loss of first phase insulin response is evident in people with impaired glucose tolerance and T2D [155] but may also predict their onset [158].

In affected skeletal and adipose cells, GLUT4 transporters are downregulated resulting in increased insulin requirements, both basal and bolus, to maintain normoglycaemia [214]. There is considerable discussion as to which body system, especially between adipose tissue and skeletal muscle cells, which then becomes the major driver for systemic metabolic disease. Given the recent advances in biochemistry and a better understanding of the pleiotropic and biochemical effects of insulin, the answer is likely multimodal with different systems, which may also include bone [168] or the central nervous system, being the catalyst for different populations.

Overall, the early stages of glycaemic stress results in compensatory hyperinsulinaemia that will maintain normoglycaemia. If not resolved sufficiently quickly, long-term/permanent changes to the mitochondria may result, leading to chronic hyperinsulinaemia with normoglycaemia. Eventually, the maintained glycaemic stress will result in β-cell failure resulting in decreased insulin secretion.

This depressed IS from pancreatic β-cells, especially in the presence of IR in the α-cells will impair glucagon suppression. This leads to excessive glucagon being released, which will raise both basal and postprandial glucose concentrations leading to hyperglycaemia [215], eventually resulting in T2D. Given that hyperglucagonaemia is associated with both type 1 and T2D, it demonstrates that diabetes mellitus is, at minimum, a bi-hormonal disorder. Therefore, it suggests that a good clinical understanding of glucagon is necessary to fully understand hyperglycaemia, but that is beyond the scope of this review.

The debate around whether T2D can be cured, reversed, or put into remission likely depends on a multitude of factors. There is evidence to demonstrate β-cell morphology with functional improvement in both α-and β-cells can occur with weight loss [166,216]. However, the changes to mitochondrial function required further investigation to determine their permanence.

1.2.2.4 *Insulin resistance or hyperinsulinaemia?*

Although the literature has traditionally discussed IR as the condition that underpins T2D, there are a number of challenges with that definition. Firstly, it ignores the role of hyperinsulinaemia. It is frequently surmised that T2D occurs when the pancreas is unable to produce sufficient compensatory insulin to overcome the defects associated with IR. Yet, as shown above, hyperinsulinaemia is an important modulator of metabolic health independently of IR. Furthermore, there needs to be a clear distinction between physiologically necessary IR_A, compared to IR_C which is almost always associated with hyperinsulinaemia under a carbohydrate load. This means that although IR and hyperinsulinaemia have distinct biochemical pathways, the two conditions are intertwined and frequently conflated, especially due to the feed-forward pathways: Chronic hyperinsulinaemia is a known driver of IR, while chronic IR causes compensatory hyperinsulinaemia (under an excessive glycaemic load).

As previously described, humans have evolved to perform well under chronic IR in the absence of excessive glycaemia. Hyperglycaemia synergistically compounds the pathophysiologies associated with hyperinsulinaemia. Given hyperglycaemia is easily measured, but hyperinsulinaemia is not, it is highly plausible that many associated pathologies, e.g. microvascular disease, commenced in the hyperinsulinaemic/ normoglycaemic state. For example, hyperinsulinaemia/IR elevates plasminogen activator inhibitor type-1 (PAI-1), which impairs the fibrinolysis processes, increasing the risk of thrombosis. This process can be induced by acute pain. So in the normoglycaemic state, it can be considered evolutionarily necessary to help survive trauma [198]. However, hyperglycaemia increases the secretion of hepatic clotting factors and the proinflammatory cytokine, interleukin-6, thus increasing the risk of microthrombi. Collectively, the increased risk of developing microthrombi combined with the decreased capacity to clear them means that people with T2D (hyperglycaemic and hyperinsulinaemic) have a significantly increased risk of microvascular disease.

Given the intertwined nature of chronic IR and pathological hyperinsulinaemia, unless otherwise specified, the two conditions will be collectively referred to as '*hyperinsulinaemia*' for the rest of this section.

1.2.2.5 *Consequences of hyperinsulinaemia*

Hyperinsulinaemia affects every cell within the body especially via mitochondrial defects and changes to fuel flux leading to increased ROS and AGE production. However, it must also be remembered that body systems do not work in isolation, and the overall impact of hyperinsulinaemia should be considered holistically. For example, IR in cardiac neurons will impair healthy function of the cardiovascular system just as vasoconstriction in cerebral capillaries will have significant effects on cerebral health.

This means that hyperinsulinaemia is directly and/or indirectly associated with many different pathologies (Fig. 1.6) both mechanistically and/or epidemiologically [217]. The main mechanisms involved are mitochondrial stress and altered substrate metabolism, ectopic lipid accumulation, increased gene transcription, vascular or neurological consequences, and by affecting different signalling pathways including intracellular pathways like PI3K or MAPK or extracellular pathways including hormones or cytokines [192,218].

1.2.2.5.1 Type 2 diabetes, metabolic syndrome, and other endocrine disorders

Type 2 diabetes As previously described, untreated chronic IR will lead to β-cell failure, hyperglucagonaemia and hyperglycaemia, which, with its feedforward cycle, will worsen with time, eventually leading to a diagnosis of T2D. Hyperglycaemia synergistically adds to damage caused by hyperinsulinaemia through the production of AGEs and other glycated proteins, stimulation of cellular growth and proliferation, especially vascular smooth muscle (via IGF-1) and increased blood coagulability (independent of insulin concentration) [219,220].

Gestational diabetes Gestational diabetes is also associated with hyperinsulinaemia. Increased pregnancy-induced insulin resistance (IRp) is a normal phenomenon of the second and third trimesters of pregnancy to ensure the developing foetus has an adequate nutrient supply [221]. However, pre-pregnancy IR_C compounded by IRp results in the foetus receiving overnutrition combined with glycaemic and oxidative stress and systemic inflammation, even if the mother does not fulfil diagnostic criteria for gestational diabetes. Insulin does not cross the placenta. However, the foetal response to this overnutrition and inflammatory environment is to develop foetal hyperinsulinaemia and excessive growth, which may present as hyperglycaemia and macrosomia at birth. As the child grows and develops, their gestational environment may result in

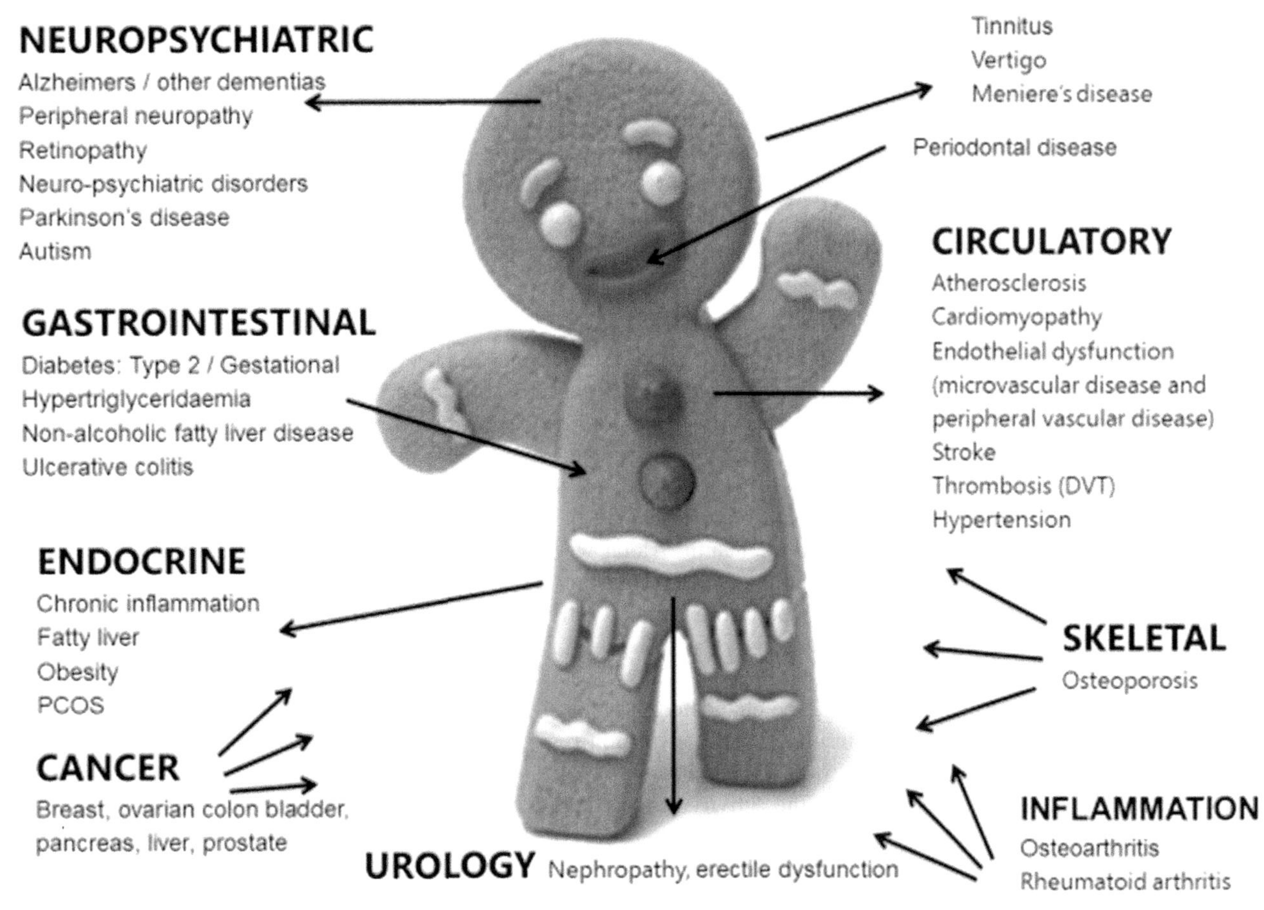

FIGURE 1.6 Complications of hyperinsulinaemia.

long-term impaired appetite regulation, mitochondrial function, and potentially brain and nerve development [221]. Consequently, the child may have increased predisposition to developing IR_C with subsequent consequences at an earlier age. Within the mother, it is believed that due to the feedforward mechanisms, IRp can increase the risk of IR_C thus explaining their increased risk of developing T2D and or other metabolic diseases later in life.

Double diabetes In recent years, there is an increasing prevalence of people with type 1 diabetes (T1D) developing IR, manifesting with increased doses of insulin (hyperinsulinaemia) to maintain glycaemic control along with other symptoms of MetS [222]. It remains uncertain whether 'double diabetes' is a separate phenotype of T1D, or simply a consequence of modern living and change of therapy guidelines over the last 20 years resulting in overnutrition and IR_C.

Polycystic ovarian syndrome Hyperinsulinaemia, hyperandrogenism, and anovulation are core pathophysiological elements of polycystic ovarian syndrome (PCOS). As hyperinsulinaemia is associated with increased androgen production and decreased sex-hormone binding globulin production thus worsening symptoms. People with PCOS have a high prevalence of MetS, with heightened hyperinsulinaemia and decreased insulin sensitivity compared to their obese peers, even during adolescence [223]. As with pregnancy, PCOS, or any condition that involves hyperinsulinaemia, will be compounded by external factors that further increase IR.

1.2.2.5.2 Hepatic disease

The liver is the major organ for controlling lipid homoeostasis and fatty acid metabolism. Despite processing large amounts of fatty acids, a healthy liver contains less than 5% triglycerides by weight [224]. However, between 50%–75% of people with either obesity and/or T2D are affected by NAFLD [225]. NAFLD describes a spectrum of hepatic fat accumulation from steatosis through fibrosis and/or cirrhosis. As described above, a combination of hyperinsulinaemia and IR increases hepatic triglyceride concentrations via overnutrition, de novo lipogenesis or systemic fatty acid metabolism. Increased lipogenesis increases endoplasmic reticulum and mitochondrial oxidative stress, which promotes further lipid accumulation in a feed-forward process [226]. Excessive fat accumulation within the liver triggers inflammatory responses within the lipocytes, which can lead to hepatocyte death and further inflammatory responses. When hepatocyte death rates surpass the processes that regenerate healthy cells, alternative pathways are initiated that result in the distorted cellular architecture found in fibrosis. If the fibrotic pathways are maintained, cirrhosis may follow.

While hyperinsulinaemia is a key driver of NAFLD, it remains uncertain whether NAFLD is a causal, or only an associative, factor for IR. However, as fibrosis develops and impairs hepatic function, this has a negative impact on many body functions including glucose and lipid homoeostasis and increased hepatic fibrinogen production [193].

1.2.2.5.3 Renal disease

Within the renal system, hyperinsulinaemia can impair renal structure and function, both directly and indirectly. As the kidneys are a highly vascular organ, hyperinsulinaemia induced vasoconstriction and/or hypercoagulability will have a profound effect on both overall kidney function and hypertension. However, the effects of insulin on the excretion rates of a variety of solutes, especially certain electrolytes, and uric acid, also have a profound effect on systemic metabolic functions.

Hyperinsulinaemia decreases renal excretion of uric acid by the kidneys. The resulting increase in uric acid has a potent, but negative, effect on overall metabolic health. Along with an increased risk of gout, hyperuricaemia is well recognised to increase hepatic lipid accumulation [227], increasing the risk of NAFLD, and also stimulates production of ROS [228], increasing oxidative stress. Hyperuricaemia also activates the renin-angiotension system [228] and independently impairs NO synthesis [229] causing vasoconstriction, thus increasing blood pressure and the risk of hypertension.

While the precise mechanisms are still to be elucidated, it is recognised that sodium retention is coupled to uric acid retention and/or mediated by a lack of insulin signalling (insulin resistance) [230]. Other electrolyte disorders can also be attributed either directly or indirectly to hyperinsulinaemia, especially potassium, magnesium, and phosphate depletion disorders. Hyperinsulinaemia increases the activity of the Na^+-K^+-ATPase pumps, which promotes potassium's entry into many cells and may induce a mild hypokalaemia. Hypokalaemia may be aggravated by hypomagnesemia, which may also be induced by an insulin mediated shift of magnesium from an extracellular to an intracellular space. Hyperinsulinaemia can also cause an intracellular shift in phosphate concentrations, which may also be compounded by hypomagnesemia. The interconnected nature of electrolyte balances may also be affected by, amongst other factors, changes in serum osmolality, renal function, or systemic acidosis [185].

Furthermore, IR is directly linked to a declining glomerular filtration rate (GFR). The glomerular endothelial cells are also significant producers of endothelial nitric oxide synthase in response to insulin, so are also markedly affected by IR. Podocytes are also highly insulin responsive to allow the kidneys manage necessary postprandial changes to GFR. Decreased insulin signalling within these cells is associated with changes associated with diabetic nephropathy, independent of changes in glucose concentrations, highlighting the importance of insulin's actions [230].

Collectively, these factors demonstrate that hyperinsulinaemia has a significant impact on renal function. Overall, the retention of uric acid has a profound impact on systemic metabolic health given the increase in ROS, and blood pressure and impact on endothelial health. However, even mild electrolyte disorders, while normally multifactorial in causation, also increase morbidity and mortality.

1.2.2.5.4 Cardiovascular disease

All forms of cardiovascular disease are aggravated by hyperinsulinaemia at the level of the macro- and micro- vasculature and the heart [202]. As previously described, insulin activates eNOS which maintains vascular tone and endothelial health [192]. However, hyperinsulinaemia in the same endothelial cells drives pro-inflammatory, pro-atherogenic, pro-thrombosis, and vasoconstrictive pathways. This increases the risk of ischaemic heart disease at both the macro- (myocardial infarction) and micro-vascular (ischaemic stroke, vascular dementia, retinopathy, nephropathy) levels. These conditions are compounded by hyperglycaemia [231]. More importantly, impaired endothelial health will impact the complete body and may act synergistically with many other pathological states, such as impaired nervous signalling, to intensify disease states such as renal disease or erectile dysfunction.

Hyperinsulinaemia also impairs many coagulation processes both directly and indirectly. Many coagulation factors, including thrombin and fibrinogen are hepatically synthesised; production is increased in the presence of hyperinsulinaemia leading to a hypercoagulable state and an increased risk of thrombi [193].

Within cardiomyocytes, IR_C results in lipotoxicity and increased myocardial oxygen consumption, which decreases cardiac efficiency and increases the risk of heart failure [232]. Although this is considered independent of myocardial ischaemia, microvascular disease and a lack of NO will cause a compounding effect.

Overall, when the effects of vasoconstriction, coagulation, hypertriglyceridaemia, and impaired endothelial surfaces are considered, hyperinsulinaemia is a leading aetiological factor for the development of cardiovascular disease.

Interestingly IR is also associated with atrial fibrillation and its arrhythmogenesis [233].

1.2.2.5.5 Nervous systems

As previously discussed, neurons are not insulin dependent; however, their high expression of INSR makes them susceptible to IR which impairs nerve signalling and communication. This can lead to a myriad of neuropathic and related disorders both centrally and peripherally. There are also many indirect mechanisms whereby hyperinsulinaemia causes significant neuronal dysfunction. Glycaemic stress will lead to an accumulation of ROS and glycaemic end-products resulting in inflammation and impaired neuronal signalling. Significant fluctuations in CNS glucose concentrations promote inflammatory processes by increasing the production of ROS and impairing glutamate activity, which can result in neurotoxicity and/or confusion or impaired memory. Endothelial damage and vasoconstriction will lead to ischaemic disease with microthrombi, potentially accelerating hypoxic damage and apoptosis. In the central nervous system this results in cerebral vascular disease and transient ischaemic attacks, ischaemic stroke, or vascular dementia. While in the peripheral system, ischaemic disease leads to the progression of microvascular disease including impaired wound healing, retinopathies, and nephropathies [234].

1.2.2.5.6 Neurological and neuropsychiatric disorders

Within the CNS, hyperinsulinaemia and/or neuronal IR can lead to systemic dysfunction including the dopaminergic systems (mood and memory disturbances), impairment of BBB insulin transport systems, reduced synaptic plasticity, and centrally driven metabolic dysfunction [191,218]. Furthermore, hyperinsulinaemia is associated with impairment of the glymphatic drainage system [213], post-INSR receptor defects, and/or reduced IGF-1 expression [235]. This means that many aspects of brain and nerve health are impaired, especially when considered alongside the previously described microvascular and mitochondrial changes leading to cerebrovascular dysfunction, including an increased risk of stroke or depression [236].

Alzheimer's disease Hyperinsulinaemia is an independent risk factor for Alzheimer's disease (AD) and increases the risk for other neurological diseases [187,213,235,237]. In fact association between T2D, a hyperinsulinaemic condition, and AD is so strong that Alzheimer's disease is being referred to as type 3 diabetes [238,239]. It is believed that IR increases tau phosphorylation and increases expression of β-amyloid peptide. When these are combined with increased expression of tumour necrosis factor-α (TNF-α), it facilitates the formation of the amyloid plaques that are the hallmark of Alzheimer's disease [239,240]. Furthermore, insulin modulates polysialylated neuronal cell adhesion molecule (PSA-NCAM) turnover. Dysregulated PSA-NCAM is associated with Alzheimer's disease and schizophrenia [241].

Mental health The impact of hyperinsulinaemia on mental health is debated, however, hyperinsulinaemia is associated with schizophrenia, and IR is a well-known consequence of many atypical antipsychotic medications [242,243]. However, increased rates of IR are being reported in first-episode, drug naïve patients with schizophrenia compared to healthy age and sex matched controls [243] suggesting a mechanism that is independent of the medications. There is some evidence to suggest that schizophrenia is associated with central oxidative stress and/or dysregulation of free radical metabolism; both would be aggravated by hyperinsulinaemia.

Neuropathies Peripheral neuropathy is an extremely complex but common consequence of both type 1 and T2D and includes both autonomic and somatic subtypes. While optimal glycaemic control is reported to reduce the relative risk of neuropathy by 78% in people with T1D, this is reduced to less than 10% in people with T2D. This highlights that the mechanism of peripheral neuropathy in people with T2D likely stems from hyperinsulinaemia, as IR, dyslipidaemia, hyperglycaemia, systemic inflammation, and mitochondrial dysfunction are all implicated [244].

Pain is common with somatic neuropathies, which, as described previously, worsens IR [198,245]. Hyperinsulinaemia can complicate somatic neuropathies by impairing the healing process following injuries, such as impaired NO preventing poor capillary circulation. Sudomotor dysfunction may be an early presentation of diabetic neuropathies. Although arising in the extremities, it may also present as proximal hyperhidrosis or gustatory sweating [244].

Autonomic neuropathies also confer significant increases in morbidity and mortality. Cardiovascular neuropathies may be associated with denervation of the vagus nerve and often result in diminished cardiac output. Gastrointestinal neuropathies can increase or decrease gastrointestinal transit times with accompanying challenges to glucose and/or electrolyte homoeostasis. Urogenital neuropathies can increase the risk of bladder and/or sexual dysfunction, with the latter being compounded by NO and/or vascular complications [244].

1.2.2.5.7 Skeletal and structural support systems

Hyperinsulinaemia affects the structural support systems, especially bone and skin, by decreasing the quality and quantity of collagen production via mitochondrial stress. Hyperinsulinaemia, compounded by hyperglycaemia, also places additional stress on all cells in the bone modelling unit (osteo -blasts, -clasts and -cytes) leading to decreased cellular differentiation and/ or early death/ apoptosis. Consequently, there is excessive bone mineralisation without the necessary underlying supporting structures, leading to normal to high bone mineral density but increased risk of fragility fractures (osteo fragalitis) [168].

1.2.2.5.8 Cancer

Hyperinsulinaemia is associated with both the development of, and the survival rates for many cancers, both directly and indirectly via obesity and increased visceral fat deposits [246,247]. These cancers include liver, bladder, colorectal, pancreatic, gastro-oesophageal, breast, endometrial and renal [231], although it must be noted that age, sex, or method of assessing visceral adiposity may influence these results [219,248]. Mechanisms include increased IGF-1, vascular endothelial growth factor (VEGF), increased mitogenic activity, decreased hepatic production of sex-hormone-binding-protein/globulin (SHBG) and increased adipokines [231]. These effects can be compounded by hyperglycaemia as most cancer cells generate ATP mostly by aerobic glycolysis (Warburg effect). Indirectly, increased ROS stimulates cell proliferation and causes structural changes to DNA, with potentially mutagenic effects [249].

Interestingly diabetes is associated with a lower incidence of prostate cancer, potentially due to lower levels of testosterone. However, no matter the type of cancer, epidemiological studies have shown that people with T2D and concomitant cancer have higher mortality rates compared to those without T2D. Whether this is due to delayed diagnosis and/or poorer treatment, or other clinical factors, or simply due to the excess age-adjusted mortality typically associated with diabetes is yet to be determined [219].

1.2.2.6 Summary

Overall, hyperinsulinaemia is connected either directly or indirectly with most, if not all, non-communicable diseases. At the cellular level, this involves impaired mitochondria, fuel use, substrate and ATP production, production of ROS, and impaired cellular signalling. While many organs and tissues are directly affected by hyperinsulinaemia and/or insulin resistance, resultant microvascular disease and impaired neuronal signalling will eventually impair all body systems.

1.3 The adoption and evolution of dietary guidelines

Timothy David Noakes

Unless care is exercised in selecting food, a diet may result which is one-sided or badly balanced - that is, one in which either protein or fuel ingredients (carbohydrate and fat) are provided in excess.... The evils of overeating may not be felt at once, but sooner or later they are sure to appear perhaps in an excessive amount of fatty tissue, perhaps in general debility, perhaps in actual disease.

W.O. Atwater, 1902 [250]

In Section 1.1 [251] we described how the species-specific human diet evolved over millions of years, gradually being adapted by distinct populations living in diverse environments where the food sources naturally differed. The knowledge of what was safe, wholesome, and had survival value in each specific environment was then handed down from generation to generation. Continuing to eat this way over millennia produced robust populations, always at risk of dying from infections and trauma [251] but which were largely free of the chronic diseases of modernity, including cancer [252].

Thus the dietary guidelines were simple: You ate the (natural and unprocessed) foods that your father hunted, your mother gathered and (probably) your mother prepared for you.

In the last decade of the 19th century and the first of the 20th century, science [253] first weighs in with advice to humans about what we should be eating. It takes the form of two publications [250,254] authored by W.O. Atwater, then the first Director of the Office of Experiment Stations in the US Department of Agriculture. The advice focused on the importance of 'variety, proportionality, and moderation in healthful eating' ([253], p. 34). At the time minerals and vitamins had not been identified; thus the advice referred only to the intakes of protein, carbohydrates, fat and 'mineral matter' (ash).

By the 1920s this advice had advanced to categorise foods into five major groups – milk and meat, cereals, vegetables and fruits, fats and fatty foods, and sugar and sugary foods – with suggested amounts of the different foods that should be purchased each week by the average family [255].

At the 1941 National Nutrition Conference for Defence, the Food and Nutrition Board of the National Academy of Sciences released the first set of Recommended Daily Allowances (RDAs) which established the recommended intakes of calories and of nine essential nutrients [256]. By 1943 the Basic 7 Food Guide had been released (Fig. 1.7).

After 1961, the campaign by the American Heart Association (AHA) and others to vigorously promote Ancel Keys' Twin Hypotheses – the Diet-Heart and Lipid Hypotheses – became the defining influence on this national US dietary advice.

As a result the concerns of those directing US nutrition policy shifted from an exclusive focus on ensuring an adequate intake of essential nutrients to one of avoiding excessive intakes of identified nutrients considered to cause specific chronic diseases. This shift was cemented with the release of what became known as the (first) US Department of Agriculture (USDA) Dietary Goals for Americans (DGA) [257,258].

Many argue that these dietary guidelines were the direct cause of the epidemics of obesity andT2D and other related chronic diseases, now reaching epidemic proportions around the globe.

1.3.1 The USDA Dietary Goals for Americans

The 1977 USDA DGA were created by Senator George McGovern's Senate Select Committee on Nutrition and Human Needs. These revolutionary guidelines [257,258] were based specifically on Keys' unproven hypotheses. They advocated replacing fat in the diet with polyunsaturated 'vegetable oils' and carbohydrate-rich cereals, grains and fruits. There were six specific goals:

Goal 1: Increase carbohydrate consumption to approximately 55%–60% of total (caloric) intake.

Goal 2: Reduce overall fat consumption from approximately 40%–30% of energy intake.

Goal 3: Reduce saturated fat consumption to account for about 10% of total energy intake; and balance that with polyunsaturated and monounsaturated fats, which should each account for about 10% of energy intake.

Goal 4: Reduce cholesterol consumption to about 300 mg a day.

Goal 5: Reduce sugar consumption by about 40% to account for about 15% of total energy.

Goal 6: Reduce salt consumption by 50%–85% to about 3 g per day.

The outcome was that the USDA DGA advised Americans to restrict their intake of saturated fats and to eat 8–12 servings of grain and cereals per day. Grains and cereals replaced the butter, lard, cheese, eggs and meat that had been

For Health...eat some food from each group...every day!
GROUP ONE
GREEN AND YELLOW VEGETABLES...
GROUP TWO
ORANGES, TOMATOES, GRAPEFRUIT...
GROUP THREE
POTATOES AND OTHER VEGETABLES AND FRUITS
GROUP FOUR
MILK AND MILK PRODUCTS...
GROUP FIVE
MEAT, POULTRY, FISH, OR EGGS...
GROUP SIX
BREAD, FLOUR, AND CEREALS...
GROUP SEVEN
BUTTER AND FORTIFIED MARGARINE
U.S. NEEDS US STRONG
EAT THE BASIC 7 EVERY DAY
U.S. GOVERNMENT CHART
IN ADDITION TO THE BASIC 7...
EAT ANY OTHER FOODS YOU WANT

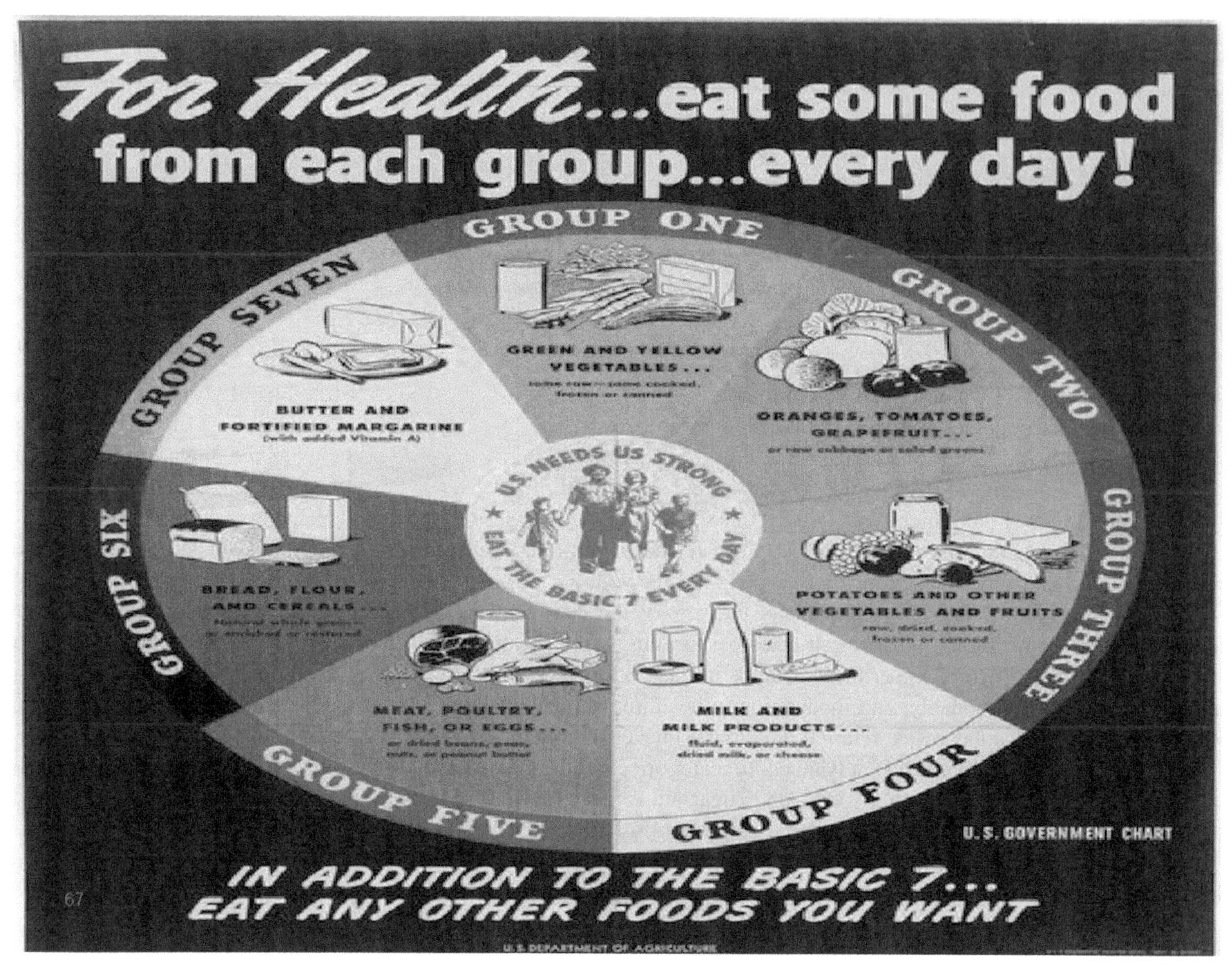

FIGURE 1.7 The Basic 7 Foods from 1943, US Department of Agriculture.

American staples for centuries [259]. It also represented a profound departure from the species-specific diet with which humans had evolved [251].

Since this represented a radical change in the way humans had acquired their knowledge about how best to feed ourselves [251], it's important to understand what drove this change.

1.3.2 The story behind the formulation and adoption of the 1977 USDA Dietary Goals for Americans

The 1972 US Presidential election contested by Californian Republican Richard Nixon and South Dakotan Democrat George McGovern provided the two key events that drove the adoption of the 1977 USDA DGA.

First, incumbent US President Richard Nixon was confronted by a losing war in Vietnam, rising food prices, unhappy housewives and a disgruntled farming community. In part this was because in 1971 Nixon ended the Bretton Woods Agreement linking the US dollar and the gold standard; consumer prices skyrocketed. Nixon appointed Earl Butz as Secretary of Agriculture, with two orders: Increase the wealth of US farmers and bring down food prices. His solution to both 'problems' was the production of maize (corn) on an industrial scale by farmers receiving large government subsidies to cultivate corn on all their available land [260].

All this newly grown maize had to be eaten. So the challenge became to convince the world that cereals and grains are healthier than natural foods high in animal fat and protein on which humans had built their health [251], and

Americans [259], their nation. The consequence was that cheap, nutrient-poor, energy-dense plant crops including corn, wheat, and soy began to replace the nutrient-dense animal foods on which America and Americans had thrived.

Nixon won the 1972 US Presidential election in a landslide. As a result of this humiliating defeat, McGovern was losing the support of his party leadership, to the point that by the end of 1972, he and his wife considered emigrating. By 1976 McGovern's sole remaining centre of political influence, the chairmanship of the Senate Select Committee on Nutrition and Human Needs, was under threat of disbandment [261] and incorporation into a nutrition subcommittee under the Senate Committee on Agriculture, resulting in a drastic reduction in the committee's budget and staff.

In an attempt to save his Committee and political career, McGovern announced a proposal for changes to the American diet in the form of *Dietary Goals for the United States* with the goal of avoiding the 'epidemic of killer diseases'. ([261], p. 1176). While the move prevented the dissolution of McGovern's committee, it still suffered major budget and staffing cuts.

McGovern fought back by shifting the focus of his Committee to the role of diet in health and, specifically, the emerging problem of obesity and coronary heart disease (CHD) in the United States.

McGovern had been strongly influenced by Dr. Jeremiah Stamler MD who, together with Dr. Henry Blackburn MD, were perhaps Keys' most ardent acolytes. In his book [262] published in 1963, Stamler had promised the following ([262], p. 5–6):

> *The definitive proof that middle-aged men who reduce their blood cholesterol will actually have far fewer heart attacks waits upon diet studies now in progress. Possibly, their diet changes will have no effect in preventing heart attacks. But massive evidence from human and animal studies gives every promise that they will.*
>
> *The vital choice and question for us all is simply this: Should we sit by and wait for the last 'i' to be dotted and 't' to be crossed before we act? Or should we begin now to adopt changes that very* probably *will protect us – changes in our way of life that cannot do any harm?*
>
> Yours is the decision.

At the time Stamler was Chairman of the 1970 Inter-Society Commission for Heart Disease Resources: Prevention of Cardiovascular Disease. Primary prevention of the atherosclerotic diseases [263]. Predictably on the basis of Stamler's personal convictions, his commission advocated that US citizens must be told to eat less fat, especially saturated fat, based on Keys' Twin Hypotheses, still unproven. The presumption at that time was clearly that this dietary change would drastically reduce the number of heart attacks and strokes amongst middle-aged US men as the fat calories removed from the diet would be replaced by an increased protein intake.

But in the seven years between 1970 and 1977, the political landscape in the United States had changed dramatically. With Butz in charge of US Agriculture, any fat removed from the diet would now have to be replaced with cheap grains, not expensive proteins.

A key belief driving the thinking of Keys, Stamler and McGovern was that the US diet had changed radically in the years immediately preceding the start of the CHD 'epidemic', usually considered to have begun in the mid- to late-1920s. They were convinced, without supporting evidence, that a dietary shift away from plant-based foods (grains, legumes, fruits and vegetables), towards animal-derived foods (meat, poultry, seafood, eggs and dairy), was driving the rise in CHD in the United States. ([264], p. 2).

Based on this untested assumption [150,259], on 27 July 1976, Senator McGovern held a Senate Select Committee meeting probing the potential role of diet in the development of CHD. The main speaker was cardiac surgeon Dr. Theodore Cooper, then Assistant Secretary for Health.

Dr. Cooper provided a body of unsubstantiated evidence that removing fat from the diet would improve the health of all Americans. He recommended that this should be achieved by reducing dietary fat (particularly saturated fat) intake which would in turn (1) lower plasma cholesterol concentrations (Key's Twin Hypotheses) and (2) reduce obesity incidence by lowering lipid-calories ([257] p. 7). He persisted: '... there is nothing that I know of (this) recommendation ... would in any sense be harmful' ([257] p. 13).

Cooper also warned of the role of carbohydrates in the causation of obesity; this was then common knowledge: 'But it is true that the consumption of high-carbohydrate sources with the induction of obesity constitutes a very serious public health problem in the underprivileged and economically disadvantaged' ([257] p. 10). He also acknowledged that personally he was carbohydrate-intolerant or insulin resistant, due to his type IV hyperlipidaemia, which is essentially carbohydrate-sensitive hypertriglyceridaemia [265]. He understood that carbohydrates posed a greater risk to his own health than did dietary cholesterol and perhaps dietary fat: 'I am classified type IV. As a type IV, my lipid levels are much more subject to elevation if I consume large amounts of carbohydrate or alcohol. I have no real problem in consuming a reasonable amount of cholesterol'. Critically Dr. Cooper failed to consider the repercussions of his dietary recommendations should a majority of Americans be insulin resistant like him.

Cooper summarised his dietary recommendations:

I think in order to have an effective reduction of weight...we have to focus on reducing fat intake (p. 19–20). ... I personally believe there is some benefit to reducing our preoccupation with sweet things .... I would recommend an appropriate amount of protein intake...A healthy intake of fresh fruits and vegetables with substantial fiber content .... It is very attractive for me to say stop eating commercially prepared foods' (p. 20).

Interestingly Cooper also confirmed the adage: 'you can't outrun a bad diet' [266]: 'Exercise, unless you are into quite heavy labor where your total energy expenditure is in the several thousands of calories like tree-chopping or lumber workers, is really not the main determinant of weight loss' (p. 33).

A year later, on 11 January 1977, Senator McGovern announced the outcome of his Committee's deliberations – the publication of the Dietary Goals for the United States [258].

In his prepared statement, Senator McGovern began:

The simple fact is that our diets have changed radically within the last 50 years, with great and often very harmful effects on our health. These dietary changes, represent as great a threat to public health as smoking. Too much fat, too much sugar or salt, can be and are linked directly to heart disease, cancer, obesity and stroke, among other killer diseases. In all, six of the ten leading causes of death in the United States have been linked to our diet.

Those of us within Government have an obligation to acknowledge this. The public wants some guidance, wants to know the truth, and hopefully today we can lay the cornerstone for the building of better health for all Americans, through better nutrition.

Last year every man, woman, and child in the United States consumed 125 pounds of fat, and 100 pounds of sugar. As you can see from our displays, that's a formidable quantity of fat and sugar.

The consumption of soft drinks has more than doubled since 1960 – displacing milk as the second most consumed beverage. In 1975, we drank on the average of 295, 12 oz. cans of soda.

In the early 1900, almost 40% of our caloric intake came from fruit, vegetables, and grain products. Today only a little more than 20% of calories comes from these sources ([258], p. 1).

McGovern indicated that his Committee would 'set forth the necessary plan of action'.

1. Six basic goals are set for changes in our national diet
2. Simple buying guides are recommended to help consumers attain these goals; and
3. Recommendations are also made for action within Government and industry to better maximise nutritional health ([258], p. 1).

The six specific 1977 USDA DGA goals were those described earlier.

1.3.3 The people behind the 1977 USDA Dietary Goals for Americans

The 1977 USDA DGA were compiled by a vegetarian Nick Mottern who had no formal training in nutrition science ([150,259], p. 45), assisted by a committee of 'lawyers and ex-journalists'. 'We were totally naïve', said the staff director Marshall Matz, 'a bunch of kids, who just thought, Hell, we should say something on this subject before we go out of business' ([150], p. 45).

Mottern and the Committee identified the six dietary goals that have fashioned the nutrition debate ever since. These remain the basis for the dietary advice provided by traditionally-trained dietitians and doctors, regardless of where they were trained.

1.3.4 How the 1977 USDA Dietary Goals for Americans were received

On their publication, the Dietary Goals were severely criticised by many including Philip Handler PhD, Pete Ahrens MD, R. Reiser MD, Alexander M. Schmidt MD, Robert E. Olson MD, George V. Mann MD, Gilbert A. Leville PhD, A.E. Harper PhD, and Eliot Corday MD.

Dr. Philip Handler, then President of the National Science Academy (NSA) posed the question ([150], p. 51):

What right has the federal government to propose that the American people conduct a vast nutritional experiment, with themselves as subjects, on the strength of so very little evidence that it will do them any good?... resolution of this dilemma turns on a value judgement. The dilemma so posed is not a scientific question; it is a question of ethics, morals, politics. Those who argue either position strongly are expressing their values; they are not making scientific judgements.

Dr. E.H. Pete Ahrens [267], known for his original work including describing the production of hypertriglyceridaemia by the ingestion of either carbohydrates or fats [268–270], noted ([267], p. 136–8):

... a trial of the low fat diet recommended by the McGovern Committee and the American Heart Association has never been carried out. It seems that the proponents of this dietary change are willing to advocate an untested diet to the nation on the basis of suggestive evidence obtained in tests of a different *diet. This illogic is presumably justified by the belief that benefits will be obtained, vis-à-vis CHD prevention, by* any *diet that causes a reduction in plasma lipid levels.*

... I believe it is anything but a service to the public to postulate one *dietary solution for hyperlipidemia, no matter how well-meaning one is in advocating it. Let us address the unanswered questions and demand the means to solve them quickly.*

His criticisms covered four subjects:

- There has been no previous test of the 'prudent diet'.
- The 'prudent diet' will have only a small effect on plasma lipid concentrations.
- Any one diet produces different results in different people.
- Crucial questions remain to be resolved. These relate specifically to the nature of the dietary fats that should be prescribed and their differential effects on the blood lipoproteins – chylomicrons; VLDL, HDL and LDL cholesterol.

George V. Mann, MD ([271], p. 23) who had resigned as Director of the Framingham Diet Heart Study when he realised that politics had trumped science [272,273], complained that:

The level of fat in the diet has not been related causally to any disease and in particular not to either obesity or to cancer. Those who contend this are adventurists .... the amount of saturated fat in the diet has not been shown causal for any disease ... The release of this document is a nutritional debacle.

Mann's scepticism arose following his discovery that the dietary findings in the Framingham Diet Heart study had been hidden when it became apparent that those with established CHD did not eat any more fat or saturated fat than did those free of CHD in the same Framingham population [273].

The submissions of Eliot Corday MD ([271], p. 13), A.E. Harper, PhD ([271], p. 20), Gilbert A. Leveille, PhD ([271], p. 22), Robert E. Olson, MD ([271], p. 23), Alexander M. Schmidt, MD, ([271], p. 24) and R. Reiser MD ([274], p. 865–7) concurred with these criticisms.

1.3.5 The Second Edition of the USDA Dietary Goals for Americans

1.3.5.1 Cautionary statements

A second Edition of the Dietary Goals was subsequently published also in 1977. An addition statement from Senators Percy, Schweiker, and Zorinsky [275] was appended indicating that they all had significant concerns about the scientific credibility of the Guidelines:

Despite the many improvements reflected in this second edition, however, I have serious reservations about certain aspects of the report... I have become increasingly aware of the lack of consensus among nutrition scientists and other health professionals regarding (1) the question of whether advocating a specific restriction of dietary cholesterol intake to the general public is warranted at this time, (2) the question of what would be the demonstrable benefits to the individual and the general public, especially in regard to coronary heart disease, from implementing the dietary practices recommended in this report, and (3) the accuracy of some of the goals and recommendations given the inadequacy of current food intake data.

On the question of whether or not a restriction of dietary cholesterol intake for the general populace 'is a wise thing to recommend at this time', the Senators wrote:

... in October 1977 the Canadian Department of National Health and Welfare reversed its earlier position and concluded in a National Dietary Position that:

Evidence is mounting that dietary cholesterol may not be important to the great majority of people .... Thus, a diet restricted in cholesterol would not be necessary for the general population.

A similar conclusion was drawn in 1974 by the Committee on Medical Aspects of Food in its report to Great Britain's Department of Health and Social Security ....

Because of these divergent viewpoints, it is clear that science has not progressed to the point where we can recommend to the general public that cholesterol intake be limited to a specified amount. The variances between different individuals are simply too great ([275], p8–9).

The Senators next questioned whether there was consensus of a causative link between a specific diet and increased risk of CHD:

For example, Dr. Jeremiah Stamler, chairman of the Department of Preventive Medicine, Northwestern School of Medicine, strongly believes thousands of premature coronary heart disease deaths can 'probably be prevented annually through dietary change'. However, Dr. E.H. Ahrens, Jr., Professor of Medicine at Rockefeller University, told the Select Committee in March: 'Advice to the public on changing its dietary habits in hope of reducing the rate of new events of coronary heart disease is premature, hence unwise' ([275], p 9).

They continued by highlighting the different opinions of those who either supported or opposed Keys' hypotheses:

The same polarity is evidenced when one compares the view of William Kannel, Framington (sic) Heart Study's Director, the Dietary Goals, 'could have a substantial effect in reducing' coronary heart disease, with the opinion of Vanderbilt University's Dr. George Mann that 'no diet therapy has been shown effective for the prevention or treatment' of that disease' ([275], p. 9).

On behalf of the three Senators, Percy concluded:

... I recognize the desirability of providing dietary guidance to the public and in helping the consumer become more responsible for every day health status. In my judgment, however, the best way to do this is to fully inform the public not only about what is known, but also about what remains controversial regarding cholesterol, the benefits of dietary change, and the reliability of current food intake data. Only then, will it be possible for the individual consumer to respond optimally to the Dietary Goals in this report ([275], p. 9–10).

1.3.5.2 Material changes

The second edition of the Dietary Goals also included some significant modifications of the original guidelines. Some suggest that the cattle industry in McGovern's home state of South Dakota was particularly unimpressed with his committee's recommendations. So the second edition no longer advised consumers to eat less meat. Instead consumers were advised to reduce their intake of animal fat 'and choose meats, poultry, and fish which will reduce saturated fat intake' ([261], p. 1177).

The revised edition also removed any reference to restricting whole milk and egg consumption by young children and increased the suggested limit for adults' salt intake from 3 to 5 g a day. This excluded 'non-discretionary' salt in processed foods. As a result the limit on salt intake was effectively increased to 8 g a day ([261], p. 1177).

Perhaps under pressure from the fast food industry, the second edition also included the suggestion that 'on the whole, quick foods are a nutritious addition to a balanced diet' ([261], p. 1177).

1.3.6 Analysis by the Task Force of the American Society for Clinical Nutrition

In July 1978, the American Society for Clinical Nutrition (ASCN) convened its own Task Force to evaluate the scientific validity of the proposed dietary interventions. Their concern was that the advice that scientists provide to government officials frequently 'takes the form of advocacy' in which those scientists 'put forth those elements of the total body of data that support the change in public policy that they favour' ([276], p. 2627).

In other words, the concern was that the scientists were 'cherry-picking' only the data that supported their particular biases. What was needed was an independent panel of experts with a wider range of opinions (and biases).

The result was that the ASCN Task Force sampled the opinions of 9 panellists who, on the basis of all the evidence – epidemiological, randomised controlled trials, animal studies, and proposed biological explanation – rated, out of a possible score of 100, ten specific issues relating specific nutrients as causative agents for specific diseases (Table 1.6).

TABLE 1.6 ASCN panellists' assessment of the evidence available in 1977 linking specific dietary factors as the cause of specific diseases.

	Issue	Mean score
1	Alcohol and liver disease	88
2	Carbohydrates and dental caries	87
3	Salt and hypertension	74
4	Dietary cholesterol and fat and CHD	73
5	Excess calories and obesity, hypertension, T2D and CHD	68
6	Dietary cholesterol and CHD	62
7	Saturated fat and CHD	58
8	Carbohydrates and T2D	13
9	Alcohol and atherosclerosis	13
10	Carbohydrates and atherosclerosis	11

Panellists considered that on the basis of the best evidence, there were only two nutrient-disease relationships for which the evidence was conclusive. These were proven relationships between alcohol and liver disease, and carbohydrates and dental caries. The evidence the panellists considered was also detailed in a series of peer-reviewed articles [277–287].

1.3.6.1 Dietary cholesterol and atherosclerosis

Henry C. McGill MD reviewed the evidence linking specifically dietary cholesterol intake and the development of atherosclerosis [281,282] whereas Charles J. Glueck MD reviewed the evidence linking dietary fat intake with atherosclerosis [277,278].

McGill concluded that it was virtually impossible to detect an independent effect of dietary cholesterol on either blood cholesterol concentrations or on the development of coronary atherosclerosis. His reasoning was that, in population studies, 'the intake of cholesterol is always associated with the intake of fat (especially saturated fat)' [281], p. 2632. He was also wary of conclusions drawn from population studies when applied to individuals: 'associations between two variables based on group means do not permit inferences to be drawn about the corresponding associations among individuals within a single group' (p. 2633). In other words, all individuals respond in their own peculiar ways to different interventions so that those individual responses cannot be predicted from observational studies of large populations.

He concluded that a reduction in dietary cholesterol intake might produce a modest reduction in total atherosclerotic disease without causing 'any other known deleterious effects' (p. 2636), a conclusion which, in retrospect, is simplistic. Because removing cholesterol from the diet requires the removal of all animal produce including eggs, a move which would be detrimental especially in more deprived communities at risk of nutritional deficiencies. McGill recognised this: 'The implementation of a low-cholesterol diet carries with it some degree of risk, however small, due to changes of food processing or food purchasing, or to unforeseeable hazards for individuals with marginally adequate diets' (p. 2636).

One 'unforeseeable' hazard was the manner in which the food processing industry would wilfully exploit this invitation to replace fat in the diet. Instead of filling this nutritional gap with an increased protein intake as Stamler and others had assumed would happen, it filled the taste gap with sugar, unleashing a global pandemic of sugar-driven, addictive eating behaviours [147,288].

In his extensive review of the literature, McGill made a few important points:

First, that in controlled experiments in humans '(dietary) cholesterol did influence serum cholesterol concentration but to a lesser degree than saturation of dietary fatty acids' ([282], p. 2685). This had been acknowledged even by Keys himself who had written: 'for all practical purposes the dietary cholesterol variable can be disregarded...' [289]. As a result, Dr. Stewart Truswell MD, another Keys' acolyte, concluded that lowering dietary cholesterol intake by reducing weekly egg intake from 5 to 2 eggs each week, would produce an effect too small to be advisable [290]. Truswell also emphasised the nutritional value of eggs.

Second, that association studies cannot prove causation but can serve only 'as suggestive evidence for a causal relationship' ([282], p. 2697). However 'numerous cross-sectional studies have failed to find a significant independent association of dietary cholesterol with either serum cholesterol concentrations or with risk of arteriosclerotic heart disease' (p. 2697).

Third, any attempt to lower blood cholesterol concentrations by simply lowering dietary cholesterol intake would be ineffective. Rather this would only be accomplished by 'changes in a variety of dietary components' (p. 2698).

1.3.6.2 Dietary fat, plasma cholesterol concentrations and atherosclerosis

In his submissions [277,278] Glueck concluded that studies of dietary fat intakes within population groups (i.e. by comparing individuals rather than population groups) 'have usually failed to show a correlation between (dietary fat) intake levels, plasma cholesterol concentrations, and incidence of atherosclerotic disease' ([277], p. 2639). He also noted that 'there are few precedents for use of diets high in polyunsaturated fats' ([277], p. 2642) and that 'the benefits that might accrue from the ingestion of a low-fat, low-saturated fat, low-cholesterol diet has never been adequately tested except in terms of reduction in plasma lipid levels' ([277], p. 2642).

Despite his inability to find any solid evidence to support Keys' Twin Hypotheses, Glueck's personal bias was clearly apparent in his second paper [278]. Thus the failure of studies to support the Lipid Hypothesis were, according to Glueck, because the studies 'began in adults whose atherosclerosis was advanced and potentially irreversible' (p. 2706). This is an example of post-hoc rationalisation: When the experiment fails to produce the desired result, the experiment, not the hypothesis, is at fault. But that is not how proper science is meant to work.

In relation to the multi-million dollar Multiple Risk Factor Intervention Trial (MRFIT) then being conducted [291], Glueck wrote: 'If MRFIT ends in a favourable conclusion we will be able to move ahead with confidence to improve the prognosis for a group of high risk patients, perhaps with a significant improvement in overall national vital statistics' ([278], p. 2708).

The reverse of this statement must equally apply. If the MRFIT (or any other similar studies) failed to show any benefit for these 'risk factor' interventions, then the NIH/AHA alliance should have declared that the interventions it tested were ineffective. Thus there was no further justification to waste more taxpayers' money exploring this blind alley.

But when the MRFIT 'failed completely' ([292], p. 45) by establishing that reducing multiple coronary 'risk factors' did not have any measurable effects on CHD outcomes [292], the alliance remained silent. Instead it invested in yet more expensive dietary intervention trials exploring the same blind alley for decades [150,259], all the time invoking the same false post-hoc rationalisations to explain why these interventions failed to produce the results that the researchers 'knew' were there, waiting to be found. But which had somehow eluded their grasp.

Indeed the post-hoc rationalisations that the NIH/AHA alliance would adopt were exactly those anticipated by Glueck: 'If the MRFIT does *not* succeed in achieving a significant reduction in events, despite a reduction in risk, the most likely explanation will be that the period of intervention was too short, and the degree of cholesterol lowering too small' ([278], p. 2708).

This was precisely the explanation used to explain, for example, why the most expensive of these trials – $700 million Women's Health Initiative Randomised Controlled Dietary Modification Trial (WHIRCDMT) – also failed to produce the expected outcomes [293,294]. Instead recent independent analyses of the WHIRCDMT have established, beyond doubt, that the authors hid evidence that the low-fat, 'heart-healthy', Prudent diet caused harm to the health of those with established CHD [295,296].

Glueck even extended his argument also to absolve the yet-to-be-released results of the Lipid Research Clinics Trial [297] of any relevance, should that trial also fail to produce the desired results. Thus ([278], p. 2708):

> *If the Lipid Research Clinics trial should end in a negative or equivocal result, the lipid hypothesis will not have been dealt a fatal blow. The atherosclerotic disease process may already have progressed too far to be arrested in these severely hypercholesterolemic subjects.*

So instead of accepting the findings from any future trials which might show that the low-fat diet does not improve health, Glueck was arguing that the NIH/AHA alliance should simply ignore any negative findings, based on their collective faith that someday Keys' Hypotheses would be proven correct.

1.3.6.3 Sugar, carbohydrates, type 2 diabetes, coronary heart disease and dental caries

Edward L. Bierman MD reviewed the evidence for links between sugar intake and T2D, CHD and dental caries [286,287]. He concluded that there was strong evidence linking sugar and dental caries but there was no such strong evidence linking sugar intake with T2D or obesity. Bierman's opinion reflects the popular idea that obesity is the cause of insulin resistance, rather than the opposite. The possibility of reverse causation – that insulin resistance precedes the development of obesity [298] had yet to be considered ([286], p. 2644–6).

> *... adiposity appears to be the major determinant of the emergence of glucose intolerance and adult-onset diabetes, not carbohydrate and particularly not sucrose intake*
>
> *... There is no known biological basis for the hypothesis that would relate higher sucrose or carbohydrate intakes to the causation of diabetes. On the contrary, a low-fat, high-carbohydrate diet, by leading to less obesity may cause a reduced prevalence of diabetes.*

Dr. Bierman did not foresee the global explosion in obesity and T2D that would be unleashed by the low-fat high-carbohydrate dietary guidelines of McGovern's Committee [299].

With regard to carbohydrates and CHD, Bierman acknowledged concerns that a high-carbohydrate diet increases blood triglyceride concentrations which 'may well represent a risk factor for the development of coronary disease in the US population [300]' ([287], p. 2713). But he discounted the importance of this effect of high-carbohydrate diets concluding that the 'atherogenic potential of these dietary manipulations has yet to be explored' (p. 2713). Any possibility that a low-fat high-carbohydrate diet might be harmful was simply implausible, given the strength of the belief in Keys' unproven hypotheses [150,259].

1.3.6.4 Energy intake and chronic disease

Theodore Van Itallie reviewed the role of excess calorie consumption as a cause of chronic disease ([279], p. 2649).

> *There is no evidence that obese individuals develop increased fat storage (i.e. obesity) owing to a high consumption of carbohydrate as compared with fat or protein...man and experimental animals more readily become obese on diets low in carbohydrates and high in fat, but this can be explained in terms of differences in palatability and a somewhat greater heat loss from carbohydrate. There is no evidence that the higher caloric density of fat .... is itself responsible for undue weight gain.*

He concluded that obesity was strongly and likely causally related to a number of chronic diseases, most especially what he termed 'carbohydrate intolerance': 'The temporal association between obesity, carbohydrate intolerance and adult-onset diabetes mellitus is very close. The association with carbohydrate intolerance is manifest in only a few weeks' ([279], p. 2651–2652).

His biological explanation for these relationships ignored the possibility of reverse causation ([279], p. 2652):

> *Increased storage of triglycerides in adipose tissue is invariably accompanied by adipocyte hypertrophy; this, in turn, leads to carbohydrate intolerance, insulin insensitivity, and hyperinsulinemia. The insulin insensitivity of hypertrophic adipose tissue as well as of other tissues of the obese has been demonstrated in various in vitro preparations. The tissue changes engendered by obesity are presumably related to the exacerbation of carbohydrate intolerance and diabetes that is observed clinically.*

What is especially interesting, in retrospect, is that Van Italie includes no mention of the nature of the diet that he believes will prevent or reverse obesity. By his reckoning it must be a low-fat high-carbohydrate diet.

1.3.6.5 Alcohol and liver disease

The reviews of the relationship between alcohol and liver disease [283,284] concluded that there is strong evidence that excessive alcohol consumption causes chronic liver disease but that there is no evidence that alcohol plays any role in coronary atherosclerosis.

1.3.6.6 Salt and hypertension

In his review of any possible relationship between dietary salt intake and the development of arterial hypertension, Tobian [285,301] concluded that 80%–91% of the US population are resistant to the development of hypertension and so have no need to lower their daily salt intake. However for those who are 'genetically susceptible to hypertension' ([301], p. 2745), 'a life-long modest restriction of NaCl intake to levels less than 60 mEq/day in adults will probably prevent the onset of hypertension indefinitely, and also prevent all subsequent hypertensive complications' (p. 2745). Identification of those at risk for the development of hypertension is key according to Tobian.

He was clearly unaware of the evidence that arterial hypertension is a key marker of insulin resistance [302,303].

1.3.7 Response of the American Medical Association to the USDA Dietary Goals for Americans

The American Medical Association (AMA) also produced a response to the Dietary Goals [304]. It began ([304], p. 576):

it would be inappropriate at this time to adopt the proposed national dietary goals as ... the evidence for assuming that benefits to be derived from adoption of such universal dietary goals...is not conclusive and there is a potential for harmful effects from a radical long term dietary change as would occur through the adoption of the proposed national goals.

The AMA presented the opinion that the evidence linking the American diet with a variety of different diseases including CHD, is 'suggestive, fragmentary, and even conflicting' ([304], p. 577):

It is not proven that dietary modifications can prevent atherosclerotic heart disease in man (sic). It is not known that the demonstration of such a proof could or would find general applicability in our society...In the absence of conclusive proof on the Diet-Heart question any dietary advice to the American public will always lack authenticity and authority, will be conducive to half-measures and will meet opposition which cannot be effectively countered.

The AMA Committee was equally unimpressed by the evidence linking high dietary fat intakes and cancer of the colon ([304], p. 579):

While epidemiological data show a correlation between high fat intake and cancer of the colon, the case against high fat intake is weak because there are populations that have a high fat intake but little bowel cancer.

The Committee also rejected any proven links between high fat diets and cancer of the breast.

Similarly the Committee found no evidence to support the reduction in salt intake to reduce the prevalence of hypertension. It argued that dietary management of T2D and obesity should both focus on calorie restriction on an individualised basis ([304], p. 580).

Adoption of national dietary goals is not an answer to obesity and could prove detrimental if followed by individuals properly requiring medical supervision for their particular condition.

So their final conclusion was that the AMA ([304], p. 580)...

does not consider it appropriate for the government to adopt national goals that specify such matters as the amount and proportions of total fat, type of fat, sugar, cholesterol or salt content in the diets of the general public as these national goals advocate.

Rather persons should be treated in individual programs that promote decreased caloric intake and increased physical activity for those with obesity or at risk of its development.

As a result '... we (the AMA Committee) urge that the Report not be adopted' (p. 581).

1.3.8 Subsequent iterations of the USDA Dietary Goals for Americans

The Dietary Goals continue to be modified every 5 years. However the advice to eat less animal fat and protein and more carbohydrate in the form of grains and cereals remains immutable. The Goals continue to attract relentless criticism.

In a hard-hitting review published in 2010, Hite et al. ([305], p. 915) concluded:

Although appealing to an evidence-based methodology, the DGAC Report demonstrates several critical weaknesses, including use of an incomplete body of relevant science; inaccurately representing, interpreting, or summarizing the literature; and drawing conclusions and/or making recommendations that do not reflect the limitations or controversies in the science. An objective assessment of evidence in the DGAC Report does not suggest a conclusive proscription against low-carbohydrate diets. The DGAC Report does not provide sufficient evidence to conclude that increase in whole grain and fiber and decrease in dietary saturated fat, salt, and animal protein will lead to positive health outcomes. Lack of supporting evidence limits the value of the proposed recommendations as guidance for consumers or as the basis for public health policy. It is time to re-examine how US dietary guidelines are created and ask whether the current process is still appropriate for our needs.

Following the publication of the 2015 Guidelines, Hite and Schoenfeld [306] again argued that the guidelines had failed to achieve 'positive health outcomes for the American public' (p. 776). Instead the authors propose that these recommendations:

- have contributed to the increase of chronic diseases, widening the health divide between minority and white Americans;
- are not compatible with adequate essential nutrition;

- 'do not reflect the biological, socioeconomic, or cultural diversity of Americans;
- are based on weak, limited, and inconclusive scientific data;
- and have expanded their purpose to issues beyond their original mandate, while failing to provide clear nutrition guidance to the general public.

Along the same lines, James DiNicolantonio, DPharm, Zoe Harcombe, PhD, and James O'Keefe, MD, [307] argued that the following four of the 2015 Dietary Guidelines lack sound scientific evidence:

- Allowing approximately half of all grains to be refined;
- The continued recommendations for fat-free or low-fat dairy and limitation of saturated fat intake to <10% of calories;
- Sodium intake <2300 mg/day; and
- Consumption of up to 27grams/day of 'oils' (high in polyunsaturated fat or monounsaturated fat).

Their specific criticisms were the following:

- Increasing the intake of grains will 'likely lead to a decrease in HDL and increase in triglycerides, small-dense LDL, insulin resistance, obesity, and hence increase in the risk of the MetS, diabetes, dyslipidaemia, obesity, atherosclerosis, and CV (cardiovascular) disease' (p. 75).
- Reducing the intake of full-fat dairy and saturated fat will likely increase the intake of refined carbohydrates and sugar, increasing the risk of diabetes, obesity, and cardiovascular disease while increasing risk for fat-soluble vitamin deficiencies.
- Reducing salt intake activates the renin-angiotensin-aldosterone system as well as the sympathetic nervous system. This effect is likely harmful.
- Rather than advising the consumption of omega-6 vegetable oils, it would be better to advise an increased intake of natural fats, nuts, and olive oil.

Their conclusion is that the best advice is to eat 'natural foods, meat, fish, eggs, dairy products, avocados, nuts and seeds, and the natural saturated and unsaturated fats contained therein' (p. 77,78).

Their predictions have all proven to be remarkably prescient. Certainly much more accurate than the incorrect 1977 guesses of Senate McGovern's Senate Committee.

Critiquing the same Guidelines, cardiologist at the Cleveland Clinic Dr. Steven E. Nissen labelled the Guidelines 'a nearly evidence-free zone' and proposed that, 'it is time to transition from the current evidence-free zone to an era where dietary recommendations are based on the same quality of evidence that we demand in other fields of medicine' ([308], p. 558–9).

Another extensive body of criticism came from Nina Teicholz, author of the pivotal book, Big Fat Surprise [259]. In an opinion piece published in the British Medical Journal, Teicholz made the following key points ([309], p. 5):

- The latest dietary guidelines for Americans are imminent and will affect the diets of millions of citizens, as well as food labelling, education, and research priorities. In the past most Western nations have adopted similar dietary advice.
- The scientific committee advising the US government has not used standard methods for most of its analyses and instead relies heavily on systematic reviews from professional bodies such as the American Heart Association and the American College of Cardiology, which are heavily supported by food and drug companies. The committee members, who are not required to list their potential conflicts of interest, also conducted ad hoc reviews of the literature, without defining criteria for identifying or evaluating studies.
- This year in its report to government, the committee largely sticks to the same advice it has given for decades—to eat less fat and fewer animal products and eat more plant foods for good health. But this decision to keep with the status quo fails to reflect much of the current, relevant science. Exceptions include a proposal for a cap on sugar intake.
- The committee recommends three diets to promote better health, again without the accompanying rigorous evidence.

Predictably there was significant academic push-back against Teicholz especially since she is not considered a qualified academic. A petition by ~180 academics [310] to have the article retracted failed, with some suggesting that many had signed the petition without bothering to read it. In response Teicholz provided a few points of clarification to answer their criticisms [311].

One consistent criticism also raised by Teicholz is that the majority of the committee members writing these guidelines have significant conflicts of interest, as did most of those who prepared the 2020 guidelines. Indeed 11 of the 20 members of 2020 Dietary Guidelines Advisory Committee, including the committee chair and vice-chair have links to the International Life Sciences Institute (ILSI) [312–314], an organisation that serves as a front organisation for the food and drug industry (Fig. 1.8) and which has captured an inordinate influence on the development of global dietary guidelines [312–318].

That the Dietary Guidelines Advisory Committee has little interest in producing dietary guidelines that reflect the totality of the modern evidence [309,311,316], continues to be an abiding concern.

1.3.8.1 Summary of the adoption and evolution of the dietary guidelines

In summary, this review of some forgotten historical material establishes that the USDA Dietary Goals for Americans were never based on hard evidence but rather, as a number of scientists and clinicians testified already in 1977, on the assumption that in the fullness of time, expensive clinical trials then being considered by the NIH and AHA, would fully vindicate Keys' Diet-Heart hypothesis.

Unfortunately that evidence has never been forthcoming. Instead, even though these guidelines have been responsible for global obesity/T2D epidemics, they have changed hardly at all in the past 44 years.

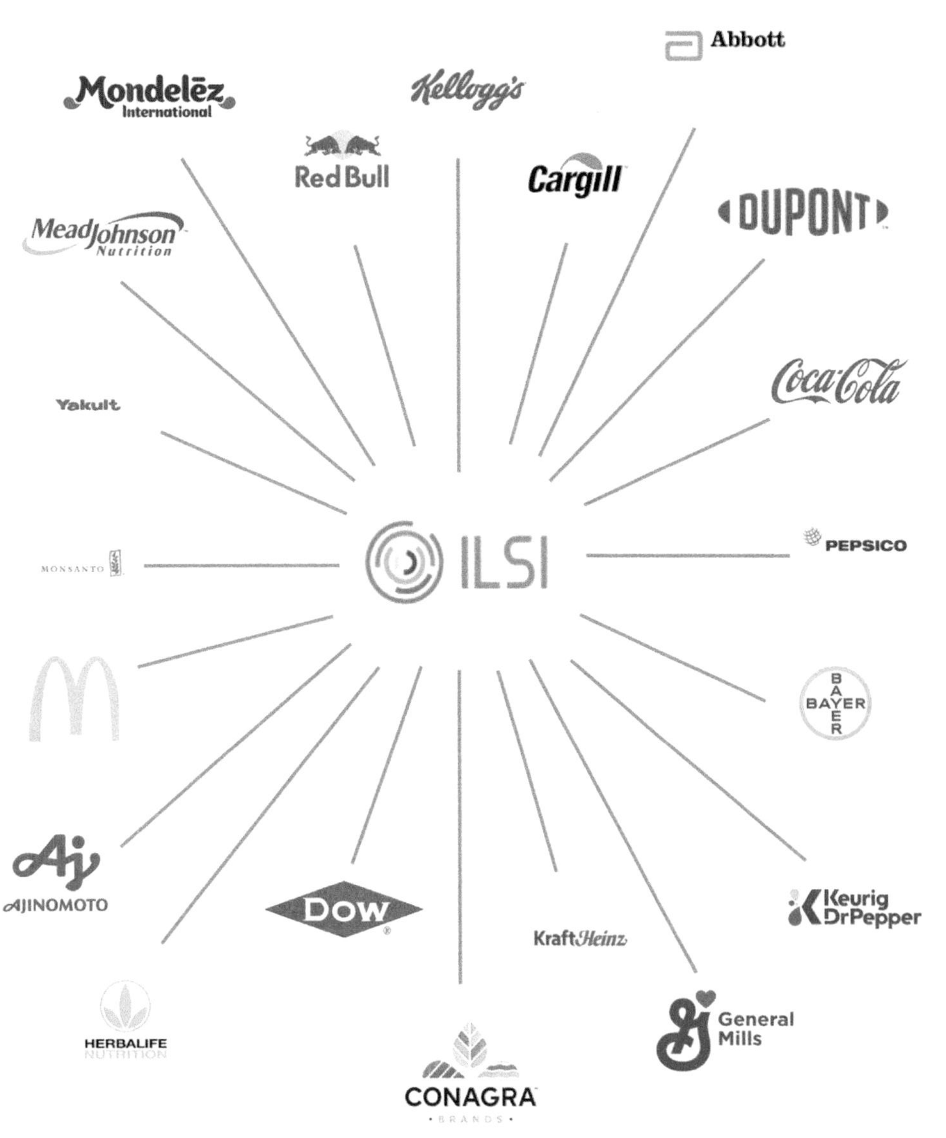

FIGURE 1.8 The International Life Sciences Institute connections. *Reproduced from the figure on page 5 of Partnership for an unhealthy planet: How big business interferes with global health policy and science. Published by Corporate Accountability 2020;1–36. Available at: https://www.corporateaccountability.org/wp-content/uploads/2020/04/Partnership-for-an-unhealthy-planet.pdf.*

The unproven, indeed disproven, belief in the Diet-Heart and Lipid Hypotheses and consequent fear that saturated fats are uniquely harmful and must be avoided, is still alive and well in 2020 [316].

1.3.9 The Six Goals proposed by the McGovern Commission

We come finally to an analysis and criticism of the Six Diet Goals which, it is argued, are the direct cause of the massive human suffering that the adoption of these guidelines have caused on a global scale. Some have even likened the consequences of this dietary advice to a form of slow 'genocide' [319].

1.3.9.1 Goal 1: Increase carbohydrate consumption to account for approximately 55%–60% of the total (caloric) intake

The problem: This change replaced dietary fat with more dietary carbohydrates.

The result: Dietary carbohydrates do not satiate; they drive hunger. Humans began to eat more calories, becoming fatter.

Once the McGovern Committee had decided that humans must eat less fat, it had to choose replacement foods for all those lost calories. The scientists of the 1960s presumed that humans would simply replace the fat with more protein since increasing carbohydrate consumption would likely promote obesity. But the unqualified enthusiasts who drew up the 1977 USDA DGA assumed they knew best. In their ignorance, they were unaware of a large body of evidence linking increased carbohydrate consumption with the development of obesity (and T2D).

For example, an editorial in *The Lancet*, in 1926, carried the statement that 'it is the starchy carbohydrate foods rather than the more quickly and readily metabolized fats which are responsible for much of the alimentary type of obesity' [320]. A leading textbook of endocrinology published in 1951 provided this dietary advice for the obese: 'complete restriction of bread (and everything made of flour), cereals, potatoes, sweets, and in general, any food containing much sugar' [321]. It continued: 'You (the obese) can eat as much as you like of the following foods: Meat, fish, birds, green vegetables, eggs, cheese and unsweetened fruit, except for bananas and grapes'.

In 1953, the *New England Journal of Medicine* included an article by the leading low-carbohydrate diet advocate of the day, New York physician Alfred Pennington [322]. He advocated treatment of obesity as 'a diet in which carbohydrate alone is restricted and protein and fat are allowed ad libitum'.

Even the AMA understood this relationship. In his chairman's address in 1957, Dr. Gerald Thorpe said: 'Evidence from widely different sources ... seems to justify the use of high-protein, high-fat, low-carbohydrate diets for successful loss of excess weight' [323].

In the same journal in 1963, Gordon et al. [324] published the paper that inspired Dr. Robert Atkins MD to develop the Atkins diet [325] based specifically on the principles that Gordon and colleagues had developed. Those authors, ignorant of the long history of low-carbohydrate diets for the management of obesity and even T2D [326], suggested (incorrectly) that they had discovered a 'new concept in the treatment of obesity'. Specifically, that a 'low carbohydrate intake tends to minimize the storage of fat' so that their diet was 'planned around the basic concept that its carbohydrate content should be low'.

They also reported that a diet that restricted carbohydrate intake to a maximum of 50 g per day, produced dramatic weight losses of up to 45 kg (100 pounds) without the development of hunger. They also noted that weight reductions reversed once subjects returned to their original high-carbohydrate diets.

But the challenge that the nutritional novices on the McGovern Committee faced was that the agricultural product it was promoting (maize) is protein-poor and carbohydrate-rich. So, it had no choice. Humans would have to eat more carbohydrates and less protein.

For three simple, biological reasons, the ultimate deleterious consequences of McGovern's Committee's dietary advice were predictable.

1.3.9.1.1 Biological reality #1: humans have no essential requirement for carbohydrate [327]

There are essential proteins and fats that humans cannot synthesise, but no essential carbohydrates. The human brain has an essential requirement for carbohydrate of between 25 and 100 g per day. But the human liver can produce more than enough glucose to cover the brain's glucose requirement without any need for ingested carbohydrate [328].

Table 1.7 extends this argument by showing the functions of the three dietary macronutrients – carbohydrates, proteins and fats. Note that carbohydrates have only **one** function, which is to act as an energy source. Carbohydrates cannot build muscles, bones, brain, liver, or heart.

TABLE 1.7 The biological functions of the three dietary macronutrients.

CARBOHYDRATES	versus PROTEIN	versus FAT
Source of energy (as glucose)	Source of energy (as glucose, amino acids)	Source of energy (as glucose, ketones and free fatty acids)
	Synthesise enzymes and antibodies	Vitamin absorption (A, D, E, K)
	Maintain acid-based balance	Structural material (for cell tissues and cell membrane)
	Repair and maintenance of tissues (hair, skin, eyes, muscles, organs)	Hormone production
	Hormones production	Chemical messengers (between cells)
	Transport of molecules (as haemoglobin)	Prostagladin formation (role in inflammation, pain, fever, and blood clotting)
	Messenger (transmit signals to coordinate biological processes)	Preserves integrity of blood brain barrier (Omega3)
		Insulation

An obvious consequence of basing a diet on a macronutrient that serves only one function in the human body is that this carbohydrate-heavy diet will be deficient in key nutrients, which will produce negative health consequences.

1.3.9.1.2 Biological reality #2: Carbohydrates do not satiate; they drive hunger

The second biological reality that McGovern's committee overlooked is that carbohydrates do not satiate [329]. Rather: 'One of the causes of failure is that the conventional low calorie diets, restricted in both fat and carbohydrate, usually lead to hunger which the patient is unable, or unwilling, to tolerate' [330]. This is especially true for a sugar-rich, ultra-processed food diet [147,148,288,331–338], for which the low-carbohydrate ketogenic diet may be helpful in alleviating symptoms [339].

Already in 1960 Yudkin and Carey wrote ([330], p. 941):

> *It would seem from this that carbohydrate does not satisfy the appetite; it may even increase it, because more dietary carbohydrate may lead to more dietary fat. This conclusion is supported by the observation that the addition of glucose to a reducing diet led to a decreased loss of weight; this could not be accounted for by the calories from the glucose, and suggests that the glucose stimulated the appetite*

As a result, the natural tendency for people eating diets high in sugar and other addictive foodstuffs, is to eat more calories, what has been termed carbohydrate-induced hyperphagia. This is precisely what seems to have happened in the United States after 1977 (Fig. 1.9).

Fig. 1.9 shows that after 1976 to 1980, both US men and women increased their energy intake from carbohydrates while reducing their intakes of total and saturated fats. The result: total energy intake increased by 6.8% in men and 21.7% in women. This increase is more than sufficient to explain the dramatic increase in obesity (and subsequent T2D) rates in US men and women beginning after 1980.

1.3.9.1.3 Biological reality #3: High-carbohydrate diets produce a cataclysmic metabolic storm in those with insulin resistance

The final biological reality of which McGovern's Committee was understandably unaware was perhaps predictable since it was only just beginning to be studied. It is that high-carbohydrate, low-fat diets produce a cataclysmic metabolic storm in those with IR. See also Section 1.2 Insulin resistance: a unifying feature of chronic disease.

Unfortunately, in 1977, the condition of IR and its relationship to dietary carbohydrate excess was only just beginning to be studied. Even the man considered the Father of IR and of the MetS, Professor Gerald Reaven MD of Stanford University School of Medicine [340] who had begun also to identify the curative effects of carbohydrate-restricted diets in those with his syndrome [341–344], eventually capitulated to a growing academic pressure to demonise fats and ignore any possible role for carbohydrates in the causation of CHD.

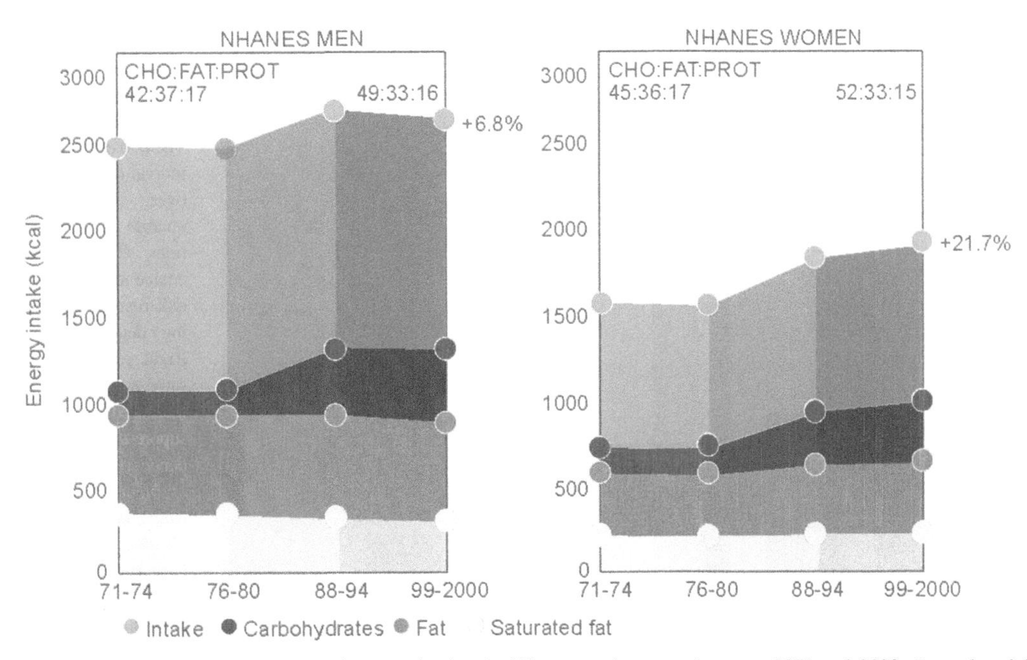

FIGURE 1.9 Changes in dietary macronutrient and energy intakes in US men and women between 1971 and 2000. *Reproduced from Hite, AH, Feinman RD, Guzman GE, et al. In the face of contradictory evidence: Report of the Dietary Guidelines for Americans Committee. Nutrition 2010; 26:915–924.*

So after publishing those studies showing the benefits of a degree of carbohydrate-restriction as low as 17% of calories, Reaven inexplicably changed course. Instead of continuing to study truly low carbohydrate diets of 5%–10% of calories, he reversed direction and began to promote a hybrid low-fat high-carbohydrate diet [345] that *sort of* addressed the IR problem, while *sort of* keeping so-called 'bad' (LDL) blood-cholesterol concentrations low. It seems he never could quite accept the obvious and powerful message of his own research findings.

It's possible that Reaven may have wished to avoid the fate of British Professor John Yudkin, who besides his novel studies of the low-carbohydrate diet for management of obesity [329,330] was amongst the first to warn of the dangers of sucrose (sugar) [346,347]. Instead Reaven began to distrust his own findings; specifically that he had discovered an ultimate truth: that IR, not elevated LDL cholesterol concentration, is driving CHD [348] and other chronic diseases [349]. Instead it seems that near the end of his career he chose to ignore [345] all the evidence he had painstakingly collected over four decades of meticulous research.

In one study (Fig. 1.10) Reaven's group followed a larger group of about 600 apparently healthy individuals over five or more years to determine whether hyperinsulinaemia could predict CHD risk [348].

In a second study shown in Fig. 1.11, Reaven and colleagues [349] measured the level of IR in 208 initially healthy Californians whose health was followed over the next 4–11 years. To measure their levels of IR, the researchers subjected study participants to the most specific and intensive testing ever devised requiring constant infusion of glucose, insulin, and somatostatin.

Note also, hypertension was the most common disease, followed by cancer, CHD, and T2D in about equal numbers, with stroke the least common.

Clearly, for those with IR, future risk is not confined to heart attack or cancer – another reason to take it seriously. Note also the strong relationship between hypertension and IR [302,303]. See also Section 1.2 Insulin resistance: a unifying feature of chronic disease.

1.3.9.1.4 How hyperinsulinaemia produces the visceral obesity that is the key to the pathology of the insulin resistance syndrome

High-carbohydrate diets produce persistently abnormal elevations in blood insulin concentrations (hyperinsulinaemia) in those with IR.

Persistent hyperinsulinaemia in turn partitions ingested fat and excess carbohydrate into subcutaneous and visceral fat stores. Included in visceral fat is fat accumulated ectopically in muscles, the pancreas and the liver, the latter causing

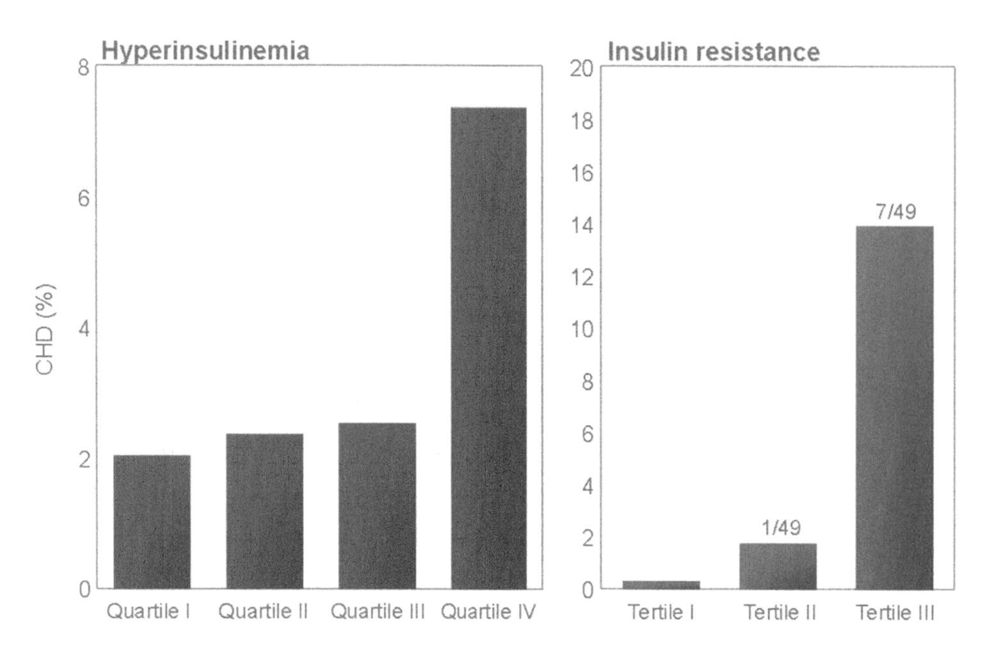

FIGURE 1.10 The percentage of apparently healthy individuals who developed coronary heart disease (CHD) over ~5 years. Left panel. The percentage of apparently healthy individuals who developed CHD over ~5 years ranked according to quartile of blood-insulin concentrations achieved during a glucose tolerance test (GTT) showing that CHD risk rose progressively with increasing degrees of hyperinsulinaemia. Right panel. The percentage of the same subjects in three tertiles of IR measured with the insulin-suppression test, who developed evidence of CHD. *Predictably, testing of blood cholesterol concentrations would never have shown this clear distinction between those at low and high risk for future development of CHD. Reproduced from Reaven G. Insulin resistance and coronary heart disease in nondiabetic individuals. Arterioscler Thromb Vasc Biol 2012; 32:1754–1759.*

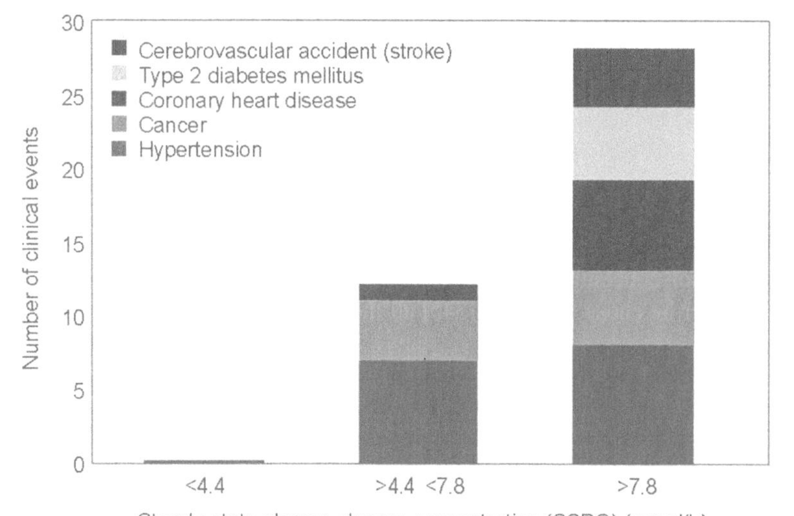

FIGURE 1.11 Number of clinical events observed over 4–11 years as a function of insulin resistance at baseline. The 208 subjects in the study [349] were divided into three tertiles on the basis of their steady state plasma glucose (SSPG) concentration infusions during the laboratory experiment. They were followed for between 4 and 11 years to determine who developed any of five listed chronic diseases. The number of clinical events experienced increased dramatically in those with mild to severe IR. *Adapted from fig. 1.1 of Facchini FS, Hua N, Abbasi F, et al. Insulin resistance as a predictor of age-related disease.* J Clin Endocrinol Metab *2001; 86:3574–3578.*

NAFLD. Some believe that once ectopic fat content of the liver and pancreas exceeds an individual's personal fat threshold (PFT), T2D becomes inevitable [350].

Fig. 1.12 illustrates the process as currently understood [351,352].

The key driver of this ectopic fat accumulation, especially in the liver [351,353–359], is increasing IR in an expanding mass of adipose tissue cells (1, 7, 8 in Fig. 1.12). But once these fat cells become insulin-resistant, free fatty acids (FFA) accumulate in the bloodstream [351,360–363], ready to be deposited as ectopic fat in skeletal muscles (2 in Fig. 1.12), the pancreas (3 in Fig. 1.12) and the liver (4 in Fig. 1.12).

Ectopic fat accumulation in skeletal muscles impairs their ability to serve as a reservoir for any diet-induced increase in blood-glucose concentrations. As a result, blood-glucose concentrations remain elevated after eating (5 in Fig. 1.12), stimulating further IS (6 in Fig. 1.12).

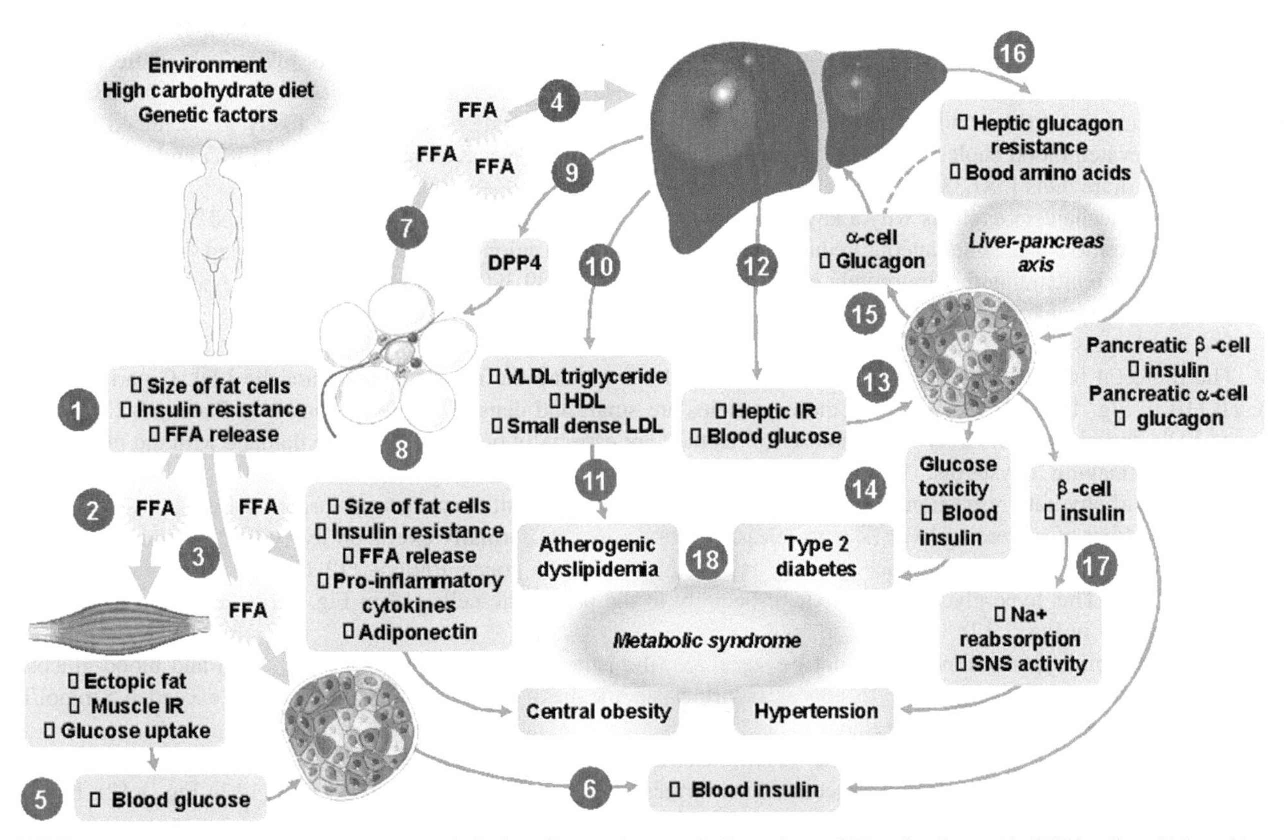

FIGURE 1.12 How insulin resistance and high-carbohydrate diets produce metabolic syndrome. FFA = free fatty acids; DPP4 = dipeptidyl peptidase 4; SNS = sympathetic nervous system; VLDL = very low-density lipoprotein; HDL = high-density lipoprotein; LDL = low-density lipoprotein. *Modified and re-drawn from fig. 1.1 in Godoy-Matos AF, Silva Junior WS, Valerio CM. NAFLD as a continuum: form obesity to metabolic syndrome and diabetes.* Diabetol Metab Syndr *2020; 12:60; and reproduced from Noakes TD, Sboros M.* The Eat Right Revolution. *Penguin Books, Cape Town, RSA, 2021.*

Even as they release free fatty acids (7 in Fig. 1.12), the increasingly insulin-resistant adipose cells retain their ability to grow yet fatter. But to avoid developing the MetS including IR, T2D, and CHD [364,365], it's critical that this fat is stored in many small (hyperplastic) fat cells rather than in fewer but much larger (hypertrophic) adipose cells.

But as fat cells grow, they accumulate two chemicals – 4-hydroxynonenal (4-HNE) and ceramide 1-phosphate (C1P) – that prevent their division into more, smaller cells [366], worsening the problem.

These larger fat cells promote the secretion of a range of inflammatory molecules [351,354,357,367–375], including the cytokines (8 in Fig. 1.12) which act on the liver, pancreas, skeletal muscles, and brain to interfere with insulin signalling, worsening IR, and producing central obesity.

Insulin-resistant fat cells also reduce their secretion of the hormone adiponectin (8 in Fig. 1.12), which would normally reduce circulating free-fatty-acid concentrations, increase tissue glucose uptake and reduces ectopic fat deposition in the liver and skeletal muscles [376,377]. Instead reduced adiponectin concentrations worsen ectopic fat deposition.

The liver worsens the inflammatory state by secreting dipeptidyl peptidase 4 (DPP4) (9 in Fig. 1.12), which enhances inflammatory secretions of macrophages in the fat tissue, further contributing to IR.

The liver attempts to cope (4 in Fig. 1.12) by exporting fat in the form of VLDL-C (triglyceride) (10 in Fig. 1.12) – the other 'bad cholesterol' to which few refer. Excretion of VLDL-C (triglyceride) limits the extent to which liver IR increases, since liver IR increases progressively with increasing ectopic fat content [351].

The enzyme, lipoprotein lipase, in blood capillaries clears the VLDL-C (triglyceride) that the liver secretes (10 in Fig. 1.6) from the bloodstream. But IR reduces the activity of this enzyme. Instead, the VLDL-lipoprotein transfers its triglyceride cargo to HDL-C lipoproteins. This produces HDL-C particles that are more rapidly cleared from the bloodstream [370]. As a result, blood HDL-C concentrations fall; an undesirable result according to the model that HDL-C is the 'good' cholesterol.

This effect explains why Reaven was amongst the first to identify that a high-carbohydrate diet may be detrimental for those with insulin resistance [378] because it raises blood triglyceride concentrations [379–382] while lowering blood HDL-C concentrations. LCHF diets do the opposite [341–344]. Already in the late 1950s Albrink [383–386] had drawn attention to the finding that high blood triglyceride concentrations were more likely to be linked to CHD than were elevated blood cholesterol concentrations; a contention that Peter Kuo had also found [387] and had linked to high-carbohydrate diets [387,388].

Thus this mechanism explains why a key diagnostic marker of IR severity is an increase in blood VLDL-C (triglyceride) concentration and simultaneous reduction in HDL-C concentration. Together with T2D and other markers of insulin resistance including the lipoprotein insulin resistance score [389,390], that ratio is one of the best markers of the extent to which coronary atherosclerosis develops [391].

But it only gets worse.

The more fat in the liver, the more insulin-resistant the liver, and the more damaged are the LDL-C particles that result (10 in Fig. 1.12). The majority of those particles are small and dense [392,393], known as Pattern B [394,395]. These LDL particles are the truly 'bad cholesterol' as they are especially prone to oxidative damage with the production of arterial-damaging oxysterols. These particles place anyone with IR at greater risk of CHD [396,397] (11 in Fig. 1.12). Carbohydrate restriction on the other hand produces the opposite pattern with larger LDL particles [398].

Another effect of increasing liver IR is to release the brake insulin normally exerts on liver glucose production. As a result, the liver begins to overproduce glucose, raising blood-glucose concentrations (12 in Fig. 1.12), the diagnostic feature of T2D. This hyperglycaemia is toxic, especially to the pancreatic-cells (13 in Fig. 1.12) and is known as glucose toxicity (14 in Fig. 1.12).

Ultimately this hyperinsulinemia cannot be sustained; the pancreatic-cells fail (14 in Fig. 1.12) and blood-glucose concentrations rise, causing glucose to appear in urine and the fasting glucose concentration to exceed 6.5 mmol/L (117 mg/dL). When this happens, the diagnosis is full-blown T2D.

Pancreatic IR also removes the brake insulin exerts on glucagon secretion from the pancreatic-cells (15 in Fig. 1.12). Increasing blood glucagon concentrations further increases liver glucose production (12 in Fig. 1.12), blood-glucose concentrations rise further stimulating yet more insulin secretion.

In time, the fatty liver also becomes glucagon-resistant. The ultimate effect is to increase blood-amino acid concentrations that feedback to the pancreas (16 in Fig. 1.12) – the liver pancreas axis – to further increase pancreatic glucagon secretion. This stimulates further glucagon secretion, causing liver glucose production, establishing a vicious cycle.

Finally, insulin increases secretion of aldosterone, which increases sodium retention in the kidneys, increasing water retention and potentially increasing blood pressure. Insulin activates the sympathetic nervous system, which may further raise blood pressure by promoting vasoconstriction in arteriolar blood vessels (17 in Fig. 1.12). Inflammatory damage to the lining cells of the blood vessels, the endothelium, compounds this, causing reduced ability to secrete the vasodilator substance, nitric oxide.

Not shown in Fig. 1.12, the brain may also become insulin-resistant with consequences for food intake, reward, and mood. Brain insulin resistance causes hyperphagia, anxiety, and depressive-like behaviour and compromises the dopaminergic system. Such effects can induce reduced compliance to medical treatment' ([332], p 83).

The end result is MetS (18 in Fig. 1.12) that comprises T2D, arterial hypertension, atherogenic dyslipidaemia and central obesity.

In contrast to these examples, other cells retain their normal responsiveness to insulin.

1.3.9.2 Goal 2: Reduce overall fat consumption from approximately 40%–30% of energy intake

The problem: This change increased consumption of dietary carbohydrates and polyunsaturated vegetable oils (Goal 3).

The result: The higher carbohydrate consumption drove the obesity epidemic that in turn unleashed the cataclysmic metabolic storm in those with insulin resistance (IR).

The intended purpose of this Goal was twofold. First, to reduce the risk of heart disease according to Ancel Keys' theory that dietary fat, especially saturated fat, is a direct cause of heart disease.

Second, to prevent and reverse obesity according to the theory that since fat provides more than twice the number of calories than an equal amount of carbohydrate – 9 versus 4 calories/g – then clearly, replacing dietary carbohydrates with fat will cure obesity.

The unanticipated outcome was that Goal 2 caused the increase in carbohydrate consumption that led to the global obesity epidemic by exposing those with IR to the cataclysmic metabolic storm shown in Fig. 1.12.

With regard to removing dietary fat to prevent obesity, in 1977, when this goal was first promoted, the popular understanding was that an imbalance between the number of calories ingested in food and expended in daily living, including during exercise, caused obesity. According to this model, subsequently named the Calories-In, Calories-Out (CICO) model, it seemed logical to suggest the restriction of calorie-dense fat in the diet. The theory goes that if you take calorie-laden-fat out of the diet, everyone should eat fewer calories and lose all their excess weight.

Problem solved. Or so the McGovern Committee believed.

The Committee did not foresee that removing fat from the diet would take with it both taste and the special texture – the mouthfeel – that its fat content adds to food. Food manufacturers soon realised the difficulty of selling fat-free, high-carbohydrate foods that taste little better than cardboard. They soon discovered the solution: simply add some sugar for taste, then more and more for a few reasons.

Firstly, because sugar is cheap and became cheaper with the discovery and production of high-fructose corn syrup (HFCS), a by-product of the waste was generated in the growing of maize (corn).

Secondly, because sugar is one of the most addictive drugs on planet Earth [331,333,334]. The addition of sugar to essentially all processed foods currently on the market produced the perfect plague – a pandemic of sugar addiction [147,288]. That plague would help drive the consumption of highly processed, sugar-saturated modern 'foods' – actually food-like substances. In turn, these would become key drivers of the modern T2D and obesity epidemics that the McGovern Committee's dietary guidelines unleashed.

To defend itself against clear evidence that these processed foods drive the obesity epidemic ([148,335–337]), the food industry took action. Following an initiative that the International Life Sciences Institute (ILSI) directed [399], the industry shifted the focus of blame away from the addictive foods they produce, and onto their customers and the consumers.

They did this by moving the emphasis from food (the toxic food environment) to physical activity. Thus, at one secret ad hoc meeting in 1999, '... the CEOs (of major US food manufacturers) rejected collective action, agreeing only to support the promotion of physical activity among children, a comforting plan that required little of them [288]. For ILSI, a company-funded and company-driven non-profit (group), physical activity thus became the only politically viable strategy to 'make industry part of the solution' [399].

The key driver of this covert strategy became Coca-Cola [400], through its front organisation, ILSI. Published evidence exposes the extent of ILSI involvement [317,399–403] and the goal: to control national dietary and exercise policies globally.

'Emails reveal a pattern of activity in which ILSI sought to exploit the credibility of scientists and academics to bolster industry positions and to promote industry-devised content in its meetings, journals and other activities' ([402], p. 1).

Inadvertently, I had also attracted ILSI's attention [352,404].

In 2015, after he had read our article [266], *New York Times* journalist Anahad O'Connor decided to investigate [405]. He found that Coca-Cola was promoting 'a new 'science-based' solution to the obesity crisis: 'To maintain a healthy weight, get more exercise and worry less about cutting calories''. To drive this message, Coca-Cola financed a new non-profit organisation, the Global Energy Balance Network (GEBN). Its vice-president was then highly respected health epidemiologist Dr. Steven Blair PhD.

Blair, a life-long exerciser with a life-long weight problem, justified GEBN's focus thus: 'Most of the focus in the popular media ... is, 'Oh they're eating too much',... – blaming fast food blaming sugary drinks and so on... there's virtually no compelling evidence that that, in fact is the cause' [405]. By the time he made these remarks, Blair had received $3.5 million from Coca-Cola for his research and GEBN president, Dr. James Hill, just $1 million [405]. In his defence, through his life work, Blair has produced a mountain of evidence for the value of physical activity in improving health. In fact he is currently the most-cited living sports scientist. But his linkage to Coca-Cola ultimately proved a poor choice.

The upshot of O'Connor's investigation was that Coca-Cola released a list of all the organisations and individuals it was funding in 2015. The list included $21.8 million on research that favoured the industry; $96.8 million on partnerships with health organisations, including $2.1 million paid directly to 115 individuals considered health 'experts', most of whom (63%) were active on social media, either on Twitter or Facebook [406]. But even that list was incomplete as it did not include funding of the Center for Disease Control (CDC) and the US National Institutes of Health (NIH) [407].

But what does the science say? Is it impossible to 'outrun a bad diet'? The evidence appears clear. A meta-analysis of 80 studies published between 1997 and 2004 produced findings shown in Fig. 1.13 [408]. This study found that advice and exercise alone were essentially useless in producing any weight loss.

The most recent meta-analysis [409] found that low-carbohydrate ketogenic diets outperform low-fat diets for weight loss for both those with and without T2D. This matches our 'anecdotal' clinical experience [410,411] that the low-carbohydrate ketogenic diet outperforms the low-fat diet in the real world. And that those self-administering this diet can achieve substantial weight losses, in some cases as much as 80–100 kilograms [410].

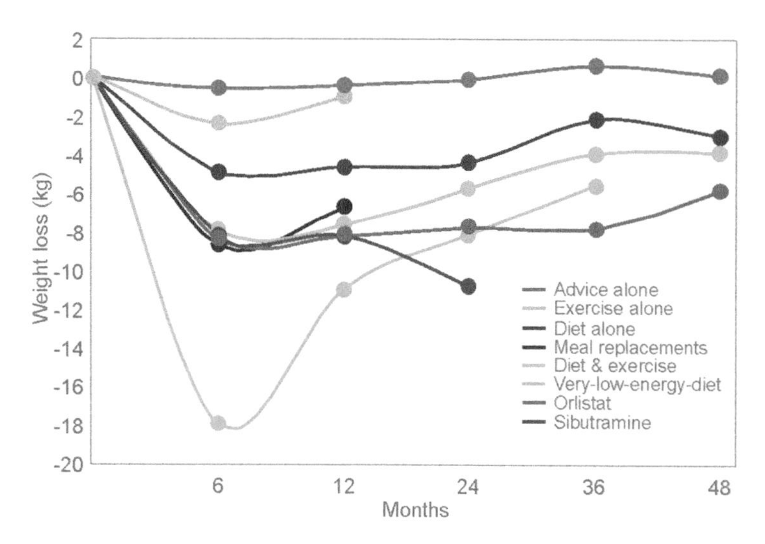

FIGURE 1.13 **Average weight loss of subjects completing a minimum 1-year weight management intervention.** Comparison of average weight losses produced by eight different interventions lasting from 12 to 48 months. Advice alone and exercise alone were the two least effective interventions. Orlistat and sibutramine are prescription drugs. Sibutramine was removed from the market because it caused cardiovascular complications, including deaths. Graph reflects that the initial efficacy of the very-low-energy diet is unable to be sustained. *Reproduced from fig. 1.1 of Franz MJ, VanWormer JJ, Crain L, et al. Weight-loss outcomes: a systematic reviewand meta-analysis of weight-loss clinical trials with a minimum of 1-year follow up. J Am Diet Assoc 2007;107:1755–1767.*

1.3.9.3 Goal 3: Reduce saturated fat consumption to about 10% of total energy intake; balance that with polyunsaturated and monounsaturated fats to about 10% of energy intake each

The problem: This change reduced consumption of nutrient-dense animal products and increased consumption of polyunsaturated 'vegetable oils'.

The result: The increased consumption of polyunsaturated vegetable oils has contributed to the burden of ill-health.

Goal 3 is the single piece of dietary advice that has caused the most uncertainty and disagreement. Because everyone 'knows' that dietary saturated fat causes 'bad' blood LDL-cholesterol concentrations to increase in everyone (the Diet-Heart hypothesis of Ancel Keys). Everyone also 'knows' that this increase clogs the coronary arteries (Key's lipid hypothesis). Everyone also 'knows' that 'bad' (LDL) cholesterol explains why dementia and cancers are rising worldwide.

Hopefully, once you've read this book, you will no longer be captured by the 'greatest scam in the history of medicine' – as a growing body of scientists and doctors has labelled it [412–415].

1.3.9.3.1 What of advice to increase polyunsaturated fat (PUFA) intake?

The single greatest change in the US diet over the past century has not been an increase in carbohydrate and sugar consumption. Rather, it has been increased consumption of vegetable oils, especially soybean oil and most especially, soy oil. This increase accelerated in 1961, when the American Heart Association (AHA) [416] finally bought into Keys' Diet-Heart Hypothesis and began to promote the substitution of dietary saturated fat with polyunsaturated fats. The fact that the AHA had recently received a large financial windfall from Procter and Gamble, manufacturers of the original polyunsaturated vegetable oil/shortening, Crisco, was clearly simply co-incidental. This change in the AHA advice had a profound effect on the consumption of 'vegetable oils' in the United States (Fig. 1.14). It would naturally have been ideal if the AHA's decision had been based on hard scientific evidence available at the time rather than on what now appears to have been a bribe from the processed food industry [259].

Both Keys and Stamler knew that to test the Diet-Heart hypothesis properly, they would need to conduct a randomised controlled trial (RCT) involving the substitution of dietary saturated fat with a polyunsaturated fat. The money for just such a study, The Minnesota Coronary Experiment (MCE) which ran from 1968 to 1973, was subsequently raised. The tested dietary intervention was the substitution of saturated fat with the poly-unsaturated fatty acid (PUFA), linoleic acid. The initial results were first published only in 1989 [418], 15 years after the trial had been completed.

The reason for this publication delay became apparent in 2016, when the original data were re-discovered, re-analysed and reported [127], 48 years after the study began. The properly analysed data uncovered some extremely inconvenient findings: Persons randomised to the intervention diet were at 22% higher risk of death for each 0.78 mmol/L (30 mg/dL) reduction in blood cholesterol concentrations, an effect that was especially apparent in those over 65 years of age.

Running somewhat concurrently with the MCE was the Sydney Diet Heart Study (SDHS) [419] which was conducted between 1966 and 1971. In that study, men with myocardial infarction were randomised to either a control group

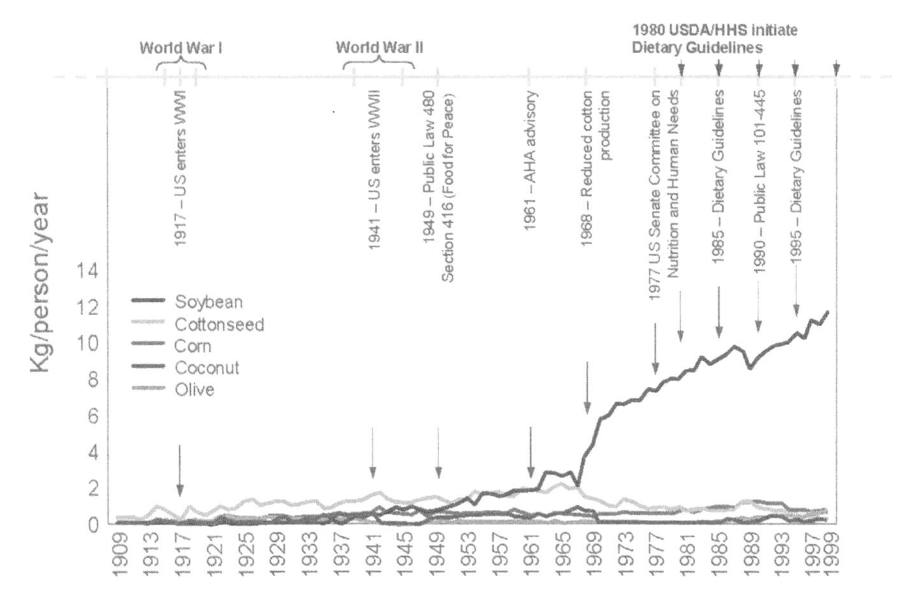

FIGURE 1.14 **The historical event immediately preceding the largest increase in apparent consumption of soy in the United States was 1961 American Heart Association (AHA) central committee advisory statement advising Americans to replace their saturated fat intake with poly-unsaturated vegetable oils.** Annual consumption of polyunsaturated 'vegetable' oils in the United States from 1909 to 1999. Note that there has been relatively little change in the annual consumption of cottonseed, corn, coconut, and olive oil. However a dramatic and progressive increase in soybean oil consumption began after publication of the 1961 AHA Advisory which advocated 'the reduction or control of fat consumption under medical supervision with reasonable substitution of poly-unsaturated fats for saturated fats ...' ([416], p. 390). *USDA*, United States Department of Agriculture; *HHS*, Health and Human Services. *Figure redrawn from Blasbalg TL, Hibbeln JR, Ramsden CE, et al. Changes in consumption of omega-3 and omega-6 fatty acids in the United States during the 20th century. Am J Clin Nutr 2011;93:950–962.*

which continued to eat its usual diet, or an intervention group which replaced dietary saturated fat with the linoleic acid from safflower oil and sunflower oils.

The original study concluded that the intervention diet had little effect, either harmful of detrimental so that 'none of the dietary factors were significantly related to survival' ([419], p. 317). Despite this there were significantly more deaths in the intervention group.

As in the MCE when the data were re-analysed and republished as the Recovered Sydney Diet Heart Study (RSDHS) [126] it was again found that replacement of dietary saturated fat with linoleic acid was associated with increased all-cause mortality and with increased deaths from both cardiovascular disease and CHD.

In reviewing all the current evidence, Lawrence [137] has concluded that:

> *PUFAs are unstable to chemical oxidation and their oxidation products are harmful in a variety of ways. PUFAs also form powerful signalling agents that can initiate inflammation which can have dire health consequences…If saturated fats are replaced by carbohydrates in the diet, there would be no significant improvement in serum cholesterol, and it can result in a more atherogenic lipoprotein profile. When looking at much of the data in the context of known biochemical and physiological mechanisms, it appears that saturated fats are less harmful than the common alternatives.*

1.3.9.4 Goal 4: Reduce cholesterol consumption to about 300 milligrams a day

The problem: Already by 1950, Ancel Keys had established that an increased intake of dietary cholesterol does not increase blood-cholesterol concentrations.

The result: Since cholesterol is present only in animal produce, this advice further increased bias against consumption of animal products for those wishing to reduce their CHD risk.

This advice was already dated in 1950. In that year, Keys published a study showing that the amount of cholesterol in the diet did not influence blood-cholesterol concentrations [420]. Two subsequent publications from the same group over the next 15 years confirmed this conclusion [421,422].

Since cholesterol is present only in animal produce, an interpretation advanced by Harcombe [423] could be that, if the consumption of animal foods containing cholesterol does not raise the blood-cholesterol concentration, then according to Keys' twin hypotheses, eating animal produce cannot cause CHD. This point is seldom appreciated.

One effect of Goal 4 was to target eggs as dangerous since they contain substantial amounts of cholesterol – about 200 milligrams per egg – or 67% of the daily allowed cholesterol intake.

Numerous studies have since shown that eggs are one of the most nutrient-dense foods on the planet. They are rich sources of high-quality protein, iron, phosphorus, riboflavin, vitamin B_{12} (especially), pantothenic acid, biotin, choline, vitamin D (especially) and Vitamin E [424]. Eating up to 14 eggs per week does not increase blood-cholesterol concentrations [425]. One case report of a healthy 88-year old male who eats 25 eggs a day shows normal blood-cholesterol concentration [426]. Egg consumption is also not linked to increased CHD risk in the long term [427]. In fact eating more than one egg per day may have a protective effect [428].

It took some time but the 2015 US Dietary Guidelines reversed the McGovern Committee's advice and reported that dietary cholesterol is no longer a 'nutrient of concern' [429]. Similarly, a series of articles in the *Annals of Internal Medicine* in 2020 concluded that the overall association of meat consumption, another major source of dietary cholesterol, with adverse outcomes is marginal. The quality of the studies suggest little or no effect [430–435].

1.3.9.5 Goal 5: Reduce sugar consumption by about 40% to account for about 15% of total energy

The problem: First, sugar is one of the most addictive products known to humans. Second, the fructose in sugar is metabolised to produce NAFLD.

The result: Obesity and diabetes epidemics.

Thus, Goal 5 is nonsensical for two reasons. First, sugar is one of the most addictive, socially acceptable drugs available [331,333,334]. And like all addictive products, most people cannot eat it 'in moderation'. Second, the fructose in sugar is metabolised differently from glucose and is specifically converted to triglyceride (fat) in the liver. This produces NAFLD [144] and all the complications, including atherogenic dyslipidaemia and increased whole body IR [436].

Since fructose produces a different hormonal response from that of glucose, one hypothesis is that it stimulates food intake, increasing the probability of calorie overconsumption and weight gain. Thus, overconsumption of fructose, especially in sugar - or HFCS-sweetened beverages, may be the key driver of the global obesity pandemic [437]. This is not a novel concept.

Chapter 1.2 introduced the work of Cleave and Campbell in reviewing what they described as the Saccharine Diseases [102,103].

Cleave, in particular, promoted the idea that sugar and refined carbohydrates are the real drivers of T2D [438] and that, in turn, T2D is the root cause of CHD [439,440]. This would be in line with Albrink's [383–386] and Kuo's [387,388] foundational studies linking carbohydrate-induced hypertriglyceridaemia with increased CHD risk.

Thus Cleave wrote ([439], p. 109–10).:

> *For an unnaturally high blood-sugar, constantly impinging on the endothelial lining of the arteries, over many years, might cause degenerative changes in this endothelium, and, by diffusion, in the arterial wall, too, especially at the sites of greatest strain ... This degeneration could then initiate the thrombosis. ... Of one thing the author is very confident; the key to causation of coronary thrombosis lies in the causation of diabetes (and also of obesity)*

That Cleave is most likely correct is confirmed by the recent finding from the Women's Health Study (WHS).

The WHS was initially designed as a clinical trial to evaluate the effects of vitamin E or low-dose aspirin on the risk of developing CHD or cancer in initially healthy women free from cardiovascular disease and cancer at baseline. Those studies found no overall benefit for either intervention. But a subsequent 21.4-year-long, prospective follow-up cohort study of 28,024 of these women evaluated the predictive value of more than 50 clinical, lipid, inflammatory and metabolic risk factors and biomarkers for the subsequent development of CHD [389]. Fig. 1.15 shows the key findings of the study.

The LPIR score is based on lipoprotein subclass and size information measured with nuclear magnetic resonance (NMR) imaging. It has strong associations with multiple markers of IR and 'may represent a simple means to identify individuals with IR' ([390], p422). The score is based on studies showing changes in lipoproteins in persons with IR. In particular, those with IR show the following characteristic NMR lipoprotein patterns [390,395,441–443]:

- Greater number of the large subclass of very low-density lipoprotein (VLDL) particles.
- Greater number of the small subclass of low-density lipoprotein (LDL) particles.
- Lower number of the large subclass of high-density lipoprotein (HDL) particles.
- In addition, mean VLDL particle sizes are generally larger and mean LDL and HDL particle sizes usually smaller in persons with IR [442,443] or pre-diabetes [441].
- In contrast serum LDL-cholesterol concentration—the principal target of the low-fat heart-healthy intervention diets in trials like the WHIRCDMT [293,294] was of little predictive value (1.38-fold increased risk) (Fig. 1.15).

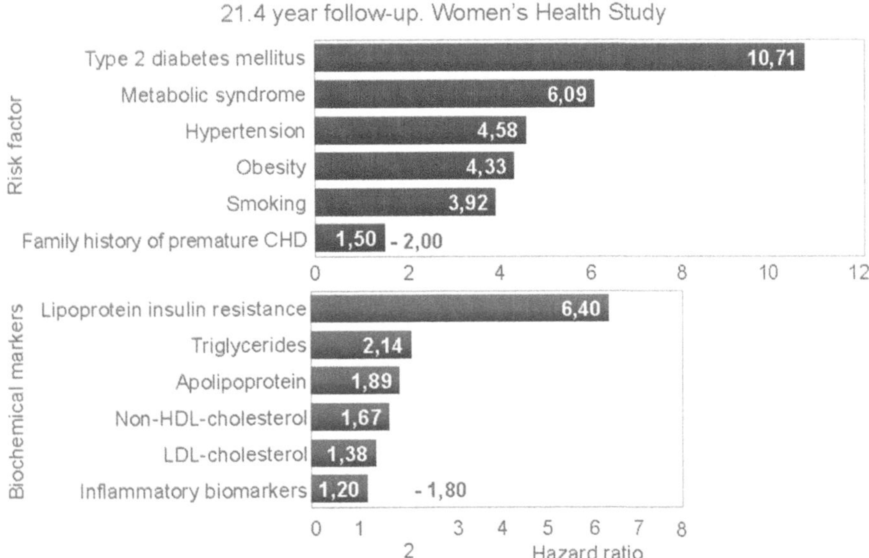

FIGURE 1.15 Hazard ratios for development of coronary heart disease in the Woman's Health Study. Hazard ratios (HR) for the six most important risk factors and the six biochemical markers for the development of CHD in 28,024 postmenopausal women who were healthy on entry to the Women's Health Study. It shows that the strongest predictors of future CHD development in these women are all the classic clinical markers of IR, most especially T2D, MetS, hypertension, and obesity with the most important metabolic risk marker being the lipoprotein insulin resistance (LPIR) score. *CHD*, coronary heart disease; *HDL*, high-density lipoprotein; *LDL*, low-density lipoprotein. *Drawn from data from Dugani SB, Moorthy MV, Li C, et al. Association of lipid, inflammatory, and metabolic biomarkers with age at onset for incident coronary heart disease in women. JAMA Cardiol 2021;6:437–447. Reproduced from fig. 1.3 of Noakes TD. Hiding unhealthy heart outcomes is a low-fat diet trial: the Women's Health Initiative Randomized Controlled Dietary Modification Trial finds that post-menopausal women with established coronary heart disease were at increased risk of an adverse outcome if they consumed a low-fat 'heart-healthy' diet. Open Heart 2021;e001680.*

Accordingly a low-fat diet, which may indeed lower blood LDL-cholesterol concentrations but at the cost of an increasing atherogenic dyslipidaemia [444–446] especially in those with IR [447–450], would be expected to worsen CHD outcomes, precisely as happened in the subgroup of postmenopausal women with prior CHD in the WHIRCDMT [296].

1.3.9.6 *Goal 6: Reduce salt consumption by 50%–85% to about 3 g per day*

The problem: There was never any scientific evidence supporting this advice.

The result: Low salt intakes are associated with the increased production of the hormone aldosterone, which raises blood pressure and is associated with higher death rates. The advice has also prevented identification of the real causes of elevated blood pressure: IR, sugar and high-carbohydrate diets.

This is another piece of advice that sounds reasonable but turns out to be hopelessly wrong. As we reviewed in detail in *Real Food on Trial* ([451], p. 75), there is evidence that those with established hypertension may benefit from sodium restriction to less than five grams per day, but in those who are healthy, lower intakes are associated with increased risk for cardiovascular events and death [452–457].

The focus on salt has shifted attention from the wrong white crystal (sugar) in causing high blood pressure [458]. Anyone with hypertension should avoid sugar, not salt, because IR is the major driver of most cases of high blood pressure [302,303].

1.3.10 Summary

It is clear that the 1977 Dietary Guidelines were written by an unqualified group with the transparent goal of extending Senator George McGovern's ailing political career. The guidelines were based on the false theory that the US diet had changed radically from a cereal-based to a meat-based diet in the early 1900s and that this abrupt change had caused the sudden appearance of the CHD epidemic. According to this logic, now clearly shown to be false, simply reversing this change (by replacing animal-based foods with cereals and grains) would reverse the CHD epidemic and, at the same time, prevent any future increases in rates of T2D and obesity.

The 45 years since 1977 have proved that this theory was hopelessly wrong. The proof that there never was any hard scientific evidence to support this hypothesis has now been clearly described [150,259,352,451].

Indeed this textbook provides all the evidence we will ever need, finally to lay the 1977 US Dietary Guidelines to rest.

References

[1] Garland T. Trade-offs. Curr Biol 2014;24:R60–1.
[2] Hunt KD. The evolution of human bipedality: ecology and functional morphology. J Hum Evol 1994;26:183–202.
[3] Stanford CB, Bunn HT. Meat-eating & human evolution. Oxford: Oxford University Press; 2001.
[4] Aiello LC, Wheeler P. The expensive-tissue hypothesis: the brain and the digestive system in human and primate evolution. CurrAnthr 1995;36:199–221.
[5] Conklin-Brittain NL, Wrangham RW, Smith CC. A two-stage model of increased dietary quality in early hominid evolution: the role of fiber. In: Ungar PS, Teaford MF, editors. Human Diet: Its Origin and Evolution. Greenwood Publishing Group; 2002. p. 61–76.
[6] Watkins PA, et al. Identification of differences in human and great ape phytanic acid metabolism that could influence gene expression profiles and physiological functions. BMC Physiol 2010;10:19.
[7] Owens FN, Basalan M. Ruminal fermentation. Rumenology. Springer; 2016. p. 63–102.
[8] Kelly RL. The Lifeways of Hunter-Gatherers: The Foraging Spectrum. Cambridge: Cambridge University Press; 2013.
[9] Faith JT, Rowan J, Du A. Early hominins evolved within non-analog ecosystems. Proc Natl Acad Sci 2019;21478–83.
[10] Gurven M, Kaplan H. Longevity among hunter-gatherers: a cross-cultural examination. Popul Dev Rev 2007;33:321–65.
[11] Eaton SB, Konner M. Paleolithic nutrition - a consideration of its nature and current implications. New Engl J Med 1985;312:283–9. Available from https://doi.org/10.1056/nejm198501313120505.
[12] Konner M, Eaton SB. Paleolithic nutrition twenty-five years later. Nutr Clin Pract 2010;25:594–602.
[13] Kuipers RS, Joordens JC, Muskiet FA. A multidisciplinary reconstruction of Palaeolithic nutrition that holds promise for the prevention and treatment of diseases of civilisation. Nutr Res Rev 2012;25:96–129.
[14] Lee RB. What hunters do for a living, or, how to make out on scarce resources. In: Lee RB, DeVore I, editors. Man the Hunter. Chicago: Aldine Publishing Company; 1968. p. 30–47.
[15] Marlowe FW. Hunter-gatherers and human evolution. Evol Anth: Issues News Rev 2005;14:54–67.
[16] Stahl AB, et al. Hominid dietary selection before fire [and Comments and Reply]. Curr Anthr 1984;25:151–68.
[17] Ströhle A, Hahn A. Diets of modern hunter-gatherers vary substantially in their carbohydrate content depending on ecoenvironments: results from an ethnographic analysis. Nutr Res 2011;31:429–35.
[18] Cordain L, Miller JB, Eaton SB, Mann N, Holt SHA, Speth JD. Plant-animal subsistence ratios and macronutrient energy estimations in worldwide hunter-gatherer diets 1, 2. Am J Clin Nutr 2000;71:682–92.
[19] Ben-Dor M, Barkai R. The importance of large prey animals during the Pleistocene and the implications of their extinction on the use of dietary ethnographic analogies. JAnthArch 2020;59:101192.
[20] Ben-Dor M, Barkai R. Prey size decline as a unifying ecological selecting agent in Pleistocene human evolution. Quarternary 2021;4:7.
[21] Ben-Dor M, Sirtoli R, Barkai R. The evolution of the human trophic level during the Pleistocene. Yearbook of Physical Anthrology 2021;1–30.
[22] Sepkoski D. Rereading the fossil record: the growth of paleobiology as an evolutionary discipline. University of Chicago Press; 2012.
[23] Pontzer H, et al. Metabolic acceleration and the evolution of human brain size and life history. Nature 2016;533:390.
[24] DeCasien AR, Williams SA, Higham JP. Primate brain size is predicted by diet but not sociality. Nature ecology & evolution 2017;1:0112.
[25] Leonard WR, Snodgrass JJ, Robertson ML. Effects of brain evolution on human nutrition and metabolism. Annu Rev Nutr 2007;27:311–27. Available from https://doi.org/10.1146/annurev.nutr.27.061406.093659.
[26] Bednarik RG. Doing with less: hominin brain atrophy. Homo 2014;65:433–49.
[27] Cahill Jr GF, Owen OE. Starvation and survival. Trans Am Clin Climatol Assoc 1968;79:13.
[28] Mathias RA, et al. Adaptive evolution of the FADS gene cluster within Africa. PLoS One 2012;7:e44926.
[29] Vining AQ, Nunn CL. Evolutionary change in physiological phenotypes along the human lineage. Evol Med Public Health 2016;2016:312–24.
[30] Swain-Lenz D, Berrio A, Safi A, Crawford GE, Wray GA. Comparative analyses of chromatin landscape in white adipose tissue suggest humans may have less beigeing potential than other primates. Genome Biol Evol 2019;11:1997–2008.
[31] Hancock AM, et al. Human adaptations to diet, subsistence, and ecoregion are due to subtle shifts in allele frequency. Proceedings of the National Academy of Sciences 2010;107:8924–30.
[32] Beasley DE, Koltz AM, Lambert JE, Fierer N, Dunn RR. The evolution of stomach acidity and its relevance to the human microbiome. PLoS One 2015;10:e0134116.
[33] Ségurel L, et al. Positive selection of protective variants for type 2 diabetes from the Neolithic onward: a case study in Central Asia Europ. J Hum Genet 2013;21:1146–51.
[34] Brand-Miller JC, Griffin HJ, Colagiuri S. The carnivore connection hypothesis: revisited. J Obes 2011;2012.
[35] Milton K. Primate diets and gut morphology: implications for hominid evolution. In: Harris M, Ross E, editors. Food and evolution: toward a theory of human food habits. Philadelphia: Temple University Press; 1987. p. 93–115.
[36] Zink KD, Lieberman DE. Impact of meat and Lower Palaeolithic food processing techniques on chewing in humans. Nature 2016;531:500.

[37] Foley RA. The evolutionary consequences of increased carnivory in hominids. Meat-eating and human evolution. Oxford University Press; 2001. p. 305–31.

[38] Bramble DM, Lieberman DE. Endurance running and the evolution of Homo. Nature 2004;432:345–52.

[39] Churchill SE, Rhodes JA. The evolution of the human capacity for "killing at a distance": The human fossil evidence for the evolution of projectile weaponry. In: Hublin JJ, Richards MP, editors. The evolution of hominin diets. Springer; 2009. p. 201–10.

[40] Pond CM, Mattacks CA. Body mass and natural diet as determinants of the number and volume of adipocytes in eutherian mammals. J Morphol 1985;185:183–93.

[41] Psouni E, Janke A, Garwicz M. Impact of carnivory on human development and evolution revealed by a new unifying model of weaning in mammals. PLoS One 2012;7:e32452.

[42] Kaplan H, Gangestad S, Gurven M, Lancaster J, Mueller T, Robson A. The evolution of diet, brain and life history among primates and humans. In: Roebroeks W, editor. Guts and brains: An integrative approach to the hominin record. Leiden University Press; 2007. p. 47–8.

[43] Bar-Yosef O. Upper Paleolithic hunter-gatherers in Western Asia. In: Cummings V, Jordan P, Zvelebil M, editors. The Oxford handbook of the archaeology and anthropology of hunter-gatherers. Oxford: Oxford University Press; 2014. p. 252–78.

[44] Blasco R, Rosell J, Arsuaga JL, de Castro JMB, Carbonell E. The hunted hunter: the capture of a lion (Panthera leo fossilis) at the Gran Dolina site, Sierra de Atapuerca. Spain JAS 2010;37:2051–60.

[45] Bunn HT, Gurtov AN. Prey mortality profiles indicate that Early Pleistocene Homo at Olduvai was an ambush predator. Quat Int 2014;322:44–53.

[46] Outram AK. Identifying dietary stress in marginal environments: bone fats, optimal foraging theory and the seasonal round. In: Miondini M, Munoz S, Wickler S, editors. Colonisation, migration and marginal areas: A zooarchaeological approach. Oxford Books; 2004. p. 74–85.

[47] Ben-Dor M, Gopher A, Hershkovitz I, Barkai R. Man the fat hunter: The demise of Homo erectus and the emergence of a new hominin lineage in the Middle Pleistocene (ca. 400 kyr) Levant. PLoS One 2011;6:e28689. Available from https://doi.org/10.1371/journal.pone.0028689.

[48] Richards M, Trinkaus E. Isotopic evidence for the diets of European Neanderthals and early modern humans. Proceedings of the National Academy of Science 2009;106:16034–9.

[49] Humphrey LT, De Groote I, Morales J, Barton N, Collcutt S, Ramsey CB, et al. Earliest evidence for caries and exploitation of starchy plant foods in Pleistocene hunter-gatherers from Morocco. Proceedings of the National Academy of Sciences 2014;111:954–9.

[50] Arcadi AC. Species resilience in Pleistocene hominids that traveled far and ate widely: an analogy to the wolf-like canids. J Hum Evol 2006;51:383–94.

[51] Werdelin L, Lewis ME. Temporal change in functional richness and evenness in the eastern African Plio-Pleistocene carnivoran guild. PLoS One 2013;8:e57944.

[52] Smith FA, Smith REE, Lyons SK, Payne JL, Villaseñor A. The accelerating influence of humans on mammalian macroecological patterns over the late Quaternary. Quat Sci Rev 2019;211:1–16.

[53] Van Valkenburgh B, Hayward MW, Ripple WJ, Meloro C, Roth VL. The impact of large terrestrial carnivores on Pleistocene ecosystems. Proceedings of the National Academy of Sciences 2016;113:862–7.

[54] Van Valkenburgh B, Wayne RK. Carnivores. Curr Biol 2010;20:R915–19.

[55] Macdonald ML, Rogers QR, Morris JG. Nutrition of the domestic cat, a mammalian carnivore. Annu Rev Nutr 1984;4:521–62.

[56] Speth JD, Spielmann KA. Energy source, protein metabolism, and hunter-gatherer subsistence strategies. J Anth Arch 1983;2:1–31. Available from https://doi.org/10.1016/0278-4165(83)90006-5.

[57] Jochim MA. Strategies for Survival: Cultural Behavior in an Ecological Context. NY: Academic Press; 1981.

[58] Tindale NB. The Pitjandjara. In: Bicchieri MG, editor. Hunters and Gatherers Today. New York: Holt, Rinehart and Winston; 1972. p. 217–68.

[59] Coote J, Shelton A. Anthropology, Art, and Aesthetics. Clarendon Press; 1992.

[60] Pitts GC, Bullard TR. Some interspecific aspects of body composition in mammals. Body Composition in Animals and Man. Washington DC: National Academy of Sciences; 1967. p. 45–70.

[61] Morin E, Ready E. Foraging goals and transport decisions in western Europe during the Paleolithic and early Holocene. Zooarchaeology and Modern Human Origins. Springer; 2013. p. 227–69.

[62] Speth JD. Bison Kills and Bone Counts: Decision Making by Ancient Hunters. Chicago: University of Chicago Press; 1983.

[63] Stiner MC. Carnivory, coevolution, and the geographic spread of the genus Homo. J Archaeol Res 2002;10:1–63.

[64] Brink J. Imagining Head-Smashed-in Aboriginal Buffalo Hunting on the Northern Plains. Edmonton: Athabasca University Press; 2008.

[65] Lev-Yadun S, Gopher A, Abbo S. The cradle of agriculture. Science 2000;288:1602–3.

[66] Diamond JM. The Worst Mistake in the History of the Human Race. Oplopanax Publishing; 2010.

[67] Debo A. A History of the Indians of the United States. University of Oklahoma Press; 2013.

[68] Lipski E. Traditional non-Western diets. Nutr Clin Pract 2010;25:585–93.

[69] Steckel RH, Prince JM. Tallest in the world: Native Americans of the Great Plains in the nineteenth century. Am Econ Rev 2001;91 (1):287–94.

[70] Narayan KV. Diabetes mellitus in Native Americans: The problem and its implications. Popul Res Policy Rev 1997;16:169–92.

[71] Ellison R. Methods of food preparation in Mesopotamia (c.3000–600 BC). J Econ Soc Hist Orient 1984;89–98.

[72] Cohen MN, Armelagos GJ, Larsen CS. Paleopathology at the Origins of Agriculture. University Press of Florida; 2013.

[73] Steckel RH, Rose JC, Spencer Larsen C, Walker PL. Skeletal health in the Western Hemisphere from 4000 BC to the present Evolutionary Anthropology: Issues. News, and Reviews: Issues, News, and Reviews 2002;11:142–55.

[74] Orr JB, Gilks JL. Studies of nutrition. The physique and health of two African tribes. London: H.M. Stationary Office; 1931. 155.
[75] Forshaw R. Dental health and disease in ancient Egypt. Br Dent J 2009;206:421–4.
[76] Nerlich AG, Haas CJ, Zink A, Szeimies U, Hagedorn HG. Molecular evidence for tuberculosis in an ancient Egyptian mummy. The Lancet 1997;350:1404.
[77] Ragheb M. Schistosomiasis of the liver: clinical, pathologic and laboratory studies in Egyptian cases. Gastroenterology 1956;30:631–60.
[78] Rowling JT. Pathological changes in mummies. SAGE Publications; 1961.
[79] Zink A, et al. Malignant tumors in an ancient Egyptian population. Anticancer Res 1999;19:4273.
[80] Cockburn A, Cockburn E, Reyman TA. Mummies, disease and ancient cultures. Cambridge University Press; 1998.
[81] Rowbotham J, Clayton P. An unsuitable and degraded diet? Part three: Victorian consumption patterns and their health benefits. J R Soc Med 2008;101:454–62.
[82] Clayton P, Rowbotham J. An unsuitable and degraded diet? Part one: public health lessons from the mid-Victorian working class diet. J R Soc Med 2008;101:282–9.
[83] Clayton P, Rowbotham J. An unsuitable and degraded diet? Part two: realities of the mid-Victorian diet. J R Soc Med 2008;101:350–7.
[84] Clayton P, Rowbotham J. How the mid-Victorians worked, ate and died. Int J Env Res Public Health 2009;6:1235–53.
[85] Yellowlees W. A Doctor in the Wilderness. Pioneer Associates (Graphic) Limited; 1993.
[86] Boyd JD, Drain CL. The arrest of dental caries in childhood. J Am Med Assoc 1928;90(23):1867–9.
[87] Price WA. New light on the etiology and control of dental caries. J Dent Res 1932;12:540–4.
[88] Dreyer TF. Dental caries in prehistoric South Africans. Nature 1935;136(3434):302–3.
[89] Price WA. Nutrition and physical degeneration: a comparison of primitive and modern diets and their effects. 8th edition Price-Pottenger Nutrition Foundation; 1939. edn.
[90] Stefansson V. The Fat of the Land. The Macmillam Cpmpany; 1960.
[91] Stefansson V. Cancer: Disease of Civilization?: An Anthropological and Historical Study. New York: Hill and Wang; 1960.
[92] Ames BN, Profet M, Gold LS. Dietary pesticides (99.99% all natural). Proc Natl Acad Sci 1990;87:7777–81.
[93] Mithöfer A, Maffei ME. General mechanisms of plant defense and plant toxins. In: Gopalakrishnakone P., Carlini C., Ligabue-Braun R. (eds) Plant Toxins: Toxicology. 2016, pp. 1–22. Springer.
[94] Fabbri AD, Crosby GA. A review of the impact of preparation and cooking on the nutritional quality of vegetables and legumes. Int J Gastron Food Sci 2016;3:2–11.
[95] Larbey C, Mentzer SM, Ligouis B, Wurz S, Jones MK. Cooked starchy food in hearths ca. 120 kya and 65 kya (MIS 5e and MIS 4) from Klasies River Cave, South Africa. J Hum Evol 2019;131:210–27.
[96] Henry AG, Brooks AS, Piperno DR. Plant foods and the dietary ecology of Neanderthals and early modern humans. J Hum Evol 2014;69:44–54. Available from https://doi.org/10.1016/j.jhevol.2013.12.014.
[97] Barkai R, Rosell J, Blasco R, Gopher A. Fire for a reason: barbecue at Middle Pleistocene Qesem Cave. Israel CurrAnthr 2017;58:S314–28.
[98] Wiest M, Schindler B. Remembering lessons from the past: fermentation and the restructuring of our food system. In: Saberi H (ed) Cured, Smoked, and Fermented: Proceedings of the Oxford Symposium on Food and Cookery, 2010, 2011. Prospect Books.
[99] Chaves-López C, Rossi C, Maggio F, Paparella A, Serio A. Changes occurring in spontaneous maize fermentation: An overview Fermentation 2020;6:36.
[100] Sinclair HM. The Work of Sir Robert McCarrison. London: Faber and Faber Ltd; 1953.
[101] McCarrison R. Nutrition and National Health being The Cantor Lectures Delivered Before the Royal Society of Arts 1936. London: Faber and Faber Ltd; 1936. p. 51–70. Available from https://mccarrison.com/wp-content/uploads/2016/04/National-Health-and-Nutrition-Cantor-Lectures-scan-smaller-version.pdf, http://journeytoforever.org/farm_library/McC/McCToC.html.
[102] Cleave TL. The Saccharine Disease, Conditions Caused by the Taking of Refined Carbohydrates, such as Sugar and White Flour. Bristol: John Wright and Sons Ltd; 1974.
[103] Cleave TL, Campbell GD. Diabetes, Coronary Thrombosis, and the Saccharine Disease. 1st Ed. Bristol, UK: John Wright and Sons Limited; 1966.
[104] O'Dea K, Trainedes K, Hopper JL, et al. Impaired glucose tolerance, hyperinsulinemia, and hypertriglyceridemia in Australian Aborigines from the desert. Diabetes Care 1988;11(1):23–9.
[105] O'Dea K. Westernization, insulin resistance and diabetes in Australian aborigines. Medical Journal of Australia 1991;155(4):258–64.
[106] O'Dea K. Marked improvement in carbohydrate and lipid metabolism in diabetic Australian aborigines after temporary reversion to traditional lifestyle. Diabetes 1984;33(6):596–603.
[107] Wtebe N, Ye F, Crumley ET, et al. Temporal associations among body mass index, fasting insulin, and systemic inflammation. A systematic review and meta-analysis. J Am Med Assoc Network Open 2021;4(3):e211263.
[108] Yudkin J. Patterns and trends in carbohydrate consumption and their relation to disease. Proc Nutr Soc 1964;23:149–62.
[109] Yudkin J. Pure, white and deadly. London: Penguin Books; 1972.
[110] Taubes G. The case against sugar. New York: Alfred A. Knopf; 2016.
[111] Cleave TL. Overconsumption, now the most dangerous cause of disease in western countries. Public Health London 1977;91:127–31.
[112] Monteiro CA. Nutrition and health. The issue is not food but nutrients, as much as processing. Public Health Nutr 2009;12(5):729–31.
[113] Monteiro CA, Cannon G, Levy RB, et al. Ultra-processed foods: what they are and how to identify them. Public Health Nutr 2019;22(5):936–41.
[114] Monteiro CA, Moubarac JC, Cannon G, Ng SW, Popkin B. Ultra-processed products are becoming dominant in the global food system. Obes Rev 2013;14:21–8.

[115] Steele EM, Baraldi LG, de Costa Louzada ML, et al. Ultra-processed foods and added sugars in the US diet: evidence from a nationally representative cross-sectional study. BMJ Open 2016;6:e009892.

[116] Pagliai G, Dinu M, Madarena M, Bonaccio M, Iacoviello L, Sofi F. Consumption of ultra-processed foods and health status: a systematic review and meta-analysis. Br J Nutr 2020;1 1.

[117] Levy RB, Rauber F, Chang K, et al. Ultra-processed food consumption and type 2 diabetes incidence: A prospective cohort study. Clinical Nutrition 2020;0. Available from https://doi.org/10.1016/j.clnu.2020.12.018.

[118] Zhong G-C, Gu H-T, Peng Y, et al. Assocation of ultra-processed food consumption with cardiovascular mortality in the US population: long-term results from a large prospective multicenter study. Int J Behav Nutr Phys Act 2021;18:21.

[119] Bonaccio M, Castelnuovo AD, Costanzo S, et al. Ultra-processed food consumption is associated with increased risk of all-case and cardiovascular mortality in the Moli-sani Study. Am J Clin Nutr 2020;0:1–10.

[120] Koiwai K, Takemi Y, Hayashi F, et al. Consumption of ultra-processed foods and relationship between nutrient intake and obesity among participants undergoing special health checkups provided by National Health Insurance. Nihon Koshu Eisei Zasshi 2020;. Available from https://doi.org/10.11236/jph.20-044 Dec 26.

[121] Konieczna J, Morey M, Abete I, et al. Contribution of ultra-processed foods in visceral fat deposition and other adiposity indicators: Prospective analysis nested in the PREDIMED-Plus trial. Clin Nutr 2021;. Available from https://doi.org/10.1016/j.clnu.2021.01.019 S0261–5614(21)00029-7.

[122] Zaretsky J, Griess-Fisheimer S, Carmi A, et al. Ultra-processed food targets bone quality via endochondral ossification. Bone Research 2021;9:14.

[123] Ben-Dor M. Use of animal fat as a symbol of health in traditional societies suggests humans may be well adapted to its consumption. J Evol Health 2015;1:10.

[124] Belury MA, Cole RM, Snoke DB, Banh T, Angelotti A. Linoleic acid, glycemic control and Type 2 diabetes prostaglandins. Leukotrienes and Essential Fatty Acids 2018;132:30–3.

[125] Bjermo H, et al. Effects of n-6 PUFAs compared with SFAs on liver fat, lipoproteins, and inflammation in abdominal obesity: a randomized controlled trial. Am J Clin Nutr 2012;95:1003–12.

[126] Ramsden CE, Zamora D, Leelarthaepin B, et al. Use of dietary linoleic acid for secondary prevention of coronary heart disease and death. Evaluation of recovered data from the Sydney Diet Heart Study and updated meta-analysis. BMJ 2013;346:e8707170.

[127] Ramsden CE, Zamora D, Majchrzak-Hong S, et al. Re-evaluation of the traditional diet-heart hypothesis: analysis of recovered data from Minnesota Coronary Experiment (1968–73). BMJ 2016;353:i1246.

[128] Sadeghi M, Simani M, Mohammadifard N, et al. Longitudinal association of dietary fat intake with cardiovascular events in a prospective cohort study in Eastern Mediterranean region. Int J Food Sci Nutr 2021;. Available from https://doi.org/10.1080/09637.2021.1895725.

[129] Ordoñez M, Presa N, Dominguez-Herrera A, Trueba M, Gomez-Muñoz A. Regulation of adipogenesis by ceramide 1-phosphate. Exp Cell Res 2018;372:150–7.

[130] Schneider C, Porter NA, Brash AR. Routes to 4-hydroxynonenal: fundamental issues in the mechanisms of lipid peroxidation. J Biol Chem 2008;283:15539–43.

[131] D'Angelo S, Motti ML, Meccariello R. ω-3 and ω-6 polyunsaturated fatty acids. Obes Cancer Nutr 2020;12:2751.

[132] Kiyabu GY, et al. Fish, n − 3 polyunsaturated fatty acids and n − 6 polyunsaturated fatty acids intake and breast cancer risk: The J apan P ublic H ealth C enter-based prospective study. Int J Cancer 2015;137:2915–26.

[133] Okuyama H, et al. Medicines and vegetable oils as hidden causes of cardiovascular disease and diabetes. Pharmacology 2016;98:134–70.

[134] Simopoulos AP. An increase in the omega-6/omega-3 fatty acid ratio increases the risk for obesity. Nutrients 2016;8:128.

[135] Tangvarasittichai S. Oxidative stress, insulin resistance, dyslipidemia and type 2 diabetes mellitus. World J Diabetes 2015;6:456.

[136] Tsai S, Clemente-Casares X, Revelo XS, Winer S, Winer DA. Are obesity-related insulin resistance and type 2 diabetes autoimmune diseases? Diabetes 2015;64:1886–97.

[137] Lawrence GD. Perspective: the saturated fat-unsaturated oil dilemma: relations of dietary fatty acids and serum cholesterol, atherosclerosis, inflammation, cancer, and all-cause mortality. Adv Nutr 2021;12:647–56.

[138] Kucek LK, Veenstra LD, Amnuaycheewa P, Sorrells ME. A grounded guide to gluten: how modern genotypes and processing impact wheat sensitivity. Compr Rev Food Sci Food Saf 2015;14:285–302.

[139] Hotz C, Gibson RS. Traditional food-processing and preparation practices to enhance the bioavailability of micronutrients in plant-based diets. J Nutr 2007;137:1097–100.

[140] Lerner A, Jeremias P, Matthias T. The world incidence and prevalence of autoimmune diseases is increasing. Int J Celiac Dis 2015;3:151–5.

[141] Lohi S, et al. Increasing prevalence of coeliac disease over time. Aliment Pharmacol Ther 2007;26:1217–25.

[142] Rubio–Tapia A, et al. Increased prevalence and mortality in undiagnosed celiac disease. Gastroenterology 2009;137:88–93.

[143] Buhler S, Raine KD, Arango M, Pellerin S, Neary NE. Building a strategy for obesity prevention one piece at a time: the case of sugar-sweetened beverage taxation. Canadian journal of diabetes 2013;37:97–102.

[144] Jegatheesan P, De Bandt JP. Fructose and NAFLD: the multifaceted aspects of fructose metabolism. Nutrients 2017;9:230.

[145] Gearhardt AN, Hebebrand J. The concept of "food addiction" helps inform the understanding of overeating and obesity: Debate consensus. American Journal of Clinical Nutrition 2021;113:274–6.

[146] Lustig RH. Ultraprocessed food: Addictive, toxic, and ready for regulation. Nutrients 2020;12:3401.

[147] Moss M. Hooked: Food, Free Will, and How the Food Giants Exploit Our Addictions. New York, NY: Random House; 2021.

[148] Hall KD, Ayuketah A, Brychta R, et al. Ultra-processed diets cause excess calorie intake and weight gain: An inpatient randomized controlled trial of ad libitum food intake. Cell Metab 2019;30(1):67–77.
[149] Steele EM, Raubenheimer D, Simpson SJ, et al. Ultra-processed foods, protein leverage and energy intake in the USA. Public Health Nutr 2017;21(1):114–24.
[150] Taubes G. Good Calories Bad Calories. Fats, carbs, and the Controversial Science of Diet and Health. New York, NY: Anchor Books; 2008.
[151] Dobzhansky T. Nothing in biology makes sense except in the light of evolution. Am Biol Teach 1973;35:125–9.
[152] Harris S. Hyperinsulinism and dysinsulinism. J Am Med Assoc 1924;83(10):729–33.
[153] Reaven GM. Why Syndrome X? From Harold Himsworth to the insulin resistance syndrome. Cell Metab 2005;1(1):9–14. Available from https://doi.org/10.1016/j.cmet.2004.12.001.
[154] Reaven GM. Insulin resistance and human disease: a short history. J Basic Clin Physiol Pharmacol 1998;9(2–4):387–406.
[155] Crofts C, Schofield G, Zinn C, Wheldon M, Kraft J. Identifying hyperinsulinaemia in the absence of impaired glucose tolerance: An examination of the Kraft database. Diabetes Res Clin Pract 2016;118:50–7. Available from https://doi.org/10.1016/j.diabres.2016.06.007.
[156] World Health Organization. Definition, diagnosis and classification of diabetes mellitus and its complications 1999. Retrieved from Geneva: http://whqlibdoc.who.int/hq/1999/WHO_NCD_NCS_99.2.pdf.
[157] Crofts C, Schofield G, Wheldon M, Zinn C, Kraft JR. Determining a diagnostic algorithm for hyperinsulinaemia. Journal of Insulin Resistance 2019;4(1). Available from https://doi.org/10.4102/jir.v4i1.49.
[158] Hayashi T, Boyko EJ, Sato KK, McNeely MJ, Leonetti DL, Kahn SE, et al. Patterns of insulin concentration during the OGTT predict the risk of type 2 diabetes in Japanese Americans. Diabetes Care 2013;36(5):1229–35. Available from https://doi.org/10.2337/dc12-0246.
[159] Wilcox G. Insulin and insulin resistance. Clinical Biochemist Reviews 2005;26(2):19–39. Available from http://www.ncbi.nlm.nih.gov/pmc/articles/PMC1204764/.
[160] Action to Control Cardiovascular Risk in Diabetes Study Group. Effects of intensive glucose lowering in type 2 diabetes. New England journal of medicine 2008;358(24):2545–59. Available from https://www.nejm.org/doi/pdf/10.1056/NEJMoa0802743?articleTools = true.
[161] Crofts, C. (2015). Understanding and diagnosing hyperinsulinaemia. (PhD). AUT, Retrieved from http://aut.researchgateway.ac.nz/handle/10292/9906.
[162] Cleeman J. National Cholesterol Education Program ATP III Guidelines At-A-Glance Quick Desk Reference. 6. https://www.nhlbi.nih.gov/files/docs/guidelines/atglance.pdf.
[163] Consensus statements [International Diabetes Federation (IDF)]. [cited 2022 Jun 14]. Available from: https://www.idf.org/e-library/consensus-statements/60-idfconsensus-worldwide-definitionof-the-metabolic-syndrome.html.
[164] Reaven GM. The metabolic syndrome: Requiescat in pace. Clin Chem 2005;51(6):931–8. Available from https://doi.org/10.1373/clinchem.2005.048611.
[165] Braun M, Ramracheya R, Rorsman P. Autocrine regulation of insulin secretion. Diabetes, Obesity and Metabolism 2012;14:143–51.
[166] Seino S, Shibasaki T, Minami K. Dynamics of insulin secretion and the clinical implications for obesity and diabetes. J Clin Invest 2011;121(6):2118–25. Available from https://www.ncbi.nlm.nih.gov/pmc/articles/PMC3104758/pdf/JCI45680.pdf.
[167] Meloni AR, DeYoung MB, Lowe C, Parkes DG. GLP-1 receptor activated insulin secretion from pancreatic β-cells: mechanism and glucose dependence. Diabetes Obes Metab 2013;15(1):15–27. Available from https://doi.org/10.1111/j.1463-1326.2012.01663.x.
[168] Cooper I, Brookler K, Crofts C. Rethinking fragility fractures in type 2 diabetes: The link between hyperinsulinaemia and osteofragilitas. Biomedicines 2021;9(9). Available from https://doi.org/10.3390/biomedicines9091165.
[169] Petersen MC, Shulman GI. Mechanisms of insulin action and insulin resistance. Physiol Rev 2018;98(4):2133–223. Available from https://doi.org/10.1152/physrev.00063.2017.
[170] Svendsen B, Larsen O, Gabe MBN, Christiansen CB, Rosenkilde MM, Drucker DJ, et al. Insulin secretion depends on intra-islet glucagon signaling Cell Reports 2018;25(5):1127–34e1122. Available from https://www.cell.com/cell-reports/pdf/S2211-1247(18)31594-8.pdf.
[171] Kanazawa I. Osteocalcin as a hormone regulating glucose metabolism. World Journal of Diabetes 2015;6(18):1345–54. Available from https://doi.org/10.4239/wjd.v6.i18.1345.
[172] Seino Y, Fukushima M, Yabe D. GIP and GLP-1, the two incretin hormones: Similarities and differences. Journal of Diabetes Investigation 2010;1(1-2):8–23. Available from https://doi.org/10.1111/j.2040-1124.2010.00022.x.
[173] Molina J, Rodriguez-Diaz R, Fachado A, Jacques-Silva MC, Berggren P-O, Caicedo A. Control of insulin secretion by cholinergic signaling in the human pancreatic islet. Diabetes 2014;63(8):2714–26. Available from https://doi.org/10.2337/db13-1371.
[174] Thams P, Capito K. L-arginine stimulation of glucose-induced insulin secretion through membrane depolarization and independent of nitric oxide. European Journal of Endocrinology 1999;140(1):87–93. Available from https://doi.org/10.1530/eje.0.1400087.
[175] Peterhoff M, Sieg A, Brede M, Chao CM, Hein L, Ullrich S. Inhibition of insulin secretion via distinct signaling pathways in alpha2-adrenoceptor knockout mice. European Journal of Endocrinology 2003;149(4):343–50. Available from https://doi.org/10.1530/eje.0.1490343.
[176] Strowski MZ, Parmar RM, Blake AD, Schaeffer JM. Somatostatin inhibits insulin and glucagon secretion via two receptors subtypes: an in vitro study of pancreatic islets from somatostatin receptor 2 knockout mice. Endocrinology 2000;141(1):111–17. Available from https://doi.org/10.1210/endo.141.1.7263.
[177] Cooper I, Brookler K, Kyriakidou Y, Elliott BT, Crofts C. Metabolic phenotypes and step by step evolution of type 2 diabetes: A new paradigm. Biomedicines 2021;9(7):800. Available from https://www.mdpi.com/2227-9059/9/7/800.
[178] Ritzel, R., Michael, D., & Butler, P. Insulin Secretion 2003. In (pp. 384-390).
[179] Shannahoff-Khalsa DS, Kennedy B, Yates FE, Ziegler MG. Low-frequency ultradian insulin rhythms are coupled to cardiovascular, autonomic, and neuroendocrine rhythms. American Journal of Physiology - Regulatory Integrative and Comparative Physiology 1997;272(3):R962–8.

[180] Satin LS, Butler PC, Ha J, Sherman AS. Pulsatile insulin secretion, impaired glucose tolerance and type 2 diabetes. Mol Aspects Med 2015;42:61–77. Available from: http://ac.els-cdn.com/S0098299715000047/1-s2.0-S0098299715000047-main.pdf?_tid = e859b332-2e1b-11e7-b3d9-00000aab0f26&acdnat = 1493608485_7ad840e7c1fe07ae75b0e05d6d9dcb06.

[181] Rorsman P, Braun M. Regulation of insulin secretion in human pancreatic islets. Annu Rev Physiol 2013;75:155–79. Available from https://www.annualreviews.org/doi/10.1146/annurev-physiol-030212-183754?url_ver = Z39.88-2003&rfr_id = ori%3Arid%3Acrossref.org&rfr_-dat = cr_pub%3Dpubmed.

[182] Crofts C, Neill A, Campbell A, Bartley J, White DE. Sleep architecture, insulin resistance and the nasal cycle: Implications for positive airway pressure therapy. Journal of Insulin Resistance 2018;3(1):6.

[183] Chourpiliadis C, Mohiuddin SS. Biochemistry, gluconeogenesis. StatPearls 2020; [Internet].

[184] Abdulla H, Smith K, Atherton PJ, Idris I. Role of insulin in the regulation of human skeletal muscle protein synthesis and breakdown: a systematic review and meta-analysis. Diabetologia 2016;59(1):44–55. Available from https://doi.org/10.1007/s00125-015-3751-0.

[185] Liamis G, Liberopoulos E, Barkas F, Elisaf M. Diabetes mellitus and electrolyte disorders. World journal of clinical cases 2014;2 (10):488–96. Available from https://doi.org/10.12998/wjcc.v2.i10.488.

[186] DeFronzo RA, Cooke CR, Andres R, Faloona GR, Davis PJ. The effect of insulin on renal handling of sodium, potassium, calcium, and phosphate in man. J Clin Invest 1975;55(4):845–55. Available from https://doi.org/10.1172/JCI107996.

[187] Grote CW, Wright DE. A role for insulin in diabetic neuropathy. Frontiers in Neuroscience 2016;10:581. Available from https://www.ncbi.nlm.nih.gov/pmc/articles/PMC5179551/pdf/fnins-10-00581.pdf.

[188] Kim B, Feldman E. Insulin resistance in the nervous system. Trends in Endocrinology & Metabolism 2012;23:133–41.

[189] Milstein JL, Ferris HA. The brain as an insulin-sensitive metabolic organ. Mol Metab. 2021;52:101234. Available from https://doi.org/10.1016/j.molmet.2021.101234 Epub 2021 Apr 15. PMID: 33845179.

[190] Nguyen TT, Ta QTH, Nguyen TKO, Nguyen TTD, Giau VV. Type 3 diabetes and its role implications in Alzheimer's disease. Int J Mol Sci. 2020;21(9):3165. Available from https://doi.org/10.3390/ijms21093165 PMID: 32365816.

[191] Spinelli M, Fusco S, Grassi C. Brain insulin resistance and hippocampal plasticity: mechanisms and biomarkers of cognitive decline. Frontiers in Neuroscience 2019;13:788. Available from https://doi.org/10.3389/fnins.2019.00788.

[192] Dongerkery SP, Schroeder PR, Shomali ME. Insulin and its cardiovascular effects: what is the current evidence? Curr Diab Rep 2017;17 (12):120. Available from https://doi.org/10.1007/s11892-017-0955-3.

[193] Li X, Weber NC, Cohn DM, Hollmann MW, DeVries JH, Hermanides J, et al. Effects of hyperglycemia and diabetes mellitus on coagulation and hemostasis. J Clin Med 2021;10(11):2419. Available from https://www.mdpi.com/2077-0383/10/11/2419.

[194] Stegenga ME, van der Crabben SN, Levi M, de Vos AF, Tanck MW, Sauerwein HP, et al. Hyperglycemia stimulates coagulation, whereas hyperinsulinemia impairs fibrinolysis in healthy humans. Diabetes 2006;55(6):1807–12. Available from http://diabetes.diabetesjournals.org/content/55/6/1807.full.pdf.

[195] Barbour LA, McCurdy CE, Hernandez TL, Kirwan JP, Catalano PM, Friedman JE. Cellular mechanisms for insulin resistance in normal pregnancy and gestational diabetes. Diabetes Care 2007;30(Supplement 2):S112–19. Available from https://doi.org/10.2337/dc07-s202.

[196] Jensen J, Rustad PI, Kolnes AJ, Lai Y-C. The role of skeletal muscle glycogen breakdown for regulation of insulin sensitivity by exercise. Frontiers in physiology 2011;2:112. Available from https://doi.org/10.3389/fphys.2011.00112.

[197] Dankner R, Chetrit A, Shanik MH, Raz I, Roth J. Basal-state hyperinsulinemia in healthy normoglycemic adults is predictive of type 2 diabetes over a 24-year follow-up: A preliminary report. Diabetes Care 2009;32(8):1464–6. Available from https://doi.org/10.2337/dc09-0153.

[198] Li L, Messina JL. Acute insulin resistance following injury. Trends Endocrinol Metab 2009;20(9):429–35. Available from https://doi.org/10.1016/j.tem.2009.06.004.

[199] Jamerson KA, Julius S, Gudbrandsson T, Andersson O, Brant DO. Reflex sympathetic activation induces acute insulin resistance in the human forearm. Hypertension 1993;21(5):618–23. Available from https://doi.org/10.1161/01.HYP.21.5.618.

[200] Vendelbo MH, Clasen BFF, Treebak JT, Møller L, Krusenstjerna-Hafstrøm T, Madsen M, et al. Insulin resistance after a 72-h fast is associated with impaired AS160 phosphorylation and accumulation of lipid and glycogen in human skeletal muscle. Am J Physiol Endocrinol Metab 2012;302(2):E190–200. Available from https://doi.org/10.1152/ajpendo.00207.2011.

[201] Sun Q, Li J, Gao F. New insights into insulin: The anti-inflammatory effect and its clinical relevance. World Journal of Diabetes 2014;5 (2):89–96. Available from https://doi.org/10.4239/wjd.v5.i2.89.

[202] Martin SD, McGee SL. The role of mitochondria in the aetiology of insulin resistance and type 2 diabetes. Biochimica et Biophysica Acta (BBA)-General Subjects 2014;1840(4):1303–12. Available from https://www.sciencedirect.com/science/article/abs/pii/S0304416513004005?via%3Dihub.

[203] Aronoff S, Bennett M, Gorden P, Rushforth N, Miller M. Unexplained hyperinsulinemia in normal and "prediabetic" Pima Indians compared with normal Caucasians: An example of racial differences in insulin secretion. Diabetes 1977;26(September):827–40.

[204] McAuley KA, Williams SM, Mann JI, Goulding A, Murphy E. Increased risk of type 2 diabetes despite same degree of adiposity in different racial groups. Diabetes Care 2002;25(12):2360–1.

[205] Mente A, Razak F, Blankenberg S, Vuksan V, Davis AD, Miller R, et al. Ethnic Variation in Adiponectin and Leptin Levels and Their Association With Adiposity and Insulin Resistance. Diabetes Care 2010;33(7):1629–34. Available from https://doi.org/10.2337/dc09-1932.

[206] Campbell GD, McKechnie J. Recent observations on Zulu and Natal Indian diabetics in Durban. South African Medical Journal 1961;35:1008–11.

[207] Campbell L. The thrifty gene hypothesis: maybe everyone is right? Int J Obes 2008;32(4):723–4. Available from https://doi.org/10.1038/sj.ijo.0803772.

[208] Reardon T, Tschirley D, Liverpool-Tasie LSO, Awokuse T, Fanzo J, Minten B, et al. The processed food revolution in African food systems and the double burden of malnutrition. Global Food Security 2021;28:100466. Available from https://doi.org/10.1016/j.gfs.2020.100466.
[209] Schnabel, L, Kesse-Guyot, E, Allès, B, Touvier, M, Srour, B, Hercberg, S, et al. Association Between Ultraprocessed Food Consumption and Risk of Mortality Among Middle-aged Adults in FranceAssociation of Ultraprocessed Foods With Mortality Risk Among French AdultsAssociation of Ultraprocessed Foods With Mortality Risk Among French Adults 2019. Available from: https://doi.org/10.1001/jamainternmed.2018.7289.
[210] Parildar H, Cigerli O, Unal D, Gulmez O, Demirag N. The impact of Vitamin D Replacement on Glucose Metabolism. Pakistan journal of medical sciences 2013;29(6):1311–14. Available from https://doi.org/10.12669/pjms.296.3891.
[211] Setola E, Monti LD, Galluccio E, Palloshi A, Fragasso G, Paroni R, et al. Insulin resistance and endothelial function are improved after folate and vitamin B12 therapy in patients with metabolic syndrome: relationship between homocysteine levels and hyperinsulinemia. European journal of endocrinology 2004;151(4):483–90.
[212] McEwen BS. Stressed or stressed out: what is the difference? Journal of Psychiatry and Neuroscience 2005;30(5):315. Available from https://www.ncbi.nlm.nih.gov/pmc/articles/PMC1197275/pdf/20050900s00002p315.pdf.
[213] Kim Y-K, Nam KI, Song J. The Glymphatic System in Diabetes-Induced Dementia. Frontiers in Neurology 2018;9(867). Available from https://doi.org/10.3389/fneur.2018.00867.
[214] Chareyron I, Christen S, Moco S, Valsesia A, Lassueur S, Dayon L, Wiederkehr A, et al. Augmented mitochondrial energy metabolism is an early response to chronic glucose stress in human pancreatic beta cells. Diabetologia 2020;. Available from https://doi.org/10.1007/s00125-020-05275-5.
[215] Honzawa N, Fujimoto K, Kitamura T. Cell Autonomous dysfunction and insulin resistance in pancreatic α cells. International J Mol Sci 2019;20(15):3699. Available from https://doi.org/10.3390/ijms20153699.
[216] Al-Mrabeh A, Hollingsworth KG, Shaw JAM, McConnachie A, Sattar N, Lean MEJ, et al. 2-year remission of type 2 diabetes and pancreas morphology: a post-hoc analysis of the DiRECT open-label, cluster-randomised trial. The Lancet Diabetes & Endocrinology 2020;. Available from https://doi.org/10.1016/S2213-8587(20)30303-X.
[217] Crofts C, Zinn C, Wheldon M, Schofield G. Hyperinsulinemia: A unifying theory of chronic disease? Diabesity 2015;1(4):34–43. Available from https://doi.org/10.15562/diabesity.2015.19.
[218] Lee S-H, Zabolotny JM, Huang H, Lee H, Kim Y-B. Insulin in the nervous system and the mind: Functions in metabolism, memory, and mood. Molecular Metabolism 2016;5(8):589–601. Available from https://doi.org/10.1016/j.molmet.2016.06.011.
[219] Giovannucci E, Harlan DM, Archer MC, Bergenstal RM, Gapstur SM, Habel LA, et al. Diabetes and cancer: a consensus report. CA Cancer J Clin 2010;60(4):207–21. Available from https://doi.org/10.3322/caac.20078.
[220] Stegenga ME, van der Crabben SN, Blümer RM, Levi M, Meijers JC, Serlie MJ, et al. Hyperglycemia enhances coagulation and reduces neutrophil degranulation, whereas hyperinsulinemia inhibits fibrinolysis during human endotoxemia. Blood 2008;112(1):82–9.
[221] Hernandez TL, Friedman JE, Barbour LA. Insulin resistance in pregnancy: implications for mother and offspring. Insulin Resistance. Springer; 2020. p. 67–94.
[222] Merger SR, Kerner W, Stadler M, Zeyfang A, Jehle P, Mueller-Korbsch M, et al. Prevalence and comorbidities of double diabetes. Diabetes Res Clin Pract 2016;119:48–56. Available from https://www.diabetesresearchclinicalpractice.com/article/S0168-8227(16)30153-X/fulltext.
[223] Chen ME, Hannon TS. Clinical Manifestations of Insulin Resistance in Youth. Insulin Resistance. Springer; 2020. p. 3–17.
[224] Alves-Bezerra M, Cohen DE. Triglyceride metabolism in the liver. Compr Physiol 2017;8(1):1–8. Available from https://doi.org/10.1002/cphy.c170012.
[225] Utzschneider KM, Kahn SE. The role of insulin resistance in nonalcoholic fatty liver disease. The Journal of Clinical Endocrinology & Metabolism 2006;91(12):4753–61.
[226] Hodson L, Gunn PJ. The regulation of hepatic fatty acid synthesis and partitioning: the effect of nutritional state. Nat Rev Endocrinol 2019;15:689–700. Available from https://doi.org/10.1038/s41574-019-0256-9.
[227] Sirota JC, McFann K, Targher G, Johnson RJ, Chonchol M, Jalal DI. Elevated serum uric acid levels are associated with non-alcoholic fatty liver disease independently of metabolic syndrome features in the United States: Liver ultrasound data from the National Health and Nutrition Examination Survey. Metabolism 2013;62(3):392–9. Available from https://doi.org/10.1016/j.metabol.2012.08.013.
[228] Borghi C, Agabiti-Rosei E, Johnson RJ, Kielstein JT, Lurbe E, Mancia G, et al. Hyperuricaemia and gout in cardiovascular, metabolic and kidney disease. Eur J Intern Med 2020;80:1–11. Available from https://doi.org/10.1016/j.ejim.2020.07.006.
[229] Choi Y-J, Yoon Y, Lee K-Y, Hien TT, Kang KW, Kim K-C, et al. Uric acid induces endothelial dysfunction by vascular insulin resistance associated with the impairment of nitric oxide synthesis. FASEB J 2014;28(7):3197–204.
[230] Hale LJ, Coward RJ. The insulin receptor and the kidney. Curr Opin Nephrol Hypertens 2013;22(1):100–6. Available from https://doi.org/10.1097/MNH.0b013e32835abb52.
[231] Wojciechowska J, Krajewski W, Bolanowski M, Kręcicki T, Zatoński T. Diabetes and cancer: a review of current knowledge. Experimental and Clinical Endocrinology & Diabetes 2016;124(05):263–75.
[232] Riehle C, Abel ED. Insulin signaling and heart failure. Circ Res 2016;118(7):1151–69. Available from https://www.ahajournals.org/doi/pdf/10.1161/CIRCRESAHA.116.306206?download = true.
[233] Chan YH, Chang GJ, Lai YJ, Chen WJ, Chang SH, Hung LM, et al. Atrial fibrillation and its arrhythmogenesis associated with insulin resistance. Cardiovasc Diabetol 2019;18(1):125. Available from https://doi.org/10.1186/s12933-019-0928-8.
[234] Quincozes-Santos A, Bobermin LD, de Assis AM, Goncalves C-A, Souza DO. Fluctuations in glucose levels induce glial toxicity with glutamatergic, oxidative and inflammatory implications. Biochimica et Biophysica Acta (BBA)-Molecular Basis of Disease 2017;1863(1):1–14.

[235] Castilla-Cortázar I, Aguirre GA, Femat-Roldán G, Martín-Estal I, Espinosa L. Is insulin-like growth factor-1 involved in Parkinson's disease development? J Transl Med 2020;18(1):70. Available from https://doi.org/10.1186/s12967-020-02223-0.

[236] van Sloten TT, Sedaghat S, Carnethon MR, Launer LJ, Stehouwer CDA. Cerebral microvascular complications of type 2 diabetes: stroke, cognitive dysfunction, and depression. The Lancet Diabetes & Endocrinology 2020;8(4):325–36. Available from https://doi.org/10.1016/S2213-8587(19)30405-X.

[237] Qiu WQ, Folstein MF. Insulin, insulin-degrading enzyme and amyloid-β peptide in Alzheimer's disease: review and hypothesis. Neurobiol Aging 2006;27(2):190–8. Available from https://doi.org/10.1016/j.neurobiolaging.2005.01.004.

[238] de la Monte SM, Wands JR. Alzheimer's Disease Is Type 3 Diabetes–Evidence Reviewed. J Diab Sci Technol 2008;2(6):1101–13. Available from http://www.ncbi.nlm.nih.gov/pmc/articles/PMC2769828/.

[239] Blázquez E, Velázquez E, Hurtado-Carneiro V, Ruiz-Albusac JM. Insulin in the brain: its pathophysiological implications for States related with central insulin resistance, type 2 diabetes and Alzheimer's disease. Frontiers in Endocrinology 2014;5:161. Available from https://doi.org/10.3389/fendo.2014.00161.

[240] Humpel C. Chronic mild cerebrovascular dysfunction as a cause for Alzheimer's disease? Experimental gerontology 2011;46(4):225–32. Available from: http://ac.els-cdn.com/S0531556510004420/1-s2.0-S0531556510004420-main.pdf?_tid = 9b18ad02-1fb3–11e6–9f40-00000aab0f02&acdnat = 1463876874_87596f847c8266a66b644e98ead7a5f3.

[241] Monzo HJ, Park TI, Dieriks VB, Jansson D, Faull RL, Dragunow M, et al. Insulin and IGF1 modulate turnover of polysialylated neuronal cell adhesion molecule (PSA-NCAM) in a process involving specific extracellular matrix components. J Neurochem 2013;. Available from https://doi.org/10.1111/jnc.12363.

[242] Miller DD, Ellingrod VL, Holman TL, Buckley PF, Arndt S. Clozapine-induced weight gain associated with the 5HT2C receptor -759C/T polymorphism. American Journal of Medical Genetics. Part B, Neuropsychiatric Genetics 2005;133B(1):97–100. Available from https://doi.org/10.1002/ajmg.b.30115.

[243] Ryan MC, Collins P, Thakore JH. Impaired fasting glucose tolerance in first-episode, drug-naive patients with schizophrenia. American Journal of Psychiatry 2003;160(2):284–9.

[244] Gibbons CH. Diabetes and metabolic disorders and the peripheral nervous system. CONTINUUM: Lifelong Learning in Neurology 2020;26(5):1161–83.

[245] Greisen J, Juhl CB, Grøfte T, Vilstrup H, Jensen TS, Schmitz O. Acute Pain Induces Insulin Resistance in Humans. Anesthesiology 2001;95(3):578–84.

[246] Iwase T, Sangai T, Fujimoto H, Sawabe Y, Matsushita K, Nagashima K, et al. Quality and quantity of visceral fat tissue are associated with insulin resistance and survival outcomes after chemotherapy in patients with breast cancer. Breast Cancer Res Treat 2020;179(2):435–43. Available from https://link.springer.com/content/pdf/10.1007/s10549-019-05467-7.pdf.

[247] Pan K, Chlebowski RT, Mortimer JE, Gunther MJ, Rohan T, Vitolins MZ, et al. Insulin resistance and breast cancer incidence and mortality in postmenopausal women in the Women's Health Initiative. Cancer. 2020.

[248] Silveira EA, Kliemann N, Noll M, Sarrafzadegan N, de Oliveira C. Visceral obesity and incident cancer and cardiovascular disease: An integrative review of the epidemiological evidence. Obesity Reviews 2020.

[249] Wiseman H, Halliwell B. Damage to DNA by reactive oxygen and nitrogen species: Role in inflammatory disease and progression to cancer. Biochem J 1996;313:17–29.

[250] Atwater WO. Principles of Nutrition and Nutritive Value of Food. US Department of Agriculture. Farmer's Bulletin 1902;142:1–8.

[251] Ben-Dor M, Noakes T.D. Understanding human diet and disease – the scientific and evolutionary evidence.

[252] Noakes TD. Cancer as a modern disease.

[253] Atwater WO. *Principles of Nutrition and Nutritive Value of Food.* US Department of Agriculture. Farmer's Bulletin 1894;23:1–357.

[254] Davis C, Saltos E. Dietary recommendations and how they have changed over time. Chapter 2: Available at: https://www.ers.usda.gov/webdocs/publications/42215/5831_aib750b_1_.pdf.

[255] Hunt CL. *Good Proportions in the Diet.* US Department of Agriculture. Farmer's Bulletin 1923;1313:18.

[256] National Nutrition Conference for Defense. Proceedings of the National Nutrition Conference for Defense. Washington DC: Federal Security Agency; 1941.

[257] Anon. Diet related to killer diseases. Hearings before the Select Committee on Nutritional and Human Needs of the US Senate. Washington, DC: *US Government Printing Office*; 1976. p. 1–42.

[258] Select Committee on Nutrition and Human Needs United States Senate. Dietary goals for the United States. Washington, DC: *US Government Printing Office*; 1977. p. 1–79.

[259] Teicholz N. The Big Fat Surprise. Why butter, meat and cheese belong in a heathy diet. New York, NY: Simon and Schuster; 2014.

[260] Peretti J. Why our food is making us fat. The Guardian [homepage on the Internet]. 2012. Available from: http://www.theguardian.com/business/2012/jun/11/why-our-food-is-making-us-fat.

[261] Anon. News and Comment. NIH deals gingerly with diet-disease link. Federal dietary guidelines for disease prevention have scant support from NIH, but pressure to take a stand is building. Science 1979;204:1175–8.

[262] Blakeslee A, Stamler J. Your heart has nine lives. New York, NY: Pocket Books; 1966.

[263] Stamler J, Beard RR, Connor WE, et al. Report of Inter-Society Commission for Heart Disease Resources. Prevention of Cardiovascular Disease. Primary prevention of the atherosclerotic diseases. Circulation 1970;42:A55–95.

[264] Brody J. Jane Brody's Good Food Book: *Living the High-Carbohydrate Way.* New York, NY: WW Norton; 1985.

[265] Levy RI, Fredrickson DS. Diagnosis and management of hyperlipoproteinemia. Am J Cardiol 1968;22:576–83.
[266] Malhotra A, Noakes TD, Phinney S. It is time to bust the myth of physical inactivity and obesity: you cannot outrun a bad diet. Br J Sports Med 2015;49:967–8.
[267] Ahrens EH. Dietary fats and coronary heart disease: unfinished business. Lancet 1979;2:1345–8.
[268] Ahrens EH, Hirsch J, Insull W, et al. Dietary control of serum lipids in relation to atherosclerosis. JAMA 1957;164:1905–11.
[269] Ahrens EH, Hirsch J, Oette K, et al. Carbohydrate-induced and fat-induced lipemia. Trans Assoc Am Physicians 1961;74:134–46.
[270] Ahrens EH. Carbohydrates, plasma triglycerides and coronary heart disease. Nutr Rev 1986;44:60–4.
[271] Anon. Responses to dietary goals for the United States. Nutr Today 1977;12(10-13):20–7.
[272] Mann GV. Diet-Heart: End of an era? N Engl J Med 1977;297:644–50.
[273] Mann GV. A short history of the diet/heart hypothesis. In: Mann GV, editor. Coronary Heart Disease. The dietary sense and nonsense. An evaluation by scientists. London, England: Janus Publishing Company; 1993. p. 1–7.
[274] Reisser R. Oversimplification of diet:coronary heart disease relationships and exaggerated diet recommendations. Am J Clin Nutr 1978;31:865–75.
[275] Select Committee on Nutrition and Human Needs United States Senate. Dietary goals for the United States In: Schweiker, Zorinsky, editors. Supplementary Foreword by Senators Percy. 2nd Edition Washington, DC: *US Government Printing Office*; 1977Available at. Available from https://traningslara.se/wp-content/uploads/2018/09/McGovern1977v1.pdf.
[276] Ahrens EH. Introduction. Am J Clin Nutr 1979;32:2627–31.
[277] Glueck CJ. Appraisal of dietary fat as a causative factor in atherogenesis. Am J Clin Nutr 1979;32:2637–43.
[278] Glueck CJ. Dietary fat and atherosclerosis. Am J Clin Nutr 1979;32:2703–11.
[279] Van Italie TB, Hirsch J. Appraisal of excess calories as a factor in the causation of disease. Am J Clin Nutr 1979;32:2648–53.
[280] Van Italie TB. Obesity:adverse effects on health and longevity. Am J Clin Nutr 1979;32:2723–33.
[281] McGill HC. Appraisal of cholesterol as a causative factor in atherogenesis. Am J Clin Nutr 1979;32:2632–6.
[282] McGill HC. The relationship of dietary cholesterol to serum cholesterol concentration and to atherosclerosis in man. Am J Clin Nutr 1979;32:2664–702.
[283] Spritz N. Appraisal of alcohol consumption as a causative factor in liver disease and atherosclerosis. Am J Clin Nutr 1979;32:2654–8.
[284] Spritz N. Review of the evidence linking alcohol consumption with liver disease and atherosclerotic disease. Am J Clin Nutr 1979;32:2734–8.
[285] Tobian L. Dietary salt (sodium) and hypertension. Am J Clin Nutr 1979;32:2659–62.
[286] Bierman EL. Carbohydrate and sucrose intake in the causation of atherosclerotic heart disease, diabetes mellitus, and dental caries. Am J Clin Nutr 1979;32:2644–7.
[287] Bierman EL. Carbohydrates, sucrose, and human disease. Am J Clin Nutr 1979;32:2712–22.
[288] Moss M. Salt, sugar, fat. How the food giants hooked us. New York, NY: Random House; 2013.
[289] Keys A. Diet and the epidemiology of coronary heart disease. JAMA 1957;164:1912–19.
[290] Truswell AS. Diet in the pathogenesis of ischaemic heart disease. Postgrad Med J 1976;52:424–32.
[291] Anon. The multiple risk factor intervention trial (MRFIT). A national study of primary prevention of coronary heart disease. JAMA 1976;23:825–7.
[292] Moore TJ. Heart Failure: A Critical Inquiry into American Medicine and the Revolution in Heart Care. New York, NY: Simon and Schuster; 1989.
[293] Howard BV, Van Horn L, Manson JE, et al. Low-fat dietary pattern and risk of cardiovascular disease. The Women's Health Initiative Randomized Controlled Dietary Modification Trial. JAMA 2006;295:655–66.
[294] Prentice RL, Aragaki AK, Howard BV, et al. Low-fat dietary pattern and cardiovascular disease: results from the women's health initiative randomized controlled trial. Am J Clin Nutr 2017;106:35–43.
[295] Noakes TD. The Women's Health Initiative Randomized Controlled Dietary Modification Trial: An inconvenient finding and the diet-heart hypothesis. S Afr Med J 2013;103:824–5.
[296] Noakes TD. Hiding unhealthy heart outcomes is a low-fat diet trial: the Women's Health Initiative Randomized Controlled Dietary Modification Trial finds that post-menopausal women with established coronary heart disease were at increased risk of an adverse outcome if they consumed a low-fat 'heart-healthy' diet. Open Heart 2021;0:e001680.
[297] The Lipid Research Clinics Program Epidemiology Committee. Plasma lipid distributions in selected North Armerican populations: The Lipid Research Clinics Program Prevalence Study. Circulation 1979;60:427–39.
[298] Wiebe N, Ye F, Crumley ET, et al. Temporal associations among body mass index, fasting insulin, and systemic inflammation. A systematic review and meta-analysis. JAMA Network Open 2021;4(3):e211263.
[299] Mitchell N, Catenacci V, Wyatt HR, et al. Obesity: Overview of an epidemic. Psychiatr Clin North Am 2011;34:717–32.
[300] Ginsberg H, Olefsky JM, Kimmerling G, et al. Induction of hypertriglyceridemia by a low-fat diet. J Clin Endocrinol Metab 1976;42:729–35.
[301] Tobian L. The relationship of salt to hypertension. Am J Clin Nutr 1979;32:2739–48.
[302] Jung C-H, Jung SH, Lee B, et al. Relation among age, insulin resistance, and blood pressure. J Am Soc Hypertens 2017;11:359–65.
[303] Reaven GM, Lithell H, Landsberg L. Hypertension and associated metabolic abnormalities – the role of insulin resistance and the sympathoadrenal system. N Engl J Med 1996;334:374–81.
[304] American Medical Association. Dietary Goals for the United States. Statement of the American Medical Association to the Select Committee on Nutrition and Human Needs, United States Senate. R I Med J 1977;60:576–81.

[305] Hite AH, Feinman RD, Guzman GE, et al. In the face of contradictory evidence: report of the Dietary Guidelines for Americans Committee. Nutrition 2010;26:915–24.

[306] Hite A, Schoenfeld P. Open letter to the Secretaries of the U.S. Departments of Agriculture and Health and Human Services on the creation of the 2015 Dietary Guidelines for Americans. Nutrition 2015;31:776–9.

[307] DiNicolantonio JJ, Harcombe Z, O'Keefe JH. Problems with the 2015 Dietary Guidelines for Americans: An Alternative. Missouri Med 2016;113:74–8.

[308] Nissen SE. U.S. Dietary Guidelines: an evidence-free zone. Ann Intern Med 2016;164:558–9.

[309] Teicholz N. The scientific report guiding the US dietary guidelines: Is it scientific. BMJ 2015;351:h4962. Available from https://www.bmj.com/content/351/bmj.h4962.

[310] Liebman B. Rapid Response: The scientific report guiding the US dietary guidelines: is it scientific. BMJ 2015;351:h4962. Available from https://www.bmj.com/content/351/bmj.h4962/rr-36.

[311] Teicholz N. The scientific report guiding the US dietary guidelines: is it scientific. BMJ 2016;355:i6061. Available from https://www.bmj.com/content/351/bmj.h4962/rr-32.

[312] Anon. Partnership for an unhealthy planet: How big business interferes with global health policy and science. Published by Corporate Accountability 2020;1-36. Available at: https://www.corporateaccountability.org/wp-content/uploads/2020/04/Partnership-for-an-unhealthy-planet.pdf.

[313] Malkan S. The International Life Science Institute (ILSI) is a food industry lobby group. US RIght to Know 2022. Available from https://usrtk.org/our-investigations/ilsi-is-a-food-industry-lobby-group/.

[314] Nutrition Coalition. The 2020 Dietary Guidelines Committee: Who will stand up for rigorous science over industry interests and – really – religion? March 6 2019. Available at: https://www.nutritioncoalition.us/news/2020-dietary-guidelines-committee.

[315] Dyer O. International Life Sciences Institute is advocate for food and drink industry, say researchers. BMJ 2019;365:14037.

[316] Nutrition Coalition. Dietary Guidelines experts again condemn saturated fats, ignore rigorous evidence. June 1 2020. Available at: https://www.nutritioncoalition.us/news/experts-again-condemn-saturated-fats.

[317] Steele S, Ruskin G, Sarcevic L, et al. Are industry-funded charities promoting "advocacy-led" studies or "evidence-based science"?: a case study of the International Life Sciences Institute. Globalization Health 2019;15:36.

[318] Steele S, Ruskin G, Stuckler D. Pushing partnerships: corporate influence on research and policy via the International Life Sciences Institute. Pub Health Nutr 2019. Available from https://doi.org/10.1017/S1368980019005184 Published 25 November.

[319] Fuhrman J, Phillips R. Fast food genocide: How processed food is killing us and what we can do about it. San Francisco, CA: Harper One; 2017.

[320] Anon. The menace of obesity. Lancet 1926;2:561–2.

[321] Green R. The Practice of Endocrinology. Philadelphia, PA: Lippincott; 1951.

[322] Pennington AW. A reorientation on obesity. New Engl J Med 1953;23:959–64.

[323] Thorpe GL. Treating overweight patients. JAMA 1957;165:1361–6 <I>JAMA<I> 1963; 186:156–166.

[324] Gordon ES, Goldberg M, Chose GJ. A new concept in the treatment of obesity. JAMA 1963;186:156–66.

[325] Atkins RC. Dr. Atkins' Diet Revolution: The high calorie way to stay thin forever. New York: David McKay Company Inc.; 1972.

[326] Henderson G. Court of last appeal – the early history of the high-fat diet for diabetics. J Diabetes Metab 2016;7:8.

[327] Westman E. Is dietary carbohydrate essential for human nutrition? Am J Clin Nutr 2002;75:951–3.

[328] Webster CC, Noakes TD, Chacko SK, et al. Gluconeogenesis during endurance exercise in cyclists habituated to a long-term low carbohydrate high-fat diet. J Physiol 2016;594:4389–405.

[329] Stock AL, Yudkin J. Nutrient intake of subjects on low carbohydrate diet used in treatment of obesity. Am J Clin Nutr 1970;23:948–52.

[330] Yudkin J, Carey M. The treatment of obesity by the "high-fat" diet. The inevitability of calories. Lancet 1960;ii:939–41.

[331] DiNicolantonio JJ, O'Keefe JH, Wilson WL. Sugar addiction: is it real? A narrative review. Brit J Sports Med 2017;0:1–5.

[332] Kleinridders A, Pothos EN. Impact of brain insulin signalling on dopamine function, food intake, reward, and emotional behaviour. Curr Nutr Reports 2019;8:83–91.

[333] Lennerz B, Lennerz JK. Food addiction, high-glycemic-index carbohydrates, and obesity. Clin Chem 2018;64:64–71.

[334] Olszweski PK, Wood EL, Klockar A, et al. Excessive consumption of sugar: an insatiable drive for reward. Curr Nutr Reports 2018;8:120–8.

[335] Canhada SL, et al. Ultra-processed foods, incident overweight and obesity, and longitudinal changes in weight and waist circumference: the Brazilian Longitudinal Study of Adult Health (ELSA-Brasil). Public Health Nutr 2020;23:1076–86.

[336] Juul F, Martinez-Steele E, Parekh N, Monteiro CA, Chang VW. Ultra- processed food consumption and excess weight among US adults. Br J Nutr 2018;120:90–100.

[337] Machado PP, Steele EM, Levy RB, et al. Ultra-processed food consumption and obesity in the Australian adult population. Nutr Diabetes 2020;10:39.

[338] Gearhardt AN, Schulte EM. Is food addictive? A review of the science. Annu Rev Nutr 2021;.

[339] Dalai SS, Sinha A, Gearhardt AN. Low carbohydrate ketogenic therapy as a metabolic treatment for binge eating and ultraprocessed food addiction. Curr Opin Endocrinol Diabetes Obes 2020;27:275–82.

[340] Kraemer FB, Ginsberg HN. Gerald M. Reaven, MD: Demonstration of the central role of insulin resistance in type 2 diabetes and cardiovascular disease. Diab Care 2014;37:1178–81.

[341] Garg A, Bantle JP, Henry RR, et al. Effects of varying carbohydrate content of diet in patients with non-insulin-dependent diabetes mellitus. JAMA 1994;271:1421–8.

[342] Garg A, Grundy SM, Unger RH. Comparison of effects of high and low carbohydrate diets on plasma lipoproteins and insulin sensitivity in patients with mild NIDDM. Diabetes 1992;41:1278–85.

[343] Coulson AM, Hollenbeck CB, Swislocki ALM, et al. Deleterious metabolic effects of high-carbohydrate, sucrose-containing diets in patients with non-insulin-dependent diabetes mellitus. Am J Med 1987;82:213–20.

[344] Coulson AM, Hollenbeck CB, Swislocki ALM, et al. Persistence of hypertriglyceridemic effects of low-fat high-carbohydrate diets in NIDDM patients. Diabetes Care 1989;12:94–101.

[345] Reaven G, Strom TK, Fox B. Syndrome X: The Silent Killer. The New Heart Disease Risk. New York, NY: Simon and Shuster; 2001.

[346] Leslie I. The sugar conspiracy. The Guardian. 7th April 2016.

[347] Yudkin J. Pure, White and Deadly. How Sugar Is Killing Us and What We Can Do To Stop It. London: Penguin Books; 1986.

[348] Reaven G. Insulin resistance and coronary heart disease in nondiabetic individuals. Arterioscler Thromb Vasc Biol 2012;32:1754–9.

[349] Facchini FS, Hua N, Abbasi F, et al. Insulin resistance as a predictor of age-related disease. J Clin Endocrinol Metab 2001;86:3574–8.

[350] Taylor R, Holman RR. Normal weight individuals who develop type 2 diabetes: the personal fat threshold. Clin Sci 2015;128:404–10.

[351] Godoy-Matos AF, Silva Junior WS, Valerio CM. NAFLD as a continuum: form obesity to metabolic syndrome and diabetes. Diabetol Metab Syndr 2020;12:60.

[352] Noakes TD, Sboros M. The Eat Right Revolution. Cape Town, RSA: Penguin Books; 2021.

[353] Gaggini M, Morelli M, Buzzigoli E, et al. Non-alcoholic fatty liver disease (NAFLD) and its connection with insulin resistance, dyslipidemia, atherosclerosis and coronary heart disease. Nutrients 2013;5:1544–60.

[354] Khan RS, Bril F, Cusi K, et al. Modulation of insulin resistance in fatty liver disease. Hepatology 2019;70:711–24.

[355] Lomonaco R, Bril F, Portillo-Sanchez P, et al. Metabolic impact of nonalcoholic steatohepatitis in obese patients with type 2 diabetes. Diab Care 2016;39:632–8.

[356] Ortiz-Lopez C, Chang Z, Lomonaco R, et al. Prevalence of prediabetes and diabetes and metabolic profile of patients with nonalcoholic fatty liver disease (NAFLD). Diab Care 2012;35:873–8.

[357] Rotman Y, Neuschwander-Tetri BA. Liver fat accumulation as a barometer of insulin responsiveness again points to adipose tissue as the culprit. Hepatology 2017;65:1088–90.

[358] Zhang Q-Q, Lu L-G. Nonalcoholic fatty liver disease: dyslipidemia, risk for cardiovascular complications, and treatment strategy. J Clin Translation Hepatol 2015;3:78–84.

[359] Bril F, Sninsky JJ, Baca AM, et al. Hepatic steatosis and insulin resistance, but not steatohepatitis, promote atherogenic dyslipidemia in NAFLD. J Clin Endocrinol Metab 2016;101:644–52.

[360] McGary JD. What if Minkowski had been ageusic? An alternative angle on diabetes. Science 1992;258:766–70.

[361] Pooliso G, Tataranni PA, Foley JE, et al. A high concentration of fasting plasma non-esterified fatty acids is a risk factor for the development of NIDDM. Diabetalogia 1995;38:1213–17.

[362] Rossetti L, Giaccari A, DeFonzo RA. Glucose toxicity. Diab Care 1990;13:610–30.

[363] Boden G. Role of fatty acids in the pathogenesis of insulin resistance and NIDDM. Diabetes 1997;46:3–10.

[364] Gustafson B, Hedjazifar S, Gogg S, et al. Insulin resistance and impaired adipogenesis. Trends Endocrinol Metab 2015;26:193–200.

[365] Tandon P, Wafer R, Minchin JEN. Adipose morphology and metabolic disease. J Exp Biol 2018;221:jeb164970.

[366] Bikman B. Why we get sick: The hidden epidemic at the root of most chronic disease – and how to fight it. Dallas, TX: Benbella Books, Inc; 2020.

[367] Esser N, Legrand-Poels S, Piette J, et al. Inflammation as the link between obesity, metabolic syndrome and type 2 diabetes. Diab Res Clin Pract 2014;105:141–50.

[368] Lumeng CN, Saltiel AR. Inflammatory links between obesity and metabolic disease. J Clin Invest 2011;121:2111–17.

[369] Rifai N, Ridker PM. High-sensitivity C-reactive protein: a novel and promising marker of coronary heart disease. Clin Chem 2001;47:403–11.

[370] Semenkovich CF. Insulin resistance and atherosclerosis. J Clin Invest 2006;116:78–84.

[371] Shoelson SE, Lee J, Goldfine AB. Inflammation and insulin resistance. J Clin Invest 2006;116:1793–801.

[372] Torres-Leal FL, Fonseca-Alaniz MH, Rogero MM, et al. The role of inflamed adipose tissue in the insulin resistance. Cell Biochem Funct 2010;28:623–31.

[373] Visser M, Bouter LM, McQuillan GM, et al. Elevated C-reactive protein levels in overweight and obese adults. JAMA 1999;282:2131–5.

[374] Bril F, Barb D, Portillo-Sanchez P, et al. Metabolic and histological implications of intrahepatic triglyceride content in Nonalcoholic Fatty Liver Disease. Hepatology 2017;65:1131–44.

[375] Chen L, Chen R, Wang H, et al. Mechanisms linking inflammation to insulin resistance. Int J Epidemiol 2015; Article ID 508409, 9 pages.

[376] Diez JJ, Iglesias P. The role of the novel adipocyte-derived hormone adiponectin in human disease. Europ J Epidemiol 2003;148:293–300.

[377] Nedvidkova J, Smitka K, Kopsky V, et al. Adiponectin, an adipocyte-derived protein. Physiol Res 2005;54:133–40.

[378] Reaven G, Calciano A, Cody R, et al. Carbohydrate intolerance and hyperlipidemia in patients with myocardial infarction with known diabetes mellitus. J Clin Endocrinol Metab 1963;23:1013–23.

[379] Farquhar JW, Frank A, Gross RC, et al. Glucose, insulin and triglyceride responses to high and low carbohydrate diets in man. J Clin Invest 1966;45:1648–56.

[380] Olefsky JM, Farquhar JW, Reaven GM. Reappraisal of the role of insulin in hypertriglyceridemia. Am J Med 1974;57:551–60.

[381] Reaven GM, Hill DB, Gross RC, et al. Kinetics of triglyceride turnover of very low density lipoproteins of human plasma. J Clin Invest 1965;44:1826–33.
[382] Reaven GM, Lerner RL, Stern MP, et al. Role of insulin in endogenous hypertriglyceridemia. J Clin Invest 1967;46:1756–67.
[383] Albrink MJ, Lavietes PH, Man EB. Vascular disease and serum lipids in diabetes mellitus: observations over thirty years (1931-1961). Ann Intern Med 1963;58:305–23.
[384] Albrink MJ, Man EB. Serum triglycerides in coronary artery disease. Arch Intern Med 1959;103:4–8.
[385] Albrink MJ, Meigs JW, Man EB. Serum lipids, hypertension and coronary artery disease. Am J Med 1961;31:4–23.
[386] Albrink MJ. Triglycerides, lipoproteins, and coronary artery disease. Arch Intern Med 1962;109:345–59.
[387] Kuo PT. Hyperglyceridemia in coronary artery disease and its management. JAMA 1967;201:101–8.
[388] Kuo PT, Feng L, Cohen NN, et al. Dietary carbohydrates in hyperlipemia (hyperglyceridemia); hepatic and adipose tissue lipogenic activities. Am J Clin Nutr 1967;20:116–25.
[389] Dugani SB, Moorthy MV, Li C, et al. Association of lipid, inflammatory, and metabolic biomarkers with age at onset for incident coronary heart disease in women. JAMA Cardiol 2021;6:437–47.
[390] Shalaurova I, Kwon S, Zheng D, et al. Lipoprotein insulin resistance index: a lipoprotein particle-derived measure of insulin resistance. Metab Syndr Relat Disord 2014;12:422–9.
[391] Da Luz PL, Favarato D, Faria-Neto Junior JR, et al. High ratio of triglycerides to HDL-Cholesterol predicts extensive coronary artery disease. Clin Sci 2008;64:427–32.
[392] Dreon DM, Fernstrom HA, Campos H, et al. Change in dietary saturated fat intake is correlated with change in mass of large low-density-lipoprotein particles in men. Am J Clin Nutr 1998;67:828–36.
[393] Krauss RM. Atherogenic lipoprotein phenotype and diet-gene interactions. J Nutr 2001;131:340S–3S.
[394] Faghihnia N, Tsimakis S, Miller ER, et al. Changes in lipoprotein(a), oxidized phospholipids, and LDL subclasses with a low-fat high-carbohydrate diet. J Lipid Res 2010;51:3324–30.
[395] Reaven GM, Ida Chen Y-D, Jepperson J, et al. Insulin resistance and hyperinsulinemia in individuals with small, dense, low density lipoprotein particles. J Clin Invest 1993;92:141–6.
[396] Austin MA, Breslow JL, Hennekens CH, et al. Low-density lipoprotein subclass patterns and risk of myocardial infarction. JAMA 1988;260:1917–21.
[397] Austin MA, King M-C, Vranizan KM, et al. Atherogenic lipoprotein phenotype. A proposed genetic marker for coronary heart disease risk. Circulation 1990;82:495–506.
[398] Falkenhain K, Roach LA, McCreary S, et al. Effect of carbohydrate-restricted dietary interventions on LDL particle size and number in adults in the context of weight loss or weight maintenance: a systematic review and meta-analysis. Am J Clin Nutr 2021;nqab212. Available from https://doi.org/10.1093/ajcn/nqab212 Online ahead of print.
[399] Greenhalgh, S. Inside ILSI: How Coca-Cola, working through its scientific nonprofit, created a global science of exercise for obesity and got it embedded in Chinese Policy (1995–2015). J Health Politics Policy Law. Duke University Press DOI: 10.1215/03616878-8802174.
[400] Sacks G, Swinburn BA, Cameron AJ, et al. How food companies influence evidence and opinion – straight from the horse's mouth. Crit Public Health 2017;28:253–6.
[401] Dwyer O. International Life Sciences Institute is advocate for food and drink industry, say researchers. BMJ 2019;365:14037.
[402] Jacobs, A. A shadowy industry group shapes food policy around the globe. *New York Times*, 16 September 2019.
[403] Steele S, Ruskin G, Stuckler D. Pushing partnerships: corporate influence on research and policy via the International Life Sciences Institute. Publ Health Nutr 2020;23:2032–40.
[404] The Russells. Big Food vs. Tim Noakes: The final crusade. Available at: https://keepfitnesslegal.crossfit.com/2017/01/05/big-food-vs-tim-noakes-the-final-crusade/.
[405] O'Connor, A. Coca-Cola funds scientists who shift blame for obesity away from bad diets. *New York Times*, 9 August 2015.
[406] Pfister, K. The new faces of Coke. Medium, 28 September 2015. Available at: https://medium.com/cokeleak/the-new-faces-of-coke-62314047160f.
[407] The Russells. Coke's "partnership" with the CDC and NIH Foundations. Available at: keepfitnesslegal.crossfit.com/2016/04/05/cokes-partnership-with-the-cdc-and-nih-foundations/.
[408] Franz MJ, VanWormer JJ, Crain L, et al. Weight-loss outcomes: A systematic review and meta-analysis of weight-loss clinical trials with a minimum of 1-year follow up. J Am Diet Assoc 2007;107:1755–67.
[409] Choi YJ, Jeon S-M, Shin S. Impact of a ketogenic diet on metabolic parameters in patients with obesity or overweight and with or without type 2 diabetes: a meta-analysis of randomized controlled trials. Nutrients 2020;12:2005.
[410] Noakes TD. Low-carbohydrate and high-fat intake can manage obesity and associated conditions: Occasional survey. S Afr Med J 2013;103:826–30.
[411] Webster CC, Murphy TE, Larmuth KM, et al. Diet, diabetes status, and personal experiences of individuals with type 2 diabetes who self-selected and followed a low carbohydrate high fat diet. Diab Metab Syndr Obes Targets Ther 2019;12:2567–82.
[412] Ravnskov U. The Cholesterol Myths: Exposing the fallacy that saturated fat and cholesterol cause heart disease. Washington, DC: New Trends Publishing, Inc; 2000.
[413] Smith RL, Pinckney ER. The Cholesterol Conspiracy. St Louis, Missouri: Warren H. Green, Inc; 1991.

[414] THINCS. In: Rosch PJ, editor. Fat and cholesterol don't cause heart attacks and statins are not the solution. UK: Columbus Publishing Ltd; 2016.

[415] Colpo A. *The Great Cholesterol Con: Why everything you've been told about cholesterol, diet and heart disease is wrong!*. Anthony Colpo 2006.

[416] Central Committee for Medical and Community Program of the American Heart Association. Dietary fat and its relation to heart attacks and strokes. JAMA 1961;175:389–91.

[417] Blasbalg TL, Hibbeln JR, Ramsden CE, et al. Changes in consumption of omega-3 and omega-6 fatty acids in the United States during the 20th century. Am J Clin Nutr 2011;93:950–62.

[418] Frantz ID, Dawson EA, Ashman PL, et al. Test of effect of lipid lowering by diet on cardiovascular risk. The Minnesota Coronary Survey. Arteriosclerosis 1989;9:129–35.

[419] Woodhill JM, Palmer AJ, Leelarthaepin B, et al. Low fat, low cholesterol diet in secondary prevention of coronary heart disease. Adv Exper Med Biol 1978;109:317–31.

[420] Keys A, Mickelsen O, Miller EVO. The relation in man between cholesterol levels in the diet and in the blood. Science 1950;113:79–81.

[421] Keys A, Anderson JT, Grande F. Serum cholesterol response to changes in the diet: II. The effect of cholesterol in the diet. Metabolism 1965;14:759–65.

[422] Keys A, Anderson JT, Mickelsen O, et al. Diet and serum cholesterol in man: lack of effect of dietary cholesterol. J Nutr 1956;59:39–56.

[423] Harcombe, Z. *An examination of the randomized controlled trial and epidemiological evidence for the introduction of dietary fat recommendations in 1977 and 1983: A systematic review and meta-analysis*. PhD thesis. University of the West of Scotland, March 2016.

[424] Vorster HH, Beynen AC, Berger GMB, et al. Dietary cholesterol – the role of eggs in the prudent diet. S Afr Med J 1995;85:253–6.

[425] Vorster HH, Benade AJ, Barnard HC, et al. Egg intake does not change plasma lipoprotein and coagulation profiles. Am J Clin Nutr 1992;55:400–10.

[426] Kern F. Normal plasma cholesterol in an 88-year-old man who eats 25 eggs a day – mechanisms of adaptation. N Engl J Med 1991;324:896–9.

[427] Godos J, Micek A, Brzotek T, et al. Egg consumption and cardiovascular risk: a dose-response meta-analysis of prospective cohort studies. Europ J Nutr 2020;. Available from https://doi.org/10.1007/s00394-020-02345-7.

[428] Krittanawong C, Narasimhan B, Wang Z, et al. Association between egg consumption and risk of cardiovascular outcomes: a systematic review and meta-analysis. Am J Med 2021;134:76–83.

[429] Mozaffarian D, Ludwig DS. The 2015 US Dietary Guidelines – Ending the 35% limit on total dietary fat. JAMA 2015;313:2421–2.

[430] Han MA, Zeraatkar D, Guyatt GH, et al. Reduction of processed meat intake and cancer mortality and incidence. A systematic review and meta-analysis of cohort studies. Ann Intern Med 2019;. Available from https://doi.org/10.7326/M19.0699.

[431] Johnston BC, Zeraatkar D, Han MA, et al. Unprocessed red meat and processed meat consumption: Dietary guideline recommendations from the NutriRECS consortium. Ann Intern Med 2019;. Available from https://doi.org/10.7326/M19.1621.

[432] Vernooij RWM, Zeraatkar D, Han MA, et al. Patterns of red and processed meat consumption and risk for cardiometabolic and cancer outcomes. A systematic review and meta-analysis of cohort studies. Ann Intern Med 2019. Available from https://doi.org/10.7326/M19.1583.

[433] Zeraatkar D, Han MA, Guyatt GH, et al. Red and processed meat consumption and risk for all-cause mortality and cardiometabolic outcomes. A systematic review and meta-analysis of cohort studies. Ann Intern Med 2019. Available from https://doi.org/10.7326/M19.0655.

[434] Zeraatkar D, Johnson BC, Bartoszko J, et al. Effect of lower versus higher red meat consumption on cardiometabolic and cancer outcomes. A systematic review of randomized trials. Ann Intern Med 2019. Available from https://doi.org/10.7326/M19.0622.

[435] Zheng Y, Li Y, Satija A, et al. Association of changes in red meat consumption with total and cause specific morality among US women and men: two prospective cohort studies. BMJ 2019;365:12110.

[436] Stanhope KL, Schwarz JM, Keim NL, et al. Consuming fructose-sweetened, not glucose-sweetened beverages increases visceral adiposity and decreases insulin sensitivity in overweight/obese humans. J Clin Invest 2009;119:1322–34.

[437] Bray GA, Nielsen SJ, Popkin BM. Consumption of high-fructose corn syrup in beverages may play a role in the epidemic of obesity. Am J Clin Nutr 2004;79:537–43.

[438] Cleave TL. On the Causation of Diabetes. Chapter VII. The Saccharine Disease. Bristol, UK: John Wright and Sons Limited; 1974. p. 80–96.

[439] Cleave TL. Coronary Disease. Chapter VIII. *The Saccharine Disease*. Bristol, UK: John Wright and Sons Limited; 1974. p. 97–119.

[440] Cleave TL. Coronary disease and diabetes. Lancet 1973;2:1320–1.

[441] Festa A, Williams K, Hanley AJG, et al. Nuclear magnetic resonance lipoprotein abnormalities in prediabetic subjects in the insulin resistance atherosclerosis study. Circulation 2005;111:3465–72.

[442] Garvey WT, Kwon S, Zheng D, et al. Effects of insulin resistance and type 2 diabetes on lipoprotein subclass particle size and concentration determined by nuclear magnetic resonance. Diabetes 2003;52:453–62.

[443] Goff DC, D'Agostino RB, Haffner SM, et al. Insulin resistance and adiposity influence lipoprotein size and subclass concentrations. results from the insulin resistance atherosclerosis study. Metabolism 2005;54:264–70.

[444] Kuipers RS, de Graaf DJ, Luxwolda MF, et al. Saturated fat, carbohydrates and cardiovascular disease. Neth J Med 2011;69:372–8.

[445] Siri-Tarino PW, Sun Q, Hu FB, et al. Saturated fat, carbohydrate, and cardiovascular disease. Am J Clin Nutr 2010;91:502–9.

[446] Volk BM, Kunces LJ, Freidenreich DJ, et al. Effects of step-wise increases in dietary carbohydrate on circulating saturated fatty acids and palmitoleic acid in adults with metabolic syndrome. PLoS One 2014;9:e113605.

[447] Hyde PN, Sapper TN, Crabtree CD, et al. Dietary carbohydrate restriction improves metabolic syndrome independent of weight loss. JCI Insight 2019;4:e128308.

[448] Volek JS, Feinman RD. Carbohydrate restriction improves the features of metabolic syndrome. metabolic syndrome may be defined by the response to carbohydrate restriction. Nutr Metab 2005;2:31.

[449] Volek JS, Fernandez ML, Feinman RD, et al. Dietary carbohydrate restriction induces a unique metabolic state positively affecting atherogenic dyslipidemia, fatty acid partitioning, and metabolic syndrome. Prog Lipid Res 2008;47:307–18.

[450] Volek JS, Phinney SD, Forsythe CE, et al. Carbohydrate restriction has a more favorable impact on the metabolic syndrome than a low fat diet. Lipids 2009;44:297–309.

[451] Noakes TD, Sboros M. Real Food on Trial: How The Diet Dictators Tried to Take Down a Top Scientist. UK: Columbus Publishers; 2019.

[452] Gaudal N, Jurgens G, Baslund B, et al. Compared with usual sodium intake, low and excessive-sodium diets are associated with increased mortality: a meta-analysis. Am J Hypert 2014;27:1129–37.

[453] Husken L. Lancet paper adds to evidence that reducing salt to very low levels may be dangerous Cardiobrief 2018;9 August. Available from http://www.cardiobrief.org/2018/08/09/lancet-paper-adds-to-evidenc.

[454] Mente A, O'Donnell M, Rangarajan S, et al. Association of urinary sodium excretion with cardiovascular events in individuals with and without hypertension: A pooled analysis of data from four studies. The Lancet 2016;388:465–75.

[455] Messerli F, Hofstetter L, Bangalore S. Salt and heart disease: a second round of "bad science.". The Lancet 2018;392:456–8.

[456] O'Brien E. Salt: Too much or too little? The Lancet, 388. 2016. p. 439–40.

[457] O'Donnell M, Mente A, Alderman MH, et al. Salt and cardiovascular disease: insufficient evidence to recommend low sodium intake. Europ Heart J 2020;ehaa586. Available from https://doi.org/10.1093/eurheartj/ehaa586.

[458] DiNicolantonio JJ, Lucan SC. The wrong white crystals: not salt but sugar as aetiological in hypertension and cardiometabolic disease. Open Heart 2014;1:e000167. Available from https://doi.org/10.1136/openhrt-2014-000167.

Chapter 2

Nutritional aspects

Amber O'Hearn[1], Eric C. Westman[2], William S. Yancy, Jr.[2,3,4] and Neville Wellington[5]

[1]*Independent Researcher, Toronto, Canada,* [2]*Division of General Internal Medicine, Department of Medicine, Duke University Medical Centre, Durham, NC, United States,* [3]*Center of Innovation to Accelerate Discovery and Practice Transformation, Durham Veterans Affairs Medical Centre, Durham, NC, United States,* [4]*Duke Diet and Fitness Centre, Duke University Health System, Durham, NC, United States,* [5]*Nutrition Network, Cape Town, Western Cape, South Africa*

2.1 Introduction

With evidence pointing to the efficacy of therapeutic carbohydrate restriction (TCR), official protocols for implementation into clinical practice are required. During the metabolic transition from a high-carbohydrate to a TCR diet, clinical considerations and patient guidance are required. Aside from the formulation and prescription of TCR, clinicians must be familiar with the precautions, assessment, and monitoring of clinical outcomes associated with this intervention. Nutritional ketosis is a physiological ketosis of the fed state with specific biochemical and nutritional aspects that must be taken into account in TCR. Understanding this metabolic state, as well as the biochemistry and physiology of ketone metabolism, is critical. When prescribing TCR, the clinician must also understand the context of nutrient requirements, as well as the differences between animal and plant nutrition. This chapter discusses the most important nutritional aspects to consider and comprehend when prescribing TCR.

2.2 Therapeutic carbohydrate restricted dietary intervention

2.2.1 Formulating a therapeutic carbohydrate restricted diet

Eric C. Westman and William S. Yancy Jr.

2.2.1.1 Definition of low carbohydrate high fat diets and therapeutic carbohydrate restriction

Dietary patterns have been described in many ways: by historical description (hunter-gatherer, paleo), by geographical use (Mediterranean), by diet book or company name or author (South Beach, WW, Atkins), by prominent type of food source (vegetarian), by what nutrient is limited (gluten-free, low-glycaemic, low-FODMAP), by the disease it is treating (Dietary Approach to Stop Hypertension [DASH]) or by level of macronutrient composition (ultra-low fat, low-fat, low-carbohydrate). Most diet research studies will include the distribution of three macronutrients, with an assumption that the essential vitamins and minerals are provided. The three macronutrients (carbohydrates, protein and fat) are typically given as a percentage of the total daily energy (caloric) intake.

Over the last 15 years, multiple independent groups have examined low-carbohydrate diets in human clinical trials, and given them the name of 'therapeutic carbohydrate restricted' or 'carbohydrate-restricted' diets (TCR) [1]. TCR diets are classified into several groups based on the amount of carbohydrate consumed per day, which is typically expressed in grammes of carbohydrate per day rather than percentages of caloric intake, owing to the fact that this is how the dietary pattern is taught. A low carbohydrate diet is defined as having below 130 g of carbohydrate per day [2]. If the dietary carbohydrate is sufficiently low to cause an increase in blood or urine ketone bodies, typically less than 50 g of total dietary carbohydrate per day, then the diet is called a very-low carbohydrate or ketogenic diet. In the medical setting, some ketogenic programs begin at 20 g total carbohydrate per day, while some programs begin at 30 g total carbohydrate per day [3,4]. TCR diets fall in the macronutrient ranges of 5%–30% carbohydrate, 20%–40% protein, and 30%–70% fat of daily energy intake. TCR, ketogenic diets (KD) typically fall in the macronutrient ranges of 0%–10% carbohydrate, 20%–35% protein, 55%–80% fat, with a daily caloric intake range from 1200 to 2000 Calories [4,5].

Ketogenic. DOI: https://doi.org/10.1016/B978-0-12-821617-0.00002-4

Defining Therapeutic carbohydrate restriction.

Neville Wellington

Low carbohydrate levels of intake have been defined by Feinman et al. as follows [2]:

1. Very low carbohydrate (VLC), VLC high fat (VLCHF) or ketogenic (KD) diets
   a. 20–50 g/day or <10% of a 2000Cal diet. Usually the level of carbohydrates that may induce ketosis in most people (>0.5 mmol/L of ketones, or 2.9 mg/dL)
2. Low carbohydrate (LCD), low carbohydrate high fat (LCHF) or therapeutic carbohydrate restricted (TCR) diets
   a. <130 g/day or less than 26% of total energy. The American Diabetic Association has previously accepted this as the lower limit.
3. Moderate carbohydrate diet
   a. 130–225 g/day or 26%–45% of a 2000Cal diet. This was the usual upper limit of carbohydrates before the obesity epidemic.
4. High carbohydrate diet
   a. >225 g/day or >45% of total energy intake.

This textbook follows common practice in using the terms LCD, LCHF, or TCR to refer to a variety of carbohydrate-reduction therapies implemented in clinical settings that fall below 130 g of dietary carbohydrate per day. A VLC, VLCHF or ketogenic diet (below 50 g carbohydrate per day) may represent a more effective treatment for certain conditions (e.g., T2D). Notably, other therapeutic dietary interventions, such as very low-calorie diets or intermittent fasting, effectively reduce carbohydrate intake as part of overall energy intake reduction.

In general, when patients reduce carbohydrates they tend to substitute it with fat, resulting in a higher ratio of energy intake from fat relative to carbohydrate, thus the term low-carbohydrate high-fat diets (LCHF). However, due to the frequent spontaneous reduction in energy intake on TCR diets, absolute increases in energy intake from fat is often minimal [2]. Recommendations for energy restriction are not typically part of TCR clinical interventions, but may be used in research protocols.

The term 'LCHF' stands for 'low-carbohydrate, high-fat' and is a popular way to describe TCR or 'carbohydrate restricted' diets, which is the term used in research papers. TCR is taught by giving a maximum limit of daily carbohydrate grams without explicitly limiting energy intake (calories). The TCR limit in carbohydrates leads to a reduction in hunger and as a result individuals consume approximately 500–1000 fewer Calories than before diet initiation without having to explicitly limit energy calories [4].

The ketogenic threshold is the level of daily carbohydrate intake at which there is an increase in measurable ketone production in the blood, urine and/or breath. This ketogenic threshold is variable, but the percentage of individuals with an elevation in ketones increases as the amount of carbohydrate in the diet decreases. When the daily total carbohydrate intake is below 20 g per day, nearly everyone will have an elevation in ketone concentrations. This increase in measurable ketones is called 'nutritional ketosis'. [5,6] So, there is TCR with nutritional ketosis, and TCR without nutritional ketosis. When reading nutritional research studies, TCR with nutritional ketosis is most similar to an LCHF ketogenic diet. TCR without nutritional ketosis is comparable to a low carbohydrate, low glycaemic or Mediterranean dietary pattern.

While most research studies of carbohydrate-restricted diets have used total carbohydrate (in grammes) in their teaching, TCR is commonly taught using net (glycaemic) carbohydrate (in grammes) as the method of counting carbohydrates. Total carbohydrate refers to all nutrients on a nutrition facts label that are labelled as carbohydrate (including net or glycaemic carbohydrate, as well as fibre and nonsugar sweeteners). Net (glycaemic) carbohydrate is calculated by subtracting carbohydrates from total carbohydrate that are in the form of fibre and nonsugar sweeteners. The rationale for subtracting out (or 'not counting') the fibre and nonsugar sweetener carbohydrates is that they have very little effect on the blood glucose concentrations compared to sugars and starches (net or glycaemic carbohydrate). Counting net (glycaemic) rather than total carbohydrate allows an individual to consume more carbohydrates: 20 g of net (glycaemic) carbohydrate may represent 40 g of total carbohydrate, because the fibre and nonsugar sweeteners have been subtracted. However, many sugar alcohols have one to two calories per gramme (compared with sugars, which have four Calories per gram). There have been no studies comparing total carbohydrate to net (glycaemic) carbohydrate for the treatment of obesity and diabetes. Total carbohydrate has been used in most research studies. A popular instructional TCR website uses net (glycaemic) carbohydrate, advising only to subtract the fibre grammes from the total carbohydrate in the net (glycaemic) carbohydrate calculation [7]. This website categorises TCR or 'LCHF' into 'strict LCHF' (<20 g net or glycaemic carbohydrate daily), 'moderate LCHF' (20–50 g net or glycaemic carbohydrate daily), and 'liberal LCHF' (50–100 g net or glycaemic carbohydrate daily).

These categories are similar to the categorisation of TCR diets used in clinical research studies, but the use of net (glycaemic) carbohydrate is different.

2.2.1.2 Nutritional sufficiency in therapeutic carbohydrate restriction

In formulating any nutritional approach, the first consideration is to ensure the provision of all of the known substances that the human body needs but cannot make on its own, known as 'essential nutrients' [8]. In other words, it is 'essential' that these substances are in the nutritional intake because they are necessary for normal human physiology and the body is unable to make them on its own (Table 2.1). Essential nutrients include amino acids, fatty acids, vitamins, minerals and an energy source. It is noteworthy that carbohydrates, sugars and starches are not on the list of essential nutrients.

In a generally healthy population, the human body is capable of endogenous carbohydrate synthesis and does not exhibit signs of deficiency in the absence of dietary carbohydrates [9]. Nutritional ketosis may even be considered an alternate 'normal' state due to its occurrence in infants who have very low carbohydrate intakes [9]. However, in certain genetic defects, such as glycogen storage disease type I, a lack of dietary carbohydrates results in abnormalities that can be corrected with carbohydrate supplementation. Dietary carbohydrates can thus be classified as conditionally essential nutrients because they are nutrients that are not required in the diet for the general population but are required for specific subpopulations.

Concerns about nutritional inadequacy of TCR diets often stem from nutrition inadequacies observed in therapeutic KD used for the treatment of childhood epilepsy [10]. However, there are several key differences between TCR diets used for other applications and the KD used for epilepsy. The KD used for epilepsy has a ketogenic level of carbohydrate restriction, protein intake is limited (thus limiting nutrient dense animal foods, which usually supply the majority of the micronutrients in carbohydrate restricted diets) [11] and fat intake is usually very high, to meet energy requirements. The ratio of macronutrients is controlled at every meal (See Chapter 2.2, Meeting micronutrient requirements). When using TCR, with or without ketosis for non-epilepsy applications (e.g., obesity and diabetes), it is not critical to be 'in nutritional ketosis' at all times, the carbohydrate intake does not have to be ketogenic, and animal food intake can be more plentiful, allowing for more liberal intake of a variety of nutrient dense foods to meet nutrient requirements.

Indeed research shows that carbohydrate restricted diets can meet micro- and essential nutrient requirements for adults [12] and adolescents [13]. In fact, due to superior bioavailability of many nutrients in TCR diets (due to the heavy reliance on minimally-processed animal-based foods), TCR nutrition may even exceed requirements [11,12]. It's also important to remember that nutritional guidelines reflect expert opinion and do not account for the possibility of different vitamin and mineral needs under varying caloric and metabolic conditions, calling the relevance of concerns about TCR meeting conventional dietary guidelines into question (See Chapter 2.2, Meeting

TABLE 2.1 Formulating a healthy diet: list of essential nutrients.

Water
Energy
Amino acids
Isoleucine, leucine, lysine, methionine, phenylalanine, threonine, tryptophan, tyrosine, valine
Fatty acids
Linoleic acid, linolenic acid
Vitamins
Water soluble: thiamine (B1), riboflavin (B2), pyridoxine (B6), cobalamine (B12), niacin, pantothenic acid, folic acid, biotin, lipoic acid, vitamin C
Fat soluble: vitamins A, D, E, K
Mineral elements
Major: calcium, phosphorus, potassium, sulphur, sodium, chlorine, magnesium
Trace: iron, iodine, copper, zinc, manganese, cobalt, chromium, selenium, molybdenum, fluorine, tin, silicon, vanadium
Other
Inositol, choline, carnitine

From Harper, A. (1999). Defining the essentiality of nutrients. In Modern nutrition in health and disease (9th ed., pp. 3–10). WIlliam & WIlkins. https://doi.org/10.1123/ijsnem.2017-0273.

micronutrient requirements). There have been no reports of micronutrient deficiencies in clinical trials of TCR diets, with or without nutritional ketosis, regardless of whether they follow expert recommendations. Although a low-carbohydrate, high-fat diet is nutritious, many experts advise taking a multivitamin to ensure adequate vitamin and mineral intake.

2.2.1.2.1 Macronutrient provision

TCR diets meet or, more often, exceed US DRI for protein (46 and 56 g per day for women and men respectively; the Acceptable Macronutrient Distribution Range (AMDR) is 10%–35% of daily energy) [12,14]. However, TCR does not comply with the US guidelines for recommended daily reference intake (DRI) for carbohydrate (130 g/day). Nutrient Recommendations: Dietary Reference Intakes DRI [14]. This carbohydrate recommendation, however, is based on the amount of energy that the brain needs to function, and that energy may also be adequately supplied endogenously by glycogenolysis, gluconeogenesis and ketogenesis [15].

The US DRI for fat is not determined but the AMDR is 20%–35% of daily energy. Nutrient Recommendations: Dietary Reference Intakes DRI [14] TCR diets exceed this AMDR, with over 60% of daily energy coming from fat [2].

2.2.1.3 Nutritional ketosis in the clinical context

In the context of TCR, nutritional ketosis simply means that the body is burning fat for fuel. Nutritional ketosis is frequently confused with 'ketoacidosis', a serious condition that can occur in people with diabetes. While ketone measurement has not been a common requirement in obesity and T2D studies, the clinical use of urine, blood, and breath ketones is increasing. In clinical practise, not everyone has measurable ketones in the urine or elevated blood ketones even when they are successfully losing weight, so the absence of an increase in ketones does not imply that the person is not losing adipose tissue.

2.2.1.4 Therapeutic carbohydrate restriction instruction

There are numerous ways to provide instruction on how to follow TCR, including books, videos, handouts, computer and smartphone apps, and classes. The typical TCR instruction allows for the restriction of dietary sugars and starches while allowing unrestricted consumption of very low carbohydrate foods containing protein and fat. Meat, poultry, fish, shellfish, and eggs are the main sources of nutrition. Vegetables and leafy greens are encouraged but limited to the point where each meal has a very low or negligible effect on postprandial rise in blood glucose. Although this is not always the case, it is necessary to keep total carbohydrate intake under 20–50 g per day in order to achieve ketosis. In practise, asking patients to select foods from a list of very low glycaemic foods that they enjoy works well.

There is no restriction on saturated fat or cholesterol in the diet, in part because the body is metabolising the dietary fat differently [17]. Carbohydrate-restriction reduces the cardiac risk factors by lowering blood triglycerides and increasing the HDL cholesterol (See Chapter 4, CVD) [18]. Some programs limit non-nutritive sweeteners, others do not. Foods and beverages that are sweetened with an alternative sweetener can be helpful to treat cravings for sugar and other sweet whole foods (fruit, etc.) [19]. Some programs restrict alcohol, and others allow for a small amount of alcohol consumption.

2.2.1.5 Long-term effects of therapeutic carbohydrate restriction

There are very few long-term prospective clinical trials of any dietary pattern; this is also true for TCR [20]. In the studies of TCR over a one to two year period, there were no concerning issues that arose in that CVD risk profiles improved [21]. The clinical experience is way ahead of the published studies in that many practitioners have monitored patients who have followed TCR for years and observed no adverse outcomes. To date some outcomes have been published of these experiences at five [22,23] and six [24] years respectively. A long-term outcome study comparing TCR to other diets with clinical endpoints of cardiovascular disease, cancer, and other health conditions is needed.

Example information sheet for patients: introduction to therapeutic carbohydrate restriction.

This way of eating is a diet low in sugary and starchy foods. Because starches are easily digested to sugar, starchy foods are similar to sugar, and must be avoided as well. This way of eating focuses on eating 'real' food and includes meat, fish, cheese, eggs, salads, and vegetables.

Sugars and starches are also known as carbohydrates, or 'carbs', and can be measured in 'grams'. To maximise fat burning, your carbohydrate intake will be 20 g or less per day. This means that you will need to avoid sugar, bread, fruit, flour, pasta, or any other sugary/starchy food that has a lot of carbohydrates. When you limit the carbohydrate intake, your hunger will go away, and if you have extra weight on your body, you will eat less and lose weight.

Once you start eating this way, you must stick to it religiously. If you consume carbohydrates, even in small amounts, the weight loss process may be halted for up to three days. This means you will exit ketosis (fat burning) and may even gain several pounds of water weight. The most important thing to remember if you do consume carbohydrates is to get right back on track with your next meal.

1. Medical supervision: Medical supervision is recommended for any dietary change if you have a medical problem or are currently taking medications. As your health and medical conditions improve, medications will probably have to be adjusted.
2. Beverages: It is important to drink an adequate amount of fluid per day—preferably water or another non-caffeinated beverage.
3. Constipation: It doesn't matter how often you go to the bathroom for a bowel movement, but if you are experiencing constipation (hard stools or hard-to-pass stools), there are a number of ways that you may address the issue.
   a. use 1 teaspoon of milk of magnesia at bedtime daily
   b. add ½ cup of fibre-rich vegetables to your diet per day
   c. have 1 to 2 servings per day of sugar-free gum or sugar-free candy that contains sorbitol or another sugar alcohol
   d. use sugar-free psyllium supplement twice a day
4. Muscle cramps: Any effective diet programme can lead to occasional muscle cramps. A tablespoon of mustard or pickle juice is an effective home remedy. If they are persistent:
   a. use 1 teaspoon of milk of magnesia at bedtime daily
   b. use 1 to 2 servings of bouillon daily (if you do not have high blood pressure or a history of heart failure or kidney failure)

   Keep the dietary carbohydrate to less than 20 total (not net/glycaemic) grams per day (not per meal).
   It doesn't matter how the food is cooked, just be sure any coating is low in sugar or starch.

When hungry, eat as much as you want of these foods, until you are comfortably full:

1. Meat: beef, pork, ham, bacon, lamb, sausage, pepperoni, hot dogs, or other meats.
2. Poultry: chicken, turkey, duck, or other fowl.
3. Fish and shellfish: any fish including tuna, salmon, catfish, tilapia, trout, shrimp, scallops, crab, and lobster.
4. Eggs: whole eggs, including yolks and whites.

Eat a limited amount of salad greens and nonstarchy vegetables every day:

1. Leafy greens: 2 cups (measured uncooked) a day. Includes: arugula, bok choy, cabbage (all varieties), chard, chives, endive, greens (including beet greens, collards, mustard, and turnip greens), kale, lettuce (all varieties), parsley, spinach, radicchio, radishes, scallions, and watercress. (If it is a leaf—you can eat it.)
2. Nonstarchy vegetables: 1 cup (measured uncooked) a day. Includes: artichokes, asparagus, broccoli, Brussels sprouts, cauliflower, celery, cucumber, eggplant, green beans (string beans), jicama, leeks, mushrooms, okra, onions, peppers, pumpkin, rhubarb, shallots, snow peas, sprouts (bean and alfalfa) sugar-snap peas, summer squash, tomatoes, wax beans, zucchini.

Foods that are allowed in limited amounts:

1. Cheese: up to 4 ounces a day. Includes: hard, aged cheeses such as Swiss, cheddar, brie, camembert, bleu, mozzarella, Gruyere, cream cheese, goat cheeses. Be sure to check the carbohydrate count.
2. Cream and oils: up to 2 tablespoons a day. Includes butter, half and half, whipping, light, or sour cream.
3. Mayonnaise: up to 2 tablespoons a day.
4. Olives: up to 6 a day.
5. Avocado: up to 1/2 of a fruit a day.
6. Lemon/lime juice: up to 2 teaspoons a day.
7. Soy sauce: up to 2 tablespoons a day.
8. Pickles, dill or sugar-free: up to 2 servings a day.
9. Zero carb snacks (unlimited): Sugar-free jello, pork rinds, pepperoni slices, beef jerky, boiled eggs.
10. Take a daily multivitamin without iron (unless your doctor recommends that you take iron) Yancy et al. [3].

2.2.2 Assessment and monitoring of therapeutic carbohydrate restriction

Eric C. Westman, and William S. Yancy Jr.

2.2.2.1 Introduction

Carbohydrate-restricted diets have been followed by many populations for centuries without any specialised monitoring. The traditional diets of several indigenous peoples (Inuit, Masai) were so low in carbohydrate that they may have lived in nutritional ketosis. Some experts argue that the most common nutritional pattern for humans for a long period of time, the hunter-gatherer or palaeolithic diet, was a carbohydrate-restricted diet [25]. From this point of view, it was only recently that humans consumed carbohydrates (first agricultural revolution, c. 10,000 BCE), or sugar (c. 1800 BCE.). So, while a low carbohydrate diet may have been the most common dietary pattern, if someone is only eating an LCHF diet, there may be no need for special monitoring above and beyond what one would do for any dietary pattern. Low carbohydrate diets have been studied in the context of obesity and diabetes treatment over the last 20 years, and as such, have recently become known as therapeutic carbohydrate restricted (TCR) diets. Most experts agree that assessment and monitoring for low carbohydrate diets are required in this context of being used as a therapeutic treatment [26].

The level of pretreatment medical evaluation for an obesity medicine treatment depends upon the presence of prior medical problems and the risk of the intervention chosen. [26]. For example, dietary programs that confer little risk will require less intensive preliminary assessment than interventions that convey higher risk such as medications, very low-calorie diets, or weight loss surgery. If TCR is considered generally healthy eating, providing all the essential nutrients, then no extra assessment or monitoring needs to be done unless there are medical problems or medications involved. [12].

2.2.2.2 Pretreatment assessment

The purpose of the pretreatment assessment is to ensure a healthy, or at least medically stable, baseline state, rule out a metabolic cause for weight gain, and provide a baseline level for comparison to monitor progress [26]. In the context of a medical setting, this includes a complete medical history, physical examination, blood tests, and some sort of anthropometric and/or body composition measurement (bioimpedance, DEXA) (Table 2.2). If symptoms of heart disease are present, an electrocardiogram or more thorough heart evaluation may be performed.

Blood testing generally includes a complete blood count, serum electrolytes/renal function/glucose, liver function tests, fasting serum lipid profile, serum thyroid function tests (TSH, free T4). If prediabetes, diabetes, or metabolic syndrome is present, then HbA1c, insulin, and c-peptide concentrations might be performed. If there is suspicion for other commonly associated conditions, an ultrasound might be done to assess for fatty liver or polycystic ovarian syndrome. If there is a suspicion for sleep apnoea, then a polysomnogram could be ordered.

2.2.2.3 During-treatment (deprescribing phase) monitoring

At each return visit, a history focused on symptoms of hunger and adverse effects, blood pressure, pulse and brief physical examination are performed (Table 2.3). In a clinical setting, the expected weight loss is half to one kilogramme (1 to 2 pounds) per week. A review of medications, particularly diabetes and hypertension medications, is required to reduce the negative effects of overmedication. Follow-up clinic visits are typically scheduled at monthly or more frequent intervals until the patient's health measures have stabilised and the patient has successfully adapted to the lifestyle change. Some clinics measure body composition to determine fat mass and water weight.

TABLE 2.2 Recommended medical evaluation prior to use of therapeutic carbohydrate restriction.

Complete medical history
Physical examination (including weight, waist circumference, neck circumference (for sleep apnoea risk), blood pressure, pulse, and body composition measurement if available.)
Complete blood count, serum electrolytes/renal function/glucose, liver function tests, fasting serum lipid profile
Serum thyroid function tests (TSH, free T4)
Electrocardiogram if symptoms for heart disease
HgbA1c, insulin (screen for pre-diabetes, diabetes, especially if metabolic syndrome is present)

TABLE 2.3 Follow-up medical evaluation for therapeutic carbohydrate restriction.

Focused history (adverse effect symptoms, hunger level) and physical exam (heart, lungs, waist, peripheral oedema)
Vital signs (blood pressure, pulse)
Serum chemistry panel (electrolytes, renal function, glucose, liver function)
Fasting serum lipid profile
HbA1c
Review of medications, especially diabetes and hypertension medications

Depending upon the clinical circumstances, periodic blood tests may be performed (electrolytes, renal function, liver function, fasting serum lipid profile, HbA1c). Because the process of weight loss may increase total cholesterol and LDL cholesterol concentrations, some experts argue that the measurement of serum lipids should be delayed until the weight loss goals have been achieved [27]. In the case of hypertriglyceridaemia, it may be useful to repeat serum triglycerides in 4 weeks to document improvement.

2.2.2.3.1 Keto-adaptation side effects

During the first few days of the diet change, there may be mild symptoms of fatigue or headache, popularly known as 'keto flu', which can be prevented or minimised by adequate fluid and sodium intake. If there is no history of hypertension or heart failure, we recommend consuming two to three litres (64-100 ounces) of water plus one or two bouillon cubes (or the sodium equivalent) per day for the first week to reduce the likelihood of these symptoms. Constipation and muscle cramps are the most common side effects of TCR adaptation during the first few weeks to months. Many people have fewer bowel movements, and confuse this with constipation (hard stools or hard-to-pass stools).

2.2.2.3.1.1 Prevention or treatment of keto-adaptation side effects in clinical practice Constipation is usually resolved by increasing fluid intake and reinforcing the consumption of greens and vegetables. Docusate twice a day, one teaspoon of milk of magnesia at bedtime for one week, bouillon supplementation, or a sugar-free fibre supplement are some other remedies for constipation. Patients may occasionally experience diarrhoea, which may be caused by metformin or excessive use of sugar substitutes, particularly sugar alcohols.

Muscle cramps typically resolve with supplementation of one teaspoon of milk of magnesia at bedtime for one week or 200 mEq/d of slow-release magnesium chloride daily. Hypokalaemia can occur if someone is taking a potassium-wasting diuretic, but the baseline assessment should detect this. If these side effects are not improved by sodium and magnesium repletion, then checking the potassium concentration is recommended.

2.2.2.3.2 Deprescribing medication

Healthy lifestyles, including TCR, can be as effective as multiple prescription medications. As a result, combining TCR with prescription medication can result in medication overdose. Common medications that may result in overdose if not adjusted include diabetes and hypertension medications, which may require a rapid reduction (days to weeks) to avoid hypoglycaemia and hypotension. Refer to Chapter 3.3, Adapting medication for type 2 diabetes in the context of Therapeutic Carbohydrate Restriction for guidelines on deprescribing diabetes medication.

2.2.2.3.2.1 Antihypertensives Blood pressure monitoring at home or at the clinic is important because a drop in blood pressure is common after starting a diet. It is critical to enquire about symptoms of orthostatic hypotension (dizziness or lightheadedness upon standing) as well as new or worsening fatigue at follow-up visits. If home or clinic blood pressures are consistently less than 110 mmHg systolic, or if symptoms of orthostatic hypotension occur, antihypertensives should be tapered or discontinued. If the patient does not become hypotensive, a low dose of renal protective blood pressure medication can be continued until the microalbuminuria is resolved.

2.2.2.3.2.2 Other medication considerations Several other medications may no longer be needed as improvements in heartburn (GERD), irritable bowel syndrome (IBS) (diarrhoea predominant), and polycystic ovarian syndrome (PCOS) are commonly seen. When treating PCOS, nonhormonal contraception should be used to avoid an unwanted pregnancy.

In general, dietary restrictions for other conditions must be maintained in the context of TCR. Sodium restriction, for example, should be maintained if there is salt-sensitive hypertension or a history of heart failure. If a vitamin K antagonist is being used for anticoagulation, vitamin K restriction should be maintained. If there has been a change in intake of leafy greens or other vitamin K-containing foods, more frequent monitoring may be required. If someone is on dialysis, dietary phosphate restriction should be maintained. Although TCR is already low in gluten, gluten restriction should be maintained if coeliac disease is present.

2.2.2.3.3 Is monitoring ketones necessary for safety?

Nutritional ketosis indicates that the body is burning fat. While it is frequently confused with ketoacidosis, nutritional ketosis is distinguished by normal blood pH and much lower serum ketones concentrations than ketoacidosis. It is now possible to monitor urine, blood, and breath ketones at home. Monitoring ketones is not required for safety, but it may help with adherence.

2.2.2.4 Long-term monitoring

Following the deprescribing phase, TCR monitoring is the same for any dietary pattern. Most experts recommend a periodic assessment of body weight, predictors of cardiometabolic risk, and adherence to other accepted disease prevention strategies (vaccines, colonoscopy). Most people on TCR see improvements in all measures of cardiometabolic risk, but a small percentage may see increases in some (total cholesterol, LDL-cholesterol). Direct arterial measurement of the carotid, aorta, and heart, as well as coronary artery calcium score, may be useful in these patients to further stratify risk and aid decision-making regarding lipid-lowering agents. TCR with or without nutritional ketosis resulted in either improvement or no change in carotid artery thickness in two two-year studies [28,29]. For more on TCR, cholesterol and cardiovascular disease risk refer to Chapter 4: CVD.

2.2.3 Cautions, contraindications and troubleshooting when prescribing therapeutic carbohydrate restriction

William S. Yancy Jr. and Eric C. Westman

2.2.3.1 Introduction

TCR has demonstrated many beneficial health effects in research and clinical settings. However, there are several cautions, a few relative contraindications and various strategies for troubleshooting in these situations that practitioners should know when prescribing these eating plans. Some of the adverse health effects can occur acutely while others are more long-term issues. Likewise, some of the potential adverse effects can be serious whereas others are mild. Most importantly, TCR can effectively lower blood glucose and blood pressure in people with diabetes and/or hypertension who are taking certain medications for these health problems. Therefore medication deprescribing is required, often at initiation of the diet plan, to prevent these iatrogenic complications (See Chapter 3.3, Adapting medication for type 2 diabetes in the context of therapeutic carbohydrate restriction).

2.2.3.2 Contraindications

Carbohydrates are not essential nutrients, but may be conditionally essential [9]. They provide energy but are not required for a healthy person to consume unless they have a rare metabolic abnormality. At the same time, some rare conditions that were previously thought to be contraindications may turn out not to be contraindications [30]. Because some tissues require carbohydrate, it has been assumed that it must be consumed without taking into account the ability to produce glucose endogenously via a process known as gluconeogenesis.

Other common misconceptions include thinking that the absence of dietary carbohydrates will cause keto-acidosis. The terms 'ketosis' and 'nutritional ketosis' (normal physiological states) are often erroneously confused with 'keto-acidosis', a dangerous condition.

The only absolute contra-indications are porphyria and inborn errors of metabolism (Table 2.4). Relative contraindications include coexisting conditions such as pregnancy or kidney or liver disease, which may require additional dietary changes or even interdict certain regimens. In these instances of potentially relative contraindications, the frequency of monitoring may be increased to assess the effects of the diet, until further research has been done.

TABLE 2.4 Absolute contraindications of therapeutic carbohydrate restriction, Watanabe et al. [31].

Contraindication	Complications
Carnitine deficiency and carnitine associated enzyme deficiency	Defective ketogenesis—fatal hypoglycaemia
Acute intermittent porphyria	Carbohydrate restriction induces relapse of the condition
Mitochondrial fatty acid B-oxidation disorders	Defective ketogenesis—fatal hypoglycaemia
Pyruvate carboxylase deficiency	Defective ketogenesis—fatal hypoglycaemia

2.2.3.3 Potentially serious adverse effects and troubleshooting

2.2.3.3.1 Dehydration and loss of sodium and potassium

TCR can initially cause water loss, with concomitant loss of sodium, potassium, and magnesium. This contributes to weight loss in the first one to two weeks but can also lead to dehydration, fatigue, hypotension, lightheadedness, headaches, difficulty concentrating and muscle cramping, also known as the 'keto flu' [3]. Water loss is caused in part by increased glycogen use because glycogen is stored with water and water is released during glycogenolysis. The other part is due to lower insulin concentrations, which signal the kidneys to retain water and sodium [32].

In those with medical conditions, especially those taking diuretic medications, it is important to be sure that blood electrolyte concentrations (sodium, potassium) are normal before initiating a change in diet [26]. Replenishing water and sodium adequately can prevent and/or minimise the above 'keto flu' symptoms. For hydration, a rule of thumb is to drink about one litre of water for every 32 kg of body weight (or half one's weight in pounds, in ounces of fluid per day up to approximately 100 ounces).

For electrolyte replacement, bouillon or broth is an efficient source of water *and* sodium. One to two cups daily is recommended. No calorie sports drinks and other no calorie electrolyte solutions are alternatives. Certain patients, however, should avoid drinking broth or other high sodium electrolyte solutions. In patients with congestive heart failure, uncontrolled hypertension or chronic kidney disease additional sodium could exacerbate their chronic conditions. In these unique cases, reduction of diuretic medication, instead of increased salt intake, is preferable for preventing dehydration. For patients taking larger doses of diuretics, in-person or virtual clinic visits every one to two weeks may be necessary at the beginning to minimise the risk for dehydration.

Symptoms of 'keto flu' typically resolve in seven to ten days whether or not these preventive measures are used. During this transition stage, heavy exercise should be avoided, and exercise can be resumed thereafter. Adequate hydration should be emphasised regularly. Increased sodium intake may only be necessary in some individuals, and may be continued as long as elevated blood pressure and swelling do not occur.

2.2.3.3.2 Overmedication in individuals with diabetes and hypertension

People with diabetes can benefit greatly from TCR including improved glycaemic control, reduced medication requirements, fewer hypoglycaemic events and lower distress related to diabetes [33–35]. These improvements can occur in people with type 1 and type 2 diabetes, but there are precautions that practitioners should take to reduce the risk of hypoglycaemia in anyone taking insulin or insulin secretagogues (sulfonylureas and meglitinides). To reduce the risk of hypoglycemia, doses of these specific medications should be reduced on the same day as diet initiation in comparison to recent glycaemic concentrations. (see Chapter 3.3, Adapting medication for type 2 diabetes in the context of therapeutic carbohydrate restriction). Patients taking these medications should monitor serum glucose (see Chapter 3.2, T2D where structured glucose monitoring is detailed) on a regular basis and be able to easily access their health care team for assistance with medication adjustments if necessary. For patients taking higher doses of insulin, in-person or virtual clinic visits every one to two weeks may be required at first to ensure safety. When blood glucose levels are under control, weight loss has slowed, and hypoglycaemic episodes are rare, visits may become less frequent. While patients are adapting to TCR and losing weight, blood glucose concentrations in the 8.4–13.9 mmol/L (150–250 mg/dl) range can be tolerated soon after medications are reduced in order to provide a cushion from hypoglycaemia episodes.

2.2.3.3.3 Elevation in total cholesterol and LDL cholesterol

TCR has had a variable impact on LDL cholesterol (LDL-c) in clinical trials. On average, low carbohydrate nutritional interventions used for weight loss do not increase LDL-c from baseline [36] but increases have been reported in some trials, particularly in comparison to low fat eating patterns, and in individuals [37]. There are physiological reasons for the uncertain effects. Firstly, low carbohydrate eating patterns are typically high in saturated fat, and saturated fat intake is an important modifiable predictor of LDL-c elevation [38]. On the other hand, lower carbohydrate intake decreases insulin concentrations, which in turn inhibits HMG-CoA reductase and therefore, cholesterol synthesis [39]. Given the amelioration effects of low carbohydrate nutrition on serum triglycerides and HDL cholesterol (HDL-c), particularly when compared to high carbohydrate low fat eating patterns, the overall impact on risk appears to be a reduction, but this will not be known definitively until a clinical outcomes study is performed [37,40].

If LDL-c rises significantly, calculating the Atherosclerosis Cardiovascular Disease (ASCVD) risk score, which includes HDL-c, blood pressure, and other risk factors that may improve with low carbohydrate nutrition, can help determine whether overall risk has increased. In individuals without known cardiovascular disease, the ASCVD risk score is now the primary consideration when deciding on lipid-lowering medication therapy. Furthermore, lipid subfraction analysis (e.g., NMR cholesterol profile) may be useful in further defining risk. Prior research has shown that low carbohydrate nutrition typically leads to increases in the less risky large LDL-c subfraction and a significant decrease in the riskier small LDL subfraction [29]. Other tests such as c-reactive protein and coronary artery calcium (CAC) score may contribute to the risk assessment and inform the shared decision making process with the individual.

If a rise in LDL-c is a concern, then the eating plan can be adjusted to increase intake of nonstarchy vegetables, leaner proteins, and unsaturated fats (e.g., olive oil, avocado, nuts) while reducing foods high in saturated fat (e.g., full-fat dairy products, processed and fatty meats, poultry skin). Initiating medical management is an additional consideration. Partly because highly trained, keto-adapted athletes have been found to have elevated LDL cholesterol concentrations, it has been argued that the LDL elevation in the context of low carbohydrate and ketogenic nutrition does not confer the same cardiometabolic risk as for those who consume higher levels of carbohydrates [41,42]. See Chapter 4, CVD for further discussion around the relationship between LDL-c and CVD.

2.2.3.4 *Mild side effects and troubleshooting*

2.2.3.4.1 Constipation and muscle cramps

Constipation and muscle cramping are the most common adverse effects that occur with TCR [3]. Not to be confused with just having less frequent stools, which is common when eating less carbohydrate, constipation is defined by hard stools or hard-to-pass stools. Contributing factors include dehydration and some may argue, decreased fibre intake (See Chapter 8, Gastrointestinal for further discussion around the conflicting evidence for fibre in constipation). Adequate hydration and sodium intake can frequently effectively prevent or treat constipation. Regular weight-bearing activity is also recommended. Insoluble fibre from low carbohydrate vegetables, avocado, berries, nuts and seeds, or fibre supplements like psyllium may or may not help with constipation. Stool softeners and osmotic laxatives are other options (e.g., milk of magnesia, magnesium citrate, polyethylene glycol, lactulose). Stimulant laxatives (e.g., bisacodyl, sennosides) should be used sparingly due to the risk of bowel hypotonia and dependency with prolonged use.

2.2.3.4.2 Food cravings

Cravings for carbohydrate-rich foods are common upon cessation. For some individuals the cravings may be very strong which has led to the concept of processed food addiction (Chapter 11.3.2, Processed food addiction) [43]. Most foods can be accommodated in small or very small amounts within the overall macronutrient goal. While most milk and dairy products such as low-fat (non-Greek) yoghurt have significant amounts of carbohydrate, milk substitutes like coconut, almond or ultrafiltered milks or Greek yoghurt are useful substitutes.

2.2.3.4.3 Halitosis

Halitosis, in the form of 'keto breath' due to exhalation of acetone (a ketone), can occur with TCR, but is uncommon. Recommendations to prevent and/or mitigate halitosis should include increased water intake, maintaining good oral hygiene and use of parsley or sugarless mints or chewing gum. In some cases, modification of macronutrient intake to increase carbohydrate consumption above 50 g per day may be helpful.

2.2.3.5 *Conclusion*

Most troubleshooting on TCR, while common, is easily remedied with simple dietary changes. Contraindications are relatively uncommon (i.e., inborn errors of metabolism), but they are still important to avoid patient complications, and the majority revolve around careful monitoring and/or discontinuation of medications such as insulin and inulin secretagogues. Importantly, LDL-c increases in many patients, if observed, do not inherently translate to atherogenic risk due to the myriad significant improvements in other risk avenues (i.e. coronary artery calcium, glycaemic control, HDL-c and triglyceride concentrations, blood pressure, etc.) and require careful assessment to avoid unnecessary and/or deleterious modification. These warnings should be weighed against the significant benefits of TCR.

2.3 Physiological ketosis of the Fed State: biochemical and nutritional aspects

Amber O'Hearn

Ketogenic diets (KDs) are often compared to fasting, and even said to mimic fasting. But the ketogenic state does not require abstaining from food, or malnutrition of any kind. Given that infants and young children are often in ketosis even without dietary restrictions [44–47], ketosis is completely compatible with growth and high levels of nutrient intake. In this chapter, we will begin by orienting ourselves in the fasting phases, beginning before fasting begins and assuming a glucose-based metabolism. Following that, we will go over ketone bodies in greater detail, including how they are produced biochemically, in what concentrations and proportions, and what they are used for. Some implications of various energy substrates and fat and protein proportions will be identified.

2.3.1 Ketogenic diets and fasting: similarities and differences

2.3.1.1 A ketogenic metabolism is more general than fasting

Ketosis is defined by rising serum ketone body concentrations that exceed a clinically defined threshold (see below). Ketosis occurs consistently in some metabolic conditions and can serve as a marker for them. While some of these conditions, such as diabetic or alcoholic ketoacidosis, are pathological, in others, ketosis is physiological. That is, it is benign and serves a purpose. The study of fasting or starvation has contributed significantly to our understanding of physiological ketogenic metabolism. However, complete abstinence from food is only one way, and an unnecessary extreme one, to induce this metabolic state. Ketosis is the normal metabolic response to a prolonged demand for glucose that exceeds what is available from exogenous (dietary) and endogenous (synthesised in the body) sources combined, in the presence of adequate fat. Simply minimising carbohydrate intake and moderating protein intake are normally sufficient to induce ketosis in humans (Fig. 2.1). When ketosis is maintained nutritionally rather than through fasting, the dire consequences of total starvation do not apply. Some of the concerns about the safety of KDs stem from starvation rather than ketogenic metabolism. Nonetheless, fasting metabolism is a good place to start for comparison and contrast.

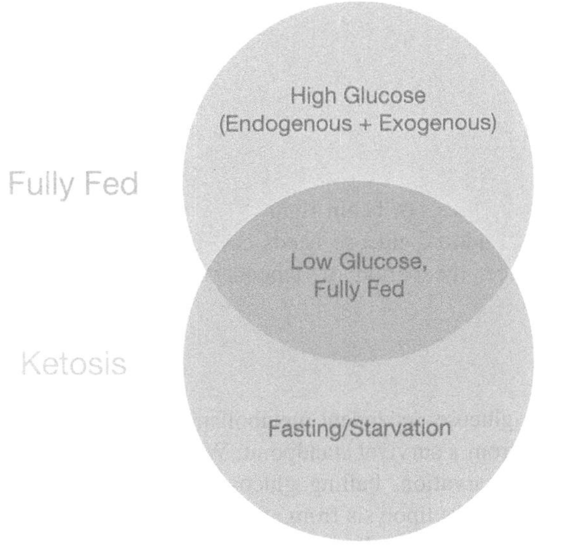

FIGURE 2.1 Ketosis in humans requires low glucose, but does not require caloric or nutrient insufficiency.

2.3.1.2 *In the animal kingdom, endogenous glucose production is the norm for meeting glucose needs*

Glucose requirements in mammals are frequently met indirectly, because the amount of digestible carbohydrate in the habitual diet of many mammals does not meet whole body glucose requirements. Rather, many animals routinely synthesise the majority of the glucose they need by the process of gluconeogenesis (GNG) [48]. Because glucose synthesis is very important, many diverse substrates can be used for GNG. In primarily herbivorous animals such as ruminants and hindgut fermenters, gluconeogenic substrate comes largely from short-chain fatty acids (SCFAs, also called volatile fatty acids) derived from microbial fermentation of fibre in the gastrointestinal tract in herbivorous animals such as ruminants and hindgut fermenters. In primarily carnivorous animals, such as felines and canines, amino acids from dietary protein serve as the primary gluconeogenic substrate. Both of these are used in more omnivorous species, as well as some exogenous glucose from digestible carbohydrates. It is a characteristic trait of omnivores to have some flexibility in adapting the rate of GNG in response to dietary carbohydrate, less when carbohydrate intake is high, and more when carbohydrate intake is low [48]. Because GNG is the typical way many animals manage glucose requirements, including the herbivorous primates with which we share ancestry, we can dismiss concerns that having to continuously provide for glucose needs by GNG, as is the case on a KD, would impose undue stress on the human body.

2.3.1.3 *Ketosis normally happens only when gluconeogenesis is insufficient*

Ketosis normally happens to a more than negligible degree only when glucose demands exceed the combination of dietary carbohydrate and gluconeogenic capacity. This means that even a diet low in digestible carbohydrate, as is common in many mammals, does not normally result in ketosis if sufficient fibre or protein is available. As a result, most animals only experience ketosis when they are malnourished. As we will see, humans are an exception to this rule.

Humans today diverge from the common pattern of meeting most energy needs from glucose derived by GNG. This is partly because we have a limited ability to get enough substrate. Compared with herbivores, our colons and caecum, the parts of the gut devoted to housing bacteria that generate SCFAs, are drastically smaller [49], leaving us with less than 10% of calories derivable this way. And compared with typical carnivores, we have limited capacity to metabolise protein, because of the detoxification of metabolites required [50,51]. These combined limits constrain gluconeogenic substrates. Moreover, humans have exceptionally large brain size requiring exceptionally large amounts of energy [52]. Brain tissue is unable to use fat for energy directly. This is thought to be because brain tissue is highly susceptible to damage from reactive oxygen species (ROS) [53]. Fatty acid oxidation generates high levels of ROS, making it more dangerous than other potential fuels [53]. Whether or not this is the reason for the physiological constraint on brains, the inability of a tissue that is relatively enlarged in humans to use fat means that the demand for glucose is also relatively intensified. To meet their entire body needs with glucose, humans would appear to need to either maximise GNG through a combination of maximum protein and fibre intake and eating only as much carbohydrate as is required to make up the difference, or simply increase carbohydrate intake. However, another solution to this metabolic quandary is to use ketone bodies, which are produced from fat. By partially metabolising fat in the liver, and sending the metabolites, ketone bodies, to the brain, we allow some of the ROS generation to occur outside of the brain. Moreover, we partially relieve the need for glucose which is difficult for humans to obtain in sufficient quantities via fibre or protein.

2.3.2 The phases of fasting

2.3.2.1 *Phase I*

When glucose and gluconeogenic substrates stop coming in, ketogenesis does not begin right away because there are glucose stores, mostly liver glycogen, that act as a buffer. In sedentary adults, glucose needs can be met for several days at a time between meals. In the context of total food abstinence, the period of dependence on glycogen is sometimes called Phase I starvation.

2.3.2.2 *Phase II*

When glycogen stores are depleted, the only way to maintain a highly glucose-dependent metabolism is to begin catabolising muscle tissue. Obviously, this is unsustainable and undesirable from a survival standpoint. When possible, muscle catabolism is reduced by utilising fat and thus entering Phase II starvation. Falling glucose concentrations are followed by falling insulin concentrations, and this lowered insulin state allows lipolysis from adipose tissue to increase. At the same time, lower insulin levels increase fatty acid oxidation in the liver. If all signals are functioning properly

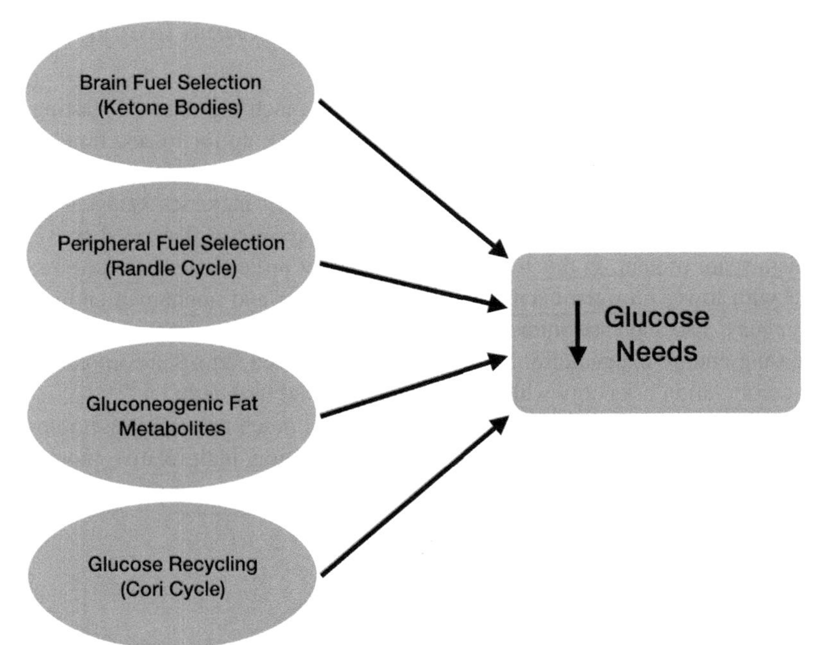

FIGURE 2.2 Factors reducing glucose needs in a ketogenic state.

and adipose tissue is of sufficient mass, the increase in free fatty acids will result in a ketogenic metabolism, which reduces reliance on glucose metabolism throughout the body in a variety of ways.

First, tissues that can use a combination of glucose and fat reduce their use of the former in favour of the latter. This fuel selection change, known as the Randle Cycle, occurs at the cellular level simply as a result of the relative availability of the two alternatives. It is a dynamic adaptation that occurs in addition to and in coordination with hormonal control, and can therefore be described as 'nutrient-mediated fine tuning' [54]. In other words, hormones such as insulin affect what fuel is available, while muscle tissue then optimises to take up what is there.

The Cori cycle is also upregulated [55]. During this cycle, glucose is only partially metabolised in peripheral tissue, resulting in a build-up of lactate, which returns to the liver to provide GNG substrate. The conversion of lactate to glucose can be accomplished with fat-derived energy. In this way, glucose is recycled using fat, making it similar to a rechargeable battery that can maintain glucose supply using fat rather than using up glucose and then requiring more [56].

Fat metabolism itself can also supply substrate for GNG. Glycerol, the backbone leftover from the metabolism of triglycerides, is one such example. Acetone, a ketone body that is continuously spontaneously generated in a ketogenic state, is another. Finally, and crucially, the brain, which accounts for a plurality of energetic use in humans, begins to use ketone bodies for the majority of its fuel (Fig. 2.2).

In addition to lowering glucose requirements, ketone bodies themselves send an anticatabolic signal. Taken together, these various aspects of ketogenic metabolism reduce the amount of glucose used during this phase. Muscle catabolism is thus reduced, but it is not completely avoided in Phase II starvation because base protein requirements continue.

2.3.2.3 Phase III

2.3.2.3.1 Phase II reduces glucose use, Phase III raises it again

When adipose tissue is depleted sufficiently, the only option is to revert to a glucose-centric metabolism. In animals that reach this phase, Phase III, resting metabolic rate increases and corticosterone levels rise sharply, inducing hunger and food seeking behaviour as well as increasing GNG by promoting muscle catabolism and activating GNG enzymes [57]. If food is not obtained, death normally occurs within days [58].

Importantly, some animals, including obese humans, do not normally reach Phase III starvation. It is thought that because there is so much fat available, the gradual but persistent loss of lean mass leads to organ failure before Phase III occurs [59]. This means that prolonged ketosis, either from fasting or nutritionally sustained, carries the risk of fatal organ tissue damage if adequate provision of protein is not provided. There are historical examples of such deaths in humans [58].

2.3.2.4 In nutritionally sustained ketosis, fuel mix can be anywhere on the spectrum from the end of Phase I through the beginning of Phase III

Nutritionally sustained ketosis with high fat intake (or high body fat access) is metabolically much like Phase II fasting, except that malnutrition is averted by supplying adequate protein, vitamins, and minerals to make up for losses. In addition, fat serves two further functions. In the case of a lean human, fat intake sustains ketosis by making up for inadequate adipose tissue. Whatever the source, higher circulating fat maximises hepatic fat oxidation which increases ketogenesis. This is of particular importance when the therapeutic effects of ketone bodies are desirable. Moreover, as described above, ketone bodies and other products of fat metabolism spare protein. In this way, it is possible that protein needs are lowered when fat is increased. This would be consistent with lower nitrogen excretion in fasting human and nonhuman animals with higher body fat [59]. Higher fat oxidation may also increase mitochondrial uncoupling and substrate cycles, for example via re-esterification [60], thereby increasing energy expenditure. So nutritionally sustained ketosis incorporating high levels of fat avoids the potential metabolic conservation of energy which may be detrimental long-term.

On the other hand, a carbohydrate restricted diet with high levels of protein intake and not much fat, more resembles Phase III starvation in fuel use patterns. With lower glucose-sparing metabolites from fat oxidation, high relative protein intake begets high protein need. High levels of protein intake also induce higher cortisol [61] which may also reflect a parallel to Phase III starvation.

A summary of the fasting phases is charted in Table 2.5.

2.3.2.5 Low glucose and high fat together stimulate ketogenesis

As previously discussed, endogenous glucose production serves as the primary fuel source for many mammals. Despite thousands of years of grain agriculture, a relatively short time in evolutionary terms, human gluconeogenic capacity is still fully functional. When fat from food or adipose tissue is the primary fuel source, the liver easily provides a steady supply of endogenous glucose from a small amount of protein and other sources, but it also provides ketone bodies. To occur, there must be more available fat than can be used for fatty acid oxidation at any given time, allowing it to accumulate into the secondary, ketogenesis pathway. Because GNG and fatty acid oxidation compete for the substrate oxaloacetate, this accumulation is accelerated (Fig. 2.3). The more oxaloacetate GNG consumes, the less available for fatty acid oxidation via the tricarboxylic acid cycle (TCA) cycle. Low glucose promotes ketogenesis in one way. Another benefit of low glucose is that it requires less insulin, allowing insulin concentrations to drop. Lower insulin levels then allow for more fat release from adipose tissue, providing enough to surpass fatty acid oxidation rate limits.

2.3.2.6 Ketone bodies

As the name suggests, for a diet to be ketogenic, it must cause the generation of significant concentrations of ketone bodies. We typically use a threshold of 0.5 mmol/L (9 mg/dL) serum beta-hydroxybutyrate (BOHB) for ketosis [62,63], but values as low as 0.2 have been used [64]. BOHB is one of three types of ketone bodies. Acetoacetate (AcAc) and acetone are the other two. It is worth noting that ketone bodies are sometimes referred to as 'ketones' for short, even though this is technically incorrect. Ketones are a broad class of organic chemicals that include many that are not ketone bodies; in fact, only two of the three ketone bodies are ketones.

The reason we typically use BOHB concentrations to confirm ketosis is that it is currently the most accurate to measure, although breath acetone measuring technology is rapidly improving [65,66]. AcAc can be measured in urine but this method has two problems. The first is that measurement can be affected by urinary dilution, which fluctuates. The second is that as the kidneys adapt to ketosis they reabsorb more AcAc rather than excreting it. This is the reason that urinary AcAc testing can result in clinical false negatives for ketoacidosis [67]. Many keto-adapted individuals may be negative for AcAc in the urine, despite having measurable ketosis as defined by serum BOHB [68].

TABLE 2.5 The phases of fasting.

Phase	Dominant fuel	Source
I	Glucose	Glycogen stores
II	Fat	Adipose tissue
III	Protein	Muscle

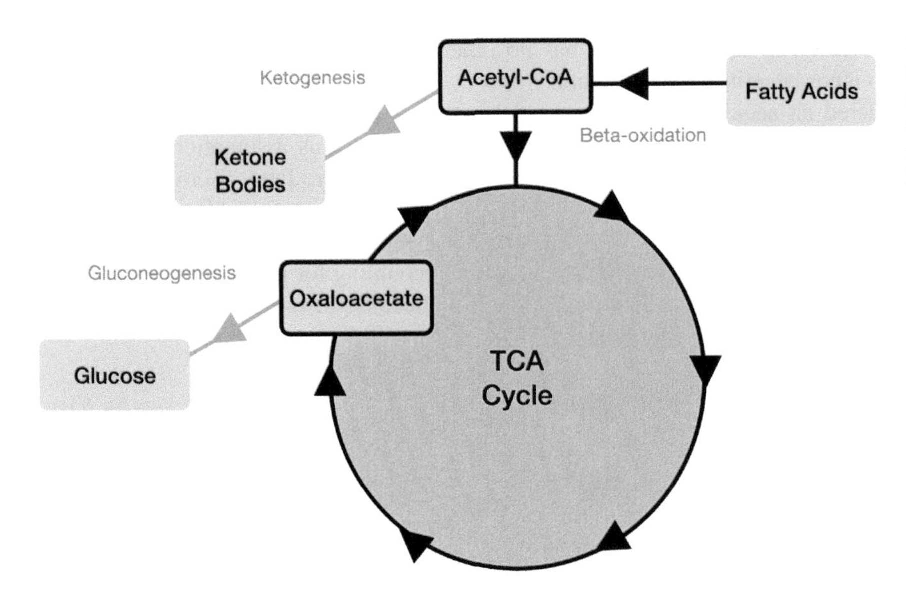

FIGURE 2.3 When the supply of oxaloacetate is diverted by use in gluconeogenesis, the acetyl-CoA that would condense with it to enter the (tricarboxylic acid) TCA cycle cannot, and instead goes into the production of ketone bodies.

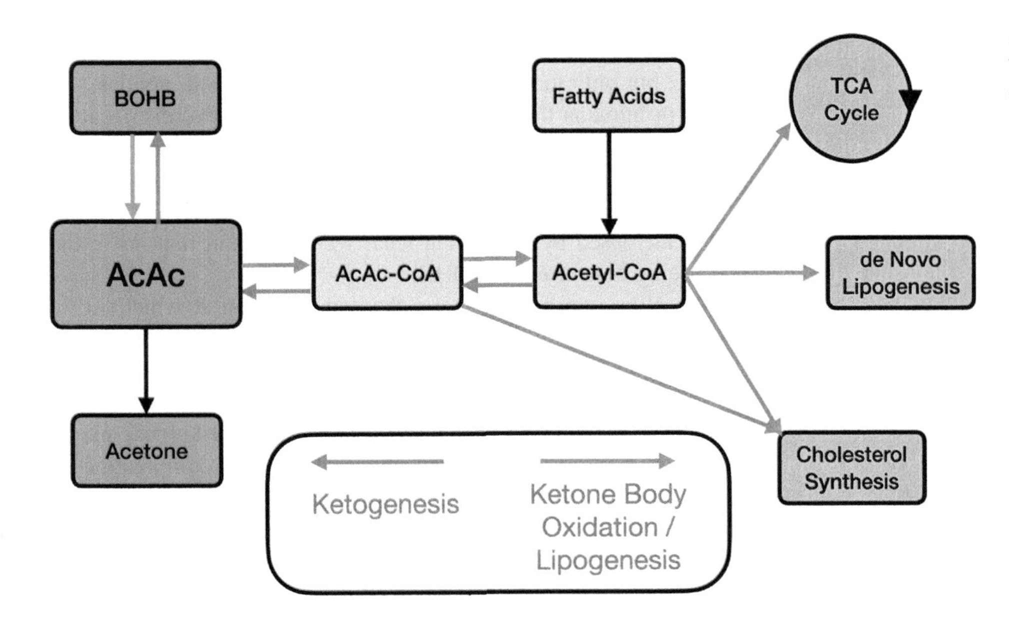

FIGURE 2.4 Ketogenesis, ketone body oxidation, and lipogenic fates of ketone bodies.

2.3.2.7 *Acetoacetate is the proto-ketone-body*

Although we use BOHB for measurement, AcAc is the central ketone body [69]. It is the 'parent', because both acetone and BOHB are derived from it. It is also the form that is used for energy and for synthesis of lipids (fat and cholesterol)—BOHB has to be reverted to AcAc before it can be used for anything. An overview of these pathways is given in Fig. 2.4. For further details, see Cotter et al. [70].

Acetone is generated spontaneously through decarboxylation. Since the generation of acetone requires no energy, AcAc may be considered 'unstable'. This instability has been proposed as a functional reason AcAc largely gets converted to BOHB in the keto-adapted: to keep it from degrading. In other words, BOHB is seen by some as a 'storage' or 'reserve' form of ketone body, keeping it for use as required [71]. Biochemically, the ratio of AcAc to BOHB is driven by redox potential (see 'NAD redox state' below). In support of the idea that BOHB is primarily a storage mechanism, studies examining high levels of ketosis show that over time serum AcAc rises, but quickly plateaus at about 1.2 mmol/L (21.6 mg/dL), whereas BOHB continues to rise passing 4 mmol (72 mg/dL) in children fed KDs [72] and over 5 mmol/L (90 mg/dL) in the ketosis of fasting [73]. In other words, after a quick initial rise, more generation of ketone bodies increases BOHB, but not AcAc. Moreover, BOHB has no other metabolic fate but to be returned to AcAc [69], so there would seem to be no other benefit to its generation.

Acetone has historically been considered an accidental waste product because it is produced spontaneously from AcAc and because it is so small in quantity. However, history warns us against making this assumption. Many substances that were once thought to be waste products, including the other ketone bodies, were later discovered to have functions. At least two proposed acetone functions call the judgement into question. First, as previously stated, animal models have shown that acetone can be a significant substrate for gluconeogenesis. Based on these experiments, it is estimated that up to 59% of all acetone produced could be used for this purpose, accounting for up to 11% of gluconeogenic needs[74]. Second, it may play a critical role in pH and fuel regulation [75]. Because metabolic routes for acetone have been described, it 'cannot further be regarded as a waste product of metabolism' [75].

2.3.2.8 In humans, the use of ketone bodies for peripheral energy proportionally decreases the more they are available

AcAc can be used to generate energy in many tissues, including skeletal muscle. However, from a functional perspective, the primary use of ketone bodies is to provide fuel for the brain in the presence of low glucose availability. As a result, it would be counterproductive for tissues that can use fat to make liberal use of ketone bodies, and we should not be surprised to see sparing effects. Indeed, the metabolic clearance rate (MCR) of ketone bodies, or the rate at which they are used by muscle tissue, decreases as concentration increases in humans [76]. This reduction appears to be exponential, dropping very quickly as ketonaemia approaches 1–2 mmol/L (18–36 mg/dL). This is consistent with an adaptation effect where higher concentrations of ketone bodies signal their preservation for the brain. In the experiments of [76], exercise did appear to raise this threshold by approximately 0.5 mmol/L (9 mg/dL), suggesting that in the context of exercise, muscles will use more ketone bodies if available, but only to a point; the pattern of sparing still applies.

This response may be unique to humans or more acute in humans than in other animals. Aerobic exercise acutely lowered both AcAc and BOHB in a study of 36-h fasted rats, which then rose again after the exercise [77]. This would imply use by muscle tissue, followed by accumulation, as the decrease in production lags slightly behind the decrease in demand. In a human study with keto-adapted athletes, however, aerobic exercise did not lower AcAc and instead acutely increased BOHB [5]. This implies that ketogenesis increased by more than what was used, and that, as in the at-rest case, AcAc concentrations plateau, with any excess being converted to BOHB.

Interestingly, in these keto-adapted athletes, both the baseline concentration and the concentration at which AcAc stabilises as BOHB rises were much lower than in the previous studies of fasted adults and children on KDs. Anecdotally, keto-adapted athletes have lower baseline ketonaemia than those who use KDs for weight loss or epilepsy. This could be explained simply by fat access levels: those losing weight will have more fat available from adipose than lean athletes, whereas those on medical KDs for epilepsy eat high levels of fat specifically to raise ketonaemia to therapeutic levels. It could also reflect a position on the MCR curve, as described above. That is, a combination of lower circulating fat due to lower fat mass and increased exercise may simply reduce skeletal muscle ketone sparing above the MCR threshold. In support of this, it should be noted that when fat intake is sufficiently high, even lean individuals can have higher ketonaemia, as evidenced by the ketogenic macronutrient ratios used for therapeutic ketosis in epilepsy. What appears to stay in common is the AcAc:BOHB ratio.

2.3.2.9 Acetoacetate is also used for lipid synthesis, but this does not appear to account for low ketonaemia in lean athletes

As mentioned above, AcAc is used for de novo lipogenesis and cholesterol synthesis. It is the preferred substrate for this in the liver [78,79] as well as in the brain, which is particularly important developmentally, given that brains are largely constructed of fat and cholesterol and that much of this is synthesised in situ [80]. This is thought to explain why the perinatal period is characterised by mild ketosis. The umbilical cord carries high concentrations of ketones [81], and breast milk is rich in medium chain triglycerides [82,83], which infants use to generate ketone bodies. Moreover, the extensive adipose tissue of human babies compared to other animals is used to support the energy and growth of our brains [80].

It is estimated that up to 75% of cholesterol synthesis can come from AcAc, and up to half of other newly synthesised lipids [84]. Synthesising lipids from AcAc, which itself is derived from lipids may seem futile, but it is important to note that so-called 'futile cycles', are not truly futile, but provide leverage for regulation [85]. Some prefer the term 'substrate cycle' for this reason. When such substrate cycles are in place, small changes in enzymatic rates can produce very large changes in the net flux of a substrate [86]. As a result, substrate cycles provide mechanical advantage. Fatty acids can also stimulate VLDL cholesterol production, which helps transport triglycerides from the liver to the periphery. Triglycerides transported by VLDL can be an important source of energy in lean individuals with low carbohydrate intake [87].

Because AcAc contributes significantly to cholesterol synthesis, one might speculate that reduced ketonaemia in ketogenic athletes is the result of increased demand for cholesterol synthesis, which would deplete the source of BOHB. This, however, does not appear to be the case. Fasting increases LDL cholesterol while lowering cholesterol synthesis [41,88]. Adding protein to the fasted condition without also adding a lot of fat, as in a lower fat KD commonly used in athletes or those who do not require high ketonaemia for medical reasons, would presumably have the same result. If cholesterol synthesis is reduced in these circumstances, the decrease in BOHB cannot be due to competition for AcAc in cholesterol synthesis. Fasting not only reduces cholesterol synthesis but also inhibits PCSK9, increasing LDL receptors and uptake [88]. Because LDL concentrations rise despite these two reducing factors of lower synthesis and higher uptake, high LDL cholesterol appears to be a result of recycling, an idea supported by concurrently high HDL concentrations.

In the case of fasting or lower fat KDs in the lean, it is possible that both cholesterol synthesis and ketogenesis are downregulated to spare fat for muscle energy use, or conversely, the use of fat by muscle simply does not leave enough for much of either of these. In this case, glucose concentrations may then need to rise to support brain function. This would increase protein requirements. As previously discussed, this would resemble Phase III fasting rather than traditional, high fat KDs, which resemble Phase II fasting. GNG and ketogenesis will occur regardless of carbohydrate intake, but substrate availability can skew the glucose-to-ketone body ratio. Some clinicians use this ratio, also known as the Glucose-Ketone-Index (GKI), in the context of cancer treatment, where the goal is a GKI close to 1.0 [89].

2.3.3 Nicotinamide adenine dinucleotide redox state

Although the lean athletes discussed above had lower baseline AcAc and BOHB, their ratio was still low, as is typical of keto-adaptation. Serum BOHB in fasted and therapeutic ketosis is typically 2-5 times that of AcAc, whereas in carbohydrate-based metabolism, BOHB is less than twice AcAc. The mitochondrial redox state of nicotinamide adenine dinucleotide (NAD+), or the ratio of the oxidised form, NAD+, to the reduced form, NADH, is a key determinant of this balance. This is because the reaction transforming AcAc to BOHB requires NADH, whereas the reverse reaction requires NAD+ [69]. When most ketone bodies are in the form of BOHB, that reflects a relative surplus of NAD+:NADH.

Equation of

$$\text{BOHB} + \text{NAD}+ <-- > \text{AcAc} + \text{NADH}$$

NAD+ was first isolated by Otto Warburg, who discovered its role in electron transfer [90]. It is essential for many metabolic processes, which is why we need the precursor, niacin (vitamin B3) [90]. In the electron transport chain (etc.) in mitochondria, NADH is used in Complex I to generate energy, leaving NAD+ (Fig. 2.5). When Complex I is dominant, as in a glucose-based metabolism, a high ratio of NAD+:NADH indicates that relatively more energy is being used than generated, which can be interpreted as a sign of energy stress. FADH2 is used for electron transfer in Complex II of the ECT instead. Both complexes are normally active, but when glucose is the primary source of energy, the ECT receives about five times as much NADH as FADH2, whereas when fat is the primary source of energy, it receives only about twice as much [91]. Thus in the context of carbohydrate metabolism, high NAD+:NADH levels can indicate a lack of energy. The ratio is higher after exercise, during fasting, and in other conditions of low glucose availability versus demand. However, high NAD+:NADH levels may simply indicate that fat metabolism is dominant. Of course, energy does not have to be scarce in this case. By providing NADH, a fat-based metabolism should shift the balance of ketone bodies towards BOHB regardless of total amount.

During exercise itself, it is not clear whether mitochondrial NAD+ or its ratio to NADH is raised. Despite the fact that we would expect this to be the case given the high energy demand, the results of human and animal studies are currently mixed [92]. Long-term adaptation to exercise, on the other hand, appears to reflect increased NAD+ in the following way. Mitochondrial biogenesis is one adaptation to exercise. Because mitochondria contain the majority of the cellular NADH pool [93], having more mitochondria may increase the total NADH available for energy generation at any given time. Sirtuins stimulate mitochondrial biogenesis via PGC-1alpha, which is boosted by NAD+ [94]. This makes functional sense. Low energy availability may stimulate the growth of new mitochondria to produce more energy. KDs, or even a high fat diet, appear to increase mitochondrial biogenesis by triggering the same signals [95–100].

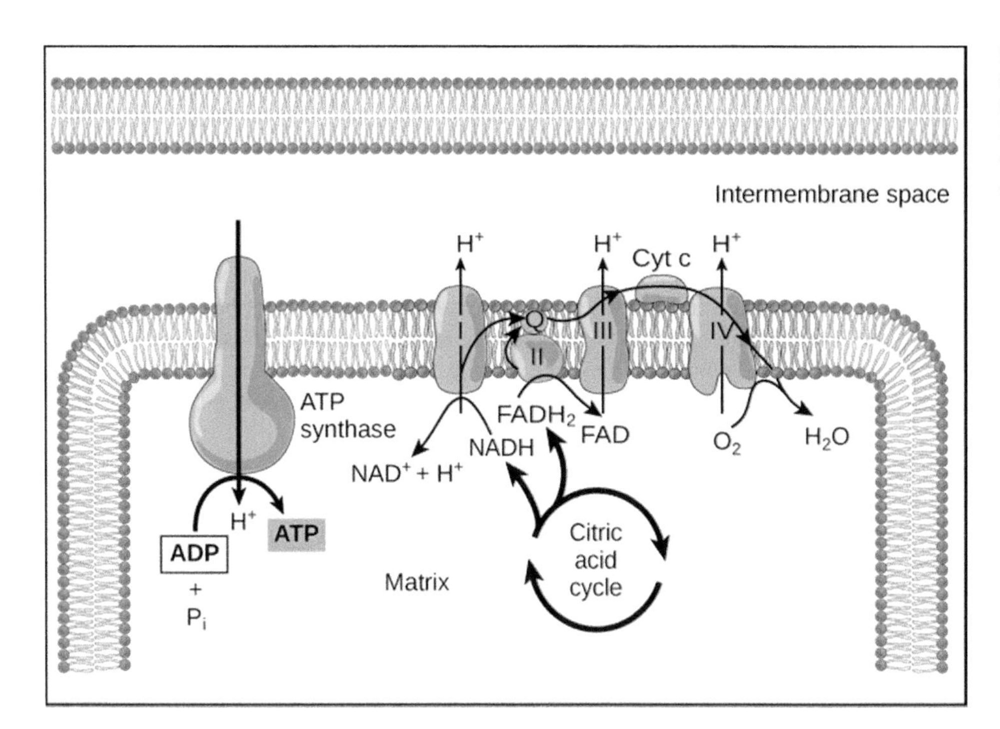

FIGURE 2.5 Electron transport chain, shows Complex I versus Complex II. *From /Rye, C. (2016).* Biology. *Houston, Texas: OpenStax. [Access for free at https://openstax.org/books/biology/].*

The increase in NAD+ from a reduction in Complex I use may be the mechanism of action of the diabetes drug Metformin which inhibits Complex I indirectly via AMPK activation ([101], but see also Fontaine [102]). Because increased NAD+ is associated with longevity [103–105], both KDs and Metformin have been proposed to be longevity enhancing interventions [106,107].

2.3.4 Conclusion

Although fasting provides much of our knowledge of ketogenic metabolism, we can see that its different phases have different properties depending on the predominant fuel available. Due to the commonality of low available glucose, some combination of GNG and ketogenesis is required to supply energy needs to tissues that cannot use fat as is. Humans have an unusual inability to process large amounts of the foods that other animals use to generate their own glucose (fibre and protein), but we can compensate by using fat to generate ketone bodies and boost GNG. As circulating fat concentrations fall due to reduced intake or fat mass, GNG must be increased to meet these demands, but its substrates are becoming more limited as the fat-based substrates glycerol and acetone are reduced. Protein is the primary source of GNG substrate in this lower fat context. When on KDs, lean athletes appear to have lower serum ketone bodies than subjects fasting or on KDs for epilepsy. This could be explained in part by athletes' low fat mass, or by skeletal muscle using ketone bodies rather than sparing them during exercise. It could also be due to a lower dietary ketogenic ratio (fat intake relative to protein and carbohydrates). Ensuring adequate protein during prolonged KDs is crucial for safety, but beyond protein adequacy, higher fat intake may be preferable for meeting remaining energy needs, depending on goals.

2.4 Implications for nutrient needs

Amber O'Hearn, M.Sc.

2.4.1 Introduction

A KD has different macronutrient needs than a high carbohydrate diet, but it may also have different micronutrient needs. This can happen in a variety of ways. Certain nutrients in the bloodstream can be altered by a KD. Different requirements can be induced by differences in the prevalence of biochemical reactions involving different coenzymes. Changes in food intake patterns can change needs through interactions at the level of digestion and absorption. A KD can also affect nutrient synthesis rates in the gut.

2.4.2 Availability

An example of nutrient availability in the bloodstream is the long chain omega-3 polyunsaturated fatty acid, docosahexaenoic acid (DHA). Either DHA or its precursor, alpha-linolenic acid (ALA), must be present in the diet to provide for the maintenance of the structural and functional integrity of the central nervous system and retina [108]. DHA is also used to make the anti-inflammatory compounds, such as docosanoids [109]. Providing DHA in the diet increases its availability for these uses. However, a KD makes all fatty acids more available, including DHA, for which we get an approximate doubling in its circulation, and a smaller, but still significant increase in its appearance in phospholipids as reported by [110]. The authors propose that this increased DHA availability could be a contributing factor to seizure resistance [110]. The rise in DHA is mostly found in triglycerides rather than free fatty acids, which suggests it is either more readily synthesised or less readily oxidised.

2.4.3 Requirements

Insofar as ketogenic diets reduce inflammation [111–113], DHA could also be less needed as a docosanoid precursor. In other words, there appears to be some efficiency induced by the KD in the use of DHA, which may impact its dietary requirement.

A related mechanism for changes in nutrient needs comes from the requirements of metabolic processes. Vitamins, technically speaking, are biochemical coenzymes. While an enzyme is used to catalyse a chemical reaction without being consumed, coenzymes are consumed or altered in the process of helping enzymes catalyse reactions. Because coenzymes are altered by the reaction, we need a continuously renewed supply. Coenzymes that we cannot synthesise ourselves are thus essential, and that's what gives them their vitamin status.

However, the metabolic processes that are dominant in a glucose-based metabolism are not all the same as those that are dominant in a fat-based metabolism, so the proportions of enzymes, cofactors, and hormones consumed can differ. One such example is the role of iodine in carbohydrate metabolism. Iodine is primarily used in the body to synthesise thyroid hormones. T3, the active thyroid hormone, is used in tandem with carbohydrate metabolism. T3 concentrations have been shown repeatedly to drop dramatically during fasting or carbohydrate restriction [114,115]. Subsequent studies show that on low carbohydrate diets over the longer term, T3 concentrations go down approximately 40%–50% [116]. This is not a sign of hypothyroidism, but rather a reflection of low need [116]. Indeed, it appears that attempting to rescue this reduction in T3 by supplementing it can interfere with the muscle sparing necessary in the low carbohydrate condition [117,118]. This reduction in T3 is reflected in rates of iodine clearance [119,120]. It has been pointed out that a lower need for thyroid hormones implies that in the preagricultural past, when carbohydrate intake was likely to have been lower, our iodine needs would also have been lower [121]. Thus the current global crisis of iodine deficiency could be less a change in soil quality, and more a change in dietary quality.

Not all such metabolic changes would favour a ketogenic diet, of course. For example, the amino acid carnitine is a requirement for fatty acid oxidation, as it is used to transport long chain fatty acids into the mitochondria. Therefore carnitine needs might be increased on ketogenic diets. There have been cases of carnitine deficiency in epileptic children treated with ketogenic diets using dietary shakes as a primary source of food [122], though a prior study with unspecified dietary intake showed carnitine deficiency to be rare [123]. Some carnitine can be synthesised endogenously, but it is usually obtained by eating meat. Adequate meat consumption could thus account for the difference and solve the problem. Low meat consumption may also put a strain on vitamin C, which is required for carnitine synthesis.

2.4.4 Interactions

A third way that low carbohydrate intake could change nutritional requirements is through food interactions at the level of absorption. Grains and legumes, which are consumed in small amounts if at all on ketogenic diets, contain phytates, which interfere with the absorption of minerals to such an extent, that it has been estimated that vegetarians may need up to 50% more zinc than nonvegetarians [124,125]. The quantitative difference between those on a grain-based diet and those eschewing grains altogether may well be similar.

2.4.5 Bacterial synthesis in the gut

Many important nutrients are produced by bacterial fermentation, which is why cheese and natto are excellent sources of vitamin K, and beer and brewers yeast are high in B vitamins. Some of these nutrients, including Vitamin K and many B vitamins such as biotin, thiamine, folate, and riboflavin, can also be synthesised by bacteria in the small and large intestines of humans and other animals [126,127]. However, the amounts of each and the extent to which they are absorbed vary and are not all well understood. Absorption is a critical component. Much of the nutritional value produced in the gut is lost in faeces in rats, so they use coprophagy (eating faeces) to recapture the nutrients they produced but did not absorb. We can see how important this is by noting that many of these vitamins can be depleted by preventing coprophagy [128]. In contrast, ruminants, having large microbial populations at the front of the digestive tract, can meet all B vitamin needs without a dietary source [129]. It has been reported that in humans, more than adequate vitamin B12 is produced intestinally to meet our needs, and yet we fail to absorb it, as evidenced, again, by deficiencies that develop [126]. This makes B12 a dietary requirement for humans and is one of the clearest points of evidence that we are evolutionarily adapted to meat eating.

The best studied of these gut-synthesised vitamins is folate. Folate, or vitamin B9, refers to a class of derivatives of tetrahydrofolic acid and include pterin, para-aminobenzoic acid (pABA), and polyglutamates [130]. It has been clearly demonstrated that folate produced in the intestines is absorbed into circulation and distributed in tissues [131]. This intestinal source has been estimated to contribute about 30% of human requirements [126].

However, it has also been shown that folate synthesis is upregulated by fasting, even the intermittent fasting of Ramadan [132], and by ketogenic diets [133,134]. In the latter study, the researchers investigated several microbial pathways. Consistent with the intermittent fasting results, they report that there was a significant increase in folate production pathways within the first day, although they continued to increase before stabilising at a new high within a week. The corresponding serum increase in folate on a KD was approximately 25% in one study [134] and over 50% in the other [133]. They note that an increase in absorption as well as synthesis could not be ruled out as a cause of the serum increase. Regardless, if the above estimate of contribution to human needs is correct, this would represent an increase of up to 45% of folate needs met this way. Alternatively, it could represent a 20% reduction in dietary requirements.

Interestingly, a cross-species analysis comparing herbivores, omnivores, and carnivores reported that on average, carnivores have one and a half times the capacity to synthesise vitamins B1 and B12 compared to the average herbivore [135]. However, it is unclear to what extent this is due to their diets as opposed to their genetics. In other words, dietary composition within a species may affect the level of production, as it does in humans with folate. Given that folate production is significantly increased in a metabolic state that is evolutionarily related to a lack of available food, one might speculate that synthesis or absorption of other B vitamins may also be increased in the ketogenic condition. This would undoubtedly be a useful adaptation, but research on this hypothesis is currently lacking.

Many of the B vitamins are essential because of their role in carbohydrate metabolism. Niacin, thiamine, and riboflavin are among these [136]. As with iodine, there is a case to be made that the RDAs for these vitamins are inflated in high carbohydrate environments. In this case, could meeting the RDAs be detrimental? What happens if you take more of a vitamin that promotes carbohydrate metabolism than you need?

2.4.6 Recommended dietary requirements

As reviewed by Mark Schatzker, fortification of feed with the B vitamins niacin, thiamine and riboflavin can be used effectively to fatten livestock [137]. Likewise, in rats, pregnant dams fed very high doses of B vitamins display more metabolic syndrome (MetS) components postweaning in response to obesogenic diets, as do their offspring [138–140]. In humans, fortification with B vitamins and infant formulas with high B vitamins are associated with higher rates of obesity, and it has been suggested that this may be due to their roles in fat storage [141]. This may interact unfortunately with the increased fattening capacity of fructose [142]. In one early experiment, rats were given diets varying in carbohydrate source and levels of niacin [143]. It was discovered that when enough niacin was provided to support a glucose-galactose carbohydrate source, the same amount of niacin was insufficient to support sucrose, fructose, starch, dextrin, or glucose. Each of these induced some degree of niacin deficiency, but especially fructose and sucrose (which contains fructose). This not only shows that certain carbohydrates can increase niacin need, but it also means that increasing available niacin allows for increased sucrose and fructose intake without symptoms of niacin deficiency. Regardless of mechanism, these findings suggest caution in treating micronutrients as if more is always better and safer.

It is important to remember that recommendations for intake of micronutrients such as the US RDAs, are not intended to apply to individuals but rather to populations, and are therefore over-estimates in the sense that they aim to be enough to cover the majority of people [144]. Since biological values such as nutrient needs tend to vary in a Gaussian pattern (normal curve), a good RDA would aim to be enough for people who need up to two standard deviations above average (ibid). That means, by definition, they are higher than necessary for most people, although the variance may be small (See Fig. 2.6). The way the quantities are estimated vary. In some cases, such as for niacin, they are

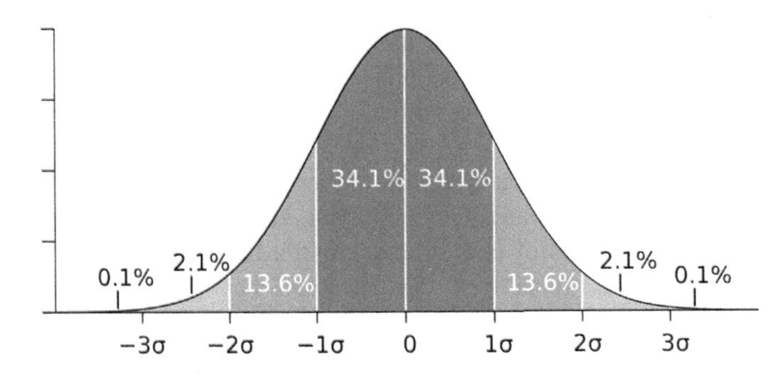

FIGURE 2.6 A Gaussian curve with mean at point 0 and standard deviation (SD) σ. Assuming that nutrient needs follow this distribution, then if an RDA value were set with the goal of meeting the requirements of everyone in the population within 2 SDs (2σ), then it would be more than enough for almost 98% of the population, potentially by a large margin, depending on the magnitude of the variance. *From M. W. Toews. "Standard Deviation Diagram." Wikimedia Commons. Based (in concept) on figure by Jeremy Kemp, CC BY 2.5. (April 7, 2007). https://commons.wikimedia.org/w/index.php?curid=1903871.*

intended to be enough to prevent frank deficiency diseases. In other cases, they are based on speculative rates to prevent metabolic disease. An example of this is the recommendation for vitamin C, which is much higher than what is needed to prevent scurvy [145]. It is based on the presumption that higher doses may reduce the risk of developing diabetes or heart disease [145]. When neither of these can be determined, for example in the case of manganese, recommendations are based on population norms [124,125]. Obviously, all of these can be affected by the baseline diet. Therefore when considering the dietary needs of individuals, we may wish to examine the assumptions behind specific recommendations before applying them.

2.4.7 Conclusion

The implications of this are far reaching. Current knowledge about nutrient needs that are based on populations eating grain-based diets, form the basis of hypotheses about our evolution. For example, it has been proposed that because the brain needs high levels of difficult-to-obtain nutrients such as iodine, zinc, and DHA, that a shore-based diet was critical for the development of the anatomically modern brain [82]. Insofar as a diet low in carbohydrates and grain in particular may have been prominent until recently, the dietary requirements for these nutrients may have been less.

In general, any diagnostic lab measurement for which we have established a normal range may need to be re-evaluated in the ketogenic context. For example, just as T3 concentrations that may be indicative of hypothyroidism on a high carbohydrate diet do not always reflect hypothyroidism on a low carbohydrate diet, mildly elevated cortisol in comparison to a high carbohydrate diet is not always indicative of MetS [146]. Indeed, to expect a value for a biological marker found on a KD to indicate the same thing it would with respect to serum ranges established in the high carbohydrate metabolic context, is the same fundamental error as conflating ketosis from diet with ketoacidosis.

2.5 Plant versus animal nutrition

Amber O'Hearn, M.Sc.

When we talk about nutrition, we frequently focus on essential micronutrients. As the phrase implies, these are minute particles of critical importance. They rose to prominence only recently, replacing the previously more acute problem of starvation due to a lack of energy or protein [147]. Protein-energy malnutrition is still common in many parts of the world, but when meeting these needs using grains and legumes micronutrition deficits remain a problem, as reflected by worldwide efforts to fortify these diets with vitamins and minerals [148].

Study of malnutrition in countries where grains and legumes form the basis of the diet reveals that all major nutrients of concern including iron, zinc, vitamin A, and B vitamins could be provided with higher intake of animal source foods [148]. This is largely because animal source foods are generally more replete with micronutrients and those micronutrients are more bioavailable when coming from animal sources than plant sources [149,150]. This increased bioavailability results either because the forms of the vitamins are more directly usable, as is the case, for example, with vitamin A, which occurs in plants only as a precursor [151], or because the plant forms are difficult to absorb, often being chemically bound such that they pass through the digestive system inaccessibly or packaged with phytates and other antinutrients that block absorption [152]. In the case of iron, there are two types: haem iron, which is found only in meat, and nonhaem iron, which is found in both plant and animal foods [153]. Haem iron is much more absorbable than nonhaem iron, a fact which is considered detrimental in cases of hemochromatosis [154]. However, it should be emphasised that hemochromatosis is not caused by high intake of iron, but rather a genetic or medically-induced disruption of hepcidin, a hormone that regulates iron absorption [154]. Another reason that simply increasing animal source foods could alleviate a variety of deficiencies is that, in general, a given animal source food has a relatively comprehensive nutrient profile when compared to plant foods, which typically need to be balanced (complemented) with intake of specific other plant foods to cover all needs [155]. These concerns make plant-based diets more nutritionally precarious, but with care and education they can be made to supply almost all essential nutrients with the exception of B12, which would have to be supplemented.

Given that energy, protein, and nearly all essential micronutrients can be obtained from either plants or animals, the choice appears to be based on personal preferences or non-nutritionally motivated factors at first. However, the components that accompany the essential nutrients, as well as the specific forms of energy and protein, have health consequences. We will look at fatty acid and amino acid profiles, as well as 'bioactives' (nutrients that have physiological effects other than nutrition) found in plant and animal foods.

We can better understand the role of different dietary components from the perspective of the immune system, which is responsible for maintaining clearly defined limits of self [156]. The immune system's primary functions are to maintain boundaries between self and nonself, deciding what to allow inside to incorporate into ourselves, and to repair and grow our tissues, deciding what to tear down, recycle, or eliminate, and what to keep and reinforce. When seen in this light, it is clear that digestion and absorption are just as much immunological functions as rejection and defence in response to unwanted components. They are, in fact, two different outcomes of the same immunological process.

With this lens in mind, two distinctions are useful for evaluating a biochemical. The first is about potential origins. An endogenous compound is one that the body creates, whereas an exogenous compound is one that comes from outside the body. If a compound cannot be produced endogenously, it must be foreign. If it can be made endogenously, we can call it 'domestic', or synthesisable, regardless of its actual origin. The body should not be able to tell the origin of a domestic compound after entry. The second distinction is between utility and requirement, as illustrated below.

With these two distinctions we can classify incoming food components into four groups (Table 2.6). The first two groups include components of food that are required or usable by the body. Food components we require and are not synthesisable are the essential nutrients. This is the definition of a vitamin—a biologically generated (i.e., nonmineral) compound we cannot make ourselves but need. A very important and underappreciated class of components are known as conditionally essential nutrients. These are required nutrients that can be obtained from food, but because we have the ability to synthesise them they are not considered essential—they are essential only conditionally upon inadequate synthesis. One issue with this classification is that adequate synthesis is not always possible. Even if a deficiency can be created by

TABLE 2.6 Types of food components. As a general goal for optimal nutrition, Quadrants I and II should be maximised as these nutrients are either not synthesised (essential nutrients) or can be inefficient when completely endogenously synthesised (conditionally essential nutrients) in some people. Meanwhile, foods fitting Quadrant IV should be minimised wherever possible—this necessarily means restricting certain plant foods with ample amounts of these compounds.

	"Domestic"	Foreign
Usable	**Conditionally essential**	**Essential Nutrients**
Unusable	**Waste Products**	**Xenobiotics / Anti-nutrients**

not consuming an exogenous source, such a nutrient will always be relegated to conditionally essential status based on the technical definition of essential. DHA is an example of this in infants. Human babies can synthesise DHA from the omega-3 precursor alpha-linolenic acid (ALA). However, infant formulas contain it because synthesis is deemed insufficient for optimal brain growth [157]. Note, however, that a Cochrane review found no difference in vision or neurodevelopment in full-term babies fed formula without added long chain polyunsaturated fatty acids compared to those fed LCPUFA supplemented formula [158]. This may be due to accessibility of stored LCPUFAs in infant adipose tissue [82].

Components of food that are not required or usable are also of two kinds. If they are synthesisable, then they are necessarily familiar to the immune system, which should already have pathways to eliminate them as waste. On the other hand, if they are foreign, they are called xenobiotics ('xeno' = foreign), and the immune system will mount a defence against them, minimising absorption and prioritising excretion should they pass through. Xenobiotics can also have antinutrient activity, meaning that their action is subtractive, resulting in a net increased need for nutritive elements.

With these conceptual distinctions, we can now make more sense of the bodily responses to animal and plant derived bioactives, depending on whether their biological effects result from immune activation, as with xenobiotics, or from nutritional enhancement, as with conditionally essential nutrients. Plant food advocates frequently cite the beneficial effects of bioactives found only in plants as evidence that plant-based foods should be included and prioritised in the human diet (see e.g., Craig [159] and Liu [160]). In accordance with the promotion of recognition of these effects there is a recent trend to rename phytochemicals ('phyto' means 'plant') as phytonutrients [161].

One early, but ultimately incorrect, idea about how plant bioactives might promote health was based on the fact that some phytochemicals exhibit antioxidant properties in vitro, which combined with the contemporaneous antioxidant theory of ageing to suggest that plant-derived antioxidants should improve health and longevity [162]. Bouayed and Bohn thus laid out a novel argument for eating plant foods specifically for antioxidation, outlined below.

1. In vitro, certain phytochemicals have prevented cell death due to excess oxidation. However, at high doses, the effect is reversed, and oxidation is actually increased.
2. In human trials, plant derived antioxidants not only did not provide benefits, but may have been detrimental.
3. Supplements have orders of magnitude higher doses of phytochemicals than what is obtained from eating plants.
4. Epidemiologically, plant-eating is associated with positive health outcomes.
5. Therefore eating plants must correspond to the beneficial, low dose case of exogenous antioxidants.

There are two problems with this argument. The first is that plant foods cannot deliver the quantities of phytochemicals clinically shown to have benefit. For example, the polyphenol resveratrol, which has been shown to increase lifespan in some (but not all) animal studies [163] is found in common foods such as grapes, chocolate, apples, and tomatoes [164]. But the amount of those foods one would need to obtain a therapeutic dose would be in the hundreds or thousands of kilograms [164]. Somewhat less dramatically, quercetin, found in highest amounts in onions and tea, has a bioavailability of about one per cent, such that supplements intended for therapeutic doses contain about 100 times the amount normally obtained in a Western diet [165] (although for residents of Japan, this factor is reduced to 10–30 [166]).

Sulforaphane is considered the most bioavailable of food-derived polyphenols with studied benefits, having orders of magnitude more bioavailability than other common polyphenols [165]. However, many factors affect its abundance in plant sources. Dietary sulforaphane comes in significant quantities from cruciferous vegetables, which are all human-bred variations of the wild mustard plant [167]. Of these, the highest in sulforaphane are raw cauliflower, cabbage, broccoli, and broccoli sprouts [168]. With a clinical dose of about 350 mg/day, this would take somewhere between 230 g (half a pound) and one and a half kilograms (three and a half pounds) of raw broccoli daily to achieve according to estimated content variation (ibid). But not only is there variability, such that a consumer cannot count on reaching this level at the lower end of intake, other components of the plant, such as myrosinase and epithiospecifier protein, can significantly affect the activation of sulforaphane, and are not quantified [165]. Moreover, cooking and even storage rapidly induce losses that would approximately double or triple the required portions (Houghton, 2016). And since raw cruciferous vegetables also contain goitrogens that may be safe in small quantities, but less safe in large doses that persist over long periods [169], even a concerted successful effort to obtain therapeutic concentrations of sulforaphane from food may cause as much harm as good.

Another way to evaluate whether a beneficial antioxidant effect can be obtained from plant foods is to look directly at concentrations of antioxidant markers after eating a diet that includes them. However, in a metastudy looking for beneficial antioxidant effects from foods rich in flavonoids and other substances thought to have antioxidant properties, most had none, leaving the evidence equivocal at best [170]. The authors speculated that this could be due to benefits only being available to those in poor health, researchers looking at the wrong markers and thus missing a benefit that existed, or simply the fact that the same substances that can have antioxidant effects can also have pro-oxidant effects. This relates to the second issue with the argument.

Although some phytochemicals have antioxidant activity in vitro, the mechanism underlying antioxidant benefit stems from immune system activation in an attempt to prevent phytochemicals from entering the body, rather than their use in essential bodily functions, as a nutrient is normally defined. This mechanism is via NF-E2-related factor 2 (Nrf2), a transcription factor involved in regulating antioxidation and detoxification, and its mammalian regulator kelch-like ECH-associated protein 1 (Keap1) [171].

Excess oxidation is indeed a problem. Many diseases are associated with it, including heart disease [172], diabetes [173], and cancer [174]. Oxidation that is not kept in balance can lead to damage of lipids, protein, and even DNA [175]. This observation led to the hypothesis that to combat these diseases we should reduce the ROS that cause oxidation (ibid). However, preventing oxidation not only doesn't always improve the diseases it was targeted for, but actually appears to have detrimental effects on insulin sensitivity and longevity [176]. The problem with the approach is that oxidation is not primarily damaging; it has a biological function (ibid). Because ROS are generated in the process of metabolism it was initially thought that this was merely an unavoidable cost or trade-off of ATP generation. And perhaps, from an evolutionary standpoint it once was [177]. Anything that is the result of a biological process, on the other hand, becomes a marker of that process, which other processes can use as information. As a result, the presence of ROS is not only a byproduct of metabolism, but also a de facto indicator of its rate. The ROS signal is used by many other processes, and it is one way biological processes are coordinated [178].

Given that ROS is a normal product of metabolism, and also an important signal, but that excess ROS can cause runaway damage, it is not surprising that in a healthy individual, ROS is very tightly regulated, such that it is neither too little nor too much. Nrf2 is an important contributor to this regulation [179]. The result of Nrf2 activation is to mitigate damage, in part by stimulating the endogenous synthesis of antioxidants [180]. In a normal, healthy person, oxidation is kept in check simply by sensing oxidation and responding with antioxidation. This system is only overwhelmed when there is a lot of damage. In this situation, external Nrf2 stimulation can promote increased defence and antioxidation. A wide range of modern medicines, both pharmaceutical and herbal, are mediated at least in part by Nrf2 stimulation [181].

An immediate problem with this strategy, however, is dose. Any medicine that works by provoking the immune system will have a hormetic pattern of effect [182]. That is, as with any toxin, exposure to a xenobiotic will be beneficial to a point, after which it overwhelms the system's ability to respond. This is exactly what we see with Nrf2 promoters in medicine, where the curve of benefit eventually becomes negative (Fig. 2.7) (Maher and Yamamoto [171]). The difficulty is in assessing at what dose each response would occur, given that the prior health of an individual and the sum of the interventions he is undergoing will determine how much more stimulation is tolerable.

The appropriate dose will depend on how much Nrf2 stimulation is already occurring from other sources. Keto-adaptation already involves Nrf2 activation. In an in vitro study of rat hippocampal mitochondria, it was discovered

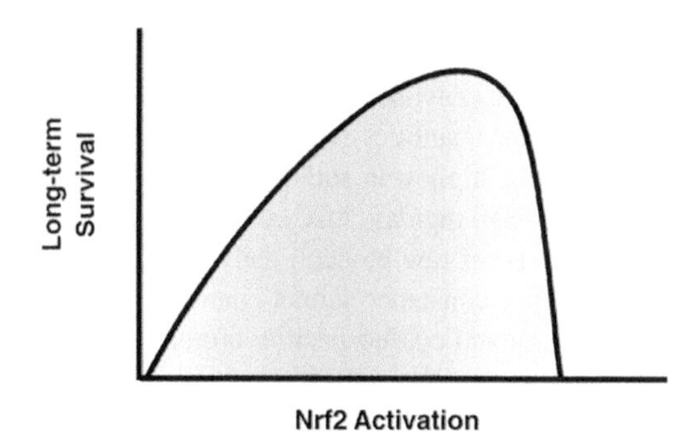

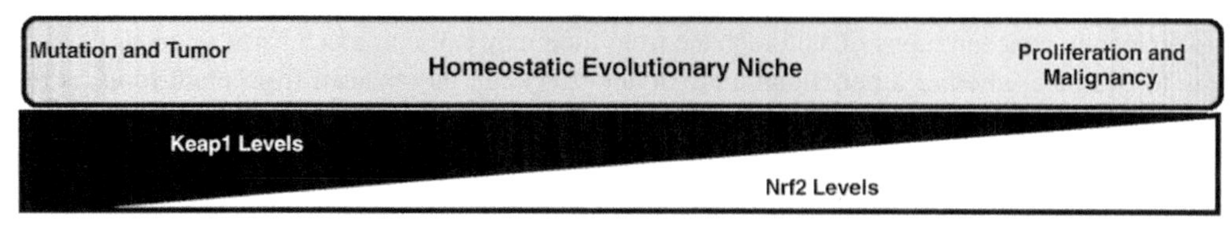

FIGURE 2.7 Theoretical Hormetic Curve for Nrf2 Activation. Activation of Nrf2 is hormetic in nature. Due to evolutionary selection, either too much or too little Nrf2 has pathological sequelae. *From Maher, Jonathan, and Masayuki Yamamoto. "The Rise of Antioxidant Signalling—The Evolution and Hormetic Actions of Nrf2." Toxicology and Applied Pharmacology 244, no. 1 (April 2010): 4–15. https://doi.org/10.1016/j.taap.2010.01.011.*

that oxidation increases over the first few days, leading to an increase in Nrf2 and enough endogenous antioxidation to compensate for this effect. After three weeks, the long-term persistent effect was a net increase in Nrf2 and a net decrease in peroxide (an ROS) concentrations when compared to the higher carb baseline [183]. One implication of this is that in the ketogenic context, the therapeutic dose of a Nrf2 promoter may be lower, as well as the threshold at which benefit gives way to detriment. On the one hand, this theoretically supports a more plausible benefit of sulforaphane derived from food in ketogenic dieters in particular. On the other hand, it raises a red flag, particularly for patients who exhibit signs of overactive immune activity for other reasons.

Does this note of caution extend to the KD itself, given that a KD may persistently activate Nrf2 relative to higher carb diets? Perhaps. However, KDs exert their benefits through multiple mechanisms, including from the ketone bodies themselves, increased circulation of highly unsaturated fatty acids (HUFAs), growth and transcription factors such as brain-derived neurotrophic factor (BDNF), and NAD + , and decreased blood glucose and inflammatory cytokines [184].

2.5.1 Animal source bioactives

If we look, in contrast, at bioactives of animal origin, they are, unsurprisingly, 'domestic', or synthesisable compounds, precisely because they were, in fact, synthesised by another animal. Therefore these are typically classifiable as conditionally essential nutrients, and they are usually amino acids or fatty acids. Correspondingly, conditionally essential nutrients are for this reason often of animal origin only, such as taurine and cholesterol, or simply more commonly found in animal source foods, such as carnitine and choline. An example that can be found in both plant and animal foods is dietary nucleotides.

Taurine is an amino acid that is high in meat and fish but absent in plants, such that plasma concentrations are low in vegetarians [185]. It is an essential nutrient for infants, who cannot synthesise it [186], but only considered conditionally essential in adults, who have limited synthesis [187]. It is the most prevalent free amino acid in tissues, especially heart, brain, and liver [188]. Given that it neither is incorporated into proteins, nor participates in many reactions, its function has been difficult to determine, and it was once considered merely an 'end-product' [188]. However, it is now known to play roles in brain and retinal development [189], calcium modulation, osmosis and electrolyte balance [187], membrane stabilisation [190], and immunity [191] and has been hypothesised to reduce advanced glycation products (AGEs) [192]. In interventional studies, supplemental taurine has shown improvement in diabetes and insulin regulation [190], cardiovascular disease prevention [193], and nonalcoholic fatty liver disease (NAFLD) [194,195]. It has even been suggested that high taurine intake is responsible for the association between longer lifespans with certain geographical regions, such as Spain, Portugal, and Japan [196].

Carnitine is also conditionally essential with limited biosynthesis. It can be found in some plant sources, but rarely, and vegetarians have lower concentrations [197], as well as reduced capacity for carnitine uptake in skeletal muscle [198]. It has important roles in fatty acid metabolism, heart function, and the immune system [199]. Echoing findings for taurine, carnitine may be fully essential in newborns [200] and relative deficiencies of it develop in association with multiple diseases, especially of the heart and liver, that in turn may benefit from its supplementation [200–202]. Carnitine requires vitamin C for its synthesis, and therefore dietary carnitine can spare vitamin C [149,150]. Because fatty acid oxidation is upregulated in KDs, carnitine may be especially needed in that context, and in fact, some studies have suggested that a KD depletes carnitine; however, as these were in the context of epilepsy treatment, and anticonvulsants can deplete carnitine, the effect of the diet alone is not clear [122,123]. Nonetheless, inclusion of carnitine sources during a KD may be warranted.

Dietary nucleotides and nucleosides are examples of bioactives found in both plant and animal source foods. Because they are components of RNA and DNA, they can be found in foods high in purines or pyrimidines, such as meat, but especially seafood and organ meats, as well as legumes and yeasts. Exogenous nucleotide sources appear to be critical for immune competence as well as intestinal development and recovery [203]. Breast milk is also high in nucleotides probably for these reasons [203,204]. In animal studies, dietary nucleotides have increased brain phosphatidylcholine, DHA, AA, and improved learning [205,206], increased longevity [207], and helped intestinal repair after varied injuries [208–212]. Purines have often been implicated in gout, because their breakdown contributes to total uric acid load. However, gout is not a necessary result of high uric acid [213] and in the absence of pre-existing gout or (MetS), high uric acid may have benefits, specifically for cognition [149,150].

When a conditionally essential substance is shown to provide medical benefit, there is an argument to be made that our bodies 'expected' those substances in food, which is why synthesis is low. Given that meat has always been an important part of the human diet, animal source bioactives may be essential in the quantitative sense, implying that synthesis is limited to suboptimal levels. Nonetheless, many of the above studies demonstrating therapeutic benefits of taurine and carnitine used quantities that exceeded plausible food intake, leaving it unclear how much benefit, if any, would be obtained at lower concentrations. For reviews including therapeutic doses used, please see [214] and [215], for taurine and carnitine respectively. Elucidating what conditions would make these nutrients essential could reveal that essentiality is for some of these the common case, not a special one. A similar argument could be, and has been, made for xenobiotics—that the body functions better with them in a way that suggests they are 'expected' evolutionarily [162]. However, as previously stated, this argument is predicated on their ability to act through food, and unlike taurine and carnitine, food-level doses are known to be ineffective. As a result of dose considerations and mechanisms of action, it appears that the role of xenobiotics is more medicinal than nutritive.

2.6 Conclusion

Animal and plant-based foods can both provide calories and essential vitamins and minerals, but the total nutritional effect of individual food items will be determined not only by their direct contributions to chemical and material needs, but also by the other components they bring with them. Other food components' biological effects can be viewed through an immunological lens to determine whether they are simply contributing more resources that the body could make itself—conditionally essential nutrients—or whether they are foreign substances that trigger a boundary challenge. Sparing functions are provided by conditionally essential nutrients, whereas xenobiotics such as phytochemicals promote improved defence and repair. Both may have a positive impact on health and are active research topics.

References

[1] Volek JS, Feinman RD. Carbohydrate restriction improves the features of metabolic syndrome. Metabolic syndrome may be defined by the response to carbohydrate restriction. Nutr Metab 2005;2(1):31. Available from: https://doi.org/10.1186/1743-7075-2-31.

[2] Feinman RD, Pogozelski WK, Astrup A, Bernstein RK, Fine EJ, Westman EC, et al. Dietary carbohydrate restriction as the first approach in diabetes management: critical review and evidence base. Nutrition 2015;31(1):1–3.

[3] McKenzie AL, Hallberg SJ, Creighton BC, Volk BM, Link TM, Abner MK, et al. A novel intervention including individualized nutritional recommendations reduces hemoglobin A1c Level, medication use, and weight in type 2 diabetes. JMIR Diabetes 2017;2(1):e5. Available from: https://doi.org/10.2196/diabetes.6981.

[4] Yancy WS, Olsen MK, Guyton JR, Bakst RP, Westman EC. A low-carbohydrate, ketogenic diet versus a low-fat diet to treat obesity and hyperlipidemia: a randomized, controlled trial. Ann Intern Med 2004;140(10):769. Available from: https://doi.org/10.7326/0003-4819-140-10-200405180-00006.

[5] Boden G, Sargrad K, Homko C, Mozzoli M, Stein TP. Effect of a low-carbohydrate diet on appetite, blood glucose levels, and insulin resistance in obese patients with type 2 diabetes. Ann Intern Med 2005;142(6):403–11. Available from: https://doi.org/10.7326/0003-4819-142-6-200503150-00006.

[6] Volek JS, Phinney SD. The art and science of low carbohydrate performance. Beyond Obesity LLC; 2012.

[7] Volek, J, Phinney MD PSD, Volek RJS, Stephen DP. The art and science of low carbohydrate living: an expert guide to making the life-saving benefits of carbohydrate restriction sustainable and enjoyable. Beyond Obesity LLC, 2011.

[8] Eenfeldt, A. How low carb is LCHF? Dietdoctor.Com, 2015, April 2. http://www.dietdoctor.com/how-low-carb-is-lchf.

[9] Harper A. Defining the essentiality of nutrients. Modern nutrition in health and disease. 9th ed. WIlliam & WIlkins; 1999. p. 3–10. Available from: https://doi.org/10.1123/ijsnem.2017-0273.

[10] Tondt J, Yancy WS, Westman EC. Application of nutrient essentiality criteria to dietary carbohydrates. Nutr Res Rev 2020;33(2):260–70. Available from: https://doi.org/10.1017/S0954422420000050.

[11] Rogovik AL, Goldman RD. Ketogenic diet for treatment of epilepsy. Can Family Phys 2010;56(6):540.

[12] Turton JL, Field RJ, Parker HM, Rooney K, Struik NA. Formulating nutritionally adequate low-carbohydrate diets-an analysis of the Australian food composition database. Biomed J Sci Techn Res 2022;44(1):35166–80.

[13] Zinn C, Rush A, Johnson R. Assessing the nutrient intake of a low-carbohydrate, high-fat (LCHF) diet: a hypothetical case study design. BMJ Open 2018;8(2):e018846. Available from: https://doi.org/10.1136/bmjopen-2017-018846.

[14] Jebeile H, Grunseit AM, Thomas M, Kelly T, Garnett SP, Gow ML. Low-carbohydrate interventions for adolescent obesity: nutritional adequacy and guidance for clinical practice. Clin Obes 2020;10(4):e12370.

[15] Nutrient Recommendations: Dietary Reference Intakes (DRI). (n.d.). https://ods.od.nih.gov/HealthInformation/Dietary_Reference_Intakes.aspx.

[16] Westman EC, Mavropoulos J, Yancy WS, Volek JS. A review of low-carbohydrate ketogenic diets. Curr Atherosclerosis Rep 2003;5(6):476–83 sity.

[17] Forsythe CE, Phinney SD, Feinman RD, Volk BM, Freidenreich D, Quann E, et al. Limited effect of dietary saturated fat on plasma saturated fat in the context of a low carbohydrate diet. Lipids 2010;45(10):947–62. Available from: https://doi.org/10.1007/s11745-010-3467-3.

[18] Volek JS, Fernandez ML, Feinman RD, Phinney SD. Dietary carbohydrate restriction induces a unique metabolic state positively affecting atherogenic dyslipidemia, fatty acid partitioning, and metabolic syndrome. Prog Lipid Res 2008;47(5):307–18. Available from: https://doi.org/10.1016/j.plipres.2008.02.003.

[19] Yang Q. Gain weight by "going diet?" Artificial sweeteners and the neurobiology of sugar cravings: Neuroscience 2010. Yale J Biol Med. 2010;83(2):101.

[20] Yancy WS, Mitchell NS, Westman EC. Ketogenic diet for obesity and diabetes. JAMA Intern Med 2019;179(12):1734. Available from: https://doi.org/10.1001/jamainternmed.2019.5148.

[21] Meng Y, Bai H, Wang S, Li Z, Wang Q, Chen L. Efficacy of low carbohydrate diet for type 2 diabetes mellitus management: a systematic review and meta-analysis of randomized controlled trials. Diabetes Res Clin Pract 2017;131:124–31.

[22] Roberts CGP, Athinarayanan SJ, Vantieghem M, Mckenzie AL, Volk BM, Adams RN, et al. 212-OR: Five-year follow-up of lipid, inflammatory, hepatic, and renal markers in people with T2 diabetes on a very-low-carbohydrate intervention including nutritional ketosis (VLCI) via continuous remote care (CRC). Diabetes 2022;71(Supplement_1) 212-OR.

[23] Athinarayanan SJ, Vantieghem M, Mckenzie AL, Hallberg S, Roberts CGP, Volk BM, et al. 832-P: five-year weight and glycemic outcomes following a very-low-carbohydrate intervention including nutritional ketosis in patients with type 2 diabetes. Diabetes 2022;71(Supplement_1) 832-P.

[24] Unwin D, Khalid AA, Unwin J, Crocombe D, Delon C, Martyn K, et al. Insights from a general practice service evaluation supporting a lower carbohydrate diet in patients with type 2 diabetes mellitus and prediabetes: a secondary analysis of routine clinic data including HbA1c, weight and prescribing over 6 years. 2020 Oct 22 [cited 2020 Oct 31]; Available from: https://www.repository.cam.ac.uk/handle/1810/312035.

[25] Cordain L, Miller JB, Eaton SB, Mann N. Macronutrient estimations in hunter-gatherer diets. Am J Clin Nutr 2000;72(6):1589–90. Available from: https://doi.org/10.1093/ajcn/72.6.1589.

[26] Steelman GM, Westman EC, editors. Obesity: evaluation and treatment essentials. 2nd ed. CRC Press, Taylor & Francis Group; 2016.

[27] Phinney SD, Tang AB, Waggoner CR, Tezanos-Pinto RG, Davis PA. The transient hypercholesterolemia of major weight loss. Am J Clin Nutr 1991;53(6):1404–10. Available from: https://doi.org/10.1093/ajcn/53.6.1404.

[28] Shai I, Spence JD, Schwarzfuchs D, Henkin Y, Parraga G, Rudich A, et al.DIRECT Group Dietary intervention to reverse carotid atherosclerosis. Circulation 2010;121(10):1200–8. Available from: https://doi.org/10.1161/CIRCULATIONAHA.109.879254.

[29] Athinarayanan SJ, Hallberg SJ, McKenzie AL, Lechner K, King S, McCarter JP, et al. Impact of a 2-year trial of nutritional ketosis on indices of cardiovascular disease risk in patients with type 2 diabetes. Cardiovasc Diabetol 2020;19(1):208. Available from: https://doi.org/10.1186/s12933-020-01178-2.

[30] Sl R, Ec W, R G, E M. Can a low-carbohydrate diet improve exercise tolerance in Mcardle disease? J Rare Disorders: Diagn Ther 2017;03(01). Available from: https://doi.org/10.21767/2380-7245.100054.

[31] Watanabe M, Tuccinardi D, Ernesti I, Basciani S, Mariani S, Genco A, et al. Scientific evidence underlying contraindications to the ketogenic diet: an update. Obes Rev 2020;21(10):e13053.

[32] DeFronzo RA. The effect of insulin on renal sodium metabolism. A review with clinical implications. Diabetologia 1981;21(3):165–71. Available from: https://doi.org/10.1007/BF00252649.

[33] Athinarayanan SJ, Adams RN, Hallberg SJ, McKenzie AL, Bhanpuri NH, Campbell WW, et al. Long-term effects of a novel continuous remote care intervention including nutritional ketosis for the management of type 2 diabetes: a 2-year non-randomized clinical trial. Front Endocrinol 2019;10:348. Available from: https://doi.org/10.3389/fendo.2019.00348.

[34] Westman EC, Yancy WS, Mavropoulos JC, Marquart M, McDuffie JR. The effect of a low-carbohydrate, ketogenic diet versus a low-glycemic index diet on glycemic control in type 2 diabetes mellitus. Nutr Metab 2008;5(1):36. Available from: https://doi.org/10.1186/1743-7075-5-36.

[35] Yancy WS, Crowley MJ, Dar MS, Coffman CJ, Jeffreys AS, Maciejewski ML, et al. Comparison of group medical visits combined with intensive weight management vs group medical visits alone for glycemia in patients with type 2 diabetes: a noninferiority randomized clinical trial. JAMA Intern Med 2019;180:70–9. Available from: https://doi.org/10.1001/jamainternmed.2019.4802.

[36] Santos FL, Esteves SS, da Costa Pereira A, Yancy WS, Nunes JPL. Systematic review and meta-analysis of clinical trials of the effects of low carbohydrate diets on cardiovascular risk factors. Obes Rev Off J Int Assoc Study Obes 2012;13(11):1048–66. Available from: https://doi.org/10.1111/j.1467-789X.2012.01021.x.

[37] Churuangsuk C, Kherouf M, Combet E, Lean M. Low-carbohydrate diets for overweight and obesity: a systematic review of the systematic reviews. Obes Rev Off J Int Assoc Study Obes 2018;19(12):1700–18. Available from: https://doi.org/10.1111/obr.12744.

[38] Mensink RP, Katan MB. Effect of dietary fatty acids on serum lipids and lipoproteins. A meta-analysis of 27 trials. Arteriosclerosis Thromb A J Vasc Biol 1992;12(8):911–19. Available from: https://doi.org/10.1161/01.atv.12.8.911.

[39] Paoli A, Rubini A, Volek JS, Grimaldi KA. Beyond weight loss: a review of the therapeutic uses of very-low-carbohydrate (ketogenic) diets. Eur J Clin Nutr 2013;67(8):789–96. Available from: https://doi.org/10.1038/ejcn.2013.116.

[40] Bueno NB, de Melo ISV, de Oliveira SL, da Rocha Ataide T. Very-low-carbohydrate ketogenic diet v. low-fat diet for long-term weight loss: a meta-analysis of randomised controlled trials. Br J Nutr 2013;110(7):1178–87. Available from: https://doi.org/10.1017/S0007114513000548.

[41] Creighton BC, Hyde PN, Maresh CM, Kraemer WJ, Phinney SD, Volek JS. Paradox of hypercholesterolaemia in highly trained, keto-adapted athletes. BMJ Open Sport Exerc Med 2018;4(1):e000429. Available from: https://doi.org/10.1136/bmjsem-2018-000429.

[42] Eisenmann JC, Womack CJ, Reeves MJ, Pivarnik JM, Malina RM. Blood lipids in young distance runners. Med Sci Sports Exerc 2001;33(10):1661–6. Available from: https://doi.org/10.1097/00005768-200110000-00008.

[43] Ifland J. Processed food addiction: foundations, assessment, and recovery. CRC Press; 2020.

[44] Medina JM, Tabernero A. Lactate utilization by brain cells and its role in CNS development. J Neurosci Res 2005;79(1–2):2–10. Available from: https://doi.org/10.1002/jnr.20336.

[45] Shambaugh GE. Ketone body metabolism in the mother and fetus. Federation Proc 1985;44(7):2347–51.

[46] Ward Platt M, Deshpande S. Metabolic adaptation at birth. SemFetal Neonatal Med 2005;10(4):341–50. Available from: https://doi.org/10.1016/j.siny.2005.04.001.

[47] Cunnane SC, Courchesne-Loyer A, Vandenberghe C, St-Pierre V, Fortier M, Hennebelle M, et al. Can ketones help rescue brain fuel supply in later life? Implications for cognitive health during aging and the treatment of Alzheimer's disease. Front Mol Neurosci 2016;9. Available from: https://doi.org/10.3389/fnmol.2016.00053.

[48] Eisert R. Hypercarnivory and the brain: protein requirements of cats reconsidered. J Comp Physiol B 2011;181(1):1–17. Available from: https://doi.org/10.1007/s00360-010-0528-0.

[49] Milton K. Nutritional characteristics of wild primate foods: do the diets of our closest living relatives have lessons for us? Nutrition 1999;15 (6):488–98. Available from: https://doi.org/10.1016/S0899-9007(99)00078-7.

[50] Ben-Dor M, Sirtoli R, Barkai R. The evolution of the human trophic level during the pleistocene. Am J Phys Anthropol 2021;. Available from: https://doi.org/10.1002/ajpa.24247 ajpa.24247.

[51] Speth JD. Early hominid hunting and scavenging: the role of meat as an energy source. J Hum Evol 1989;18(4):329–43. Available from: https://doi.org/10.1016/0047-2484(89)90035-3.

[52] Aiello LC, Wheeler P. The expensive-tissue hypothesis: the brain and the digestive system in human and primate evolution. Curr Anthropol 1995;36(2):199–221. Available from: https://doi.org/10.1086/204350.

[53] Schönfeld P, Reiser G. Why does brain metabolism not favor burning of fatty acids to provide energy? - Reflections on disadvantages of the use of free fatty acids as fuel for brain. J Cereb Blood Flow Metab 2013;33(10):1493–9. Available from: https://doi.org/10.1038/jcbfm.2013.128.

[54] Hue L, Taegtmeyer H. The Randle cycle revisited: a new head for an old hat. Am J Physiol - Endocrinol Metab 2009;297(3):E578–91. Available from: https://doi.org/10.1152/ajpendo.00093.2009.

[55] Katz J, Tayek JA. Gluconeogenesis and the Cori Cycle in 12-, 20-, and 40-h-fasted humans. Am J Physiol Endocrinol Metab 1998;275(3): E537–42. Available from: https://doi.org/10.1152/ajpendo.1998.275.3.E537.

[56] Cahill GF, Owen OE. Starvation and survival. Trans Am Clin Climatological Assoc 1968;79:13–20.

[57] Kuo T, McQueen A, Chen T-C, Wang J-C. Regulation of glucose homeostasis by glucocorticoids. Adv Exp Med Biol 2015;872:99–126. Available from: https://doi.org/10.1007/978-1-4939-2895-8_5.

[58] Lignot J-H, LeMaho Y. A history of modern research into fasting, starvation, and inanition. In: McCue Marshall D, editor. Comparative physiology of fasting, starvation, and food limitation. Berlin, Heidelberg: Springer; 2012. p. 7–23. Available from: https://doi.org/10.1007/978-3-642-29056-5_2.

[59] Cherel Y, Robin J-P, Heitz A, Calgari C, Maho Yle. Relationships between lipid availability and protein utilization during prolonged fasting. J Comp Physiol B 1992;162(4):305–13. Available from: https://doi.org/10.1007/BF00260757.

[60] Townsend LK, Knuth CM, Wright DC. Cycling our way to fit fat. Physiol Rep 2017;5(7). Available from: https://doi.org/10.14814/phy2.13247.

[61] Slag MF, Ahmed M, Gannon MC, Nuttall FQ. Meal stimulation of cortisol secretion: a protein induced effect. Metabolism 1981;30 (11):1104–8. Available from: https://doi.org/10.1016/0026-0495(81)90055-X.

[62] Gibson AA, Seimon RV, Lee CMY, Ayre J, Franklin J, Markovic TP, et al. Do ketogenic diets really suppress appetite? A systematic review and meta-analysis: do ketogenic diets really suppress appetite? Obes Rev 2015;16(1):64–76. Available from: https://doi.org/10.1111/obr.12230.

[63] Guerci B, Benichou M, Floriot M, Bohme P, Fougnot S, Franck P, et al. Accuracy of an electrochemical sensor for measuring capillary blood ketones by fingerstick samples during metabolic deterioration after continuous subcutaneous insulin infusion interruption in Type 1 diabetic patients. Diabetes Care 2003;26(4):1137–41. Available from: https://doi.org/10.2337/diacare.26.4.1137.

[64] Williamson DH, Thornton PS. Chapter 43 - Ketone body production and metabolism in the fetus and neonate. In: Polin Richard A, Fox William W, Steven HAbman, editors. Fetal and neonatal physiology. 3rd ed. W.B. Saunders; 2004. p. 419–28. Available from: https://doi.org/10.1016/B978-0-7216-9654-6.50046-1.

[65] Suntrup III DJ, Ratto TV, Ratto M, McCarter JP. Characterization of a high-resolution breath acetone meter for ketosis monitoring. PeerJ 2020;8:e9969. Available from: https://doi.org/10.7717/peerj.9969.

[66] Alkedeh O, Priefer R. The ketogenic diet: breath acetone sensing technology. Biosensors 2021;11(1):26. Available from: https://doi.org/10.3390/bios11010026.

[67] Harano Y, Suzuki M, Kojima H, Kashiwagi A, Hidaka H, Shigeta Y. Development of paper-strip test for 3-hydroxybutyrate and its clinical application. Diabetes Care 1984;7(5):481–5. Available from: https://doi.org/10.2337/diacare.7.5.481.

[68] O'Hearn LA. Evidence on chronic ketosis in traditional arctic populations. J Evol Health 2019;3(1). Available from: https://doi.org/10.15310/2334-3591.1101.

[69] White H, Venkatesh B. Clinical review: ketones and brain injury. Crit Care 2011;15(2):219. Available from: https://doi.org/10.1186/cc10020.

[70] Cotter DG, Schugar RC, Crawford PA. Ketone body metabolism and cardiovascular disease. Am J Physiol Heart Circ Physiol 2013;304(8): H1060–76. Available from: https://doi.org/10.1152/ajpheart.00646.2012.

[71] Musa-Veloso K, Likhodii SS, Cunnane SC. Breath acetone is a reliable indicator of ketosis in adults consuming ketogenic meals. Am J Clin Nutr 2002;76(1):65–70. Available from: https://doi.org/10.1093/ajcn/76.1.65.

[72] Neal EG, Chaffe H, Schwartz RH, Lawson MS, Edwards N, Fitzsimmons G, et al. A randomized trial of classical and medium-chain triglyceride ketogenic diets in the treatment of childhood epilepsy. Epilepsia 2009;50(5):1109–17. Available from: https://doi.org/10.1111/j.1528-1167.2008.01870.x.

[73] Owen OE. Ketone bodies as a fuel for the brain during starvation. Biochem Mol Biol Educ 2005;33(4):246–51. Available from: https://doi.org/10.1002/bmb.2005.49403304246.

[74] Reichard GA, Haff AC, Skutches CL, Paul P, Holroyde CP, Owen OE. Plasma acetone metabolism in the fasting human. J Clin Investig 1979;63(4):619–26. Available from: https://doi.org/10.1172/JCI109344.

[75] Kalapos MP. Possible physiological roles of acetone metabolism in humans. Med Hypotheses 1999;53(3):236–42. Available from: https://doi.org/10.1054/mehy.1998.0752.

[76] Evans M, Cogan KE, Egan B. Metabolism of ketone bodies during exercise and training: physiological basis for exogenous supplementation. J Physiol 2017;595(9):2857–71. Available from: https://doi.org/10.1113/JP273185.

[77] Boninsegna A, Federspil G, De Palo C. The effect of muscular exercise on free fatty acids, acetoacetate and 3-hydroxybutyrate blood levels. Hormone Metab Res Horm Und Stoffwechselforschung Hormones Et Metabol 1974;6(6):488–91. Available from: https://doi.org/10.1055/s-0028-1093809.

[78] Bergstrom JD, Wong GA, Edwards PA, Edmond J. The regulation of acetoacetyl-CoA synthetase activity by modulators of cholesterol synthesis in vivo and the utilization of acetoacetate for cholesterogenesis. J Biol Chem 1984;259(23):14548–53.

[79] Geelen MJH, Lopes-Cardozo M, Edmond J. Acetoacetate: a major substrate for the synthesis of cholesterol and fatty acids by isolated rat hepatocytes. FEBS Lett 1983;163(2):269–73. Available from: https://doi.org/10.1016/0014-5793(83)80833-3.

[80] Cunnane SC, Menard CR, Likhodii SS, Brenna JT, Crawford MA. Carbon recycling into de novo lipogenesis is a major pathway in neonatal metabolism of linoleate and alpha-linolenate. Prostaglandins, Leukotrienes, Essent Fat Acids 1999;60(5–6):387–92. Available from: https://doi.org/10.1016/s0952-3278(99)80018-0.

[81] Muneta T. Ketone body elevation in placenta, umbilical cord, newborn and mother in normal delivery. Glycative Stress Res 2016;3(3):133–40.

[82] Cunnane SC, Crawford MA. Energetic and nutritional constraints on infant brain development: implications for brain expansion during human evolution. J Hum Evol 2014;77:88–98. Available from: https://doi.org/10.1016/j.jhevol.2014.05.001.

[83] Delplanque B, Gibson R, Koletzko B, Lapillonne A, Strandvik B. Lipid quality in infant nutrition: current knowledge and future opportunities. J Pediatric Gastroenterol Nutr 2015;61(1):8–17. Available from: https://doi.org/10.1097/MPG.0000000000000818.

[84] Puchalska P, Crawford PA. Multi-dimensional roles of ketone bodies in fuel metabolism, signaling, and therapeutics. Cell Metab 2017;25(2):262–84. Available from: https://doi.org/10.1016/j.cmet.2016.12.022.

[85] Feinman RD. The biochemistry of low-carbohydrate and ketogenic diets. Curr OpEndocrinol Diabetes Obes 2020;27(5):261–8. Available from: https://doi.org/10.1097/MED.0000000000000575.

[86] Berg, JM, Tymoczko, JL, Stryer, L. Gluconeogenesis and glycolysis are reciprocally regulated. Biochemistry. 5th ed., 2002. https://www.ncbi.nlm.nih.gov/books/NBK22423/.

[87] Salam WH, Wilcox HG, Cagen LM, Heimberg M. Stimulation of hepatic cholesterol biosynthesis by fatty acids. Effects of oleate on cytoplasmic acetoacetyl-CoA thiolase, acetoacetyl-CoA synthetase and hydroxymethylglutaryl-CoA synthase. Biochem J 1989;258(2):563–8. Available from: https://doi.org/10.1042/bj2580563.

[88] Browning JD, Horton JD. Fasting reduces plasma proprotein convertase, subtilisin/kexin type 9 and cholesterol biosynthesis in humans. J Lipid Res 2010;51(11):3359–63. Available from: https://doi.org/10.1194/jlr.P009860.

[89] Meidenbauer JJ, Mukherjee P, Seyfried TN. The glucose ketone index calculator: a simple tool to monitor therapeutic efficacy for metabolic management of brain cancer. Nutr Metab 2015;12:12. Available from: https://doi.org/10.1186/s12986-015-0009-2.

[90] Cantó C, Menzies KJ, Auwerx J. NAD+ metabolism and the control of energy homeostasis: a balancing act between mitochondria and the nucleus. Cell Metab 2015;22(1):31–53. Available from: https://doi.org/10.1016/j.cmet.2015.05.023.

[91] Speijer D. Being right on Q: shaping eukaryotic evolution. Biochem J 2016;473(22):4103–27. Available from: https://doi.org/10.1042/BCJ20160647.

[92] White AT, Schenk S. NAD+/NADH and skeletal muscle mitochondrial adaptations to exercise. Am J Physiol Endocrinol Metab 2012;303(3):E308–21. Available from: https://doi.org/10.1152/ajpendo.00054.2012.

[93] Anderson KA, Madsen AS, Olsen CA, Hirschey MD. Metabolic control by sirtuins and other enzymes that sense NAD+, NADH, or their ratio. Biochim Biophys Acta 2017;1858(12):991–8. Available from: https://doi.org/10.1016/j.bbabio.2017.09.005.

[94] Jokinen R, Pirnes-Karhu S, Pietiläinen KH, Pirinen E. Adipose tissue NAD+-homeostasis, sirtuins and poly(ADP-ribose) polymerases -important players in mitochondrial metabolism and metabolic health. Redox Biol 2017;12:246–63. Available from: https://doi.org/10.1016/j.redox.2017.02.011.

[95] Miller VJ, Villamena FA, Volek JS. Nutritional ketosis and mitohormesis: potential implications for mitochondrial function and human health. J Nutr Metab 2018;2018. Available from: https://doi.org/10.1155/2018/5157645.

[96] Bough KJ, Wetherington J, Hassel B, Pare JF, Gawryluk JW, Greene JG, et al. Mitochondrial biogenesis in the anticonvulsant mechanism of the ketogenic diet. Ann Neurol 2006;60(2):223–35. Available from: https://doi.org/10.1002/ana.20899.

[97] Garcia-Roves P, Huss JM, Han D-H, Hancock CR, Iglesias-Gutierrez E, Chen M, et al. Raising plasma fatty acid concentration induces increased biogenesis of mitochondria in skeletal muscle. Proc Natl Acad Sci U S Am 2007;104(25):10709–13. Available from: https://doi.org/10.1073/pnas.0704024104.

[98] Hancock CR, Han D-H, Chen M, Terada S, Yasuda T, Wright DC, et al. High-fat diets cause insulin resistance despite an increase in muscle mitochondria. Proc Natl Acad Sci 2008;105(22):7815–20. Available from: https://doi.org/10.1073/pnas.0802057105.

[99] Hasan-Olive MM, Lauritzen KH, Ali M, Rasmussen LJ, Storm-Mathisen J, Bergersen LH. A ketogenic diet improves mitochondrial biogenesis and bioenergetics via the PGC1α-SIRT3-UCP2 axis. Neurochem Res 2019;44(1):22–37. Available from: https://doi.org/10.1007/s11064-018-2588-6.

[100] Hassani A, Horvath R, Chinnery PF. Mitochondrial myopathies: developments in treatment. Curr OpNeurol 2010;23(5):459–65. Available from: https://doi.org/10.1097/WCO.0b013e32833d1096.

[101] Martín-Rodríguez S, de Pablos-Velasco P, Calbet JAL. Mitochondrial complex I inhibition by metformin: drug–exercise interactions. Trends Endocrinol Metab 2020;31(4):269–71. Available from: https://doi.org/10.1016/j.tem.2020.02.003.

[102] Fontaine E. Metformin-induced mitochondrial complex i inhibition: facts, uncertainties, and consequences. Front Endocrinol 2018;9:753. Available from: https://doi.org/10.3389/fendo.2018.00753.

[103] Levine DC, Hong H, Weidemann BJ, Ramsey KM, Affinati AH, Schmidt MS, et al. NAD + controls circadian reprogramming through PER2 nuclear translocation to counter aging. Mol Cell 2020;78(5):835–49. Available from: https://doi.org/10.1016/j.molcel.2020.04.010 e7.

[104] Xie N, Zhang L, Gao W, Huang C, Huber PE, Zhou X, et al. NAD + metabolism: pathophysiologic mechanisms and therapeutic potential. Signal Transduct Target Ther 2020;5(1):1–37. Available from: https://doi.org/10.1038/s41392-020-00311-7.

[105] Connell NJ, Houtkooper RH, Schrauwen P. NAD + metabolism as a target for metabolic health: have we found the silver bullet? Diabetologia 2019;62(6):888–99. Available from: https://doi.org/10.1007/s00125-019-4831-3.

[106] Roberts MN, Wallace MA, Tomilov AA, Zhou Z, Marcotte GR, Tran D, et al. A ketogenic diet extends longevity and healthspan in adult mice. Cell Metab 2017;26(3):539–46. Available from: https://doi.org/10.1016/j.cmet.2017.08.005 e5.

[107] Romero R, Erez O, Hüttemann M, Maymon E, Panaitescu B, Conde-Agudelo A, et al. Metformin, the aspirin of the 21st century: its role in gestational diabetes, prevention of preeclampsia and cancer, and the promotion of longevity. Am J Obstet Gynecol 2017;217(3):282–302. Available from: https://doi.org/10.1016/j.ajog.2017.06.003.

[108] Mallick R, Basak S, Duttaroy AK. Docosahexaenoic acid, 22:6n-3: its roles in the structure and function of the brain. Int J Dev Neurosci 2019;79(1):21–31. Available from: https://doi.org/10.1016/j.ijdevneu.2019.10.004.

[109] Salem N, Litman B, Kim H-Y, Gawrisch K. Mechanisms of action of docosahexaenoic acid in the nervous system. Lipids 2001;36 (9):945–59. Available from: https://doi.org/10.1007/s11745-001-0805-6.

[110] Fraser DD, Whiting S, Andrew RD, Macdonald EA, Musa-Veloso K, Cunnane SC. Elevated polyunsaturated fatty acids in blood serum obtained from children on the ketogenic diet. Neurology 2003;60(6):1026–9. Available from: https://doi.org/10.1212/01.WNL.0000049974.74242.C6.

[111] Ruskin DN, Kawamura M, Masino SA. Reduced pain and inflammation in juvenile and adult rats fed a ketogenic diet. PLoS ONE 2009;4(12). Available from: https://doi.org/10.1371/journal.pone.0008349.

[112] Shen Y, Kapfhamer D, Minnella AM, Kim J-E, Won SJ, Chen Y, et al. Bioenergetic state regulates innate inflammatory responses through the transcriptional co-repressor CtBP. Nat Commun 2017;8(1):624. Available from: https://doi.org/10.1038/s41467-017-00707-0.

[113] Kim DY, Hao J, Liu R, Turner G, Shi F-D, Rho JM. Inflammation-mediated memory dysfunction and effects of a ketogenic diet in a murine model of multiple sclerosis 5In: Villoslada P, editor. PLoS ONE, 7. 2012. p. e35476. Available from: https://doi.org/10.1371/journal.pone.0035476.

[114] Spaulding SW, Chopra IJ, Sherwin RS, Lyall SS. Effect of caloric restriction and dietary composition on serum T3 and reverse T3 in man. J Clin Endocrinol Metab 1976;42(1):197–200. Available from: https://doi.org/10.1210/jcem-42-1-197.

[115] Danforth E, Horton ES, O'Connell M, Sims EA, Burger AG, Ingbar SH, et al. Dietary-induced alterations in thyroid hormone metabolism during overnutrition. J Clin Investig 1979;64(5):1336–47. Available from: https://doi.org/10.1172/JCI109590.

[116] Phinney SD, Bistrian BR, Wolfe RR, Blackburn GL. The human metabolic response to chronic ketosis without caloric restriction: physical and biochemical adaptation. Metabol Clin Exp 1983;32(8):757–68.

[117] Yang MU, van Itallie TB. Variability in body protein loss during protracted, severe caloric restriction: role of triiodothyronine and other possible determinants. Am J Clin Nutr 1984;40(3):611–22. Available from: https://doi.org/10.1093/ajcn/40.3.611.

[118] Kaptein EM, Janis SF, Duda MJ, Nicoloff JT, Drenick EJ. Relationship between the changes in serum thyroid hormone levels and protein status during prolonged protein supplemented caloric deprivation. Clin Endocrinol 1985;22(1):1–15. Available from: https://doi.org/10.1111/j.1365-2265.1985.tb01059.x.

[119] Alexander WD, Harrison MT, Harden RMG, Koutras DA. The effect of total fasting on thyroid function in man. Metabolism 1964;13 (7):587–90. Available from: https://doi.org/10.1016/0026-0495(64)90067-8.

[120] Heyden JTvan der, Docter R, van Toor H, Wilson JH, Hennemann G, Krenning EP. Effects of caloric deprivation on thyroid hormone tissue uptake and generation of low-T3 syndrome. Am J Physiol Endocrinol Metab 1986;251(2):E156–63. Available from: https://doi.org/10.1152/ajpendo.1986.251.2.E156.

[121] Kopp W. Nutrition, evolution and thyroid hormone levels – a link to iodine deficiency disorders? Med Hypotheses 2004;62(6):871–5. Available from: https://doi.org/10.1016/j.mehy.2004.02.033.

[122] Neal EG, Zupec-Kania B, Pfeifer HH. Carnitine, nutritional supplementation and discontinuation of ketogenic diet therapies. Epilepsy Res 2012;100(3):267–71. Available from: https://doi.org/10.1016/j.eplepsyres.2012.04.021.

[123] Berry-Kravis E, Booth G, Sanchez AC, Woodbury-Kolb J. Carnitine levels and the ketogenic diet. Epilepsia 2001;42(11):1445–51. Available from: https://doi.org/10.1046/j.1528-1157.2001.18001.x.

[124] Institute of Medicine (US) Panel on Micronutrients. Dietary Reference Intakes for Vitamin A, Vitamin K, Arsenic, Boron, Chromium, Copper, Iodine, Iron, Manganese, Molybdenum, Nickel, Silicon, Vanadium, and Zinc. Washington (DC): National Academies Press (US); 2001a. 12, Zinc. Available from: https://www.ncbi.nlm.nih.gov/books/NBK222317/.

[125] Institute of Medicine (US) Panel on Micronutrients. Manganese. Dietary Reference Intakes for Vitamin A, Vitamin K, Arsenic, Boron, Chromium, Copper, Iodine, Iron, Manganese, Molybdenum, Nickel, Silicon, Vanadium, and Zinc. National Academies Press (US), 2001b. https://www.ncbi.nlm.nih.gov/books/NBK222332/.

[126] Hill MJ. Intestinal flora and endogenous vitamin synthesis. Eur J Cancer Prev: Off J Eur Cancer Prevent Organ (ECP) 1997;6(Suppl 1): S43–5. Available from: https://doi.org/10.1097/00008469-199703001-00009.

[127] Klipstein FA, Michael Samloff I. Folate synthesis by intestinal bacteria. Am J Clin Nutr 1966;19(4):237–46. Available from: https://doi.org/10.1093/ajcn/19.4.237.

[128] Giovannetti PM. Effect of coprophagy on nutrition. Nutr Res 1982;2(3):335–49. Available from: https://doi.org/10.1016/S0271-5317(82)80015-8.

[129] Stevens CE, Hume ID. Contributions of microbes in vertebrate gastrointestinal tract to production and conservation of nutrients. Physiol Rev 1998;78(2):393–427. Available from: https://doi.org/10.1152/physrev.1998.78.2.393.

[130] Engevik, Melinda A, Morra CN, Röth D, Engevik K, Spinler JK, Devaraj S, et al. Microbial metabolic capacity for intestinal folate production and modulation of host folate receptors. Front Microbiol 2019;10:2305. Available from: https://doi.org/10.3389/fmicb.2019.02305.

[131] Kok DE, Steegenga WT, Smid EJ, Zoetendal EG, Ulrich CM, Kampman E. Bacterial folate biosynthesis and colorectal cancer risk: more than just a gut feeling. Crit Rev Food Sci Nutr 2020;60(2):244–56. Available from: https://doi.org/10.1080/10408398.2018.1522499.

[132] Aksungar FB, Topkaya AE, Akyildiz M. Interleukin-6, C-reactive protein and biochemical parameters during prolonged intermittent fasting. Ann Nutr Metab 2007;51(1):88–95. Available from: https://doi.org/10.1159/000100954.

[133] Mardinoglu A, Wu H, Bjornson E, Zhang C, Hakkarainen A, Räsänen SM, et al. An integrated understanding of the rapid metabolic benefits of a carbohydrate-restricted diet on hepatic steatosis in humans. Cell Metab 2018;27(3):559–71. Available from: https://doi.org/10.1016/j.cmet.2018.01.005 e5.

[134] Urbain P, Strom L, Morawski L, Wehrle A, Deibert P, Bertz H. Impact of a 6-week non-energy-restricted ketogenic diet on physical fitness, body composition and biochemical parameters in healthy adults. Nutr Metab 2017;14. Available from: https://doi.org/10.1186/s12986-017-0175-5.

[135] Alrubaye HS, Kohl KD. Abundance and compositions of B-vitamin-producing microbes in the mammalian gut vary based on feeding strategies. MSystems 2021;e0031321. Available from: https://doi.org/10.1128/mSystems.00313-21.

[136] Nutrition Division. Human vitamin and mineral requirements: Report of a joint FAO/WHO expert consultation, Bangkok, Thailand. Training Materials for Agricultural Planning 1014. Rome, Italy: FAO & WHO, 2002. https://www.fao.org/documents/card/en/c/ceec621b-1396-57bb-8b35-48a60d7faaed/.

[137] Schatzker M. The end of craving: recovering the lost wisdom of eating well. Simon and Schuster; 2021.

[138] Pannia E, Cho CE, Kubant R, Sánchez-Hernández D, Huot PSP, Chatterjee D, et al. A high multivitamin diet fed to wistar rat dams during pregnancy increases maternal weight gain later in life and alters homeostatic, hedonic and peripheral regulatory systems of energy balance. Behav Brain Res 2015;278:1–11. Available from: https://doi.org/10.1016/j.bbr.2014.09.019.

[139] Szeto IMY, Huot PSP, Reza-López SA, Jahan-mihan A, Anderson GH. The effect of high multivitamin diet during pregnancy on food intake and glucose metabolism in wistar rat offspring fed low-vitamin diets post weaning. J Dev Orig Health Dis 2011;2(5):302–10. Available from: https://doi.org/10.1017/S2040174411000523.

[140] Szeto IMY, Aziz A, Das PJ, Taha AY, Okubo N, Reza-Lopez S, et al. High multivitamin intake by wistar rats during pregnancy results in increased food intake and components of the metabolic syndrome in male offspring. Am J Physiol-Regulat Integr Comp Physiol 2008;295(2):R575–82. Available from: https://doi.org/10.1152/ajpregu.90354.2008.

[141] Zhou S-S, Zhou Y. Excess vitamin intake: an unrecognized risk factor for obesity. World J Diabetes 2014;5(1):1–13. Available from: https://doi.org/10.4239/wjd.v5.i1.1.

[142] Johnson RJ, Andrews P. Fructose, uricase, and the back-to-Africa hypothesis. Evolut Anthropol Issues, News, Rev 2010;19(6):250–7. Available from: https://doi.org/10.1002/evan.20266.

[143] Hundley JM. Influence of fructose and other carbohydrates on the niacin requirement of the rat. J Biol Chem 1949;181(1):1–9. Available from: https://doi.org/10.1016/S0021-9258(18)56617-5.

[144] Harper AE. Evolution of recommended dietary allowances–new directions? Annu Rev Nutr 1987;7:509–37. Available from: https://doi.org/10.1146/annurev.nu.07.070187.002453.

[145] Padayatty SJ, Levine M. Vitamin C physiology: the known and the unknown and goldilocks. Oral Dis 2016;22(6):463–93. Available from: https://doi.org/10.1111/odi.12446.

[146] O'Hearn LA. Ketogenic diets, caloric restriction, and hormones. J Evol Health 2018;2(3). Available from: https://doi.org/10.15310/2334-3591.1093.

[147] Mozaffarian D, Rosenberg I, Uauy R. History of modern nutrition science—implications for current research, dietary guidelines, and food policy. BMJ 2018;361:k2392. Available from: https://doi.org/10.1136/bmj.k2392.

[148] Allen, L., World Health Organization, and Food and Agriculture Organization of the United Nations. Guidelines on Food Fortification with Micronutrients. Geneva; Rome: World Health Organization; Food and Agriculture Organization of the United Nations, 2006. http://catalog.hathitrust.org/api/volumes/oclc/152582146.html.

[149] O'Hearn A. Can a carnivore diet provide all essential nutrients? Curr OpEndocrinol, Diabetes Obes 2020;27(5):312–16. Available from: https://doi.org/10.1097/MED.0000000000000576.

[150] O'Hearn LA. My case against uricase: a critical examination of hypotheses. J Evol Health: Ancestral Health Soc Publ 2020;4(1). Available from: https://doi.org/10.15310/J34145990.

[151] Scott KJ, Rodriquez-Amaya D. Pro-vitamin A carotenoid conversion factors: retinol equivalents – fact or fiction? Food Chem 2000;69:125–7.

[152] Cofnas N. Is vegetarianism healthy for children? Crit Rev Food Sci Nutr 2019;59(13):2052–60. Available from: https://doi.org/10.1080/10408398.2018.1437024.

[153] Gulec S, Gregory JA, James FC. Mechanistic and regulatory aspects of intestinal iron absorption. Am J Physiol - Gastrointest Liver Physiol 2014;307(4):G397–409. Available from: https://doi.org/10.1152/ajpgi.00348.2013.

[154] Ganz T. Hepcidin—a regulator of intestinal iron absorption and iron recycling by macrophages. Best Pract Res Clin Haematol Iron Dis 2005;18(2):171–82. Available from: https://doi.org/10.1016/j.beha.2004.08.020.

[155] Kiely ME. Risks and benefits of vegan and vegetarian diets in children. Proc Nutr Soc 2021;80(2):159–64. Available from: https://doi.org/10.1017/S002966512100001X.

[156] Pradeu T. Philosophy of immunology. 1st ed. Cambridge University Press; 2019. Available from: https://doi.org/10.1017/9781108616706.

[157] Hadley KB, Ryan AS, Forsyth S, Gautier S, Salem N. The essentiality of arachidonic acid in infant development. Nutrients 2016;8(4). Available from: https://doi.org/10.3390/nu8040216.

[158] Jasani, B, Simmer, K, Patole, SK, and Rao, SC. Long chain polyunsaturated fatty acid supplementation in infants born at Term. Edited by Cochrane Neonatal Group. Cochrane Database of Systematic Reviews, March 10, 2017. https://doi.org/10.1002/14651858.CD000376.pub4.

[159] Craig WJ. Phytochemicals: guardians of our health. J Am Dietetic Assoc 1997;97(10):S199–204. Available from: https://doi.org/10.1016/S0002-8223(97)00765-7 Supplement.

[160] Liu RH. Potential synergy of phytochemicals in cancer prevention: mechanism of action. J Nutr 2004;134(12):3479S–85S. Available from: https://doi.org/10.1093/jn/134.12.3479S.

[161] Nahar L, Xiao J, Sarker SD. Introduction of phytonutrients. In: Xiao Jianbo, Sarker Satyajit D, Asakawa Yoshinori, editors. Handbook of dietary phytochemicals. Singapore: Springer Singapore; 2020. p. 1–17. Available from: https://doi.org/10.1007/978-981-13-1745-3_2-1.

[162] Bouayed J, Bohn T. Exogenous antioxidants—double-edged swords in cellular redox state. Oxid Med Cell Longev 2010;3(4):228–37. Available from: https://doi.org/10.4161/oxim.3.4.12858.

[163] Pallauf K, Rimbach G, Rupp PM, Chin D, Wolf IMA. Resveratrol and lifespan in model organisms. Curr Med Chem 2016;23(41):4639–80. Available from: https://doi.org/10.2174/0929867323666161024151233.

[164] Weiskirchen S, Weiskirchen R. Resveratrol: how much wine do you have to drink to stay healthy?123. Adv Nutr 2016;7(4):706–18. Available from: https://doi.org/10.3945/an.115.011627.

[165] Houghton CA, Fassett RG, Coombes JS. Sulforaphane and other nutrigenomic Nrf2 activators: can the clinician's expectation be matched by the reality? Oxid Med Cell Longev 2016;(2016). Available from: https://doi.org/10.1155/2016/7857186.

[166] Nishimuro H, Ohnishi H, Sato M, Ohnishi-Kameyama M, Matsunaga I, Naito S, et al. Estimated daily intake and seasonal food sources of quercetin in Japan. Nutrients 2015;7(4):2345–58. Available from: https://doi.org/10.3390/nu7042345.

[167] Mabry ME, Turner-Hissong SD, Gallagher EY, McAlvay AC, An H, Edger PP, et al. The evolutionary history of wild, domesticated, and feral Brassica Oleracea (Brassicaceae). Mol Biol Evol 2021;38(10):4419–34. Available from: https://doi.org/10.1093/molbev/msab183.

[168] McNaughton SA, Marks GC. Development of a food composition database for the estimation of dietary intakes of glucosinolates, the biologically active constituents of cruciferous vegetables. Br J Nutr 2003;90(3):687–97. Available from: https://doi.org/10.1079/BJN2003917.

[169] Felker P, Bunch R, Leung AM. Concentrations of thiocyanate and goitrin in human plasma, their precursor concentrations in brassica vegetables, and associated potential risk for hypothyroidism. Nutr Rev 2016;74(4):248–58. Available from: https://doi.org/10.1093/nutrit/nuv110.

[170] Loft S, Møller P, Cooke MS, Rozalski R, Olinski R. Antioxidant vitamins and cancer risk: is oxidative damage to DNA a relevant biomarker? Eur J Nutr 2008;47(S2):19–28. Available from: https://doi.org/10.1007/s00394-008-2004-0.

[171] Maher J, Yamamoto M. The rise of antioxidant signaling—the evolution and hormetic actions of Nrf2. Toxicol Appl Pharmacol 2010;244(1):4–15. Available from: https://doi.org/10.1016/j.taap.2010.01.011.

[172] Peoples JN, Saraf A, Ghazal N, Pham TT, Kwong JQ. Mitochondrial dysfunction and oxidative stress in heart disease. Exp Mol Med 2019;51(12):1–13. Available from: https://doi.org/10.1038/s12276-019-0355-7.

[173] Maritim AC, Sanders RA, Watkins III JB. Diabetes, oxidative stress, and antioxidants: a review. J Biochem Mol Toxicol 2003;17(1):24–38. Available from: https://doi.org/10.1002/jbt.10058.

[174] Sosa V, Moliné T, Somoza R, Paciucci R, Kondoh H, Leonart MEL. Oxidative stress and cancer: an overview. Ageing Res Rev Spec Issue: Invertebr Model Aging 2013;12(1):376–90. Available from: https://doi.org/10.1016/j.arr.2012.10.004.

[175] Ghezzi P, Ghiara V, Davies K. Epistemological challenges of the oxidative stress theory of disease and the problem of biomarkers. Oxidative stress. Elsevier; 2020. p. 13–27. Available from: https://doi.org/10.1016/B978-0-12-818606-0.00002-X.

[176] Finkel T. Signal transduction by reactive oxygen species. J Cell Biol 2011;194(1):7–15. Available from: https://doi.org/10.1083/jcb.201102095.

[177] Speijer D, Manjeri GR, Szklarczyk R. How to deal with oxygen radicals stemming from mitochondrial fatty acid oxidation. Philos Trans R Soc B: Biol Sci 2014;369(1646):20130446. Available from: https://doi.org/10.1098/rstb.2013.0446.

[178] Thannickal VJ, Fanburg BL. Reactive oxygen species in cell signaling. Am J Physiol-Lung Cell Mol Physiol 2000;279(6):L1005–28. Available from: https://doi.org/10.1152/ajplung.2000.279.6.L1005.

[179] Kaspar JW, Niture SK, Jaiswal AK. Nrf2:INrf2 (Keap1) signaling in oxidative stress. Free Radic Biol Med Spec Issue Redox Signal 2009;47(9):1304–9. Available from: https://doi.org/10.1016/j.freeradbiomed.2009.07.035.

[180] Ma Q. Role of Nrf2 in oxidative stress and toxicity. Annu Rev Pharmacol Toxicol 2013;53:401–26. Available from: https://doi.org/10.1146/annurev-pharmtox-011112-140320.

[181] Staurengo-Ferrari L, Badaro-Garcia S, Hohmann MSN, Manchope MF, Zaninelli TH, Casagrande R, et al. Contribution of Nrf2 modulation to the mechanism of action of analgesic and anti-inflammatory drugs in pre-clinical and clinical stages. Front Pharmacol 2019;9. Available from: https://www.frontiersin.org/article/10.3389/fphar.2018.01536.

[182] Calabrese EJ. Hormesis and medicine. Br J Clin Pharmacol 2008;66(5):594–617. Available from: https://doi.org/10.1111/j.1365-2125.2008.03243.x.

[183] Milder JB, Liang L-P, Patel M. Acute oxidative stress and systemic Nrf2 activation by the ketogenic diet. Neurobiol Dis 2010;40(1):238–44. Available from: https://doi.org/10.1016/j.nbd.2010.05.030.

[184] O'Hearn LA. The therapeutic properties of ketogenic diets, slow-wave sleep, and circadian synchrony. Curr OpEndocrinol Diabetes Obes 2021;28:503–8. Available from: https://doi.org/10.1097/MED.0000000000000660.

[185] Laidlaw SA, Shultz TD, Cecchino JT, Kopple JD. Plasma and urine taurine levels in vegans. Am J Clin Nutr 1988;47(4):660–3. Available from: https://doi.org/10.1093/ajcn/47.4.660.

[186] Lourenço R, Camilo ME. Taurine: a conditionally essential amino acid in humans? An overview in health and disease. Nutr Hosp 2002;9.

[187] Stapleton PP, Charles RP, Redmond HP, Bouchier-Hayes DJ. Taurine and human nutrition. Clin Nutr 1997;16(3):103–8. Available from: https://doi.org/10.1016/S0261-5614(97)80234-8.

[188] Schuller-Levis GB, Park E. Taurine: new implications for an old amino acid. FEMS Microbiol Lett 2003;226(2):195–202. Available from: https://doi.org/10.1016/S0378-1097(03)00611-6.

[189] Sturman JA. Taurine in Development. Physiolog Rev 1993;73(1):119–47. Available from: https://doi.org/10.1152/physrev.1993.73.1.119.

[190] Schaffer S, Kim HW. Effects and mechanisms of taurine as a therapeutic agent. Biomol Therapeutics 2018;26(3):225–41. Available from: https://doi.org/10.4062/biomolther.2017.251.

[191] Bouckenooghe T, Remacle C, Reusens B. Is taurine a functional nutrient? Curr OpClNutr Metab Care 2006;9(6):728–33. Available from: https://doi.org/10.1097/01.mco.0000247469.26414.55.

[192] McCarty MF. The low-age content of low-fat vegan diets could benefit diabetics – though concurrent taurine supplementation may be needed to minimize endogenous AGE production. Med Hypotheses 2005;64(2):394–8. Available from: https://doi.org/10.1016/j.mehy.2004.03.035.

[193] Yamori Y, Taguchi T, Hamada A, Kunimasa K, Mori H, Mori M. Taurine in health and diseases: consistent evidence from experimental and epidemiological studies. J Biomed Sci 2010;17(Suppl 1):S6. Available from: https://doi.org/10.1186/1423-0127-17-S1-S6.

[194] Murakami S, Ono A, Kawasaki A, Takenaga T, Ito T. Taurine attenuates the development of hepatic steatosis through the inhibition of oxidative stress in a model of nonalcoholic fatty liver disease in vivo and in vitro. Amino Acids 2018;50(9):1279–88. Available from: https://doi.org/10.1007/s00726-018-2605-8.

[195] Zvenigorodskaia LA, Ovsiannikova ON, Noskova KK, Nilova TV, Elizarova EP. [Taurine in the treatment of non-alcoholic fatty liver disease]. Eksperimental'naia I Klinicheskaia Gastroenterol Exp Clin Gastroenterol 2010;7:43–50.

[196] Yamori Y, Liu L, Mori M, Sagara M, Murakami S, Nara Y, et al. Taurine as the nutritional factor for the longevity of the japanese revealed by a world-wide epidemiological survey In *Taurine 7*In: Azuma J, Schaffer SW, Ito T, editors. Advances in experimental medicine and biology, 643. New York, NY: Springer New York; 2009. Available from: https://doi.org/10.1007/978-0-387-75681-3_2.

[197] Lombard KA, Olson AL, Nelson SE, Rebouche CJ. Carnitine status of lactoovovegetarians and strict vegetarian adults and children. Am J Clin Nutr 1989;50(2):301–6. Available from: https://doi.org/10.1093/ajcn/50.2.301.

[198] Stephens FB, Marimuthu K, Cheng Y, Patel N, Constantin D, Simpson EJ, et al. Vegetarians have a reduced skeletal muscle carnitine transport capacity. Am J Clin Nutr 2011;94(3):938–44. Available from: https://doi.org/10.3945/ajcn.111.012047.

[199] Higdon, J. L-Carnitine. Linus Pauling Institute, April 23, 2014. https://lpi.oregonstate.edu/mic/dietary-factors/L-carnitine.

[200] Kendler BS. Carnitine: an overview of its role in preventive medicine. Preventive Med 1986;15(4):373–90. Available from: https://doi.org/10.1016/0091-7435(86)90005-8.

[201] Flanagan JL, Simmons PA, Vehige J, Willcox MDP, Garrett Q. Role of carnitine in disease. Nutr Metab 2010;7(1):30. Available from: https://doi.org/10.1186/1743-7075-7-30.

[202] Laviano A, Meguid MM, Guijarro A, Muscaritoli M, Cascino A, Preziosa I, et al. Antimyopathic effects of carnitine and nicotine. Curr OpClNutr Metab Care 2006;9(4):442–8. Available from: https://doi.org/10.1097/01.mco.0000232905.89662.60.

[203] Hess JR, Greenberg NA. The role of nucleotides in the immune and gastrointestinal systems. Nutr ClPract 2012;27(2):281–94. Available from: https://doi.org/10.1177/0884533611434933.

[204] György P. Biochemical aspects of human milk. Am J Clin Nutr 1971;24(8):970–5. Available from: https://doi.org/10.1093/ajcn/24.8.970.

[205] Sato N, Murakami Y, Nakano T, Sugawara M, Kawakami H, Idota T, et al. Effects of dietary nucleotides on lipid metabolism and learning ability of rats. Biosci Biotechnol Biochem 1995;59(7):1267–71. Available from: https://doi.org/10.1271/bbb.59.1267.

[206] Chen T-H, Huang H-P, Matsumoto Y, Wu S-H, Wang M-F, Chung S-Y, et al. Effects of dietary nucleoside-nucleotide mixture on memory in aged and young memory deficient mice. Life Sci 1996;59(21):PL325–30. Available from: https://doi.org/10.1016/0024-3205(96)00526-7.

[207] Xu M, Liang R, Guo Q, Wang S, Zhao M, Zhang Z, et al. Dietary nucleotides extend the life span in Sprague-Dawley rats. J Nutr Health Aging 2013;17(3):223–9. Available from: https://doi.org/10.1007/s12603-012-0399-z.

[208] Nunez MC, Ayudarte MV, Morales D, Suarez MD, Gil A. Effect of dietary nucleotides on intestinal repair in rats with experimental chronic diarrhea. J Parenter Enter Nutr 1990;14(6):598–604. Available from: https://doi.org/10.1177/0148607190014006598.

[209] Ogita, K, Suita, S, Taguchi, T, Yamanouchi, T, Masumoto, K, Nakao, M. Roles of nucleosides and nucleotide mixture in small bowel transplantation, 18, no. 4, 2002: 5.

[210] Ortega MA, Nuněz MC, Gil A, Sánchez-Pozo A. Dietary nucleotides accelerate intestinal recovery after food deprivation in old rats. J Nutr 1995;125(6):1413–18. Available from: https://doi.org/10.1093/jn/125.6.1413.

[211] Uauy R, Stringel G, Thomas R, Quan R. Effect of dietary nucleosides on growth and maturation of the developing gut in the rat. J Pediatric Gastroenterol Nutr 1990;10(4):497–503. Available from: https://doi.org/10.1097/00005176-199005000-00014.

[212] Bueno J, Torres M, Almendros A, Carmona R, Nuñez MC, Rios A, et al. Effect of dietary nucleotides on small intestinal repair after diarrhoea. histological and ultrastructural changes. Gut 1994;35(7):926–33.

[213] Schlesinger N, Norquist JM, Watson DJ. Serum urate during acute gout. J Rheumatol 2009;36(6):1287–9. Available from: https://doi.org/10.3899/jrheum.080938.

[214] Waldron M, Patterson SD, Tallent J, Jeffries O. The effects of oral taurine on resting blood pressure in humans: a meta-analysis. Curr Hypertension Rep 2018;20(9):81. Available from: https://doi.org/10.1007/s11906-018-0881-z.

[215] Goa KL, Brogden RN. L-carnitine. Drugs 1987;34(1):1–24. Available from: https://doi.org/10.2165/00003495-198734010-00001.

Further reading

Banting, W. Letter on corpulence, addressed to the public. (3rd ed.), Harrison, 1864.

Goff DC, Lloyd-Jones DM, Bennett G, Coady S, D'Agostino RB, Gibbons R, et al.American College of Cardiology/American Heart Association Task Force on Practice Guidelines 2013 ACC/AHA guideline on the assessment of cardiovascular risk: a report of the American College of Cardiology/American Heart Association Task Force on Practice Guidelines. Circulation 2014;129(25 Suppl 2):S49–73. Available from: https://doi.org/10.1161/01.cir.0000437741.48606.98.

Westman EC, Feinman RD, Mavropoulos JC, Vernon MC, Volek JS, Wortman JA, et al. Low-carbohydrate nutrition and metabolism. Am J Clin Nutr 2007;86(2):276–84. Available from: https://doi.org/10.1093/ajcn/86.2.276.

Part 2

Medical nutritional therapy

Chapter 3

Endocrine

Robert Cywes[1], Hassina Kajee[2], Neville Wellington[2,3,4], Mark Cucuzzella[5], Karen Riley[6], Diana Isaacs[7], Nadia Pataguana[8], Ian Lake[9,10,11], Laurie Rauch[12], Sean McKelvey[6], William S. Yancy, Jr.[13,14,15], Susan Wolver[16], Campbell Murdoch[17], Brian Lenzkes[18], Caroline Roberts[19], David Cavan[20], David Unwin[21], Eric C. Westman[22], Miriam Berchuk[23], Graham Phillips[24], Ali Irshad Al Lawati[25], Nafeeza Hj Mohd Ismail[26], Daniel Katambo[27] and Anne-Sophie Brazeau[28]

[1]JSAPA Metabolic Centre, Jupiter, FL, United States, [2]Nutrition Network, Cape Town, South Africa, [3]Private Practice, Cape Town, South Africa, [4]Kenilworth Diabetes Medical Centre, Cape Town, South Africa, [5]West Virginia University School of Medicine, Morgantown, WV, United States, [6]Institute for Personalized Nutrition Therapy, Vancouver, Canada, [7]Cleveland Clinic, Cleveland, OH, United States, [8]Public Health Collaboration, United Kingdom, [9]Aspen Medical Practice, Gloucester, United Kingdom, [10]Everyone Health, Cambridge, United Kingdom, [11]The Fasting Method, New York City, NY, United States, [12]Physiological Sciences, Faculty of Health Sciences, University of Cape Town, Cape Town, South Africa, [13]Division of General Internal Medicine, Department of Medicine, Duke University Medical Centre, Durham, NC, United States, [14]Center of Innovation to Accelerate Discovery and Practice Transformation, Durham Veterans Affairs Medical Centre, Durham, NC, United States, [15]Duke Diet and Fitness Centre, Duke University Health System, Durham, NC, United States, [16]VCU Medical Weight Loss Program, Richmond, VA, United States, [17]Millbrook Surgery, Somerset, United Kingdom, [18]Internal Medicine, San Diego, CA, United States, [19]Virta Health, Denver, CO, United States, [20]Independent consultant, London, United Kingdom, [21]Norwood Surgery, Southport, United Kingdom, [22]Division of General Internal Medicine, Department of Medicine, Duke University Medical Centre, Durham, NC, United States, [23]Alberta Health Services, Calgary, Alberta, Canada, [24]iHeart Pharmacy Group, Hertfordshire, United Kingdom, [25]Diwan of Royal Court, Muscat, Oman, [26]School of Medicine, International Medical University, Kuala Lumpur, Federal Territory of Kuala Lumpur, Malaysia, [27]Afyaplanet, Dagoretti Corner, Nairobi, Kenya, [12]McGill University, Montreal, Canada

3.1 Introduction

Endocrine dysregulation is the hallmark of modern chronic disease, with insulin resistance (IR) playing a central role. Research surrounding treatments to such disorders are complicated due to complex hormonal regulation of homoeostasis, with the liver playing a central role. Yet recognising the common pathology provides a more universally applicable approach to treatment: the target and regulation of insulin. Therapeutic carbohydrate restriction (TCR) has efficacy in regulating insulin, often without the need for, or with the deprescription of, pharmacotherapeutics. The most evidence for TCR focuses on its induced remission of metabolic syndrome (MetS), IR, and type 2 diabetes (T2D). Emerging research also supports its use for type 1 diabetes (T1D), polycystic ovarian syndrome (PCOS) and the regulation of the thyroid and the hypothalamic-pituitary-adrenal-axis. Overall, TCR is promising in the treatment of endocrine disorders, often surpassing many medications prescribed to treat them.

3.2 Liver

Robert Cywes

3.2.1 Introduction

3.2.1.1 Description – the normal human liver

The human body is driven by cellular energy demands. There are two metabolic systems: the enterohepatic portal venous system and the systemic system. The liver as the system interface has unique anatomy allowing it to fulfil this role. The liver has no sensory or motor nervous control and only minor autonomic influence. Denervation after liver transplantation does not appear to affect liver function [1,2]. It is primarily a hormonal homoeostasis organ that receives systemic hormonal feedback. The enterohepatic system accommodates ebb and flow while the systemic system demands stability, though having a degree of tolerance. However, chronic hormonal imbalance of either system causes global metabolic dysfunction.

Blood supply is critical to understand metabolism and nutrition. The liver receives 25% of the body's total blood volume per minute. All blood from the intestine, pancreas, and spleen flows via the portal vein (PV) supplying

Ketogenic. DOI: https://doi.org/10.1016/B978-0-12-821617-0.00010-3

75%–80%, while the hepatic artery provides 20%–25% nutrient-depleted blood returning from systemic circulation [3]. The liver derives oxygenation via the hepatic artery while most nutrients and gastro-intestinal hormones traffic directly to the liver from the intestine via the PV.

Adipocyte-derived fatty acids (FAs) return lipoproteins and autophaged cellular debris traffics via the hepatic artery or indirectly via the PV after filtration in the intestine. This unique vascular flow pattern makes the intestine and liver the primary regulator of nutrient production and release. Nutrient-rich blood traverses the following path throughout the body:

Liver → Heart → Dilutes with nutrient-depleted blood → Pulmonary capillary bed → Heart → Rest of body via capillary network, including intestinal/pancreatic capillaries → Liver

The greatest nutrient gradient is between the PV coming to the liver and the hepatic veins leaving the liver: rich during meals and depleted between meals. The liver is also a rich manufacturing and nutrient storage organ, including glycogen, proteins, and fats. Several somatic hormones regulate storage, production, degradation, release and uptake of nutrients by the liver following the feeding-fasting cycle as well as a circadian cycle [4]. For example, the Dawn Effect is an early morning predominantly cortisol-induced override of glycogenolysis and glucose release that results in a transient but normal blood glucose (BG) surge [5].

3.2.2 Pathophysiology

3.2.2.1 Chronic excessive carbohydrate consumption and snacking

Metabolically, the human body is regulated by a complex hormonal system influenced by nutrient demand, supply and storage. Prolonged disruption of hormonal cycling uncouples the feedback pathways leading to variable diseases. In an age of perpetual abundance, the greatest metabolic disruption to hepatic pathophysiology is driven by chronic excessive carbohydrate consumption (CECC) exacerbated by pro-inflammatory polyunsaturated fatty acids (PUFAs) common in processed foods [6].

Normally, feeding triggers insulin release enhancing global cellular glucose uptake, suppressing glucose production, activating de novo lipogenesis (DNL) in the liver and adipocytes while blocking lipoprotein lipase fat release, triggering protein, cholesterol and sterol hormone synthesis and having a general cellular anabolic effect [7]. However, dietary glucose surges and CECC overwhelms the enormous hepatic capacity for first pass monosaccharide uptake so that perpetually raised PV monosaccharide concentration spill over to systemic circulation triggering continuous hyperinsulinaemia. Elevated glucose concentration is universally toxic. Initially, the rate and concentration of BG supply is hepatically controlled by insulin, but several factors affect its availability and efficacy. Firstly, the liver utilises 40%–60% of insulin [8]. Even the liver has a peak capacity of post-prandial glucose uptake, and when reached, excess glucose spills into systemic circulation where insulin drives glucose into many cells, such as skeletal muscle, via GLUT4 [9].

High concentrations of BG drive intracellular hyperglycaemia via GLUT4. Intracellular hyperglycaemia, beyond muscular glycogen storage capacity, leads to toxic glucose concentrations and down regulation of GLUT4 receptor number and phosphorylation of the GLUT4 receptor, inducing insulin resistance (IR). In the pancreatic alpha cells this results in glucagon and insulin secretion despite elevated BG concentration with paradoxical glycogenolysis, gluconeogenesis, and hepatic release of glucose despite existing hyperglycaemia [10].

While IR results in hyperglycaemia, GLUT2 hepatic glucose uptake continues with maximum DNL regulated only by AMPK, inducing non-alcoholic fatty liver disease (NAFLD) and hyperaminoacidaemia. Glucagon concentration in the PV is 40% greater than systemic concentration [11].

Cells initially increase glycogenesis, DNL, and glycolytic pathway flux through the citric acid cycle. In the pancreas, elevated beta cell glucose concentration drive insulin release and glucagon inhibition, but reach a genetically predetermined maximum. In addition, due to high production and IR, arterial hyperinsulinaemia blocks further beta cell release. Finally, IR in pancreatic alpha cells results in paradoxical glucagon release, that together with elevated cortisol concentration and hyperglycaemia, triggers hepatic glycolysis and gluconeogenesis despite hyperglycaemia that is toxic to blood cells [12].

Under hyperglycaemia, hyperinsulinaemia and IR, hepatic VLDL production becomes continuous with significant rises in IDL and small dense LDLb, after deposition of hepatically produced lipids in adipocytes [13]. Together with hyperglycaemia-mediated endothelial injury and intrinsic clotting cascade activation without thrombolysis, LDLb particles stabilise the clots anchored by macrophages [14]. Hyperinsulinaemia-driven HDL reduction reduces transfer of hepatic apoproteins from HDL to LDLb particles, leaving them in circulation unrecognised by the liver inhibiting removal. This default leads to vascular lipid deposition resulting in atherogenic plaque rather than cyclical thrombosis-thrombolysis that occurs continually in healthy vascular systems as part of injury repair [15]. Not only does hyperglycaemia damage the vessels directly, chronic hyperglycaemia-induced hyperinsulinaemia inhibits HDL formation and plaque lysis while leading to elevated LDLb concentration. In clinical experience, low, smaller HDL correlates with higher incidence of atheroma, while a therapeutic carbohydrate restriction (TCR) increases HDL number and size, decreases free triglyceride concentration, and appears to stabilise coronary artery calcium (CAC) score.

3.2.2.2 *Obesity and type 2 diabetes*

High-carbohydrate consumption directs postprandial lipid traffic from the liver to adipocytes rather than from intestine to adipocytes as seen with TCR. This process is driven by hyperinsulinaemia and only occurs under high-carbohydrate conditions. Evolutionarily, this process of tolerance for transient seasonal hyperinsulinaemia allowed humans to store large amounts of fat before winter [16]. However, in the era of carbohydrate abundance, this process has transformed from a survival advantage to a constant state. CECC overwhelms this system and triggers progressive stages of worsening IR.

Genetically, some humans have massive insulin production capacity (as high as 90 IU – clinical data) so that hyperinsulinaemia drives DNL, even through fasting hyperglycaemia, keeping BG in relative check as measured by HbA1c < 5.9%, reducing IR but resulting in obesity. Clinical experience indicates that this 'obesogenic' pattern manifests where these patients appear spared from intravascular effects of hyperglycaemia, but have chronic fatigue issues, steroid synthesis dysfunction, cellular inflammation and higher cancer and dementia risk. Due to the weight and inflammation, orthopaedic joint degeneration is common. While reversible NAFLD is ubiquitous, they are spared from non-alcoholic steatohepatitis (NASH) and metabolic syndrome (MetS) and are relatively healthy. Fat distribution is mostly subcutaneous.

Under high-carbohydrate conditions, in patients incapable of high insulin production (<15 IU at peak – clinical data), hyperglycaemia and IR occur early. These patients gain a modest amount of weight, but due to IR, persistent intravascular hyperglycaemia occurs, raising HbA1c, but also activating white blood cells and platelets. Clinical experience indicates that this 'diabesogenic' pathway is expressed as hypertriglyceridaemia, vasculopathy, atherogenesis, thrombo-occlusion, MetS, intravascular inflammation, and increased risk for steatohepatitis and ischaemic hepatocellular dysfunction [17]. Osmotic capacity of glucose also affects blood volume, blood pressure and oedema. IR also leads to uncoupling of negative feedback control between beta and alpha cells of the pancreas, leading to paradoxical hyperglucagonaemia resulting in hepatic glucose production and release, increasing lipolysis and elevated concentration of LDLb. This progression culminates in T2D. Risk for T2D is directly related to biomarkers of hepatic DNL and palmitic and palmitoleic acid concentration [18]. Fructose has a lower GLP-1 and pancreatic insulin release stimulation further raising BG, increasing its vascular and intracellular toxicity [19].

These pathways occur in a bell curve distribution in a mixed population of high-carbohydrate consumers. In genetically similar populations, patterns of obesogenicity (e.g., Polynesian Islanders) versus diabesogenicity (e.g., East Indians) are recognisable [20,21]. Clinical observations reflect that, while the diabesogenic pathway is progressive and somewhat linear in disease spectrum and progression (as similarly seen in T1D), the obesogenic pathway stalls when insulin production capacity peaks. These patients then assume a tertiary diabesogenic pattern [22], but their disease spectrum occurs as a combination of both patterns. These crossover patients are the most difficult to treat since they are resistant to insulin therapy. Intermittent fasting (IF), or periods exceeding 12 h of fasting with 6 to 8 h eating windows or less is a useful starting therapy for these individuals.

Thus, when diagnosing CECC diseases, it is important to understand insulin production capacity since pathophysiology is predictably influenced by hyperglycaemia, hyperinsulinaemia, and IR. Measuring fasting BG, HbA1c, C-peptide, insulin, glucagon, and lipid concentration has great diagnostic value [23]. Ultimately, however, conversion to permanent TCR with IF corrects the root cause and overtime induces remission of the diabetic and obese states. Furthermore, caloric reductive TCR diets and weight loss as monitored by the scale is of greatest therapeutic benefit in obesogenic individuals, while continuous glucose monitoring and strict carbohydrate reduction with aggressive transient hypoglycaemic and possibly insulin therapy, leaning more towards a high fat TCR diet, has greater therapeutic benefit in diabesogenic individuals. GLP-1 agonist medications that treat appetite, as well as reducing gluconeogenesis and increasing insulin release, are highly beneficial in both genetic types [24]. Assigning differential insulin production capacity to genetics is probable, but epigenetic, environmental, and other lifestyle factors cannot be excluded.

The SREBP family regulates the synthesis of fatty acids (FAs), triglycerides, and cholesterol. The SREBP family consists of three isoforms: SREBP-1a, SREBP-1c, and SREBP-2. The biosynthesis of FAs and triglycerides is controlled by SREBP-1c. In obesity and T2D, insulin fails to suppress glucose production while lipogenesis is paradoxically enhanced. At the molecular level, increased lipogenesis observed in the insulin-resistant state is due, at least in part, to the dysregulation of SREBP-1c [25].

3.2.2.3 *Fatty liver – non-alcoholic fatty liver disease*

NAFLD or steatosis is accumulation of macrovesicular fatty triglyceride globules within hepatocytes. Steatosis is visible via microscopy on biopsy or visualised by radiologic imaging as a change in the density of the liver. NAFLD can progress to inflammatory fatty liver disease or NASH that results in permanent hepatic injury via fibrosis [14] (Fig. 3.1). Diagnosis is based on medical history supported by blood tests [26], medical imaging [27], and liver biopsy [28,29].

The human liver does not ordinarily store lipids so that all forms of hepatic steatosis are the consequence of pathophysiology. Although there are several contributing factors, the origin has been divided into alcoholic fatty liver disease (AFLD) and NAFLD [30]. Contributing factors include CECC, viruses such as hepatitis C, human immunodeficiency virus (HIV), inborn errors of metabolism (abetalipoproteinemia, glycogen storage diseases, lipodystrophy, Weber-Christian disease) and drugs (amiodarone, methotrexate, diltiazem, etc.). Clinical experience reflects that fatty liver is a common feature in persons who regularly consume carbohydrates as >60% of their total daily caloric intake in an acute or CECC manner [31].

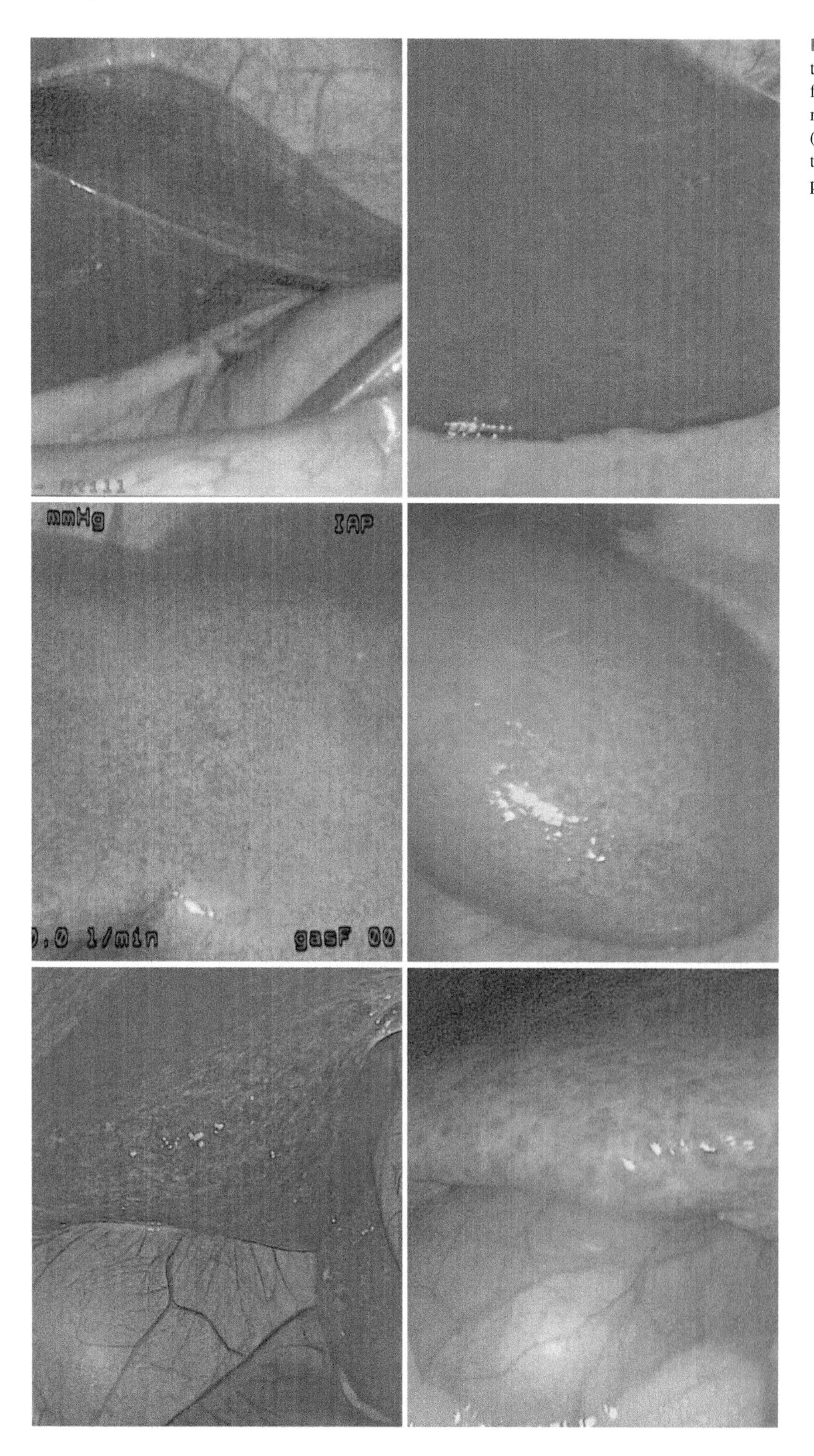

FIGURE 3.1 Intraoperative pictures taken during surgery showing stages of fatty liver disease. Top row: normal liver; middle row: non-alcoholic fatty disease (NAFLD) without fibrosis or inflammation; bottom row: non-alcoholic steatohepatitis progressing to fibrosis and cirrhosis.

NAFLD triglyceride accumulation occurs due to several factors:

1. The post-prandial liver is a primary producer of lipid (cholesterol, triglyceride, phospholipid (PL)) by DNL under the influence of insulin, and the capacity for DNL is not rate-limiting, so depending on the volume (CECC) and frequency (snacking) of substrate from the intestine, the liver can produce lipids particularly from carbohydrates. Proof comes from the high concentrations of palmitic and oleic FAs in the liver that are the direct product of glucose lipogenesis [32].
2. There is little evidence that the liver releases free triglyceride or non-esterified fatty acids (NEFA) into the blood directly [33]. The primary exit for lipids is via insulin-mediated VLDL production, and lipid accumulation results when this rate-limiting step is exceeded by DNL production.
3. Somatic lipid influx into the liver comes from chylomicron remnants, HDL, and LDL. This mechanism is the focus of most research that erroneously ignores CECC DNL and blames saturated fat intake as the cause of NAFLD [33].
4. The liver has a high capacity for free triglyceride and NEFA uptake that is blood concentration-regulated and during fasting is the most active metabolic organ to metabolise triglyceride/NEFA. This occurs via three pathways: (1) complete oxidation, producing water, carbon dioxide, and ATP (2) incomplete oxidation, producing ketones, and (3) esterification to triglycerides and phospholipids. Fasting triglyceride/NEFA concentration is normally dependent on adipocyte release. Under IR conditions, paradoxical triglyceride/NEFA and lipid-laden LDL release occurs despite post-prandial anabolic hormonal conditions. This elevates the NEFA concentration that induces hepatic gradient-based uptake, adding somatic lipids to the already lipid-laden hepatocyte. These processes culminate in NAFLD, the driving force being CECC and IR [33].

In NAFLD, BG is elevated and somatic cells lower NEFA use and increase glucose use under insulin. Thus there is greater NEFA concentration in blood, and the liver develops a futile cycle to convert NEFA to triglyceride into VLDL; thus, fatty liver is a combination of DNL and recycling of NEFA that should have gone to cells. Decreasing carbohydrate consumption decreases DNL and BG that increases cellular NEFA use, reducing fatty liver. NEFA release differs when fed (low) or fasted (high) so snacking increases DNL and lowers NEFA release until IR results in paradoxical adipocyte NEFA release despite high BG. This is likely a glucagon uncoupling effect. On a TCR diet, hepatic DNL is low even postprandially.

Clinical experience shows NAFLD is rectifiable to clinically observed remission within three to seven days of reducing carbohydrate intake to $<10\%$ of daily calories and reducing caloric intake frequency to no more than twice a day. This is true for AFLD when the person is abstinent from alcohol [34]. The position that NAFLD is a direct result of CECC is not universally accepted because of cognitive dissonance combined with erroneous assumption of hepatic triglyceride accumulation assigning 'cause' to (saturated) fat consumption [35]. Obesity does not cause NAFLD. CECC results in NAFLD that over time results in obesity as a disease continuum starting with CECC. A lack of appreciation of loss of hormonal cycling because of IR due to CECC, has led to a large body of erroneously corroborative studies performed in IR patients with NAFLD that further reinforces the role of saturated fat consumption as the cause of NAFLD. For example, tracer studies of ingested fat demonstrate that much of the fat comes from adipocytes in the form of fasting NEFA (59%) vs postprandial DNL (29%) in already IR subjects [36].

AFLD and NAFLD are caused by triglyceride overproduction. This is a protective mechanism whereby the liver accelerates triglyceride conversion of excess alcohol and glucose to protect the circulation. Normally, both glucose and ethanol are converted into cytosolic acetyl CoA and enter the Krebs Cycle via acetyl CoA carboxylase for conversion into ATP or are stored as glycogen. However, this process generates NADH, and increases the NADH/NAD+ ratio. Increased NADH blocks passage into mitochondria diverting to fatty acid synthesis, while decreased NAD+ results in decreased fatty acid oxidation under the influence of insulin. DNL occurs in the cytosol via pyruvate decarboxylase and alcohol dehydrogenase enzymes converting ethanol or pyruvate to acetaldehyde, raising NADH. Uncoupling of cytosolic to mitochondrial transfer is the key step in lipogenesis. Insulin drives this process towards lipogenesis by phosphorylation of acetyl CoA carboxylase. DNL is an intrinsic metabolic process that converts excess macronutrients to fat. Under normal physiological conditions, DNL in hepatocytes and adipocytes is synergistically regulated by signals from the peripheral tissues and the central nervous system. However, under pathophysiological conditions of CECC, the equilibration between hepatocyte and adipocyte DNL is disturbed at both a receptor phosphorylation and a transcription level, leading to increased DNL in the liver and decreased DNL in adipose tissues, which contributes to NAFLD. Under these conditions, the liver is forced into excessive DNL not only to deal with the post-prandial macronutrient load from the PV, but also as part of the systemic hyperglycaemia regulatory mechanism to take up and convert excess systemic BG to fat. Under insulin-resistant conditions, there is additional uncoupling of insulin-glucagon control, with paradoxical gluconeogenesis in the face of hyperglycaemia, and this adds to hepatic DNL and NAFLD.

Clinical experience shows the treatment of carbohydrate-induced NAFLD with strict TCR is simple and rapid (3–7 days). There is no medication therapy for self-induced lifestyle disease. While treatment with insulin-sensitising drugs transiently improves NAFLD, such therapy has poor long-term value [37]. Bariatric surgery may briefly improve

NAFLD, but unless CECC GLP-1 agonist medications, by suppressing gluconeogenesis, accelerates the process but may be used ancillary to but not as a substitute for TCR [38]. Abstinence from alcohol consumption accelerates fatty liver disease resolution [39].

3.2.2.4 Steatohepatitis and hepatic inflammation

Hepatic injury is rarely a primary presenting feature of a high carbohydrate diet. Fatty liver is so common as to be unusual if absent in untreated MetS, obese, or diabetic patients. Elevated liver enzymes, CT, and MRI are common modalities that reveal fatty liver when mildly elevated and are more predictive of NASH when levels are significantly elevated together with global inflammatory markers such as C-reactive protein (CRP), erythrocyte sedimentation rate (ESR), ferritin, and white blood cell count (WBC). Hypertriglyceridaemia, low HDL concentration, and fasting hyperglycaemia are indirect indicators of fatty liver. The only absolute way to tell the difference between NAFLD and NASH is by biopsy [28]. Criteria for NAFLD include >5% hepatic steatosis in the absence of other known causes of fatty liver, while NASH is diagnosed by added inflammation, ballooning steatohepatitis with or without fibrosis. The severity of NASH can be evaluated by the degree of fibrosis (scored via biopsy grading 1–4) and progression to cirrhosis [26].

Post-prandial PV concentration of monosaccharides and amino acids are normally high, while lipid concentration is low because chylomicron transport bypasses the PV via lymphatic absorption. Hepatocytes are commonly exposed to macronutrient fluctuations after meals and during fasting. The liver is the gatekeeper preventing these extreme nutrient concentrations from spilling into the systemic circulation and causing injury. Therefore hepatocytes, under the influence of insulin, have a rapid capacity to convert amino acids and monosaccharides to glycogen and fat, both processes protecting hepatocytes and hepatic sinusoidal endothelium against harm from hyperglycaemia and inflammation. Transient fat accumulation is normal and unlikely to result in injury.

Under certain conditions, the benign fatty liver may be subject to acute or chronic inflammatory steatohepatitis starting as injury to the hepatic sinusoidal vascular endothelium then involving hepatocytes themselves. This may be an acute hepatocellular toxic injury that is only measured by increased hepatic enzymes and resolve, but persistent sinusoidal exposure to toxic hyperglycaemia leads to vascular inflammation, endothelial injury, thickening or fibrosis of the fibronectin and collagen support system and ischaemia with hepatocellular necrosis, scarring, hepatic fibrosis. When the surviving hepatocytes regenerate, clonal regenerating nodules are seen as cirrhosis. NASH is the leading cause of chronic liver disease [40] and the second most common reason for liver transplant in the United States and Europe.

Hepatic sinusoids are arranged so that hepatocytes and endothelial cells are in single rows with every hepatocyte being directly exposed to portal blood. In addition, the flattened endothelial cells have fenestrae ('windows') exposing hepatic microvilli directly to the blood. This unique flattened shape of endothelial cells and the dynamic nature of the fenestrae are controlled by an internal microfilament cytoskeleton made up of actin and vimentin filaments that appear to be sensitive to glycosylation and insulin [41,42].

Under conditions of hyperglycaemia, in the absence of lipid infusion, when using an insulin clamp to control monosaccharide concentration, there is rapid hepatocellular glycogenesis and DNL with fatty liver accumulation and dose-dependent alteration in sinusoidal endothelial shape with rounding up due to glycosylation-induced alteration in the actin-vimentin cytoskeleton and loss of surface anticoagulant properties resulting in the expression of procoagulant surface molecules and dis-association of tight junctions creating procoagulant exposure of underlying hepatocytes and triggering the intrinsic clotting cascade – essentially microscopically visible diabetic vasculopathy in evolution [14]. Early on, if hyperglycaemic hyperinsulinaemic conditions are reversed, fibrinolysis occurs with the restoration of resting endothelial configuration; however, under continuous or repeated hyperglycaemia-hyperinsulinaemia representative of CECC, fibrin clots induce macrophage-led inflammatory cascade activating and trapping circulating platelets followed by neutrophil and leukocyte activation. This plugs the sinusoids, leading to irreversible ischaemic and cytokine-mediated injury to hepatocytes. This can be measured by rising liver enzymes in the blood that represent the transition from NAFLD to NASH. Under these ischaemic thrombo-inflammatory conditions, the hepatocellular environment is similarly affected with progression to 'foam' cell formation, hepatocellular membrane injury followed by hepatocellular apoptosis and necrosis. Hepatocellular hyperglycaemia overwhelms acetyl CoA carboxylase activity, the rate limiting step of glycogenesis and lipogenesis, damaging the cytoskeleton, representing the transition from hepatic steatosis to steatohepatitis. This is seen by ballooning hepatocyte degeneration and is associated with lipid droplets and cytoskeleton degenerative clumping seen as Mallory-Denke Bodies in the pre-apoptotic stage that eventually leads to hepatocellular necrosis [43]. While this ischaemic thrombo inflammatory injury may be reversible at first, over time the injury leads to Kupffer cell-mediated fibrosis and hepatocellular clonal regeneration and cirrhosis [14].

This cascade occurs because of CECC and earlier stages are reversible with TCR because the liver has the unique capacity to tolerate transient, but not persistent hyperglycaemia. When systemic BG increases, somatic cells use GLUT receptor phosphorylation resistance and receptor down-regulation as a protective mechanism against intracellular hyperglycaemia. Once intracellular glucose is phosphorylated to G6P, it cannot leave most cells. Hepatocytes uniquely can transport glucose bidirectionally because they have glucose-6-phosphatase that cleaves phosphate from G6P, releasing free glucose. Thus, three mechanisms protect hepatocellular hyperglycaemia: glycogenesis, DNL, and glucose release back into the systemic circulation. This is critically important because postprandial glucose concentrations are highest in hepatic sinusoids and glucose enters hepatocytes using GLUT1 transport molecules [44].

Insulin is the critical driver of these hepatocellular functions including glycogenesis, lipogenesis, VLDL formation, steroid hormone production, protein and cholesterol synthesis and glucagon suppression. In IR, simultaneous hyperinsulinaemic and hyperglucagonaemic conditions occur irrespective of feeding or fasting states affecting all hepatocellular synthetic pathways as well as release of NEFA and triglyceride from adipocytes that should be blocked by insulin. This perpetual sinusoidal hyperglycaemia prevents endothelial repair and leads to progressive fibrosis. While it appears from clinical laboratory data that insulinogenic pathways predominate, loss of nutrient-driven hormonal cycling likely drives futile cycling of gluconeogenesis-ketogenesis at the same time as glycogenesis and lipogenesis in the liver with sinusoidal and intrahepatocellular hyperglycaemia and activation of a thrombo-inflammatory cascade.

While there are association studies and mechanistic theories involving PUFA [45], there are no studies demonstrating causal proof involving PUFA without also involving carbohydrates. Indeed in our isolated clamp models of liver injury, infusion of 20% PUFA Intralipid, a lipid emulsion used in parenteral nutrition, did not demonstrate either hepatocellular or sinusoidal vascular injury at microscopy [14]. PUFAs potentially contribute to inflammation via lipid peroxidation, but carbohydrates are the cause of NAFLD. If long-chain PUFAs are implicated in NASH, they would have to come from adipocytes, as NEFA and/or in chylomicron remnants, since PUFAs are not absorbed into the PV postprandially, but travel via chylomicrons directly to adipocytes [46]. Post-prandially, the liver is exposed to PV absorbed medium chain triglycerides that paradoxically appear to have a protective effect [47]. CECC results in uncoupling of pancreatic hormonal cycling and persistent hyperglycaemia that results in NASH and leads to fibrosis and cirrhosis. NAFLD is easily reversible, but NASH to the point of fibrosis is not [48].

In obesogenic individuals, the prevalence of NAFLD is nearly ubiquitous. Higher rates of hepatic fibrosis are observed in diabetic patients (56.4%) compared with prediabetic (29.2%), and normoglycaemic patients (28.6%) ($P < .001$). Patients with NAFLD and T2D show accelerated progression to cirrhosis. NASH occurred in 59.4% of diabetics, in 49.2% of prediabetics, and in 36% of normoglycaemic obese patients ($P < .001$). Only 1.5% of diabetics had no histological hepatic alterations [49].

Several NAFLD progression and fibrosis scoring systems have been developed to determine the rate of progression and timing of possible transplantation [50–52].

Medical treatment for NAFLD or NASH requires reversal of IR. There are no medications that do this completely, but metformin and GLP-1 agonists with or without GIP receptor antagonists do have a desirable effect in reducing IR and thereby potentially the severity of NASH [38,53]. Blocking triglyceride formation and anti-inflammatory medication has failed to resolve the disease. Research into inhibiting triglyceride synthesis improves hepatic steatosis but exacerbates liver damage and fibrosis in obese mice with nonalcoholic steatohepatitis [54]. Statin therapy and low-fat high carbohydrate diets also exacerbate disease. In foregut and bariatric surgery, it is a common practice to place patients on a very low calorie diet a month prior to surgery [55]. Both the sustainability and efficacy of this diet shows poor results, however, clinical experience, using our NAFLD reduction protocol of 5 to 7 days of near total (<20 g) TCR while eating protein and fat unrestricted, results in biopsy-proven resolution of NAFLD and osmotically overloaded swollen livers [56].

NASH is more resistant to treatment but can certainly be stabilised by TCR. Adding the biguanide metformin, a glucagon suppressor, as a way to dampen glucagon-mediated paradoxical glycogenolysis and gluconeogenesis may speed up the resolution of NASH. Clinical experience indicates that IF of 48–72 h, with aggressive transient treatment of BG using continuous glucose monitors (CGM) with long and short acting insulin to maintain normoglycaemia, in combination with TCR, is the most effective way to treat NASH to biochemical and radiologic improvement.

Further evidence implicating monosaccharides but not PUFA in NAFLD and NASH comes from total parenteral nutrition (TPN) data. In long-term TPN patients there is near universal hepatic fibrosis and cirrhosis often requiring liver transplantation [57]. Standard clinical TPN macronutrients include 15%–25% dextrose solution that usually requires the addition of insulin for BG regulation, amino acids, and a 20% high PUFA low-saturated fat lipid emulsion. Standard clinical monitoring manages hyperglycaemia with insulin, not dextrose concentration reduction, as well as serial peripheral triglyceride testing with reduction in lipid emulsion infusion for high triglyceride concentration. Many studies have altered timing, cycling, altered FA, and protein mixes that only resulted in minor alterations to the inevitable hepatic cirrhosis outcome [58,59]. However, because of the common erroneous belief that carbohydrates are an essential source of energy, there are no studies eliminating dextrose from TPN. In my practice, I have not used dextrose in short- or long-term TPN in any patient over the age of 2 years for over a decade, including T1D. We have not seen any evidence of NAFLD by blood testing, imaging or biopsy, and have also not seen hypoglycaemia. This is true despite the mandatory use of high omega-6 PUFA in the lipid component, and even when triglyceride concentrations are high, there is no evidence of NAFLD. In addition, we have rarely required insulin infusion except in T1D, while maintaining normoglycaemia. Clinical experience shows the risk of catheter infections and venous thrombosis is also significantly lower. However, these data have never been accepted for publication because no international research body has given permission for such a study, and the use has always been off label. These data provide additional proof that carbohydrates, not PUFA, cause NAFLD and NASH.

Fibrosis may progress to cirrhosis and complications including hepatocellular carcinoma. Once cirrhosis has occurred, this cannot be resolved, but can be stabilised by strict TCR and aggressive medical treatment of hyperglycaemia until the patient is insulin sensitive, then potentially deprescribing the medication as warranted. Unfortunately, when end-stage NASH is treated with liver transplantation, recurrence of NASH is common since accelerated injury occurs if the diet remains high-carbohydrate particularly with the use of steroids for immunosuppression [60].

3.2.3 Managing the patient

3.2.3.1 Clinical presentation, investigation and treatment

The liver is a highly regenerative and resilient organ such that pathology usually presents with glycaemic, lipid and hormonal disruption, rather than intrinsic liver injury apart from the aforementioned NAFLD-NASH spectrum [61]. NAFLD-NASH injury is assessed by elevated lactate dehydrogenase (LDH), aspartate aminotransferase (AST) and alanine aminotransferase (ALT), gamma glutamyl transferase (GGT) concentrations, radiologic imaging, and liver biopsy if necessary. Fibrosis scores can be used to calculate severity of injury [50].

The liver is primarily responsible for nutrient substrate and energy distribution to all cells in the body. Based upon energy utilisation capacity and in particular insulin production capacity, dysfunction may be seen as a myriad of conditions:

1. hyperglycaemia due to early failure of the liver to convert glucose into fat in people with low insulin production resulting in early IR diabesogenic intravascular thrombo inflammatory vascular disruption, atherogenesis, and vascular occlusion,
2. intracellular glycaemic energy deficiency, or
3. persistent hyperinsulinaemia causing massive lipogenesis and obesogenicity with pathological adipocyte hypertrophy, steroid hormone synthetic disruption and cholesterol/protein hypersynthesis, and intracellular inflammation.

Early morning fasting blood work including lipid panels (NMR if necessary), HbA1c, BG, C-peptide, insulin, glucagon, ketones, uric acid, Vitamin D, testosterone, and inflammatory markers are needed to evaluate hepatopathology as well as determine genetic pattern. Kraft Oral Glucose Tolerance Testing is also often of value to elucidate genetic pattern and disease severity. Monitoring for auto-immune diseases is also important. A Coronary Artery Calcium Score (CAC) may assist in vascular disease risk assessment. Follow-up bloodwork every 4–6 months shows trends and return to fat-adapted insulin sensitivity that may take 6–12 months to manifest after implementing TCR.

Treatment requires addressing the root cause. There is no pill that treats a self-induced lifestyle problem. Effective treatment is with TCR, particularly low fructose, including intermittent fasting with no more than two calorie-consuming meals in a 24-h period to restore glucagon-insulin hormonal cycling. Metformin and GLP-1 agonist/GIP receptor antagonist medications that improve IR and hyperglycaemia may accelerate the restoration of this relationship, but aggressive return to normoglycaemia and insulin sensitivity is the most consistent way to reverse NAFLD and possibly early NASH, even if that requires transient use of diabetic medications. There are no other medications that have been shown to reverse NAFLD. Abstinence from alcohol is also strongly suggested during the corrective phase. Frequent physical activity to induce glycogenolysis is also strongly recommended. Use of ursodeoxycholic acid, 3-omega fatty acids, vitamin E, and thiazolidinediones have failed to show convincing therapeutic benefit. Medications transiently slow down the progression of the consequences of such lifestyle conditions, but addressing the cause requires behavioural change that cannot be outsourced, mitigated, or medicated. Only catastrophic endpoint damage such as stroke or myocardial infarction is irreversible. MetS, IR-diabetes, NAFLD and obesity are imminently reversible often to remission over time with near-abstinence from carbohydrates and snacking, but remission only remains as long as TCR is followed.

Therapy begins with physician-led education including dietary and psychologic therapy and follow-up monitoring of health, diet as well as psychological state. Dietary relapses are expected and common at first, but quitting carbohydrates repeatedly after each relapse usually leads to sustained abstinence and improved quality of life. Psychological and dietary counselling and support groups assist patients in understanding, transforming, and maintaining their diet. Patient- centred metabolic monitoring of weight, blood pressure, BG by glucometer or CGM and ketone monitoring are all of value as feedback metrics.

Disease-specific medications should definitely be used to control the results of metabolic derangement. This includes tight BG and blood pressure control by whatever medical means necessary. Metformin and GLP-1 agonist/GIP receptor antagonist medication, even in hyperinsulinaemic patients, has value in gluconeogenic suppression and hepatic glycolysis [62]. Low-dose aspirin, a thromboxane A2 inhibitor that blocks platelet activation, may be of value in hypercoagulable states. This medication, if tolerated, should be continued well into the fat- adapted state. Appetite suppression medication may be transiently valuable in helping a patient gain dietary control and may even include bariatric devices and surgery if warranted by disease and co-morbid severity since caloric reduction of any kind as well as consumption frequency reduction has transient benefit. Salt supplementation (including iodised salt up to 150–200 mcg) is essential. Vitamin and micronutrient supplementation, essential FA supplementation (fish oil particularly DHA up to 1000 mg/day) is prescribed as needed. MCT or coconut oil has early value in accelerating return to a ketogenic state and may have hepatoprotective value since these shorter chain lipids are absorbed via the PV directly to the liver [63]. Statin therapy is not warranted for patients on TCR diets and may negatively affect hepatic cholesterol handling [64]. Real unprocessed food with a preference toward animal micro and macronutrients, particularly of marine sourcing, most closely conforms to the best nutrient supply for the entire gastrointestinal tract, with the liver at the metabolic apex of the entire intestinal system. Physical activity, adequate high-quality sleep for circadian rhythm restoration and daily exposure to sunlight is of great physical and psychological value.

Every physician treating metabolic disease with TCR and IF should have a medication deprescription protocol (see Section 3.5).

3.2.4 Summary

Ultimately diseases caused by CECC, carbophilia, and lipophobia are best treated at source by removal of carbohydrates and snacking with addition of complex naturally-occurring fat. This does not seem difficult to understand, but cognitive dissonance and societal transformation is a very slow process. The best we can do is guide individual patients down their own path of recovery and remission by education and leading by example.

3.3 Metabolic syndrome

Hassina Kajee

3.3.1 Introduction

It is well documented that metabolic syndrome (MetS) is a collection of cardio metabolic risk factors. It is important to know what risk a diagnosis of MetS confers.

Many studies [65] have investigated and identified MetS as an independent risk factor for cardiovascular disease (CVD), coronary artery disease (CAD), stroke and T2D. Individuals with MetS have been shown to have an increased incidence of CVD (RR 1.53) and stroke (RR 1.76) [65]. In addition, all-cause mortality (RR 1.35) and cardiovascular mortality (RR 1.74) is also increased in individuals with MetS with women having a higher risk compared to men [65]. Individuals with MetS have also been shown to have an increased risk of developing T2D (RR of 3.5–5.2) [66]. Due to MetS increasing the risk for these, the biggest chronic diseases of our time, identifying and targeting the risk factors for MetS is essential.

The concept of MetS was first described by Swedish Physician, Kylin, over 80 years ago as a cluster of hypertension, hyperglycaemia and gout [67]. In 1947, Vague recognised upper abdominal adiposity to be associated with T2D and CVD [68]. Later Avogadro et al. described a syndrome of hyperglycaemia, hypertension, and obesity [69]. However, most people are reminded of the famous Banting lecture of 1988 [70], where Gerald Reaven drew attention to hyperinsulinaemia. He described a syndrome comprising a constellation of cardiovascular risk factors characterised by hyperinsulinaemia, glucose intolerance, dyslipidaemia, and hypertension. These symptoms, which could all be present in a single individual, is now widely referred to as MetS.

MetS is not a disease per se but a constellation of risk factors for atherosclerotic disease and T2D. It is also known as Syndrome X, insulin resistance (IR) syndrome, cardio-metabolic syndrome, dysmetabolic syndrome, and the deadly quartet syndrome [71]. The constellation includes glucose intolerance (T2D, impaired fasting glucose or impaired glucose tolerance), IR, central obesity, dyslipidaemia, and hypertension; all well-documented risk factors for CVDs [71].

3.3.1.1 Definition

Several definitions have been put forward in an attempt to describe the diagnosis from various expert perspectives. A consensus definition has been proposed by the International Diabetes Federation (IDF) as a result of a consensus workshop in 2004 (Table 3.1).

3.3.1.2 Epidemiology

As the global prevalence of MetS continues to increase at alarming rates in line with obesity and T2D [70,73], prevalence is seen to be rising in both urban populations and developing countries [74,75], where previously, MetS was thought to be an urban issue.

MetS continues to be a burgeoning problem worldwide [76–81].

In the United States, 38% of the population met the criteria for MetS in 2017–18. There is a similar prevalence in European adults as well as in Latin America [73]. East Asian countries, including China, Japan, and Korea are also seeing an increased number of cases with prevalence in East Asia in 2007 ranging from 8% to 13% in men and from 2% to 18% in women depending on diagnostic criteria used and may be as high as 30% [82–84]. In Sub-Saharan Africa, MetS ranges from 10% to 34.6% of the population depending on region and diagnostic criteria with the highest prevalence in South Africa [85–88].

MetS prevalence increases with age and 40% of people over the age of 60 have a MetS diagnosis [89]. It is disturbing to note that this diagnosis is increasingly prevalent in children and adolescents, corresponding with the rising obesity trend seen in this paediatric population [90].

Prevalence in men (24%) and women (23%) is similar when adjusted for age, putting both men and women at an increased cardiometabolic risk [91–93]. However women have several unique sex-related predisposing factors, for example, pregnancy, use of oral contraceptives, and polycystic ovarian syndrome [92,93]. In addition, breast cancer may be modestly associated with MetS in postmenopausal women [94,95]. There are also some studies that have found associations in sex hormones as independent risk factors of and MetS [96,97]. Low testosterone and low SHBG have both been found to be independent risk factors associated with MetS. However, obesity and insulin are associated with low SHBG. Low SHBG concentrations may be used as a marker to predict metabolic diseases and has a twofold increase in CVS disease [98].

TABLE 3.1 Summary of various diagnostic criteria for MetS [72].

International Diabetes Federation (IDF)	American Heart Association/ National Heart, Lung and Blood Institute (AHA/NHLBI)	National Cholesterol Education Programme Adult Treatment Panel III (NCEP ATP III)	World Health Organization (WHO) (1998)
Central obesity (defined as waist circumference with ethnicity specific values) plus any two of the following: a. Raised triglycerides ≥ 150 mg/dL (1.7 mmol/L) or specific treatment for this lipid abnormality b. Reduced HDL cholesterol < 50 mg/dL (1.3 mmol/L) or specific treatment for this lipid abnormality c. Raised blood pressure ≥ 130/85 mm Hg or treatment of chronic hypertension d. Raised fasting plasma glucose ≥ 100 mg/dL (5.6 mmol/L), or previously diagnosed type 2 diabetes mellitus	Any three of the following: a. Elevated waist circumference (according to population and country specific definitions) b. Plasma triglycerides ≥ 150 mg/dL (1.7 mmol/L) or specific treatment for this lipid abnormality c. HDL cholesterol < 50 mg/dL (1.3 mmol/L) or specific treatment for this lipid abnormality d. Blood pressure ≥ 130/85 mmHg or treatment of previously diagnosed hypertension e. Fasting plasma glucose ≥ 100 mg/dL (5.6 mmol/L) or on drug treatment for elevated glucose	Any three of the following: a. Waist circumference > 88 cm b. Plasma triglycerides > 150 mg/dL (1.7 mmol/L) c. HDL cholesterol < 50 mg/dL (1.3 mmol/L) d. Blood pressure ≥ 130/85 mmHg e. Fasting plasma glucose ≥ 110 mg/dL (6.1 mmol/L)	Presence of insulin resistance or type 2 diabetes mellitus (T2DM) or impaired fasting glucose (IFG) or impaired glucose tolerance

Adapted from Jayasinghe IU, Agampodi TC, Dissanayake AK, et al. Comparison of global definitions of metabolic syndrome in early pregnancy among the Rajarata Pregnancy Cohort participants in Sri Lanka. *Sci Rep* 12, 2009 (2022). https://doi.org/10.1038/s41598-022.

It is important to note that the original criteria for diagnosis of MetS was developed from Caucasian majority research groups. As such, there has been an argument around the modification of diagnostic criteria for specific ethnic groups, for example, a body mass index (BMI) of over 23 may suggest IR in a Japanese population [99,100] In the United States, data from 2002 showed the highest prevalence of MetS to be in Mexican Americans (31.9%) [101] and African Americans, particularly African American women have a higher prevalence of MetS [102]. However, this may not be truly representative of metabolic risk in these populations.

3.3.2 Pathophysiology

Armed with the knowledge of the importance of addressing MetS, due to its detrimental effects on human health and its pervasiveness globally, we will now move on to understanding its root cause in order to learn how best to prevent it.

The MetS cluster can all be centrally linked to IR [103]. There is a clearly defined association between IR and the individual components of MetS [103]. The consequences of IR are tissue specific. By understanding the downstream functions of an activated insulin receptor (INSR), it can be understood why IR perpetuates obesity, dysglycaemia, and diabetes, hypertension, and dyslipidaemia. Let us first discuss insulin and then IR, before moving on to the components of the MetS symptom cluster.

3.3.2.1 Insulin and insulin resistance

3.3.2.1.1 Insulin

Insulin is an endocrine peptide hormone with multiple direct and indirect physiological actions in tissues. While insulin's main role is anabolic and to regulate metabolic fluxes according to nutrient availability [103], in all animals, insulin-like peptides (ILP), and insulin-like growth factor (IGF) have been identified that promote mitogenic regulation and cell growth and differentiation input respectively. This overlap in functionality is what is thought to be responsible for the well-established relationship between insulin and several cancers [104].

Insulin binds to the INSR on target cells and can exert these metabolic effects. The INSR is a heterotetrameric receptor tyrosine kinase with two isoforms, A and B. The B isoform, is expressed primarily in liver, muscle, and white adipose tissue (WAT) and is more specific for insulin.

INSR activation results in two main functional effects, namely mitogenic (by activating mitogen activated protein kinase pathway) and metabolic (by activating the PI3 kinase pathway). It is important to note that the concentration of insulin required to activate the metabolic pathway is much lower than that required for mitogenic processes. It is also important to note that this effect is reversed in the case of the IGF-1 receptor [105].

In order to accomplish its main role of glucose homoeostasis, insulin has a direct effect on certain target tissues involved in metabolic homoeostasis, namely, the skeletal muscle, the liver, and WAT. This is for the purposes of glucose utilisation and glycogen synthesis in the skeletal muscle, glycogen synthesis, increased lipogenic gene expression, and reduced gluconeogenic gene expression in the liver and suppression of lipolysis, increased glucose transport and lipogenesis in the WAT [103].

Insulin exerts indirect effects on certain target tissues. In the brain, insulin crosses the blood brain barrier to act centrally on INSR on neurons and glial cells to suppress appetite and influence energy metabolism by: suppressing hepatic glucose production, promoting skeletal myocyte glucose uptake, and suppressing adipose lipolysis. Insulin also acts on the exocrine pancreas to suppress glucagon secretion as well as on the WAT and liver in what has been termed the adipocyte-hepatocyte axis [103].

3.3.2.1.2 Insulin resistance

Defective IR at the target cell results in an increased requirement of insulin secretion and consequent hyperinsulinaemia. Insulin-stimulated metabolic processes of suppression of glucose production as well as suppression of lipolysis, uptake of glucose by cells and net glycogen synthesis are impaired despite compensatory hyperinsulinaemia. Chronic hyperinsulinaemia in the setting of overnutrition and the biochemical and metabolic consequences thereof result in IR [106,107].

Much research has gone into the question of whether IR is due to receptor defects or post-receptor defects. It is now clear that it is both a decrease in INSR as well as defects in insulin signal transduction contribute to IR [106,108].

However central to all suggested mechanisms for IR is nutrient oversupply. Whether by increasing metabolites of overnutrition such as DAG, ceramides etc., overuse of the organelles involved in nutrient breakdown processes, for example, ER and oxidative stress or the inflammatory response to nutrient stress-mediated cellular toxicity, the model of IR seems to be one that is integrated in which several mechanisms, driven by overnutrition converge to facilitate IR in skeletal muscle and liver [103].

3.3.2.2 Insulin resistance as central to the key features of metabolic syndrome

3.3.2.2.1 Obesity and insulin resistance

The role of insulin in the skeletal muscle is predominantly glucose uptake. In the liver, the role of insulin is to regulate metabolism of all nutrients. WAT is exquisitely sensitive to insulin stimulation and seems to play a central co-ordinated role in cross talk between the various role players including liver, muscle, central and peripheral nervous system, and the gastrointestinal tract within minutes of nutrient intake.

Many studies have shown that the consumption of calories in excess of nutritional needs in a non-obese, non-diabetic person results in marked resistance to insulin action [109–111]. Insulin sensitivity has been well documented to decline with increasing body weight [112]. The resultant hyperinsulinaemia progresses to IR which further stimulates adipocyte hypertrophy, resulting in inflammation and worsening IR.

3.3.2.2.2 Dyslipidaemia and insulin resistance

Several studies highlight the relationship between carbohydrate intake and dyslipidaemia [111] with smaller denser lipid particles being directly associated with increased risk of CVD. Elevated triglyceride concentrations have been shown to promote the formation of small dense lipid particles and elevated triglycerides are associated with hyperinsulinemia [69].

Under normal circumstances, LDL cholesterol is synthesised from hepatic derived VLDL by progressive cleavage of lipids and apolipoproteins and IDL formed in this process are particularly arthrogenic [111]. It follows that factors which promote VLDL synthesis will also result in higher IDL and LDL concentrations. Plasma VLDL concentration is determined by the rate of liver VLDL synthesis and the rate of VLDL removal at the peripheral tissue level. Serum insulin concentration and nutrient substrate availability are responsible for VLDL concentration [111].

Over short periods of time and in controlled amounts, insulin suppresses VLDL production. However, in the setting of prolonged insulin secretion and hyperglycaemia, the resultant hyperinsulinemia causes hepatic IR and hepatic de-novo lipogenesis. Triglyceride synthesis is enhanced as well as raised triglyceride-rich VLDL and VLDL clearance peripherally is inhibited [113]. In addition, increased insulin and glucose concentrations upregulate HMGCoA reductase activity resulting in increased cholesterol synthesis [114].

3.3.2.2.3 Hypertension and insulin resistance

As far back as 1988 Gerald Reaven proposed a link between hypertension and hyperinsulinaemia in his Banting lecture [70]. Several studies have since shown that patients with hypertension also have hyperinsulinaemia and IR [115–121]. Moreover, when insulin sensitivity improves and serum insulin concentrations are lowered, blood pressure has been shown to reduce [122–124]. Although there is strong evidence of correlation between hyperinsulinaemia, hypertension, and IR, some population studies could not show a significant relationship [125,126].

The mechanism for hypertension in hyperinsulinaemic patients is postulated to be the direct effect of insulin on the sympathetic nervous system [122], as well as an increase in renal sodium retention. The theory of renal sodium handling is supported by many studies [127,128] including recent work by Dr. David Unwin [129]. Insulin promotes the renal reuptake of sodium and consequently fluid, at the level of the tubule [111]. Insulin is also believed to have a role in hypertrophy of vascular smooth muscle related to the mitogenic action of insulin and the mitogenic arm of the INSR. Hypertrophy via insulin action results in increased myocyte size and number as well as increases in contractile protein, collagen, and DNA. The resultant narrowing of the vascular wall has been thought to contribute to insulin-resistant hypertension [130–132].

3.3.2.2.4 Other hormones and IR

Abnormalities in other hormones namely leptin, resistin, adiponectin, amongst others, play a role in the pathophysiology of IR and MetS [133].

3.3.2.2.5 Mitochondrial dysfunction, oxidative stress and MetS

Several bodies of research have highlighted the role oxidative stress and mitochondrial dysfunction play in the pathogenesis of ageing and degenerative metabolic diseases [134].

Mitochondrial dysfunction and metabolic syndrome Mitochondria perform key biochemical functions that are essential for metabolic homoeostasis including adenosine triphosphate (ATP) production, intracellular calcium regulation,

ROS production and scavenging. Mitochondria also regulate apoptotic cell death as well as cell survival [135,136]. The primary mitochondrial function is ATP synthesis through oxidative phosphorylation via the citric acid cycle as well as beta oxidation of fats.

Evidence suggests that when there are alterations that arise in mitochondrial fission and fusion processes this inhibits mitophagy (a process responsible for the elimination of dysfunctional mitochondria). This then results in reduced mitochondrial biogenesis [137].

The mitochondria continuously metabolise oxygen and generate ROS. However, in the process of electron flow, approximately 5% of oxygen consumed is incompletely reduced [138]. This results in the production of ROS. Superoxide anions are thought to be the primary ROS and when they are generated in excess, they cross react with multiple compounds in an effort to stabilise, in turn yielding secondary ROS [138,139]. These ROS further interact with nitrogenous bases in DNA molecules thereby causing damage to the DNA backbone [139]. Excess ROS also damages vital mitochondrial enzymes and proteins thus disrupting ATP production as well as essential functions in mitochondria [137]. By the same processes, RNS are also produced which similarly cause damage to cellular organelles and potent antioxidant production is reduced.

Mitochondrial dysfunction by these mechanisms is implicated in each of the clinical conditions that make up the clinical diagnosis of MetS [140–145]. It is also important to note that various lifestyle processes contribute to ROS production and reduced antioxidants e.g., poor sleep quality and quantity, shift work, and chronic stress.

Oxidative stress Reactive species are essential signalling molecules in health. They play a physiological role in all bodily processes from cell division, growth, and differentiation to metabolic regulation (including insulin signalling) and are coupled with neutralisation factors to maintain homoeostasis.

In the physiological state, homoeostasis is maintained through highly efficient and synchronised processes of reactive species and antioxidant production, as well as the removal and repair of damaged molecules. However, in the presence of nutrient excess, all nutrient metabolic pathways are overwhelmed and the metabolic redox equilibrium is disrupted. For example, in glucose excess, the accumulation of glycolytic metabolites activates alternate pathways for glucose metabolism, namely the polyol, hexosamine and advanced glycation pathways [146]. This in turn increases ROS and nitrogen species (NS) Production [146]. With regards to the polyol pathway, nicotinamide adenine dinucleotide phosphate (NADPH) is depleted, which is associated with a reduction in glutathione [147], as well as IR (related to IRS-1 tyrosine phosphorylation, Akt phosphorylation/activation, and GLUT4 expression) [148]. Glutathione is a potent cellular antioxidant, so its reduction contributes to the overall reduction in antioxidant capacity and oxidative damage. Thus excess glucose ingestion overloads oxidation pathways by enhancing free radical production as well as impairing antioxidant defence mechanisms by reducing their availability [149]. In IR and MetS, physiological states usually characterised by excess glucose ingestion, glutathione exhaustion and oxidative stress overload are both inevitable exacerbators for these diseases.

A further metabolic consequence of glucotoxicity is the oxidative, carbonyl, and glycation stress caused by advanced glycation end products (AGE) and other metabolites such as reactive carbonyls. AGEs when bound to specific cell surface receptors of AGE (RAGE), result in alterations in signalling pathways and promote intracellular RO(N)S production [147]. There is recent evidence to suggest that common stress signalling pathways nuclear factor-kappa B and NH2-terminal JNK/SAPK are all central to the development of diabetes complications.

When WAT storage becomes overwhelmed due to excess nutrient intake, increased free fatty acids (FFA) circulate and deposit as visceral fat in the liver, muscle, pancreas as well as ectopically resulting in lipotoxicity and resultant oxidative stress and damage, as well as IR (Fig. 3.2). Aside from the obvious impairment of efficiency of each organ, FFA delivery and fatty acid oxidation in muscles have been hypothesised to increase acetyl CoA/CoA and NADH/NAD ratio. This in itself has been postulated to inactivate glucose-6-phosphate (G6P) thus inhibiting hexokinase II activity and a resultant increase in intracellular glucose, followed by reduced glucose uptake and glycogen synthesis [150]. In the setting of lipotoxicity, there is an accumulation of fatty acids and other lipid metabolites namely, diacylglycerol (DAG), ceramide, and lipid aldehydes, which increase oxidative stress via numerous intracellular mechanisms [151].

DAGs directly activate protein kinase C (PKC) and other serine/threonine kinases, which results in the impaired tyrosine phosphorylation of insulin receptor substrate (IRS) and insulin signalling.

There are numerous sources of cellular oxidative stress related to lipotoxicity and calcium signalling including mitochondrial impairment, endoplasmic reticulum stress, as well as various kinases, AGEs, iNOS, oxidases, xanthine oxidase. Likewise, as a consequence of multiple cellular oxidative stress sources, a vicious cycle of insulin insensitivity and impaired insulin secretion develops.

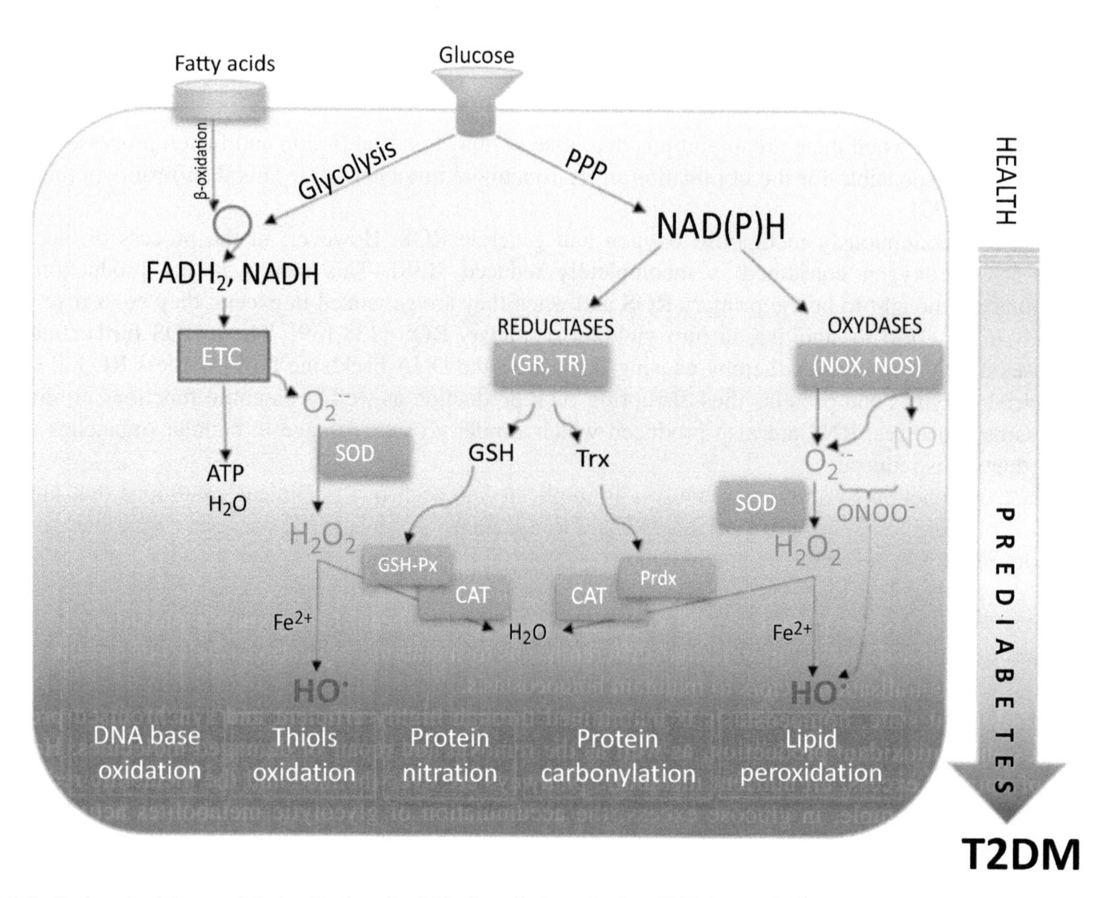

FIGURE 3.2 Redox physiology and its implications for T2D via radical production. T2DM, type 2 diabetes mellitus; etc, electron transport chain; GSH, glutathione; GSH-Px, glutathione peroxidase; GR, glutathione reductase; NOS, nitric oxide synthase; NOX, NADPH oxidase; PPP, pentose phosphate pathway; Prdx, peroxiredoxin; SOD, superoxide dismutase; TR, thioredoxin reductase; Trx, thioredoxin [134].

3.3.2.2.6 Nitric oxide and metabolic syndrome

Nitric oxide (NO) is well known as a potent vasodilator and a vital role player in endothelial tone regulation especially in the action of dilating coronary arteries. It also is known to play a role in lowering blood pressure by dilating distant arteries [152,153]. Its production is also mediated by the glycocalyx in response to sheer-stress forces [154].

Interestingly NO also plays a role in oxidative stress, mitochondrial dysfunction and IR. Excess ROS interact with NO, reducing its bioavailability due to the formation of a potent oxidant, peroxynitrate. This has downstream effects in many cells and receptors, including the insulin receptor where it disrupts the phosphorylation/dephosphorylation of the molecules within the insulin signalling cascade (Fig. 3.3) [156,157].

A further reduction in NO occurs due to the presence of pro-inflammatory cytokines found in the abundance of WAT seen in obesity [155].

So, the inflammatory and high-oxidative stress environment of MetS results in lower NO, which in turn increases blood pressure, clotting and IR, thereby creating a worsening cycle of MetS and its sequelae.

Both exercise and dietary interventions (a ketogenic diet or a diet) high in nitrite and nitrate-rich vegetables have been shown to increase NO concentrations and have beneficial effects of IR [155,158,159].

3.3.3 Managing the patient

3.3.3.1 Aims of care

Across all models of therapy, there is global agreement that early identification and management is imperative to prevent diabetes and CVD. Current management and therapeutics of MetS target risk reduction by advising lifestyle change and pharmacotherapy. Despite much ongoing research into newer drugs, the burden of disease continues to increase.

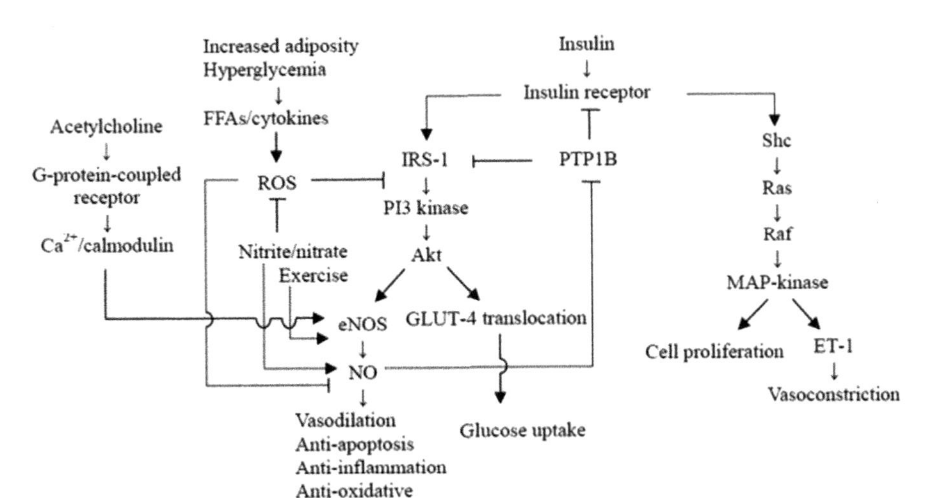

FIGURE 3.3 The insulin signalling pathway with emphasis on anti-inflammatory effects of nitric oxide and its inhibition via hyperglycaemia and elevated reactive oxygen species. ROS, reactive oxygen species; FFAs, free fatty acids; IRS-1, insulin receptor substrate-1; PI3 kinase, phosphatidylinositol 3 kinase; NO, nitric oxide; eNOS, endothelial nitric oxide synthase; GLUT4, glucose transporter 4; MAP-kinase, mitogen-activated protein kinase; PTP1B, protein tyrosine phosphatase 1B; ET-1, endothelin 1 [155].

As highlighted, central to the aetiology of the diseases associated with MetS is overnutrition and IR. Thus, all efforts to reverse MetS must address the aggressive reversal of IR. While pharmacotherapy does have a role, the role of nutrition and lifestyle warrants more attention.

3.3.3.2 Pharmacotherapy

The International Diabetes Federation (IDF) recommends aggressive treatment for those diagnosed with MetS. Weight loss is suggested as the primary intervention and drug therapy for all those in whom 'lifestyle change is not enough and who are considered to be at high risk for CVD.' The following drug therapy is recommended by the IDF for the below mentioned aspects of MetS.

3.3.3.2.1 Insulin resistance and hyperglycaemia

Metformin is recommended for people with prediabetes in order to delay the onset of diabetes. They also suggest that thiazolidinediones, acarbose, and orlistat show some efficacy in delaying and preventing diabetes in people with impaired glucose tolerance and IR.

3.3.3.2.2 Elevated blood pressure

The IDF recommend the JNC 7 recommendations for the treatment of hypertension (blood pressure of 140/90 mmHg or above). Angiotensin converting enzyme (ACE) inhibitors and angiotensin receptor blockers are recommended for people with diabetes. It is important to highlight that the main risk reduction is due to 'blood pressure lowering per se' and not to any particular drug therapy.

3.3.3.2.3 Atherogenic dyslipidaemia

With the main aim being to lower triglycerides, raise HDL cholesterol and lower LDL cholesterol, fibrate and statin therapy are what the current guidelines recommend.

Reduction in inflammation and the effect of redox imbalance are not mentioned in the IDF guidelines for MetS.

Considering the pathophysiology and the role that IR plays in raising BG concentrations, elevating blood pressure and abnormal blood lipids, as well as the effect on redox imbalance and systemic inflammation, it is clear that IR plays a central role in MetS and TCR must therefore be the primary factor in disease management.

3.3.3.3 Lifestyle factors

3.3.3.3.1 Exercise

Many studies have shown that MetS prevalence is higher in individuals with lower cardiorespiratory fitness [160]. Exercise has a complementary and an adjunctive role in metabolic health.

All forms of exercise including aerobic exercise, interval training as well as resistance training have been shown to improve insulin sensitivity [161,162]. Physical activity when compared to sedentary lifestyle is also associated with increased insulin sensitivity [163,164].

Muscle strength and lean body mass are independently associated with MetS with each of the five components of MetS showing an inverse association with muscle strength [165].

As we age, skeletal muscle shows impaired mitochondrial function. It is this impairment that contributes to age-associated atrophy as well as IR [166]. Exercise, by the process of up-regulation and expression of various enzymes including AMPK, SIRT1, SIRT3, MAPK, as well as by the increased expression of antioxidant enzymes and proteins involved in oxidative phosphorylation, results in mitochondrial adaptation in skeletal muscle [167]. By signalling bioenergetic and oxidative stressors, exercise therefore acts as a stimulator of mitohormesis, thus up regulating mitochondrial capacity [168–170].

The beneficial mitochondrial and metabolic enhancements of exercise have been shown to be enhanced on a ketogenic diet [171] (Fig. 3.4).

3.3.3.3.2 Circadian rhythm and sleep

Misalignment between the central clocks that regulate the circadian rhythm and the sleep-wake cycle, or food intake and behavioural rhythms are associated with IR, obesity, and diabetes [172–174] with shift workers being at higher risk of metabolic disease [175]. It is therefore vital to address the role of these factors in metabolic disease and to target strategies to help realign with the circadian rhythm including sleep quality improvement, time restricted eating, and adequate daylight exposure [176].

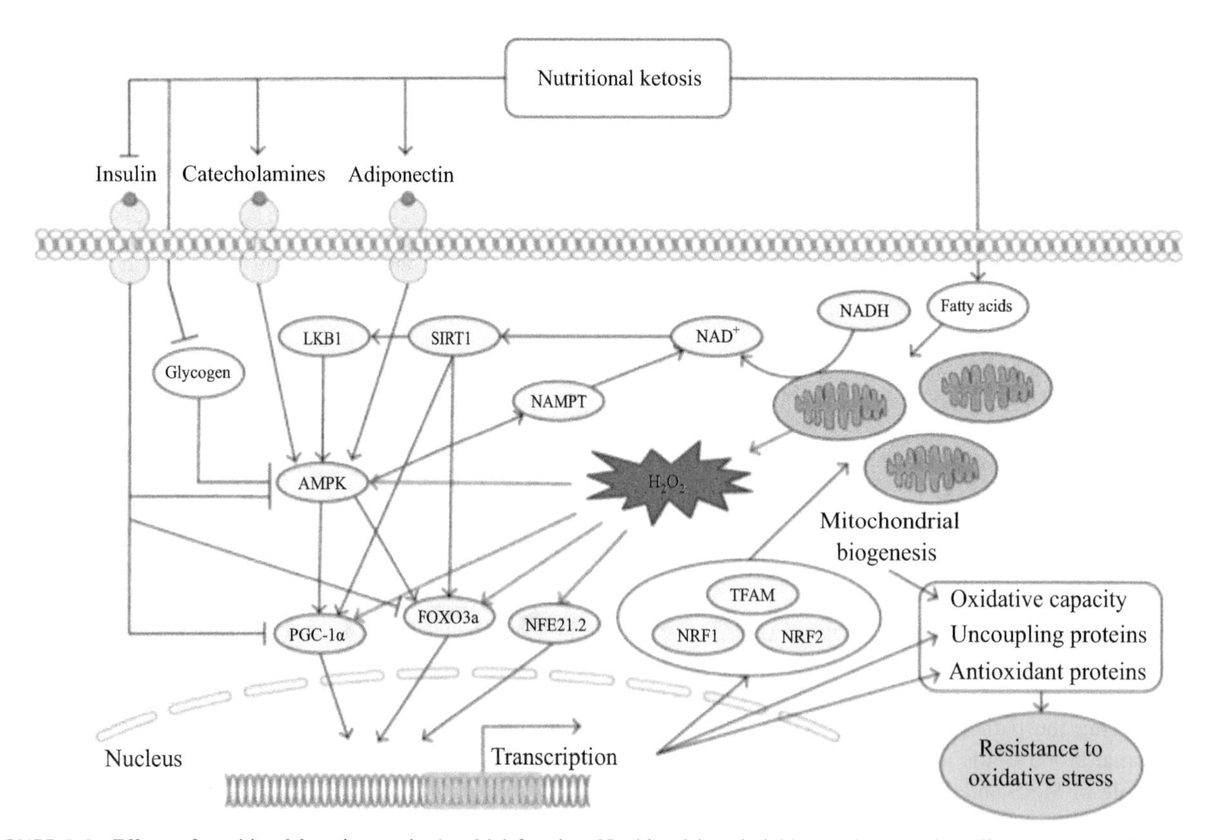

FIGURE 3.4 Effects of nutritional ketosis on mitochondrial function. Nutritional ketosis initiates mitoprotective effects against oxidative stress. NAD^+, nicotinamide adenine dinucleotide; NADH, NAD^+ hydrogen (H); LKB1, liver kinase B1; SIRT1, silent mating type information regulation 2 homologue 1; NAMPT, nicotinamide phosphoribosyltransferase; AMPK, AMP-activated protein kinase; PGC-1α, peroxisome proliferator-activated receptor γ coactivator 1α; FOXO3a, forkhead box O 3a; NFE2L2, nuclear factor erythroid-derived 2-like 2; TFAM, mitochondrial transcription factor A; NRF-1 and NRF-2, nuclear respiratory factors 1 and 2 [167].

Calorie restriction (CR) without malnutrition and exercise have been found to buffer the oxidative effects of mitochondrial dysfunction and inflammation [177]. CR and exercise increase tissue NAD^+, which activates the longevity and reparative gene, SIRT1. CR also reduces overall ROS production and enhances mitochondrial function. In addition CR substantially improves insulin sensitivity [178,179] and inhibits key nutrient sensing and inflammatory pathways [177].

3.3.3.3.3 Cold exposure

Cold exposure therapy is another modality showing promising results in the improvement of mitochondrial number and function as well as other important improvements such as reduction in inflammation, activation of antioxidant enzymes and an increase in brown fat [180–187]. To be considered under caution and supervision, this therapy form is gaining popularity by those wishing to improve athletic performance as well as cardiometabolic health.

3.3.3.3.4 Nutritional medicines

Resveratrol, vitamin C, vitamin E, curcumin as well as mitochondrial support compounds (MitoQ), have all been shown to have anti-inflammatory effects [159,177]. However, additional antioxidants and nutraceuticals are not a replacement for a poor lifestyle and should be seen only as additional supportive supplements, prescribed on an individualised basis.

3.3.3.4 Diet: Therapeutic carbohydrate restriction for reversing and reducing MetS markers

3.3.3.4.1 Evidence

MetS is a conglomerate of symptoms and biomarkers that include elevated fasting BG, raised BMI, hypertriglyceridemia and a low HDL cholesterol concentration, and hypertension. These can all be shown to be centrally linked to IR [103]. TCR improves glycaemic control [188] and results in greater long-term body weight reduction in obese patients. Additionally, it lowers triglycerides and diastolic blood pressure, and increases HDL and LDL cholesterol concentrations compared to a low-fat diet [114,188–190]. The evidence for the use of TCR and a ketogenic diet for addressing each of these hallmarks of MetS, in addition to mitochondrial dysfunction, oxidative stress, and inflammation, are discussed in more detail below.

Glycemic control Meta-analyses show that patients who were overweight or obese with pre-existing T2D show a marked improvement in HbA1c on TCR. Overall TCR is more effective at glycaemic control than other comparative diets [188].

Body weight Meta-analyses [188] show that when TCR is used in obese patients, they were more likely to experience a greater weight reduction, and this was especially significant for those with T2D (Fig. 3.5).

The current standard of practice recommends a low calorie, low-fat (high carbohydrate) diet for the treatment of obesity [191,192] in order to reduce energy intake. The replacement of fat with carbohydrate stimulates insulin secretion, which in turn increases appetite [193]. Conversely, a reduction in insulin (a consequence of TCR) results in appetite reduction and lower energy intake, particularly in insulin resistant patients [114]. Other hormones and adipokines such as leptin also play a role [193]. Additionally, basal metabolic rate [194] and lean body mass are conserved [193,194] on very low-calorie ketogenic diets, unlike caloric-restricted low-fat diets.

Lipids Study analysis of overweight or obese patients with T2D who are treated with TCR shows a greater improvement in serum triglyceride concentrations while at the same time raised HDL concentrations. For nondiabetic patients, there is a relatively higher increase in total cholesterol and LDL cholesterol. For all patients, TCR was associated with a larger reduction in serum triglyceride and an increase in serum LDL and HDL concentrations [188]. Other studies have shown a slight reduction in total and LDL cholesterol [195] or no effect [196] and clinically we see some variation in the effect on these variables. Of significance, nuclear magnetic resonance (NMR) results showed that on TCR, there was a shift in the number of small and very small atherogenic LDL particles to larger fluffier LDL particles [197]. Retinol binding protein 4 (RBP4), a marker of IR, also decreased, which further supports the role of insulin as the primary mediator of MetS. Changes in lipid profile were attributed to a reduction of insulin concentrations and were independent of fat loss [198,199].

Feinman [200] has made an argument for Apo B/Apo A-1 ratio to be considered a better indicator of risk for vascular disease [200] and this ratio was shown to improve on TCR [197,200].

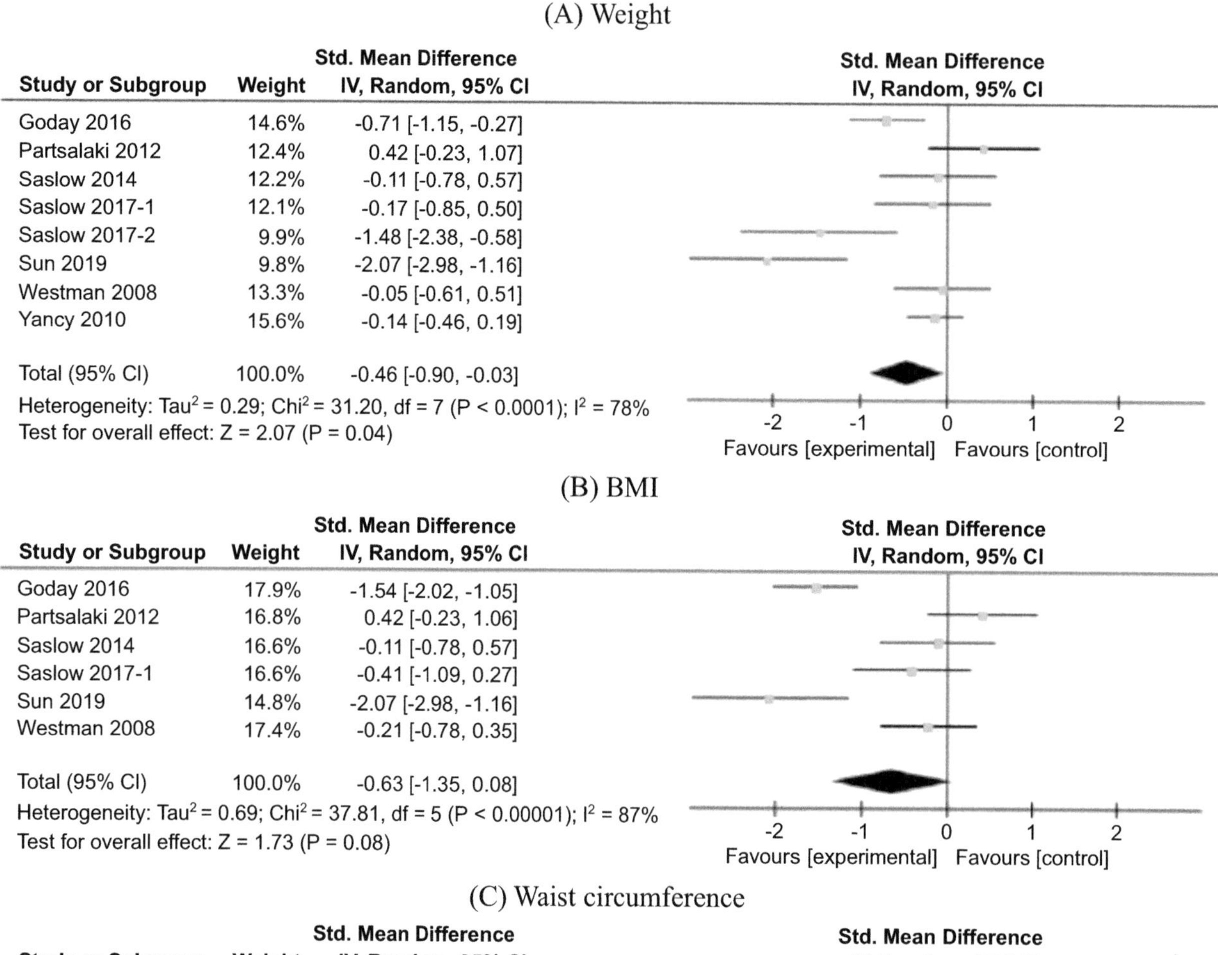

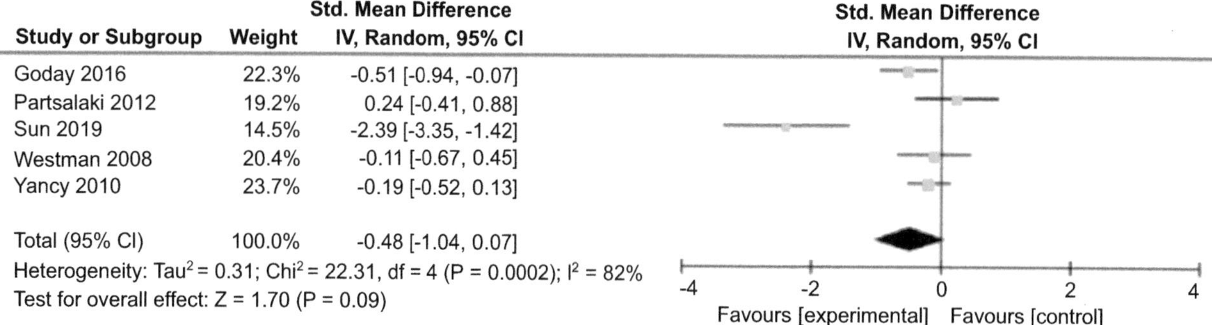

FIGURE 3.5 Forest plots indicating associations between dietary interventions (ketogenic experimental diet compared to control) and body weight (A), body mass index (BMI) (B), and waist circumference (C), respectively, in overweight or obese individuals with or without T2D [188].

Blood pressure Elevated blood pressure is a marker of MetS and while some studies show no substantial difference in DBP and SBP between low fat and TCR [188], other meta-analyses show a drop in global BP on TCR [190].

Mitochondrial health and oxidative stress Mitohormesis is an adaptive state that occurs when an organism increases reliance on mitochondrial respiration. By up-regulating mitochondrial capacity, there is enhanced resistance to the oxidative effects of mitochondrial ROS and an increase in antioxidant defence mechanisms [167,201]. The negative effect that excesses ROS has on the mitochondria is clear. However at modest concentrations, ROS stimulate biological processes such as proliferation, differentiation and immunity, as well as regulating postprandial IR and fuel influx [202].

Ketogenic diets shift metabolism towards reliance on fatty acid oxidation with a resultant increase in ketone body production [167,203–205]. This enhanced mitochondrial respiration and mitochondrial ROS production induces mitohormesis [167].

Ketone bodies play an important role in enhancing antioxidant defence mechanisms in the mitochondria through histone deacetylase inhibition [206]. This important role of BHB provides antioxidant defence protection in the cardiomyocytes of the heart [207] as well as neuronal and anti-seizure effects [208,209].

Ketone bodies can themselves have direct antioxidant capability [210]. In addition, by decreasing the duration of opening of mitochondrial permeability transition pore and by reducing mtROS production, ketone bodies have a protective role and reduce cellular injury and death [210,211].

Inflammation C-reactive protein (CRP), an inflammatory marker, is shown to be reduced on TCR [190].

3.3.3.4.2 Guiding the patient

While stricter ketogenic diets are medically prescribed for the management of conditions such as resistant seizures, a growing body of evidence attributes keto adaptation to a range of health gains [113,189,200,212–223]. A less restrictive and therefore more sustainable form of the ketogenic diet can be used for the management of metabolic diseases such as T2D and MetS. A well-formulated ketogenic diet is generally accepted as a carbohydrate intake of under 50 g per day and protein intake of around 1.5 g per kilogram of ideal body weight per day. This diet typically results in an increase in beta hydroxybutyrate and acetoacetate concentrations from 0.3 mM to what is defined as nutritional ketosis range of 0.5–3 mM [224]. This range is far below the concentrations associated with ketoacidosis (5–10 mM) [224].

3.3.4 Conclusion

Current management and therapeutics of MetS target risk reduction by advising lifestyle change and pharmacotherapy. Despite much ongoing research into newer drugs, the burden of disease continues to increase. The case has been made for a single root factor being associated with MetS: hyperinsulinaemia. It has also been shown that when this factor is reduced by the prescription of TCR, the individual diseases or risk factors associated with this syndrome also improve. This makes a powerful case for TCR as the critical, if not first, step towards treatment of MetS. TCR and nutritional ketosis, as well as lifestyle interventions such as exercise and improved circadian biorhythms, target key pathophysiological mechanisms in MetS and offer efficacious therapeutic interventions for the reversal of MetS.

3.4 Type 2 diabetes

Neville Wellington

Contributions made by:

Mark Cucuzzella, Karen Riley, Diana Isaacs

Additional authors:

International Working Group on Remission of Type 2 Diabetes

Sean McKelvey, IPTN Institute for Personalized Therapeutic Nutrition, Vancouver, BC, Canada

William Yancy Jr, Lifestyle and Weight Management Center and Department of Medicine, Duke University, United States

Susan Wolver, General Internal Medicine, Diplomate, American Board of Obesity Medicine, VCU Medical Weight Loss Program, Richmond, VI, United States

Campbell Murdoch, Millbrook Surgery, Somerset, United Kingdom

Brian Lenzkes, Internal Medicine, San Diego, CA, United States

Caroline Roberts, Virta Health, United States

David Cavan, United Kingdom

David Unwin, The Norwood Surgery, Southport, United Kingdom

Eric Westman, Department of Medicine, Duke University, United States

Miriam Berchuk, Dipl. American Board of Obesity Medicine, Canada

Graham Phillips, United Kingdom

Ali Irshad Al Lawati, Internal Medicine, Diwan of Royal Court, Oman

Nafeeza Hj Mohd Ismail, School of Medicine, International Medical University, Malaysia

Daniel Katambo, Afyaplanet, Kenya

Anne-Sophie Brazeau, McGill University, Canada

3.4.1 Introduction

T2D follows on in patients at risk who have developed insulin resistance or MetS and who continue to follow a high carbohydrate lifestyle over many years. As noted in the chapters on MetS, damage first occurs in the liver and causes non-alcoholic fatty liver disease (NAFLD), which then progresses to insulin resistance and then the overproduction of glucose from the liver and ultimately frank diabetes [225]. Here, evidence and practical information is provided for the use of low carbohydrate diets (LCDs) in the management and possible reversal of T2D.

3.4.1.1 Description

T2D is defined using any one of the following parameters:

- Fasting glucose (FG) (after an 8 h non-caloric fast) ≥7 mmol (≥126 mg/dL) OR
- 2 h oral glucose tolerance test (OGTT) (using a glucose load of 75 g) ≥11.1 mmol/L (≥200 mg/dL) OR
- Glycated Haemoglobin (HbA1c) ≥6.5% (48 mmol/mol) OR
- Random glucose ≥11.1 (≥200 mg/dL) in a patient with classic symptoms of hyperglycaemia [226].

Prediabetes is defined using the following parameters:

- FG 5.6 mmol/L (100 mg/dL) to 6.9 mmol/L (126 mg/dL)
- 2 h OGTT 7.8 mmol/L (140 mg/dL) to 11.0 mmol/L (199 mg/dL)
- HbA1c 5.7% to 6.4% (39 to 47 mmol/mol).

3.4.1.2 Clinical presentation

Patients who develop T2D may present with a whole spectrum of clinical pictures from asymptomatic, and usually only diagnosed during routine screening, to a full picture of signs and symptoms of hyperglycaemia, which may include thirst, polyuria, fatigue, weight loss, and even hyperosmolar non-ketotic acidosis (HONK), although a severe presentation is rare. In usual practice patients are screened for testing depending on a number of commonly known factors such as age (>45 years old), gender, history of gestational diabetes in women, family history of diabetes, other raised cardiovascular and metabolic conditions (e.g., raised blood pressure, raised triglycerides), physical inactivity and increased weight (BMI >25 kg/m^2). Studies have shown that patients may be pre-diabetic for many years and may decompensate to T2D within a fairly short time-frame (Fig. 3.6).

3.4.1.3 Complications of diabetes

Macrovascular (cardiovascular and peripheral vascular disease) and microvascular (retinopathy, nephropathy, and neuropathy) complications are widespread in T2D, even pre-dating the onset of diabetes. Studies have shown that even patients who have concentrations of HbA1c lower than that accepted for diabetes (i.e., <6.5%) have an increased risk of CVD [228–231], and worsening coronary artery disease [232]. Mortality rates in adult people with T2D from CHD and stroke are two to four times higher than in healthy individuals without it [233].

These complications can be explained in a large part to the glucotoxic effect of raised glucose concentrations in the bloodstream. Hyperglycaemia raises glucose concentrations in the cells of the body especially in cells like the endothelial cells and nerve cells which do not have mechanisms to reduce the uptake of glucose [234].

At a cellular level hyperglycaemia has been shown to induce four major pathways through which excess substrates of glucose metabolism will flux: the polyol pathway, the hexosamine pathway, the protein kinase C pathway and the advanced glycation endproducts (AGEs) pathway [234–236]. All these pathways are known to cause damage and increase inflammatory markers such as interleukin (IL)-1, IL-6, tumour necrosis factor-α (TNF-α), leptin, resistin, nuclear factor-kB, platelet-derived growth factor-β, transforming growth factor-β (TNF-β), plasminogen activator inhibitor-1 (PAI-1), C-reactive protein (CRP), fibrinogen, angiotensin, visfatin, retinol-binding protein-4 and many other cytokines. In the endothelium (which is where much of the damage takes place), the end result is the reduction in nitric oxide (NO) production (by inactivating endothelial nitric oxygen synthase (eNOS)) and inactivating prostacyclin synthase, and then increasing intracellular adhesion molecules (ICAM-1) and vascular cellular adhesion molecules (VCAM-1) and monocyte chemoattractant molecule-1 (MCP-1) [233,237].

In arteries the inflammatory milieu of diabetes causes changes and activation to the endothelial cells, which promote coagulation and thrombosis in the arteries. Platelets are activated, NO is depleted and angiotensin II increases,

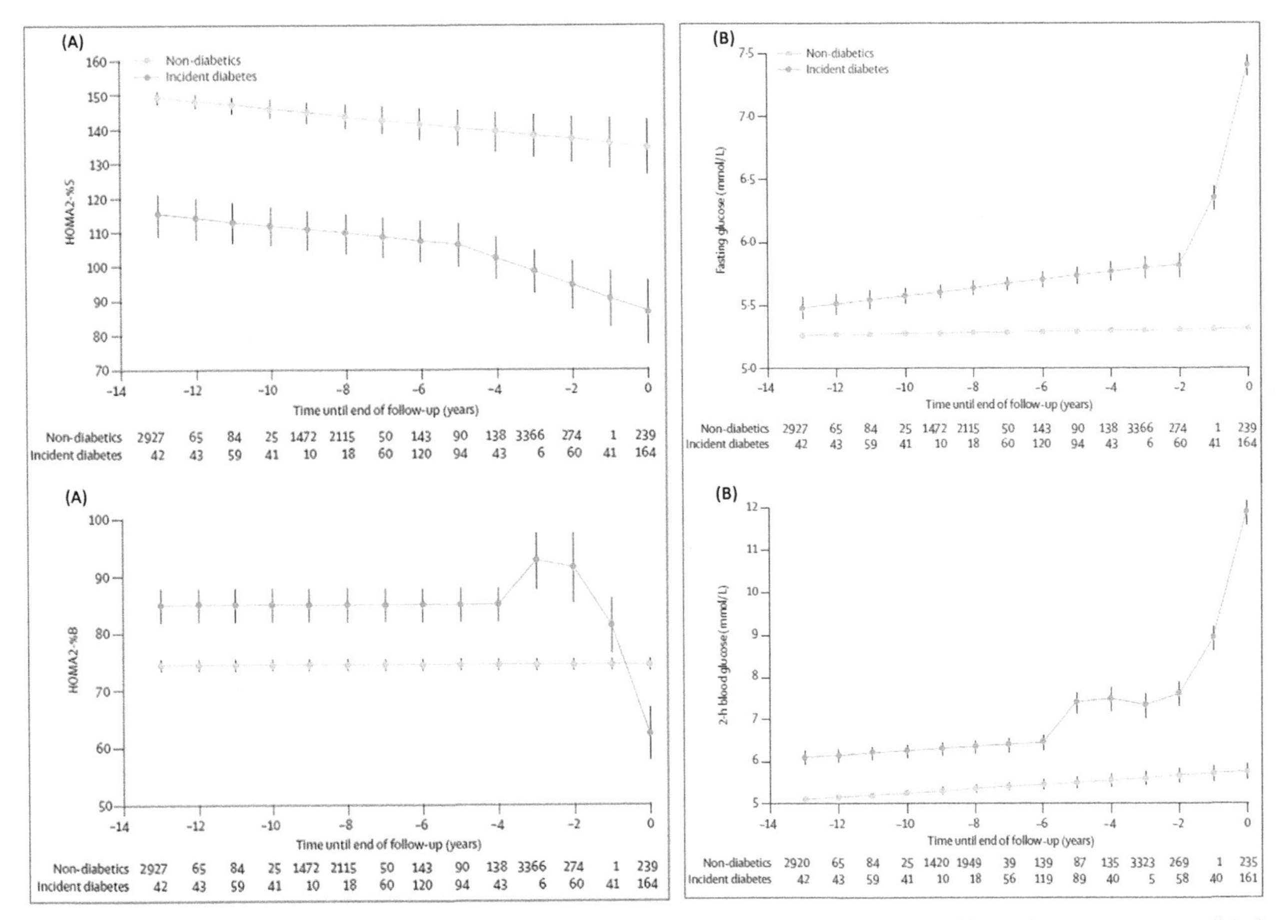

FIGURE 3.6 **Progression to T2D over time.** 505 patients who developed T2D (blue line) compared to 6033 patients who were non-diabetic. Graphs A and B on the left show increasing insulin resistance (A) and beta-cell failure (B), whereas the graphs on the right show worsening FG (A) and 2-h glucose readings on a OGTT. HOMA2-%S, homoeostasis model assessment insulin sensitivity, HOMA2-%B, homoeostasis model assessment beta cell function [227]. *From Whitehall II study.*

promoting vasoconstriction. The first step in the formation of atherosclerotic plaques is the uptake of oxidised LDL cholesterol/particles simultaneously with the adhesion and uptake of monocytes. In the subendothelial space monocytes change to macrophages which then ingest oxidised LDL cholesterol/particles eventually forming foam cells. Cytokines are released, which promote the translocation of smooth muscle cells to the area and further increase growth of the plaque [237]. Stable plaques are usually formed, but ongoing inflammation can destabilise the plaques [238]. Matrix metalloproteinases are released by the macrophages which appear to thin the fibrous cap and make it susceptible to rupture [238]. This helps to explain the proliferation of plaques that occur in diabetes and the propensity to peripheral vascular disease, coronary artery disease, cerebral artery disease, and other vascular disease processes.

Spikes of glucose that last for more than 16 h to concentrations >8.6 mmol/L (154.8 mg/dL) have been shown to cause epigenetic changes in the promoter of NF-κβ subunit p65 in the aortic endothelial cells. These effects are caused by hyperglycaemia-induced ROS formation in the mitochondria. Increased concentrations of NF-κβ p65 causes increased concentrations of MCP-1, which recruits plasma monocytes in the early stages of atherosclerosis, and VCAM-1, which promotes monocyte adhesion to the arterial endothelial cells. These changes can persist for 6 days after normalisation of glucose concentrations and highlights the dramatic and long-lasting effects even short-term hyperglycaemic spikes can have on cells [239].

Glucose toxicity is also known to occur in the insulin producing β-cells of the pancreas [240–242]. This ultimately leads to a relative reduction in insulin production, which reduces the glucose lowering ability of insulin in the liver. Hyperglycaemia may then also be explained by the inability of the pancreas to produce enough insulin to suppress glucose production from the liver.

3.4.2 Managing the patient

3.4.2.1 *Therapeutic carbohydrate restriction for type 2 diabetes*

The treatment of T2D includes any interventions that lower the glucose concentrations in patients and includes lifestyle changes, surgery, oral medications, and insulin therapy. All diabetes guidelines highlight, as a first step, the need to change lifestyles and increase exercise, and then stepwise approaches to medication use. For many years, as has been highlighted elsewhere, low-fat interventions with exercise have been used, yet the increase in global diabetes rates continues unabated [243]. Here, we will focus on TCR and evidence that may support its use in T2D.

3.4.2.2 *Evidence for therapeutic carbohydrate restriction in type 2 diabetes*

Systematic reviews of studies of TCR compared to conventional low-fat, energy-restricted diets, conclude that the lower the dietary carbohydrate the greater the improvements in glucose control and in weight loss [244–247]. This is despite many of the TCR arms not achieving a level of carbohydrate restriction that would classify them as true LCDs [248]. Most studies cited could show data up to 6 months or 12 months, so the long-term efficacy of the studies was unknown. In a review by Goldenberg et al., 57% of patients who followed LCD (<130 g/day) or VLCKD (<50 g/day) could achieve diabetes remission (defined as HbA1c <6.5%) at 6 months, although those who could stop all medication as well were a smaller group [247]. This review also highlighted the general safety of TCR, showing no worsening of CVD risk factors or adverse events. Although they noted a trend for increasing LDL cholesterol at 12 months. Benefits shown were in weight loss, reduction in medication usage and in reducing triglyceride concentration.

Feinman et al. [248] cite 12 points of the best evidence for the use of TCR in diabetes management. These points highlight that LCDs have the greatest effect on reducing hyperglycaemia (as reflected in HbA1c), a predictor of microvascular (and to some extent macrovascular) complications, Benefits of LCDs do not require weight loss, but it is often the best intervention to help with weight loss. Adherence to LCDs is as good as or better than adherence to any other diet. The intake of fat is not associated with increased risk for CVD (see Chapter 4). In fact plasma triglycerides (a key CVD risk factor) are controlled more by the intake of carbohydrates than by lowering fat intake. Patients with T2D are able to reduce medication use, thereby reducing exposure to adverse effects (see Section 3.5). Feinman et al. conclude that LCDs should be the first approach in patients with T2D due to its many benefits and few disadvantages to this approach (e.g., hypoglycaemic episodes if patients are not counselled about correctly lowering hypoglycaemic agents).

Noakes and Windt [249] have subsequently authored a narrative review showing evidence for the use of TCR for weight loss, insulin resistance, NAFLD, T2D, and atherogenic dyslipidaemia with associated CVD. They highlight the safety aspects of the diet in patients with these medical conditions, mentioning that at initiation of the diet may come with some transient side-effects linked to the natriuresis of fasting (colloquially known as 'keto-flu'), such as headache, fatigue, and muscle cramps. They also highlight the fact that as studies progress, an element of 'carbohydrate creep' may occur which often reduces the efficacy of the intervention in the long-term. However, motivated patients who remain on the diet continue to experience health benefits.

Brouns offered an alternative to these views where he looked at further evidence for or against the use of TCR in overweight or T2D patients [250]. In his review he shows evidence for good quality high carbohydrate (e.g. Paleo high fibre diets, like the Tsimane people of South America) diets being healthy in certain populations, but that when those populations introduce poor quality refined carbohydrates (sugars, etc.) into their diets, their health suffers. In overweight non-diabetes individuals, they show that low fat and LCDs seem to be equivalent in weight loss, and CVD marker improvements (except in LDL changes) and in prevention of progression from pre-diabetes to diabetes. However, he confirms the benefits for LCHF diets in diabetes patients which include weight loss, improved FG concentrations, reduction in HbA1c concentrations, reduction in medication use, reduction in hypoglycaemia and improvement in CVD markers. His final comments are cautionary and suggest that while LCHF diets in the short term are beneficial, long-term evidence is needed. He also highlights the observation seen in many studies (as well as in clinical practice by clinicians), that many patients experience 'carbohydrate creep' over time, and often end up at higher intakes of 130–160 g/day. He then recommends that a target of 100–150 g/day may be more sustainable. The major problem with the review is that he gives no alternative recommendations for controlling or reversing diabetes effectively.

There is a growing body of published literature discussing the clinical application of TCR for T2D. Virta Health's report on their novel digitally-monitored continuous care intervention at 2 years demonstrated sustained long-term beneficial effects on multiple clinical markers of diabetes and cardiometabolic health while utilising less medication [251]. While, in a primary care setting in the United Kingdom, Dr. David Unwin published on patient data over 6 years [252]. The findings from Unwin et al. [252] include (1) For those choosing a lower carbohydrate dietary approach for an average of 23 months it is possible to achieve a 46% drug-free T2D remission rate in UK primary care while achieving significant improvements in weight, blood pressure, and lipid profiles; (2) In patients with prediabetes, TCR reduced HbA1c to within a non-diabetes threshold in 93% of patients; (3) participants who started with the highest HbA1c saw the greatest improvements in glycaemic control. These clinical findings of TCR compare favourably to historical usual care for T2D. The DiRECT trial, which investigated a very low calorie formula feed in T2D found similar results, with only 4% of the usual-care control arm achieving remission (defined as A1C below 6.5% after at least 2 months off all diabetes medication) compared to 46% of the intervention arm [253].

Achieving tight glycaemic targets is important for preventing microvascular complications such as neuropathy, nephropathy, and retinopathy. However, modern treatment of T2D using pharmacological approaches does not consistently achieve HbA1c targets. Higher HbA1c is associated with more diabetes complications, morbidity, and mortality [254]. Lowering HbA1C alone does not always reduce complications. The Action to Control Cardiovascular Risk in Diabetes (ACCORD) trial demonstrated that intensive medical treatment carries an increased risk of all-cause mortality, a 35% increased risk of cardiovascular mortality, and a greater risk of hypoglycaemic events and weight gain of 10 kilograms compared to those on standard insulin therapy [255]. Other multinational, multicentre, randomised controlled trials that used medications to achieve tight glycaemic targets did not demonstrate the expected reductions in heart disease or overall mortality [256–261]. There is strong evidence for an alternative approach to treating people with T2D.

Evidence for TCR in patients with T2D continues to show improvements in glycaemic control, reduction in medication use, good safety profiles and improvement in CVD markers. Long-term outcomes in CVD improvements still need to be shown. Notably, studies in low fat diets have not yielded any beneficial improvements in CVD outcomes (see Chapter 4). There is no reason to suggest that TCR should not be offered to patients with T2D as the first line therapy and to continue to support patients who are interested in following this lifestyle or who have already started to follow it.

Despite the acceptance of reducing carbohydrates as a powerful option in T2D management, there is still a certain amount of clinical inertia and a large gap between awareness of the benefits of this intervention and practical application. Even in the recent 63-page publication in the Lancet from the Lancet Commission on Diabetes, which embodies four years of extensive work to make recommendations to improve clinical practice, carbohydrates are only mentioned once and only in relation to adjusting insulin doses [262].

3.4.2.3 Therapeutic carbohydrate restriction in type 2 diabetes: guiding the patient

Health providers who are willing to support patients with TCR should ensure they are comfortable with the guidelines and science of TCR. Interventions can either take place individually or in group settings and ideally should also have the help of diabetes nurse practitioners and, if possible, dietitians and/or health coaches, depending on the individual's needs.

There are five main areas that need to be dealt with when counselling patients about TCR in T2D:

1. Education on carbohydrates, what foods contain them and how to count carbohydrates
2. What can be eaten
3. Structured monitoring of glucose concentrations
4. De-prescribing medication
5. Common challenges encountered with TCR.

3.4.2.3.1 Education on carbohydrates

In general, patients need to understand that carbohydrates are the macronutrients that release glucose, fructose, and galactose, and these are the main monosaccharides that cause glucose concentrations to rise. They need to be educated on which foods contain them and the approximate values of carbohydrates in those foods. In this regard, a list may help them (e.g Table 3.2). From the above evidence, the aim is for patients to reduce carbohydrate consumption to about 30 g/day. All guidelines agree that refined carbohydrates (e.g., sugar and sweetened beverages) and processed foods or snacks should be avoided, and that only foods containing 'natural' carbohydrates should be eaten. However, a high intake of fruit and starchy foods may also need to be avoided, as these contain high concentrations of carbohydrates.

TABLE 3.2 Common carbohydrate-containing foods and their approximate carbohydrate content (g).

1 tsp sugar = 4–5 g
1 slice bread ≈ 15 g
1 plate cereal ≈ 23–30 g
250 mL fizzy sugary drink = 28 g
200 mL fruit juice = 28–32 g
250 mL apple juice = 24–32 g
100 g spaghetti = 75 g uncooked, 28 g cooked
1 × 100g potato/sweet potato = 21 g
1 cup cooked rice = 53 g
1 medium apple = 18 g
1 large banana = 28 g
100 mL sweetened yoghurt = 15 g
250 mL sweetened yoghurt = 37.5 g
100 g slab chocolate 62 g
1 cup whole milk = 11 g,
1 cup low fat = 12 g

Dr. Eric Westmen, author of *A New Atkins for a New You* (2010), explains [263] how dietary carbohydrate affects blood glucose in the context of T2D

An understanding of just how little glucose is contained in the bloodstream may give a better insight into the relationship between food and diabetes. The amount of glucose in the human bloodstream is very tightly regulated; the amount of serum glucose in an adult with a serum glucose concentration of 5.55 mmol/L (100 mg/dL) and 5 L of blood is about 5 g. This explains why a heaping teaspoon of table sugar or a few medium-sized strawberries (each approximately 5 g or 5000 mg of carbohydrate) can raise the BG concentration by 2.77 mmol/L (50 mg/dL), because the blood contains only about that amount of glucose (5 grams or 5000 mg) at any given moment. Normal serum glucose ranges from 80 to 99 mg/dL, and when a fasting serum glucose is elevated to 5.55–6.94 mmol/L (100–125 mg/dL), the diagnosis of impaired fasting glucose is made. These small changes in concentration in serum glucose represent changes in the amount of glucose in the blood of only a few grams. On the contrary, a meal without carbohydrate has very little effect on the BG concentration [264] (see Figs 3.7 and 3.8).

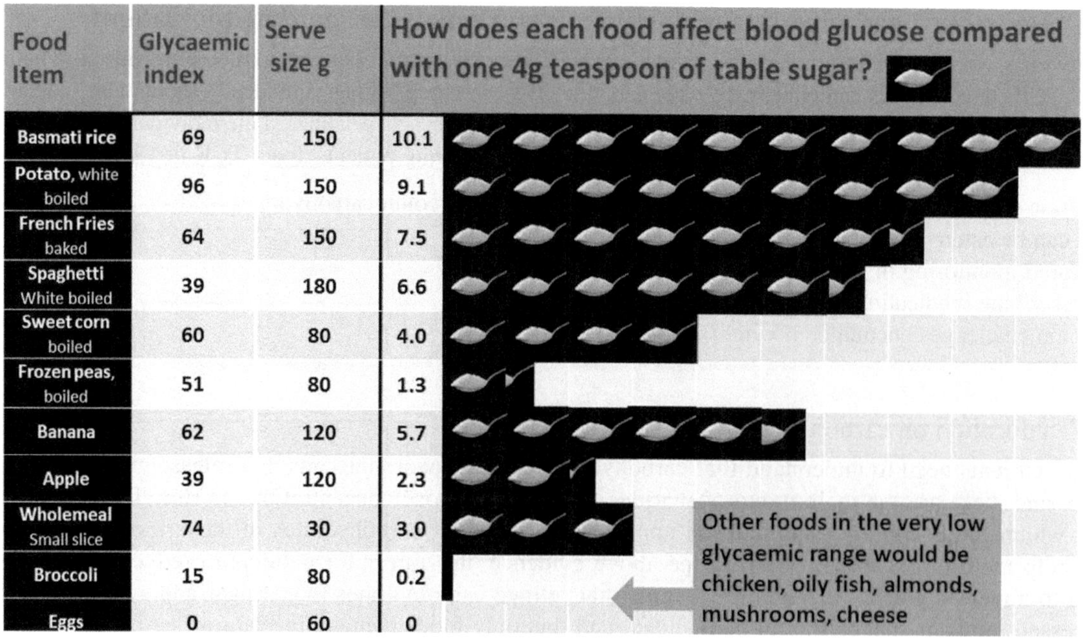

Food Item	Glycaemic index	Serve size g	How does each food affect blood glucose compared with one 4g teaspoon of table sugar?
Basmati rice	69	150	10.1
Potato, white boiled	96	150	9.1
French Fries baked	64	150	7.5
Spaghetti White boiled	39	180	6.6
Sweet corn boiled	60	80	4.0
Frozen peas, boiled	51	80	1.3
Banana	62	120	5.7
Apple	39	120	2.3
Wholemeal Small slice	74	30	3.0
Broccoli	15	80	0.2
Eggs	0	60	0

Other foods in the very low glycaemic range would be chicken, oily fish, almonds, mushrooms, cheese

FIGURE 3.7 A comparative chart of high and low-carbohydrate foods, their respective glycaemic indexes, and effects on blood glucose. Norwood infographic as per it is the glycaemic response to, not the carbohydrate content of food that matters in diabetes and obesity: The Glycaemic Index revisited (Unwin et al. [265]).

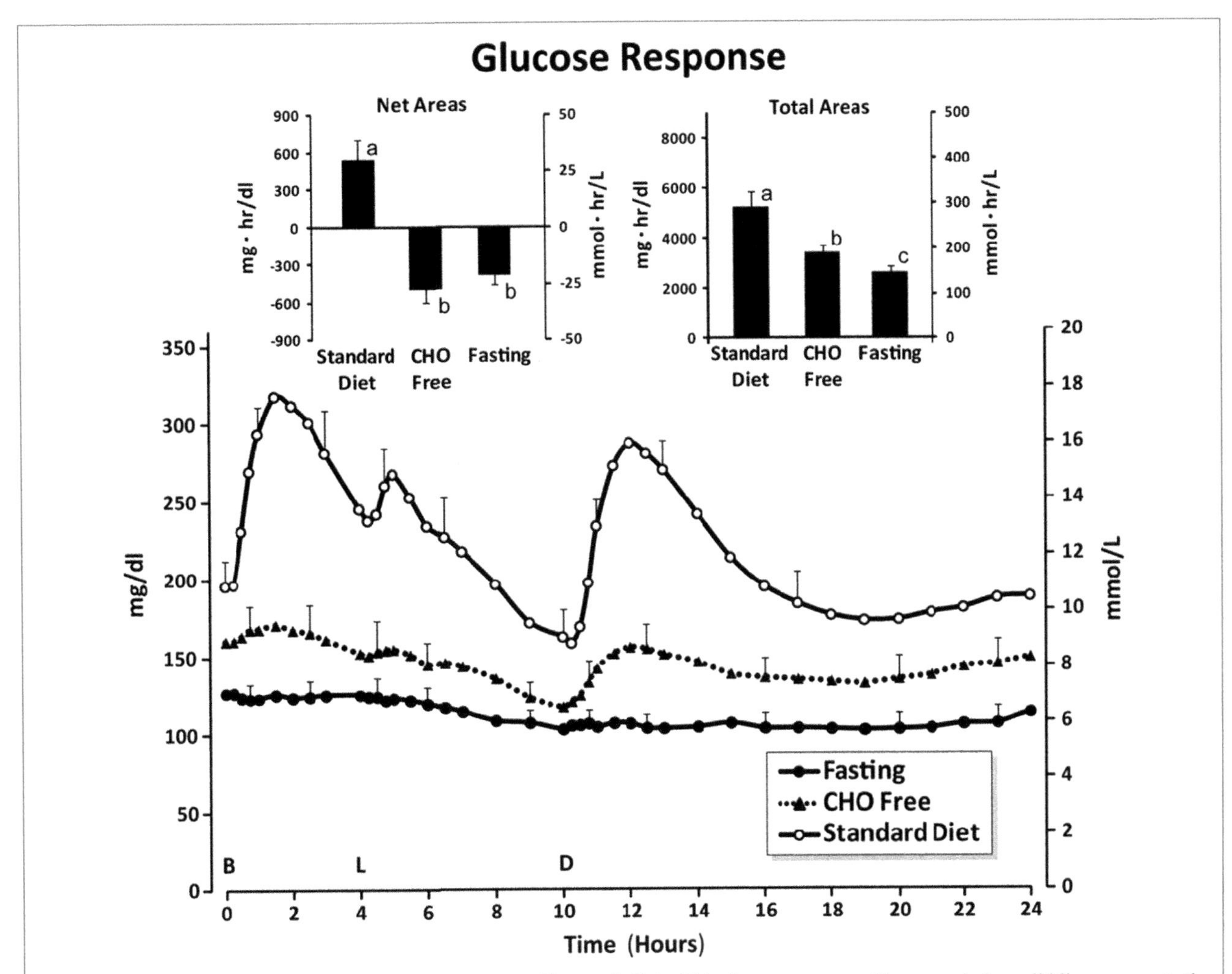

FIGURE 3.8 **Fasting and postprandial glucose response of low carb diets.** 24-h glucose response. The open circle–solid line represents the mean glucose concentration at several time points during the first 24 h of both days during which the standard diet was ingested (i.e., day 1 of each arm of the study). The triangle–dotted line represents the mean glucose concentration during the last 24 h on a carbohydrate-free diet. The closed circle–solid line represents the mean glucose concentration during the last 24 h of the fast (energy-free) diet. B, L, D, indicate the times at which breakfast, lunch, and dinner were ingested. The net area response (Left Insert) indicates the area under the curve using the fasting concentration as baseline. Different letters on bars indicate statistically significant differences (Friedman $P \leq .0012$). The total area response (Right Insert) indicates the area under the curve, using zero as baseline. Different letters on bars indicate statistically significant differences (Friedman: $P \leq .0001$) (Nuttall et al. [266]).

Other helpful resources could include books (e.g., The Drinking Man's Diet [267]), websites (e.g., http://www.carbohydrate-counter.org) or reading nutritional labels (Fig. 3.9).

3.4.2.3.2 What can be eaten

While food choices will differ based on individual preferences and cultural dictates there are general principles which can be followed to ensure low carbohydrate intake and adequate intakes of protein and fat. A simple list can be used to give broad principles (Table 3.3), or more specific lists (e.g., Fig. 3.10; or the green, orange and red lists from 'The Real Meal Revolution' [268]). Many patients may find it helpful to see a dietitian for advice on healthy LCDs. In general, unprocessed saturated or mono-unsaturated fats, from natural sources (e.g., animals or certain vegetables (olive or coconut oils)) are viewed as healthy, whereas polyunsaturated fats from seed or processed 'vegetable' oils should be avoided.

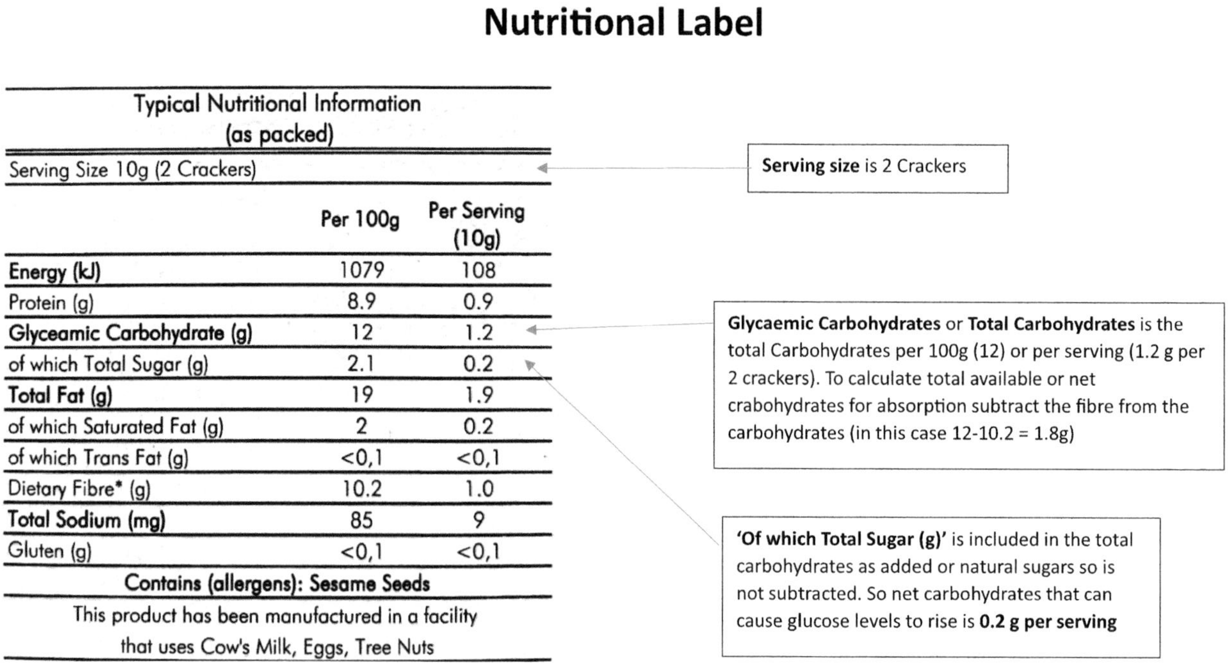

Nutritional Label

Typical Nutritional Information (as packed)

Serving Size 10g (2 Crackers)

	Per 100g	Per Serving (10g)
Energy (kJ)	1079	108
Protein (g)	8.9	0.9
Glyceamic Carbohydrate (g)	12	1.2
of which Total Sugar (g)	2.1	0.2
Total Fat (g)	19	1.9
of which Saturated Fat (g)	2	0.2
of which Trans Fat (g)	<0,1	<0,1
Dietary Fibre* (g)	10.2	1.0
Total Sodium (mg)	85	9
Gluten (g)	<0,1	<0,1

Contains (allergens): Sesame Seeds

This product has been manufactured in a facility that uses Cow's Milk, Eggs, Tree Nuts

Serving size is 2 Crackers

Glycaemic Carbohydrates or **Total Carbohydrates** is the total Carbohydrates per 100g (12) or per serving (1.2 g per 2 crackers). To calculate total available or net crabohydrates for absorption subtract the fibre from the carbohydrates (in this case 12-10.2 = 1.8g)

'Of which Total Sugar (g)' is included in the total carbohydrates as added or natural sugars so is not subtracted. So net carbohydrates that can cause glucose levels to rise is **0.2 g per serving**

FIGURE 3.9 Example resource on how to read nutritional labels.

TABLE 3.3 Examples of foods that can be eaten on an low carbohydrate diet.

Eggs
Full fat meats
Chicken with the skin
Fish
Leafy green vegetables
Avocadoes
Olive oil
Coconut and coconut oil
Fatty nuts like almonds and macadamia nuts
Cheese
Full cream milk
Butter

3.4.2.3.3 Structured monitoring of glucose concentrations

In the past, glucose monitoring in T2D has been done in an unstructured manner, mainly in the belief that monitoring is only needed in those who are on insulin [269]. In practice, many patients only measure FG concentration if they measure at all. More recently, structured monitoring, including pre- and post-meal readings have been studied and found to produce significant benefits in improving glycaemic control [270–272]. We have found that self-monitoring in patients helps patients in understanding how food affects their glucose concentrations, allowing for better choices to be made. We advocate intensive monitoring of meals especially in the first few months after starting LCDs and give handouts to patients (Fig. 3.11). Post-meal readings are best done 60–90 min after eating starts, as many studies show that the glucose spikes occur in that time frame [273–275].

Patients are also encouraged to bring in their glucometers for download purposes, or use cloud-based systems to store their data, which can be accessed by their healthcare providers. These provide valuable feedback to healthcare providers and are also used to support and encourage patients (Fig. 3.12).

A lower carb diet for type 2 diabetes:

In this condition your metabolism can no longer deal with sugar, which becomes almost a poison- so its consumption needs cutting back dramatically.

Sugar, cut it out altogether. Although it will be in the blueberries, strawberries and raspberries you are allowed to eat. Cakes and biscuits are a mixture of sugar and starch that make it almost impossible to avoid food cravings; they just make you hungrier!!

Reduce starchy carbs a lot Remember they digest down into surprising amounts of sugar). If possible cut out the 'White Stuff' like bread, pasta, rice and breakfast cereals

All green veg/salads are fine – ***eat as much as you can, turn the white stuff green***

So that you still eat a good big dinner try substituting veg such as broccoli, courgettes or green beans for your mash, pasta or rice – still covering them with your gravy, Bolognese or curry!

Tip: try home-made soup – it can be taken to work for lunch and microwaved. Mushrooms, tomatoes, and onions can be included in this. Aldi and Tesco now sell cauliflower rice!

Fruit is trickier..,

Some tropical fruits like bananas, oranges, grapes, mangoes or pineapples have too much sugar in and can set those carb cravings off. Berries are better and can be eaten; blueberries, raspberries, strawberries, apples and pears too.

Eat healthy proteins..,

Such as in meat, eggs (three eggs a day is not too much), fish – particularly oily fish such as salmon, mackerel or tuna –are fine and can be eaten freely. Plain **full fat** yoghurt makes a good breakfast with the berries. Processed meats such as bacon, ham, sausages or salami are not as healthy and should only be eaten in moderation.

Fats are fine in moderation..,

Olive oil is very useful, butter may be tastier than margarine and could be better for you! Coconut oil is great for stir fries. Four essential vitamins A, D, E and K are only found in some fats or oils. Please avoid margarine, corn oil and vegetable oil.

Beware 'low fat' foods. They often have sugar or sweeteners added to make them palatable. Full fat mayonnaise and pesto are definitely on!!

Cheese: only in moderation..,

It is a very calorific mixture of fat, and protein.

Snacks: avoid, as habit forming. But un-salted nuts such as almonds or walnuts are OK to stave off hunger. The occasional treat of strong dark chocolate 70% or more in small quantity is allowed.

EATING LOTS OF VEG WITH PROTEIN AND HEALTHY FATS LEAVES YOU PROPERLY FULL IN A WAY THAT LASTS.

Finally, about sweeteners and what to drink – sweeteners have been proven to tease your brain into being even hungrier, making weight loss more difficult – drink tea, coffee, and water or herb teas. (100mL of milk is 1 teaspoon of sugar) Alcoholic drinks are often full of carbohydrate – for example, beer is almost 'liquid toast' hence the beer belly!! Perhaps the odd glass of red wine wouldn't be too bad if it doesn't make you get hungry afterwards – or just plain or sparkling water with a slice of lemon.

On medication? Remember to check this diet with your GP or practice nurse

P.S. some folk need more salt on a lower carb diet

FIGURE 3.10 General recommendations for beginning a ketogenic diet in patients with type 2 diabetes (Unwin et al. [252]).

CGM data is particularly useful in patients as it gives constant feedback especially in those who are on insulin (Figs 3.13 and 3.14).

3.4.2.3.4 De-prescribing medication

Refer to Section 3.5.

3.4.2.3.5 Common issues

Dawn phenomenon: The dawn phenomenon describes the increase in glucose concentrations seen in most diabetes patients upon rising in the morning [276]. Many patients who start LCDs are confused by the high concentrations of their glucose in the morning, yet find their concentrations decline satisfactorily as the day progresses (and they keep the carbohydrate intake low). The cause of the dawn phenomenon is the increase in growth hormone, which increases in the early hours of the morning (usually before waking) and drives the release of glucose and insulin resistance from the liver [277,278]. Experience has shown that as patients continue the LCD, the dawn phenomenon is attenuated.

Constipation: See 'Keto-flu' below.

Keto-flu: Soon after starting an LCD, patients may experience adverse symptoms related to the change in diet, often known as 'keto-flu.' Symptoms often start in the first week and patients describe varying symptoms, but commonly headaches, nausea, light-headedness, fatigue, irritability, lack of motivation, constipation, halitosis, muscle cramps, bloating, diarrhoea, and rash [279]. These occur due to the insulin lowering effects of reducing carbohydrates, and the subsequent loss of sodium, potassium, and water (natriuresis). In general, most symptoms are transient lasting a few days, with bloating, cravings for carbohydrate foods and mood improving early in changing to LCDs [279]. In those that may experience prolonged symptoms, or even mitigate the onset of symptoms, many clinicians suggest extra intake of fluids (to thirst) and salt (0.5–1 tsp) in the early days, with or without a slight

Name: ______________________ Medication: ______________________

DIARY (with oral medication)			EARLY MORNING / BEFORE BREAKFAST	BREAKFAST MEAL (food eaten)	1 - 1.5 hours AFTER BREAKFAST	Spiking up/down	BEFORE LUNCH	LUNCH MEAL (food eaten)	1 - 1.5 hours AFTER LUNCH	Spiking up/down	BEFORE DINNER	DINNER MEAL (food eaten)	1 - 1.5 hours AFTER DINNER	Spiking up/down
Date	Day	Time												
		Reading												
		Time												
		Reading												
		Time												
		Reading												
		Time												
		Reading												
		Time												
		Reading												
		Time												
		Reading												
		Time												
		Reading												
	NOTES													

Always test 60-90 mins from START of meal.

Targets: Pre-meal <6
Post-meal <8
Spikes <1.7

1. Know your carbohydrates, i.e. which foods contain them and how much.
2. Reduce your carbohydrates to under 25g a day.
3. Monitor, monitor, monitor! Ensure that you monitor your blood glucose levels before and after meals to ensure you are eating correctly, and taking the correct medication (esp if you are taking insulin).
4. Eat whole foods (unprocessed) with healthy fats.
5. Stay motivated and don't give up!

FIGURE 3.11 Example of a patient sheet for data collection. Patients are encouraged to fill in pre- and post-meal readings and a brief description of their meals for recall purposes.

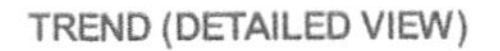

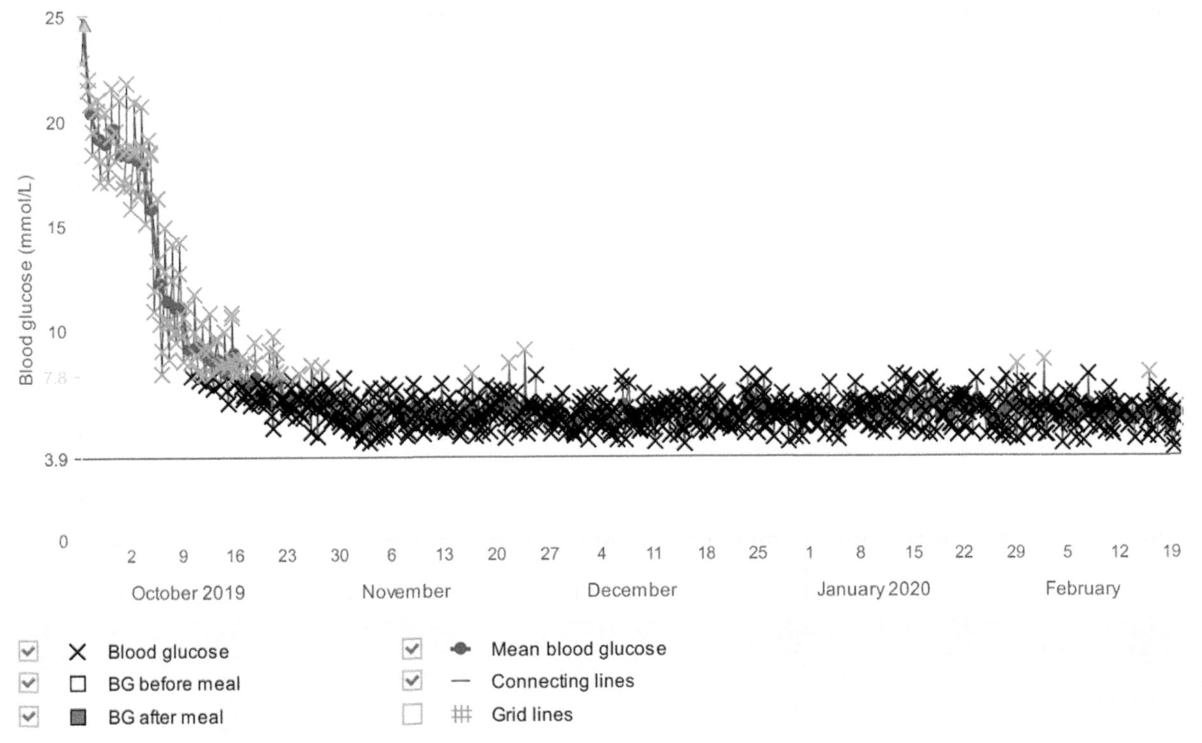

FIGURE 3.12 A glucometer download of a patient who restarted an low carbohydrate diet after a period of poor control. Within 3 weeks the patient's BG readings had normalised. HbA1c after 3 months reduced to 6.7% and after 6 months was 5.3%.

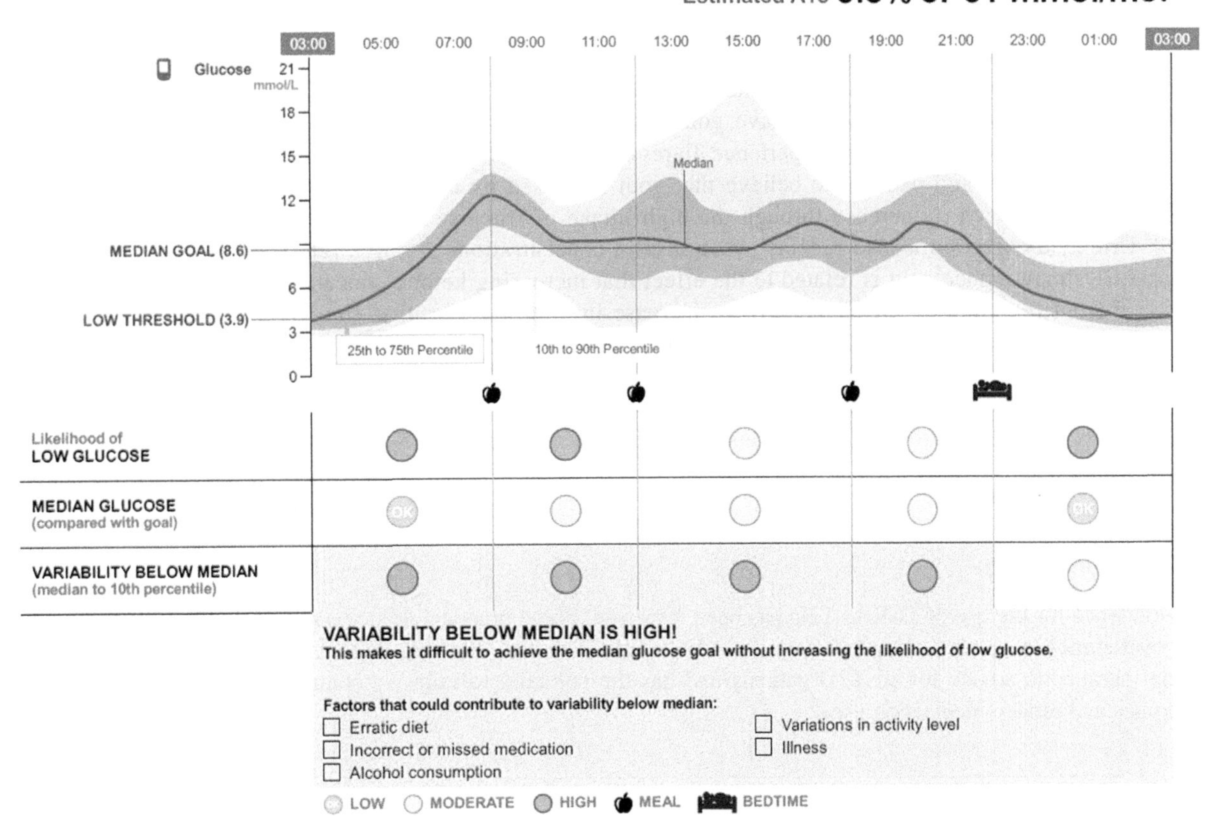

FIGURE 3.13 A patient's CGM download, before changes to his diet, while on insulin, showing glucose peaks with meals and low readings in the night.

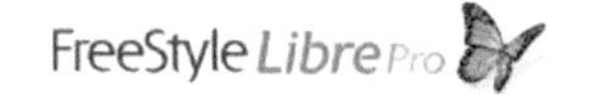

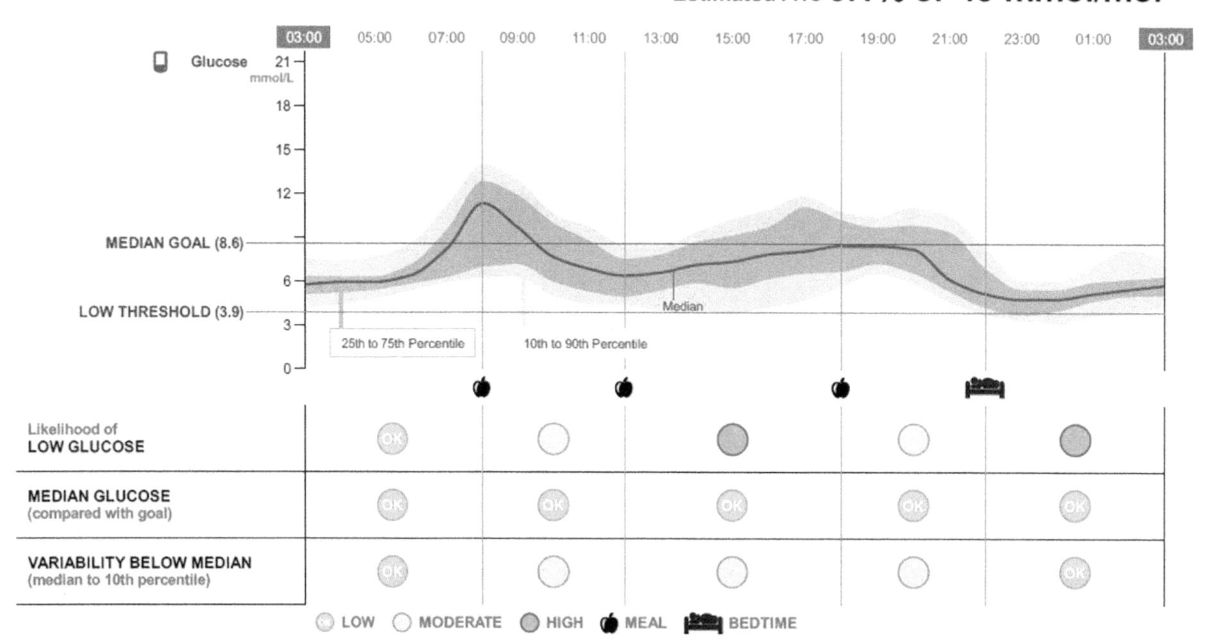

FIGURE 3.14 The same patient's CGM after changes to his diet, showing reduced glucose peaks (except at breakfast, as he still ate cereals) and also reduced lows at night as he reduced insulin doses.

increase in carbohydrate intake up to 25% of calorie intake or 130 g/day. Exercise initially may need to be reduced and, for some patients, an increase in fat intake may be required.

Gout: Patients with diabetes often have gout associated with MetS. Experience by clinicians has shown that some patients, prone to gout may experience flares of their gout attacks within weeks of starting an LCD. This may cause clinicians and patients to believe that gout is caused by carbohydrate restriction. Uric acid concentrations have been shown to increase through the high intake of fructose and its subsequent metabolism in the liver [280]. Uric acid excretion is also reduced when insulin concentrations are high [281]. However, the mechanism by which LCDs may induce gout is related to the effect that increasing ketone concentrations have on the excretion of uric acid from the kidneys. In the kidneys an increase in urate reabsorption (by Urate transporter-1) occurs from the proximal tubule when high ketone concentrations (of β-hydoxybutyrate and acetoacetate) occur [281]. This may cause hyperuricaemia, which may induce a gout attack. In clinical situations treatment for acute gout flares/attacks may be needed. However, experience has shown that if patients persist with TCR (with a reduced intake of fructose and reduced insulin concentrations) uric acid concentrations do reduce and gout attacks will attenuate with time.

3.4.3 Conclusion

The evidence for the use of TCR in T2D has been reviewed. Some practical advice on using LCDs, monitoring patients, and overcoming common issues that may arise, has been discussed. Offering patients LCDs in practice should be part of the therapeutic advice for all T2D patients and has the potential to improve control of diabetes, weight loss, CVD outcomes and reduce medication use.

3.5 Adapting medication for type 2 diabetes in the context of therapeutic carbohydrate restriction

Mark Cucuzzella, Karen Riley, Diana Isaacs
Additional authors
International Working Group on Remission of T2D
Sean McKelvey, IPTN Institute for Personalized Therapeutic Nutrition, Vancouver, BC, Canada
William Yancy Jr, Lifestyle and Weight Management Center and Department of Medicine, Duke University, United States
Susan Wolver, General Internal Medicine, Diplomate, American Board of Obesity Medicine, VCU Medical Weight Loss Program, Richmond, Virginia, United States
Campbell Murdoch, Millbrook Surgery, Somerset, United Kingdom
Brian Lenzkes, Internal Medicine, San Diego, CA, United States
Caroline Roberts, Virta Health, United States
David Cavan, United Kingdom
David Unwin, The Norwood Surgery, Southport, United Kingdom
Eric Westman, Department of Medicine, Duke University, United States
Miriam Berchuk, Dipl. American Board of Obesity Medicine, Canada
Graham Phillips, United Kingdom
Ali Irshad Al Lawati, Diwan of Royal Court, Oman
Nafeeza Hj Mohd Ismail, School of Medicine, International Medical University, Malaysia
Daniel Katambo, Afyaplanet, Kenya
Anne-Sophie Brazeau, McGill University, Canada

3.5.1 Introduction

Healthcare professionals in the primary care setting need to be competent to safely adapt diabetes medications when patients with T2D alter their diet. Safe prescribing practice is supported by an understanding of the clinical evidence, basic science, and pharmacology of medications. This review article supports clinicians in the practical application of this knowledge to achieve safe practice.

The American Diabetes Association (ADA) in their *Standards of Medical Care in Diabetes 2021* recognise low carbohydrate nutritional therapy as a viable option for the management of T2D. The publication states 'For people with T2D, low-carbohydrate and very-low-carbohydrate eating patterns, in particular, have been found to reduce A1C and the need for antihyperglycaemic medications' [282]. In addition their *Nutrition Therapy for Adults with Diabetes or Prediabetes: A Consensus Report 2019* states: [283]

> *Reducing overall carbohydrate intake for individuals with diabetes has demonstrated the most evidence for improving glycemia and may be applied in a variety of eating patterns that meet individual needs and preferences. For individuals with T2D not meeting glycemic targets or for whom reducing glucose-lowering drugs is a priority, reducing overall carbohydrate intake with a low- or very-low-carbohydrate eating pattern is a viable option…Use of organization-approved protocols for insulin and other glucose-lowering medications can help reduce therapeutic inertia and/or reduce the risk of hypoglycemia and hyperglycemia…Low-carbohydrate eating patterns, especially very low-carbohydrate (VLC) eating patterns, have been shown to reduce A1C and the need for antihyperglycemic medications. These eating patterns are among the most studied eating patterns for T2D*

The ADA publications are mirrored internationally by the European Association for the Study of Diabetes (EASD) [284] and Diabetes Canada [285].

Clinical experience finds that TCR or an LCD can be effective for all forms of diabetes mellitus, including T2D, and those characterised by a low insulin state such as T1D [286]. This review will only discuss medication adaptation for T2D. It should be noted that rapid physiological changes can be expected and close monitoring with timely communication of glucose and medication management is essential to ensure patient safety and optimal efficacy. Potential harms include hypoglycaemia due to insulins, and insulin secretagogues, and of ketoacidosis due to SGLT2 inhibitors. Equally it is important to consider that carbohydrate restriction should be tailored to the specific needs and health goals of the person living with diabetes.

Immediate diabetes and even blood pressure medication reduction or elimination is standard care for patients undergoing gastric bypass. The practice is similar in patients undergoing a VLCD protocol. An example of this was in the DiRECT trial that required all oral antidiabetic and antihypertensive drugs to be discontinued on day one of the weight management programme, with standard protocols for drug reintroduction under national clinical guidelines, if indicated by regular monitoring of BG and blood pressure. The clinical emphasis must be on glucose and blood pressure monitoring especially in the first weeks. Other examples of studies are listed in Table 3.4 that provide some guidance on the medication adjustments and frequency of monitoring for diabetes and antihypertensive medications.

3.5.2 Managing the patient

3.5.2.1 Pharmacotherapy

Categories of drugs used in type 2 diabetic patients: Specific medications and mechanisms [3]

A brief summary of various agents used for diabetes and their mechanisms and adverse effects are provided below.

1. Biguanides. Metformin is the only drug in this class. Metformin reduces liver glucose output and slightly lowers IR in muscles and adipose tissue, and can decrease intestinal glucose uptake. Adverse effects can include gastrointestinal side effects such as diarrhoea, vomiting and abdominal pain, vitamin B12 deficiency, worsening of neuropathic symptoms. Side effects can be mitigated with extended release preparation. Metformin has numerous beneficial pleiotropic actions, the consideration of which is outside the scope of this article.
2. Sulfonylureas include glyburide, glibenclamide, glipizide, glimepiride, and gliclazide. Sulfonylureas stimulate the pancreas to secrete more insulin. Adverse effects include hypoglycaemia, weight gain and potential pancreatic beta cell failure.
3. DPP-IV inhibitors include sitagliptin, saxagliptin, linagliptin, and alogliptin. These agents prevent the breakdown of the GLP-1 hormone, which lowers glucagon, increases insulin, slows gastric emptying, and reduces appetite in a glucose dependent manner. These medications have less A1C lowering ability compared with GLP-1 receptor agonists. Infrequent adverse effects are abdominal pain, diarrhoea, nausea, and headache.
4. Thiazolidinediones (TZD) include pioglitazone and rosiglitazone. These agents improve IR, but can contribute to weight gain due to insulin sensitivity in the adipose tissue. They are associated with many adverse effects such as peripheral oedema, osteoporosis, heart failure as well as a risk of developing new primary bladder cancer.
5. Meglitinides include nateglinide and repaglinide. These cause the pancreas to release more insulin. Similar to sulfonylureas but with a shorter half-life, they have more frequent dosing and slightly lower risk of hypoglycaemia.
6. Alpha glucosidase inhibitors include acarbose and miglitol. They prevent absorption of carbohydrates and can cause gastrointestinal symptoms including gas and bloating.
7. Sodium-Glucose Transporter 2 Inhibitors (SGLT2i) include canagliflozin, dapagliflozin, empagliflozin, and ertugliflozin. These agents prevent the kidneys from absorbing glucose back into the bloodstream, so that more is excreted in the urine. They can cause euglycaemic diabetic ketoacidosis (even in T2D patients), genital bacterial and fungal infections, dehydration, and hypotension. Several agents in this class have been shown to reduce the progression of chronic kidney disease and to have cardioprotective effects.
8. Glucagon Like Peptide-1 receptor agonists (GLP1-RA) include exenatide, liraglutide, dulaglutide, semaglutide, and lixisenatide. They increase GLP-1, which leads to a glucose dependent increase in insulin and decrease in glucagon, which leads to decreased glucose, including postprandial glucose. They also delay gastric emptying and enhance satiety which helps facilitate weight loss. They are more potent than DPP-4 inhibitors. Adverse effects include gastrointestinal side effects such as nausea, vomiting, diarrhoea, and pancreatitis. They are contraindicated if a patient has a personal or family history of medullary thyroid cancer.
9. Basal insulins include insulin glargine, insulin detemir, insulin glargine U300, Degludec U100, U200, Humulin U-500, and NPH. Insulin stimulates glucose to be taken up by muscle, liver and fat cells, as well as brain tissue. Insulin also inhibits glucagon action, making it anti-catabolic. Supra-physiological doses in those with IR may increase hunger and contribute to weight gain. Adverse effects include hypoglycaemia and lipodystrophy.
10. Bolus insulins include Regular, Lispro, Aspart, Glulisine, lispro-aabc, and inhaled insulin. Effects are similar to basal insulin but they are shorter acting and wear off more quickly.
11. Amylin mimetics include pramlintide which is less commonly used since it requires multiple daily injections in addition to meal-time insulin. Pramlintide is a synthetic hormone that resembles human amylin, a hormone that is produced by the pancreas and released into the blood after meals where it helps the body to regulate concentrations of BG. Amylin slows the rate at which food (including glucose) is absorbed from the intestine and reduces the

TABLE 3.4 Medication adjustments for therapeutic carbohydrate restriction: summary of studies.

Study	Type of medication	Adjustments made	Frequency of monitoring for medication adjustments
Yancy et al. [287] (*n* = 21) Single-arm pilot intervention trial T2D	Insulin	Reduced 50% upon starting the diet	Medical team access and active medication adjustments every other week for 16 weeks
	Sulfonylureas	Reduced 50% or discontinued upon starting the diet	
	Diuretics	Reduced 50%. Discontinued if on low dose (25 mg of hydrochlorothiazide or 20 mg of furosemide) upon starting the diet	
Westman et al. [288] (*n* = 49) Prospective observational study T2D	Insulin	At 24 weeks, 20 of 21 (95.2%) eliminated or reduced medication	Weekly for 3 months, then every other week for 3 months
Saslow et al. [289] (*n* = 16) Parallel-group randomised trial T2D and prediabetes	Sulfonylureas/DPP-4 inhibitors	All participants discontinued medications by 12 months post-baseline	Not specified
Athinarayanan et al. [251] (*n* = 267) Open label, non-randomized, controlled study T2D	Insulin Sulfonylureas	Total insulin reduced 62% Sulfonylureas reduced 100%	Continuous care intervention with remote patient monitoring
Saslow et al. [290] (*n* = 16) Parallel-group randomised trial T2D and prediabetes	Sulfonylureas	Doses were reduced 50% if the entry HbA1c was <7.5%; discontinued if pre-dinner glucose concentrations went below 6.11 mmol/L (110 mg/dL) in spite of prior dose reduction	Participants were asked to monitor fasting glucose and before dinner daily. Doctor visits unspecified
	Thiazolidinediones	Discontinued for those with starting HbA1c below 7%	
	Metformin	Continued	
Yabe et al. [291] (*n* = 24) Randomised, open-label, 3-arm parallel comparative exploratory study T2D	SGLT2 inhibitors	N/A. Study reflects risk of SGLT2i associated DKA using a low carb approach Discontinuation recommended due to risk of euglycemic DKA	Weekly
Unwin et al. [252] (*n* = 54 on DM meds) Ongoing audit of service provision	Sulfonylureas, insulin, metformin, SGLT2i, GLP1a	Discontinued completely in 19 (35%)	Regular office visits with general practitioner offices

(*Continued*)

TABLE 3.4 (Continued)

Study	Type of medication	Adjustments made	Frequency of monitoring for medication adjustments
Lean et al. [253] DiRECT ($n = 148$) 111 on DM meds, 12 mos. Open-label, cluster-randomised trial	Not specified	Approx 75% taking meds in both groups at start. Approx 74% off all meds intervention group, 18% controls	Regular office visits with general practitioner offices

Abbreviations: T2D, type 2 diabetes; DKA, diabetic ketoacidosis; meds, medications; DM, diabetes melitus; SGLT2i, sodium-glucose transport protein 2 inhibitors; GLP1a, glucagon-like peptide-1 receptor agonist; HbA1c, haemoglobin A1c; DPP-4, dipeptidyl peptidase 4.

production of glucose by the liver by inhibiting the action of glucagon. Adverse effects include nausea, vomiting, and hypoglycaemia.

12. Other agents with T2D indications. Bromocriptine and bile acid sequestrants have also been used with some efficacy in management of T2D.

3.5.2.2 *Diabetes medications and therapeutic carbohydrate restriction*

Diabetes medications work by different mechanisms of action and vary based on their benefits and risks. This is important to consider in light of new evidence for various diabetes agents. A summary of risks to benefits can be found in Table 3.5.

Importantly, BG concentrations typically fall rapidly and substantially when an individual adopts TCR. It is therefore essential that medications are adjusted in order to prevent hypoglycaemia. The following recommendations are based on combined clinical expertise, clinical trials, and from current published guidelines on TCR and medications.

When deciding the safety and appropriateness of T2D medications with TCR there are three key clinical considerations:

1. Is there a risk of the drug causing hypoglycaemia or other adverse events?
2. What is the degree of carbohydrate restriction?
3. Once carbohydrates are reduced, does the drug continue to provide health benefits, and if so, are the potential benefits greater than or less than the possible risks and side effects?

The preferences of the person with diabetes should be taken into account in all decisions on medication changes. Clinicians must support patients by balancing the pros and cons of different approaches. Cost is an issue that may influence medication choice in many health care systems. Medication costs are a large burden to individuals and the health systems so it is advisable before prescribing expensive medication that all other options have been considered. Cardiovascular and renal benefits of certain medications should be taken into consideration and may warrant continued use even when a person has met their A1C target. An easy approach to consider when adjusting medications is using a stoplight approach (see Fig. 3.15).

3.5.2.2.1 Medications that create a risk of hypoglycaemia

A risk of hypoglycaemia exists with sulfonylureas, meglitinides, and exogenous insulins. When carbohydrate intake is reduced, these medications need to be reduced or stopped, with adjustment being individualised to patient circumstances. The authors recommend at least a 50% reduction in dose of insulin while stopping the sulfonylureas and meglitinides. Further reductions in insulin may be necessary according to the BG response. There may be a period of short-term hyperglycaemia while the individual adapts to a lower carbohydrate intake. This is preferable to the risk of hypoglycaemia from not reducing doses. These patients benefit from reducing hyperinsulinaemia as this is thought to contribute to many of the metabolic and other abnormalities seen in T2D. Hypoglycaemia can contribute to increased hunger, making it more difficult to lose weight [294].

Sulfonylureas and meglitinides: The absence of long-term health benefits of these drugs provides reassurance that stopping them will not adversely affect long-term health. Sulfonylureas as second line drugs may increase the risk of

TABLE 3.5 Summary of T2D medication benefits and risks [284,292,293].

	Biguanides	Secretagogues	DPP4is	GLP1RAs	SGLT2i	TZD	Insulin
Agents	Metformin	Sulfonylureas Glyburide Glibenclamide Glipizide Glimepiride Gliclazide Meglitinides Nateglinide Repaglinide	Sitagliptin Saxagliptin Linagliptin Alogliptin	Exenatide Liraglutide Dulaglutide Lixisenatide Semaglutide	Canagliflozin Dapagliflozin Empagliflozin Ertugliflozin	Pioglitazone Rosiglitazone	Rapid-acting insulin Basal insulins
Mechanism of action	Decreases hepatic gluconeo-genesis, decreases intestinal absorption of glucose, improves insulin sensitivity by increasing peripheral glucose uptake	Stimulates pancreatic islet cells which causes an increase in insulin secretion. These drugs are not effective in the absence of functioning beta cells	Slows the inactivation of incretin hormones GLP-1 and GIP	Increase GLP-1 →glucose dependent ↑ in insulin & ↓ in glucagon & ↓ glucose. Benefits of delayed gastric emptying & enhanced satiety	Reduces reabsorption of filtered glucose and lowers the renal threshold for glucose thereby increasing urinary glucose excretion	Enhances insulin sensitivity in adipose tissue, skeletal muscle and liver to decrease plasma glucose, insulin concentrations	
Hypoglycaemia	Neutral	Moderate-severe ([a]mild glinide)	Neutral	Neutral	Neutral	Neutral	Moderate-severe
Weight	Slight loss	Gain	Neutral	Loss	Loss	Gain	Gain
Renal/GU	Not for EGFR < 30	Hypoglycaemic risk	Renal dosing except linagliptin	No exenatide for CrCL < 30	Reduce progression of CKD	Neutral	More hypoglycaemia risk
GI ADR	Moderate	Neural	Neutral	Moderate	Neutral	Neutral	Neutral
Cardiac/CHF	Neutral	More CHF risk	Possible with saxagliptin, alogliptin	Possible benefit liraglutide	Reduced risk hospitalisation for heart failure	Moderate	More CHF risk
Cardiac/ASCVD	Neutral	?	Neutral	Benefit liraglutide, semaglutide, dulaglutide, albiglutide	Benefit empagliflozin, canagliflozin	May reduce stroke risk	Neutral
Bone	Neutral	Neutral	Neutral	Neutral	Canagliflozin warning	Moderate fracture risk	Neutral
ketoacidosis	Neutral	Neutral	Neutral	Neutral	DKA in T2D in stress	Neutral	Neutral

Abbrveiations: DPP4is, dipeptidyl peptidase 4 inhibitors; GLP1Ras, glucagon-like-peptide-1 receptor agonists; SGLT2i, sodium = glucose cotransporter 2 inhibitors; TDZ, thiazolidinediones.
[a] *mild with glinide; Mod/severe with sulfonylurea.*

CAUTION

- When reducing medication, patients must be checking blood glucose frequently and have immediate communicating with their clinician.

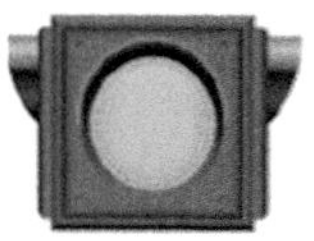

- Biguanides
- GLP1 Agonists
- DPP4 Inhibitors

REDUCE

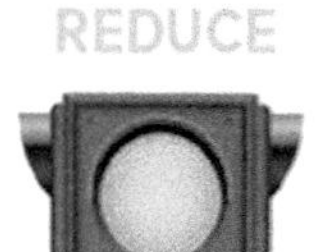

- Basal long acting insulins— may need to reduce dose by up to 50%. Follow blood sugars and adjust as needed
- Thiazolidinediones

STOP

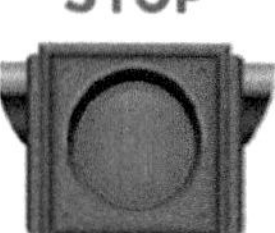

- Sulfonylureas
- Meglitinides
- SGLT2 inhibitors
- Bolus meal time insulin. *Might need small amounts to correct high blood sugar.*
- Combination insulins (70/30) — switch to basal long acting
- Alpha-glucosidase inhibitors

FIGURE 3.15 Stoplight approach to medication management with therapeutic carbohydrate reduction.

myocardial infarction, all-cause mortality, and severe hypoglycaemia especially in the elderly, compared with remaining on metformin monotherapy [295]. Glucose variability and glucose spikes may also be associated with increased cardiovascular risk [296,297].

Insulins: Unless embarking on an 800 kcal/day very low calorie and LCD similar to the one used in DiRECT, practical expertise suggests a 50% reduction of total daily insulin dose at initiation of TCR is appropriate in most cases. In individuals whose HbA1c is markedly elevated, a smaller reduction (e.g., of 30%) may be appropriate, with further reductions over time. In individuals on a basal bolus regimen, it is advised to preferentially reduce or stop bolus insulin. As glucose concentration improves, basal insulin can then be reduced. Mixed insulin should be stopped and switched to basal insulin alone and the daily dose can be reduced by 30%–50% at the start of TCR. If on a single dose of long-acting insulin with a peak, the preferred timing is to administer it in the morning to coincide with higher insulin concentrations with normal circadian physiology of daytime feeding and a reduction of circulating insulin with a nighttime fast. Many basal insulins do not have a high peak especially with reduced doses, allowing them to be administered at any time of day. Some patients can expect to eliminate the need for insulin completely over the next few days or months, as IR resolves.

It should be cautioned that some people diagnosed with T2D may in fact have an insulin deficiency form of diabetes, such as Latent Autoimmune Diabetes of Adults (LADA) or Maturity Onset Diabetes of Youth (MODY). These patients should not have their insulin stopped completely. Endogenous insulin insufficiency is more likely in patients who were not overweight at the time of their diagnosis of diabetes or who required insulin earlier in the course of diagnosis [298]. They are also likely to be more insulin sensitive, requiring smaller insulin doses than typically used in T2D. Over-reduction in insulin dosage in these patients would lead to significant hyperglycaemia, and further dosage reduction should be avoided. It is recommended that expert advice and additional testing such as c-peptide and GAD antibodies is sought in cases of doubt.

3.5.2.2.2 Medications that increase ketoacidosis risk

SGLT2 inhibitors: These medications carry a risk of euglycaemic ketoacidosis. TCR alone cannot cause ketoacidosis, but it may enhance the risk posed by SGLT2i by lowering insulin concentrations because insulin inhibits ketone formation. SGLT2i-induced ketoacidosis may occur with normal BG concentrations, and this heightens the risk of ketoacidosis going unrecognised. It is worth noting that a VLCD (typically less than 50 g of carbohydrate a day) can produce a physiologically normal state of ketosis, that should not be confused with the pathological state of diabetic ketoacidosis. Despite recent literature supporting slight cardiovascular risk reduction and renal protection of SGLT2i, it is recommended that SGLT2i are used with caution in those adhering to a low carbohydrate eating plan. It is appropriate to stop SGLT2i in many cases, particularly in those adhering to a VLCD (30–50 g/day). A GLP-1 agonist is a safer choice as a second-line agent after metformin. See Murray et al. [299] for an excellent review of the physiology of an LCD mimicking many effects of SGLT2i.

3.5.2.2.3 Medications with minimal risk but little to no benefit

Thiazolidinediones: These agents are safe to continue from a short-term perspective as they do not cause hypoglycaemia. Concerns exist over their long-term safety, including risks of bladder cancer [300], heart failure [301] and reduced bone mineral density [302]. It is recommended to stop thiazolidinediones (TZD) as soon as glucose concentrations allow. TZD are also known to cause weight gain [303].

Acarbose: Although acarbose is safe to continue while on an LCD, the benefits are much less pronounced because of reduced starch ingestion so the patient can usually stop the medication.

3.5.2.2.4 Medications that pose no excess risk with therapeutic carbohydrate restriction and may have benefit

Metformin is safe to continue and in some patients continues to offer favourable benefits. There is no hypoglycaemia associated with metformin and neutral or minor weight loss. However, up to 25% of people experience gastrointestinal side effects from metformin [304].

GLP-1 agonists: Safe to continue. Benefits with TCR include increased satiety, slowed gastric emptying [305] and cardiovascular benefits [306]. With sustained TCR, people may be able to stop their GLP-1 agonist. However, guidelines encourage continued use for those with atherosclerotic cardiovascular disease (ASCVD) or high ASCVD risk independent of A1C. For a detailed review of the multiple mechanisms of this class of medications refer to the full review from Drucker [307].

DPP4 inhibitors are less potent than GLP-1 agonists but safe to continue as they do not cause hypoglycaemia and are weight neutral. Clinical experience from the International group of authors agrees that these seem to have little BG lowering effect in the context of TCR.

A summary of medications for diabetes can be found in Table 3.5. Box 3.1 is a list of current published clinical guidelines on TCR with medication reduction suggestions.

BOX 3.1 Current published clinical guidelines on LCDs with medication reduction.

- Guideline Central: Low-Carbohydrate Nutrition Approaches in Patients with Obesity, Prediabetes and T2D
  http://eguideline.guidelinecentral.com/i/1180534-low-carb-nutritional-approaches-guidelines-advisory/0?
  UK version: http://eguideline.guidelinecentral.com/i/1183584-low-carb-nutrition-queens-units/0?
- Adapting diabetes medication for low carbohydrate management of T2D: a practical guide
  https://bjgp.org/content/69/684/360
- A clinician's guide to inpatient low carbohydrate diets for remission of T2D: toward a standard of care protocol
  https://www.openaccessjournals.com/articles/a-clinicians-guide-to-inpatient-lowcarbohydrate-diets-for-remission-of-type-2-diabetes-toward-a-standard-of-care-protocol-12898.html
- Clinical Guidelines For the Prescription of Carbohydrate Restriction as a Therapeutic Intervention/Low Carb USA International Scientific and Clinical Advisory
  https://thesmhp.org/clinical-guidelines/

3.5.2.2.5 Individualisation of therapy and the role of blood glucose monitoring

For those individuals who wish to adopt a VLCD or ketogenic diet (less than 50 g of carbohydrate/day), a significant reduction or complete discontinuation of insulin may be required. Self-monitoring of BG or continuous glucose monitoring (CGM) can be very helpful in providing rapid feedback on how foods affect BG as a person adopts an LCD, and to inform whether medication doses can be reduced further. There is evidence that frequent paired glucose testing is effective in supporting appropriate food choices, regardless of the type of diabetes treatment [270,308]. Patients on drugs that increase the risk of hypoglycaemia should have access to rescue therapies (glucose tablets, gel, or glucagon), an adequate supply of testing strips, and immediate access to a member of the healthcare team. This is especially important at the initiation of carbohydrate reduction. Checking BG for the purpose of feedback and behaviour change can be extremely effective [309].

It can be highly educational for patients to see how their own glycaemic response to food correlated with how they feel. This is now possible with CGM technology, and has recently become more accessible and affordable with improved CGM technology. Such systems can show the large post-meal glucose spikes and increased glucose variability that are common in patients who have standard high carbohydrate dietary patterns, are insulin-resistant, and in later-stage T2D with beta cell insufficiency. The CGM can also show the impact of TCR on reducing glucose spikes after meals [309,310].

3.5.2.2.6 Anti-hypertensive medication adjustment

It is important to review the medication list for anti-hypertensives. Blood pressure will need to be monitored either at home or in the clinic during the initiation of the dietary intervention. Patients should be shown how to self-monitor their blood pressure and made aware of symptoms of low blood pressure, such as orthostatic hypotension (light-headedness upon standing) or severe fatigue. These symptoms and/or systolic blood pressure below 120 mmHg should prompt reduction of anti-hypertensive medication. Hyponatraemia may be exacerbated by SGLT2i, thiazides, or loop diuretics. The initiation of the diet is associated with diuresis and natriuresis; therefore, adequate sodium intake is emphasised to prevent dehydration and hypotension. A review in the *Journal of Hypertension*, states 'Our analysis suggests that insulin plays a primary role in hypertension, highlighting the tight link between essential hypertension and diseases associated with the metabolic syndrome' [311].

Broth with sodium is a good remedy as well as preventive measure in the initiation phase of the diet. Some patients with heart failure are salt sensitive so monitor this subgroup closely or reduce diuretics judiciously instead of advising sodium-rich broths or foods. Tailor any reduction in anti-hypertensives to the patient's comorbidities. Results of Dr. David Unwin's six year observational trial showed a 10.9 mmHg reduction in systolic blood pressure (SBP) and 6.3 mmHg diastolic blood pressure reduction despite a 20% reduction in anti-hypertensive medication [129].

3.5.2.2.7 Other medications needing adjustment

If there is a significant change in intake of leafy greens or other foods containing vitamin K, vitamin K antagonists (i.e., warfarin) will need frequent monitoring. Improvements in heartburn (gastroesophageal reflux disease) may allow reduction or elimination of proton pump inhibitors (PPIs) or H2 Blockers. Diarrhoea predominant irritable bowel syndrome (IBS) may also improve with more bioavailable foods containing essential proteins and fats. Patients with polycystic ovary syndrome (PCOS) may see an improvement in their condition with a return of fertility so advice on contraception may be required. Migraines and inflammatory joint pains also may also improve and require medication adjustments. Due to the natural diuresis that occurs with insulin reduction, if loop diuretics are given for oedema these can be safely reduced or removed as the oedema is monitored.

3.5.2.2.8 Other lifestyle interventions to affect IR and aid in medication reduction

Physical activity of all forms can assist insulin sensitivity. This can be just the general movement of walking and having an active day, to directed aerobic type activity, as well as high intensity activity and strength training. Adequate sleep, reducing stress, emerging data on the microbiome, time restricted eating, Vitamin D status, genetics, and multiple other modulators of IR and sensitivity are now being discovered and individually tailored by clinicians and patients.

A summary of considerations given to T2D medications under an LCD or a KD is given in Table 3.6.

TABLE 3.6 T2D: Diabetic medications on an LCD: summary and suggestions [305].

There are three considerations with the use of diabetic medications in type 2 diabetes when on a low carbohydrate diet:

- Is there a risk of hypoglycaemia?
- What is the degree of carbohydrate restriction?
- Does the medication provide any benefit, and if so, do any potential benefits outweigh any side effects and potential risks?

Drug Group	Action	Hypo risk?	Suggested action (to continue/stop)
Sulfonylureas	Increase pancreatic insulin secretion	YES	**STOP** (or if gradual carbohydrate restriction then wean by e.g. halving dose successively)
Insulins	Exogenous insulin	YES	**REDUCE/STOP** (Change to basal only and wean appropriately, e.g. successive 30-50% reductions, towards elimination) *see below
Meglitinides	Increase pancreatic insulin secretion	YES	**STOP** (or if gradual carbohydrate restriction then wean by e.g. halving dose successively)
Biguanides	Reduces insulin resistance	No	Optional, consider clinical pros/cons.
GLP-1 agonists	Slow gastric emptying. Glucose dependent pancreatic insulin secretion.	No	Optional, consider clinical pros/cons (expensive).
SGLT-2 inhibitors	Increase renal glucose secretion	No	Usually stop. Concern over possible risk of ketoacidosis (though this risk may be with LADA that has been misdiagnosed as T2DM). Use in selected patients may be beneficial in early reversal.
Thiazolidinediones	Reduce peripheral insulin resistance	No	Usually stop. Concern over risks usually outweighs benefits.
DPP-4 inhibitors	Inhibit DPP-4 enzyme	No	Stop. No significant risk, but no benefit in most cases.
Alpha-glucosidase inhibitors	Delay digestion of starch and sucrose	No	Stop. No benefit on a low carbohydrate diet.

*Insulin reduction suggestion Tailor to individual. If using basal-bolus regime convert to long-acting insulin only, BD in equal doses (OD may suit some people). If a very low carbohydrate diet is planned any bolus insulin dosing can simply be eliminated. On commencing low carbohydrate diet reduce insulin by 30-50%. Monitor QDS initially for hypoglycaemia (rescue glucose if required). Continue down-titration of insulin as insulin resistance improves (can take months). Goal for most can be to eliminate insulin.

Caution: Some people with T2DM may have pancreatic insufficiency. Also people with other forms or pancreatic insufficiency (e.g. LADA or T3c) may have been misdiagnosed as T2DM. Consider this if rapidly increasing HbA1c, thirst, polydipsia, weight loss, low C-peptide. Insulin should not be eliminated in this cohort.

3.5.3 Summary

TCR is an increasingly popular and effective option for managing T2D and can lead to an improvement in the condition, reduced medication burden, and contribute to significant weight loss. A recent qualitative review reports medication reduction to be a primary reason for patients to start TCR, even more important than weight loss [312]. Safe initiation of TCR in patients on medications requires significant monitoring and medication adjustments to decrease and eliminate the risk of hypoglycaemia and hypotension. The healthcare team, including clinicians in primary care, nursing, pharmacy, and nutrition needs to be competent in adjusting or recognising the need for adjustment of diabetes and antihypertensive medications to achieve safe and effective care. The most immediate and important adjustments are to insulin, sulfonylureas, SGLT2i, blood pressure medications, and diuretics. Interdisciplinary care teams can individualise therapy while following the guidance above, which includes monitoring BG and blood pressure closely, decreasing medications that can cause hypoglycaemia and hypotension, evaluating BG and blood pressure responses regularly, and open access communication with the team.

Medical education and practise for decades has focused almost exclusively on prescribing and intensifying medical therapy as chronic disease progresses. Our international team of clinician authors hopes for a day when medical education and practise will invest as much time, thought, and effort into safely de-prescribing medications as then do in helping our patients restore health.

3.6 Type 1 diabetes

Neville Wellington
Ian Lake

3.6.1 Introduction

T1D results from autoimmune destruction of the pancreatic β-cells and an almost complete loss of insulin production [313]. This results in hyperglycaemia with its concomitant symptoms and signs, and if left untreated can lead to diabetic ketoacidosis (DKA) and death. All patients with T1D will require some form of insulin therapy.

For every year a person with either T1D or T2D has an HbA1c above 7.5% they lose 100 days of life [314]. This equates to 70% of people in England and Wales with T1D ending their year on the 23rd of September. It is around 8 years of loss of life for someone with T1D. Clearly the importance of achieving normoglycemia in diabetes is paramount.

T1D not only reduces length or life, it negatively impacts quality of life too. In a questionnaire of 180 people with T1D between ages 18 and 35 the following conclusions were drawn: [315]

> *Although participants demonstrated appropriate self-management behaviours and moderate self-efficacy, on the Diabetes Quality of Life Instrument, they reported high dissatisfaction with the burden that diabetes places on their families and the amount of time it takes to manage their diabetes. Quality of life was significantly positively correlated with fear of hypoglycemia and fear of complications. Quality of life was significantly negatively correlated with self-efficacy. These observations suggest that, as fear of hypoglycemia and fear of complications increase, quality of life decreases, and as self-efficacy increases, so does the quality of life.*

In this section, we will look at the use of TCR in T1D to control glycaemia, reduce diabetic and insulin-treatment-related complications and improve health and quality of life.

3.6.2 Pathophysiology

T1D is an autoimmune disease where progressive destruction of the beta cells of the pancreas occurs over a variable period of time. It can present at any age but is commoner in childhood with two peaks at ages 4–7 and 10–14 years old. There is no known causative agent and multiple aetiologies have been proposed: genetics, lack of vitamin D [316], milk casein, infection, and geographical location.

3.6.3 Managing the patient

3.6.3.1 Background

In the pre-insulin era the only form of treatment for T1D was a carbohydrate restricted diet which showed variable success, depending on the proportions of protein and fat [317]. Once insulin was discovered, this allowed an increase in carbohydrate consumption, eventually increasing to more than 50% of energy intake in the 1960s when low-fat diets were introduced [318]. While the use of insulin in patients with T1D has prolonged their lives, the increase in carbohydrates and increased doses of insulin have caused a number of related conditions. These include greater risks of hypoglycaemia, hyperglycaemia, DKA, and obesity. Added to this are the ongoing increased cardiovascular complications associated with diabetes, which are related in a linear fashion to increasing HbA1 concentrations [319]. Maintaining glucose concentrations in a normal range remains a lifelong challenge for many patients. Data from T1D registries show that only 17% of children and adolescents, and 21% of adult patients achieve HbA1c targets of less than 7.5% and 7%, respectively [318,320]. Despite the introduction of newer insulins, greater use of insulin pumps and increased glucose monitoring with continuous glucose monitors, no improvements in these data has been shown over an 8-year period [318,320].

Patients are taught to match insulin dosage with carbohydrate intake, yet few are able to achieve adequate control. A typical patient's journey includes high BG variability and poor control as shown in glucometer downloads from two patients shown in (Fig. 3.16A and B). Constant BG fluctuations mean greater risk of severe hypoglycaemic episodes, which often lead to rebound hyperglycaemia and greater risks of DKA.

3.6.3.2 Aims of care

The ultimate aim in treating patients with T1D, is to achieve glucose concentrations (and Hba1c) as close as possible to normal, reduce hypoglycaemia, reduce BG variability (see Figs 3.16 vs 3.17), and improve quality of life. A small percentage of people can achieve normoglycaemia using a guideline diet that is high in carbohydrates. For the vast majority of people though, carbohydrate restriction will be the most appropriate dietary contribution to normoglycaemia. The evidence to date suggests that the lower the number of carbohydrates, the better the BG control [321,322].

As highlighted in the studies discussed below, there is even a possibility of inducing a remission of T1D. Many diabetologists have, in the past, observed that patients who achieve control of their glucose concentrations soon after diagnosis enter a 'honeymoon phase' during which they need little or no insulin for extended periods. It now seems possible from the studies that by using TCR soon after diagnosis that the 'honeymoon phase' could be prolonged indefinitely in some patients, thereby achieving remission.

3.6.3.3 Lifestyle-related considerations

Lifestyle management is fundamental to holistic health. Dietary management is the most significant strategy in T1D management and physiological concentrations of glucose can be routinely achieved, with TCR in particular.

3.6.3.3.1 Exercise

T1D management extends to physical activity, which should be thought of as integral to managing this condition. The gut-liver-brain axis of glucose control plays a major role in glucose metabolism. But the contribution of muscle to glucose regulation should not be underestimated.

Exercise increases GLUT-4 transporter translocation to the cell surface and consequent glucose uptake, independent of insulin [323]. Skeletal muscle is one of the few organs to increase in mass as a result of regular exercise, and this increases the number of GLUT 4 transporters and hence the ability of the body to take up glucose. In cases of high BG, an alternative to insulin injection is physical activity to increase the absorption of glucose.

In addition to its ability to increase the rate of glucose uptake into muscle cells, and the ability to metabolise glucose anaerobically in muscle, glucose is the only fuel available for anaerobic respiration and even though it has a poor net gain in ATP, the rate of reaction in anaerobic conditions is 100 times that of aerobic respiration. The effect of this is a relative fivefold increase in glucose use. So, it is good to encourage a mix of aerobic and anaerobic activity regularly throughout the day where possible in people with T1D.

3.6.3.3.2 Sunlight

For people who live in temperate and northern latitudes, it is good practice to recommend oral vitamin D supplements for the winter months. There is a wide range of dose recommendations with 1000–4000 IU being the safe upper limit depending on a number of factors including age [324]. Vitamin D has been shown to improve BG, and HbA1c, and decrease insulin resistance in T2D [325], and low vitamin D concentrations are associated with the aetiology of T1D [316].

3.6.3.4 Pharmacotherapy

Insulin is effectively a hormone replacement therapy in the context of its lack in T1D. The clinical challenge is to provide insulin in the amount needed and with effective timing to balance the effect of diet on glucose control. In the short term, the issue of hypoglycaemia is significant. In the longer term, a failure to keep glucose concentrations in the physiological range will expose the person with T1D to the risk of complications.

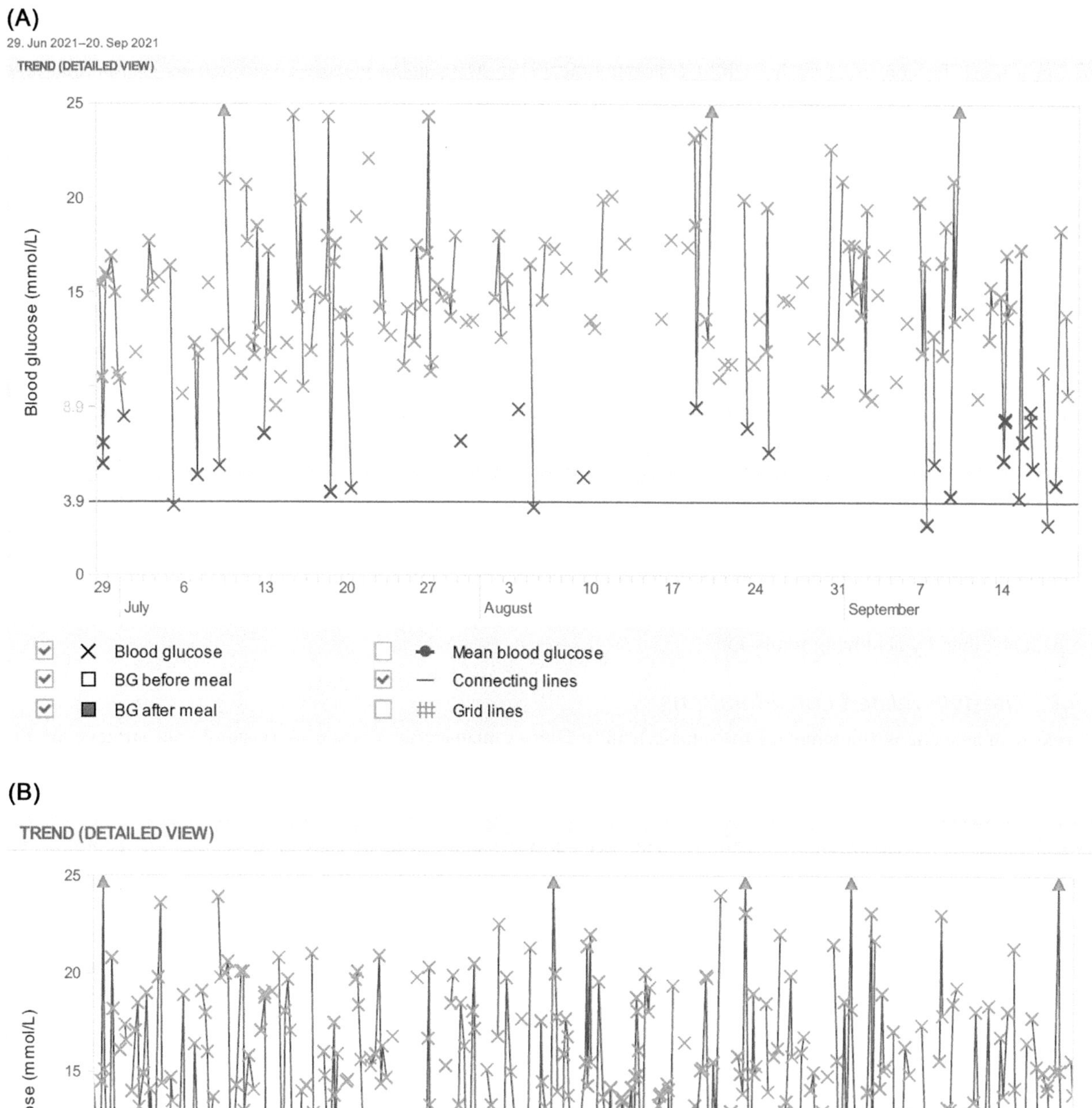

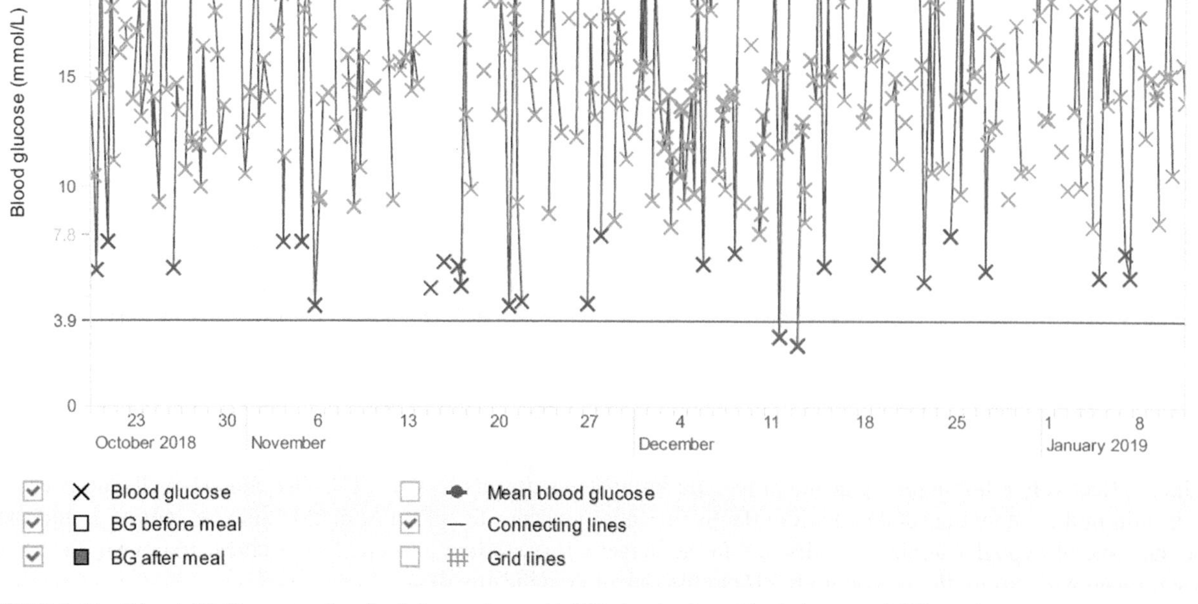

FIGURE 3.16 (A) and (B) Glucometer downloads from patients with T1D showing large blood glucose variability and poor control when using standard dietary advice.

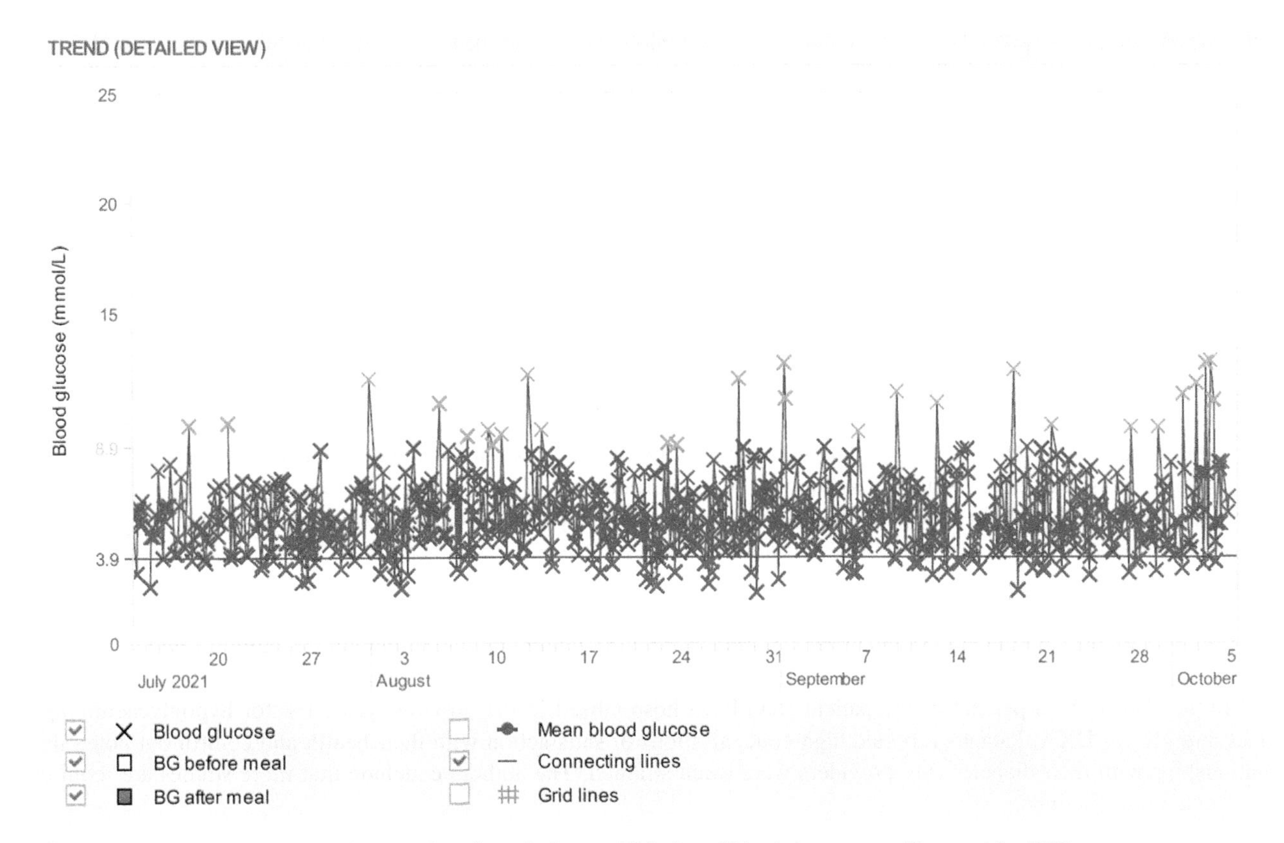

FIGURE 3.17 Glucometer readings from a T1D patient who has established good blood glucose control by practicing TCR.

3.6.3.4.1 Basal insulin adjustment

Whichever type of diet is chosen, the fundamentals of T1D management are to establish the timing and amount of basal insulin when the person is in a fasted state. It can be done in one 24-h fast or two 12-h fasts that cover the full 24-h period. Even though most basal insulins have a 24-h time of action, insulin sensitivity differs throughout the day and splitting the dose might be advised. People who use pumps can refine their basal dose to cover the times of insulin resistance and sensitivity hourly throughout the day if needed and a pump system will benefit those who find basal control difficult to achieve. Once a flat trace in the physiological range has been established, then the person has flexibility over eating times and will bolus for carbohydrates and protein as needed.

Time restricted eating can benefit people with T1D and a carbohydrate restricted diet facilitates this process by removing the need for snacking, which is typically needed with high volumes of insulin.

Time-restricted eating has many benefits in T1D management, as it improves insulin sensitivity, allows for cell repair through autophagy, and means less time is spent with dysregulated physiology caused by peripheral insulin [326].

People who are approaching TCR and who have diabetes complications will be advised by their clinician to transition at a pace suited to their existing complications. Typically this involves an extended transition phase over weeks to months.

3.6.3.5 Therapeutic carbohydrate restriction

3.6.3.5.1 Evidence for the use of therapeutic carbohydrate restriction

The American Diabetes Association Standards of Care in Diabetes for 2021 states that 'There is inadequate research in T1D to support one eating pattern over another at this time' [327]. However, they do concede that 'Reducing overall carbohydrate intake for individuals with diabetes has demonstrated the most evidence for improving glycemia and may be applied in a variety of eating patterns that meet individual needs and preferences' [327]. Numerous case studies, clinical trials and review articles have shown benefits in patients who use low carbohydrate lifestyles in T1D. Here we mention some of these for reference.

Intervention studies In a 1-year study, 24 patients with T1D were enrolled; of which 22 completed the study [328]. Patients reduced their carbohydrate intakes to 70–90 g per day, were encouraged to monitor glucose concentrations at least four times daily and insulin doses were adapted to the new regimen. Follow-up measurements were done at three and 12 months. The average HbA1c lowered from 7.5% to 6.4%. Mealtime insulin dosage reduced from 21.1 to 12.4 units and the total daily dose of insulin reduced from 0.5 u/kg/day to 0.4 u/kg/day. Total cholesterol and LDL cholesterol concentrations were unchanged, whereas blood triglyceride concentrations reduced by 16%. Hypoglycaemic episodes reduced by 94% at three months and 84% by one year. The authors conclude that for motivated T1D patients this approach to therapy is feasible.

In a 12-week randomized crossover study of 14 T1D patients, of whom 10 completed the study, the intake of 98 g carbohydrate was compared to 246 g carbohydrate per day [329]. Results showed reduced variability and less hypoglycaemia in the lower carbohydrate arm, and weight loss of 2 kg in LCD compared to a gain of 2.6 kg in the higher carbohydrate diet group. There was no effect on HbA1c or on the CVD risk markers, but the total daily dose of insulin was reduced from 43.2 to 33.6 units. The authors concluded that a reduction in carbohydrate intake helped to reduce weight, glucose variability and hypoglycaemic events.

In a one-year retrospective study, 33 patients self-selected to follow a very low carbohydrate diet (<50 g/day) which was designed to be eucaloric. The number of patients achieving an HbA1c of <7% rose from 12% to 57% and there was a statistically significant decrease in the number of units of daily insulin used and hypoglycaemic episodes experienced. There was incidental weight loss among some participants. The authors conclude that a low-carbohydrate approach appears safe and effective with medical supervision and appropriate adjustments in insulin dose [330].

Cross-sectional observational studies In one study, T1D patients who were participants in the Facebook group, TypeOneGrit, responded to an online survey. The study evaluated glycemic control among children and adults who consumed a VLCD or a KD [321]. There were 316 respondents, of whom 131 were parents of children with T1D. The study found that the average use of LCDs was 2.2 years. The mean carbohydrate intake was 36 g daily and the mean HbA1c was 5.7%. Two percent of the patients had been hospitalised in the previous year, 1% for hypoglycaemic episodes and 1% for DKA. Patients reported high concentrations of satisfaction with their health and control but noted that relationships with their diabetes care providers were often strained. The authors conclude that more studies are required to validate these findings.

Most studies look at CVD risk factors and in general tend to find that total, LDL and HDL cholesterol concentrations may increase, but that blood triglyceride concentrations tend to reduce in T1D patients who use LCDs. However, very few studies report on actual CVD outcomes. In an interesting study, Ahola et al. evaluated a subset of T1D patients (69 (7.6%) of 902) who follow a Low carbohydrate (<130 g/day) diet and compared them to a matched population of 69 patients from the study [331]. They compared the CVD risk factors and showed that the patients in the LCD arm had lower body mass index (BMI), reduced BG variability, and lower diastolic blood pressure values. Women had higher HDL cholesterol concentrations. Men had slightly raised total and non-HDL cholesterol concentrations in comparison to women. However, the data indicate that the rate of CVD events in the LCD arm was lower than the high carbohydrate diet arm (10.1% vs 17.6%), but this was not reported in the discussion. This study seems to confirm that LCDs are safe from a CVD perspective.

Case reports A patient who had T1D for 41 years started an LCD after visiting Dr. Bernstein in New York in 1998 and was able to reduce and stabilise his BG concentrations, reduce HbA1c to 5.6%, have fewer hypoglycaemic episodes, lose weight, and experience less hunger and a better quality of life. At the time of publishing the article in 2003, he had maintained the regimen for four years [332].

A case report from 2014 describes a 19 year old with T1D who starts a palaeolithic-ketogenic diet 20 days after diagnosis and rapidly normalized BG concentrations and came off insulin therapy [333]. After 6 months, he still did not require insulin therapy, but unfortunately no further follow-up was provided.

A case report of three older patients (aged 36, 40 and 38 years, respectively) who started an LCD soon after T1D diagnosis (confirmed with antibody positive results), reports T1D remission [334]. The patients all achieved adequate BG control, allowing them to stop insulin therapy: one for 4 years of follow-up and one for 15 months of follow-up. The third was still able to maintain control after 4 years of follow-up even though he had restarted insulin therapy after 2 years.

In another case report, a 37-year-old man with a history of 20 years of T1D and of 4 years following a KD (average HbA1c 5%, no DKA, no severe hypoglycaemic events), completed a 4011 km cycle ride in 20 days but was still able to maintain glycaemic stability [335]. The authors reported that his diet on the ride contained carbohydrates 11%, protein 31% and fat 58%. He used a continuous glucose monitor (CGM) which showed he maintained his glucose concentration at an average of 6.1 mmol/L (110 mg/dL) with a standard deviation of 2.1 mmol/L (37.8 mg/dL) for the 10 days. He experienced one episode of symptomatic hypoglycaemia which he reversed by ingesting 9.9 g of glucose.

Review articles A number of reviews have examined the use of TCR in patients with T1D. Turton et al.'s [336] systematic review of LCDs for T1D included nine studies. Unfortunately they found that due to the heterogeneity of the studies, they were unable to determine any significant outcome differences between LCD and high carbohydrate diets. However, they did note that in all studies the total daily dose of insulin was reduced in those following the LCDs. They conclude that more studies are needed to evaluate LCDs in T1D patients and that these should evaluate five specific outcomes namely, a reduction in HbA1c, no increase in hypoglycaemia, a reduction in total daily insulin use, a reduction in BMI, and improving quality of life.

Bolla et al. [337] reviewed low-carbohydrate and KDs in T1D and T2D; the review included many of the studies discussed above. Their conclusions are cautiously optimistic about the use of LCDs in T1D. They tend to emphasise the quality of carbohydrate (advocating low GI/GL foods), although they do suggest that quantity is also relevant. They suggest that in motivated patients and informed, motivated medical professionals, LCDs are a great tool to use to achieve adequate control and reduce long-term complications in T1D patients. As is usual, in all the trials reviewed, there is concern about the increase in LDL cholesterol concentrations; yet no trials show actual evidence that CVD worsens with increased LDL cholesterol concentrations in T1D patients who use LCDs.

An excellent review by Scott et al. [318] discusses the use of LCDs in T1D patients and evaluated potential benefits (weight loss, reduced hypoglycaemia, less hyperglycaemia, reduced insulin doses and reduced insulin resistance) and potential risks (increased DKA, increased total and LDL cholesterol concentrations, possible nutritional deficiencies, growth abnormalities in children, eating and psychological disorders). They review the use of LCDs in athletes without T1D and provide some evidence for the use of LCDs in athletes with T1D. Some physiological mechanisms are provided, which suggest that LCD may be effective in T1D patients especially in lowering glycaemic concentrations and enhancing the use of adipose stores for energy during exercise. They show intriguing evidence that training in the fasted state may actually have overall benefits in lowering BG concentrations. They also promote the use of regular monitoring and even CGMs usage. They note that more evidence for LCD use is needed in T1D but indicate that LCDs (<130 g/day carbohydrates) is a viable option to help control BG concentrations in T1D patients.

On a cautionary note, De Bock et al. highlight six cases of children (and some families) who followed LCDs after a diagnosis of T1D [338]. At the outset the paper states that 'endocrinologists and dietitians across Australia and New Zealand were invited to describe T1D cases where adherence to a restricted carbohydrate diet was believed to result in endocrine and metabolic consequences.' They reported that these children were found to have a failure to grow and also worsened CVD risk factors. It is also clear that all patients were actually on low calorie diets or underfed and would have benefitted from sympathetic help and advice on how to improve their energy and nutritional intake, while remaining on a relatively lower carbohydrate diet. The only advice given was to counsel the patients to increase their carbohydrate intakes. Two families were clearly upset with the services, and one even left the clinic and was lost to follow up.

However, in an overview Gallagher et al. reviewed the medical and psychological considerations for LCDs in youth with T1D [339]. They evaluated the potential benefits and risks and highlighted the need for individualised and family dietary habits to be aligned, and for healthcare providers to be thoughtful and supportive to families who may choose TCR. They highlight the potential for eating disorders, which is an area all providers should be aware of when advising youth with T1D.

Overall, the evidence shows that for motivated patients and healthcare providers, it is possible to control T1D, safely achieving almost normal glycaemia, using TCR. All healthcare providers should be prepared to offer this lifestyle therapy to patients, and to support patients who wish to follow this therapy.

3.6.3.6 *Therapeutic carbohydrate restriction dietary intervention*

TCR is about the reduction of carbohydrates to a level that will enable someone with T1D to have normal glucose concentrations (a good place to start may be around 70–90 g of carbohydrate per day). A typical TCR diet will importantly be from sources of food that are real and unprocessed. It is well known that ultra-processed food is directly harmful to health and this should be discouraged in all diets [340].

The object of dietary choices in T1D is to maximise the health gain from unprocessed food, enable near physiological concentrations of BG, and reduction in hypoglycaemic episodes. Real foods in a typical TCR diet will be leafy vegetables, ideally seasonal, locally sourced and organic, tree nuts (reduce or avoid peanuts and cashews), berry fruits in small amounts, full-fat dairy products, eggs, all meats (with fatty cuts preferable), all fish, cooking oils not derived from seeds and that is cold-pressed rather than processed industrially with solvents. This is a VLCD or KD (less than 50 g carbohydrate per day). A higher carbohydrate diet in TCR will include more root vegetables, pulses, and possibly limited grains.

An often overlooked part of all dietary recommendations is enjoyment. The perception of TCR diets as being bland and unsustainable is outdated and represents individual clinician bias and possibly their own personal behaviours around food, rather than any evidence-based assessment. There are thousands of recipes that suit a TCR diet that is healthy, visually appealing, and highly palatable.

With all chronic diseases, there is a big learning curve when starting out on a TCR lifestyle. Clinician support and simple messaging can go a long way towards successful dietary intervention and clinical outcomes. Below are some guides to help patients with this lifestyle.

1. It is important that all patients understand which foods contain carbohydrates, so that when they reduce their carbohydrate intakes, they understand how to match insulin doses to the reduced carbohydrate intakes. In most cases, the basal insulin regime may be maintained, but the bolus doses will need to be reduced.
2. Monitoring BG concentrations is extremely important and, at a minimum, should be performed pre- and post-meals. Ideally, if patients can afford it, patients should use CGM devices, but they may still need to record pre-and post-meal concentrations to ensure that insulin doses are correct and that meals eaten are not high in carbohydrates, producing high postprandial BG concentrations.
3. Patients should try to stick to a maximum of three meals a day and minimise (or stop) snacking between meals. This allows glucose and insulin concentrations to reduce and stabilise. The lower blood insulin concentrations will allow adipose tissue lipolysis increasing energy utilisation from fat oxidation. Unfortunately, when snacking, patients tend not to dose with insulin for the snack, which makes it difficult to control BG concentrations.
4. Treat protein with insulin. As protein conversion to glucose takes longer, patients may find that glucose concentrations spike later after a protein meal. This may require a prolonged bolus on a pump or a longer acting bolus insulin (e.g., Humulin R).
5. Use slow-acting carbohydrates to counteract exercise associated hypoglycaemia (e.g., superstarch). Exercise can induce a late hypoglycaemic event, so to prevent this may require some slow-release complex carbohydrates to counteract the late dip.
6. Ensure that patients are willing to eat more fat. As patients reduce carbohydrates, they will need to increase healthy fat intakes. If they do not, they will find that they become hungry and will be tempted to snack more which will affect glucose concentrations abnormally.
7. Following a low carbohydrate high-fat lifestyle may induce nutritional ketosis. This is often a target for many patients, but it is important for patients to understand the concentration of ketones they can achieve safely. For this reason, it would be advisable to have a ketone metre to measure the concentration of ketones (β-hydroxybutyrate) in their blood. Acceptable concentrations range from 0.5 mmol/L to 3 mmol/L. Ketone metres are also helpful when patients are unwell and may even develop euglycaemic DKA, an important condition to be aware of.
8. Consider using insulin pumps if it is affordable. Many pumps now have feedback loops that can prevent patients from 'overdosing' on insulin and have a suspend function if glucose concentrations are reducing and the pump senses that hypoglycaemia may ensue.
9. Patients are advised to plan some time out (e.g., a weekend) where they can concentrate on an LCD and see the effects on their glucose concentrations and insulin doses. At these times, it is incredibly helpful to keep a diary of readings, food intake, and insulin doses.
10. Beware of keto-related hypoglycaemic unawareness. This is when many patients, including non-TCR type 1 patients, develop unawareness of low glucose concentrations due to frequent hypoglycaemic episodes. This can lead to them losing the compensatory mechanisms and symptoms that warn them that they are going 'low,' such as sweating, dizziness, tachycardia, aggressiveness, etc. In effect, this leads them to have severe hypoglycaemic episodes without initially being aware of them, and by the time, they (or others) realise they are 'low' they may already be in a coma, and will need outside help. Some patients who are in nutritional ketosis may develop hypoglycaemic unawareness, which may have serious effects. Be aware that these patients will have to monitor more frequently and, if possible, should use a CGM.
11. Encourage patients to be compassionate towards themselves. They need to listen to their bodies, listen to their mind and realise that they will need to take their time to develop the learning, the skills, and the confidence to control their BG concentrations. Encourage them and celebrate small successes with them. Remind them to be kind to themselves even when things don't go well.

Help them to be part of a community, including other patients, their family and their team of healthcare providers.

3.6.3.6.1 Guiding the patient

Unless patients are in DKA at diagnosis, it is possible to treat patients at an outpatient level. This may be the best opportunity to introduce the concepts of TCR and the careful use of insulin.

People might be at any stage of their diabetes journey, some will be newly diagnosed, others will have complications, and some are potentially advanced. Others will be at a stage where chronic hyperinsulinaemia of peripherally administered insulin has led to a type 2 insulin-resistant pattern, adding co-morbidity to T1D. This will guide the clinician in recommending the amount of carbohydrate restriction and the timing of the transition, immediate, weeks, or months.

However, the technique of transitioning to a lowered carbohydrate or even a KD is familiar to clinicians. It applies to pumps or pens and follows existing teaching. Firstly, adjust the basal insulin dose until the patient achieves fasting normoglycaemia, then count the carbohydrates and use the required bolus insulin dose with meals. The only addition to this practice is to count protein and add a bolus dose for protein, possibly at a delayed timing peri-prandially.

Dietary education is hampered by current guidelines, which have been slow to adapt to research findings and present a confusing message to people needing appropriate dietary information. Clinical knowledge tends to favour guideline recommendations, which have become a poor information source for patients and clinicians.

It is important therefore to accurately assess the needs of someone wanting to transition to a TCR diet. What is their motivation? How determined are they to succeed? What are the barriers to success, and how can they be negotiated? What does success look like for a patient? What personal and other resources do they have? It is likely to be appropriate to plan a series of incremental steps towards a goal and recognise when those milestones are achieved? This is based on the GRIN (Goals, Resources, Increments, Noticing) model of motivation to bring about change (see Chapter 11.2.2.2) [341].

It is necessary to understand the types of macronutrients and the effects they have on metabolism and how insulin fits into this. This step might be challenging for a patient who finds it difficult to learn concepts and relies on word of mouth and popular articles and advertising for their information. But managing T1D is mostly a practical skill, and a simple prescriptive diet sheet with recipes suited to the person's budget will help a great deal.

3.6.3.6.2 Monitoring

A clinician should provide patients with a glucometer, and a continuous glucose metre (CGM) is preferable to a finger prick glucometer. Learning is more rapid, and there is an element of safety during the transition when trends of glucose can be visualised and alarms set if available. Finger prick metres should be made available also for calibration of CGMs and for sensor failure. Some countries require finger-prick tests to be carried in motor vehicles in order to comply with driving laws.

Blood ketone metres are an essential part of T1D management whether on a TCR diet or not. Nutritional ketosis is not a risk factor for DKA. But people with T1D, however it is managed, are still at risk of DKA. It is important for the patient to regularly test blood ketone concentrations during the transition to a TCR diet, in order to get the ketone concentrations that are normal for them (clinical experience with 120 individuals with T1D on a KD suggests that 75% fall in the range 0.6–1.5 mmol/L (3.5–8.7 mg/dL)). This will aid clinicians to care for patients at those times when DKA might be more likely, such as during a severe infection. HbA1c is still widely used as a marker for medium term control. With the increasing use of CGMs, time in range (TIR) is becoming a useful marker. The ranges for TIR are typically set between 4 mmol/L and 10 mmol/L (72–180 mg/dL). The achievement percentage changes with age, with those under 25 years old being set a lower target, but 70% TIR is considered a good level of control for adults.

The TIR target is calibrated for people on high-carbohydrate diets as is evident from the relaxed targets for those considered to be more at risk of hypoglycaemic episodes. Patients on a KD diet should easily reach and exceed these targets and might want to work within a tighter range, which can then be adjusted to obtain the comparison figures for a clinic. It has been mentioned before that even though hypoglycaemia risk still exists, the frequency is reduced approximately fivefold with therapeutic restriction to 75–90 g of carbohydrate per day [328]. TIR target setting is a decision of clinical judgement made between clinicians and patients.

3.6.4 Conclusion

We have looked at the evidence for the use of TCR in T1D. While the evidence for TCR is compelling, all healthcare providers should be aware of the pitfalls that may occur. This lifestyle should be offered to all T1D patients as part of their treatment and patients who are already following this lifestyle should continue to be supported and not discouraged. Some guidelines are offered to help patients on this journey.

3.7 Polycystic ovarian syndrome and infertility

Nadia Pataguana

3.7.1 Introduction

Polycystic ovarian syndrome (PCOS) is the most common reproductive disorder in the world. It affects an estimated 8 to 20% of women of reproductive age globally, depending upon the specific diagnostic criteria used [342]. Forty percent of patients diagnosed with PCOS suffer from infertility, and 90%–95% of women in infertility clinics who cannot conceive due to lack of ovulation suffer from PCOS.

3.7.1.1 History

PCOS, conceived as a disease of modernity, is actually ancient. Originally described as a gynaecological curiosity, it is now the most common endocrine disorder in young women, involving multiple organ systems.

3.7.1.2 Early definitions

PCOS was recognised as early as Hippocrates (460–377 BC), who defined it as 'women whose menstruation is less than three days or is meagre, are robust, with a healthy complexion and a masculine appearance; yet they are not concerned about bearing children nor do they become pregnant' [343]. The ancient Greek gynaecologist Soranus of Ephesus (c.98–138 AD) made a similar observation. French obstetrician Ambroise Paré (1510–1590) corroborated that these women were 'manly' and 'become bearded.' Italian scientist Antonio Vallisneri (1661–1730) connected these features into a single disease when he described several young infertile women whose ovaries were white, shiny, and the size of pigeon eggs [344].

In 1921 French doctors Émile Charles Achard and Joseph Thiers described a syndrome that included masculinising features and T2D. Further cases in 1928 cemented the link between what is now called PCOS and T2D, and these were described in the article 'Diabetes of Bearded Women' [345]. Careful observation had revealed to these clinicians common pathology beneath menstrual irregularities, infertility, masculine features, and obesity-coupled T2D. The only feature differing from the modern definition of PCOS was the ovarian cysts, which were understandably missed due to a lack of non-invasive imaging.

3.7.1.3 Clinical presentation

3.7.1.3.1 The PCOS spectrum: What PCOS is and is not

To confirm a diagnosis of PCOS, clinicians must confirm the presence of two of three of the following conditions:

1. hyperandrogenism,
2. menstrual irregularities, and
3. polycystic ovaries.

Because some women will present with all three criteria and others will have only two, PCOS represents a spectrum of disease.

The Rotterdam criteria recognised this continuum and grouped patients into four different phenotypes:

- Frank or classic polycystic ovary PCOS (chronic anovulation, hyperandrogenism, and polycystic ovaries—3/3 criteria)
- Classic non-polycystic ovary PCOS (chronic anovulation, hyperandrogenism, and normal ovaries—2/3 criteria)
- Nonclassic ovulatory PCOS (regular menstrual cycles, hyperandrogenism, and polycystic ovaries—2/3 criteria)
- Nonclassic, mild PCOS (chronic anovulation, normal androgens, and polycystic ovaries—2/3 criteria)

The frank phenotype represents the most severe disease and is associated with metabolic diseases like obesity and T2D and with cardiovascular risk factors like high blood pressure and triglyceride concentration. In contrast, women with nonclassic, mild PCOS are at the lowest risk of metabolic disease [346]. Why some women with PCOS present with hyperandrogenism as opposed to anovulatory cycles is unknown.

3.7.1.3.2 Hyperandrogenism

Male sex hormones, called androgens, are normally present in both men and women, but the normal concentrations for men are far higher than for women. Testosterone is the best-known androgen and contributes to many of the physical factors that distinguish men from women. It is produced in the testes of men and in the ovaries of women. Small amounts are also produced in the adrenal glands that sit above the kidneys. Testosterone helps regulate sex drive, fat distribution, and bone mass. More than 80% of women who present with symptoms of hyperandrogenism will eventually be diagnosed with PCOS [347].

Common features of hyperandrogenism include:

- increased facial and body hair growth (hirsutism)
- male-pattern baldness
- acne
- lowered tone of voice
- menstrual irregularities
- clitoral enlargement (in severe cases)

3.7.1.3.3 Menstrual irregularities

Irregular, absent, or rare menstrual cycles are all common symptoms of PCOS. An estimated 85% of women with PCOS suffer menstrual irregularities [348]. During the normal menstrual cycle, the human egg develops from the primordial follicle. It grows during the first half of the menstrual cycle and then is released into the fallopian tubes to be carried to the uterus, where it awaits fertilisation by the sperm. Ovulation is the release of the egg inside the ovary. Irregular menstrual cycles are caused by the failure of ovulation. In PCOS, the main menstrual problems are anovulation and oligo-ovulation. Anovulation means a complete lack of ovulation and oligo-ovulation refers to a lower-than-normal rate of ovulation.

When normal ovulation does not occur, menstrual cycles may be completely absent (amenorrhoea) or may last longer than usual (oligomenorrhea). However, having a regular cycle does not mean that ovulation has occurred normally, especially in women with other evidence of hyperandrogenism. Of note, 20%–50% of women with signs of excess testosterone and regular periods still have evidence of anovulation. This lack of ovulation will result in difficulty conceiving and infertility. PCOS is associated with recurrent miscarriages, and it is the most common cause of infertility in industrialised nations.

3.7.1.3.4 Polycystic ovaries

Follicles are collections of cells in the ovary. During normal menstruation, many follicles begin to develop, and one eventually becomes the human egg that is released into the uterus at the time of ovulation. The other follicles usually shrivel up and are reabsorbed into the body. When these follicles fail to shrivel up, they become cystic and show up on an ultrasound as ovarian cysts.

The Rotterdam criteria define polycystic ovaries as being the presence of twelve or more follicles measuring 2–9 mm in diameter in each ovary. Two main factors influence the number of cysts. Small (2–5 mm) follicles are related to the serum androgen concentration and larger (6–9 mm) follicles are related to both serum testosterone and fasting insulin concentration. Of note, 20%–30% of otherwise normal women may have multiple cysts on their ovaries, consequently, the mere presence of cysts is not enough to make the diagnosis of PCOS. Additionally, there is no correlation between the number of cysts and the severity of PCOS.

3.7.1.4 Investigations

3.7.1.4.1 Differential diagnoses

Hyperandrogenism and polycystic ovaries are not exclusive to PCOS; thus other diseases that mimic PCOS must be excluded by history or by physical or laboratory examination before the diagnosis can be confirmed. While most of these conditions are rare, they may be serious and require entirely different treatments, which makes the distinction important. The list of similar conditions includes:

- pregnancy,
- hyperprolactinemia (prolactin excess),
- thyroid disorders,
- nonclassic congenital adrenal hyperplasia (NCAH),
- Cushing's syndrome, and
- hyperandrogenemia (androgen excess, tumour/drug-induced).

3.7.2 Health risks associated with polycystic ovarian syndrome

If PCOS were just about acne and a few missing periods, then it would not be so bad. Unfortunately, PCOS is associated with many health concerns, reproductive as well as general [349]. The reproductive issues include

- anovulatory cycles,
- infertility,
- disorders of pregnancy, and
- Foetal concerns.

Other significant health concerns include

- CVD,
- NAFLD,
- sleep apnoea,
- anxiety and depression,
- cancer,
- T2D, and
- MetS.

These are some of the deadliest conditions in the world, including the top two causes of death in America, cardiovascular disease, and cancer. PCOS is not merely a nuisance; it is an important warning of risk. For this reason, it's worth taking a closer look at each of these conditions in more detail to try to understand their link with PCOS.

3.7.2.1 Understanding the link between polycystic ovarian syndrome and its associated risks

PCOS must be considered more than merely a disorder of excess facial hair, acne, and abnormal reproduction. Patients with PCOS have double the chance of being hospitalised compared with those without the disease. The United States spent an estimated $4 billion in 2004 on healthcare related to treating PCOS [350], an amount equal to the entire gross domestic product of Barbados. Much of this cost (40.4%) is due to the associated T2D [351].

Even more sobering, this number likely underestimates the true costs, because it takes into account only the reproductive years and not the associated health risks such as T2D, heart attacks, strokes, and cancer that may arise in the future. These diseases typically occur in a woman's post-menopausal years and are many, many times more expensive than simply treating PCOS.

Furthermore, PCOS is one of the leading causes of infertility and in vitro fertilisation (which is its own multi-billion-dollar industry), and as we've seen, women with PCOS who do become pregnant are at increased risk of obstetrical complications such as gestational diabetes, pregnancy-induced hypertension, and pre-eclampsia.

Though they are not part of the formal definition of PCOS, obesity leading to MetS and IR leading to T2D have been frequently noted in patients and affect an estimated 50%–70% of women with PCOS. The close link between obesity and T2D suggests that all three conditions have the same underlying root cause. All three are now understood as metabolic diseases, putting women with PCOS at high risk later in life for cardiovascular disease, strokes, and cancer (Fig. 3.18).

Perhaps the most important associated disease is a history of weight gain that often precedes the diagnosis of PCOS. Of the obese women referred to one clinic, 28.3% were diagnosed with PCOS [352]. PCOS can be more common as severity of obesity increases, but more importantly, weight loss has also been proven to reduce testosterone, improve T2D, and decrease hirsutism (more on this later).

3.7.3 Pathophysiology

While there is a genetic predisposition to developing PCOS [353], endocrine factors (insulin) in response to diet (carbohydrates and eating) can determine who develops PCOS and who does not.

3.7.3.1 Insulin: the energy storage and energy use hormone

The body set weight (BSW) sets an ideal body fat percentage that it defends just like our house thermostat. Below this set point, the body attempts to gain weight. Above this set point, the body attempts to lose weight. The body seeks homoeostasis, which is why counting calories is futile. The body can burn more or fewer calories depending on the

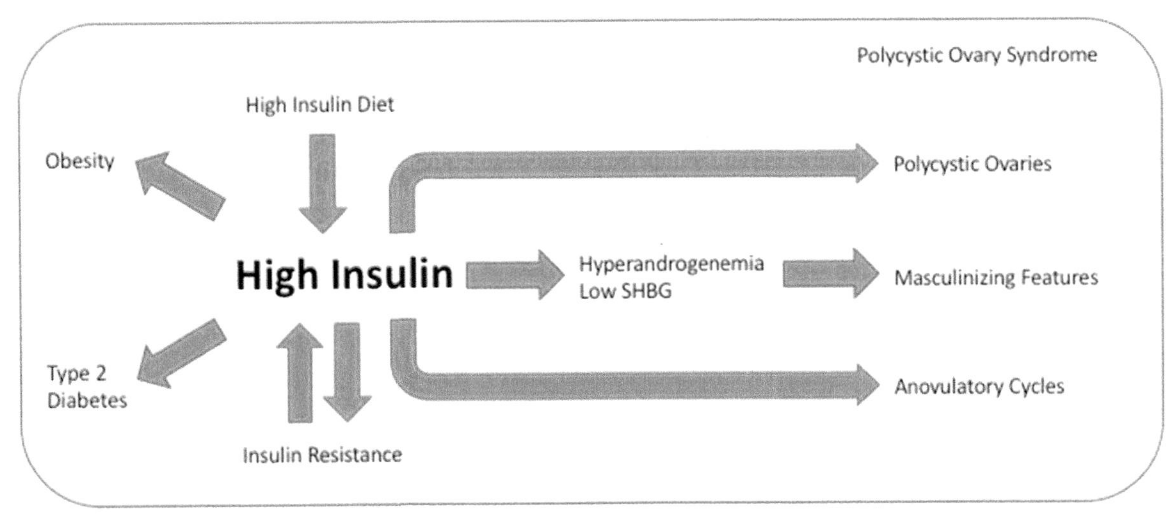

FIGURE 3.18 **IR as the root cause of chronic disease.** In the predisposed, diet-induced hyperinsulinaemia results in T2D, IR and obesity, as well as the three defining features of PCOS: polycystic ovaries, masculinising features and anovulatory cycles. SHBG, sex hormone binding globulin.

situation. The hormone insulin instructs the body to gain body fat. If you keep feeding the body, it will continue to gain body fat. Insulin will keep directing the body to convert the food energy to glycogen and body fat. This is the reason that snacking continuously leads to weight gain. It is also the reason that insulin injections lead to weight gain. Your body has no mechanism to count calories (see Section 3.8).

3.7.3.2 *Insulin is the common link*

Given that obesity is a hormonal imbalance that results in the gradual increase of the BSW thermostat over time, it is likely that the root cause of PCOS is also hormonal.

But is insulin the other factor? In the study of a disease, the most crucial piece of information is its aetiology. If you know that a virus causes hepatitis C, you can prescribe an antiviral that kills the virus and cures the disease. If you understand that smoking causes lung cancer, you can prevent much of this disease by introducing smoking-cessation programs. We can get a hint of PCOS's aetiology by looking at its associated conditions.

3.7.3.2.1 Insulin and hyperandrogenism

Excessive insulin causes both:

1. overproduction of testosterone and
2. decreased sex hormone binding globulin (SHBG) concentration that leads to increased testosterone effect.

The striking correlation between blood concentrations of insulin and testosterone was noted as far back as 1980 [354]. When ovarian cells are purified and bathed in insulin, they increase testosterone production significantly [355]. Insulin is the major regulator of SHBG production in the liver. The higher the insulin, the lower the SHBG production. This relationship holds true not just in women but also in men [356]. Decreasing insulin concentration through weight loss increases SHBG production.

3.7.3.2.2 The surprising link between insulin and reproduction

The ovary itself is particularly rich in insulin receptors [357], which seems rather strange at first glance because insulin is most commonly associated with digestion, BG and body fat. Why would the ovaries carry insulin receptors? In fact, the pathways that link reproductive function and metabolism are seen in virtually every living animal, from fruit flies to roundworms to human beings. Why?

The answer is that all animals need to know that food is available before committing to reproduction. Raising children requires a good deal of resources, including adequate food supplies for both the expectant mother and the developing baby.

We can therefore conclude that a high insulin concentration is the primary factor stimulating excessive ovarian production of testosterone and that this increased androgen (hyperandrogenism) is responsible for the masculinising features of PCOS, including acne and hirsutism [358]. Hyperinsulinemia is the root cause of hyperandrogenism. Too much insulin causes too much testosterone. Is insulin responsible for the lack of ovulation and polycystic ovaries, too?

In 1982, it was first observed that the ovaries of women with PCOS contain two to three times the number of small primary follicles measuring 2–5 mm [359]. More recent studies suggest up to six times the usual number. The small ovarian follicles are rich in testosterone receptors, and it was determined that high testosterone concentration was forcing too many primordial follicles from the resting phase to become primary follicles [360].

Hyperinsulinemia causes premature response to luteinising hormone (LH) which stops further follicular development.

In PCOS, the many small follicles do not mature to become eggs that can be pushed out into the uterus for fertilisation. This failure of ovulation causes anovulatory cycles and menstrual irregularities. And the excessive numbers of small follicles fill with fluid and are visible as polycystic ovaries.

3.7.3.3 The insulin connection

High insulin concentratiosn are predominantly responsible for the follicular arrest [361] by disturbing the delicate balance of follicle stimulating hormone (FSH) to LH ratio that triggers the correct follicular development (Fig. 3.19) [361]. During normal development, FSH encourages the growth of primordial follicles into primary follicles, and a surge of LH selects the dominant follicle, which leads to proper ovulation. In women with PCOS, the high insulin concentration promotes the transition of primordial follicles to primary follicles [362]. They also increase testosterone concentration, making the receptors on the primary follicles overly sensitive to LH.

The primary follicles respond too early in the menstrual cycle, and stop growing when they are still small and not yet ready for ovulation. Consequently, no single dominant follicle is selected and no signal is given for involution (shrivelling up). The many small follicles simply accumulate fluid, and it is these numerous small fluid-filled cysts that are visible on ultrasound and clinch the diagnosis of PCOS.

In women with PCOS, insulin sends its 'stop growing' message to the follicles much too early. These immature follicles cannot be expelled as mature eggs, nor can they involute. Eventually they just become cysts. Lots and lots of cysts. Insulin causes this follicular arrest, which results in polycystic ovaries.

During follicular arrest, no dominant follicle grows large enough to ovulate. The result is a menstrual cycle in which no ovulation occurs (anovulatory cycle). No ovulation, no egg, no baby.

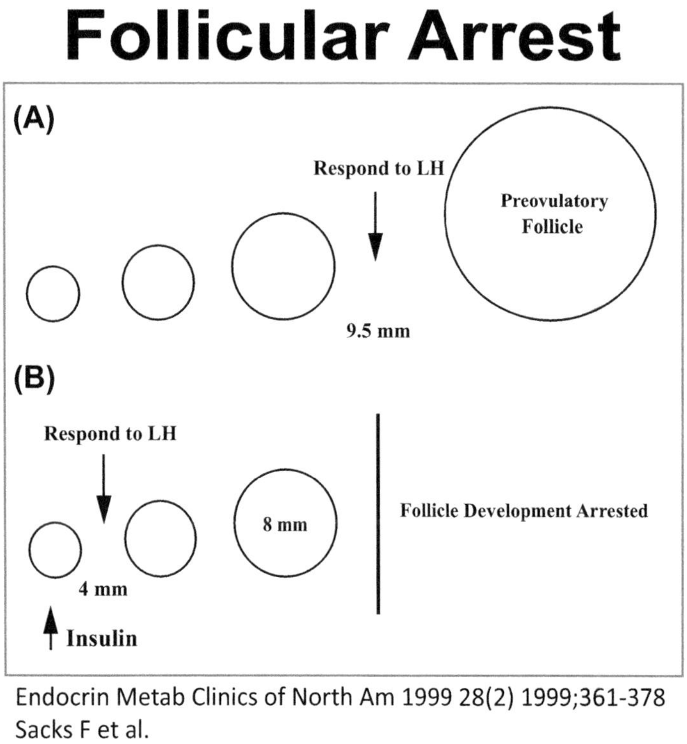

FIGURE 3.19 Normal ovulation in response to luteinizing hormone (LH).

Almost all women will experience a few anovulatory cycles in their lifetimes, especially during puberty and menopause. However, the excessive insulin and testosterone in PCOS cause recurrent anovulatory cycles. Since testosterone is overproduced due to high insulin, the single-most important cause of anovulatory cycles is high insulin. Both weight loss and the insulin-lowering drug metformin lower plasma testosterone and improve ovulatory rates [363]. Indeed, all known treatments to reduce insulin, including weight loss, bariatric surgery, and the drugs somatostatin and metformin, significantly improve ovulatory function and reduce the symptoms of PCOS. Interestingly, patients with T1D who use high doses of injected insulin also have an increased risk of PCOS.

The bottom line then, is that the three defining features of PCOS (hyperandrogenism causing masculine features, polycystic ovaries and anovulatory cycles) all reflect the same pathophysiology: too much testosterone, ultimately caused by too much insulin.

In other words, too much insulin causes PCOS. Like obesity, PCOS is best understood as a disease of hyperinsulinemia. Although obesity and PCOS do not always occur together, they are both manifestations of an underlying hyperinsulinemia.

The eponymous criterion of PCOS is the presence of multiple cysts in the ovaries, which are derived from the multitude of small follicles. Many women have a few cysts on their ovary, but the sheer number of cysts distinguishes this syndrome from virtually all others. Almost no other much insulin and too much testosterone human disease causes polycystic ovaries. Ultimately, these polycystic ovaries are caused by too.

Both the cysts on the ovaries and the hyperandrogenism are caused by the same underlying problem: too much insulin.

3.7.3.3.1 Hyperinsulinemia, insulin resistance, and polycystic ovarian syndrome

All known forms of IR are associated with PCOS. By 1980, hyperinsulinemia and IR were noted in obese PCOS patients [354]. Hyperinsulinaemia is independent of the degree of obesity [364].

The conclusion is that hyperinsulinemia drives PCOS. Moreover, the phenomenon known as IR *causes* hyperinsulinemia. IR is a factor in T2D and a risk factor for MetS. It is this association with hyperinsulinemia and IR that firmly established PCOS as a metabolic disorder and accounts for the increased prevalence of T2D, central adiposity, and metabolic disease in women with PCOS. MetS affects an estimated one-third of adolescents and half of all adults with PCOS [365].

3.7.3.3.2 The link between diet, insulin resistance, and polycystic ovarian syndrome

The overflow paradigm (Fig. 3.18) explains perfectly the selective IR seen in PCOS, T2D, and obesity. If you eat a diet that is very high in sugar and refined carbohydrates and if you eat frequently throughout the day, you are constantly stimulating insulin, leading to hyperinsulinemia.

In other words, all the related metabolic diseases of obesity, T2D, PCOS, and fatty liver disease are caused by the same underlying condition: too much insulin. In PCOS without T2D, you most often find normal BG, but high blood insulin concentration. This situation is often called IR. That is, insulin has succeeded in pushing glucose into the overflowing cell. But the situation has not been fixed, because the moment insulin concentration reduces, glucose will rise. Hyperinsulinaemia is a temporary band-aid.

This is the key to understanding PCOS, and indeed, all the metabolic diseases. The underlying problem is the same: *too much insulin*. The solution then becomes immediately obvious: we need to lower insulin.

While women may have genetic or other factors that predispose them to PCOS, lifestyle, and particularly their body mass index (BMI), likely determine their position on the spectrum. Weight gain moves women towards the severe end of the spectrum [366]. Weight loss, in contrast, moves women toward the less severe end of the spectrum by improving fertility, ovulatory cycles, and hirsutism [367].

3.7.4 Managing the patient

3.7.4.1 Aims of care

The primary aim of care should be addressing the underlying cause of PCOS.

3.7.4.2 Pharmacotherapy

Refer to the recommendations from the international evidence-based guideline for the assessment and management of polycystic ovary syndrome (2018) [368]. Most PCOS treatments with the exception of metformin do not treat the underlying pathology of hyperinsulinaemia in PCOS and should be adjunct treatments. By focusing efforts on serum insulin reduction, not only do we address the symptomatic relief of PCOS as well as infertility, we also reduce the risk of the metabolic consequences of IR in patients with this condition. It is incomprehensible that this is not the focus of current medical therapies for PCOS and begs further consideration, as many of the current treatments are insufficient:

1. symptomatic treatments
2. fertility treatments

3.7.4.2.1 Symptomatic treatments

The methods in this category are prescribed to treat symptoms of PCOS.

The birth control pill The birth control pill (BCP) is a hormonal contraceptive containing oestrogen and progestin hormones in a variety of formulations to improve menstrual irregularities, reduce androgen concentration, and increase liver production of SHBG [369], which reduces symptoms such as acne and hair loss [370]. There are also side effects to consider, including the higher risk of blood clots [370].

Spironolactone Spironolactone is a diuretic drug introduced in the 1960s that blocks the actions of androgens at the level of the receptor. It does not reduce androgen concentration, but it alleviates symptoms such as excessive hair growth and acne [371]. Hair may be reduced by up to 40% with this drug [370].

Important side effects include hyperkalaemia and probable teratogenicity and thus must always be used with birth control to prevent pregnancy and the possibility of birth defects [372].

Metformin The American Association of Clinical Endocrinologists suggests that metformin be considered an initial therapy for women with PCOS, particularly obese women [373]. It improves insulin sensitivity and reduces the hyperinsulinemia behind T2D and PCOS. Lower insulin concentration reduces ovarian production of androgens, the hallmark of PCOS [374].

Metformin taken at least 3 months prior to conception increases pregnancy rates, reduces miscarriage [375], lowers rates of other pregnancy complications, including gestational diabetes and pre-eclampsia [376]. Like any other drug, metformin has the potential for side effects (mild to severe gastrointestinal discomfort) but these are negligible compared to benefits for PCOS [377].

Surgery Surgery, like the ovarian wedge resection performed by Drs. Stein and Leventhal in 1935, was successful [378] but is rarely used today due to high complication risk. Doctors may use the less invasive laparoscopic ovarian drilling (LOD) method, to reduce ovary testosterone production, as a last resort [379]. LOD is not always successful, with conception rates similar to the medical (oral) therapy treatments listed above [380]. Surgical complications include excessive scar tissue and decrease in ovarian reserve and function.

3.7.4.2.2 Fertility treatments

In 1961 the first drugs were developed to promote ovulation, and the era of fertility medicine began [381].

Clomiphene citrate Clomiphene citrate (CC) affects oestrogen receptors to stimulate ovulation in up to 75%–80% of women, resulting in a live birth rate of 20%–50%. CC revolutionized fertility treatment because it is both inexpensive and effective. If no effects occur within 3 months, other treatments must be considered. CC is also not synergistic with metformin.

Letrozole Letrozole is an aromatase inhibitor, which blocks androgen conversion into oestrogen to produce follicle-stimulating hormone (FSH) and induce ovulation. Compared with CC, letrozole produces a more physiological hormonal stimulation that results in a lower rate of multiple births, fewer side effects and a higher rate of live births. Some studies, however, elucidate higher risk of serious birth defects (though not statistically significant) advising caution in its use [382].

Gonadotropins Gonadotropins stimulate ovulation by mimicking FSH and luteinizing hormone (LH), to increase ovulation change. The PCOS ovulation rate using gonadotropins is approximately 70% and the pregnancy rate is approximately 20% [383]. Gonadotropins carry the risk of multiple pregnancies and mild to severe ovarian hyperstimulation syndrome (OHSS).

Intrauterine insemination and in vitro fertilisation Both intrauterine insemination (IUI) in vitro fertilisation (IVF) involve injecting gonadotropins to stimulate ovulation. At ovulation, in IUI sperm is inserted directly into the uterus, while in IVF, mature eggs are retrieved surgically, combined with sperm and successful fertilisations are transferred back into the uterus. Success rates with IUI are slightly lower than IVF. IVF comes with physical discomfort from self-injecting gonadotropins, a rare chance of infection and high cost.

3.7.4.3 Diet

3.7.4.3.1 The optimal diet for polycystic ovarian syndrome

PCOS requires a low-insulin-stimulating diet, which is not necessarily low in calories. Knowing which foods affect insulin concentrations and when to eat them is necessary.

3.7.4.3.2 What to eat

All carbohydrates will produce an insulin response but the biggest culprit is the refined carbohydrates, such as sweets, white bread, and flour. Unprocessed carbohydrates, such as legumes and tubers, have much lower insulin stimulation compared to processed carbohydrates such as bread or sugar. The standard low-fat, calorie-reduced diet is typically high in carbohydrates because it follows the original 1977 Dietary Guidelines for Americans, which suggested carbohydrates constitute 55%–60% of the diet. This amount might be okay if people were eating a lot of sweet potatoes like the Okinawans, but the guidelines recommend eating 6–11 servings of highly refined grains in the bread, cereal, rice, and pasta group per day, which will raise insulin tremendously.

Refined carbohydrates generate the largest insulin response; dietary protein, particularly animal protein, also has an insulin response (but less than carbohydrate); and dietary fat, almost none at all. Protein, however, has the greatest effect on satiety, which makes us feel full. Thus, the optimal diet for reducing insulin, limits refined carbohydrates because the body does not need carbohydrate for good health. Include a moderate amount of dietary protein, since we need a certain amount to maintain health. But because it can also cause a significant insulin response and because the body cannot store excess dietary protein, eating more than is needed is not recommended. Dietary fat, on the other hand, should not be feared and should be included.

3.7.4.3.3 The ketogenic diet

A KD for adults typically allows less than 50 g per day. In practice a very low carbohydrate, moderate protein, high healthy fat diet, restricting carbohydrate to less than 20 g per day is effective.

An optimal low-insulin diet consists of the following steps:

1. Severely restrict added sugars
2. Severely restrict refined carbohydrates, particularly grains
3. Moderate intake of dietary protein
4. Eat natural fats liberally

3.7.4.3.4 When to eat

Eating, by its very nature, raises insulin. The mixture of carbohydrate, fat, and protein in the food determines to what degree. Eating continuously keeps your insulin concentration high, which in turn stimulates appetite, which makes snacking more prevalent. In contrast, not eating (fasting), allows your insulin to fall. Eating raises insulin and fasting drops insulin. Thus, to lower insulin concentration to treat PCOS, simply spend more time fasting and less time eating by:

- Skipping the snacks
- Eating earlier in the day and avoiding late night eating
- Incorporating intermittent fasting (IF) and or time-restricted eating (TRE)

Refer to Chapter 10 for more details on fasting.

3.7.5 Conclusion

PCOS remains the most common and problematic reproductive health disorder in women globally, despite current treatment methods and billions invested in research. PCOS's pathophysiological commonalities with IR, T2D, obesity, and other metabolic maladies, coupled with the documented inefficacy of current standards of care, require that PCOS is examined from an alternative disease standpoint (a metabolic one), with the concurrent option of alternative treatment modalities (primarily diet). TCR (a KD) combined with insulin sensitising medication might just prove to be the best treatment.

3.8 Body weight

Robert Cywes

3.8.1 Introduction: normal physiology and metabolism

Normal physiological body weight is a function of growth, seasonal opportunistic energy reserve storage and physical activity – cellular hyperplasia (increase in number) and cellular hypertrophy (increase in size). Fat distribution is hormonally dependent and regulated by genetics.

3.8.1.1 Measuring body weight

Body weight can be standardised by using BMI calculation (weight in kg/height in m^2) that allows equilibration irrespective of height or age. While BMI correlates most often with fat mass and is used predictively in this regard, it does not accommodate for specific body weight make-up, for example, a body builder may have a BMI of 32 kg/m^2, putting him in the obese category, but his body fat percent age may only be 3%–15%. 'Normal' BMI tables exist for all ages and sexes and are currently the most beneficial office-based measure of (excess) weight [384]. Body composition includes bone, muscle, fat, water and organs. A better way to define body weight is structural lean mass versus stored energy mass (fat). Body fat percentage can be indirectly assessed by calliper skinfold testing, bioelectrical impedance, dual energy x-ray absorptiometry (DEXA scan) or most accurately by underwater or hydrostatic weighing, however, all metrics are calculated not absolute [385]. The simplest most common current determinant of excess body fat remains the scale and mirror.

3.8.1.2 Fat distribution

Monosaccharides, protein, fat, and water are the four elements that are included in every cell in the body and, together with bone, make up the majority of body weight. Water, protein, and fat consumption are essential nutrient elements for both lean structural mass and stored energy mass. Fat is an essential component of every cell membrane (including organelles) and in larger quantities makes up additional structural mass such as in the central nervous system. Fat is the primary energy mass exclusively stored in adipocytes (healthy humans do not store energy fat in organs). Consumed and recycled protein contributes to lean structural mass since there is no primary protein energy store. Excess protein must be converted to glucose or ketones and stored as glycogen or fat. Monosaccharides contribute to structural mass (e.g., glycosylated proteins, DNA and RNA) as well as energy mass stored as glycogen in muscles, liver and other organs, but with a very limited and fixed storage capacity. Excess monosaccharides are converted to fat stored in adipocytes via DNL primarily in the liver and fat cells, but also in other organs for local structural use such as the brain.

3.8.1.3 Body weight regulation

Modern human thinking about nutrition is erroneous when it separates macronutrients into energy or calories and nutrients for tissue building, repair, and function. Almost all substrate nutrients are interchangeable and can perform energy or nutrient functions. In commonly held caloric or thermodynamic theories of body weight change, body weight is gained or lost by the balance of energy consumption versus energy utilisation driven by a set point. Energy consumption comes from fat, protein, and carbohydrates. The amount, ratio, and frequency are determined by set points such as genetics, hormonal homoeostasis, environment including seasonality, culture, physical activity, disease, food group circumstantial availability and psychological preference. Energy utilisation is determined by physical, cerebral, and metabolic activity. Body weight gain, growth and obesity are a direct consequence of chronic excessive energy consumption greater than energy utilisation, while weight loss is a direct consequence of consumed caloric reduction less than energy utilisation. The thermodynamic theory does not account for nutrient recycling and turnover and supposes interchangeability between energy substrates as well as substrates exercising autonomy over their use. The popular premise of the word 'diet' as a simile for weight loss, is principled on calorie-based mathematical formulae that define nearly every calorie-reductive diet that usually advocates for exercise as a way to 'burn off' calories (calories in-calories out CICO) [386,387].

This simplistic understanding of body weight regulation fails to recognise the most fundamental rule of human nutrition: nutrient (caloric) impact is always purpose driven and is regulated by anabolic or catabolic by hormonal dominance. All body weight changes are demand driven and genetically/hormonally controlled responses to physiological requirements induced by growth, pregnancy and menstrual cycling, exercise (increase muscle and decrease stored fat) and environmentally/seasonally driven storage fat accumulation or starvation, none of which are harmful except starvation due to food scarcity. Even body weight changes related to pathological alterations induced by inflammation, autoimmune diseases, trauma, communicable diseases, somatic diseases (acute and chronic), anasarca, pathological hormonal over- or under- production (e.g., pituitary adenomas), are demand-driven and hormonally controlled. This includes pre-death sarcopenia and cachexia [388,389].

However, the purpose of body weight change (increase or decrease) related to mental health disturbances are primarily and intentionally supply-driven and hormonally disruptive.

3.8.2 Body weight pathophysiology

3.8.2.1 Underweight

Lifetime prevalence rates of anorexia nervosa are increasing. Up to 4% among females and 0.3% among males. Bulimia nervosa rates are declining with 3% of females and 1% of males suffering from this disorder during their lifetime [390]. Anorexia nervosa has the highest mortality rate among all psychiatric illnesses, as it can result in significant psychopathology along with life-threatening medical complications [391]. In anorexia and bulimia nervosa, neuropsychological and neurochemical factors are prevalent such as serotonin, noradrenaline (norepinephrine) and dopamine dysfunction; depression and anxiety; poor stress and emotional-management skills; excessive worrying and fear or doubt about the future; authoritarian perfectionism (setting strict, demanding goals or standards, emotional restraint with an externalised locus of validation); and often tending toward obsessive-compulsive behaviour for instant emotional restitution. Skinniness and vomiting are the visible result of anorexia and bulimia (the condition). While distorted body image, dysfunctional/deficient emotion management skill sets (psychopathology) are the causes [392–395].

Ultimately, a comprehensive deficiency of effective emotion management strategies results in the use of starvation or binge eating followed by self-induced purging or vomiting as a self-inflicted, distorted, and dysfunctional form of instant gratification from intense emotional distress, be that anxiety, stress, depression, fear, sadness, anger, frustration, exhaustion, boredom, or pleasure. These are collectively referred to as emotional tension, and fall in line with other forms of self-harm for distorted emotional gratification. Such short-lived but powerful instant gratification emotional restitution has profound consequences including negativity, guilt and remorse that are erosive to already fragile self-esteem, self-confidence and self-respect [395,396]. Physiological harm is another consequence (e.g., anaemia; cardiovascular disturbance such as mitral valve prolapse, arrhythmias, or heart failure; bone demineralisation, osteopenia and the risk of fractures later in life; hormonal disturbances such as amenorrhoea and low testosterone; gastrointestinal problems, such as constipation, bloating or nausea; electrolyte abnormalities, such as low potassium, sodium, and chloride; renal failure; and sudden death) [392,394].

In these individuals, the cause of body weight changes is driven by psychological disturbance and a lack of nutrient-caloric supply or nutrient-caloric purging as opposed to being demand-driven by physiological need. Such psychological nutrient deprivation supersedes biological need and demand, resulting in loss of intrinsic homoeostatic hormonal energy flux control and profound decreases in body weight [392,394]. Anorexic and bulimic individuals progressively migrate away from nutritionally and hormonally driven satiety as a stopping point for eating, towards a lifestyle of psychologically driven starvation and purging. It is well accepted that primary treatment consists of psychotherapy and psychological restitution, with slow steady nutrient supply, not forced caloric refeeding that has often been attempted with disastrous consequences [397]. As psychological restitution evolves, the patient vicariously transitions from not eating primarily for emotion management, towards eating for nutritional fulfilment. Intentional refeeding rarely lasts as a primary therapeutic intervention and usually results in greater psychopathology, profound metabolic risk, and often self-harm.

While still in its infancy, research into employing KDs for safely refeeding anorexia patients, attending to the omega 3:6 ratio of PUFAs in the refeeding diet, similar to the refeeding protocols recommended for fast-breaking after extended intentional fasting periods used as part of the currently fashionable 'intermittent fasting' diet protocols has shown promise over refeeding using standard calorie-balanced diets [398–401].

3.8.2.2 Overweight – excessive body fat percentage

The WHO 2022 global adult obesity prevalence is estimated at 32% with the highest incidence occurring in genetically homogeneous populations such as South Sea Islanders (led by Nauru at 61%) [402,403]. For comparison, the age-adjusted prevalence of obesity among US adults was 42.4% in 2017–18 without significant differences between men and women among all adults or by age group [404].

A large meta-analysis examined relative all-cause mortality risk in overweight (BMI of 25 to <30), obesity (BMI of ≥30), grade 1 obesity (BMI of 30 to <35), and grades 2 and 3 obesity (BMI of ≥35) relative to normal weight (BMI of 18.5 to <25): [405].

Relative to normal weight, both obesity (all grades) and grades 2 and 3 obesity were associated with significantly higher all-cause mortality. Grade 1 obesity overall was not associated with higher mortality, and overweight was associated with significantly lower all-cause mortality.

Obesity defined by BMI is generally but erroneously accepted as a strong predictor of overall early mortality. An inverse association between BMI and mortality, called obesity-survival paradox, occurs clinically in a number of diseases including: haemodialysis, cardiovascular diseases, diabetes, chronic obstructive pulmonary disease, and surgery. The concept of metabolically healthy obesity and metabolically obese normal weight is perplexing when the pathophysiology is not understood. Metabolically healthy obesity is characterised by a phenotype with a BMI of 30 or above, but no metabolic syndrome component and a homoeostasis model assessment of IR (HOMA-IR) below 2.5. Metabolically obese normal weight individuals, popularly called 'TOFI' phenotype (Thin Outside, Fat Inside), have a normal BMI and yet display obesity-related phenotypic characteristics and a HOMA-IR above 2.5. The genetically predetermined and lifestyle impacted hormonal milieu linking body composition, fat distribution, ageing and cardiorespiratory fitness is critical to our evolving understanding that weight gain and obesity is not causal to metabolic derangement, but merely one possible associated outcome consequential to IR [406].

3.8.2.3 Pathophysiology of obesity and obesity-related metabolic disturbance

In obesity and obesogenic metabolic health disturbances associated with or preceded by increased body weight, particularly body fat percentage, the current established belief doctrine of causation is: energy (calories) in must exceed energy (calories) out (the 'calories in, calories out' or CICO model). The logical treatment based on this model is to eat less (reduce calories in) and do more (increase calories out). Current thinking considers obesity itself to be the cause of metabolic derangements and diseases (e.g., T2D is caused by obesity, thus weight loss will control T2D), therefore weight reduction is considered to be curative of the so-called obesity-related co-morbidities. This model fails to consider that nutrient-caloric impact is always purpose driven. Significant body fat weight gain is always preceded by disruption of insulin-glucagon anabolic-catabolic cycling with hyperinsulinaemia, then graded IR, sometimes ending with insulin failure and paradoxical hyperglucagonemia [407].

Human adaptive evolution towards higher cerebral function at the cost of less robust musculoskeletal performance capacity is reflected in evolutionary changes to nutrient substrate requirement with small intestinal elongation toward enzymatic over fermentation digestion. Shoreline evolution towards greater cerebration is evidenced by high requirements for marine fats, particularly 3- and 6-omega fatty acids [408]. Almost half of the brain's membrane phospholipid fatty acids are DHA, which together with eicosapentaenoic acid (EPA) affects membrane receptor function, as well as neurotransmitter generation and metabolism [409].

Accounting for water weight, most food is either carbohydrate-protein plant-based or protein-fat carnivore-based with a relatively similar protein base around 15%–20% [410,411]. When examining the life-patterns of animals based upon diet, vegetarian animals require 12–16 hs per day to ingest a nutrient-sparse vegetarian diet accompanied by 12 h a day of sleep with little cerebration other than instinctive behaviour. Vegetarian animals tend to be carbohydrate-insulin dominant due to slow continuous nutrient supply from grazing, with ketones coming from intestinal fermentation [412]. Pure carnivores consume massive nutrient-dense foods episodically with days between meals followed by prolonged periods of rest, often sleeping 18–20 h per day, with short bursts of intense physical activity. Glycogen stores are replenished by gluconeogenesis and carnivores are hormonally predominantly glucagon-based [413]. Human anatomic and hormonal metabolic evolution is consistent with an episodic high-fat, high-salt, protein-based diet with (starchy) carbohydrate supplementation for short periods of anabolic nutrient supply/storage. This is followed by long periods of non-consumption (fasted) catabolic store utilisation and redistribution, during which time humans are cerebrally and physically active with relatively shorter periods of rest (8 h per day). This includes complete micro- and macronutrient provision. Human hormonal homoeostatic feedback cycling further corroborates this way of eating. Healthy humans cycle through brief insulin-dominant anabolic phases of nutrient-supplying meals per day with prolonged glucagon-dominant catabolic phases where nutrient needs are met from internal stores. Glucagon, not insulin, is the dominant energy substrate-regulating hormone [414].

Healthy human nutrition involves brief periods of eating, creating a portal venous and systemic BG dominant state with hepatic and adipocyte DNL; storage of lipids in adipocytes; storage of monosaccharides as glycogen; protein, VLDL, steroid hormone and cholesterol synthesis under the anabolic influence of incretins (insulin, human growth hormone, testosterone and thyroid hormones). Between meals, under catabolic glucagon, IGF-1 (somatomedin), and cortisol dominance, non-essential fatty acids and triglyceride-cholesterol-rich LDLa are released from adipocytes as the dominant energy substrate, with hepatic glycogenolysis, protein gluconeogenesis, HDL synthesis, and ketogenesis [415]. Such diurnal cycling takes about 8 to 24 h so that healthy meal frequency is one to three meals per day [416,417]. Between meals only water for hydration is required. No adult mammalian species other than modern humans drink anything but water and only humans routinely have dilute urine indicative of overhydration.

Historically, food scarcity and insecurity dominated the human experience. Transient autumnal overeating dominated by carbohydrate-rich plants, seeds and fruits, resulted in intentional brief systemic IR, driving hepatic and adipocyte glucose to triglyceride denovo lipogenesis for fat storage, while protecting somatic cells from intracellular hyperglycaemia, similar to that seen in hibernating animals [418,419], allowing seasonal unidirectional fat weight gain, systemic tolerance of hyperglyacaemia and storage of fat for winter survival [420]. This form of transient IR results in fat weight gain without pathophysiological disturbance since it is primarily related to portal hyperglycaemia-hyperinsulinaemia with a high hepatic first pass effect for insulin. Persistent systemic hyperinsulinaemia (without glucagon cycling) maintains relative normoglycaemia, particularly since this diet is high in carbohydrate but low in fat. This is Kraft pattern 2 on oral glucose tolerance testing [421] and is historically associated with survival benefit.

However, the modern era's food environment is dominated by non-seasonal ubiquitous high-carbohydrate food availability, snacking (increased frequency of caloric consumption), binge or overeating (caloric quantity excess) in defiance of hormonal satiety feedback signals (mediated by PYY, GIP, GLP-1, CCK, Somatostatin, Apo A-IV and leptin [422]), and a shift toward chronic excessive carbohydrates, often combined with industrial hydrogenated polyunsaturated fat (PUFA) consumption. These result in disturbance to healthy human anabolic-catabolic nutritional homoeostasis, shifting the system toward higher and prolonged hyperinsulinaemia and insulin-glucose dominance, measured as continuous Kraft pattern 2, even prior to weight gain [407]. At first, humans may purposefully exchange dietary fat for dietary carbohydrates, shifting from an animal-based towards a plant-based diet, because of misguided societal lipophobia and the erroneous lipid-heart hypothesis of cardiovascular disease entrenched in the US dietary Guidelines [423].

This way of eating may have transient benefits in terms of human physical and cerebral productivity and performance [406,424], but over time, persistent Kraft pattern 2 leads to substrate surplus, systemic hyperglycaemia, weight gain and a transition from physiological enhancement toward pathophysiological inflammatory liability, negatively affecting every cell system.

Systemic hyperglycaemia causes cerebral hyperglycaemia triggering a profound instant endorphin hormonal cascade, similar to all other psychotropic drugs such as opioids, cocaine, methamphetamines, nicotine, and alcohol [425–427]. Instant massive endorphin activation produces profound emotional gratification, tranquillity and restitution, numbing, soothing, and obliterating emotional tension and stress. Instant gratification is an intermittent readily available mechanism used by all humans to manage episodic emotional tension. On a biochemical level, dopamine concentrations continuously build in the cerebrally focused brain. At a critical threshold, serotonin release triggered by an endorphin-activating substance or behaviour is required to dissipate the dopamine concentration. Every human has a set of instant serotonin-releasing behaviours that control this cyclical pattern of intense cerebral concentration [428–430]. Usually carbohydrates, not other macronutrients, trigger this endorphin response [431]. The unnatural combination of high glycaemic index carbohydrate, PUFA and salt, as seen in many manufactured foods, is the most potent trigger of such endorphin activation that can be measured in all humans [425].

Physiologically, excessive carbohydrate intake in a person that is already Kraft pattern 2 produces immediate systemic hyperglycaemia followed by a delayed hyperinsulinaemic response that causes a rapid plummet of BG concentration. This triggers intense somatic, as well as psychological hunger, so that the person develops a continuous repetitive habit of snacking for both psychological and physiologic reasons, maintaining a state of chronic hyperglycaemia-hyperinsulinaemia and progressing to a Kraft 3 pattern [432]. Snacking (eating frequently), particularly carbohydrates, prolongs the anabolic state and transforms humans from a healthy catabolic state to a predominantly anabolic state. This perpetual flooding of the intracellular cytoplasm with excessive glucose, reduces insulin membrane receptor expression, resulting in further IR and systemic hyperglycaemia, Kraft pattern 3. Such IR induces the liver and adipocytes to increase DNL resulting in significant weight gain as a protective mechanism against the inflammatory harm caused by constant hyperglycaemia. Adipocytes are equally affected by IR, reducing DNL, but the liver does not require insulin for glucose uptake. Kraft pattern 3 therefore results in hepatic steatosis, increased VLDL, increased triglyceride and cholesterol production, decreased HDL and ketone production and transfer of triglyceride-laden VLDL to adipocytes, causing obesity. Psychologically, carbohydrate snacking is similar to smoking. Nicotine or sugar are the drugs and repetitively lighting up or snacking to support fluctuating nicotine or BG concentrations are the pattern. The sole purpose of smoking is endorphin activation and dysfunctional emotion management, the hormonal driver in snacking is Kraft pattern 3 and the consequence is obesity. Obese people have insidiously transitioned from primarily eating for the nutritional value, towards eating for endorphin relief; carbohydrates being used as a psychoactive drug rather than a nutrient.

Cutting is the psychopathological practice of intentionally making small cuts on your body [433,434], triggering an intense endogenous opioid release for endorphin relief from intense psychological distress. Less dramatic forms of this habit such as nail-biting and self-pinching become increasingly frequent and routine over time. Similarly, overeating, and rapid binge eating substantially beyond satiety-hormonal-signalling, triggers a painful visceral response of gastric distention, queasiness, pain, and discomfort that has a bizarre sense of psychological comfort on the back end. Humans have become increasingly pre-emptive in deciding much is needed per meal, with a bizarre fear of undereating. Our portion sizes and frequency of eating have grown significantly since the 1970s [435,436], overriding any hormonal satiety feedback, resulting in an endorphin-releasing discomfort that has become foundational to our emotive management system. Overeating is further reinforced by caloric nutritional formulas that seldom consider the purpose of each meal in the context of the individual and foster fears of nutritional deficit. Similar to cutting, humans have habituated towards overeating by volume, further disrupting anabolic-catabolic homoeostasis prolonging the insulinergic response, and thereby driving obesity [437].

As nutrient-caloric impact is always purpose driven, under modern conditions of ubiquitous abundance and availability, the purpose of eating has transitioned away from episodic nutrient supply, toward continuous endorphin release and emotion management involving carbohydrates, snacking and binge overeating. All modern humans USE eating for endorphin relief on occasion. Most humans abuse endorphin-eating occasionally, as part of a comprehensive diverse emotion-management system. However, more and more humans are being raised with a comprehensive deficiency of effective emotion-management strategies and decaying mental health strategies, creating increased vulnerability to instant gratification addictive behaviour that tends to enlist the most readily available endorphin-activating substances and dysfunctional behaviours – currently carbohydrate-dominant processed foods driven by lipophobia and a societal push back towards plant-based eating [438]. With the enormous instant gratification from carbohydrates (which can act like a psychoactive drug) being so readily available, there is little need to expand the diversity of emotion-management strategies. This results in chronic excessive carbohydrate snacking to the point of physiological harm and psychosomatic dependence via IR. This in turn requires distortion of the reality of such harm to justify and allow ongoing beneficial use of the relationship with carbohydrates to the point of addiction defined by the inability to control the relationship despite tangible harm namely, obesity, IR/diabetes, metabolic syndrome, and psychopathology (see Section 11.3.2). Thus, CECC, snacking and binge overeating for the purpose of psychological restitution from emotional tension causes IR and results in obesity, T2D and metabolic derangement.

3.8.3 Managing the patient

3.8.3.1 Aims of care

The aim of care in body weight management is generally to achieve a normal body weight, indicated by a normal BMI. However, as already established body fat percentage, as well as metabolic health, measured by blood laboratory parameters, are often far more valuable indicators of metabolic health and the risk of disease. As such basing patient goals on these parameters is superior to BMI.

Dietary intervention, in combination with physical activity, is generally accepted as the first line intervention for controlling body weight, based on the calorie-in, calorie-out model. Medications and surgery are usually only considered when diet and exercise have failed, in the context of morbid obesity or comorbidities.

While almost all calorie-reductive diets reduce weight, when used as an exclusive strategy, only approximately 25% of participants across a range of diet types sustain meaningful adherence [439]. Even bariatric surgery, the most calorie-restrictive approach to weight loss after intentional extended fasting [398], has up to 59% weight regain [440]. Intentional caloric reduction, changing what we eat, transiently results in weight loss and improvement of most metabolic pathophysiology. Caloric reduction is necessary for weight loss, but may not restore insulin sensitivity. By definition, obesity is always preceded and dominated by IR, and exclusively, carbohydrate reduction restores insulin sensitivity. However, no caloric reduction diet via substrate elimination or global reduction, treats the underlying root cause of why the person became obese. Effective treatment of obesity for sustainable remission requires changing what, who and why we eat: an addiction approach as opposed to a diet approach [441].

3.8.3.2 Pharmacotherapy and surgery

Any form of caloric reduction induces transient weight loss. Innumerable calorie-reductive weight loss programmes exist that often employ a variety of drugs, devices, injections, supplements, shakes, shots, potions, powders [442] that all have very plausible stories using pseudoscience or scientific manipulation to sell their benefits, but there is no outsourcing or substitute for the slow, steady hard work required to initiate and maintain lifestyle change. Appetite suppressing and IR-inducing medications, supplements, psychotropic medications, weight loss surgery, and devices may be useful aids along the journey towards metabolic and emotion management health, but are not surrogates or alternatives.

Metabolic change requires treating restoration of insulin sensitivity and the paradoxical hyperglucagonaemia that co-exists with hyperinsulinaemia in Kraft pattern 3, by lowering BG using ketogenic or VLCHF diet (<30 g carbohydrate per day total non-vegetable carbohydrates) higher fat diet, with long periods of eating abstinence. Pharmacologically reducing gluconeogenesis and glycogenolysis with the biguanide metformin, assists in lowering BG and restoring insulin sensitivity. Newer insulinergic medications such as GLP-1 agonists [443] and dipeptidyl peptidase 4 inhibitors or glipins [444] that block the enzyme that breaks down GLP-1, increase early insulin release and block glucagon release, while profoundly reducing appetite. These work effectively to restore insulin sensitivity, reduce caloric intake and increase weight loss.

While some anti-depressants may induce weight gain, many psychotropic medications such as antidepressants of various classes, as well as medications that treat attention deficit hyperactivity disorder (ADHD) are also effective as appetite suppressants since they regulate the endorphin response mechanism [445,446].

Capitalising on such anorectic neuromodulatory effects, specific drugs and drug combinations have been developed to aid weight loss directly. However, since the fenfluramine/phentermine (Fen-Phen) cardiopulmonary disaster [447], that class of specific appetite suppression medications has been so dose-restricted to be of little sustainable effective weight loss value. This is despite multibillion dollar marketing campaigns and the medication being widely prescribed by practitioners, in conjunction with calorie-restrictive weight loss methodology, for many years to reduce weight, with early success and common relapse, while having high risk profiles precluding adequate dosing or long-term use [448]. This class of medications is best avoided since it inhibits root cause cognitive behavioural therapy (CBT) and often triggers psychopathology when patients regain their weight.

The single most effective weight loss intervention is bariatric surgery [449]. There is an extended history of procedural interventions involving three principles:

1. reduction in gastric volume: 'quantity restriction' devices and surgeries, such as intragastric balloons and space-occupying pills, fixed and adjustable gastric band devices, gastric reductive surgeries such as sleeve gastrectomy
2. malabsorptive products such as intestinal tubes and procedures like Roux-en-Y gastric bypass, duodenal switch [450]
3. neuromodulatory devices and implants such as gastric pacemakers, vagal stimulators, intracerebral probes [451].

It is beyond the scope of this chapter to discuss outsourcing of weight loss methodology. However, the degree of excess BMI, the age of the patient and the severity of comorbid disease should be considered in the use of effective adjunctive therapies, pharmacological or surgical, and none should be excluded because of the bias of the practitioner or because the method has a high rate of recidivism. The emphasis of sustainable treatment is cognitive-behavioural transformation addressing the reason the patient gained the weight. The backbone of therapy should be TCR, with consideration of any and all forms of adjunctive weight loss interventions as needed towards sustainable lifestyle change (see Section 11.1).

3.8.3.3 Lifestyle-related considerations

Obesity is a lifestyle, a pattern of living that has to fundamentally change in order to be sustained. Diets use a deprivation approach that requires strict control. By definition, addiction defies control capacity and the method should be empowering, non-mathematical but binary, focusing on nutrient-based eating, and effort-based emotion management. The principles of addiction management require breaking habits and relationships that are harmful and replacing them with new habits and relationships that are beneficial without causing harm. Harmful habits/relationships cannot be broken if you are still engaged, and healthy habits/relationships cannot be developed if you do not engage with them every day [452].

3.8.3.4 Diet: Guiding the patient

3.8.3.4.1 Stage 1

What you eat includes anything that is not a carbohydrate with one exception. All animal products are fine to eat, the broader the range the better, focusing on micronutrients (the macronutrients will always be adequate). Dairy is an acceptable choice. All vegetables are carbohydrates. Because addiction considers the addict's relationship with the drug rather than demonising the drug, all vegetables are fine to eat, even starchy vegetables like pulses and squashes. There are three absolute exceptions: no rice, no potatoes, and no grain products of any kind. No fruit including berries, avocados excepted. Starchy (carbohydrate-rich) food substitutes should be avoided. It is irrelevant if a manufactured food sports the word 'keto.' Ice cream is ice cream with an exclusive endorphin rationale no matter what it is made of. Ideally, all meals should be fortified with some soluble fat to trigger an early hormonal satiety response. Salt should also be added as a hygroscopic replacement for hydrophilic glucose.

All fluids should be calorie-free, but artificial sweeteners are allowed as long as they don't trigger the addiction. Developing a relationship with a sugar-free fluid has enormous snack-replacement value: Instead of a cigarette, a recovering smoker may use gum. Instead of a snack, a carbohydrate-addict may use a sugar-free 'bridge' drink, which is readily available at a mind-cleansing moment and coincidentally also provides hydration.

Changing how one eats requires consistent pre-emptive meal planning to restore hormonal cycling. Planning a maximum of two meals a day in a 6–8 h window is ideal (Intermittent Fasting) (see Chapter 10). When you eat is irrelevant and personal, but should be relatively consistent. Breakfast is usually the least important meal of the day and there is no metabolic reason not to eat just before bedtime [453]. Intermittent daily fasting is essential, but extended fasts beyond 36 h may be of value early in recovery of insulin sensitivity but are not necessary [398]. No snacking, even if it involves non-carbohydrate calories. A calorie-containing snack is always an emotional event, a 'bridge' drink is a non-calorie-containing snack.

Meals should be an exclusive event, sitting at a table with a plate of food and eating utensils. The default option is to skip that meal. Eating sequentially treats overeating and binge eating. Start with an empty plate with food in serving dishes that can go back to storage if unfinished. Start with a small amount. It is then a conscious decision to dish up more based on satiety. This is eating sequentially until beginning to feel full, as opposed to starting with a loaded plate and deciding when to stop (which usually results in overeating). After a meal, replace a carbohydrate-laden dessert with an emotional relaxation activity.

A dietitian has value in guiding patients back toward a nutritional LCHF pattern of eating. However, specific unnatural mathematical formulae of micro- and macro- nutrient consumption, the cornerstone of most dietary recommendations and programs, should be avoided. It is far more important to entrench and reinforce the dietary and nutritional concepts outlined above. Dietary prescription rigidity usually leads to failure and relapse because it is focused on weight loss rather than eating behavioural change. The emotion management toolkit of most obese people is stocked with carbohydrates, snacks, and emotional and psychological issues that need to be worked through. Dietary failure almost always involves sudden, unexpected emotional events that trigger the carbohydrate-addict to relapse back to an emotive way of eating, validated by the stress-inducing event. Addiction is managed according to permission. 'Cheating' is always a sophisticated way of granting permission to relapse for emotional restitution.

3.8.3.4.2 Stage 2

In parallel to treating carbohydrate addiction, replacing carbohydrates and snacking with effort-based emotion management strategies is essential to sustain change and treat the reason behind the person eating to the point of obesity and comorbid disease, and continuing to do so. Guiding a patient using a staged cognitive behavioural therapy (CBT) approach is far more sustainable over time than any dietary approach. A therapist, coach, or counsellor trained in addiction methodology (and familiar with diet) is of far greater value for long-term sustainability than dietary management based on the calorie-in-calorie-out model. Changing for good [452] requires stepwise transition through stages of contemplative ownership of the broken relationship with carbohydrates and eating as an emotion management system followed by a stage of planning and preparing mentally and environmentally to initiate change prior to initiating change itself.

3.8.3.4.3 Stage 3

Stage three involves active engagement in a stepwise removal and breaking of addictive eating patterns and behaviours, replacing them with a nutritional pattern of eating while habituating to effort-based emotion management strategies for mental well-being. Encourage consciously forcing the establishment of daily self-care routines until those new behaviours become subconscious daily go-to habits. This requires time, repetition, and routine. The pillars of healthy effort-based, as opposed to short-lived instant gratification, habits include physical activity, creative arts, spirituality and meditation, empathetic human connection, and safe sexuality. Such behaviours take effort and time to perform and establish as routines, but allow unconditional self-affirmation that restores the self-esteem, self-confidence and self-respect, absent in addicts. They act as a healthy emotional replacement for the 'high' from carbohydrates used as an emotional drug. A healthy, diverse, effort-based emotion management system, with a return to nutritional eating and restoration of insulin sensitivity is the most effective way to lose excess body weight and restore healthy hormonal anabolic-catabolic homoeostasis, free of metabolic disease.

3.8.3.4.4 Stage 4

Once the pattern is changed, relapses are inevitable. Stage four defines strategies that recognise and treat relapses. This stage is essential if the behavioural change, restoration of insulin sensitivity and weight loss is to become a lifelong journey with milestones but no endpoints. Ownership of the relapse, Analysis of how and why it occurred, and development of a Corrective action plan for future similar situations (OAC) is part of a process of changing for good.

3.8.3.5 Monitoring

Weight loss monitoring is vital to evaluation and affirmation of methodology, as well as consideration toward additional intervention strategies. The scale, a direct measure of body weight, is the most commonly used monitoring device and has both asset and liability value. Weight loss is not linear but the scale creates expectations of immediate cause and effect that are not biological, may be psychologically destructive, and may lead to abandonment of the weight loss methodology. Periodic use of the scale to monitor long term weight loss is appropriate, but daily use should be discouraged [454]. Body composition monitoring such as impedance and DEXA scans may be useful as motivational tools, but have limited monitoring value [455]. The most overlooked yet psychologically valuable weight loss monitoring strategies involve the mirror, tape measure and a notebook record of daily dietary and selfcare performance.

Biofeedback devices are the most effective immediate forms of behavioural change that directly address IR and indirectly address weight loss. Monitoring BG and ketone concentrations by fingerstick or using continuous glucose monitoring (CGM) devices transform the educated patient's selection of food, quantity and frequency [456]. Smart devices that track biometrics may have value in disease states, particularly cardiovascular, but are usually a psychological liability in weight loss. The number of steps you take is far less important than going for a walk.

Metabolic blood work is the most beneficial method of engaging patients and ensuring healthy and enduring change. However, it is most commonly misused by practitioners for therapeutic medication prescription. While medications and supplements may be transiently necessary, the primary value of bloodwork is for 'metabolic storytelling' and tracking the transformation of IR to insulin sensitivity while avoiding 'insulin suppression' when KDs are taken too far.

Regular ongoing support that offers empathetic human connection through social media and telehealth groups, a therapist or group therapy, or a ketogenic clinical practice is invaluable in the sustainability of change. Relapses are inevitable and support groups assist in ownership and getting back on track. Support groups are also invaluable in monitoring for psychopathology and 'drug transfer,' where patients may become depressed or transfer to a different but equally toxic instant gratification drug or methodology.

3.8.4 Summary

Current established treatment doctrine for overweight is a structured but transient consumed calorie reduction program of intentional energy deficit via some theoretical mathematical calorie-reduction formula or food group elimination diet and forced increased caloric utilisation: diet and exercise. There may also be the use of 'energy-burning,' 'metabolism stimulating' medications, appetite suppression medications or calorie-restrictive or calorie-malabsorbtion devices or surgeries. This strategy works. Nearly everyone who engages in intentional caloric reduction transiently loses weight and transiently improves obesity-related comorbidities but it is impossible to sustain such caloric deficit. For people who have gained less than 7 or 8 kg in excess fat without measurable metabolic harm, this minor weight gain does not represent a lifestyle shift and any form of intentional caloric reduction works well. For those who can, sustaining a balanced diet is an appropriate intervention.

However, for people with greater than 20–25 kilograms in excess fat weight, typically with biochemical evidence of early metabolic derangement, 'balanced' diet methodology is a failed dogma that may result in transient weight loss, but fails to keep the weight off and the comorbidities in remission about 98% of the time, because intentional caloric reduction cannot be sustained lifelong.

The current calorie-reductive diet paradigm is flawed in that obesity is not the problem. Caloric reduction strategies address what you are eating to lose weight, they do not address why you gained the weight in the first place. Excess body weight and obesity are the result of the problem. Obesity is not causal to metabolic comorbidities for the most part. It is itself a comorbidity. Treating a consequence without understanding or treating the cause always results in failure, unless the patient vicariously also treats the cause.

Pathological body fat increase is the result of a metabolic change from insulin sensitivity to IR. IR is the driver of metabolic derangement of all types and is exclusively caused by CECC and snacking despite multiple contributing and confounding factors. In the modern era, the combination of ubiquitous availability of abundant processed high carbohydrate foods driven by societal lipophobia, coupled with an increasingly dysfunctional requirement for emotional management, transitions humans from eating for primary nutritional repletion toward eating for primary emotional restitution. The root cause is a comprehensive deficiency of effective effort-based emotion management strategies. The consequence is IR, weight gain, and metabolic comorbidity. Weight loss, restoration of metabolic and emotional well-being, is a journey measured in milestones without ever having goals of completion. The restorative process only ends after death. Healthy metabolic longevity is more about the prevention of harm than about achieving some unattainably high health status. Contentment, compassion, and humble self-approval are far more important than metabolic perfection. Understanding that nutrient impact is always purpose-driven, being attuned to the body's nutritional metabolic needs, separately and distinctly from the mind's emotional needs, is the best life any human can live.

3.9 Thyroid health and insulin resistance

Hassina Kajee

3.9.1 Introduction

The thyroid gland is one of the key regulators of metabolism. Thyroid hormones (TH) play an important role in regulating glucose and lipid metabolism, blood pressure as well as energy consumption. Evidence based medicine links the clinical conditions of hypothyroidism and subclinical hypothyroidism with an increased risk of MetS [457,458]. Studies also show that people with thyroid stimulating hormone (TSH) concentrations at the upper limit of the normal range (2.5–4.5 mU/L), have higher rates of obesity, raised triglyceride (TG) concentrations, and are at a higher risk of MetS [459]. Obesity has been shown to affect thyroid function and is associated with an increased risk of hypothyroidism [460]. There is also an increasing body of evidence demonstrating that thyroid dysfunction has an impact on the various metabolic parameters associated with MetS and may lead to the development or aggravation of MetS.

With rising rates of thyroid disease (including autoimmune thyroid disease (AITD), cancer, and thyroid diseases of childhood), and an equally alarming rise in obesity in all age groups, it is not surprising that evidence links obesity with thyroid disease. It is well known that thyroid disease can negatively impact weight, and if obesity worsens thyroid disease in turn, we need to pay even closer attention to the factors that cause weight gain in order to stem the tide and hopefully reverse the double burden of obesity and thyroid disease.

3.9.1.1 Epidemiology

The prevalence of thyroid diseases varies based on iodine nutrition [461]. Approximately one third of the global population reside in areas of iodine deficiency [462]. In these areas, where daily intake is generally below 50 μg, goitre is endemic. Populations at risk generally reside in remote and mountainous regions in South-East Asia, Latin America, and Central Africa. In these cases, iodisation programs are successful in reducing and preventing goitre. However, even within endemic regions goitre rates vary, emphasising the equal importance of environmental goitrogens and antithyroid agents in food and water [463].

In iodine replete areas, AITD is the predominant form of thyroid disease ranging from Hashimoto's thyroid disease to Graves disease and primary atrophic hypothyroidism. Globally, the annual incidence of Hashimoto's thyroiditis is estimated to be 0.8 and 3.5 cases per 1000 persons and Graves' disease (GD), 0.1 and 0.4 per 1000 persons in men and women respectively [464]. Women, aged 30–50, seem to be at a higher risk of AITD with a risk of 10:1 female to male [461].

3.9.1.2 *Thyroid hormone physiology*

THs are essential for cellular development and differentiation and act on nearly every cell in the human body (Fig. 3.20). THs increase basal metabolic rate (BMR) leading to heat generation. They regulate protein, fat, and carbohydrate metabolism and have an effect on protein synthesis. They play a role in bone growth and skeletal development and promote brain development and have chronotropic effects in the cardiac muscle by increasing the number and affinity of beta adrenergic receptors and inotropic effects by enhancing the response to catecholamines [465].

The thyroid gland is a ductless, butterfly-shaped structure located in the anterior neck. Its main role, via the thyroid follicular cells, is the synthesis and secretion of TH, as well as iodine homoeostasis in the body. In between the follicular cells are the parafollicular cells of the thyroid. These cells are responsible for calcium homoeostasis in the body [466].

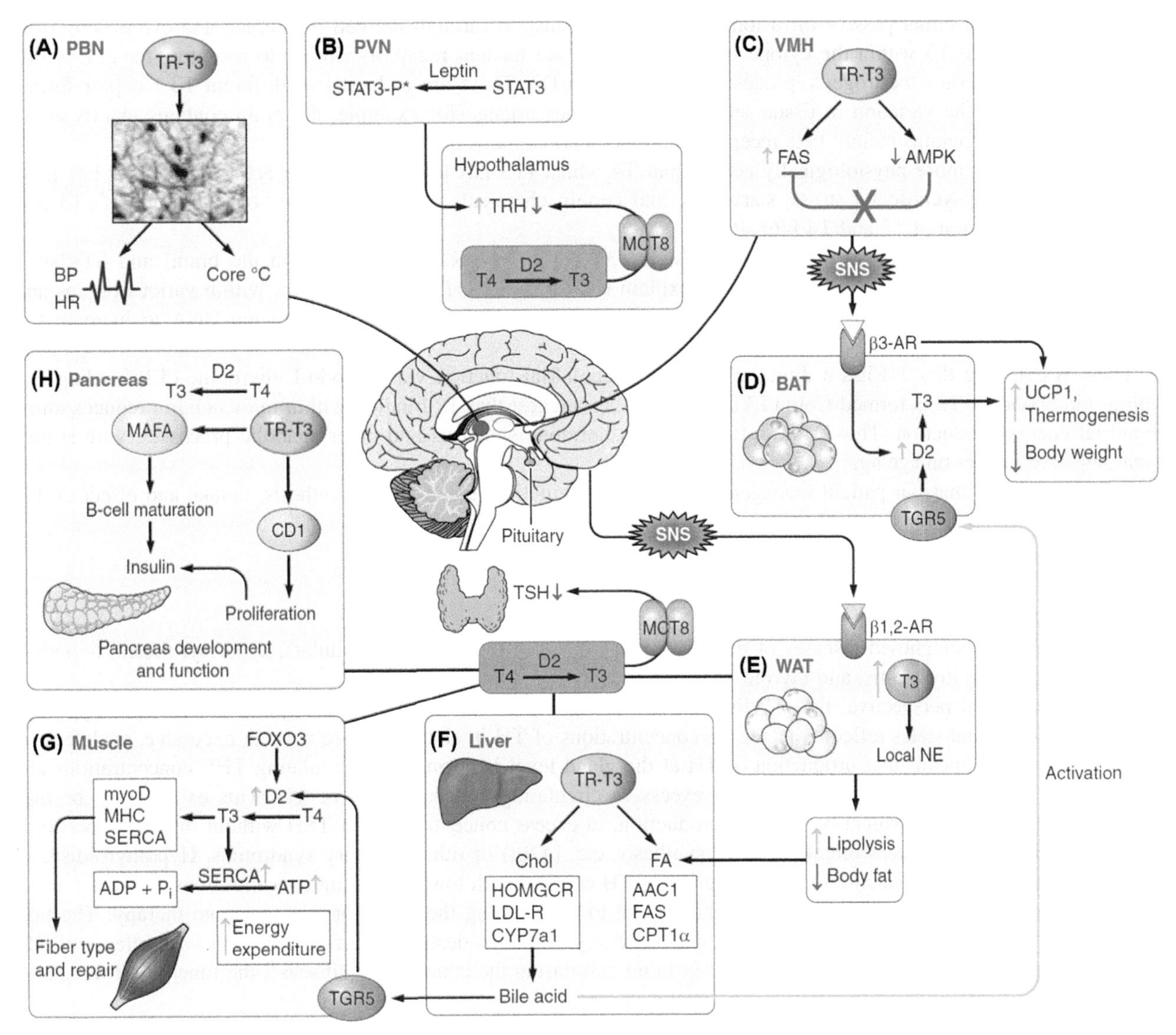

FIGURE 3.20 **Thyroid regulation of metabolism.** The thyroid hormones T3 and T4 have a near global hormonal impact, stimulating a variety of physiological processes, and its homoeostatic balance is thus important [465].

When iodine is first ingested in food, it is converted to iodide and then taken up by the thyroid gland where the follicular cells transport the iodine through an iodine pump into the colloid of the thyroid gland. This active transport process is known as 'iodine trapping' and stimulated by TSH.

The thyroid follicles consist of colloid, a proteinaceous material composed mainly of thyroglobulin.

Thyroglobulin is the precursor of all TH. On entering the colloid, iodine is rapidly bound to tyrosine molecules attached to thyroglobulin, forming monoiodotyrosine (MIT), which is further iodinated to form diiodotyrosine (DIT). Two DIT condense to form thyroxine (T4). A small amount of T3 is formed as well as a small amount of reverse T3 (rT3). The normal thyroid has on average a distribution of 23% MIT, 33% DIT, 35% T4, 7% T3, and 2% rT3. Inactive thyroxin or T4 is a prohormone of triiodothyronine, T3 [466].

Secretion of T4 (and to a lesser extent T3) is dependent upon stimulation of the thyroid gland by TSH, which is produced by the pituitary gland. The pituitary gland is in turn regulated by thyrotropin releasing hormone (TRH) which is secreted by the hypothalamus in a negative feedback loop that is dependent on serum concentrations of TH.

The thyroid gland secretes 90% of its hormones in the inactive form, T4, which can be deiodinated by deiodinase enzymes in the peripheral tissues (primarily the liver). The process of deiodination can occur via either a type 1 or type 2 deiodinase, resulting in the active T3, or via a type 3 deiodinase resulting in rT3 [467]. Of clinical importance is that type 1 deiodinase is a selenoenzyme, hence requiring adequate selenium for its activity. Selenium deficiency has been shown to be associated with impaired functionality of TH deiodinases.

TH enter cells by either passive diffusion or by specific transport through the cell membrane and cytoplasm. Most of T4 is converted to T3 within the cytoplasm. TH receptors are nuclear receptors similar to receptors for glucocorticoids, mineralocorticoids, oestrogens, progestins, and vitamin D3. There are at least two different T3 receptor forms, which may explain the variation in tissue sensitivity by various organs (for example, the brain contains mainly alpha receptors, the liver contains mainly beta receptors, and the heart contains both) [466].

T3 is four times more physiologically active than T4 whilst rT3 has less than 1% the activity of T4. It has been shown that illness, psychosocial stress, starvation, and certain chemicals can increase the concentrations of rT3 and decreased concentration of T3 and T4 [468,469].

T3 binding may occur via two different types of T3 receptors, hTRalpha1 (mainly in the brain) and hTRbeta2 (mainly found in the liver). These receptor types explain the variation in TH responsiveness within various organs and tissues. T3 must first bind to its receptor and then the T3-receptor complex must bind to the DNA to increase the expression of specific genes [466].

There is evidence that TH has a direct effect on mitochondrial function via a diiodo-L-thyronine (T2) binding site within mitochondria. T2 is formed from rT3 and T3. Studies suggest that T2 binding within mitochondria reduces mitochondrial energy production. This in turn affects growth hormone synthesis and other anabolic processes, with subsequent negative impact on ageing.

It is thus critical that our patient management promotes regulation, metabolism, synthesis, uptake and effect of TH at a cellular level, as well as optimal ratios of T4, T3, rT3, and T2 (Table 3.7).

3.9.1.3 Clinical presentation and classification of thyroid disease

The most commonly diagnosed diseases of the thyroid gland are goitre (diffuse or nodular), hyperthyroidism, hypothyroidism, autoimmune thyroiditis, and thyroid neoplasm.

From a functional perspective, thyroid diseases can be classified into euthyroidism, hyperthyroidism and hypothyroidism. These clinical states reflect whether the concentrations of TH in circulation are normal, excessive, or defective [470]. Euthyroidism means that production of TH at the gland level is normal and circulating THE concentrations are normal. Hyperthyroidism means that there are excessive circulating concentrations of TH. This excess may be due either to thyroid gland hyperfunction and overproduction, to excess concentrations of TSH without thyroid hyperfunction (i.e., excess intake, excess release without synthesis, etc. [470]) or other pituitary syndromes. Hypothyroidism is almost always due to hypo-functioning and secretion of TH coupled with low circulating concentrations of TH.

The type of thyroid gland dysfunction is fundamental to determining the basis for diagnosis and therapy. The primary biosynthetic problem of the thyroid gland may vary (e.g., immune destruction of thyroid cells with release of TH or iatrogenic causes). It is also important to bear in mind that during the course of the disease, the function of the gland may change.

The pathophysiology of the different forms of thyroid disease may vary widely and will be reflected in the management of the different forms of disease.

TABLE 3.7 Sites of thyroid hormone action in metabolic regulation.

Process	Elements That regulate metabolism	Basic mechanisms	Examples of physiological actions	References
Thyroid hormone action	TR isoforms Corepressor action (NcoR and SMRT) Nutrient feedback Nongenomic action Tissue-selective thyroid hormone transport	TR isoform specificity Histone modification Sumoylation Corepressor interactions Modulation of signal Transduction pathways Stimulation of Na −K+ -ATPase and SERCA1	Increased basal metabolic rate (BMR) Stimulate lipolysis/ lipogenesis Increase in adaptive thermogenesis Stimulate β-oxidation of fatty acids	27, 39, 159, 232
Central regulation of TRH/TSH	T4/T3 Feedback Leptin AMPK activation Oxrexigenic / anorectic peptides / appetite regulation Thyronamines (T1AM) Circadian rhythms	Integration of TRH/TSH regulation with metabolic signals Thyroid hormone transport into the hypothalamus and pituitary (e.g., by MCTB) Integration of adrenergic signalling	TSH measurement for the diagnosis of thyroid disease And to monitor treatment Central adaptation to fasting, illness and obesity	117, 163
Local ligand activation by D2	D2 expression and activity D2 polymorphisms Selenium requirement for deiodinase activity	Regulation of D2 ubiquitination /deubiquitination Increase in D2 activity with reduction in serum T4 concentration Developmental and tissue selective deiodinase expression	TSH/T4 set point T4/T3 replacement therapy of hypothyroidism Stimulates adaptive thermogenesis	90, 149
Thermogenesis and body weight	Basal metabolic rate Adaptive thermogenesis Body weight and body composition Appetite	Integration of adrenergic signalling Central and local adrenergic actions Stimulation of CP1a expression Stimulation of UP1 expression	Reduces body fat Increases β-oxidation of fatty acids Stimulates adaptive thermogenesis	229

(Continued)

TABLE 3.7 (Continued)

Process	Elements That regulate metabolism	Basic mechanisms	Examples of physiological actions	References
Cholesterol and triglycerides	Cholesterol synthesis Reverse cholesterol transport Lipolysis/ lipogenesis Hepatic steatosis	Stimulates LDL-R Stimulates ABCA 1	Reduces serum cholesterol Reduces serum triglycerides Reduces hepatic steatosis	145, 157, 270
Carbohydrate metabolism	Pancreatic islet development Pancreatic islet proliferation Insulin production Gluconeogenesis Insulin sensitivity Insulin metabolism	TR expression in developing islets D2 required for developing islets and islet function Insulin signalling Stimulation of mitochondrial respiration Increase in expression of ChREBP, GLUT4, ACC1	Stimulates gluconeogenesis Reduces insulin sensitivity Increase insulin metabolism	49

Abbreviations: ABCA1, ATP-binding cassette transporter AT; ACC1, acetyl CoA carboxylase; ChREBP. Carbohydrate response element binding protein; CPT-Ia, carnitine palmitoyltransferase Ia; CYP7A1, cholesterol 7-hydroxylase; D2, 5′-deiodinase type 2; GLUT4, glucose transporter 4; LDL-R, low-density lipoprotein receptor; LXR, liver X receptor; NcoR, nuclear corepressor; PPARa, peroxisome proliferator-activated receptor; RXR, retinoid X receptor; SERCA, sarcoplasmic reticulum calcium ATPase, SMRT, silencing mediator for retinoic and thyroid hormone receptor; T3, triiodothyronine; T4 thyroxine; TGR5. G-Protein-coupled receptor bile acid receptor; TRH, thyrotropin-releasing hormone; TSH, thyroid-stimulating hormone; UCP. Uncoupling protein.

The entire hypothalamic-pituitary-thyroid (HPT) axis and the feedback mechanisms determine whether the condition is at a subclinical or clinical level. Patent symptomatology, a good relationship with the patient, and history taking are key to determining the diagnosis. A review by Monaco gives a more thorough functional classification (see Table 3.8) [470].

3.9.1.3.1 Autoimmune thyroid disease

The most common AITDs include Grave's disease and Hashimoto's thyroiditis, as well as non-endemic goitre [461]. AITDs are polygenic and result from complex interactions between environmental and genetic factors in a genetically susceptible individual. Iodine, certain medications, infection, smoking, and stress are some of the well-described environmental triggers for the development of AITD [471,472].

Alarming data suggest that up to 40% of healthy women have lymphocytic infiltration of the thyroid gland, and there is a prevalence of 10% of anti-thyroglobulin antibody (TgAb). Thyroid peroxidase (TPOAb) antibodies are detectable in 12% of the general population. In some, a suggestive ultrasound pattern of AITD may precede anti-TPOAb positivity but in 20% of cases, ultrasound evidence of disease is present without evidence of thyroid autoantibodies [473]. TPOAb, in the case of hypo functioning of the thyroid gland, are usually due to anti-thyroid antibodies that impair TH metabolism and sensitivity.

3.9.1.3.2 Thyroid hormone resistance

Resistance to TH can occur at multiple points and is referred to as thyroid resistance. Resistance may be due to genetic polymorphisms of the thyroid receptor [474,475]. Variation may also occur due to polymorphisms in deiodinase enzymes [476,477]. It is important to recognise the existence of polymorphisms in order to improve our management of

TABLE 3.8 Functional classification of thyroid diseases.

I. Diseases characterised by (tissue) euthyroidism
  A. Euthyroid goiter
    1. Diffuse (chronic)
    2. Nodular (chronic)
    3. Diffuse (transient)
  B. Tumours
    1. Benign (single nodule)
    2. Malignant
      a. Differentiated (papillary and follicular)
      b. Undifferentiated (anaplastic)
      c. Medullary
  C. Thyroiditis
    1. Acute thyroiditis
    2. Subacute thyroiditis (De Quervain's) (in the euthyroid phase: polar disease)
    3. Chronic autoimmune thyroiditis or Hashimoto's disease (in the euthyroid phase: polar disease)
    4. Postpartum and silent thyroiditis (in the euthyroid phase: polar disease)
    5. Riedel's thyroiditis
II. Diseases characterised by (tissue) hyperthyroidism
  A. With thyroid gland hyperfunction
    1. Hyperthyroid goitre with thyroid-associated ophthalmopathy or Basedow-Graves' disease
    2. Multinodular hyperthyroid goitre or Plummer's disease
    3. Autonomous nodule (hyperthyroid)
    4. Rare forms: excessive exogenous iodine, hyperthyroidism due to Hashimoto's disease (Hashitoxicosis), postpartum thyroiditis (in the hyperthyroid phase), pituitary resistance to thyroid hormones, TSH-secreting pituitary adenoma, chorionic gonadotropin-secreting tumour, adenoma, or carcinoma (follicular) of the thyroid
  B. Thyrotoxicosis (without thyroid gland hyperfunction)
    1. Excessive, exogenous thyroid hormones (thyrotoxicosis actitial and iatrogenic)
    2. Post-inflammatory or from destruction of the thyroid
    3. Amiodarone-induced
  C. Transient hyperthyroidism
III. Diseases characterised by (tissue) hypothyroidism
  A. With thyroid gland hypofunction
    1. Primary hypothyroidism
      a. Adult (iatrogenic surgery, ^{131}I therapy, external radiotherapy), chronic autoimmune thyroiditis (in the hypothyroid phase), Graves' disease (end-stage), diffuse and nodular goitre, iodine deficiency
      b. Neonatal congenital (ectopia, agenesis, dyshormonogenesis)
    2. Secondary: hypothalamic-pituitary hypothyroidism (or central)
    3. Dyshormonogenetic congenital goitre
  B. Without hypothyroidism
    1. Generalised and peripheral resistance to thyroid hormones (receptor and post-receptor defects)
  C. Transient hypothyroidism
IV. Thyroid-associated ophthalmopathy
V. Abnormal thyroid parameters without thyroid diseases (nonthyroidal illness, deficit of TBG, etc.)

From F. Monaco, Classification of thyroid diseases: suggestions for a revision. *J Clin Endocrinol Metabol*, 88 (4), (2003), 1428–1432.

the various ways in which thyroid diseases present. In many instances, resistance may be seen as 'euthyroid sick syndrome' where the patient presents with symptoms of thyroid dysfunction but serum concentrations of hormones are mildly abnormal or even all within normal parameters.

3.9.1.3.3 Subclinical hypothyroidism

A wide range of clinical illnesses may have subclinical hypothyroidism as an underlying abnormality including cardiovascular disease, depression, memory and cognitive disorders, sleep disorders especially obstructive sleep apnoea, and musculoskeletal disorders [478–483]. Since thyroid dysfunctions are closely associated with secondary metabolic dysfunction and share similar exacerbating factors with IR, such as chronic stress and chronic inflammation which worsen and drive each other, it is important to consider this as an underlying issue where suggestive. Reports indicate that thyroxine replacement therapy in symptomatic patients may be of benefit [484,485].

3.9.2 Pathophysiological links between thyroid dysfunction and conditions related to insulin resistance

3.9.2.1 Metabolic syndrome and thyroid diseases

As TH are known to have multiple effects on glucose and lipid metabolism, as well as blood pressure and energy regulation, it should come as no surprise that hypothyroidism and subclinical hypothyroidism are associated with an increased risk of MetS [457–459]. The risk is higher in women than men, particularly in postmenopausal women. Early surveillance is critical [486]. Data indicate that TH are related with the majority of MetS parameters and that the correlation is stronger with T3 and TSH.

3.9.2.2 Insulin resistance, glycaemia, and diabetes as a normal consequence of thyroid disease

Thyroid function and glycaemic control appear to be interrelated. The increased prevalence of AITD in T1D is well described [487] and both autoimmune diseases have a similar genetic susceptibility. Some associations between T2D and thyroid dysfunction have also been noted, but without consistency. In one study, 30% of participants with poorly controlled T2D had abnormal TSH concentrations which, for the most part, once corrected, were associated with improved glycaemic control [488]. Conversely, thyrotoxicosis has also been associated with hyperglycaemia (explained below) [489].

TH exert different actions on different tissues [490]. While in the muscle TH function as insulin agonists, they perform an opposite action as insulin antagonists in the liver. It is hypothesised that abnormal TH concentrations result in simultaneously increased glucose output, glycogenolysis, and hepatic IR [490]. TH have a wide range of genomic and non-genomic actions across liver, skeletal muscle, WAT, and pancreas that has effects on glucose concentrations, as well as insulin sensitivity. Indeed, the effect of TH to reduce mitochondrial activity has been linked to T2M. TH also induce hypoxia-inducible factor-1 alpha (HIF-1α), thereby stimulating target genes GLUT1, phosphofructokinase (PFKP) and monocarboxylate transporter 4 (MCT4). These genes control glucose uptake, glycolysis and lactate transport and are key in cellular glucose metabolism.

At physiological concentrations and in the hyperthyroid state, T3 stimulates gluconeogenesis. This is due to T3's actions in the liver where it stimulates genes that regulate glycogenolysis and gluconeogenesis, particularly phosphoenolpyruvate carboxykinase (PEPCK), which is a rate-regulating enzyme for gluconeogenesis. The rate of peripheral uptake is then also adjusted when TH stimulates GLUT-4 mRNA in skeletal muscle to maintain euglycemia. The opposite holds true for hypothyroidism where gluconeogenesis is reduced.

T3 also plays a role in the maturation of insulin-secreting islet cells in the pancreas and high TH concentrations can impair islet function, resulting in reduced insulin release despite higher glucose concentrations. However at physiological T3 concentrations, islet cell integrity is maintained.

As alluded to above, a paradox in glucose homoeostasis is seen in severely thyrotoxic patients. This is because, in thyrotoxic states, there is a profound effect on endogenous glucose production, as well as hyperglucagonaemia, by mechanisms described above. At the same time, there is reduced plasma insulin as well as enhanced insulin clearance [465]. Thyronamines (physiologically occurring TH analogues) may play a role, as they were found to rapidly increase the endogenous production of glucose, glucagon, and corticosterone without a concurrent increase in plasma insulin [465,491].

There appears to be an inter-relation between the HPT and insulin axes in obesity. One mechanism suggested is that in the IR state, the activity of deiodinase 2, which converts T4 into T3 in the thyrotropic cells, is reduced, resulting in stimulation of TSH [492]. Raised TSH and T4 are associated in turn with reduced insulin sensitivity in obese children [493]. Baseline glucose concentration was shown in particular to correlate with TSH, and glucose intake is shown to promote an additional increase in TSH.

Additionally, IR has been cited as a major driver of increased thyroid volume [494], which is in turn associated with autoantibodies (i.e. AITD) in those with an elevated TSH [495].

3.9.2.3 Obesity and thyroid diseases

There seems to be a bidirectional and causal relationship between obesity and thyroid disorders [460]. Meta-analyses show an increased risk (OR 3.21) of overt hypothyroidism in people with a body mass index (BMI) over 28 kg/m^2 with a 70% increased risk of subclinical hypothyroidism [460]. Obesity is associated with hormonal changes, especially in women, including raised TSH concentrations and decreased TH concentrations [496,497].

TH regulates and maintains BMR as well as appetite and body weight. BMR is a key source of energy expenditure in humans and central to weight regulation, with changes in BMR being responsible for weight gain or weight loss. TH increases BMR by increasing production of ATP through stimulation of sodium-potassium (Na/K) as well as Na/K ATPase gradients in cellular organelles, particularly sarcoplasmic and endoplasmic reticulum in skeletal and cardiac muscle [465]. Unsurprisingly then, subclinical hypothyroidism impairs resting energy expenditure (REE) in obese subjects [498].

TH is known to regulate adipose tissue mass and function. The direct evidence for this is the presence of TH receptors in human adipocytes. In addition, adipocytes are one of the non-thyroid tissues that contain TSH receptors. Other tissues include the liver, ovaries, immune cells, ocular muscles, and erythrocytes [499–504]. TSH receptor numbers increase as BMI increases and TSH-bound receptors seem to play a regulatory role in adipogenesis. Increased adiposity results in an increased TSH secretion due to the effect of adipokines on the HPT axis. This raised TSH is not always clinically significant (i.e., results in variable TH concentrations).

In obesity, T3 receptors are also decreased as is the negative feedback loop with TSH. The hormones and neurotransmitters involved in regulation of body weight and satiety also affect TSH production. Some studies [505] show decreased concentrations of free T4 and free T3 with increasing adiposity, suggestive of peripheral hypometabolism.

3.9.2.3.1 Obesity and autoimmune thyroid disease

In obese patients with high TSH, 60% tested positive for AITD, suggesting an underlying autoimmune thyroid disorder [505]. A hypothesis has been described linking obesity, leptin, autoimmunity, and hypothyroidism [505] suggesting that obesity is a risk factor for thyroid autoimmunity. This is supported by other studies that suggest a bidirectional role in AITD and obesity [506].

Despite this the link between AITD and obesity remains unclear. The prevalence of AITD in childhood obesity is 12.4% with a wide variance of between 10% and 16% in obese adults [505]. Interestingly, the relationship between AITD and obesity is only statistically significant in Hashimoto's thyroiditis, not in Grave's disease. Additionally, there seems to be a significant association between TPOAb positivity and obesity but not between a positive TgAb and obesity [460].

3.9.2.3.2 Proposed mechanisms for obesity-related thyroid diseases

Chronic inflammation Obesity is a chronic inflammatory disorder with raised cytokines and inflammatory markers such as interleukin one (IL-1) and six (IL-6) and tumour necrosis factor alpha (TNFα) [507]. A proposed mechanistic link between obesity and hypothyroidism is that increased inflammatory cytokines possibly inhibit the mRNA expression of the sodium/iodine symporter thus affecting iodide uptake in thyroid cells [508].

A second proposed link is that cytokines result in vasodilation and increased thyroid vascular permeability which may account for morphological and functional thyroid changes [492,508].

There is also a role for the chronic inflammatory status in obesity which is thought to affect thyroid function by modulating the activity and expression of deiodinases [509,510].

Leptin The role of leptin, an adipokine secreted by adipocytes, has been described as a contributing factor in TH abnormalities (Fig. 3.21; [511]). In obese patients, there is a tendency towards a mild increase in TSH and decrease in TH concentrations [506]. However in extremely obese patients, raised leptin concentrations act centrally by stimulating the HPT axis, thus regulating the activity of neurons in the hypothalamus with both direct and indirect effects on TRH–TSH secretion. In short, leptin directly stimulates TRH neurons in the paraventricular nucleus, which leads to raised concentrations of TSH [506,512]. Even subtle increases in TSH concentrations have been associated with a measurable decrease in REE and increased body weight [506,513].

Leptin is also thought to restrict the expression of the sodium/iodide symporter as well as of thyroglobulin, the protein from which TH are produced [514].

IL-6 and leptin inhibit regulatory T-cells. In obesity there is an altered cell-mediated Th-1 immune response generating defects in T-suppressor/cytotoxic cells [515–517]. Leptin has a regulatory role in the Th-1 response [505,518] and has been shown to regulate the proliferation of CD4and CD25T cells, a cell line involved in apoptosis in AITD [519]. Leptin concentrations have been found to remain high up to six months postpartum in a clinical study of women with postpartum thyroiditis [520]. Based on these findings, it is hypothesised that leptin has a role in thyroid autoimmunity, especially in a patient who is genetically and environmentally predisposed to a Th-1 immune response [505].

It is important to note that while the above mechanisms, unearthed by good quality meta-analyses, shed some light on possible mechanisms, the pathophysiology still needs to be researched in further in-depth studies.

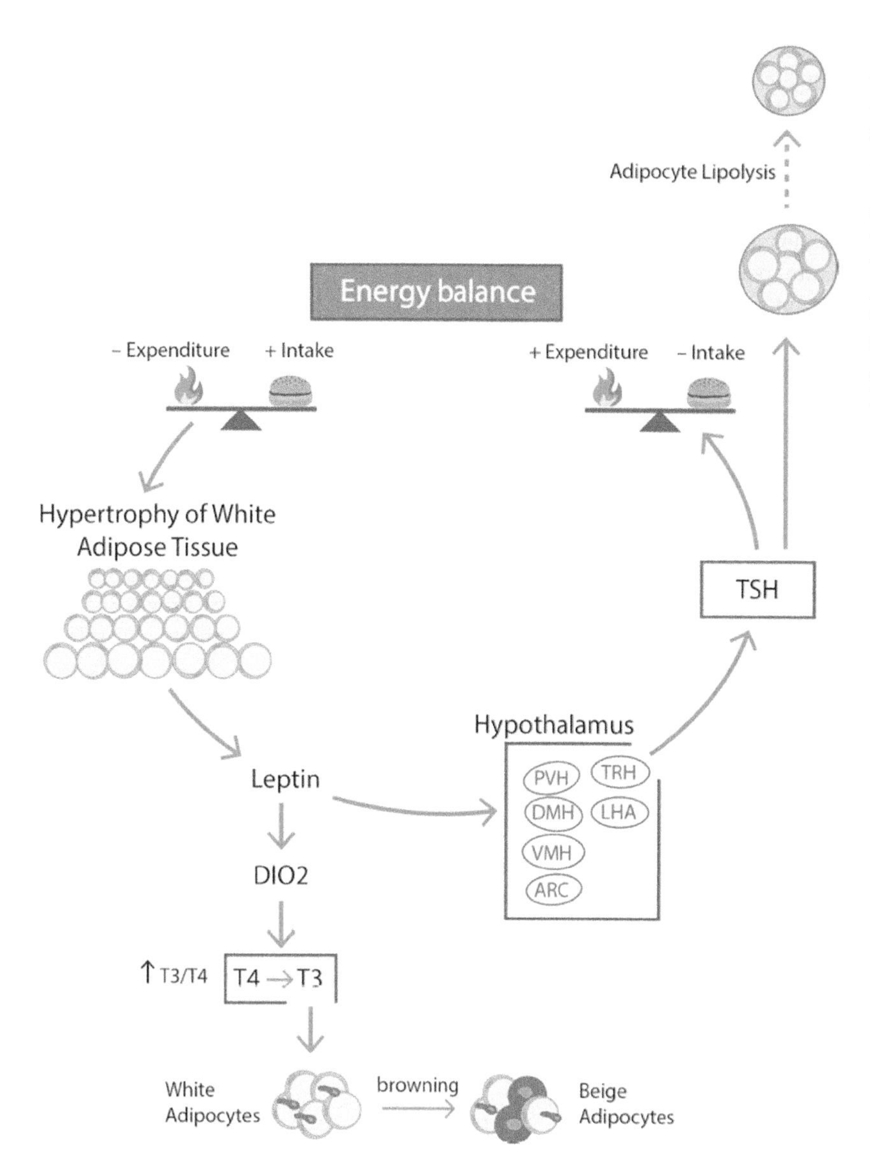

FIGURE 3.21 **Roles of leptin in thyroid synthesis and regulation.** In conditions of excess caloric supply, leptin activates thyrotropin-releasing hormone (TRH) expression and then synthesis of thyroid stimulating hormone (TSH) and THs. It suppresses appetite and promotes energy expenditure by increasing lipolysis and thermogenesis. In obese people, leptin can activate iodothyronine deiodinase (DIO) expression and can increase conversion of thyroxine (T4) to triiodothyronine (T3). THs play a role in the browning of adipose tissue. *From Walczak K, Sieminska L. Obesity and thyroid axis.* Int J Environ Res Public Health, *18 (18) (2021), 9434.*

3.9.2.4 *The thyroid-gut axis*

A healthy gut microbiome is beneficial for the immune system and in particular for AITD. It is known that the prevalence of AITD co-existing with coeliac disease is high [521]. Dysbiosis is also commonly found in thyroid disorders. Dysbiosis not only promotes inflammation and reduces immune tolerance, it also results in local inflammation with increased intestinal permeability and a resultant higher exposure to potential antigens. Dysbiosis also has a direct impact on TH concentrations by microbes' deiodinase activity, which results in the inhibition of TSH (Fig. 3.22). The absorption of important thyroid minerals including iodine, selenium, zinc, and iron may also be altered [521]. Probiotic supplementation has shown a beneficial effect on TH and function [521].

Dysbiosis has been linked to diets high in ultra-processed foods especially those high in sugar [522]. A ketogenic diet has been shown to have metabolic, glycaemic as well as gut microbe benefits [194].

3.9.2.5 *Thyroid cancer*

Thyroid cancers are reportedly increasing in prevalence and studies link obesity and IR to thyroid cancers. The mechanisms have been linked to altered TH, IR, raised adipokines, chronic inflammation, and female sex hormones [523].

Several studies have also shown that dysbiosis of the microbiota could be linked to certain cancer types [524–526].

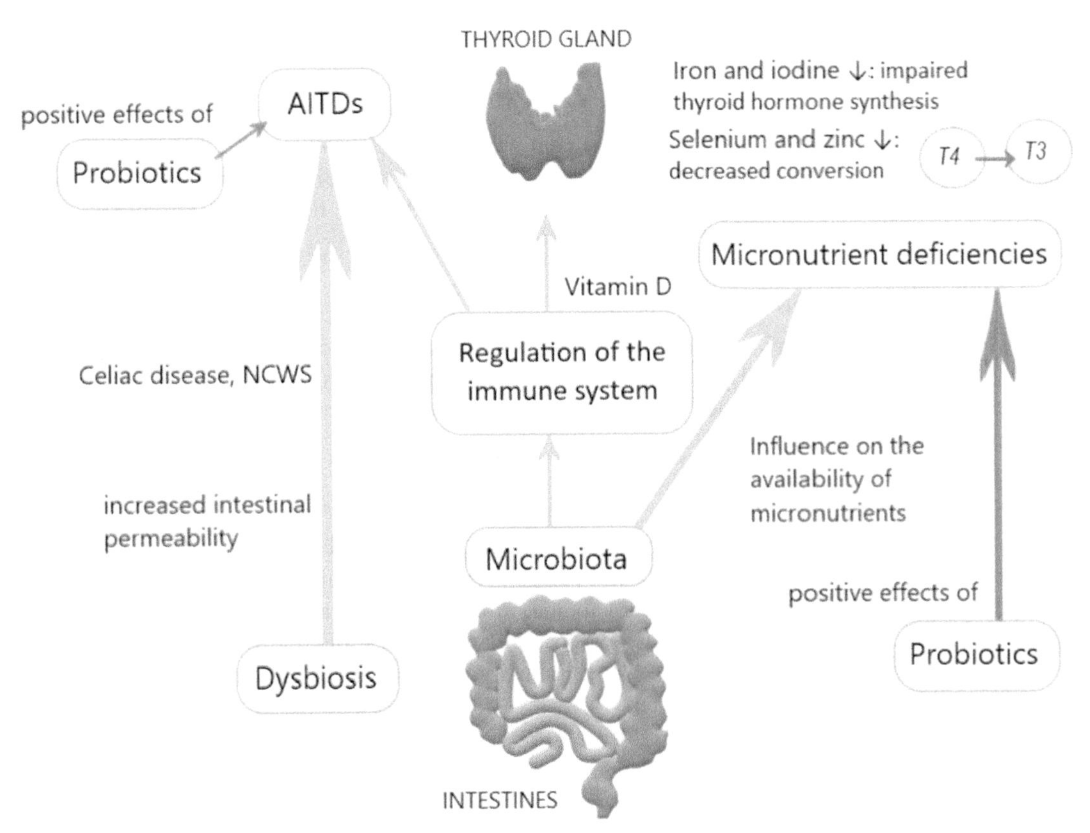

FIGURE 3.22 **Overview of the influence of the gut on the thyroid.** Autoimmune thyroid diseases (AITDs); thyroxine (T4); triiodothyronine(T3). *From Knezevic J, Starchl C, Tmava Berisha A, Amrein K. Thyroid-gut-axis: how does the microbiota influence thyroid function?* Nutrients*12 (6) (2020), 1769.*

In addition, altered iodide concentrations have been associated with tumour development and iodide has been shown to be an antioxidant as well as anti-neoplastic, anti-proliferative, and cytotoxic in human cancer [527].

3.9.3 Managing the patient

3.9.3.1 Aims of care

The traditional first approach in modern health care, once the diagnosis of thyroid disease has been made, is to replace or reduce TH pharmacologically or via other treatment modalities, including radiation ablation therapies. This may be required and helpful in many, but other factors are also an important part of therapy. Take into account the multiple physiological concentrations and inter-relations in the patient and begin by supporting imbalances in the HPT axis.

3.9.3.2 Assessment

3.9.3.2.1 Patient evaluation

The patient's history is critical to evaluation. A patient may have symptoms of thyroid disease without impaired thyroid function. Careful family and genetic history, clinical and symptom history along with a timeline, as well as the emotional, environmental, genetic, and nutritional predisposition towards a subclinical autoimmune thyroid condition is critical. Careful history taking will be helpful to decide which patients require further antibody testing and which patients require regular follow-up. Many patients have lost faith in medicine due to not being believed by their doctor, only to deteriorate further down the line or, if they are lucky, to find an empathetic doctor who does further testing and diagnoses the condition that was subclinical and already present.

Clinical experience suggests that all individuals with obesity be screened for thyroid dysfunctions and optimum control of hypothyroidism should be considered an integral part of obesity management.

3.9.3.2.2 Thyroid function evaluation

General principles of testing include running a TSH, free T3, free T4 and in some cases TPOAb activity. There is some controversy around the question of whether laboratory testing can define borderline thyroid dysfunction. A study evaluating 56,000 tests in a population of 471,000 people and using TSH concentrations as a first line test, found that while in most cases TSH is useful for evaluating pituitary function, secondary thyroid diseases and TH resistance were missed in 17 patients [528]. It is therefore important to understand the limitations of testing and to employ patient history, symptoms and clinical acumen in evaluation [529].

3.9.3.3 Lifestyle related considerations

The individual psychosocial, nutritional, emotional, and behavioural history as well as environmental exposure is key to be able to work towards a bio-individual patient plan. Healthy thyroid function depends on the synergy and optimal levels of multiple role players. Starting at the central regulating level, all stressors that influence the HPT axis can have an effect on TH production and metabolism.

3.9.3.3.1 Environmental thyroid antagonists

Xenobiotics such as organochlorine compounds, found in pesticides, plastics and many other industrial chemicals, have an effect on TH metabolism and can act as agonists and antagonists on thyroid nuclear receptors [530]. Mechanisms of injury to the thyroid gland include impaired uptake of iodine, inhibition of TH activity, coupling of iodothyronines to thyroxine, as well as production of thyroid antibodies. Exposure is particularly of concern in infants and young children though it has an impact on adults as well [531–534]. Elimination of xenobiotics including support of phase I and II detoxification processes in the liver is recommended.

3.9.3.3.2 Stress

Chronic stress is a powerful carcinogen, it increases chronic inflammation, has a negative impact on the immune system, the gut microbiome, as well as glucose homoeostasis and the HPT axis, by promoting cortisol production [535]. Guiding the patient towards processes that balance lifestyle to better manage chronic stressors, including mental/emotional, physical and environmental stressors and living within circadian clocks [536], is suggested.

3.9.3.4 Diet

3.9.3.4.1 Nutrients for thyroid health

Iodide deficiency is a key limiting factor to thyroid health and care must be taken to ensure adequate dietary intake of this important nutrient. Selenium supports intracellular deiodination [484]. Zinc has been shown to be an important cofactor for the thyroid receptor. Zinc supplementation in patients with deficiency, has been shown to improve T3, reduce rT3, and normalise TSH [537]. Vitamin A has a role in T3 receptor binding. Adequate vitamin A along with omega 3 fatty acids helps improve TH activity [484]. Vitamin E, selenium, and vitamin C have been shown to have important antioxidant effects and a role in mitochondrial function [538–541]. Ensuring adequate levels of Vitamin D for immune support may also be required [542].

3.9.3.4.2 Antagonists to thyroid function

Certain dietary compounds, in very high amounts, have been shown to block the iodination of thyroglobulin (e.g., thiocyanate and sulfhydryl compounds found in the Brassica family of vegetables). It is important to note that general consumption of Brassica family vegetables will not be sufficient to reach goitrogenic levels and that most studies are animal studies using uncooked vegetables [484,543,544].

Soya has been implicated as a goitrogenic food due to the ability of genistein, a soy isoflavone, to compete with TPO. Though studies are inconclusive on the effect of dietary soya on thyroid health [545,546], there is still concern with regards to its effect. Data suggest that when dietary soya isoflavones are increased, iodide intake should be increased and particular care to maintain adequate selenium levels should be taken too [547]. A suggestion to monitor TH concentrations in patients on exogenous thyroid supplements has also been made.

Other specific bioflavonoids that antagonise both TPO and iodinate enzymes are some plant- derived bioflavonoids such as fisetin and quercetin. L-carnitine has also been identified as a thyroid antagonist and can lower TH entry into the nucleus of hepatocytes, neurons, and fibroblasts [484]. Consequently L-carnitine has successfully been used in the treatment of patients with hyperthyroidism [548]. As such, be cautious of L-carnitine intake in hypothyroid patients.

3.9.3.4.3 Reduce inflammation

Inflammation plays an important role in the pathogenesis of obesity and its related illnesses as well as diseases of the thyroid. Ultra-processed foods, exposure to preservatives and additives, poor circadian rhythms, high-sugar diets, obesity, prolonged chronic stress, and isolation have all been shown to promote inflammation. A structured and holistic approach to processes that reduce inflammation is critical [549].

3.9.3.4.4 Gastrointestinal health

The role of the microbiome in disease has been well established [522]. Many books [535] cover this topic's association with disease in elegant detail. An approach using targeted nutrition practice as well as limiting compounds that are detrimental to the gut microbiome is key to its recovery (refer to chapter 8 Gastrointestinal). Carnivore diets have garnered interest as a form of elimination diet for patients with autoimmune diseases (refer to section on autoimmunity). Gastrointestinal disease can also affect absorption of key nutrients. For example this study [550] suggests a causal relationship between absorption and metabolism of vitamin A and zinc and low T3 syndrome.

3.9.3.4.5 Addressing obesity and insulin resistance

By now the clear interrelation between obesity and IR and diseases of the thyroid has been shown. TCR has been shown to be successful in the reversal of obesity (Section 3.8), as well as the successful management of IR (Sections 3.3 and 3.4). A well-structured ketogenic diet or other TCR approach can be used as a treatment modality in the management of thyroid diseases [551,552] (also see Section 1.2).

3.9.3.4.6 Reduction of antithyroid antibodies

As explained earlier, AITD has a complex aetiology. Comprehensive risk reduction is suggested, including reduction of antithyroid antibodies. Foods that induce antibodies and cross react with the thyroid gland, a diet free of gluten, grains, and dairy and indeed an elimination diet may need to be employed.

3.9.4 Conclusion

TH play a central role in regulating energy balance, metabolism of glucose, and lipids. The bidirectional role between obesity and thyroid disorders has been described. MetS prevalence is increasing, as is the prevalence of diseases of the thyroid, and patients with thyroid disease have an increased risk for metabolic disease.

Nutrition is key in maintaining thyroid health, as well as overall health, including optimal gastrointestinal and metabolic health. TCR has a beneficial role in reversing obesity, reducing inflammation, improving immunity, enhancing mitochondrial health, and improving gastrointestinal health, all key factors in improving metabolic health as well as thyroid functionality. It is critical that we review our approach to health and disease and consider TCR as a treatment and support modality for thyroid health and chronic diseases.

3.10 Adrenals and the hypothalamic-pituitary-adrenal (HPA) axis

Laurie Rauch

3.10.1 Introduction

Corticosteroids (cortisol in humans, corticosterone in the rat and mouse) are steroid hormones that are released into the bloodstream from the adrenal cortex zona fasiculata upon adrenocorticotropin (ACTH) binding to melanocortin receptors 2 (MCR2). ACTH is a posttranslational product of the proopiomelanocortin prohormone that is produced in the anterior pituitary. ACTH is in turn released from the anterior pituitary gland into the circulation upon activation by corticotropin-releasing hormone (CRH) that is produced in parvocellular neuroendocrine cells in the paraventricular hypothalamus (PVH) [553,554]. Given that glucocorticoids have pervasive genomic and non-genomic effects, it is crucial that blood cortisol concentration be maintained at optimal concentrations [555]. Cortisol acts as its own negative feedback signal to the brain where it binds to glucocorticoid receptors (GR) to facilitate optimal cortisol release from the adrenals [556]. Too much cortisol release leads to, amongst others, hyperphagia, hyperglycaemia, insulin resistance and visceral adiposity, while too little cortisol release leads to hypoglycaemia, weight loss and fatigue [556,557].

3.10.2 Pathophysiology

Thomas Addison was the first to describe a disorder known as adrenal insufficiency (AI) in 1855. AI can be (1) primary (Addison disease or autoimmune adrenalitis), when insufficient glucocorticoids/mineralocorticoids/aldosterone are produced in the adrenal cortex; (2) secondary, if the anterior pituitary produces insufficient ACTH or (3) tertiary, if the PVH produces insufficient CRH. AI disorder was fatal until Kendall, Sarett, and Reichstein synthesised cortisone in the laboratory in 1949 [558,559].

Cushing's disease (CD) has the opposite effect in that a pituitary tumour induces excessive ACTH production and attendant chronic hypercortisolism. CD is associated with co-morbidities like visceral obesity, diabetes, dyslipidaemia, hypertension, all features of metabolic syndrome, and can also bring about reproductive/sexual, neuropsychiatric, and skeleto-muscular disorders [560].

3.10.2.1 The stress of being born

Being born is a more stress inducing and alerting experience than what we will ever encounter as an adult [561]. One moment the intrauterine baby is basking in bliss, the next both its oxygen and its nutrient supplies are severed. Cortisol and catecholamines (adrenaline and noradrenaline) flood the new-born's bloodstream to kick its heart, lungs, and muscles into full alert, to ensure that enough resources are released so that feeding behaviour can be engaged. Innate reflexes (such as the breathing reflex), neural responses, and behavioural programmes subsumed in the new-born's hypothalamus-brainstem-spine take full control.

The orienting response [562] increases bodily arousal, tunes in to environmental signals and activates motor responses. The mother's reassuringly familiar smell and skin-to-skin touch send chemical signals to the infant's hypothalamus-brainstem so that the potentially harmful effects of excessive cortisol and adrenaline are neutralised with chemicals like oxytocin.

Feeding behaviour also involves smell, the newborn is guided to the breast by the smell of colostrum. Cortisol is required to drive the feeding behaviour [563] to enable the newborn baby to crawl against gravity, for the very first time, to latch on to the breast. More reflexes like chewing and swallowing are involved with consuming breast milk [564,565].

A newborn requires massive amounts of cortisol and catecholamines to provide the required resources for the infant to take its first breath and to latch on to the breast. As adults we don't require nearly as much cortisol and catecholamines to engage feeding behaviour, though it is still a requirement.

3.10.3 Managing the patient

3.10.3.1 Lifestyle-related considerations

Indeed, we also require cortisol to help us through our daily workloads. The increased prefrontal cortex (PFC) processing required to manage our daily list of tasks will signal the parvocellular nuclei in the PVH to upregulate the release of CRH into the anterior pituitary gland [556,566,567]. This then increases pituitary ACTH release and ultimately increases adrenal cortisol release to provide the additional resources necessary to complete our daily tasks. If this elevated cortisol release from the adrenal cortex becomes chronic though, the brain will start down regulating the release of CRF and ACTH, to thereby dampen down adrenal cortisol release [568].

This downregulation of CRH and ACTH release, to maintain blood cortisol at optimal concentrations, will only succeed if the signalling from the PFC, hippocampal, amygdala, etc to the parvocellular nuclei in the PVH is also decreased [569,570]. However, if the higher brain centres continue to activate the parvocellular nuclei in the PVH, CRH release will remain upregulated, more ACTH will be released into the circulation, and more cortisol will be produced by the adrenals [569,571].

3.10.3.1.1 Cortisol-insulin antagonism

Both cortisol and insulin have powerful but opposing central and peripheral effects. Cortisol drives feeding behaviour and releases glucose into the blood; insulin inhibits feeding behaviour and it removes glucose out of the blood [563]. If cortisol and insulin concentrations are both low and/or balanced their mutual antagonism will ensure optimal BG/weight regulation, but if both are elevated it will bring about severe disruptions of the same [572].

Goal-directed behaviours, such as appetitive feeding behaviour, are associated with elevated cortisol concentration [573] that serves to increase the gluconeogenic rate in the liver, inhibit insulin-mediated glucose uptake in muscle and adipose tissue, and inhibit insulin release. The overall effect being that the exercising musculature needed for hunting/foraging now has a rich supply of BG to fuel insulin-independent muscle contraction.

In sharp contrast, consummatory behaviour that generally follows immediately after appetitive behaviour, is associated with elevated insulin (and decreased cortisol) concentrations. Insulin has the opposite effect to that of cortisol, it inhibits liver glucose output, enhances muscle and adipose tissue glucose uptake, and inhibits feeding behaviour [556,557].

However, when both cortisol and insulin concentrations are elevated in the bloodstream the cortisol-insulin antagonism favours cortisol and the increased glucose output from the liver combined with the insulin resistant muscle will further stimulate insulin release and eventually redistribute fat from peripheral to central sites (i.e., increased visceral fat) [556,574].

3.10.3.2 Therapeutic intervention

Like the newborn infant that needs cortisol to latch on to the breast to feed, we need cortisol to complete our daily list of tasks. If our to do lists become excessive, more and more CRH will be released from the hypothalamus that will then serve to release greater amounts of ACTH from the pituitary gland, that will then result in excessive cortisol release into the bloodstream from the adrenal cortex [575,576]. The resultant hypercortisolaemia would then induce insulin resistance in both muscle and adipose tissue, increase the gluconeogenic and lipogenic rates in the liver and inhibit insulin release from the pancreatic β cells [556,557,577]. Two things are needed to break this vicious cycle. (1) reduce brain activity or stress to dampen down activation of the parvocellular nuclei in the PVH to thereby produce less CRH and (2) introduce TCR restriction to dampen down insulin release from the pancreatic β cells.

3.10.3.3 Therapeutic carbohydrate restriction

The same balance that exists in the bloodstream between the stress needed to drive feeding behaviour as mediated by e.g., cortisol [573], and the energy needed to fuel feeding behaviour (e.g., from glucose, free fatty acids (FFA) and ketone bodies) also exists in every mitochondrial cell in the body [578]. If the stress inside our mitochondria (measured as reactive oxygen species (ROS)) and the energy (ATP) produced in our mitochondria from glucose, FFA and ketone bodies are out of kilter, our energy, and weight regulation abilities would become impaired [167,578].

The same oxidative processes that generate ATP in the mitochondria also produce free radicals that contain oxygen, known as ROS [167]. If the oxygen containing free radicals are effectively neutralised, mitochondrial function will not be impaired. Adaptive mitochondrial responses known as mitohormesis, that can be induced by exercise and/or diet, enables cells to better tolerate ROS [167,579]. A good way to bring about a protective anti-oxidative mitohormesis response is via increasing the circulating ketone bodies, such as D-β-hydroxybutyrate (βOHB) and acetoacetate, via a low carbohydrate, high fat diet [167] (see Section 3.3 for more information on mitohormesis). Increased ketone bodies in the blood are indicative of fat breakdown and low carbohydrate availability, and hence lower insulin concentrations [294]. Ketone bodies are produced in the liver when acetyl-CoA is converted to acetoacetate and then reduced by mitochondrial βOHB dehydrogenase to βOHB. Small amounts of acetoacetate also decarboxylates into acetone and carbon dioxide. Once released into the circulation the above-mentioned three ketone bodies are taken up by other tissues, such as the brain and heart, via monocarboxylate transporters 1 and 2 as an alternative source of energy [580]. βOHB can meet two-thirds of the energy requirements of the brain during fasting/starvation. The heart also makes greater use of fatty acid oxidation that can account for 60%–85% of ATP produced during fasting [581].

3.10.3.3.1 Guiding the patient

Glucocorticoid feedback to the brain targets the hypothalamus, hippocampus, and the PFC [568,571]. This enables the hypothalamus to regulate cortisol concentrations during everyday predictable circumstances, but when unexpected environmental or psychosocial stresses occur, input from higher brain centres like the hippocampus, amygdala, and PFC are necessary [566,567]. Cortisol concentrations also change according to ultradian (pulsatile) and circadian (24 h) rhythms, when sleeping vs. awake, and even when asleep during the day it will influence cortisol concentrations [582]. Cortisol concentration is usually at its lowest between 11 pm and 1 am and then starts rising to reach its highest point just after getting up in the morning (8–9 am) to help prepare for the day [583].

A good way to start the day is to do some rhythmic rotational movement [584] around the spine and to restrict breakfast carbohydrate intake or preferably extend your overnight fast until lunchtime. Also, focusing on one task at a time can help quieten thoughts.

3.10.4 Summary/conclusion

The HPA-axis ensures that enough cortisol is produced in the adrenal cortex to drive goal directed behaviour, but feedback regulation can become dysregulated when daily workloads/stressors become unmanageable. There are two ways to regain optimal cortisol release from the adrenal gland: (1) decrease cortical information processing (busy brain) to thereby dampen down CRH production in the PVH parvocellular nuclei that will serve to decrease cortisol release from the adrenal cortex and (2) introduce TCR to decrease insulin release into the bloodstream.

References

[1] Jensen KJ, Alpini G, Glaser S. Hepatic nervous system and neurobiology of the liver. Compr Physiol 2013;3(2):655–65.

[2] Dicostanzo CA, Dardevet DP, Neal DW, Lautz M, Allen E, Snead W, et al. Role of the hepatic sympathetic nerves in the regulation of net hepatic glucose uptake and the mediation of the portal glucose signal. Am J Physiol Endocrinol Metab 2006;290(1):E9–16. 2005.

[3] Hsieh PS, Moore MC, Neal DW, Cherrington AD. Importance of the hepatic arterial glucose level in generation of the portal signal in conscious dogs. Am J Physiol Endocrinol Metab 2000;279(2):E284–92.

[4] Moore MC, Coate KC, Winnick JJ, An Z, Cherrington AD. Regulation of hepatic glucose uptake and storage in vivo. Adv Nutr 2012;3 (3):286–94.

[5] Atiea JA, Aslan SM, Owens DR, Luzio S. Early morning hyperglycaemia "dawn phenomenon" in non-insulin dependent diabetes mellitus (NIDDM): effects of cortisol suppression by metyrapone. Diabetes Res 1990;14(4):181–5. PMID: 2132191.

[6] Hodson L, Rosqvist F, Parry SA. The influence of dietary fatty acids on liver fat content and metabolism Proc Nutr Soc 2020;79(1):30–41. Available from: https://doi.org/10.1017/S0029665119000569. Epub 2019 Apr 3. Erratum in: Proc Nutr Soc. 2019 Aug;78(3):473. PMID: 30942685.

[7] Titchenell PM, Lazar MA, Birnbaum MJ. Unraveling the regulation of hepatic metabolism by insulin. Trends Endocrinol Metab 2017;28 (7):497–505. Available from: https://doi.org/10.1016/j.tem.2017.03.003. Epub 2017 Apr 14. PMID: 28416361. PMCID: PMC5477655.

[8] Asare-Bediako I, Paszkiewicz RL, Kim SP, Woolcott OO, Kolka CM, Burch MA, et al. Variability of directly measured first-pass hepatic insulin extraction and its association with insulin sensitivity and plasma insulin. Diabetes. 2018;67(8):1495–503. Available from: https://doi.org/10.2337/db17-1520. PMID: 29752425. PMCID: PMC6054441.

[9] Richter EA, Hargreaves M. Exercise, GLUT4, and skeletal muscle glucose uptake. Physiol Rev 2013;93(3):993–1017. Available from: https://doi.org/10.1152/physrev.00038.2012. PMID: 23899560.

[10] Salehi A, Vieira E, Gylfe E. Paradoxical stimulation of glucagon secretion by high glucose concentrations. Diabetes. 2006;55(8):2318–23.

[11] Gerich JE. Physiology of glucagon. Int Rev Physiol 1981;24:243–75. PMID: 7021445. Hayashi Y. Glucagon regulates lipolysis and fatty acid oxidation through inositol triphosphate receptor 1 in the liver. *J Diabetes Investig*. 2021;12(1):32–34.

[12] Santoleri D, Titchenell PM. Resolving the paradox of hepatic insulin resistance. Cell Mol Gastroenterol Hepatol 2019;7(2):447–56. Available from: https://doi.org/10.1016/j.jcmgh.2018.10.016. Epub 2018 Nov 3. PMID: 30739869. PMCID: PMC6369222.

[13] Gormsen LC, Jensen MD, Schmitz O, Møller N, Christiansen JS, Nielsen S. Energy expenditure, insulin, and VLDL-triglyceride production in humans J Lipid Res 2006;47(10):2325–32. Available from: https://doi.org/10.1194/jlr.M600175-JLR200. Epub 2006 Jul 18. PMID: 16849776.

[14] Cywes, R. Doctoral Thesis. The role of platelets in hepatic allograft preservation-reperfusion injury. Univ of Toronto, 1995.

[15] Hoffman M. Remodeling the blood coagulation cascade. J Thrombosis Thrombolysis 2003;16(1–2):17–20.

[16] Szosland K, Lewinski A. Insulin resistance – "the good or the bad and ugly." Neuro Endocrinol Lett 2018;39(5):355–62PMID. PMID: 30664340.

[17] Rohli KE, Boyer CK, Blom SE, Stephens SB. Nutrient regulation of pancreatic islet β-cell secretory capacity and insulin production. Biomolecules 2022;12(2):335. Available from: https://doi.org/10.3390/biom12020335. PMID: 35204835. PMCID: PMC8869698.

[18] Jackson KH, Harris WS. Blood fatty acid profiles: new biomarkers for cardiometabolic disease risk. Curr Atheroscler Rep 2018;20(5):22 20.

[19] Losada-Barragán M. Physiological effects of nutrients on insulin release by pancreatic beta cells Mol Cell Biochem 2021;476(8):3127–39. Available from: https://doi.org/10.1007/s11010-021-04146-w. Epub 2021 Apr 12. PMID: 33844157.

[20] Sundborn G, Metcalf PA, Gentles D, Scragg R, Dyall L, Black P, et al. Overweight and obesity prevalence among adult Pacific peoples and Europeans in the Diabetes Heart and Health Study (DHAHS) 2002–2003, Auckland New Zealand. N Z Med J 2010;123(1311):30–42. PMID. PMID: 20360794.

[21] Pandya A, Mehta M, Sankavaram K. The relationship between macronutrient distribution and type 2 diabetes in Asian Indians. Nutrients. 2021;13(12):4406. Available from: https://doi.org/10.3390/nu13124406. PMID: 34959958. PMCID: PMC8704419.

[22] Krishnan M, Major TJ, Topless RK, Dewes O, Yu L, Thompson JMD, et al. Discordant association of the CREBRF rs373863828 A allele with increased BMI and protection from type 2 diabetes in Māori and Pacific (Polynesian) people living in Aotearoa/New Zealand. Diabetologia. 2018;61(7):1603–13. Available from: https://doi.org/10.1007/s00125-018-4623-1. Epub 2018 May 2. PMID: 29721634. PMCID: PMC6434933.

[23] Park SE, Park CY, Sweeney G. Biomarkers of insulin sensitivity and insulin resistance: Past, present and future Crit Rev Clin Lab Sci 2015;52 (4):180–90. Available from: https://doi.org/10.3109/10408363.2015.1023429. Epub 2015 Jun 4. PMID: 26042993.

[24] Brown E, Cuthbertson DJ, Wilding JP. Newer GLP-1 receptor agonists and obesity-diabetes. Peptides. 2018;100:61–7. Available from: https://doi.org/10.1016/j.peptides.2017.12.009. PMID: 29412833.

[25] Takashi Matsuzaka T, Hitoshi Shimano H. Insulin-dependent and -independent regulation of sterol regulatory element-binding protein-1c. J Diabetes Investig 2013;4(5):411–12.

[26] Lassailly G, Caiazzo R, Hollebecque A, Buob D, Leteurtre E, Arnalsteen L, et al. Validation of noninvasive biomarkers (FibroTest, SteatoTest, and NashTest) for prediction of liver injury in patients with morbid obesity. Eur J Gastroenterol Hepatol 2011;23(6):499–506.

[27] Schwenzer NF, Springer F, Schraml C, Stefan N, Machann J, Schick F. Non-invasive assessment and quantification of liver steatosis by ultrasound, computed tomography and magnetic resonance. J Hepatol 2009;51:433–45.

[28] Chalasani N, Younossi Z, Lavine JE, Charlton M, Cusi, et al. The diagnosis and management of nonalcoholic fatty liver disease: Practice guidance from the American Association for the Study of Liver Diseases. Hepatology. 2018;67(1):328–57.

[29] Brunt EM, Janney CG, Di Bisceglie AM, Neuschwander-Tetri BA, Bacon BR. Nonalcoholic steatohepatitis: a proposal for grading and staging the histological lesions. Am J Gastroenterol 1999;94:2467–74.

[30] Zhang P, Wang W, Mao M, Gao R, Shi W, Li D, et al. Similarities and differences: a comparative review of the molecular mechanisms and effectors of NAFLD and AFLD. Front Physiol 2021;12:710285. Available from: https://doi.org/10.3389/fphys.2021.710285. PMID: 34393826. PMCID: PMC8362097.

[31] Hudgins LC, et al. Relationship between carbohydrate-induced hypertriglyceridemia and fatty acid synthesis in lean and obese subjects. J Lipid Res 2000;41:595–604.

[32] Lee JJ, Lambert JE, Hovhannisyan Y, Ramos-Roman MA, Trombold JR, Wagner DA, et al. Palmitoleic acid is elevated in fatty liver disease and reflects hepatic lipogenesis. Am J Clin Nutr 2015;101(1):34–43.

[33] Donnelly KL, Smith CI, Schwarzenberg SJ, Jessurun J, Boldt MD, Parks EJ. Sources of fatty acids stored in liver and secreted via lipoproteins in patients with nonalcoholic fatty liver disease. J Clin Invest 2005;115(5):1343–51. Available from: https://doi.org/10.1172/JCI23621. PMID: 15864352. PMCID: PMC1087172.

[34] Suk KT, Kim MY, Baik SK. Alcoholic liver disease: treatment. World J gastroenterology 2014;20(36):12934–44.

[35] Nakamura A, Terauchi Y. Lessons from mouse models of high-fat diet-induced NAFLD. Int J Mol Sci 2013;14(11):21240–57.

[36] Timlin MT, Parks EJ. The temporal pattern of de novo lipogenesis in the postprandial state. Am J Clin Nutr 2005;81:35–42.

[37] Promrat K, et al. A pilot study of pioglitazone treatment for nonalcoholic steatohepatitis. Hepatology. 2004;39:188–96.

[38] Lamos EM, Kristan M, Siamashvili M, Davis SN. Effects of anti-diabetic treatments in type 2 diabetes and fatty liver disease Expert Rev Clin Pharmacol 2021;14(7):837–52. Available from: https://doi.org/10.1080/17512433.2021.1917374. Epub 2021 Apr 22. PMID: 33882758.

[39] Suk KT, Kim MY, Baik SK. Alcoholic liver disease: treatment. World J gastroenterology 2004;20(36):12934–44.

[40] Younossi Z, Anstee QM, Marietti M, Hardy T, Henry L, Eslam M, et al. Global burden of NAFLD and NASH: trends, predictions, risk factors and prevention. Nat Rev Gastroenterology & Hepatology 2018;15(1):11–20.

[41] Wang H, Wang AX, Barrett EJ. Insulin-induced endothelial cell cortical actin filament remodeling: a requirement for trans-endothelial insulin transport. Mol Endocrinol 2012;26(8):1327–38.

[42] Kemeny SF, Figueroa DS, Clyne AM. Hypo- and hyperglycemia impair endothelial cell actin alignment and nitric oxide synthase activation in response to shear stress. PLoS One 2013;8(6):e66176.

[43] Caldwell S, Ikula Y, Dias D, et al. Hepatocellular ballooning in NASH. J Hepatol 2010;53(4):719–23.

[44] Bell GI, Kayano T, Buse JB, Burant CF, Takeda J, Lin D, et al. Molecular biology of mammalian glucose transporters. Diabetes Care 1990;13 (3):198–208. Available from: https://doi.org/10.2337/diacare.13.3.198. PMID: 2407475.

[45] Khadge S, Sharp JG, Thiele GM, McGuire TR, Klassen LW, Duryee MJ, et al. Dietary omega-3 and omega-6 polyunsaturated fatty acids modulate hepatic pathology. J Nutr Biochem 2018;52:92–102. Available from: https://doi.org/10.1016/j.jnutbio.2017.09.017. Epub 2017 Oct 4. PMID: 29175671. PMCID: PMC5996979.

[46] Kohan AB, Qing Y, Cyphert HA, Tso P, Salati LM. Chylomicron remnants and non-esterified fatty acids differ in their ability to inhibit genes involved in lipogenesis in rats. J Nutr 2011;141(2):171–6.

[47] Ronis MJ, Baumgardner JN, Sharma N, Vantrease J, Ferguson M, Tong Y, et al. Medium chain triglycerides dose-dependently prevent liver pathology in a rat model of non-alcoholic fatty liver disease. Exp Biol Med (Maywood) 2013;238(2):151–62. Available from: https://doi.org/10.1258/ebm.2012.012303. PMID: 23576797.

[48] Schuster S, Cabrera D, Arrese M, Feldstein AE. Triggering and resolution of inflammation in NASH. Nat Rev Gastroenterol Hepatol 2018;15 (6):349–64. Available from: https://doi.org/10.1038/s41575-018-0009-6. PMID: 29740166.

[49] Souto KP, Meinhardt NG, Ramos MJ, Ulbrich-Kulkzynski JM, Stein AT, Damin DC. Nonalcoholic fatty liver disease in patients with different baseline glucose status undergoing bariatric surgery: analysis of intraoperative liver biopsies and literature review. SOARD 2018;14(1):66–73.

[50] Ekstedt M, Hagstrom H, Nasr P, et al. Fibrosis stage is the strongest predictor for disease-specific mortality in NAFLD after up to 33 years of follow-up. Hepatology. 2015;61:1547–54.

[51] Angulo P, Hui JM, Marchesini G, et al. The NAFLD fibrosis score: a noninvasive system that identifies liver fibrosis in patients with NAFLD. Hepatology. 2007;45:846–54.

[52] Czul F, Bhamidimarri KR. Noninvasive markers to assess liver fibrosis. J Clin Gastroenterol 2016;50:445–57.

[53] Boland ML, Laker RC, Mather K, Nawrocki A, Oldham S, Boland BB, et al. Resolution of NASH and hepatic fibrosis by the GLP-1R/GcgR dual-agonist Cotadutide via modulating mitochondrial function and lipogenesis. Nat Metab 2020;2(5):413–31. Available from: https://doi.org/10.1038/s42255-020-0209-6. Epub 2020 May 21. PMID: 32478287. PMCID: PMC7258337.

[54] Tiniakos DG, Vos MB, Brunt EM. Nonalcoholic fatty liver disease: pathology and pathogenesis. Annu Rev Pathol 2010;5:145–71.

[55] Lewis MC, Phillips ML, Slavotinek JP, Kow L, Thompson CH, Toouli J. Change in liver size and fat content after treatment with Optifast very low calorie diet. Obes Surg 2006;16(6):697–701.

[56] Tendler D, Lin S, Yancy Jr WS, Mavropoulos J, Sylvestre P, Rockey DC, et al. The effect of a low-carbohydrate, ketogenic diet on nonalcoholic fatty liver disease: a pilot study. Dig Dis Sci 2007;52(2):589–93.

[57] Mitra A, Ahn J. Liver disease in patients on total parenteral nutrition. ClLiver Dis 2017;21(4):687–95.

[58] Golucci APBS, Morcillo AM, Hortencio TDR, Ribeiro AF, Nogueira RJN. Hypercholesterolemia and hypertriglyceridemia as risk factors of liver dysfunction in children with inflammation receiving total parenteral nutrition Clin Nutr ESPEN 2018;23:148–55. Available from: https://doi.org/10.1016/j.clnesp.2017.10.010. Epub 2017 Nov 20. PMID: 29460791.

[59] Kelly DA. Preventing parenteral nutrition liver disease. 2010;86(11), 683–687. Available from: https://doi.org/10.1016/j.earlhumdev.2010.08.012.

[60] Germani G, Laryea M, Rubbia-Brandt L, Egawa H, Burra P, O'Grady J, et al. Management of recurrent and de novo NAFLD/NASH after liver transplantation. Transplantation. 2019;103(1):57–67. Available from: https://doi.org/10.1097/TP.0000000000002485. PMID: 30335694.

[61] Mao SA, Glorioso JM, Nyberg SL. Liver regeneration. Transl Res 2014;163(4):352–62. Available from: https://doi.org/10.1016/j.trsl.2014.01.005. Epub 2014 Jan 16. PMID: 24495569. PMCID: PMC3976740.

[62] He L, Sabet A, Djedjos S, Miller R, et al. Metformin and insulin suppress hepatic gng through phosphorylation of CREB binding protein. Cell. 2009;137(4):635–46.

[63] Juárez-Hernández E, Chávez-Tapia NC, Uribe M, Barbero-Becerra VJ. Role of bioactive fatty acids in nonalcoholic fatty liver disease. Nutr J 2016;15(1):72.

[64] Diamond DM, Bikman BT, Mason P. Statin therapy is not warranted for a person with high LDL-cholesterol on a low-carbohydrate diet. Curr Opin Endocrinol Diabetes Obes. 29(5):497-511. Available from: https://doi.org/10.1097/MED.0000000000000764.

[65] Galassi A, Reynolds K, He J. Metabolic syndrome and risk of cardiovascular disease: a meta-analysis. Am J Med 2006;119(10):812–19. Available from: https://doi.org/10.1016/j.amjmed.2006.02.031. PMID: 17000207.

[66] Ford ES, Li C, Sattar N. Metabolic syndrome and incident diabetes: Current state of the evidence Diabetes Care 2008;31:1898–904PMID. PMID: 18591398.

[67] Kylin E. Studien uber das Hypertonie-Hyperglyka 'mie-Hyperurika' miesyndrom. Zentralbl Inn Med 1923;44:105–27.

[68] Vague J. La differenciation sexuelle, facteur determinant des formes de l'obesité. Presse Medl 1947;53:339–40.

[69] Avogaro P, Crepaldi G. Essential hyperlipidemia, obesity and diabetes. Diabetologia 1965;1:137.

[70] Reaven GM. Banting lecture 1988. Role of insulin resistance in human disease. Diabetes 1988;37(12):1595–607. Available from: https://doi.org/10.2337/diab.37.12.1595. PMID: 3056758.

[71] Oladejo AO. Overview of the metabolic syndrome; an emerging pandemic of public health significance. Ann Ib Postgrad Med 2011;9(2):78–82.

[72] Jayasinghe IU, Agampodi TC, Dissanayake AK, et al. Comparison of global definitions of metabolic syndrome in early pregnancy among the Rajarata Pregnancy Cohort participants in Sri Lanka. Sci Rep 2022;12:2009. Available from: https://doi.org/10.1038/s41598-022-05919-z.

[73] Grundy SM. Metabolic syndrome pandemic. Arterioscler Thromb Vasc Biol 2008;28(4):629–36 [Medline].21.

[74] Xu H, Li X, Adams H, Kubena K, Guo S. Etiology of metabolic syndrome and dietary intervention. Int J Mol Sci 2018;20(1) [Medline]. [Full Text].

[75] Saklayen MG. The global epidemic of the metabolic syndrome. Curr Hypertens Rep 2018;20(2):12.

[76] Kolovou GD, Anagnostopoulou KK, Salpea KD, et al. The prevalence of metabolic syndrome in various populations. Am J Med Sci 2007;333(6):362–71 [Medline].

[77] Hu G, Lindstrom J, Jousilahti P, et al. The increasing prevalence of metabolic syndrome among Finnish men and women over a decade. J Clin Endocrinol Metab 2008;93(3):832–6 [Medline].

[78] Erem C, Hacihasanoglu A, Deger O, et al. Prevalence of metabolic syndrome and associated risk factors among Turkish adults: Trabzon MetS study. Endocrine. 2008;33(1):9–20 [Medline].

[79] Mahadik SR, Deo SS, Mehtalia SD. Increased prevalence of metabolic syndrome in non-obese Asian Indian-an urban-rural comparison. Metab Syndr Relat Disord 2007;5(2):142–52 [Medline].

[80] Mokan M, Galajda P, Pridavkova D, et al. Prevalence of diabetes mellitus and metabolic syndrome in Slovakia. Diabetes Res Clin Pract 2008;81(2):238–42 [Medline].

[81] Malik M, Razig SA. The prevalence of the metabolic syndrome among the multiethnic population of the United Arab Emirates: a report of a national survey. Metab Syndr Relat Disord 2008;6(3):177–86 [Medline].

[82] Hoang KC, Le TV, Wong ND. The metabolic syndrome in East Asians. J Cardiometab Syndr 2007;2(4):276–82 [Medline].34.

[83] Hwang LC, Bai CH, Chen CJ. Prevalence of obesity and metabolic syndrome in Taiwan. J Formos Med Assoc 2006;105(8):626–35 [Medline].

[84] Nestel P, Lyu R, Low LP, et al. Metabolic syndrome: recent prevalence in East and Southeast Asian populations. Asia Pac J Clin Nutr 2007;16(2):362–7 [Medline].

[85] Dalal S, Beunza JJ, Volmink J, et al. Non-communicable diseases in sub-Saharan Africa: what we know now. Int J Epidemiol 2011;40:885–901.

[86] Oguoma VM, Nwose EU, Richards RS. Prevalence of cardio-metabolic syndrome in Nigeria: a systematic review. Public Health 2015;129:413–23.

[87] Ofori-Asenso R, Agyeman AA, Laar A. Metabolic syndrome in apparently "healthy" Ghanaian adults: a systematic review and meta-analysis. Int J Chronic Dis 2017;2017:1–9.

[88] Kaduka LU, Kombe Y, Kenya E, et al. Prevalence of metabolic syndrome among an urban population in Kenya. Diabetes Care 2012;35:887–93.
[89] Ford ES, Giles WH, Mokdad AH. Increasing prevalence of the metabolic syndrome among U.S. adults. Diabetes Care 2004;27(10):2444–9 [Medline].
[90] De Ferranti SD, Osganian SK. Epidemiology of paediatric metabolic syndrome and type 2 diabetes mellitus. Diab Vasc Dis Res 2007;4 (4):285–96 [Medline].
[91] Lovre D, Mauvais-Jarvis F. Trends in prevalence of the metabolic syndrome. JAMA. 2015;314(9):950 [Medline].
[92] Cussons AJ, Stuckey BG, Watts GF. Metabolic syndrome and cardiometabolic risk in PCOS. Curr Diab Rep 2007;7(1):66–73.
[93] Bentley-Lewis R, Koruda K, Seely EW. The metabolic syndrome in women. Nat Clin Pract Endocrinol Metab 2007;3(10):696–704 [Medline].
[94] Xue F, Michels KB. Diabetes, metabolic syndrome, and breast cancer: a review of the current evidence. Am J Clin Nutr 2007;86(3):s823–35 [Medline].
[95] Srinivasan M, Arzoun H, Gk LB, Thangaraj SR. A systematic review: does insulin resistance affect the risk and survival outcome of breast cancer in women? Cureus [Internet] 2022;14(1). Available from: https://www.cureus.com/articles/84608-a-systematic-review-does-insulin-resistance-affect-the-risk-and-survival-outcome-of-breast-cancer-in-women.
[96] Bhasin S, Jasjua GK, Pencina M, et al. Sex hormone-binding globulin, but not testosterone, is associated prospectively and independently with incident metabolic syndrome in men: the framingham heart study. Diabetes Care 2011;34(11):2464–70 [Medline]. [Full Text].
[97] Tsujimura A, Miyagawa Y, Takezawa K, et al. Is low testosterone concentration a risk factor for metabolic syndrome in healthy middle-aged men? Urology. 2013;82(4):814–19 [Medline].
[98] Xargay-Torrent S, Carreras-Badosa G, Borrat-Padrosa S, Prats-Puig A, Soriano P, ÁlvarezCastaño E, et al. Circulating sex hormone binding globulin: An integrating biomarker for an adverse cardio-metabolic profile in obese pregnant women. PLoS One 2018;13(10):e0205592. Available from: https://doi.org/10.1371/journal.pone.0205592.
[99] Banerjee D, Misra A. Does using ethnic specific criteria improve the usefulness of the term metabolic syndrome? Controversies and suggestions. Int J Obes (Lond) 2007;31(9):1340–9 [Medline].
[100] Okura T, Nakamura R, Fujioka Y, Kawamoto-Kitao S, Ito Y, Matsumoto K, et al. Body mass index ≥23 is a risk factor for insulin resistance and diabetes in Japanese people: A brief report. PLoS One 2018;13(7):e0201052.
[101] Ford ES, Giles WH, Dietz WH. Prevalence of the metabolic syndrome among US adults: findings from the third National Health and Nutrition Examination Survey. JAMA. 2002;287(3):356–9 [Medline].
[102] Clark LT, El-Atat F. Metabolic syndrome in African Americans: implications for preventing coronary heart disease. Clin Cardiol 2007;30 (4):161–4 [Medline].
[103] Petersen MC, Shulman GI. Mechanisms of insulin action and insulin resistance. Physiol Rev 2018;98(4):2133–223. Available from: https://doi.org/10.1152/physrev.00063.2017. PMID: 30067154. PMCID: PMC6170977.
[104] Perseghin G, Calori G, Lattuada G, Ragogna F, Dugnani E, Garancini MP, et al. Insulin resistance/hyperinsulinemia and cancer mortality: the Cremona study at the 15th year of follow-up. Acta Diabetol 2012;49:421–8. Available from: https://doi.org/10.1007/s00592-011-0361-2. PMID: 22215126. [CrossRef: 10.1007/s00592-011-0361-2].
[105] Bedinger DH, Adams SH. Metabolic, anabolic, and mitogenic insulin responses: a tissue-specific perspective for insulin receptor activators. Mol Cell Endocrinol 2015;415:143–56. Available from: https://doi.org/10.1016/j.mce.2015.08.013. PMID: 26277398. [CrossRef: 10.1016/j.mce.2015.08.013].
[106] Olefsky JM, Kolterman OG, Scarlett JA. Insulin action and resistance in obesity and noninsulindependent type II diabetes mellitus. Am J Physiol Endocrinol Metab 1982;243:E15–30. PMID: 7046470.
[107] Samuel VT, Shulman GI. Mechanisms for insulin resistance: common threads and missing links. Cell 2012;148:852–71. Available from: https://doi.org/10.1016/j.cell.2012.02.017. PMID: 22385956. [CrossRef: 10.1016/j.cell.2012.02.017].
[108] Kolterman OG, Gray RS, Griffin J, Burstein P, Insel J, Scarlett JA, et al. Receptor and postreceptor defects contribute to the insulin resistance in noninsulin-dependent diabetes mellitus. J Clin Invest 1981;68:957–69. Available from: https://doi.org/10.1172/JCI110350. PMID: 7287908. [CrossRef: 10.1172/JCI110350].
[109] Sims EAH, Danford E, Horton ES, Bray GA, Glennon JA, Salans LB. Endocrine and metabolic effects of experimental obesity in man. Recent Prog Horm Res 1973;29:457–96 11.
[110] DeFronzo RA, Tobin JD, Andres R. The glucose clamp technique: a method for quantifying insulin secretion and resistance. Am J Physiol 1979;6:E214–23.
[111] Ralph AD, Eleuterio F. Insulin resistance: a multifaceted syndrome responsible for NIDDM, obesity, hypertension, dyslipidemia, and atherosclerotic cardiovascular disease. Diabetes Care 1 1991;14(3):173–94. Available from: https://doi.org/10.2337/diacare.14.3.173.
[112] Erdmann J, Kallabis B, Oppel U, Sypchenko O, Wagenpfeil S, Schusdziarra V. Development of hyperinsulinemia and insulin resistance during the early stage of weight gain. Am J Physiology-Endocrinology Metab 2008;294(3):E568–75.
[113] Paoli A, Rubini A, Volek JS, Grimaldi KA. Beyondweight loss: a review of the therapeutic uses of very-lowcarbohydrate (ketogenic) diets. Eur J Clin Nutr 2013;67(8):789–96.
[114] Gershuni V, Yan S, Medici V. Nutritional ketosis for weight management and reversal of metabolic syndrome. Curr Nutr Rep 2018;7:97–106.
[115] Landsberg L, Krieger DR. Obesity, metabolism, and the sympathetic nervous system. Am J Hypertens 1989;2:1255–325.
[116] Lucas CP, Estigarribia JA, Darga LL, Reaven GM. Insulin and blood pressure in obesity. Hypertension. 1985;7:702–6.

[117] Modan M, Halkin H, Almog S, Lusky A, Eshkil A, Shefi M, et al. Hyperinsulinemia: a link between hypertension, obesity and glucose intolerance. J Clin Invest 1985;75:809−17.
[118] Ferrannini E, Buzzigoli G, Bonadona R. Insulin resistance in essential hypertension. N Engl J Med 1987;317:350−7.
[119] Shen DC, Shieh SM, Fuh M, Wu DA, Chen YD, Reaven GM. Resistance to insulin-stimulated glucose uptake in patients with hypertension. J Clin Endocrinol Metab 1988;66:580−3.
[120] Swislocki ALM, Hoffman BB, Reaven GM. Insulin resistance, glucose intolerance and hyperinsulinemia in patients with hypertension. Am J Hypertens 1989;2:419−23.
[121] Tarray R, Saleem S, Afroze D, Yousuf I, Gulnar A, Laway B, et al. Role of insulin resistance in essential hypertension. Cardiovascular Endocrinol 2014;3(4):129−33. Available from: https://doi.org/10.1097/XCE.0000000000000032.
[122] Ikeda T, Gomi T, Hirawa N, Sakurai J, Yoshikawa N. Improvement of insulin sensitivity contributes to blood pressure reduction after weight loss in hypertensive subjects with obesity. Hypertension. 1996;27(5):1180−6.
[123] Krotkiewski M, Mandroukas K, Sjostrom L, Sullivan L, Wetterqvist H, Bjorntorp P. Effects of long-term physical training on body fat, metabolism, and blood pressure in obesity. Metabolism 1979;28:650−8.
[124] DeFronzo RA. Insulin secretion, insulin resistance, and obesity. Int I Obes 1982;6(1):72−82.
[125] Silva A, Carmo J, Li X, Wang Z, Mouton A, Hall J. Role of hyperinsulinemia and insulin resistance in hypertension: metabolic syndrome revisited. Can J Cardiology 2020;36 Feb 1.
[126] Zhou MS, Wang A, Yu H. Link between insulin resistance and hypertension: What is the evidence from evolutionary biology? Diabetology & Metab Syndrome 2014;6(1):12.
[127] Brands Michael W. Role of insulin-mediated antinatriuresis in sodium homeostasis and hypertension. Hypertension. 2018;72(6):1255−62.
[128] DeFronzo RA. The effect of insulin on renal sodium metabolism. Diabetologia. 1981;21(3):165−71.
[129] Unwin DJ, Tobin SD, Murray SW, Delon C, Brady AJ. Substantial and sustained improvements in blood pressure, weight and lipid profiles from a carbohydrate restricted diet: an observational study of insulin resistant patients in primary care. Int J Env Res Public Health 2019;16 (15):2680. Available from: https://doi.org/10.3390/ijerph16152680. PMID: 31357547. PMCID: PMC6695889.
[130] Cruz AB, Amatuzio DS, Grande F, Hay LJ. Effect of intraarterial insulin on tissue cholesterol and fatty acids in alloxan-diabetic dogs. Ore Res 1961;9:39−43.
[131] Brayden JE, Halpern W, Brann LR. Biochemical and mechanical properties of resistance arteries from normotensive and hypertensive rats. Hypertension 1983;5:17−25.
[132] Ooshima A, Fuller GC, Cardinale GJ, Spector S, Udenfriend S. Increased collagen synthesis in blood vessels of hypertensive rats and its reversal by antihypertensive agents. Proc Natl Acad Sci USA 1974;71:3019−23.
[133] Mir MM, Mir R, Alghamdi MAA, Wani JI, Sabah ZU, Jeelani M, et al. Differential association of selected adipocytokines, adiponectin, leptin, resistin, visfatin and chemerin, with the pathogenesis and progression of type 2 diabetes mellitus (T2DM) in the asir region of Saudi Arabia: a case control study. J Personalized Med 2022;12(5):735.
[134] Korac B, Kalezic A, Pekovic-Vaughan V, Korac A, Jankovic A. Redox changes in obesity, metabolic syndrome, and diabetes. Redox Biol 2021;42:101887. Available from: https://doi.org/10.1016/j.redox.2021.101887. Epub 2021 Feb 4. PMID: 33579666. PMCID: PMC8113039.
[135] Kim JA, Wei Y, Sowers JR. Role of mitochondrial dysfunction in insulin resistance Circulation Res 2008;102:401−14PMID. PMID: 18309108.
[136] Halliwell B, Gutteridge JMC. Free Radicals in Biology and Medicine. 4th ed. Oxford: Oxford University Press; 2007.
[137] Chistiakov DA, Sobenin IA, Revin VV, Orekhov AN, Bobryshev YV. Mitochondrial aging and age-related dysfunction of mitochondria BioMed Res Int 2014;2014. PMID: 238463. PMID: 24818134.
[138] Valko M, Rhodes CJ, Moncol J, Izakovic M, Mazur M. Free radicals, metals and antioxidants in oxidative stress-induced cancer. Chemico-biological Interact 2006;160:1−40. PMID: 16430879.
[139] Youle RJ, van der Bliek AM. Mitochondrial fission, fusion, and stress. Science 2012;337(6098):1062−5. Available from: https://doi.org/10.1126/science.1219855. PMID: 22936770. PMCID: PMC4762028.
[140] Barnham KJ, Masters CL, Bush AI. Neurodegenerative diseases and oxidative stress. Nat Rev Drug discovery 2004;3:205−14. PMID: 15031734.
[141] Roberts CK, Sindhu KK. Oxidative stress and metabolic syndrome. Life Sci 2009;84:705−12. PMID: 19281826.
[142] Nojiri H, Shimizu T, Funakoshi M, Yamaguchi O, Zhou H, Kawakami S, et al. Oxidative stress causes heart failure with impaired mitochondrial respiration. J Biol Chem 2006;281:33789−801. PMID: 16959785.
[143] Otani H. Oxidative stress as pathogenesis of cardiovascular risk associated with metabolic syndrome. Antioxid & redox Signal 2011;15:1911−26. PMID: 21126197.
[144] Ozgen IT, Tascilar ME, Bilir P, Boyraz M, Guncikan MN, Akay C, et al. Oxidative stress in obese children and its relation with insulin resistance. J pediatric Endocrinol & metabolism: JPEM 2012;25:261−6. PMID: 22768654.
[145] Poitout V, Tanaka Y, Reach G, Robertson RP. Stress oxydatif, insulinosécrétion, et insulinorésistance [Oxidative stress, insulin secretion, and insulin resistance]. Journ Annu Diabetol Hotel Dieu. 2001:75−86. French. PMID: 11565471.
[146] Zephy D, Ahmad J. Type 2 diabetes mellitus: role of melatonin and oxidative stress. Diabetes & Metab syndrome: Clin Res & Rev 2015;9 (2):127−31.
[147] Cumbie BC, Hermayer KL. Current concepts in targeted therapies for the pathophysiology of diabetic microvascular complications. Vasc Health Risk Manag 2007;3:823−32.

[148] Lastra G, Whaley-Connell A, Manrique C, Habibi J, Gutweiler AA, Appesh L, et al. Low-dose spironolactone reduces reactive oxygen species generation and improves insulin-stimulated glucose transport in skeletal muscle in the TG (mRen2) 27 rat. Am J Physiology-Endocrinology Metab 2008;295(1):E110–16.

[149] Marí M, Morales A, Colell A, García-Ruiz C, Fernández-Checa JC. Mitochondrial glutathione, a key survival antioxidant. Antioxid & Redox Signal 2009;11(11):2685–700. Available from: https://doi.org/10.1089/ars.2009.2695.

[150] Randle PJ, Garland PB, Hales CN, Newsholme EA. The glucose fatty-acid cycle its role in insulin sensitivity and the metabolic disturbances of diabetes mellitus. Lancet 1963;281:785–9. Available from: https://doi.org/10.1016/S0140-6736(63). 91500-9.

[151] Evans JL, Goldfine ID, Maddux BA, Grodsky GM. Oxidative stress and stress-activated signaling pathways: a unifying hypothesis of type 2 diabetes. Endocr Rev 2002;23:599–622. Available from: https://doi.org/10.1210/er.2001-0039.

[152] Liu VW, Huang PL. Cardiovascular roles of nitric oxide: a review of insights from nitric oxide synthase gene disrupted mice. Cardiovasc Res 2008;77(1):19–29. Available from: https://doi.org/10.1016/j.cardiores.2007.06.024. PMID: 17658499. PMCID: PMC2731989.

[153] Kelly RA, Balligand JL, Smith TW. Nitric oxide and cardiac function. Circulation Res 1996;79(3):363–80.

[154] https://derangedphysiology.com/required-reading/infectious-diseases-antibiotics-and-sepsis/Chapter%20131/significance-endothelial-glycocalyx.

[155] Kobayashi Jun. Nitric oxide and insulin resistance. Immunoendocrinology 2015;2657. Available from: https://doi.org/10.14800/Immunoendocrinology.657.

[156] Hartge MM, Unger T, Kintscher U. The endothelium and vascular inflammation in diabetes. Diabetes Vasc Dis Res 2007;4(2):84–8.

[157] Litvinova L, Atochin DN, Fattakhov N, Vasilenko M, Zatolokin P, Kirienkova E. Nitric oxide and mitochondria in metabolic syndrome. Front Physiol 2015;6:20 Feb 17.

[158] Greco T, Glenn TC, Hovda DA, Prins ML. Ketogenic diet decreases oxidative stress and improves mitochondrial respiratory complex activity. J Cereb Blood Flow Metab 2016;36(9):1603–13.

[159] Tabassum H, Parvez S. Chapter 20 – Curcumin and mitochondria In: de Oliveira MR, editor. Mitochondrial Physiology and Vegetal Molecules [Internet]. Academic Press; 2021. p. 439–54[cited 2022 Jun 20]. Available from: https://www.sciencedirect.com/science/article/pii/B9780128215623000502.

[160] Lakka TA, Laaksonen DE, Lakka HM, Mannikko N, Niskanen LK, Rauramaa R, et al. Sedentary lifestyle, poor cardiorespiratory fitness, and the metabolic syndrome. Med Sci Sports Exerc 2003;35:1279–86. PMID: 12900679.

[161] Poehlman ET, Dvorak RV, DeNino WF, Brochu M, Ades PA. Effects of resistance training and endurance training on insulin sensitivity in nonobese, young women: A controlled randomized trial. J Clin Endocrinol Metab 2000;85:2463–8. PMID: 10902794.

[162] Polak J, Moro C, Klimcakova E, Hejnova J, Majercik M, Viguerie N, et al. Dynamic strength training improves insulin sensitivity and functional balance between adrenergic alpha 2A and beta pathways in subcutaneous adipose tissue of obese subjects. Diabetologia. 2005;48:2631–40. PMID: 16273345.

[163] Kriska AM, Pereira MA, Hanson RL, de Courten MP, Zimmet PZ, Alberti KG, et al. Association of physical activity and serum insulin concentrations in two populations at high risk for type 2 diabetes but differing by BMI. Diabetes Care 2001;24:1175–80. PMID: 11423498.

[164] Roberts CK, Hevener AL, Barnard RJ. Metabolic syndrome and insulin resistance: underlying causes and modification by exercise training. Compr Physiol 2013;3(1):1–58. Available from: https://doi.org/10.1002/cphy.c110062. PMID: 23720280. PMCID: PMC4129661.

[165] Jurca R, Lamonte MJ, Church TS, Earnest CP, Fitzgerald SJ, Barlow CE, et al. Associations of muscle strength and fitness with metabolic syndrome in men. MedSci Sports Exerc 2004;36:1301–7. PMID: 15292736.

[166] Dai DF, Chiao YA, Marcinek DJ, Szeto HH, Rabinovitch PS. Mitochondrial oxidative stress in aging and healthspan. Longev & Healthspan 2014;3(1):6.

[167] Miller VJ, Villamena FA, Volek JS. Nutritional ketosis and mitohormesis: potential implications for mitochondrial function and human health. J Nutr Metab 2018;2018:5157645. Available from: https://doi.org/10.1155/2018/5157645. PMID: 29607218. PMCID: PMC5828461.

[168] Tapia PC. Sublethal mitochondrial stress with an attendant stoichiometric augmentation of reactive oxygen species may precipitate many of the beneficial alterations in cellular physiology produced by caloric restriction, intermittent fasting, exercise and dietary phytonutrients: "Mitohormesis" for health and vitality. Med Hypotheses 2006;66(4):832–43.

[169] Ristow M, Zarse K. How increased oxidative stress promotes longevity and metabolic health: the concept of mitochondrial hormesis (mitohormesis). Exp Gerontology 2010;45(6):410–18.

[170] Ristow M, Schmeisser K. Mitohormesis: promoting health and lifespan by increased levels of Reactive Oxygen Species (ROS). Dose Response 2014;12(2):288–341.

[171] Simi B, Sempore B, Mayet MH, Favier RJ. Additiveeffects of training and high-fat diet on energy metabolism during exercise. J Appl Physiol 1991;71(1):197–203.

[172] Stenvers DJ, Scheer FAJL, Schrauwen P, la Fleur SE, Kalsbeek A. Circadian clocks and insulin resistance. Nat Rev Endocrinol 2019;15:75–89. Available from: https://doi.org/10.1038/s41574-018-0122-1.

[173] Kolbe I, Leinweber B, Brandenburger M, Oster H. Circadian clock network desynchrony promotes weight gain and alters glucose homeostasis in mice. Mol Metab 2019;30:140–51. Available from: https://doi.org/10.1016/j.molmet.2019.09.012.

[174] Chaix A, Lin T, Le HD, Chang MW, Panda S. Time-restricted feeding prevents obesity and metabolic syndrome in mice lacking a circadian clock. Cell Metab 2019;29:303–19. Available from: https://doi.org/10.1016/j.cmet.2018.08.004. e4.

[175] Garbarino S, Magnavita N. Sleep problems are a strong predictor of stress-related metabolic changes in police officers. A prospective study. PLoS One 2019;14(10):e0224259. Available from: https://doi.org/10.1371/journal.pone.0224259.

[176] Panda, S.: The Circadian Code: Lose weight, supercharge your energy and sleep well every night. Random House; 2018.

[177] Bhatti JS, Bhatti GK, Reddy PH. Mitochondrial dysfunction and oxidative stress in metabolic disorders – A step towards mitochondria based therapeutic strategies. Biochim Biophys Acta Mol Basis Dis 1863;2017(5):1066–77. Available from: https://doi.org/10.1016/j.bbadis.2016.11.010.

[178] Sharma N, Arias EB, Bhat AD, Sequea DA, Ho S, Croff KK, et al. Mechanisms for increased insulin-stimulated Akt phosphorylation and glucose uptake in fast- and slow-twitch skeletal muscles of calorie-restricted rats. Am J Physiol Endocrinol Metab 2011;300:E966–78. PMID: 21386065.

[179] Kemnitz JW, Roecker EB, Weindruch R, Elson DF, Baum ST, Bergman RN. Dietary restriction increases insulin sensitivity and lowers blood glucose in rhesus monkeys. Am J Physiol 1994;266:E540–7. PMID: 8178974.

[180] Chung N, Park J, Lim K. The effects of exercise and cold exposure on mitochondrial biogenesis in skeletal muscle and white adipose tissue. J Exerc Nutr Biochem 2017;21(2):39–47. Available from: https://doi.org/10.20463/jenb.2017.0020.

[181] Ihsan M, Markworth JF, Watson G, Choo HC, Govus A, Pham T, et al. Regular postexercise cooling enhances mitochondrial biogenesis through AMPK and p38 MAPK in human skeletal muscle. Am J Physiol Regulatory Integr Comp Physiol 2015;309(3):R286–94. Available from: https://doi.org/10.1152/ajpregu.00031.2015.

[182] Liang H, Ward WF. PGC-1: a key regulator of energy metabolism. Adv Physiol Educ 2006;30(4):145–51. Available from: https://doi.org/10.1152/advan.00052.2006.

[183] Jansk L, ?avlkov J, Vybral S. Human physiological responses to immersion into water of different temperatures. Eur J Appl Physiol 2000;81(5):436–42. Available from: https://doi.org/10.1007/s004210050065.

[184] Sidossis L, Kajimura S. Brown and beige fat in humans: thermogenic adipocytes that control energy and glucose homeostasis. J Clin Investigation 2015;125(2):478–86. Available from: https://doi.org/10.1172/jci78362.

[185] Ruiz, Jonatan R, Martinez-Tellez Borja, Sanchez-Delgado Guillermo, Osuna-Prieto Francisco J, Rensen Patrick CN, et al. Role of human brown fat in obesity, metabolism and cardiovascular disease: strategies to turn up the heat. Prog Cardiovascular Dis 2018;61(2):232–45. Available from: https://doi.org/10.1016/j.pcad.2018.07.002.

[186] Yoneshiro T, Aita S, Matsushita M, Kayahara T, Kameya T, Kawai Y, et al. Recruited brown adipose tissue as an antiobesity agent in humans. J Clin Investigation 2013;123(8):3404–8. Available from: https://doi.org/10.1172/jci67803.

[187] Hanssen MJW, van der Lans AAJJ, Brans B, Hoeks J, Jardon KMC, Schaart G, et al. Short-term cold acclimation recruits brown adipose tissue in obese humans. Diabetes 2015;65(5):1179–89. Available from: https://doi.org/10.2337/db15-1372. December.

[188] Choi YJ, Jeon SM, Shin S. Impact of a ketogenic diet on metabolic parameters in patients with obesity or overweight and with or without type 2 diabetes: a meta-analysis of randomized controlled trials. Nutrients 2020;12(7). Available from: https://doi.org/10.3390/nu12072005. 2005. Published 2020 Jul 6.

[189] Bueno NB, de Melo IS, de Oliveira SL, da Rocha Ataide T. Very-low-carbohydrate ketogenic diet v. low-fat diet for long-term weight loss: a meta-analysis of randomised controlled trials. Br J Nutr 2013;110(7):1178–87.

[190] Santos FL, Esteves SS, da Costa Pereira A, Yancy Jr. WS, Nunes JP. Systematic review and meta-analysis of clinical trials of the effects of low carbohydrate diets on cardiovascular risk factors. Obes Rev 2012;13:1048–66.

[191] Yumuk V, Tsigos C, Fried M, Schindler K, Busetto L, Micic D, et al. European Guidelines for obesity management in adults. Erratum in: Obes Facts 2015;8(6):402–24. Available from: https://doi.org/10.1159/000442721. Epub 2015 Dec 5. PMID: 26641646. PMCID: PMC5644856.

[192] Strychar I. Diet in the management of weight loss. CMAJ 2006;174:56–63.

[193] Westman EC, et al. Low-carbohydrate nutrition and metabolism. Am J Clin Nutr 2007;86:276–84.

[194] Dowis K, Banga S. The potential health benefits of the ketogenic diet: a narrative review. Nutrients 2021;13(5):1654. Available from: https://doi.org/10.3390/nu13051654. PMID: 34068325. PMCID: PMC8153354.

[195] Yuan X, Wang J, Yang S, Gao M, Cao L, Li X, et al. Effect of the ketogenic diet on glycemic control, insulin resistance, and lipid metabolism in patients with T2DM: a systematic review and meta-analysis. Nutr & Diabetes 2020;10(1):1–8.

[196] Meng Y, Bai H, Wang S, Li Z, Wang Q, Chen L. Efficacy of low carbohydrate diet for type 2 diabetes mellitus management: A systematic review and meta-analysis of randomized controlled trials. Diabetes Res Clin Pract 2017;131:124–31 Sep 1.

[197] Volek JS, Phinney SD, Forsythe CE, et al. Carbohydrate restriction has a more favorable impact on the metabolic syndrome than a low fat diet. Lipids 2009;44:297–309.

[198] Gavidia K, Kalayjian T. Treating diabetes utilizing a low carbohydrate ketogenic diet and intermittent fasting without significant weight loss: a case report. Front Nutr 2021;8:687081.

[199] Krauss RM. Dietary and genetic probes of atherogenic dyslipidemia. Arterioscler Thromb Vasc Biol 2005;25(11):2265–72.

[200] Feinman RD, Pogozelski WK, Astrup A, et al. Dietarycarbohydrate restriction as the 8rst approach in diabetes management: critical review and evidence base. Nutrition 2015;31(1):1–13.

[201] Hamanaka RB, Chandel NS. Mitochondrial reactive oxygen species regulate cellular signaling and dictate biological outcomes. Trends Biochemical Sci 2010;35(9):505–13.

[202] Besse-Patin A, Estall JL. An intimate relationship between ROS and insulin signalling: implications for antioxidant treatment of fatty liver disease. Int J Cell Biol 2014;2014:e519153 Feb 12.

[203] Schrauwen P, van Marken Lichtenbelt WD, Saris WH, Westerterp KR. Role of glycogen-lowering exercise in the change of fat oxidation in response to a high-fat diet. Am J Physiology-Endocrinology Metab 1997;273(3):E623–9.

[204] Garcia-Roves P, Huss JM, Han DH, et al. Raising plasma fatty acid concentration induces increased biogenesis of mitochondria in skeletal muscle. Proc Natl Acad Sci 2007;104(25):10709–13.

[205] Deleted in review.

[206] Shimazu T, Hirschey MD, Newman J, et al. Suppression of oxidative stress by β- hydroxybutyrate, an endogenous histone deacetylase inhibitor. Science 2013;339(6116):211–14.

[207] Nagao M, Toh R, Irino Y, et al. β-Hydroxybutyrate elevation as a compensatory response against oxidative stress in cardiomyocytes. Biochemical Biophysical Res Commun 2016;475(4):322–8.

[208] Tanegashima K, Sato-Miyata Y, Funakoshi M, Nishito Y, Aigaki T, Hara T. Epigenetic regulation of the glucose transporter gene Slc2a1 by β-hydroxybutyrate underlies preferential glucose supply to the brain of fasted mice. Genes Cell 2017;22(1):71–83.

[209] Simeone TA, Simeone KA, Rho JM. Ketone bodies as anti-seizure agents. Neurochem Res 2017;42(7):2011–18.

[210] Haces ML, Hernandez-Fonseca K, Medina-Campos ON, Montiel T, Pedraza-Chaverri J, Massieu L. Antioxidant capacity contributes to protection of ketone bodies against oxidative damage induced during hypoglycemic conditions. Exp Neurol 2008;211(1):85–96.

[211] Kim DY, Davis LM, Sullivan PG, et al. Ketone bodies are protective against oxidative stress in neocortical neurons. J Neurochemistry 2007;101(5):1316–26.

[212] Paoli A. Ketogenic diet for obesity: friend or foe? Int J Environ Res Public Health 2014;11(2):2092–107.

[213] McKenzie AL, Hallberg SJ, Creighton BC, et al. A novel intervention including individualized nutritional recommendations reduces hemoglobin A1c level, medication use, and weight in type 2 diabetes. JMIR Diabetes 2017;2(1):14.

[214] Feinman RD, Volek JS. Carbohydrate restriction as the default treatment for type 2 diabetes and metabolic syndrome. Scand Cardiovascular J 2008;42(4):256–63.

[215] Cotter DG, Schugar RC, Crawford PA. Ketone body metabolism and cardiovascular disease. Am J Physiol-Heart Circulatory Physiology 2013;304(8):H1060–76.

[216] Branco AF, Ferreira A, Simoes RF, et al. Ketogenic diets: from cancer to mitochondrial diseases and beyond. Eur J Clin Investigation 2016;46 (3):285–98.

[217] Oliveira CL, Mattingly S, Schirrmacher R, Sawyer MB, Fine EJ, Prado CM. A Nutritional perspective of ketogenic diet in cancer: a narrative review. J Acad Nutr Dietetics 2017; in press.

[218] Simone BA, Champ CE, Rosenberg AL, et al. Selectively starving cancer cells through dietary manipulation: methods and clinical implications. Future Oncol 2013;9(7):959–76.

[219] Seyfried TN, Marsh J, Shelton LM, Huysentruyt LC, Mukherjee P. Is the restricted ketogenic diet a viable alternative to the standard of care for managing malignant brain cancer? Epilepsy Res 2012;100(3):310–26.

[220] Fine EJ, Feinman RD. Insulin, carbohydrate restriction, metabolic syndrome and cancer. Expert Rev Endocrinol & Metab 2014;10(1):15–24.

[221] Moreno CL, Mobbs CV. Epigenetic mechanisms underlying lifespan and age-related eects of dietary restriction and the ketogenic diet. Mol Cell Endocrinol 2017;455:33–40.

[222] Edwards C, Copes N, Bradshaw PC. D-β-hydroxybutyrate: an anti-aging ketone body. Oncotarget 2015;6(6):3477–8.

[223] Veech RL, Bradshaw PC, Clarke K, Curtis W, Pawlosky R, King MT. Ketone bodies mimic the life span extending properties of caloric restriction. IUBMB Life 2017;69(5):305–14.

[224] Volek JS, and Phinney SD, The Art and Science of Low Carbohydrate Performance, Beyond Obesity, LLC, Miami, FL, USA, 2012.

[225] Rizza RA. Pathogenesis of fasting and postprandial hyperglycemia in type 2 diabetes: implications for therapy. Diabetes 2010;59 (11):2697–707.

[226] American Diabetes Association. Classification and diagnosis of diabetes: standards of medical care in diabetes-2020. Diabetes Care 2020;43 (Suppl 1):S14–31.

[227] Tabak AG, Jokela M, Akbaraly TN, Brunner EJ, Kivimaki M, Witte DR. Trajectories of glycaemia, insulin sensitivity, and insulin secretion before diagnosis of type 2 diabetes: an analysis from the Whitehall II study. Lancet 2009;373(9682):2215–21.

[228] Khaw KT, Wareham N, Luben R, Bingham S, Oakes S, Welch A, et al. Glycated haemoglobin, diabetes, and mortality in men in Norfolk cohort of european prospective investigation of cancer and nutrition (EPIC-Norfolk). BMJ 2001;322(7277):15–18.

[229] Khaw KT, Wareham N, Bingham S, Luben R, Welch A, Day N. Association of hemoglobin A1c with cardiovascular disease and mortality in adults: the European prospective investigation into cancer in Norfolk. Ann Intern Med 2004;141(6):413–20.

[230] Selvin E, Coresh J, Golden SH, Brancati FL, Folsom AR, Steffes MW. Glycemic control and coronary heart disease risk in persons with and without diabetes: the atherosclerosis risk in communities study. Arch Intern Med 2005;165(16):1910–16.

[231] Barr EL, Boyko EJ, Zimmet PZ, Wolfe R, Tonkin AM, Shaw JE. Continuous relationships between non-diabetic hyperglycaemia and both cardiovascular disease and all-cause mortality: the Australian Diabetes, Obesity, and Lifestyle (AusDiab) study. Diabetologia 2009;52 (3):415–24.

[232] Garg N, Moorthy N, Kapoor A, Tewari S, Kumar S, Sinha A, et al. Hemoglobin a1c in nondiabetic patients: an independent predictor of coronary artery disease and its severity. Mayo Clin Proc Mayo Clin 2014;89(7):908–16.

[233] Matheus AS, Tannus LR, Cobas RA, Palma CC, Negrato CA, Gomes MB. Impact of diabetes on cardiovascular disease: an update. Int J hypertension 2013;2013:653789.

[234] Brownlee M. The pathobiology of diabetic complications: a unifying mechanism. Diabetes. 2005;54(6):1615–25.

[235] Giugliano D, Ceriello A, Esposito K. Glucose metabolism and hyperglycemia. Am J Clin Nutr 2008;87(1):217S–222SS.

[236] Giacco F, Brownlee M. Oxidative stress and diabetic complications. Circulation Res 2010;107(9):1058–70.

[237] Faxon DP, Fuster V, Libby P, Beckman JA, Hiatt WR, Thompson RW, et al. Atherosclerotic Vascular Disease Conference: Writing Group III: pathophysiology. Circulation 2004;109(21):2617–25.

[238] Hansson GK, Libby P, Tabas I. Inflammation and plaque vulnerability. J Intern Med 2015;278(5):483–93.

[239] El-Osta A, Brasacchio D, Yao D, Pocai A, Jones PL, Roeder RG, et al. Transient high glucose causes persistent epigenetic changes and altered gene expression during subsequent normoglycemia. The Journal of experimental medicine 2008;205(10):2409–17.

[240] Rossetti L, Giaccari A, DeFronzo RA. Glucose toxicity. Diabetes Care 1990;13(6):610–30.

[241] Robertson RP, Harmon J, Tran PO, Poitout V. Beta-cell glucose toxicity, lipotoxicity, and chronic oxidative stress in type 2 diabetes. Diabetes 2004;53(Suppl 1):S119–24.

[242] Giaccari A, Sorice G, Muscogiuri G. Glucose toxicity: the leading actor in the pathogenesis and clinical history of type 2 diabetes - mechanisms and potentials for treatment. Nutr Metab Cardiovasc Dis 2009;19(5):365–77.

[243] Saeedi P, Petersohn I, Salpea P, Malanda B, Karuranga S, Unwin N, et al. Global and regional diabetes prevalence estimates for 2019 and projections for 2030 and 2045: Results from the International Diabetes Federation Diabetes Atlas, 9(th) edition. Diabetes Res Clin Pract 2019;157:107843.

[244] Sainsbury E, Kizirian NV, Partridge SR, Gill T, Colagiuri S, Gibson AA. Effect of dietary carbohydrate restriction on glycemic control in adults with diabetes: A systematic review and meta-analysis. Diabetes Res Clin Pract 2018;139:239–52.

[245] Snorgaard O, Poulsen GM, Andersen HK, Astrup A. Systematic review and meta-analysis of dietary carbohydrate restriction in patients with type 2 diabetes. BMJ open diabetes Res & care 2017;5(1):e000354.

[246] van Zuuren EJ, Fedorowicz Z, Kuijpers T, Pijl H. Effects of low-carbohydrate- compared with low-fat-diet interventions on metabolic control in people with type 2 diabetes: a systematic review including GRADE assessments. Am J Clin Nutr 2018;108(2):300–31.

[247] Goldenberg JZ, Day A, Brinkworth GD, Sato J, Yamada S, Jonsson T, et al. Efficacy and safety of low and very low carbohydrate diets for type 2 diabetes remission: systematic review and meta-analysis of published and unpublished randomized trial data. BMJ 2021;372:m4743.

[248] Feinman RD, Pogozelski WK, Astrup A, Bernstein RK, Fine EJ, Westman EC, et al. Dietary Carbohydrate restriction as the first approach in diabetes management. Critical review and evidence base. Nutrition 2014.

[249] Noakes TD, Windt J. Evidence that supports the prescription of low-carbohydrate high-fat diets: a narrative review. Br J Sports Med 2016;51:133–9.

[250] Brouns F. Overweight and diabetes prevention: is a low-carbohydrate-high-fat diet recommendable? Eur J Nutr 2018;57(4):1301–12.

[251] Athinarayanan SJ, Adams RN, Hallberg SJ, McKenzie AL, Bhanpuri NH, Campbell WW, et al. Long-term effects of a novel continuous remote care intervention including nutritional ketosis for the management of type 2 diabetes: a 2-year non-randomized clinical trial. Front Endocrinol 2019;10:348.

[252] Unwin D, Khalid AA, Unwin J, et al. Insights from a general practice service evaluation supporting a lower carbohydrate diet in patients with type 2 diabetes mellitus and prediabetes: a secondary analysis of routine clinic data including HbA1c, weight and prescribing over 6 years. BMJ Nutr Prev Health 2020;3(2):285–94. Available from: https://doi.org/10.1136/bmjnph-2020-000072.

[253] Lean M, Leslie WS, Barnes AC, et al. Primary care-led weight management for remission of type 2 diabetes (DiRECT): an open-label, cluster-randomised trial. Lancet 2018;10391(10120):541–51. Available from: https://doi.org/10.1016/S0140-6736(17)33102-1. Epub 2017 Dec 5.

[254] Stratton IM. Association of glycaemia with macrovascular and microvascular complications of type 2 diabetes (UKPDS 35): prospective observational study. BMJ 2000;321(7258):405–12. Available from: https://doi.org/10.1136/bmj.321.7258.405.

[255] Action to Control Cardiovascular Risk in Diabetes Study Group. Effects of intensive glucose lowering in type 2 diabetes. N Engl J Med 2008;358(24):2545–59. Available from: https://doi.org/10.1056/NEJMoa0802743.

[256] Zoungas S, Chalmers J, Neal B, et al. Follow-up of blood-pressure lowering and glucose control in type 2 diabetes. N Engl J Med 2014;371 (15):1392–406. Available from: https://doi.org/10.1056/NEJMoa1407963.

[257] Hayward RA, Reaven PD, Wiitala WL, et al. Follow-up of glycemic control and cardiovascular outcomes in type 2 diabetes. N Engl J Med 2015;372(23):2197–206. Available from: https://doi.org/10.1056/NEJMoa1414266.

[258] Gerstein HC, Bosch J, Dagenais GR, et al. Basal insulin and cardiovascular and other outcomes in dysglycemia. N Engl J Med 2012;367 (4):319–28. Available from: https://doi.org/10.1056/NEJMoa1203858.

[259] Green JB, Bethel MA, Armstrong PW, et al. Effect of sitagliptin on cardiovascular outcomes in type 2 diabetes. N Engl J Med 2015;373 (3):232–42. Available from: https://doi.org/10.1056/NEJMoa1501352.

[260] Hirshberg B, Katz A. Insights from cardiovascular outcome trials with novel antidiabetes agents: What have we learned? An industry perspective. Curr Diab Rep 2015;15(11):87. Available from: https://doi.org/10.1007/s11892-015-0663-9.

[261] Scirica BM, Bhatt DL, Braunwald E, et al. Saxagliptin and cardiovascular outcomes in patients with type 2 diabetes mellitus. N Engl J Med 2013;369(14):1317–26. Available from: https://doi.org/10.1007/s11892-015-0663-9.

[262] Chan JCN, Lim L-L, Wareham NJ, et al. The Lancet Commission on diabetes, using data to transform diabetes care and patient lives. Lancet 2021;396(10267):2019–82. Available from: https://doi.org/10.1016/S0140-6736(20)32374-6.

[263] Westman EC, Volek JS, Phinney SD. New Atkins for a NEW You: The Ultimate Diet for Shedding Weight and Feeling Great. Random House; 2010.

[264] Nuttall FQ, Gannon MC. Metabolic response of people with type 2 diabetes to a high protein diet. Nutr & Metab 2004;1:6. Available from: https://doi.org/10.1186/1743-7075-1-6.

[265] Unwin D, Haslam D, Livesey G. It is the glycaemic response to, not the carbohydrate content of food that matters in diabetes and obesity: The glycaemic index revisited. J Insulin Resistance 2016;1(1):9.

[266] Nuttall F, Almokayyad R, Gannon M. Comparison of a carbohydrate-free diet vs. fasting on plasma glucose, insulin and glucagon in type 2 diabetes. Metabolism. 2014;64 Oct 8.

[267] Jameson GW E. The Drinking Man's Diet. Cameron & Co: San Francisco; 1964.

[268] Noakes TDC SA, Proudfoot J, Greer D. The Real Meal Revolution. 2nd Edn ed Cape Town, South Africa: Quivertree Publications; 2013. p. 293.

[269] Farmer AJ, Perera R, Ward A, Heneghan C, Oke J, Barnett AH, et al. Meta-analysis of individual patient data in randomised trials of self monitoring of blood glucose in people with non-insulin treated type 2 diabetes. BMJ. 2012;344:e486.

[270] Polonsky WH, Fisher L, Schikman CH, Hinnen DA, Parkin CG, Jelsovsky Z, et al. Structured self-monitoring of blood glucose significantly reduces A1C levels in poorly controlled, noninsulin-treated type 2 diabetes: results from the Structured Testing Program study. Diabetes Care 2011;34 (2):262–7.

[271] Polonsky WH, Fisher L, Schikman CH, Hinnen DA, Parkin CG, Jelsovsky Z, et al. A structured self-monitoring of blood glucose approach in type 2 diabetes encourages more frequent, intensive, and effective physician interventions: results from the STeP study. Diabetes Technol & therapeutics 2011;13(8):797–802.

[272] Bosi E, Scavini M, Ceriello A, Cucinotta D, Tiengo A, Marino R, et al. Intensive structured self-monitoring of blood glucose and glycemic control in noninsulin-treated type 2 diabetes: the PRISMA randomized trial. Diabetes Care 2013;36(10):2887–94.

[273] Krezowski PA, Nuttall FQ, Gannon MC, Billington CJ, Parker S. Insulin and glucose responses to various starch-containing foods in type II diabetic subjects. Diabetes Care 1987;10(2):205–12.

[274] Gannon MC, Nuttall FQ. Control of blood glucose in type 2 diabetes without weight loss by modification of diet composition. Nutr & Metab 2006;3:16.

[275] Nuttall FQ, Schweim K, Hoover H, Gannon MC. Effect of the LoBAG30 diet on blood glucose control in people with type 2 diabetes. Br J Nutr 2008;99(3):511–19.

[276] Bolli GB, Gerich JE. The "dawn phenomenon" – a common occurrence in both non-insulin-dependent and insulin-dependent diabetes mellitus. N Engl J Med 1984;310(12):746–50.

[277] Porcellati F, Lucidi P, Bolli GB, Fanelli CG. Thirty years of research on the dawn phenomenon: lessons to optimize blood glucose control in diabetes. Diabetes Care 2013;36(12):3860–2.

[278] Reyhanoglu G, Rehman A. Somogyi Phenomenon StatPearls [Internet]. Treasure Island (FL). StatPearls Publishing; 2022[cited 2022 Jun 27]. Available from: http://www.ncbi.nlm.nih.gov/books/NBK551525/.

[279] Harvey Cjdc SG, Zinn C, Thornley S. Effects of differing levels of carbohydrate restriction on mood achievement of nutritional ketosis, and symptoms of carbohydrate withdrawal in healthy adults: A randomized clinical trial. Nutrition: X 2019;.

[280] Hannou SA, Haslam DE, McKeown NM, Herman MA. Fructose metabolism and metabolic disease. J Clin investigation 2018;128(2):545–55.

[281] Mount DB, Kwon CY, Zandi-Nejad K. Renal urate transport. Rheum Dis Clin North Am 2006;32(2):313–31 vi.

[282] American Diabetes Association. Facilitating behavior change and well-being to improve health outcomes: standards of medical care in diabetes—2021. Diabetes Care 1 January 2021;44(Supplement_1):S53–72. Available from: https://doi.org/10.2337/dc21-S005.

[283] Evert A, et al. Nutrition therapy for adults with diabetes or prediabetes: a consensus report. Diabetes Care 2019;42(5):731–54. Available from: https://doi.org/10.2337/dci19-0014.

[284] Davies M, et al. Management of hyperglycemia in type 2 diabetes, 2018. A consensus report by the American Diabetes Association (ADA) and the European Association for the Study of Diabetes (EASD). Diabetes Care 2018;41(12):2669–701. Available from: https://doi.org/10.2337/dci18-0033.

[285] Diabetes Canada Position. Statement on low-carbohydrate diets for adults with diabetes: a rapid review. Can J Diabetes 2020;44(4):295–9. Available from: https://doi.org/10.1016/j.jcjd.2020.04.001. Epub 2020 Apr 24.

[286] Lennerz BS, Barton A, Bernstein RK, et al. Management of type 1 diabetes with a very low–carbohydrate diet. Pediatrics 2018;141(6): e20173349.

[287] Yancy Jr WS, Foy M, Chalecki AM, Vernon MC, Westman EC. A low-carbohydrate, ketogenic diet to treat type 2 diabetes. Nutr Metab (Lond) 2005;1(2):34. Available from: https://doi.org/10.1186/1743-7075-2-34.

[288] Westman EC, Yancy Jr WS, Mavropoulos JC, Marquart M, McDuffie JR. The effect of a low-carbohydrate, ketogenic diet versus a low-glycemic index diet on glycemic control in type 2 diabetes mellitus. Nutr Metab (Lond) 2008;5:36. Available from: https://doi.org/10.1186/1743-7075-5-36.

[289] Saslow LR, Daubenmier JJ, Moskowitz JT, et al. Twelve-month outcomes of a randomized trial of a moderate-carbohydrate versus very low-carbohydrate diet in overweight adults with type 2 diabetes mellitus or prediabetes. Nutr Diabetes 2017;7(12):304. Available from: https://doi.org/10.1038/s41387-017-0006-9.

[290] Saslow LR, Kim S, Daubenmier JJ, et al. A randomized pilot trial of a moderate carbohydrate diet compared to a very low carbohydrate diet in overweight or obese individuals with type 2 diabetes mellitus or prediabetes. PLoS One 2014;9(4):e91027. Available from: https://doi.org/10.1371/journal.pone.0091027.

[291] Yabe D, Iwasaki M, Kuwata H, et al. Sodium-glucose co-transporter-2 inhibitor use and dietary carbohydrate intake in Japanese individuals with type 2 diabetes: A randomized, open-label, 3-arm parallel comparative exploratory study. Diabetes Obes Metab 2017;19:739–43. Available from: https://doi.org/10.1111/dom.12848. Epub 2017 Feb 21.

[292] Murdoch C, Unwin D, Cavan D, Cucuzzella M, Patel M. Adapting diabetes medication for low carbohydrate management of type 2 diabetes: a practical guide. Br J Gen Pract 2019;69(684):360–1.

[293] Garber A, et al. Consensus Statement by the American Association of Clinical Endocrinologists and American College of Endocrinology on the Comprehensive type 2 Diabetes Management Algorithm – 2017 Executive Summary. Endocr Pract 2017;23(2):207–38.

[294] Kolb H, Kempf K, Röhling M, et al. Insulin: too much of a good thing is bad. BMC Med 2020;18(1):224. Available from: https://doi.org/10.1186/s12916-020-01688-6.

[295] Douros A, et al. Sulfonylureas as second line drugs in type 2 diabetes and the risk of cardiovascular and hypoglycemic events: population based cohort study. BMJ 2018;18:362. Available from: https://doi.org/10.1136/bmj.k2693. k2693.

[296] Jiang J, et al. Postprandial blood glucose outweighs fasting blood glucose and HbA1c in screening coronary heart disease. Sci Rep 2017;7(1):14212. Available from: https://doi.org/10.1038/s41598-017-14152-y.

[297] Sourij H, et al. Post-challenge hyperglycaemia is strongly associated with future macrovascular events and total mortality in angiographied coronary patients. Eur Heart J 2010;31(13):1583–90. Available from: https://doi.org/10.1093/eurheartj/ehq099. Epub 2010 Apr 30.

[298] Nambam B, et al. Latent autoimmune diabetes in adults: A distinct but heterogeneous clinical entity. World J Diabetes 2010;1(4):111–15. Available from: https://doi.org/10.4239/wjd.v1.i4.111.

[299] Murray SW, McKelvey S, Heseltine TD, et al. The "discordant doppelganger dilemma": SGLT2i mimics therapeutic carbohydrate restriction - food choice first over pharma? J Hum Hypertens 2021;. Available from: https://doi.org/10.1038/s41371-021-00482-y. Feb 9. Online ahead of print.

[300] Bosetti C, et al. Cancer risk for patients using thiazolidinediones for type 2 diabetes: a meta-analysis. Oncologist 2013;18(2):148–56. Available from: https://doi.org/10.1634/theoncologist.2012-0302.

[301] Singh S, et al. Thiazolidinediones and heart failure: a teleo-analysis. Diabetes Care 2007;30:2148–53. Available from: https://doi.org/10.2337/dc07-0141. Aug.

[302] McDonough AK, et al. The effect of thiazolidinediones on BMD and osteoporosis. Nat Clin Pract Endocrinol Metab 2008;4(9):507–13. Available from: https://doi.org/10.1038/ncpendmet0920. Sep.

[303] Fonseca V. Effect of thiazolidinediones on body weight in patients with diabetes mellitus. Am J Med 2003;115(Suppl 8):A:42S–48S42S. Available from: https://doi.org/10.1016/j.amjmed.2003.09.005.

[304] McCreight LJ, et al. Metformin and the gastrointestinal tract. Diabetologia 2016;59(3):426–35. Available from: https://doi.org/10.1007/s00125-015-3844-9.

[305] Dailey M, Moran T. Glucagon-like peptide 1 and appetite. Trends Endocrinol Metab 2013;24(2):85–91. Available from: https://doi.org/10.1016/j.tem.2012.11.008.

[306] Scheen AJ. Cardiovascular outcome studies in type 1 diabetes: Comparison between SGLT2 inhibitors and GLP-1 receptor agonists. Diabetes Res Clin Pract 2018;143:88–100. Available from: https://doi.org/10.1016/j.diabres.2018.06.008.

[307] Drucker D. Mechanisms of action and therapeutic application of glucagon-like peptide-1. Cell Metab 2018;27(4):740–56. Available from: https://doi.org/10.1016/j.cmet.2018.03.001.

[308] Franciosi M, et al. ROSES: role of self-monitoring of blood glucose and intensive education in patients with Type 2 diabetes not receiving insulin. A pilot randomized clinical trial. Diabet Med 2011;28(7):789–96. Available from: https://doi.org/10.1111/j.1464-5491.2011.03268.x.

[309] Zhu H, et al. Is self-monitoring of blood glucose effective in improving glycaemic control in type 2 diabetes without insulin treatment: a meta-analysis of randomized controlled trials. BMJ Open 2016;6(9):e010524. Available from: https://doi.org/10.1136/bmjopen-2015-010524.

[310] Muneta T, Kawaguchi E, Hayashi M, et al. Normalized glucose variability by low carbohydrate diet (LCD) in CGM study. Asp Biomed Clin Case Rep 2019;2(1):22–7.

[311] Botzer A, Grossman E, Moult J, Unger R. A system view and analysis of essential hypertension. J Hypertens 2018;36(5):1094–103. Available from: https://doi.org/10.1097/HJH.0000000000001680.

[312] Wong K, Raffray M, Blunden S, Roy-Fleming A, Brazeau AS. The ketogenic diet as a normal way of eating for people with diabetes: a qualitative study. Can J Diabetes 2021;45(2):137–43. Available from: https://doi.org/10.1016/j.jcjd.2020.06.016.

[313] American Diabetes Association. Classification and diagnosis of diabetes: standards of medical care in diabetes-2020. Diabetes Care 2020;43(Suppl 1):S14–31.

[314] Heald AH, Stedman M, Davies M, Livingston M, Alshames R, Lunt M, et al. Estimating life years lost to diabetes: outcomes from analysis of National Diabetes Audit and Office of National Statistics data. Cardiovasc Endocrinol Metab 2020;9(4):183–5.

[315] Kent DA, Quinn L. Factors that affect quality of life in young adults with type 1 diabetes. Diab Educ 2018;44(6):501–9. Available from: https://doi.org/10.1177/0145721718808733.

[316] Hyppönen E, Läärä E, Reunanen A, Järvelin MR, Virtanen SM. Intake of vitamin D and risk of type 1 diabetes: a birth-cohort study. Lancet. 2001;358(9292):1500–3.

[317] Henderson G. Court of last appeal - the early history of the high-fat diet for diabetes. J Diabetes Metab 2016;7(8).

[318] Scott SN, Anderson L, Morton JP, Wagenmakers AJM, Riddell MC. Carbohydrate restriction in type 1 diabetes: a realistic therapy for improved glycaemic control and athletic performance? Nutrients. 2019;11(5).

[319] Lind M, Svensson AM, Kosiborod M, Gudbjornsdottir S, Pivodic A, Wedel H, et al. Glycemic control and excess mortality in type 1 diabetes. N Engl J Med 2014;371(21):1972–82.

[320] Foster NC, Beck RW, Miller KM, Clements MA, Rickels MR, DiMeglio LA, et al. State of type 1 diabetes management and outcomes from the T1D exchange in 2016-2018. Diabetes Technol & therapeutics 2019;21(2):66–72.

[321] Lennerz BS, Barton A, Bernstein RK, Dikeman RD, Diulus C, Hallberg S, et al. Management of type 1 diabetes with a very low-carbohydrate diet. Pediatrics. 2018;141(6).

[322] Nielsen JV, Gando C, Joensson E, Paulsson C. Low carbohydrate diet in type 1 diabetes, long-term improvement and adherence: A clinical audit. Diabetol Metab Syndr 2012;4:23 May 31.

[323] Vargas E, Podder V, Carrillo Sepulveda MA. Physiology, glucose transporter type 4 StatPearls [Internet]. Treasure Island, FL: StatPearls Publishing; 2022Available from:http://www.ncbi.nlm.nih.gov/books/NBK537322/.

[324] Office of Dietary Supplements – Vitamin D [Internet]. [cited May 27, 2022]. Available from: https://ods.od.nih.gov/factsheets/VitaminD-Consumer/.

[325] Sahebi R, Rezayi M, Emadzadeh M, Salehi M, Tayefi M, Parizadeh SM, et al. The effects of vitamin D supplementation on indices of glycemic control in Iranian diabetics: A systematic review and meta-analysis. Complementary Therapies ClPract 2019;34:294–304. Available from: https://pubmed.ncbi.nlm.nih.gov/11705562/.

[326] Edgerton DS, Moore MC, Gregory JM, Kraft G, Cherrington AD. Importance of the route of insulin delivery to its control of glucose metabolism. Am J Physiology-Endocrinology Metab 2021;320(5):E891–7.

[327] American Diabetes Association. Facilitating behavior change and well-being to improve health outcomes: standards of medical care in diabetes-2021. Diabetes Care 2021;44(Suppl 1):S53–72.

[328] Nielsen JV, Jonsson E, Ivarsson A. A low carbohydrate diet in type 1 diabetes: clinical experience—a brief report. Upsala J Med Sci 2005;110 (3):267–73.

[329] Schmidt S, Christensen MB, Serifovski N, Damm-Frydenberg C, Jensen JB, Floyel T, et al. Low versus high carbohydrate diet in type 1 diabetes: A 12-week randomized open-label crossover study. Diabetes, Obes & Metab 2019;21(7):1680–8.

[330] Kleiner A, Cum B, Pisciotta L, Cincione IR, Cogorno L, Prigione A, et al. Safety and efficacy of eucaloric very low-carb diet (EVLCD) in type 1 diabetes: a one-year real-life retrospective experience. Nutrients. 2022;14(15):3208.

[331] Ahola AJ, et al. Dietary carbohydrate intake and cardio-metabolic risk factors in type 1 diabetes. Diabetes Res Clin Pract 2019;107818. Available from: https://doi.org/10.1016/j.diabres.2019.107818.

[332] Raab R. The low carbohydrate/low insulin regimen - personal experience in type 1 diabetes. Practical Diabetes Int 2003;20(4):140–2.

[333] Toth CC Z. Type 1 diabetes mellitus successfully managed with the paleolithic ketogenic diet. Int J Case Rep Images 2014;4(10):699–703.

[334] Bouillet B. A Low-carbohydrate high-fat diet initiated promptly after diagnosis provides clinical remission in three patients with type 1 diabetes. Diabetes & Metab 2019.

[335] Nolan J, Rush A, Kaye J. Glycaemic stability of a cyclist with Type 1 diabetes: 4011 km in 20 days on a ketogenic diet. Diabet Med: a J Br Diabet Assoc 2019.

[336] Turton JL, Raab R, Rooney KB. Low-carbohydrate diets for type 1 diabetes mellitus: A systematic review. PLoS One 2018;13(3):e0194987.

[337] Bolla AM, Caretto A, Laurenzi A, Scavini M, Piemonti L. Low-carb and ketogenic diets in type 1 and type 2 diabetes. Nutrients. 2019;11(5).

[338] de Bock M, Lobley K, Anderson D, Davis E, Donaghue K, Pappas M, et al. Endocrine and metabolic consequences due to restrictive carbohydrate diets in children with type 1 diabetes: An illustrative case series. Pediatric diabetes 2018;19(1):129–37.

[339] Gallagher KAS, DeSalvo D, Gregory J, Hilliard ME. Medical and psychological considerations for carbohydrate-restricted diets in youth with type 1 diabetes. Curr diabetes Rep 2019;19(6):27.

[340] Chen X, Zhang Z, Yang H, et al. Consumption of ultra-processed foods and health outcomes: a systematic review of epidemiological studies. Nutr J 2020;19:86.

[341] Unwin J, Unwin D. A simple model to find patient hope for positive lifestyle changes: GRIN [Internet]. British Holistic Medical Association. [cited 2022 May 27]. Available from: https://bhma.org/a-simple-model-to-find-patient-hope-for-positive-lifestyle-changes-grin/.

[342] Sirmans SM, Pate KA. Epidemiology, diagnosis, and management of polycystic ovary syndrome. Clin Epidemiol 2014;6:1–13.

[343] This quote and the ones in the next paragraph from Azziz R, et al. Polycystic ovary syndrome: an ancient disorder? Fertil Steril 2011;95 (5):1544–8.

[344] Insler V, Lunesfeld B. Polycystic ovarian disease: a challenge and controversy. Gynecol Endocrinol 1990;4:51–69.

[345] Brown WH. A case of pluriglandular syndrome: "diabetes of bearded women.". Lancet 1928;212(5490):1022–3.

[346] El Hayek S, et al. Poly cystic ovarian syndrome: an updated overview. Front Physiol 2016;7:124.

[347] Azziz R, et al. Androgen excess in women: experience with over 1000 consecutive patients. J Clin Endocrinol Metab 2004;89(2):453–62.

[348] Azziz R, et al. The androgen excess and PCOS society criteria for the polycystic ovary syndrome: the complete task force report. Fertil Steril 2009;91(2):456–88.

[349] Carmina E, et al. Polycystic ovary syndrome (PCOS): arguably the most common endocrinopathy is associated with significant morbidity in women. J Clin Endocrinol Metab 1999;84(6):1897–9.

[350] Azziz R, et al. Health care-related economic burden of the polycystic ovary syndrome during the reproductive life span. J Clin Endocrinol Metab 2005;90:4650–8.

[351] Deleted in review.

[352] Alvarez-Blasco F, et al. Prevalence and characteristics of the polycystic ovary syndrome in overweight and obese women. Arch Intern Med 2006;166:2081–6.

[353] Ajmal N, Khan SZ, Shaikh R. Polycystic ovary syndrome (PCOS) and genetic predisposition: A review article. Eur J Obstet Gynecol Reprod Biol X 2019;3:100060. Available from: https://doi.org/10.1016/j.eurox.2019.100060. Published 2019 Jun 8.

[354] Burghen GA, et al. Correlation of hyperandrogenism with hyperinsulinism in polycystic ovarian disease. J Clin Endocrinol Metab 1980;50:113–16.

[355] Willis D, et al. Modulation by insulin of follicle-stimulating hormone and luteinizing hormone actions in human granulosa cells of normal and polycystic ovaries. Clin Endocrinol Metab 1996;81:302–9.

[356] Strain G, et al. The relationship between serum levels of insulin and sex hormone-binding globulin in men: the effect of weight loss. J Clin Endocrinol Metab 1994;79(4):1173–6.
[357] Franks S, et al. Insulin action in the normal and polycystic ovary. Endocrinol Metab Clin North Am 1999;28(2):361–78.
[358] Baillargeon JP, et al. Commentary: polycystic ovary syndrome: a syndrome of ovarian hypersensitivity to insulin? J Clin Endocrinol Metab 2006;91(1):22–4.
[359] Hughesdon PE. Morphology and morphogenesis of the Stein-Leventhal ovary and of so-called "hyperthecosis.". Obstet Gynecol Surv 1982;37 (2):59–77. Available from: https://doi.org/10.1097/00006254-198202000-00001. PMID: 7033852.
[360] Webber LJ, et al. Formation and early development of follicles in the polycystic ovary. Lancet 2003;362:1017–21.
[361] Franks S, et al. Etiology of anovulation in polycystic ovary syndrome. Steroids 1998;63:306–7.
[362] Kezele PR, Nilsson EE, Skinner MK. Insulin but not insulin-like growth factor-1 promotes the primordial to primary follicle transition. Mol Cell Endocrinol 2002;192:37–43.
[363] Creanga AA, et al. Use of metformin in polycystic ovary syndrome: a meta-analysis. Obstet Gynecol 2008;111(4):959–68.
[364] Dunaif A, et al. Profound peripheral insulin resistance, independent of obesity, in polycystic ovary syndrome. Diabetes 1989;38:1165–74.
[365] Rosenfield RL, et al. The pathogenesis of polycystic ovary syndrome (PCOS): the hypothesis of PCOS as functional ovarian hyperandrogenism revisited. Endocr Rev 2016;.
[366] Homburg R, et al. Polycystic ovary syndrome: from gynaecological curiosity to multisystem endocrinopathy. Hum Reprod 1996;11:29–39.
[367] Kiddy DS, et al. Improvement in endocrine and ovarian function during dietary treatment of obese women with polycystic ovary syndrome. Clin Endrocrinol (Oxf) 1992;36:105–11.
[368] Teede HJ, Misso ML, Costello MF, Dokras A, Laven J, Moran L, et al. International PCOS Network, Recommendations from the international evidence-based guideline for the assessment and management of polycystic ovary syndrome. Hum Reprod 2018;33(9):1602–18. Available from: https://doi.org/10.1093/humrep/dey256.
[369] de Melo AS, et al. Hormonal contraception in women with polycystic ovary syndrome: choices, challenges, and noncontraceptive benefits. Open Access J Contracept 2017;8:13–23.
[370] Bargiota A, Diamanti-Kandarakis E. The effects of old, new and emerging medicines on metabolic aberrations in PCOS. Ther Adv Endocrinol Metab 2012;3(1):27–47.
[371] Evans, et al. Spironolactone in the treatment of idiopathic hirsutism and the polycystic ovary syndrome. J R Soc Med 1986;79(8):451–3.
[372] Agrawal NK. Management of hirsutism. Indian J Endocrinol Metab 2013;17(Suppl1):S77–82.
[373] Polycystic Ovary Syndrome Writing Committee. American Association of Clinical Endocrinologists position statement on metabolic and cardiovascular consequences of polycystic ovary syndrome. Endocr Pract 2005;11:126–34.
[374] Nestler JE, Jakubowicz DJ. Decreases in ovarian cytochrome P450c17α activity and serum free testosterone after reduction in insulin secretion in polycystic ovary syndrome. N Engl J Med 1996;335:617–23.
[375] Morin-Papunen, et al. Metformin improves pregnancy and live-birth rates in women with polycystic ovary syndrome (PCOS): a multicenter, double-blind, placebo-controlled randomized trial. J Clin Endocrinol Metab 2012;97(5):1492–500.
[376] Vanky, et al. Metformin reduces pregnancy complications without affecting androgen levels in pregnant polycystic ovary syndrome women: results of a randomized study. Hum Reprod 2004;19(8):1734–40.
[377] Rafieian-Kopaei, et al. Metformin: current knowledge. J Res Med Sci 2014;19(7):658–64.
[378] Hasner E, et al. Long-term clinical effects of ovarian wedge resection in polycystic ovarian syndrome. Acta Obstet Gynecol Scand 1983;62 (1):55–7.
[379] Hendriks ML, et al. Why does ovarian surgery in PCOS help? Insight into the endocrine implications of ovarian surgery for ovulation induction in polycystic ovary syndrome. Hum Reprod Update 2007;13(3):249–64.
[380] Mitra, et al. Laparoscopic ovarian drilling: An alternative but not the ultimate in the management of polycystic ovary syndrome. J Nat Sci Biol Med 2015;6(1):40–8.
[381] Panidis D, et al. Anovulation and ovulation induction. Hippokratia 2006;10(3):120–7.
[382] Legro, et al. Letrozole versus clomiphene for infertility in the polycystic ovary syndrome. N Engl J Med 2014;371:119–29.
[383] Tarlatzis, et al. Consensus on infertility treatment related to polycystic ovary syndrome. Fertil Steril 2008;89:505–22.
[384] CDC BMI charts. Department of Health and Human Services, Centers for Disease Control and Prevention, revised 2013.
[385] Katherine M, Flegal KM, Shepherd JA, Looker AC, Graubard BI, et al. Comparisons of percentage body fat, body mass index, waist circumference, and waist-stature ratio in adults. Am J Clin Nutr 2009;89(2):500–8.
[386] Ludwig DS, Ebbeling CB. The carbohydrate-insulin model of obesity: beyond "Calories In, Calories Out.". JAMA Intern Med 2018;178 (8):1098–103.
[387] Howell S, Kones R. "Calories in, calories out" and macronutrient intake: the hope, hype, and science of calories. Am J Physiol Endocrinol Metab 2017;313(5):E608–12.
[388] Molfino A, Amabile MI, Rossi Fanelli F, Muscaritoli M. Novel therapeutic options for cachexia and sarcopenia. Expert Opin Biol Ther 2016;16(10):1239–44.
[389] Sanford AM. Anorexia of aging and its role for frailty. Curr Opin Clin Nutr Metab Care 2017;20(1):54–60.
[390] van Eeden AE, van Hoeken D, Hoek HW. Incidence, prevalence and mortality of anorexia nervosa and bulimia nervosa. Curr Opin Psychiatry 2021;34(6):515–24.
[391] Moskowitz L, Weiselberg E. Anorexia nervosa/atypical anorexia nervosa. Curr Probl Pediatr Adolesc Health Care 2017;47(4):70–84.

[392] Schorr M, Miller KK. The endocrine manifestations of anorexia nervosa: mechanisms and management. Nat Rev Endocrinol 2017;13 (3):174–86.
[393] Berner LA, Brown TA, Lavender JM, Lopez E, Wierenga CE, Kaye WH. Neuroendocrinology of reward in anorexia nervosa and bulimia nervosa: beyond leptin and ghrelin. Mol Cell Endocrinol 2019;497:110320.
[394] Misra M, Klibanski A. Endocrine consequences of anorexia nervosa. Lancet Diabetes Endocrinol 2014;2(7):581–92.
[395] Lavender JM, Wonderlich SA, Engel SG, Gordon KH, Kaye WH, Mitchell JE. Dimensions of emotion dysregulation in anorexia nervosa and bulimia nervosa: a conceptual review of the empirical literature. Clin Psychol Rev 2015;40:111–22 Aug.
[396] Oldershaw A, Startup H, Lavender T. Anorexia nervosa and a lost emotional self: a psychological formulation of the development, maintenance, and treatment of anorexia nervosa. Front Psychol 2019;10:219 Mar 4.
[397] Skowrońska A, Sójta K, Strzelecki D. Refeeding syndrome as treatment complication of anorexia nervosa. Psychiatr Pol 2019;53(5):1113–23.
[398] Jason Fung J, Moore J. The complete guide to fasting: heal your body through intermittent, alternate-day, and extended fasting. 2016.
[399] Parker EK, Flood V, Halaki M, Wearne C, Anderson G, Gomes L, et al. A standard enteral formula versus an iso-caloric lower carbohydrate/high fat enteral formula in the hospital management of adolescent and young adults admitted with anorexia nervosa: a randomised controlled trial. J Eat Disord 2021;9(1):160.
[400] Scolnick B. Hypothesis: Clues from mammalian hibernation for treating patients with anorexia nervosa. Front Psychol 2018;9:2159.
[401] Scolnick B, Zupec-Kania B, Calabrese L, Aoki C, Hildebrandt T. Remission from chronic anorexia nervosa with ketogenic diet and ketamine: case report. Front Psychiatry 2020;11:763.
[402] Mean body mass index trends among adults, age-standardized (kg/m^2) by country. World Health Organization 2022.
[403] Prevalence of obesity among adults, BMI $>$ 30, age-standardized by country. World Health Organization 2022.
[404] Hales CM, Carroll MD, MSPH, Fryar CD, Ogden CL. CDC epidemiology: prevalence of obesity and severe obesity among adults: United States, 2017–2018. NCHS Data Brief No. 360, 2020.
[405] Flegal KM, Kit BK, Orpana H, Graubard BI. Association of all-cause mortality with overweight and obesity using standard body mass index categories: a systematic review and meta-analysis. JAMA 2013;309(1):71–82.
[406] Bosello O, Donataccio MP, Cuzzolaro M. Obesity or obesities? Controversies on the association between body mass index and premature mortality. Eat Weight Disord 2016;21(2):165–74.
[407] Pennings N, Jaber J, Ahiawodzi P. Ten-year weight gain is associated with elevated fasting insulin levels and precedes glucose elevation. Diabetes Metab Res Rev 2018;34(4):e2986.
[408] Cunnane SC, Crawford MA. Survival of the fattest: fat babies were the key to evolution of the large human brain. Comp Biochem Physiol A Mol Integr Physiol 2003;136(1):17–26.
[409] Simopoulos AP. Evolutionary aspects of diet: the omega-6/omega-3 ratio and the brain. Mol Neurobiol 2011;44(2):203–15.
[410] Wardlaw G, Smith A. 7th ed. Contemporary Nutrition, 10. McGraw Hill; 2009. p. 2008.
[411] Dehghan M, Mente A, Zhang X, et al. Prospective Urban Rural Epidemiology (PURE) study investigators. Associations of fats and carbohydrate intake with cardiovascular disease and mortality in 18 countries from five continents (PURE): a prospective cohort study. Lancet 2017;390(10107):2050–62.
[412] Brockman RP. Roles for insulin and glucagon in the development of ruminant ketosis – a review. Can Vet J 1979;20(5):121–6.
[413] Verbrugghe A, Hesta M, Daminet S, Janssens GP. Nutritional modulation of insulin resistance in the true carnivorous cat: a review. Crit Rev Food Sci Nutr 2012;52(2):172–82.
[414] El K, Capozzi ME, Campbell JE. Repositioning the alpha cell in postprandial metabolism. Endocrinology. 2020;161(11):bqaa169.
[415] Vázquez-Borrego MC, del Rio-Moreno M, Kineman RD. Towards understanding the direct and indirect actions of growth hormone in controlling hepatocyte carbohydrate and lipid metabolism. Cells 2021;10(10):2532.
[416] Konturek PC, Brzozowski T, Konturek SJ. Gut clock: implication of circadian rhythms in the gastrointestinal tract. J Physiol Pharmacol 2011;62(2):139–50.
[417] Paoli A, Tinsley G, Bianco A, Moro T. The influence of meal frequency and timing on health in humans: the role of fasting. Nutrients 2019;11(4):719. Available from: https://doi.org/10.3390/nu11040719. PMID: 30925707. PMCID: PMC6520689.
[418] Wu CW, Biggar KK, Storey KB. Biochemical adaptations of mammalian hibernation: exploring squirrels as a perspective model for naturally induced reversible insulin resistance. Braz J Med Biol Res 2013;46(1):1–13.
[419] Rigano KS, Gehring JL, Evans Hutzenbiler BD, Chen AV, Nelson OL, Vella CA, et al. Life in the fat lane: seasonal regulation of insulin sensitivity, food intake, and adipose biology in brown bears. J Comp Physiol B 2017;187(4):649–76.
[420] Martin SL. Mammalian hibernation: a naturally reversible model for insulin resistance in man? Diab Vasc Dis Res 2008;5(2):76–81.
[421] Crofts C, Schofield G, Zinn C, Wheldon M, Kraft J. Identifying hyperinsulinaemia in the absence of impaired glucose tolerance: An examination of the Kraft database. Diabetes Res Clin Pract 2016;118:50–7.
[422] D'Alessio D. Intestinal hormones and regulation of satiety: the case for CCK, GLP-1, PYY, and Apo A-IV. JPEN J Parenter Enter Nutr 2008;32(5):567–8.
[423] Carson JAS, Lichtenstein AH, Anderson CAM, et al. Dietary cholesterol and cardiovascular risk: a science advisory from the American Heart Association. Circulation. 2020;141(3):e39–53.
[424] Gibson EL. Carbohydrates and mental function: feeding or impeding the brain? Nutr Bull 2007;32(s1):71–83.
[425] Schulte EM, Avena NM, Gearhardt AN. Which foods may be addictive? The roles of processing, fat content, and glycemic load. PLoS One 2015;10(2):e0117959.

[426] Guterstam J, Jayaram-Lindström N, Cervenka S, Frost JJ, Farde L, Halldin C, et al. Effects of amphetamine on the human brain opioid system – a positron emission tomography study. Int J Neuropsychopharmacol 2013;16(4):763–9.

[427] Gudehithlu KP, Duchemin AM, Tejwani GA, Neff NH, Hadjiconstantinou M. Nicotine-induced changes of brain β-endorphin. Neuropeptides. 2012;46(3):125–31.

[428] Meguid MM, Fetissov SO, Varma M, Sato T, Zhang L, Laviano A, et al. Hypothalamic dopamine and serotonin in the regulation of food intake. Nutrition. 2000;16(10):843–57.

[429] Tulloch AJ, Murray S, Vaicekonyte R, Avena NM. Neural responses to macronutrients: hedonic and homeostatic mechanisms. Gastroenterology. 2015;148(6):1205–18.

[430] Lee PC, Dixon JB. Food for thought: reward mechanisms and hedonic overeating in obesity. Curr Obes Rep 2017;6(4):353–61.

[431] Avena NM, Rada P, Hoebel BG. Evidence for sugar addiction: behavioral and neurochemical effects of intermittent, excessive sugar intake. Neurosci Biobehav Rev 2008;32(1):20–39.

[432] Kraft JR, Wehrmacher WH. Diabetes – a silent disorder. Compr Ther 2009;35(3-4):155–9.

[433] Klonsky ED. The functions of deliberate self-injury: a review of the evidence. Clin Psychol Rev 2007;27(2):226–39.

[434] Nock MK. Self-injury. Annu Rev Clin Psychol 2010;6:339–63.

[435] Young LR, Nestle M. The contribution of expanding portion sizes to the US obesity epidemic. Am J Public Health 2002;92(2):246–9. Available from: https://doi.org/10.2105/ajph.92.2.246. PMID: 11818300. PMCID: PMC1447051.

[436] Evans EW, Jacques PF, Dallal GE, Sacheck J, Must A. The role of eating frequency on total energy intake and diet quality in a low-income, racially diverse sample of schoolchildren Public Health Nutr 2015;18(3):474–81. Available from: https://doi.org/10.1017/S1368980014000470. Epub 2014 Apr 29. PMID: 24780506. PMCID: PMC4471996.

[437] Avena NM, Bocarsly ME, Hoebel BG. Animal models of sugar and fat bingeing: relationship to food addiction and increased body weight. Methods Mol Biol 2012;829:351–65.

[438] Bou Khalil R, Sleilaty G, Richa S, Seneque M, Iceta S, Rodgers R, et al. The impact of retrospective childhood maltreatment on eating disorders as mediated by food addiction: a cross-sectional study. Nutrients. 2020;12(10):2969.

[439] Dansinger ML, Gleason JA, Griffith JL, Selker HP, Schaefer EJ. Comparison of the Atkins, ornish, weight watchers, and zone diets for weight loss and heart disease risk reduction: a randomized trial. JAMA 2005;293(1):43–53.

[440] Velapati SR, Shah M, Kuchkuntla AR, Abu-Dayyeh B, Grothe K, Hurt RT, et al. Weight regain after bariatric surgery: prevalence, etiology, and treatment. Curr Nutr Rep 2018;7(4):329–34.

[441] Fauconnier M, Rousselet M, Brunault P, Thiabaud E, Lambert S, Rocher B, et al. Food addiction among female patients seeking treatment for an eating disorder: prevalence and associated factors. Nutrients. 2020;12(6):1897.

[442] Velazquez A, Apovian CM. Updates on obesity pharmacotherapy. Ann N Y Acad Sci 2018;1411(1):106–19.

[443] Secher A, Jelsing J, Baquero AF, Hecksher-Sørensen J, Cowley MA, Dalbøge LS, et al. The arcuate nucleus mediates GLP-1 receptor agonist liraglutide-dependent weight loss. J Clin Invest 2014;124(10):4473–88.

[444] Ahmadieh H, Azar ST. The role of incretin-based therapies in prediabetes: a review. Prim Care Diabetes 2014;8(4):286–94.

[445] Johnson RJ, Gold MS, Johnson DR, Ishimoto T, Lanaspa MA, Zahniser NR, et al. Attention-deficit/hyperactivity disorder: is it time to reappraise the role of sugar consumption? Postgrad Med 2011;123(5):39–49.

[446] Gill H, Gill B, El-Halabi S, Chen-Li D, Lipsitz O, Rosenblat JD, et al. Antidepressant medications and weight change: a narrative review. Obesity. 2020;28(11):2064–72.

[447] Voelker R. The problem with Fen-Phen. JAMA 1998;280(12):1041. Available from: https://doi.org/10.1001/jama.280.12.1041-JQU80006-2-1.

[448] Tak YJ, Lee SY. Long-term efficacy and safety of anti-obesity treatment: where do we stand? Curr Obes Rep 2021;10(1):14–30.

[449] Courcoulas AP, King WC, Belle SH, Berk P, Flum DR, Garcia L, et al. Seven-year weight trajectories and health outcomes in the longitudinal assessment of bariatric surgery (LABS) study. JAMA Surg 2018;153(5):427–34.

[450] Buchwald H. The evolution of metabolic/bariatric surgery. Obes Surg 2014;24(8):1126–35.

[451] Nicolaidis S. Neurosurgery of the future: Deep brain stimulations and manipulations. Metabolism. 2017;69S:S16–20.

[452] Prochaska JO, Norcross JC, DiClemente CC. Changing for Good. New York: Avon Books; 1994.

[453] Kinsey AW, Ormsbee MJ. The health impact of nighttime eating: old and new perspectives. Nutrients 2015;7(4):2648–62. Available from: https://doi.org/10.3390/nu7042648. PMID: 25859885. PMCID: PMC4425165.

[454] Ross KM, Qiu P, You L, Wing RR. Week-to-week predictors of weight loss and regain. Health Psychol 2019;38(12):1150–8.

[455] Holmes CJ, Racette SB. The utility of body composition assessment in nutrition and clinical practice: an overview of current methodology. Nutrients. 2021;13(8):2493.

[456] Hegedus E, Salvy SJ, Wee CP, Naguib M, Raymond JK, Fox DS, et al. Use of continuous glucose monitoring in obesity research: A scoping review. Obes Res Clin Pract 2021;15(5):431–8.

[457] Erdogan M, Canataroglu A, Ganidagli S, Kulaksızoglu M. Metabolic syndrome prevalence in subclinic and overt hypothyroid patients and the relation among metabolic syndrome parameters. J Endocrinol Invest 2011;34(7):488–92. Available from: https://doi.org/10.3275/7202.

[458] Waring AC, Rodondi N, Harrison S, Kanaya AM, Simonsick EM, Miljkovic I, et al. Thyroid function and prevalent and incident metabolic syndrome in older adults: the Health, Ageing and Body Composition Study. Clin Endocrinol 2012;76(6):911–18. Available from: https://doi.org/10.1111/j.1365-2265.2011.04328.x.

[459] Ruhla S, Weickert MO, Arafat AM, Osterhoff M, Isken F, Spranger J, et al. A high normal TSH is associated with the metabolic syndrome. Clin Endocrinol 2010;72(5):696–701. Available from: https://doi.org/10.1111/j.1365-2265.2009.03698.x.

[460] Song RH, Wang B, Yao QM, Li Q, Jia X, Zhang JA. The impact of obesity on thyroid autoimmunity and dysfunction: a systematic review and meta-analysis. Front Immunol 2019;10:2349. Available from: https://doi.org/10.3389/fimmu.2019.02349.

[461] Vanderpump MP. The epidemiology of thyroid disease. Br Med Bull 2011;99:39–51. Available from: https://doi.org/10.1093/bmb/ldr030. PMID: 21893493.

[462] Zimmerman MB. Iodine deficiency. Endocr Rev 2009;30:376–408.

[463] Gaitan E. Goitrogens in food and water. Annu Rev Nutr 1990;10:21–39.

[464] Mincer DL, Jialal I. Hashimoto thyroiditis StatPearls [Internet]. Treasure Island (FL): StatPearls Publishing; 2022. [cited 2022 Jun 23]. Available fromhttp://www.ncbi.nlm.nih.gov/books/NBK459262/.

[465] Mullur R, Liu YY, Brent GA. Thyroid hormone regulation of metabolism. Physiol Rev 2014;94(2):355–82. Available from: https://doi.org/10.1152/physrev.00030.2013. PMID: 24692351. PMCID: PMC4044302.

[466] William F, McPhee SJ, G.. Lange Medical Books Pathophysiology of Disease: An Introduction to Clinical Medicine. 5th edition McGraw-Hill; 2006.

[467] Peeters RP, Visser TJ. Metabolism of thyroid hormone In: Feingold KR, Anawalt B, Boyce A, Chrousos G, de Herder WW, Dhatariya K, et al., editors. Endotext [Internet]. South Dartmouth (MA): MDText.com, Inc.; 2000[cited 2022 Jun 23]. Available from: http://www.ncbi.nlm.nih.gov/books/NBK285545/.

[468] Wittekind DA, Kratzsch J, Mergl R, Baber R, Witte V, Villringer A, et al. Free triiodothyronine (T3) is negatively associated with fasting ghrelin serum levels in a population sample of euthyroid subjects. J Endocrinol Invest 2021;44(12):2655–64.

[469] Helmreich DL, Tylee D. Thyroid hormone regulation by stress and behavioral differences in adult male rats. Hormones Behav 2011;60 (3):284–91. Available from: https://doi.org/10.1016/j.yhbeh.2011.06.003.

[470] Monaco F. Classification of thyroid diseases: suggestions for a revision. J Clin Endocrinol & Metab 2003;88(4):1428–32.

[471] Tomer Y, Huber A. The etiology of autoimmune thyroid disease: a story of genes and environment. J Autoimmunity 2009;32(3-4):231–9.

[472] Iddah MA, Macharia BN. Autoimmune thyroid disorders. ISRN Endocrinol 2013;2013:509764 http://doi.org/10.1155/2013/509764.

[473] Biondi B, Cooper DS. The clinical significance of subclinical thyroid dysfunction. Endocr Rev 2008;29:76–131.

[474] Gurnell M, Rajanayagam O, Barbar I, Jones MK, Chatterjee VK. Reversible pituitary enlargement in the syndrome of resistance to thyroid hormone. Thyroid. 1998;8(8):679–82. Available from: https://doi.org/10.1089/thy.1998.8.679. PMID: 9737363.

[475] Sørensen HG, van der Deure WM, Hansen PS, Peeters RP, Breteler MM, Kyvik KO, et al. Identification and consequences of polymorphisms in the thyroid hormone receptor alpha and beta genes. Thyroid. 2008;18(10):1087–94. Available from: https://doi.org/10.1089/thy.2008.0236. PMID: 18844476.

[476] Lazar MA. Thyroid hormone receptors: multiple forms, multiple possibilities. Endocr Rev 1993;14(2):184–93. Available from: https://doi.org/10.1210/edrv-14-2-184. PMID: 8325251.

[477] Williams GR, Franklyn JA, Neuberger JM, Sheppard MC. Thyroid hormone receptor expression in the "sick euthyroid" syndrome. Lancet. 1989;2(8678-8679):1477–81. Available from: https://doi.org/10.1016/s0140-6736(89)92930-9. PMID: 2574767.

[478] Serter R, Demirbas B, Korukluoglu B, Culha C, Cakal E, Aral Y. The effect of L-thyroxine replacement therapy on lipid based cardiovascular risk in subclinical hypothyroidism. J Endocrinol Invest 2004;27(10):897–903. Available from: https://doi.org/10.1007/BF03347530. PMID: 15762035.

[479] Adlin V. Subclinical hypothyroidism: deciding when to treat. Am Fam Physician 1998;57(4):776–80. PMID: 9491000.

[480] McDermott MT, Ridgway EC. Subclinical hypothyroidism is mild thyroid failure and should be treated. J Clin Endocrinol & Metab 2001;86 (10):4585–90.

[481] Bahammam SA, Sharif MM, Jammah AA, BaHammam AS. Prevalence of thyroid disease in patients with obstructive sleep apnea. Respiratory Med 2011;105(11):1755–60.

[482] Song L, Lei J, Jiang K, Lei Y, Tang Y, Zhu J, et al. The association between subclinical hypothyroidism and sleep quality: a population-based study. Risk Manag Healthc Policy 2019;12:369–74.

[483] Loh HH, Lim LL, Yee A, Loh HS. Association between subclinical hypothyroidism and depression: an updated systematic review and meta-analysis. BMC Psychiatry 2019;19(1):12.

[484] Jones DS. Textbook of Functional Medicine. The Institute of Functional Medicine; 2010.

[485] Monzani F, Caraccio N, Del Guerra P, Casolaro A, Ferrannini E. Neuromuscular symptoms and dysfunction in subclinical hypothyroid patients: beneficial effect of L-T4 replacement therapy. Clin Endocrinol (Oxf) 1999;51(2):237–42. Available from: https://doi.org/10.1046/j.1365-2265.1999.00790.x. PMID: 10468996.

[486] He J, Lai Y, Yang J, Yao Y, Li Y, Teng W, et al. The relationship between thyroid function and metabolic syndrome and its components: a cross-sectional study in a Chinese population. Front Endocrinol 2021;12:661160. Available from: https://doi.org/10.3389/fendo.2021.661160.

[487] Tomer Y, Menconi F. Type 1 diabetes and autoimmune thyroiditis: the genetic connection. Thyroid 2009;19:99–102.

[488] Celani MF, Bonati ME, Stucci N. Prevalence of abnormal thyrotropin concentrations measured by a sensitive assay in patients with type 2 diabetes mellitus. Diabetes Res 1994;27:15–25.

[489] Hage M, Zantout MS, Azar ST. Thyroid disorders and diabetes mellitus. J Thyroid Res 2011;2011:439463. Available from: https://doi.org/10.4061/2011/439463.

[490] Brenta G. Why can insulin resistance be a natural consequence of thyroid dysfunction. J Thyroid Res 2011;2011:152850. Available from: https://doi.org/10.4061/2011/152850.

[491] Scanlan TS. Minireview: 3-iodothyronamine (T1AM): a new player on the thyroid endocrine team? Endocrinology 2009;150:1108–11.

[492] Fontenelle LC, Feitosa MM, Severo JS, Freitas TE, Morais JB, Torres-Leal FL, et al. Thyroid function in human obesity: underlying mechanisms. Horm Metab Res 2016;48:787–94. Available from: https://doi.org/10.1055/s-0042-121421.

[493] Brufani C, Manco M, Nobili V, Fintini D, Barbetti F, Cappa M. Thyroid function tests in obese prepubertal children: Correlations with insulin sensitivity and body fat distribution. Horm Res Paediatr 2012;78:100–5. [CrossRef] [PubMed].

[494] Rezzonico J, Rezzonico M, Pusiol E, Pitoia F, Niepomniszcze H. Introducing the thyroid gland as another victim of the insulin resistance syndrome. Thyroid 18:461–464T cells. Endocrinology 2008;150:2000–7.

[495] Bülow Pedersen I, Laurberg P, Knudsen N, Jørgensen T, Perrild H, Ovesen L, et al. A population study of the association between thyroid autoantibodies in serum and abnormalities in thyroid function and structure. Clin Endocrinol (Oxf) 2005;62:713–20.

[496] Wang B, Song R, He W, Yao Q, Li Q, Jia X, et al. Sex differences in the associations of obesity with hypothyroidism and thyroid autoimmunity among chinese adults. Front Physiol 2018;9:1397. Available from: https://doi.org/10.3389/fphys.2018.01397.

[497] Matzen LE, Kvetny J, Pedersen KK. TSH, TH and nuclear-binding of T3 in mononuclear blood cells from obese and non-obese women. Scand J Clin Lab Invest 1989;49:249–53. Available from: https://doi.org/10.1080/00365518909089090.

[498] Tagliaferri M, Berselli ME, Calò G, Minocci A, Savia G, Petroni ML, et al. Subclinical hypothyroidism in obese patients: relation to resting energy expenditure, serum leptin, body composition, and lipid profile. Obes Res 2001;9:196–201.

[499] Crisp MS, Lane C, Halliwell M, Wynford-Thomas D, Ludgate M. Thyrotropin receptor transcripts in human adipose tissue. J Clin Endocrinol Metab 1997;82:2003–5.

[500] Lu S, Guan Q, Liu Y, Wang H, Xu W, Li X, et al. Role of extrathyroidal TSHR expression in adipocyte differentiation and its association with obesity. Lipids Health Dis 2012;11:17.

[501] Aghajanova L, Lindeberg M, Carlsson IB, Stavreus-Evers A, Zhang P, Scott JE, et al. Receptors for thyroid-stimulating hormone and thyroid hormones in human ovarian tissue. Reprod Biomed Online 2009;18(3):337–47. Available from: https://doi.org/10.1016/s1472-6483(10)60091-0. PMID: 19298732.

[502] Kloprogge SJ, Busuttil BE, Frauman AG. TSH receptor protein is selectively expressed in normal human extraocular muscle. Muscle Nerve 2005;32(1):95–8. Available from: https://doi.org/10.1002/mus.20315. PMID: 15779008.

[503] Bağriaçik EU, Klein JR. The thyrotropin (thyroid-stimulating hormone) receptor is expressed on murine dendritic cells and on a subset of CD45RB high lymph node T cells: functional role for thyroid-stimulating hormone during immune activation. J Immunol 2000;164(12):6158–65. Available from: https://doi.org/10.4049/jimmunol.164.12.6158. PMID: 10843665.

[504] Balzan S, Nicolini G, Forini F, Boni G, Del Carratore R, Nicolini A, et al. Presence of a functional TSH receptor on human erythrocytes Biomed Pharmacother 2007;61(8):463–7. Available from: https://doi.org/10.1016/j.biopha.2007.04.009. Epub 2007 May 25. PMID: 17570630.

[505] Marzullo P, Minocci A, Tagliaferri MA, Guzzaloni G, Di Blasio A, De Medici C, et al. Investigations of thyroid hormones and antibodies in obesity: leptin levels are associated with thyroid autoimmunity independent of bioanthropometric, hormonal, and weight-related determinants J Clin Endocrinol Metab 2010;95(8):3965–72. Available from: https://doi.org/10.1210/jc.2009-2798. Epub 2010 Jun 9. PMID: 20534769.

[506] Verma A, Jayaraman M, Kumar HK, Modi KD. Hypothyroidism and obesity. Cause or effect? Saudi Med J 2008;29(8):1135–8. PMID: 18690306.

[507] Falagas ME, Kompoti M. Obesity and infection. Lancet Infect Dis 2006;6:438–46.

[508] Longhi S, Radetti G. Thyroid function and obesity. J Clin Res Pediatr Endocrinol 2013;5(Suppl. 1):40–4. Available from: https://doi.org/10.4274/jcrpe.856.

[509] Jakobs TC, Mentrup B, Schmutzler C, Dreher I, Köhrle J. Proinflammatory cytokines inhibit the expression and function of human type I 5′-deiodinase in HepG2 hepatocarcinoma cells. Eur J Endocrinol 2002;146:559–66. Available from: https://doi.org/10.1530/eje.0.1460559.

[510] Kwakkel J, Surovtseva OV, Vries EM, Stap J, Fliers E, Boelen A. A novel role for the thyroid hormone-activating enzyme type 2 deiodinase in the inflammatory response of macrophages. Endocrinology 2014;155:2725–34. Available from: https://doi.org/10.1210/en.2013-2066.

[511] Walczak K, Sieminska L. Obesity and thyroid axis. Int J Env Res Public Health 2021;18(18):9434.

[512] Pinkney JH, Goodrick SJ, Katz J, et al. Leptin and the pituitary-thyroid axis: a comparative study in lean, obese, hypothyroid and hyperthyroid subjects. Clin Endocrinol (Oxf) 1998;49:583–98.

[513] Al Adsani H, Hoffer LJ, Silva JE. Resting energy expenditure is sensitive to small dose changes in patients on chronic thyroid hormone replacement. J Clin Endocrinol Metab 1997;82:1118–25.

[514] Isozaki O, Tsushima T, Nozoe Y, Miyakawa M, Takano K. Leptin regulation of the thyroids: negative regulation on thyroid hormone levels in euthyroid subjects and inhibitory effects on iodide uptake and Na + /I- symporter mRNA expression in rat FRTL-5 cells. Endocr J 2004;51:415–23. Available from: https://doi.org/10.1507/endocrj.51.415.

[515] Tanaka S, Inoue S, Isoda F, Waseda M, Ishihara M, Yamakawa T, et al. Impaired immunity in obesity: suppressed but reversible lymphocyte responsiveness. Int J Obes Relat Metab Disord 1993;17:631–6.

[516] Tanaka S, Isoda F, Ishihara Y, Kimura M, Yamakawa T. T lymphopaenia in relation to body mass index and TNF- in human obesity: adequate weight reduction can be corrective. Clin Endocrinol (Oxf) 2001;54:347–54.

[517] Yang H, Youm YH, Vandanmagsar B, Rood J, Kumar KG, Butler AA, et al. Obesity accelerates thymic aging. Blood 2009;114:3803–12.

[518] Lord GM, Matarese G, Howard JK, Baker RJ, Bloom SR, Lechler RI. Leptin modulates the T-cell immune response and reverses starvation-induced immunosuppression. Nature 1998;394:897–901.

[519] Wang SH, Chen GH, Fan Y, Van Antwerp M, Baker Jr. JR. Tumor necrosis factor-related apoptosis-inducing ligand inhibits experimental autoimmune thyroiditis by the expansion of CD4 + CD25 + regulatory T cells. Endocrinology 2009;150(4):2000–7. Available from: https://doi.org/10.1210/en.2008-1389.

[520] Mazziotti G, Parkes AB, Lage M, Premawardhana LD, Casanueva FF, Lazarus JH. High leptin levels in women developing postpartum thyroiditis. Clin Endocrinol (Oxf) 2004;60(2):208–13. Available from: https://doi.org/10.1046/j.1365-2265.2003.01966.x. PMID: 14725682.

[521] Knezevic J, Starchl C, Tmava Berisha A, Amrein K. Thyroid-gut-axis: how does the microbiota influence thyroid function? Nutrients 2020;12 (6):1769. Available from: https://doi.org/10.3390/nu12061769. Published 2020 Jun 12.

[522] Zinöcker MK, Lindseth IA. The Western diet-microbiome-host interaction and its role in metabolic disease. Nutrients 2018;10(3):365. Available from: https://doi.org/10.3390/nu10030365.

[523] Marcello MA, Cunha LL, Batista FA, Ward LS. Obesity and thyroid cancer. Endocrine-related cancer 2014;21(5):T255–71.

[524] Zitvogel L, Ayyoub M, Routy B, Kroemer G. Microbiome and anticancer immunosurveillance. Cell 2016;165:276–87. [CrossRef] [PubMed].

[525] Rajagopala SV, Vashee S, Oldfield LM, Suzuki Y, Venter JC, Telenti A, et al. The human microbiome and cancer. Cancer Prev Res 2017;10:226–34 [CrossRef] [PubMed].

[526] Meng S, Chen B, Yang J, Wang J, Zhu D, Meng Q, et al. Study of microbiomes in aseptically collected samples of human breast tissue using needle biopsy and the potential role of in situ tissue microbiomes for promoting malignancy. Front Oncol 2018;8:1–10.

[527] De La Vieja A, Santisteban P. Role of iodide metabolism in physiology and cancer. Endocr Relat Cancer 2018;25:R225–45. [CrossRef] [PubMed].

[528] Wardle CA, Fraser WD, Squire CR. Pitfalls in the use of thyrotropin concentration as a first-line thyroid-function test. Lancet. 2001;357 (9261):1013–14. Available from: https://doi.org/10.1016/S0140-6736(00)04248-3. PMID: 11293597.

[529] Downing D. Hypothyroidism: treating the patient not the laboratory. J Nutr Environ Med 2000;10:101–3.

[530] Diamanti-Kandarakis E, Bourguignon JP, Giudice LC, et al. Endocrine-disrupting chemicals: an Endocrine Society scientific statement. Endocr Rev 2009;30(4):293–342. Available from: https://doi.org/10.1210/er.2009-0002.

[531] Capen CC. Mechanisms of chemical injury of thyroid gland. Prog Clin Biol Res 1994;387:173–91. PMID: 7526405.

[532] McKinney JD, Pedersen LG. Do residue levels of polychlorinated biphenyls (PCBs) in human blood produce mild hypothyroidism? J Theor Biol 1987;129(2):231–41. Available from: https://doi.org/10.1016/s0022-5193(87)80015-2. PMID: 3138502.

[533] Brucker-Davis F. Effects of environmental synthetic chemicals on thyroid function. Thyroid. 1998;8(9):827–56. Available from: https://doi.org/10.1089/thy.1998.8.827. PMID: 9777756.

[534] Cheek AO, Kow K, Chen J, McLachlan JA. Potential mechanisms of thyroid disruption in humans: interaction of organochlorine compounds with thyroid receptor, transthyretin, and thyroid-binding globulin. Environ health Perspect 1999;107(4):273–8. Available from: https://doi.org/10.1289/ehp.99107273.

[535] Winters N. The Metabolic Approach to Cancer.

[536] Panda S. The Circadian Code.

[537] Nishiyama S, Futagoishi-Suginohara Y, Matsukura M, Nakamura T, Higashi A, Shinohara M, et al. Zinc supplementation alters thyroid hormone metabolism in disabled patients with zinc deficiency. J Am Coll Nutr 1994;13(1):62–7. Available from: https://doi.org/10.1080/07315724.1994.10718373. PMID: 8157857.

[538] Venditti P, Daniele MC, Masullo P, Di Meo S. Antioxidant-sensitive triiodothyronine effects on characteristics of rat liver mitochondrial population. Cell Physiol Biochem 1999;9(1):38–52. Available from: https://doi.org/10.1159/000016301. PMID: 10352343.

[539] Meydani SN, Meydani M, Rall LC, Morrow F, Blumberg JB. Assessment of the safety of high-dose, short-term supplementation with vitamin E in healthy older adults. Am J Clin Nutr 1994;60(5):704–9. Available from: https://doi.org/10.1093/ajcn/60.5.704. PMID: 7942576.

[540] Traber MG, Stevens JF. Vitamins C and E: beneficial effects from a mechanistic perspective. Free Radic Biol Med 2011;51(5):1000–13.

[541] Tapiero H, Townsend DM, Tew KD. The antioxidant role of selenium and seleno-compounds. Biomed Pharmacother 2003;57(3–4):134–44.

[542] Cantorna MT. Vitamin D and autoimmunity: is vitamin D status an environmental factor affecting autoimmune disease prevalence? Proc Soc Exp Biol Med 2000;223(3):230–3. Available from: https://doi.org/10.1046/j.1525-1373.2000.22333.x. PMID: 10719834.

[543] de Groot AP, Willems MI, de Vos RH. Effects of high levels of brussels sprouts in the diet of rats. Food Chem Toxicol 1991;29(12):829–37. Available from: https://doi.org/10.1016/0278-6915(91)90110-s. PMID: 1765328.

[544] McMillan M, Spinks EA, Fenwick GR. Preliminary Observations on the Effect of Dietary Brussels Sprouts on Thyroid Function. Hum Toxicol 1986;5(1):15–19. Available from: https://doi.org/10.1177/096032718600500104.

[545] Ishizuki Y, Hirooka Y, Murata Y, Togashi K. [The effects on the thyroid gland of soybeans administered experimentally in healthy subjects] Nihon Naibunpi Gakkai Zasshi 1991;67(5):622–9. Japanese.. Available from: https://doi.org/10.1507/endocrine1927.67.5_622. PMID: 1868922.

[546] Chang HC, Doerge DR. Dietary genistein inactivates rat thyroid peroxidase in vivo without an apparent hypothyroid effect. Toxicol Appl Pharmacol 2000;168(3):244–52. Available from: https://doi.org/10.1006/taap.2000.9019. PMID: 11042097.

[547] Bruce B, Messina M, Spiller GA. Isoflavone supplements do not affect thyroid function in iodine-replete postmenopausal women J Med Food 2003;6(4):309–16. Winter. Available from: https://doi.org/10.1089/109662003772519859. PMID: 14977438.

[548] Benvenga S, Ruggeri RM, Russo A, Lapa D, Campenni A, Trimarchi F. Usefulness of L-carnitine, a naturally occurring peripheral antagonist of thyroid hormone action, in iatrogenic hyperthyroidism: a randomized, double-blind, placebo-controlled clinical trial. J Clin Endocrinol Metab 2001.

[549] Furman D, Campisi J, Verdin E, Carrera-Bastos P, Targ S, Franceschi C, et al. Chronic inflammation in the etiology of disease across the life span. Nat Med 2019;25(12):1822–32. Available from: https://doi.org/10.1038/s41591-019-0675-0.

[550] Morley JE, Russell RM, Reed A, Carney EA, Hershman JM. The interrelationship of thyroid hormones with vitamin A and zinc nutritional status in patients with chronic hepatic and gastrointestinal disorders. Am J Clin Nutr 1981;34(8):1489–95. Available from: https://doi.org/10.1093/ajcn/34.8.1489. PMID: 7196691.

[551] Krysiak R, Szkróbka W, Okopień B. The effect of gluten-free diet on thyroid autoimmunity in drug-naïve women with Hashimoto's thyroiditis: a pilot study. Exp Clin Endocrinol Diabetes 2019;127(07):417–22.

[552] Esposito T, Lobaccaro JM, Esposito MG, Monda V, Messina A, Paolisso G, et al. Effects of low-carbohydrate diet therapy in overweight subject with autoimmune thyroiditis: possible synergism with ChREBP. DDDT. 2016;10:2939–46.

[553] Gjerstad JK, Lightman SL, Spiga F. Role of glucocorticoid negative feedback in the regulation of HPA axis pulsatility Stress 2018;21 (5):403–16. Available from: https://doi.org/10.1080/10253890.2018.1470238. Epub 2018 May 15. PMID: 29764284. PMCID: PMC6220752.

[554] Rousseau K, Kauser S, Pritchard LE, Warhurst A, Oliver RL, Slominski A, et al. Proopiomelanocortin (POMC), the ACTH/melanocortin precursor, is secreted by human epidermal keratinocytes and melanocytes and stimulates melanogenesis FASEB J 2007;21(8):1844–56. Available from: https://doi.org/10.1096/fj.06-7398com. Epub 2007 Feb 22. PMID: 17317724. PMCID: PMC2253185.

[555] Nicolaides NC, Charmandari E, Kino T, Chrousos GP. Stress-related and circadian secretion and target tissue actions of glucocorticoids: impact on health. Front Endocrinol (Lausanne) 2017;8:70. Available from: https://doi.org/10.3389/fendo.2017.00070. PMID: 28503165. PMCID: PMC5408025.

[556] Chrousos GP. The glucocorticoid receptor gene, longevity, and the complex disorders of Western societies. Am J Med 2004;117(3):204–7. Available from: https://doi.org/10.1016/j.amjmed.2004.05.006. PMID: 15300973.

[557] Andrews RC, Walker BR. Glucocorticoids and insulin resistance: old hormones, new targets. Clin Sci (Lond) 1999;96(5):513–23. Available from: https://doi.org/10.1042/cs0960513. PMID: 10209084.

[558] Charmandari E, Nicolaides NC, Chrousos GP. Adrenal insufficiency. Lancet 2014;383(9935):2152–67.

[559] Huecker MR, Bhutta BS, Dominique E. Adrenal insufficiency [Updated 2022 Mar 7] StatPearls [Internet]. Treasure Island (FL): StatPearls Publishing; 2022.

[560] Pivanello R. Medical treatment of Cushing's disease: an overview of the current and recent clinical trials. Front Endocrinol (Lausanne) 2020;11:648.

[561] Lagercrantz H, Slotkin TA. The "stress" of being born. Sci Am 1986;254(4):100–7. Available from: https://doi.org/10.1038/scientificamerican0486-100. PMID: 3961465.

[562] Jacobs B, Fornal C. Activity of serotonergic neurons in behaving animals. Neuropsychopharmacol 1999;21:9–15. Available from: https://doi.org/10.1016/S0893-133X(99)00012-3.

[563] Strack AM, Sebastian RJ, Schwartz MW, Dallman MF. Glucocorticoids and insulin: reciprocal signals for energy balance. Am J Physiol 1995;268(1 Pt 2):R142–9. Available from: https://doi.org/10.1152/ajpregu.1995.268.1.R142. PMID: 7840315.

[564] Azuma K, Zhou Q, Niwa M, Kubo KY. Association between mastication, the hippocampus, and the HPA axis: a comprehensive review. Int J Mol Sci 2017;18(8):1687. Available from: https://doi.org/10.3390/ijms18081687. PMID: 28771175. PMCID: PMC5578077.

[565] Delaney AL, Arvedson JC. Development of swallowing and feeding: prenatal through first year of life. Developmental disabilities Res Rev 2008;14(2):105–17.

[566] Mizoguchi K, Ishige A, Aburada M, Tabira T. Chronic stress attenuates glucocorticoid negative feedback: involvement of the prefrontal cortex and hippocampus. Neuroscience. 2003;119(3):887–97. Available from: https://doi.org/10.1016/s0306-4522(03)00105-2. PMID: 12809708.

[567] Sullivan RM, Gratton A. Prefrontal cortical regulation of hypothalamic-pituitary-adrenal function in the rat and implications for psychopathology: side matters. Psychoneuroendocrinology 2002;27(1-2):99–114. Available from: https://doi.org/10.1016/S0306-4530(01)00038-5.

[568] Sandström A, Peterson J, Sandström E, Lundberg M, Nystrom IL, Nyberg L, et al. Cognitive deficits in relation to personality type and hypothalamic-pituitary-adrenal (HPA) axis dysfunction in women with stress-related exhaustion Scand J Psychol 2011;52(1):71–82. Available from: https://doi.org/10.1111/j.1467-9450.2010.00844.x. Epub 2010 Oct 22. PMID: 20964695.

[569] Herman JP, McKlveen JM, Ghosal S, Kopp B, Wulsin A, Makinson R, et al. Regulation of the hypothalamic-pituitary-adrenocortical stress response. Compr Physiol 2016;6(2):603–21.

[570] McEwen BS. Physiology and neurobiology of stress and adaptation: central role of the brain. Physiol Rev 2007;87(3):873–904. Available from: https://doi.org/10.1152/physrev.00041.2006. PMID: 17615391.

[571] Starkman MN, Giordani B, Gebarski SS, Berent S, Schork MA, Schteingart DE. Decrease in cortisol reverses human hippocampal atrophy following treatment of Cushing's disease. Biol Psychiatry 1999;46(12):1595–602. Available from: https://doi.org/10.1016/s0006-3223(99)00203-6. PMID: 10624540.

[572] Van Cauter E, Blackman JD, Roland D, Spire JP, Refetoff S, Polonsky KS. Modulation of glucose regulation and insulin secretion by circadian rhythmicity and sleep. J Clin Invest 1991;88(3):934–42. Available from: https://doi.org/10.1172/JCI115396. PMID: 1885778. PMCID: PMC295490.

[573] Torres SJ, Nowson CA. Relationship between stress, eating behavior, and obesity Nutrition. 2007;23(11-12):887–94. Available from: https://doi.org/10.1016/j.nut.2007.08.008. Epub 2007 Sep 17. PMID: 17869482.

[574] Kolb H, Stumvoll M, Kramer W, Kempf K, Martin S. Insulin translates unfavourable lifestyle into obesity. BMC Med 2018;16(1):232. Available from: https://doi.org/10.1186/s12916-018-1225-1. PMID: 30541568. PMCID: PMC6292073.

[575] Wirtz PH, Ehlert U, Kottwitz MU, La Marca R, Semmer NK. Occupational role stress is associated with higher cortisol reactivity to acute stress. J Occup Health Psychol 2013;18(2):121–31. Available from: https://doi.org/10.1037/a0031802. PMID: 23566275.

[576] Wong JD, Mailick MR, Greenberg JS, Hong J, Coe CL. Daily work stress and awakening cortisol in mothers of individuals with autism spectrum disorders or fragile X syndrome. Fam Relat 2014;63(1):135–47. Available from: https://doi.org/10.1111/fare.12055. PMID: 25313265. PMCID: PMC4192722.

[577] Delaunay F, Khan A, Cintra A, Davani B, Ling ZC, Andersson A, et al. Pancreatic beta cells are important targets for the diabetogenic effects of glucocorticoids. J Clin Invest 1997;100(8):2094–8. Available from: https://doi.org/10.1172/JCI119743. PMID: 9329975. PMCID: PMC508401.

[578] Kolb H, Kempf K, Röhling M, Lenzen-Schulte M, Schloot NC, Martin S. Ketone bodies: from enemy to friend and guardian angel. BMC Med 2021;19(1):313. Available from: https://doi.org/10.1186/s12916-021-02185-0. PMID: 34879839. PMCID: PMC8656040.

[579] Merry TL, Ristow M. Mitohormesis in exercise training Free Radic Biol Med 2016;98:123–30. Available from: https://doi.org/10.1016/j.freeradbiomed.2015.11.032. Epub 2015 Nov 30. PMID: 26654757.

[580] Pierre K, Pellerin L. Monocarboxylate transporters in the central nervous system: distribution, regulation and function. J neurochemistry 2005;94(1):1–4.

[581] Murashige D, Jang C, Neinast M, Edwards JJ, Cowan A, Hyman MC, et al. Comprehensive quantification of fuel use by the failing and nonfailing human heart. Science. 2020;370(6514):364–8.

[582] O'Byrne NA, Yuen F, Butt WZ, Liu PY. Sleep and circadian regulation of cortisol: A short review. Curr OpEndocr Metab Res 2021;18:178–86. Available from: https://doi.org/10.1016/j.coemr.2021.03.011.

[583] Debono M, Ghobadi C, Rostami-Hodjegan A, Huatan H, Campbell MJ, Newell-Price J, et al. Modified-release hydrocortisone to provide circadian cortisol profiles J Clin Endocrinol Metab 2009;94(5):1548–54. Available from: https://doi.org/10.1210/jc.2008-2380. Epub 2009 Feb 17. PMID: 19223520. PMCID: PMC2684472.

[584] Wallden M. Rebalancing the autonomic nervous system (ANS) with work in exercises: practical applications. J Bodyw Mov Ther 2012;16 (2):1–267. Available from: http://doi.org/10.1016/j.jbmt.2012.01.034.

Chapter 4

Cardiovascular disease and its association with insulin resistance and cholesterol

Nadir Ali[1], David M. Diamond[2] and Sarah M. Rice[3]
[1]*Webster, TX, United States,* [2]*University of South Florida, Tampa, FL, United States,* [3]*Nutrition Network, Cape Town, South Africa*

Cardiovascular disease (CVD), insulin resistance (IR), and cholesterol metabolism are intricately linked with many missing pieces of the pathophysiologic puzzle, making rendering a clear image difficult. This chapter describes the normal anatomy and physiology of the cardiovascular system, examines common cardiac diseases, and explores the interaction of the heart and major vessels in the context of IR and lipoprotein metabolism.

4.1 Anatomy and normal physiology of the cardiovascular system

The cardiovascular system consisting of the heart and blood vessels is a primary mechanism for the delivery of oxygen and nutrients to the cells of the body. In addition, it has a role in host defence, immune modulation, as well as transport of cholesterol and fat. While the heart can be described as a pump to circulate blood, it is better understood if we break it down into different components:

1. An involuntary electrical system providing approximately 60–80 beats per minute at rest without the need for any neural input.
2. A muscular pump to generate a stroke volume with each beat to sustain blood flow to the body.
3. A hormonal system that responds to blood volume shifts by producing proteins that regulate salt balance, like B type natriuretic peptide.
4. The chambers of the heart, namely the right atrium, right ventricle, left atrium and left ventricle.
5. Its own blood supply system, called the coronary arteries. The heart cannot use any of the blood in its chambers for its own energy needs. It depends, like the rest of the body, on the supply of blood through arterial blood flow. One of the aspects we will learn in this chapter is how susceptible these arteries are to the process of plaque build-up or atherosclerosis that leads to myocardial infarction or heart attack.

The left atrium receives oxygenated blood from the lungs. Through a combination of its pumping action as well as the relaxation mechanisms of the left ventricle which creates a suction effect, it can transfer blood to the later chamber. The function of the left ventricle is to act as a pump to eject blood to the rest of the body. It accomplishes this through a system of arteries, starting with the aorta, which has several branches. The coronaries supply blood to the heart. The innominate artery carries blood to the right hand and the right side of the brain. The left common carotid and the left subclavian perfuse the left side of the brain as well as the left hand, respectively. The aorta then arches downward supplying blood to the kidneys, liver, digestive system, gonads, and legs.

As they reach the cells, the arteries branch out into smaller vessels called capillaries, which are near to the cells to transfer oxygen and nutrients. Oxygen and nutrients are taken up by the cells from the capillaries. The deoxygenated blood from the capillaries is then collected by the venous system which transports blood back to the right side of the heart. The venous system interacts with the capillaries through venules, which then drain into veins that then collect blood into the inferior vena cava, from the lower part of the body, and the superior vena cava, from the head and upper extremities. The superior and inferior vena cava empty into the right atrium, the upper chamber of the right side of the heart. This is a low-pressure volume chamber that transfers blood to the right ventricle to be pumped into the lungs for

Ketogenic. DOI: https://doi.org/10.1016/B978-0-12-821617-0.00016-4

the process of oxygenation and removal of carbon dioxide in the alveoli (structures in the lungs designed for the air exchange).

The human circulatory system is a closed system in which cells in the blood remain in the vessels (Fig. 4.1). However, nutrients and molecules exit the circulation and bathe the cells via fenestra in the capillary bed. The fluid that leaves the circulatory system through these openings in the capillary bed is then collected by a different set of vessels called the lymphatics. The lymphatic system collects the fluid leaving the vascular system and then returns it back to the venous circulation.

4.1.1 Structure of the arteries

It is important to understand the artery wall architecture since their susceptibility to plaque build-up or atherosclerosis is responsible for the narrowing of these vessels leading to a reduction or cessation of blood flow to important organs like the heart, brain, and kidneys. The arteries have an inner layer called intima, which is lined by a single layer of endothelial cells. Underneath this is the subendothelial layer of the intima which contains proteoglycans, fibronectin, laminin, and collagen. This is not an exhaustive list of the components of the subendothelium. The section on atherosclerosis describes the interaction of low-density lipoprotein cholesterol particles (LDL-c) with this layer of the vessel

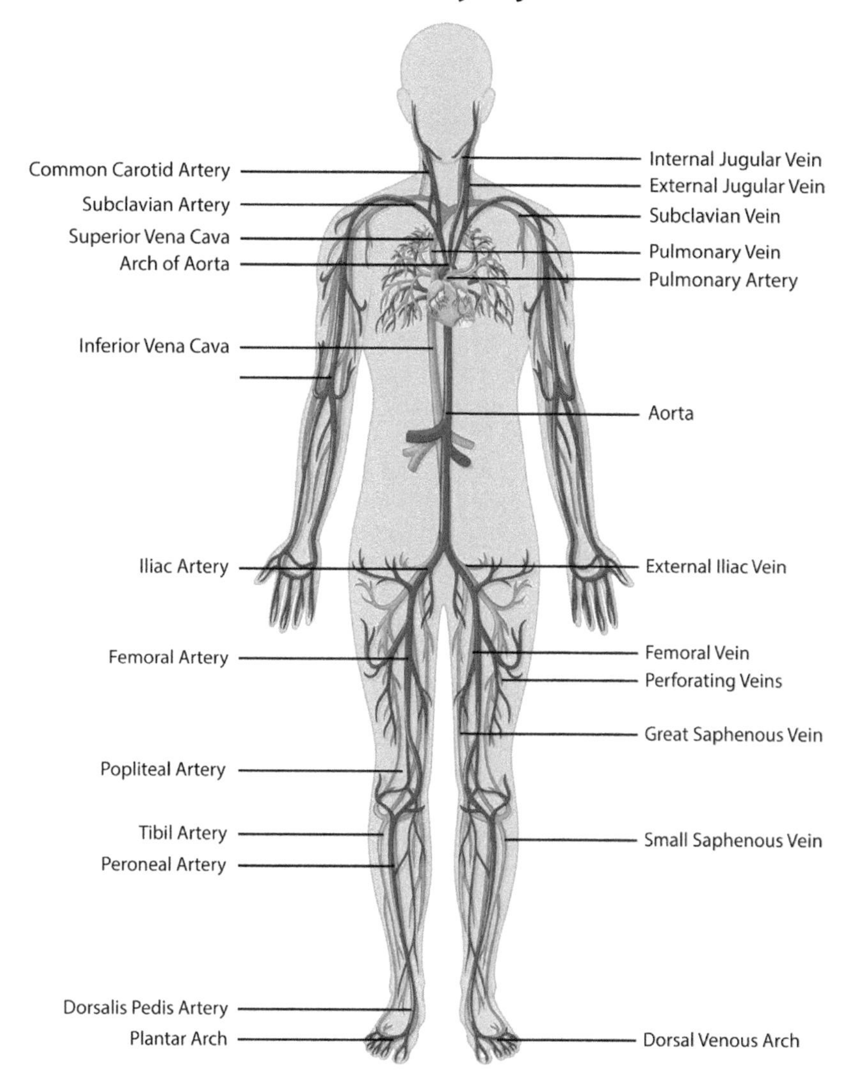

FIGURE 4.1 A basic structure of the human circulatory system. *Designed by Freepik.*

wall. The outer boundary of intima is an elastic tissue called the internal elastic lamina. Due to the interaction of the intima with blood, it is the main regulator of the response of the vessel wall to injury, inflammation, and shear stress.

The next layer is the muscular media, which has a concentric layer of vascular smooth muscle cells. It regulates the size of the blood vessels through vascular tone, which can keep the arteries in a state of vasodilatation (wide) or vasoconstriction (narrow). It interacts with the intima as well as with neural input to maintain the vascular tone. The outer boundary of the media is another elastic layer called the external elastic lamina.

The outermost layer is the adventitia, which contains connective tissue like collagen, to anchor the vessel to the adjacent tissue. The adventitia also harbours the vasa vasorum for nutrient supply as well as nerve endings to mediate vascular tone. The vasa vasorum are small blood vessels that supply oxygen and nutrients to the vessel wall itself. The arteries, like the heart, are not able to use the circulating blood in its lumen for oxygen and nutrient needs. It depends on the vasa vasorum for this function.

The primary role of adventitia is to function as a supporting tissue of the vessel wall. However, studies are beginning to reveal its participation in cell trafficking through the arterial wall, as well as signalling between the adventitia, media, and intima. There is also the concept of the 'outside-in' model of atherosclerosis in which the plaque accumulation in the arteries is proposed to be mediated by injury and inflammatory mediators carried into the vessel wall from the adventitia rather than originating in the higher LDL-c concentration of the circulating blood and its interaction with the sub endothelium [1].

4.1.1.1 The glycocalyx

While the three-layer concept of the arterial wall is well established, there is an emerging role of a fourth layer called the glycocalyx. This is a thin gel-like matrix that covers the endothelial cells and functions like a physical barrier preventing entry of molecules and pathogens into the vessel wall. It contains glycoproteins and glycolipids that mediate the interaction of this layer with cellular components of the blood to mediate vascular signalling and prevent injury. Alteration of the glycocalyx can also lead to susceptibility of the vessel wall to the process of atherosclerosis. High shear stress from arterial hypertension has been shown to reduce the thickness of the glycocalyx. Hyperglycaemia and inflammation promote dysregulation of glycocalyx-degrading-enzymes, such as hyaluronidase and heparinase, damaging the glycocalyx. Hyperglycaemia also drives the abnormal expression of matrix metalloproteinases and hyaluronic acid synthase contributing to endothelial dysfunction. The damaged glycocalyx produces fragments which include hyaluronic acid, further driving damage and inflammation. This creates a vicious cycle contributing to endothelial cell damage and a prothrombotic environment [2].

4.1.2 Role of the cardiovascular system in fluid and electrolyte balance

The circulatory system, through its interaction with the kidneys, maintains normal fluid and electrolyte balance. The kidneys receive about 20% of the cardiac output (a large amount for an organ that is small in size) primarily to maintain blood volume. The filtering unit of the kidney is a glomerulus. The volume and pressure of blood flow into the renal glomeruli is regulated by cardiac output and hormones. In situations of volume excess, the filtering by the glomeruli is increased, resulting in increased urine output. On the other hand, if there is dehydration, blood flow into the renal glomeruli is reduced along with hormonal changes that reduce the filtering and flow of urine to maintain fluid volume homoeostasis. The sodium, electrolyte and water balance of the body are similarly regulated by the blood flow to the renal glomeruli, which alters the filtration volume. In addition, the reabsorption of the filtered electrolytes is regulated to maintain plasma concentrations in a narrow range.

4.2 Cardiovascular pathophysiology

CVD is the major cause of morbidity and mortality in industrialised nations. An overconsumption of simple and refined carbohydrates is the proximate cause of increased insulin synthesis (hyperinsulinaemia) and decreased responsiveness of cells to insulin action (IR). Other factors include frequent meal consumption, caloric excess as well as reduced physical activity (where muscle sarcopenia may play a role [3]). Insulin sensitivity in most of human history was promoted by frequent periods of forced involuntary fasting. The advent of agriculture, supermarkets, personal refrigerators, and pantries has largely abolished fasting.

4.2.1 Abnormal fluid and electrolyte balance

Diabetes, hypertension, and congestive heart failure (CHF) alter blood flow to the kidneys as well as the absorption of water and electrolytes by the renal tubules. Diabetes initially increases the filtering of the renal glomeruli. This chronic glomerular hyperfiltration results in scarring of the glomeruli with kidney dysfunction. Vascular renal disease is a consequence of long-standing diabetes.

Long-standing hypertension can also cause renal dysfunction through glomerular scarring. IR also promotes hypertension by resulting in fluid and salt retention by the kidneys.

CHF, on the other hand, reduces blood flow to the renal glomeruli. A set of compensatory hormonal changes ensue from the compromised renal blood flow resulting in an increase in renin, angiotensin, and aldosterone concentrations. This so-called activation of the renin-angiotensin-aldosterone system (RAAS) axis sets in motion mechanisms to retain both sodium and water to increase cardiac output. The increase in aldosterone concentrations is responsible for sodium retention. When sodium is retained, there is a compensatory loss of potassium mediated by aldosterone. The low potassium concentrations are associated with heart rhythm disorders.

It is important to highlight fluid and electrolyte balance in the setting of a carbohydrate-restricted diet. TCR is associated with a reduction in insulin concentrations and improved insulin sensitivity resulting in decreased reabsorption of filtered sodium. There is also volume loss because sodium excretion is accompanied by water loss. Often, blood pressure improves in individuals on TCR because of urine sodium excretion in an insulin sensitive state. This may result in dizziness, light-headedness, fatigue, and tiredness if the individual on TCR fails to replenish their sodium and water loss. The so-called 'keto-flu' is related to this sodium and water depletion when one initiates a carbohydrate restricted diet. Section 2.2.3. Cautions, contraindications, and troubleshooting when prescribing therapeutic carbohydrate restriction.

4.2.2 Atherosclerosis

Atherosclerosis can be defined as plaque that leads to stenosis or blockage in the lumen of the blood vessels. This compromises blood flow to critical organs such as the heart and brain leading to heart attacks and strokes, which are the major cause of disease and death.

Atherosclerosis can cause the narrowing of the arteries supplying the heart, brain, kidneys, and other organs leading to their dysfunction. These are manifested as myocardial infarction (MI), strokes, dementia, and renal dysfunction.

High blood pressure cannot only cause all these diseases by promoting atherosclerosis but also by disrupting the integrity of blood vessels leading to their rupture with ensuing bleeding in internal organs such as haemorrhagic strokes in the case of the brain or retinal haemorrhages in the eyes.

Reduced blood supply to the heart results in heart muscle dysfunction. The pumping capacity of the heart is reduced, resulting in CHF. There is a failure to meet the oxygen and nutrient demands of the cells and the organs of the body because they are underperfused. Congestive heart failure is manifested clinically as tiredness, fatigue, reduced exercise tolerance, and oedema.

In addition, the reduction in organ perfusion from reduced pumping capacity of the left ventricle of the heart results in compensatory hormonal dysfunction. There is an increase in adrenaline and cortisol concentrations, which over time leads to further deterioration in heart muscle function and worsens atherosclerosis. This is further exacerbated by activation of the RAAS.

The process of atherosclerosis in the coronary arteries can narrow these vessels and reduce blood flow to the heart, resulting in coronary artery disease (CAD) and coronary ischaemia (a chronic process that happens over several decades). However, atherosclerosis can also weaken the endothelial layer, leading to plaque rupture and exposure of the plaque to blood flow. This initiates the coagulation cascade which at times leads to an occlusive clot, which blocks blood flow in the coronary arteries. The clinical manifestation of this is an acute MI, which is a leading cause of mortality in industrialised nations.

Acute MI causes ischaemia and resultant necrosis of a portion of the cardiac muscle. The infarcted area then heals over time into scar tissue. The presence of scar tissue in the left ventricle not only reduces its pumping capacity but alters its electrical conduction. This can lead to premature or irregular beats causing further dysfunction. In advanced cases, the heart rhythm irregularities are sustained, completely disrupting the ability of the heart to pump any blood forward. The clinical manifestation of this is an arrhythmic sudden cardiac death (SCD).

4.2.2.1 The traditional paradigm of atherosclerosis

Atherosclerosis is a process that involves the interaction between endothelial cells, the proteoglycans, collagen, and elastin of the subendothelial matrix, vascular smooth muscle cells of the media as well as the vasa vasorum of the adventitia. The first necessary step is endothelial dysfunction. Normal endothelium has tight junctions and prevents penetration of macromolecules present in circulating blood into the sub endothelium. In addition, intact endothelium prevents adhesion of circulating inflammatory cells. A variety of stimuli including hypertension, inflammation, infection, IR as well as hyperlipidaemia (specifically high LDL-c) are considered to alter endothelial permeability.

LDL-c accumulation in the subendothelial proteoglycan matrix is considered as an initial and necessary first step without which atherosclerosis cannot progress. The retained sub endothelial LDL-c then gets oxidised. There is subsequent release and expression of vascular adhesion molecules on the endothelium for monocyte recruitment, inflammation, and production of reactive oxygen species (ROS). There is associated alteration in flow dynamics of the vessel and simultaneous production of growth factors that lead to proliferation of vascular smooth muscle cells in the media. The activated monocytes express scavenger receptors to orchestrate LDL-c uptake. The resident arterial wall monocytes are now called macrophages, and when loaded with lipids and cholesterol, are called foam cells. As the hyperlipidaemia continues, there is further subendothelial recruitment and retention of LDL-c and atheroma growth. The atheroma will eventually get calcified and its growth increases vessel wall thickness. The increased thickness of the atheroma is a stimulus for neovascularization, through the adventitial vasa vasorum, to support energy needs of the vessel.

The vessel also has anti-atherogenic mechanisms. For example, the oxidised LDL-c uptake by the macrophages initiates the expression of ABCA1 transporters. These transporters mediate the efflux of cholesterol to HDL particles. A normal endothelium also produces nitric oxide (NO). The synthesised NO promotes vasodilation, increasing blood flow, thereby hampering monocyte adhesion. In addition, NO synthesis decreases the expression of adhesion molecules and growth factors for vascular smooth muscle cell proliferation. The subendothelial LDL-c is considered to reduce the synthesis of NO. Interestingly, a TCR approach that elevates ketones can increase NO by upregulating nitric oxide synthase (NOS) which promotes vasodilation, thereby supporting the cardiac patient [4].

4.2.2.2 *Alternative mechanisms of atherosclerosis*

There are a number of processes involved in vascular damage that leads to atherosclerosis. In fact, the term is unfortunate as it conjures up images of fat and cholesterol as proximate causes of the process. A microscopic evaluation of the atherosclerotic plaque demonstrates an impressive array of mediators that are associated with vascular inflammation and repair. The initiating event is most likely endothelial denudation with exposure of the sub intima. This results in degradation and removal of the underlying proteoglycans. The removal of proteoglycans exposes subendothelial fibronectin which binds with LP(a) [5]. This is followed by activation of the coagulation cascade with deposition of platelets and fibrin. There is subsequent recruitment of inflammatory cells such as leucocytes and monocytes to the area. The migration of T cells, B cells, natural killer cells from the outer layers of the vessel wall is induced by cytokines and growth factors elaborated by the preceding inflammatory cells. The process of injury and repair is orchestrated by innumerable growth factors, cytokines, and inflammatory and anti-inflammatory mediators that are summoned by precise signals to the damaged area of the vessel.

There is no question that LDL-c, HDL-c, and specifically LP(a) are present in the vascular lesion, but their temporal presence in the process from injury, coagulation, inflammation, and repair is by no means well defined. The concept that high cholesterol concentrations promote sub-endothelial deposition of LDL-c in a normal vessel has no actual factual data [6–9]. This concept is derived from in vitro models demonstrating binding of LDL-c to collagen [8] or animal studies, where the extent, type and cause of endothelial injury is not well defined. It is not a matter of debate that there is deposition of LDL-c and more specifically LP(a) to the sub endothelial matrix, but this requires preceding injury or inflammation-induced endothelial dysfunction. The LDL-c and LP(a) may well be a part of the healing process as seen with elegant studies on wound healing [10,11], rather than the proximate cause of vascular damage and plaque progression. The LDL-c in particular and the LDL-HDL-c combination may be a part of our antioxidant defence. Afterall, these lipoproteins are endowed not only with potent antioxidants, CoQ10, tocopherol, and beta-carotene, but also have an array of proteins such as paraoxonase and clusterin which have antioxidant properties [12]. Their involvement in the process may be modulation of inflammation rather than the inciting event in plaque formation.

The LDL-c at the site of vascular injury undergoes oxidative modification. This oxidised LDL is necessary for migration of bone marrow-derived mesenchymal stem cells to the site of injury, a process necessary for vascular repair [9,13,14]. Similar mechanisms orchestrated by oxidised LDL-c have also been elucidated for the neuronal cells' repair after damage to their myelin sheath [9].

The Virchow's triad, although used to explain thrombosis, is a good framework to evaluate the proximate cause of atherosclerosis. The components of the triad are vessel flow dynamics, coagulability of blood and endothelial injury. The latter can perhaps be mediated by shear stress from abnormal flow (hypertension) or by an inflammatory state induced by metabolic syndrome (MetS) and IR. The flow dynamics at arterial bifurcations along with abnormal flow states induced by worsening compliance of the vessel with age along with hypertension can cause endothelial disruption. Finally, coagulability of blood is altered with inflammation, infection, and autoimmune disease. All these pathological states can initiate and propagate the process of atherosclerosis. The lipid, cellular, and humoral factors implicated in plaque formation are perhaps a response to an insult that goes through stages of inflammation and uneventful repair in many situations. It is only when the injury is extensive and repeated that the process goes unchecked and leads to plaque growth, rupture and, in some instances, complete occlusion of the artery, leading to an ischaemic event like MI or stroke.

To manipulate lipids with pharmacological interventions based on an imperfect understanding of the process must be viewed with a critical lens. The number of trials of statins and PCSK9 inhibitors that reduce LDL-c have shown a minor or no reduction in mortality (see Section 4.3.2.6.2). In addition, these trials have a major drawback of conflict of interest and lack transparent review by an impartial third party for data fidelity.

4.2.2.2.1 Evidence that LDL-c and oxidised LDL-c are firefighters rather than arsonists

The prevailing wisdom is that LDL-c is atherogenic. However, if for a moment we suspend this paradigm and evaluate that LDL has several antioxidants [15]. When exposed to oxidant injury, such as injured or dysfunctional endothelium, the antioxidants of the LDL are first consumed [16,17]. If the oxidative process exceeds the capacity of the resident antioxidants present in the LDL, then the phospholipid bilayers are oxidised [17]. This LDL-c is now termed the oxidised LDL-c (oxLDL) and is unsuitable for uptake by the liver or endothelial cells via the LDL receptor (LDLR) and must thus be processed differently.

The mechanisms for uptake of oxidised LDL-c at the site of inflammation/damage is orchestrated by a remarkable set of cellular events. The inflammatory cytokines present at the site of injury activate vascular smooth muscle cells (vSMCs) mediated release of PCSK9. Studies have shown that PCSK9 is present in atherosclerotic plaques and is elaborated by several different cells locally rather than being derived from soluble PCSK9 that is secreted by the hepatocytes [18]. Local sources of PCSK9 are vascular smooth muscle cells (vSMCs), intestines, certain neurons, as well as pancreas. There is controversy if macrophages themselves are a source of PCSK9. The elaboration of PCSK9 at the site of vascular injury has been shown to down-regulate the LDLR and upregulate receptors like LOX-1, scavenger receptor A (SRA) and CD36, on macrophages to facilitate the uptake of oxLDL. There is also laboratory evidence that this process directly results in uptake of oxLDL by macrophages [19]. What this implies is that macrophages are programmed to clear oxLDL as a part of the repair and healing process. If the injury is finite and within the capabilities of the repair mechanisms, the macrophages would then be able to clear the damaged proteins and lipids through lysosomal degradation. A portion of the cholesterol from the oxLDL can be recycled through efflux via the ATP binding cassette A1 (ABCA1) to a nascent HDL particle to mediate reverse cholesterol transport (RCT). What is perplexing is the unchallenged hypothesis that LDL-c is the culprit in atherosclerosis, despite the presence of contradictory and conflicting information on its role as an antioxidant amongst its many functions as well as interplay between vSMCs, PCSK9, macrophages, LDLR, and scavenger receptors in the milieu of an injured vessel wall.

4.2.2.2.2 Reverse cholesterol transport and HDL functionality

The cellular content of cholesterol is maintained in a narrow range. This is essential for normal cellular function. Since cholesterol is not a metabolic fuel, excess cholesterol must be eliminated, rather effluxed from cells by a process termed RCT. The effluxed cholesterol is picked up by HDL, taken directly to the liver or via LDL for elimination either as free cholesterol or converted to bile salts for excretion to maintain cholesterol balance. Another pathway for cholesterol balance is trans-intestinal cholesterol elimination (TICE), which is also mediated by both LDL and HDL. In this process, HDL is involved in about 30%–35% of cholesterol elimination directly into the intestines, bypassing the liver altogether.

While all cells require cholesterol homoeostasis, perhaps the cells where it is of primary importance are the macrophages in the vessel wall, responsible for plaque formation or atherosclerosis. The process of vascular injury by inflammation or hypertension leads to release of inflammatory cytokines attracting monocytes and lipoproteins for healing and repair. The LDL-c at the site of vascular damage functions as an antioxidant, and if the oxidative damage is severe, can itself get oxidised. This oxLDL is phagocytosed by resident monocytes (macrophages) in the injured vessel wall [17,20]. Exploring the process of RCT in macrophages that have acquired oxLDL is perhaps of primary importance in understanding the factors that prevent atherosclerosis. A properly functioning RCT would lead to prevention of macrophages from becoming foam cells with overloaded sterol content. It is the rupture of foam cells with release of their cholesterol and fat content that is proposed as a mechanism for not only compromise in vascular lumen but also in mediation of vascular thrombotic events leading MI and strokes (Fig. 4.2).

The macrophages deal with excess cholesterol by converting it to CE and storing them in lipid droplets or by promoting cholesterol efflux through ABCA1, G1/G5, in their cell membranes. Only free cholesterol can be effluxed and thus the CE present in the lipid droplets needs to undergo hydrolysis. The cholesterol efflux from macrophages is a rate limiting step in RCT. Experimental evidence indicates that activation of autophagy is an important process in promoting cholesterol efflux [21]. The lipid droplet is taken up by autophagosomes, which fuse with the lysosome for hydrolysis of CE. In addition, there is increased synthesis of ABCA1 and other cholesterol efflux receptors along with their translocation to the cell membrane as part of the autophagic process. It is thus possible that intermittent and long-term fasting, as well as endurance exercise, mediate their CV benefit by enhancing the process of macrophage autophagy and RCT.

The process of vascular RCT can be broadly divided into three overlapping steps:

1. cholesterol efflux,
2. translocation of cholesterol though HDL and other interacting lipoproteins in circulation, and
3. cholesterol elimination through the liver or directly via TICE.

The cholesterol efflux is primarily directed by the ABCA1 to pre-HDL (HDL-3) but there is also contribution of passive diffusion to the mature large HDL particle (HDL-2). The vascular smooth muscle cells (VSMC) can also

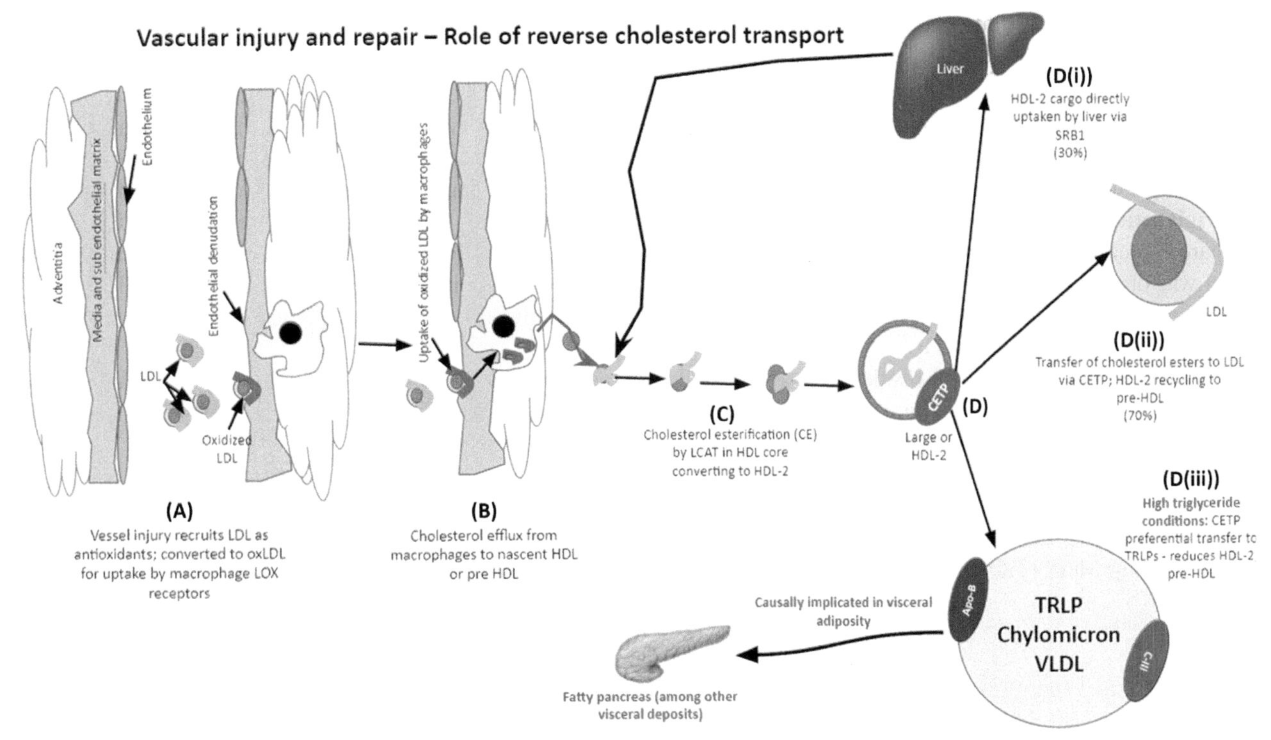

FIGURE 4.2 **Role of reverse cholesterol transport (RCT) in vascular injury and repair.** (A) Vessel injury with denudation of endothelium from hypertension or inflammation with recruitment of LDL (as firefighters) to function as antioxidants and repair mechanisms. The LDL in this process gets oxidised and taken up by special LOX receptors in macrophages. The macrophages are attracted to the area by inflammatory mediators present at the site of vascular injury. (B) Repair involves reverse cholesterol transport from the macrophages that has taken up the oxidised LDL. There is free cholesterol efflux medicated by ATP-binding cassette on to a nascent Apo A-I (pre HDL). (C) As the pre HDL takes up free cholesterol, there is conversion of cholesterol to CE by action of lyso-lecithin cholesterol ester transferase (LCAT) in the core of the HDL molecule. This is now called large HDL or HDL-2. (D) HDL-2 (large HDL) has one of three possible fates depending on the prevailing metabolic conditions. (D(i)) About 30% of HDL-2's cargo is taken up by the liver directly by scavenger receptor B1 (SRB1). (D(ii)) The major pathway for RCT is however through LDL (70%). This process involves the transfer of CE to LDL by the action of cholesterol ester transfer protein (CETP). After the HDL-2 unloads the CE, it can then recycle and become pre-HDL ready to pick up free cholesterol effluxed by the macrophages. (D(iii)) If the prevailing metabolic conditions are one of high triglycerides or Triglyceride rich lipoproteins (TRLP), then CETP will preferentially transfer CE to TRLPs, bypassing RCT. TRLPs have an extended plasma half-life and are causally related to ectopic fat deposition in visceral tissue such as the pancreas (fatty pancreas), liver (NAFLD), or in vascular tissue. These conditions reduce both large HDL as well as pre HDL reducing cholesterol efflux and RCT, leading to sterol and fat accumulation in the macrophages (foam cells). See text for details.

acquire macrophage-like capabilities and take up oxidised lipoproteins [22]. There is also a role of the lymphatic vessels present in the adventitia for movement of HDL-c and cholesterol out of the media of the vessel wall. Finally, there is reverse transmigration of the monocyte-macrophages out to the media into circulation.

The translocation of free cholesterol in HDL after initial efflux involves its esterification by the enzyme lecithin cholesterol acyl transferase (LCAT), as well as the exchange of CE between lipoproteins mediated by CETP. The large HDL-2 can be taken up directly by the liver via scavenger receptor B1 (SRB1). The CE acquired in this process is eliminated as cholesterol in bile or converted to bile salts. Alternatively, CETP mediates the transfer of CE to apo-B-containing lipoproteins, LDL and VLDL/chylomicrons. The transfer of CE to LDL as an intermediate step illustrates the importance of this lipoprotein in the process of RCT (Fig. 4.1).

In the setting of metabolic health and insulin sensitivity transfer of CE to chylomicrons/VLDL and their remnants, collectively labelled under the category of triglyceride rich lipoproteins (TRLP), is minor. However, in the setting of MetS and adipose tissue IR there are persistent high concentrations of triglycerides (TRLP), especially in the postprandial state. The concentration of HDL-c is dependent on the metabolism of TRLP. In the setting of disturbed triglyceride metabolism, such as the genetic deficiency of lipoprotein lipase (LPL), an enzyme response for de-lipidation of chylomicrons and VLDL in adipose tissue, triglyceride concentrations rise, and HDL concentrations consistently decrease. The factors underlying the metabolic dependence of HDL on TRLP is the equilibration of CE and triglycerides between lipoproteins in all plasma lipoprotein classes. This process is mediated by CETP. A persistence rise in the concentration of TRLP allows increased translocation of CE from HDL to chylomicrons and VLDL, while increasing the triglyceride content of HDL. Therefore, all classes of HDL decrease with the preponderant reduction in large HDL (HDL-2). Thus, persistent elevation of triglyceride concentrations is a driving force for not only reducing HDL concentrations and thereby reducing RCT but diverting CE from RCT to TRLP, which are implicated in promoting ectopic fat deposition. The half-life of an HDL particle exceeds that of chylomicron by a factor of ~ 1000 and of $\sim$VLDL by a factor of 50. An HDL particle is therefore exposed to several generations of TRLP and serves as a marker of triglyceride metabolism and residence time. Fasting triglyceride concentration does not provide the temporal persistence and magnitude of postprandial lipaemia and offers an imperfect picture of triglyceride metabolic capacity. Thus, investigators used postprandial triglyceride values to assess the alteration in RCT as predictors of CAD [23]. Patients with established CAD were compared to controls in terms of post prandial persistence of high triglycerides. A pattern of persistent hypertriglyceridemia was observed, especially in the 4–8-h post-meal window in patients with CAD compared to controls (Fig. 4.3).

This was accompanied by a significant reduction in HDL-2, an indication that the RCT was compromised, and the CE diverted to TRLP (Table 4.1).

These TRLP have prolonged residence time in circulation, are not cleared by adipose tissue or the liver and lead to ectopic visceral fat deposition. The ectopic fat deposition is implicated in fatty liver and pancreas and causes hepatic IR and pancreatic beta-cell dysfunction.

A group of investigators have shown the extent of alteration and reduction in HDL-c is dependent on the severity of MetS [24]. When more variables that define higher grades of MetS are present, the reduction in large HDL (HDL-2) is higher compared to HDL-3. However, it should be noted that there is a reduction in concentrations of all HDL particles with worsening MetS (Table 4.2; Fig. 4.4).

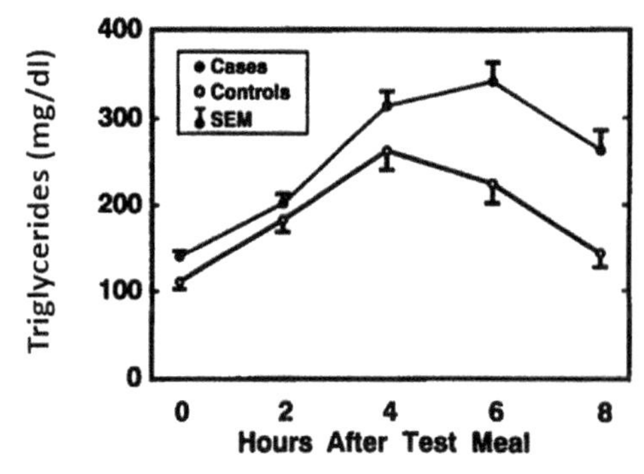

FIGURE 4.3 **Postprandial triglyceride kinetics in coronary artery disease (CAD) patients and control subjects.** There is a marked persistent elevation in triglycerides in patients with CAD from 4–8 h post-meal. *Figure extracted from Patsch JR, Miesenböck G, Hopferwieser T, Mühlberger V, Knapp E, Dunn JK, et al. Relation of triglyceride metabolism and coronary artery disease. Studies in the postprandial state. Arterioscler Thromb. 1992;12(11):1336–1345.*

TABLE 4.1 Fasting plasma lipid, lipoprotein, and apolipoprotein concentrations in control patients and patients with coronary artery disease (CAD).

	Cases (coronary score > 50)	Controls (coronary score = 0)	*P*
n	61	40	
Age (years)	54.1 (0.7)	50.5 (1.2)	.0140
BMI (kg/m^2)	25.5 (0.3)	25.1 (0.3)	.4930
Plasma cholesterol	263.1 (5.2)	250.9 (8.0)	.1850
Plasma triglycerides*	139.7 (6.9)	111.1 (8.6)	.0098
HDL cholesterol	45.4 (1.4)	51.2 (2.1)	.0211
HDL_2 cholesterol	11.7 (0.8)	17.6 (1.7)	.0002[†]
HDL_3 cholesterol	33.8 (1.1)	33.8 (1.2)	.9899
LDL cholesterol	189.7 (5.1)	177.4 (7.0)	.1521
ApoA-I	130.2 (2.9)	134.2 (3.7)	.3985
ApoB*	100.9 (3.1)	84.7 (3.3)	.0002[†]
ApoA-II	44.1 (1.7)	41.4 (1.6)	.0404
Cholesterol/HDL cholesterol	5.8 (0.3)	4.9 (0.2)	.0055

BMI, Body mass index; *HDL*, high-density lipoprotein; *LDL*, low-density lipoprotein; *Apo*, apolipoprotein. Results are mean and SEM.
**Probability value obtained by the two-sample Wilcoxon rank-sum test.*
[†]Statistically significant difference, using restrictions (see paper).
Source: Figure extracted from Patsch JR, Miesenböck G, Hopferwieser T, Mühlberger V, Knapp E, Dunn JK, et al. Relation of triglyceride metabolism and coronary artery disease. Studies in the postprandial state. Arterioscler Thromb. 1992;12(11):1336–1345.

TABLE 4.2 Marked reduction in HDL-2 (large HDL) and mild reduction in HDL-3 (pre-HDL), as well as increase in small dense LDL in patients with metabolic syndrome compared to controls.

	Controls	Metabolic syndrome	*P*
sdLDL (mg/dL)	4 (0–50)	12 (0–79)	<.001
sdLDL (%)	3 (0–28)	9 (0–56)	<.001
HDL-2 (mg/dL)	21 (6–44)	12 (4–37)	<.001
HDL-2 (%)	35 (16–62)	26 (9–52)	<.001
HDL-3 (mg/dL)	37 (18–47)	34 (14–43)	<.05
HDL-3 (%)	66 (38–84)	74 (48–91)	<.001

Source: Taken from Lagos KG, Filippatos TD, Tsimihodimos V, Gazi IF, Rizos C, Tselepis AD, et al. Alterations in the high density lipoprotein phenotype and HDL-associated enzymes in Subjects with metabolic syndrome. Lipids. 2009;44(1):9.

It is enticing and overly simplistic to assume that higher HDL-c concentrations are a marker of robust RCT and protection from atherosclerosis. Such a mistake has been made in trials of CETP inhibition [25]. The Illuminate trial with a synthetic CETP inhibitor was launched with the hypothesis that high HDL-c concentrations as a result of blockade of CE transfer to LDL-c would be beneficial. The concentrations of HDL-c in this study increased by 72% with a robust reduction in LDL-c (Fig. 4.5).

However, this was most likely at the cost of RCT mediated via the LDL pathway and its uptake by the liver through the LDLR. The use of CETP inhibitor was associated with a statistically increased risk of death and other adverse events in this study leading to premature discontinuation of the trial (Table 4.3).

Clinical trials with both PCSK9 inhibitors as well as statins show a modest (PCSK9 inhibitors) and mild (statins) increase in HDL-c, respectively [26]. This may be at the cost of reducing RCT. The PCSK9 inhibitors lead to

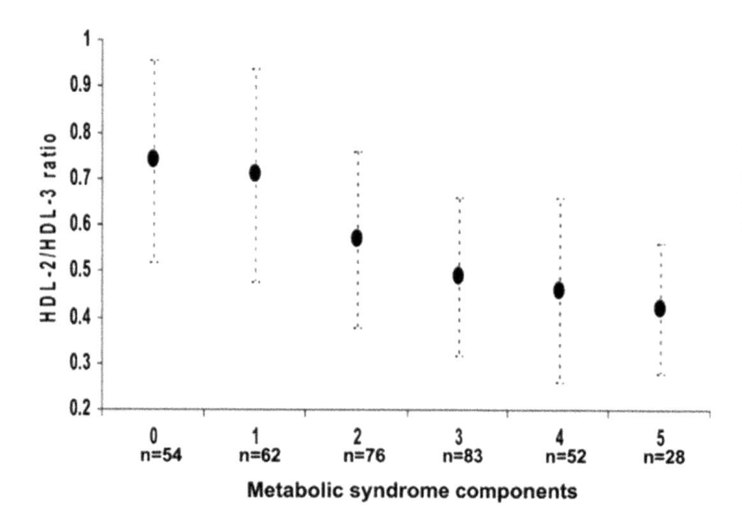

FIGURE 4.4 Alterations of HDL-2/HDL-3 ratio according to the number of components of metabolic syndrome (Kruskal–Wallis, P for trend <.001). Values are given as means ± SD. n = number of subjects. *Figure extracted from Lagos KG, Filippatos TD, Tsimihodimos V, Gazi IF, Rizos C, Tselepis AD, et al. Alterations in the high density lipoprotein phenotype and HDL-associated enzymes in Subjects with metabolic syndrome. Lipids. 2009;44(1):9.*

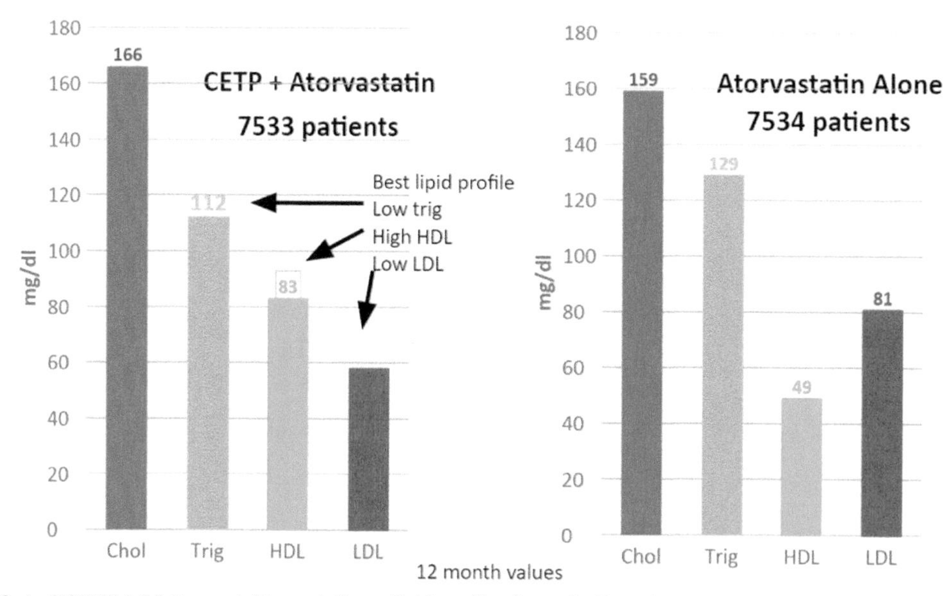

FIGURE 4.5 **Effect of CETP inhibitor and Atorvastatin on lipid profiles from the Investigation of Lipid Level Management to Understand its Impact on Atherosclerotic Events (ILLUMINATE) trial.** This trial was structured with the hypothesis that addition of a CETP inhibitor would improve overall lipid profiles, operating on traditional conceptions of LDL-c and HDL-c as 'good' and 'bad' cholesterol respectively. These patterns were indeed observed via triglyceride and LDL-c reductions coupled with HDL-c increases. *Figure adapted from results of Barter PJ, Caulfield M, Eriksson M, Grundy SM, Kastelein JJP, Komajda M, et al. Effects of torcetrapib in patients at high risk for coronary events. N Engl J Med. 2007;357 (21):2109–2122.*

a 70% reduction in LDL-c concentrations, which markedly reduces the exchange of CE between HDL-2 and LDL, compromising RCT. Statins reduce LDL-c by a modest 30%–50% leading perhaps to a lower impact on RCT. Thus, the increase in HDL-c associated with both statins and PCSK9 may be at the cost of HDL functionality. Nevertheless, the unintended consequences of pharmaceutical interventions on RCT should be considered and explored in more detail.

Since HDL-c concentrations do not correlate with either subclinical atherosclerosis or outcomes, a measure of HDL functionality, that is the ability to carry out RCT, was investigated by Anand Rohatgi and co-workers [27]. They measured the cholesterol efflux capacity of whole serum in 2924 individuals free of CVD at baseline and followed them for a median of 9.4 years. They found a significant inverse association between cholesterol efflux capacity and incident CV events (i.e. high cholesterol efflux capacity was associated with a better outcome).

TABLE 4.3 Effect of CETP inhibitor and Atorvastatin on mortality from the Investigation of Lipid Level Management to Understand its Impact on Atherosclerotic Events (ILLUMINATE) trial.

	CETP + Atorvastatin	Atorvastatin alone
7533 patients		**7534 patients**
Total mortality	93	59
Cancer mortality	24	14
Hospital for CHF	84	50
Infections	9	0
Stroke	6	0

Hosp, Hospitalisations; *CHF*, congestive heart failure.
Source: Figure adapted from results of Barter PJ, Caulfield M, Eriksson M, Grundy SM, Kastelein JJP, Komajda M, et al. Effects of torcetrapib in patients at high risk for coronary events. N Engl J Med. 2007;357(21):2109–2122.

4.2.2.3 Insulin resistance as a proximate cause of atherosclerosis

It will be useful at this point to explain the mechanisms by which IR promotes vascular disease.

- Insulin not only regulates glucose homoeostasis but is intricately involved in lipid metabolism. LPL is an insulin sensitive enzyme that transfers the absorbed dietary fat into adipose tissue. Decreased responsiveness of LPL is a hallmark of IR and leads to a longer residence time of circulating triglyceride-rich lipoproteins (TRL) in the blood [28]. The dyslipidaemia of IR is high TRL along with a reduction in HDL-c. This lipoprotein profile is associated with an increased prevalence of atherosclerosis [29].
- IR leads to hyperglycaemia and glycation of proteins in the body (glycated haemoglobin (HbA1c) is usually as a proxy measure for this). An increase in glycated proteins has been demonstrated to increase atherosclerosis [30].
- IR causes an increase in arterial blood pressure. Hypertension is known to cause endothelial damage leading to vascular injury and atherosclerosis [31].
- IR and hyperinsulinaemia results in sodium retention by the kidneys, leading to intravascular volume overload with ensuing arterial hypertension [32].
- IR has been demonstrated to cause hunger, leading to a vicious cycle of hyperinsulinaemia, hunger, caloric-overconsumption (see Chapter 11.3.1. Hunger)
- Hyperinsulinaemia and IR are associated with redox imbalance and inflammation, which contributes to impaired vascular function and the development of CVD [33].

4.3 Cholesterol

4.3.1 Biology of cholesterol

Cholesterol is essential for life. In the human body, cholesterol is an integral part of the phospholipid bilayer cell membrane, imparting it with fluidity, flexibility, and reinforcement. The membrane permeability is controlled by cholesterol. The cholesterol is also a key ingredient of the lipid rafts and caveolae, part of the cell membrane where protein receptors are anchored in an orientation to facilitate signalling and trafficking between cells. Even a cursory examination of the role of cholesterol in animal and human biology will reveal that it is an integral part of neural function, nerve conduction, precursor of steroid hormones like testosterone, oestrogens, and cortisol, and essential in the synthesis of vitamin D in the skin [34]. This list is by no means complete.

Both cholesterol and fat (triglycerides) are fatty waxy substances. Biological organisms from single cellular bacteria to humans operate in an essentially aqueous medium. Since fat does not dissolve in an aqueous environment, provisions were made early in evolution to carry these vital molecules within the organism through macromolecules that dissolve in aqueous transport media. This transport medium over millions of years of evolution has specialised into blood. There are many cholesterol and lipid transport molecules, called lipoproteins. Each lipoprotein has an identifying protein and a phospholipid bilayer that makes it water soluble. The internal cargo of these transport molecules are not just cholesterol and triglycerides, but also other molecules with biological activity, such as fat-soluble vitamins and antioxidants.

4.3.1.1 Cell membrane, cholesterol content, lipid rafts and membrane receptor function

Cholesterol has a four-ring structure along with a flexible tail. The tail is hydrophobic and associated with the polar interior of the cell membrane phospholipid bilayer. There is a 3β OH group that is polar and oriented towards the aqueous phase of the cell membrane. The cholesterol content of a red blood cell membrane is about 45%. The cholesterol in the cell membrane is distributed in a non-uniform fashion. There are sections of the cell membrane called lipid rafts that are cholesterol rich. These rafts contain membrane proteins such as the insulin receptor. The proper functioning of the insulin receptor requires the appropriate cholesterol content of the lipid rafts [35]. The alteration of the membrane sterol content by pharmacological manipulation has been shown to disrupt the function of these receptors [36]. This is perhaps a mechanism for IR associated with statin use. The cholesterol content and location are also determinants of membrane permeability and fluidity.

4.3.1.2 Absorption of fat- and fat-soluble vitamins

Bile salts are synthesised in the liver from cholesterol. They are stored in the gallbladder. The bile salts enter the intestines after ingestion of a fatty meal. They are essential for the absorption of fat- and fat-soluble vitamins. The bile salt synthesis is precisely regulated by their rate of reabsorption in the distal ileum [37] after it aids in the absorption of fat- and fat-soluble vitamins by micelle formation.

4.3.1.3 Brain function, neurological development, and peripheral nervous system

The human brain is only 2% of body weight yet has 25% of body cholesterol. Cholesterol is present in myelin (70%) and the rest is a part of glial and neuronal cell membranes [6]. The cholesterol in membranes is involved in lipid raft-mediated neuroreceptor orientation [6]. The brain cannot utilise either the ingested cholesterol or cholesterol synthesised by the liver because the blood brain barrier prevents the exchange or entry of lipoproteins present in systemic circulation [6]. So, the entirety of the brain's cholesterol is synthesised in situ, from basic materials like acetyl-CoA [38].

The synthesis of cholesterol is at its peak during early development, while the neuronal axons that transmit nerve impulses are being myelinated. The cholesterol for myelination is produced by supporting glial cells called oligodendrocytes. This formation of myelin in the central and peripheral nervous system during development means that there is a dramatic increase in the cholesterol content of the brain from infancy to adulthood [39].

After development, cholesterol synthesis continues at low concentrations for repair of neural cell membranes [40]. Most of the cholesterol from neuronal cell use is synthesised by supporting central nervous system (CNS) cells, called astrocytes. The neurons themselves synthesise very little, but neural damage such as strokes, neurodegenerative disorders and traumatic brain injury, has the capability to reactivate cholesterol synthesis [40].

The cholesterol synthesised in the astrocytes is distributed to the neurons by cholesterol efflux to apolipoprotein E (ApoE), which is the predominant lipoprotein in the CNS. ApoE is synthesised in the glial cells including the astrocytes and lipidated by cholesterol efflux mechanisms, namely the ATP binding cassette A1 (ABCA1) and other cholesterol effluxers [40].

CNS cholesterol is homeostatically regulated: [41–43]

1. Excess cholesterol is hydroxylated in the brain through a cytochrome P450 enzymes, converting cholesterol 24-hydroxylase (CYP46A1) to 24s-hydroxycholesterol. Unlike cholesterol, 24s-hydroxycholesterol can cross the lipophilic blood brain barrier, is picked up by the LDL lipoprotein, transported to the liver where it is either eliminated as such or converted to bile acid.
2. Conversion it to cholesterol esters and storage it in lipid droplets (LD) in neurons. The LD are also a storage form for fat in the liver.
3. Cholesterol efflux to the apolipoprotein A1 in the cerebrospinal fluid. While the CNS cells themselves make no apolipoprotein A1, the predominant apoprotein of HDL, the choroid plexus responsible for interfacing the cerebrospinal fluid with systemic circulation transports this protein into the cerebrospinal fluid (CSF). The lipidated apolipoprotein A1 in the CSF is an HDL-like particle that is taken up by brain capillary endothelial cells via their scavenger receptor B1 or LDL receptor related protein (LRP).

The receptors of neurotransmitters are located in cholesterol rich lipid rafts. Statins, especially the lipophilic ones, alter the cholesterol content of lipid rafts and can adversely alter neuronal signal transduction [44].

While neuronal cholesterol synthesis and elimination is shielded by dietary cholesterol intake or hepatic synthesis, its regulation is altered by cerebral IR as well as by statins that readily cross the blood brain barrier [45]. While alteration in CNS cholesterol regulation is a hallmark of neuro degenerative disease like Alzheimer's and Parkinson's disease, the exact biochemical abnormalities are not well understood [40]. Pharmaceutical interventions aimed at reducing cholesterol have so far shown no significant benefit in randomised trials (see Statin box). At present the best strategy is prevention of neuronal IR through lifestyle changes such as low carbohydrate diets, intermittent and long-term fasting as well as exercise [46–49].

4.3.1.4 Precursor for vitamin D

Vitamin D is not only involved in calcium regulation of bone, but also regulates immune response to viral and bacterial infections [50]. Low vitamin D concentrations are associated with higher risk and greater intensity of Sars-COVID infections [51]. The synthesis of vitamin D from UVB sun rays is directly proportional to cholesterol concentration [52]. The synthesis of vitamin D is initiated by conversion of absorbed or synthesised cholesterol to 7-dehydrocholesterol which is then transported to the epidermis layer of the skin when in it undergoes isomerization under UVB exposure to pre-vitamin D3 or cholecalciferol [53].

It is interesting to note that cholesterol and vitamin D have the same precursor, namely 7-dehydrocholesterol. Statins inhibit the synthesis of 7-dehydrocholesterol by inhibiting HMG Coenzyme A reductase. It might therefore be expected that there would be a reduction of vitamin D synthesis and it is perhaps strange that this has never been reported clinically. There is no biochemical explanation for this finding and may relate to modulation of inflammation with statins that alters the degradation of vitamin D or an area that needs further detailed exploration [54].

4.3.1.5 Host defence

While our focus has been on hyperlipidaemia and its association with atherosclerosis, we have neglected the downside of hypolipidaemia in predisposing the individual to bacterial lung infections. Severe hypolipidemia has been associated with septic shock and burn injury. Both states are characterised by a cytokine storm and extensive inflammation [55,56].

4.3.1.6 Cellular repair and growth

Growing cells and tissues require cholesterol. This is either synthesised de novo or acquired from external sources through receptor mediated endocytosis, mediated by the LDL receptor (LDLR) on the cell membrane. Specialised cells are not able to meet the demands of cholesterol for either growth or injury and repair by de novo synthesis. The liver is thus the primary supply of cholesterol to tissue through the synthesis and export of LDL. The liver itself will either synthesise the cholesterol to be packaged into the LDL or may prefer to acquire dietary cholesterol via the chylomicron remnant receptor. There are many putative receptors implicated in remnant particle metabolism, the principal amongst these is the LDLR related protein (LRP1) [57]. The chylomicron remnant acquires an apo E from the HDL to facilitate its interaction with LRP1.

The neonatal brain is undergoing rapid growth and cholesterol is required. While neuronal cells like peripheral cells have machinery to synthesise cholesterol, the demand cannot be met from this source alone. The function of exogenous cholesterol supply to neurons is met by astrocytes. The astrocytes package cholesterol in a lipoprotein molecule with apoE as its principal structural lipoprotein. This apoE-mediated cholesterol delivery is orchestrated through LRP1 and other LDL family of receptors in neuronal cells. Defects in these receptors have been shown to impair neuronal growth.

Relatively few studies have been done to evaluate the role and requirement of cholesterol for cell growth. This is perhaps because of its demonisation and postulated role in CVD. This is unfortunate, because the source of cholesterol for tissues undergoing growth or repair is most likely LDL [58].

4.3.1.7 Steroid hormone biosynthesis

The endocrine glands, adrenal cortex, ovaries, and testes are involved in steroid hormone synthesis. There are five major classes of steroid hormones: oestrogens for development of female sexual characteristics; progestins, which are necessary for reproduction; testosterone, involved in male sexual development; mineralocorticoids, to mediate sodium/potassium and volume balance; and glucocorticoids, that have a variety of functions including glucose regulation, protein metabolism and modulation of inflammation. These classes of hormones are derived from a common precursor, which is cholesterol. Human steroidogenic endocrine glands are not bestowed with the capacity to make all cholesterol needed for hormone synthesis by de novo cholesterol synthesis. They depend on LDLR mediated endocytosis of LDL for cholesterol uptake [59].

4.3.2 Regulation of cholesterol synthesis and elimination (cholesterol balance)

Cholesterol is essential for life in all eukaryotic cells [60]. In fact, sterols are present in all living organisms in some form [61]. Fungi make ergosterol, plants synthesise phytosterol, and humans produce cholesterol and absorb it from the gastrointestinal tract [61,62]. Since cholesterol is not a metabolic fuel, its regulation is orchestrated by adjusting de novo synthesis, absorption, and elimination [62].

Making cholesterol is energy expensive and requires an array of enzymes. Synthesis of a single cholesterol molecule consumes ~100 ATP molecules [63]. A simplified cholesterol synthesis pathway is shown in Fig. 4.6.

Approximately, 1000 mg (about the weight of a small paper clip) of cholesterol is produced endogenously in humans in a day [65]. An average human ingests about 300 mg (30%, about the weight of 10 grains of rice) from their diet [65]. The remaining 700 mg (70%) is synthesised in various tissues, predominantly in the liver, but also in intestines and skin [64,66]. The absorption and synthesis of this sterol is tightly coupled with elimination in faeces, such as in bile acid or biliary cholesterol [65]. There has been the discovery of a novel pathway of cholesterol removal, the trans intestinal cholesterol elimination (TICE), which is described later in this chapter. Even though most cells synthesise cholesterol de novo, this is insufficient to meet the need for formation of new membrane or steroid hormone production in specialised cells such as the adrenal cortex, testes, and ovaries [67]. Consequently, to meet demand, cells rely on HDL-c and LDL-c for supply, through the process of receptor-mediated endocytosis [67]. An exception to this

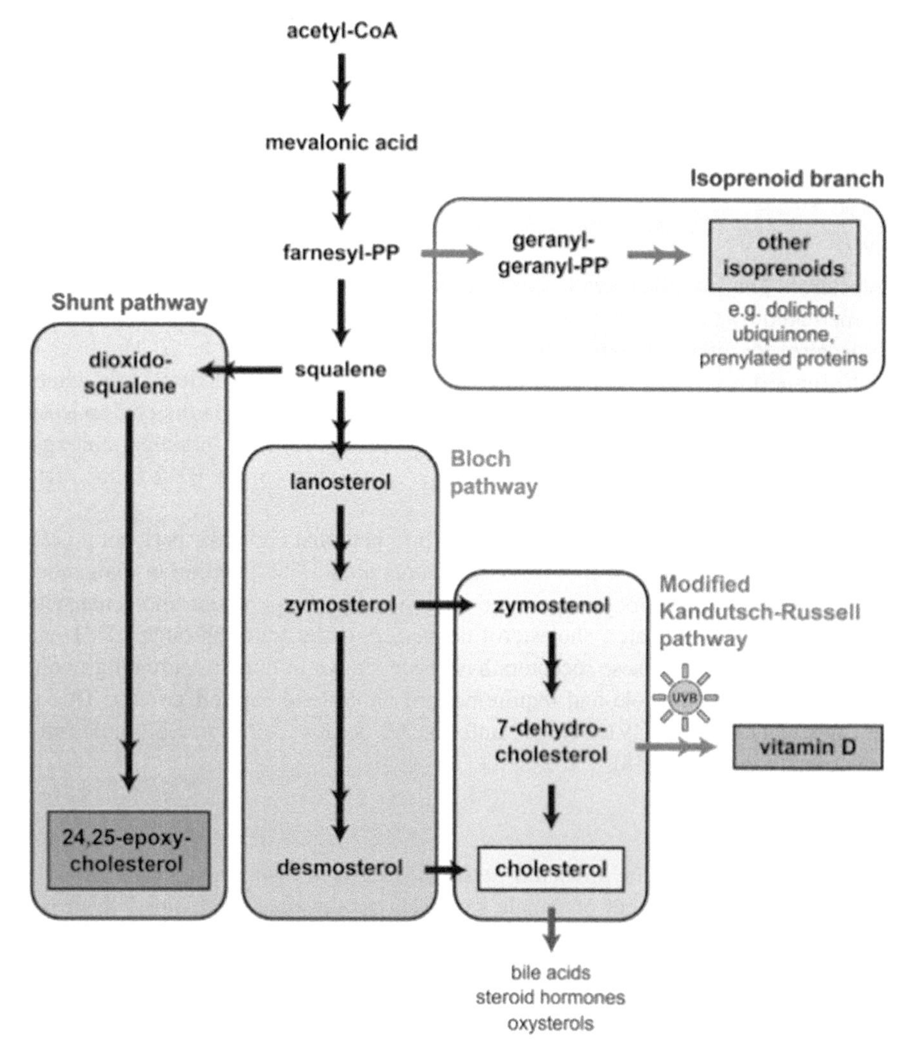

FIGURE 4.6 **A simplified cholesterol synthesis pathway.** The basic initial molecule is acetyl CoA, which is subsequently enzymatically processed into intermediate compounds hydroxymethylglutaryl-CoA (HMG CoA), mevalonic acid, squalene and lanosterol. The pathway for synthesis then diverges into two pathways that make different intermediates but their final enzymatic step results in the formation of cholesterol. These are the Bloch pathway with an intermediary desmosterol and the Kandutsch-Russell pathway with 7-dehydrochlolesterol synthesis [64]. The final step in both pathways is cholesterol synthesis.

is the human brain, which acquires all its cholesterol needs through de novo synthesis because LDL-c is not able to cross the blood brain barrier [67,68].

Cholesterol homoeostasis is finely controlled by cells [64]. If it is unable to obtain cholesterol from the receptor-mediated endocytosis of LDL-c, it upregulates synthesis through transcription factors called sterol regulatory element binding proteins (SREBPs) [67]. The SREBPs not only upregulate cholesterol synthesising enzymes like HMG CoA reductase (the target of statins) but also increase the production and expression of LDLR to take-up cholesterol from LDL. Since cholesterol is present in the membranes of the cell and is an insoluble lipid, it cannot directly regulate its biosynthesis and uptake via cytoplasmic sensors [69]. Its sensor, the SREBP, is membrane bound and can gauge the concentration of sterols in endoplasmic reticulum and other intracellular membranes, and thus serve this role of regulating cholesterol homoeostasis (Fig. 4.7).

The finely tuned regulation of cholesterol synthesis by SREBPs is demonstrated in cultured human fibroblast experiments [71]. In cholesterol-depleted serum, SREBP demonstrates nuclear localisation in order to upregulate genes for cholesterogenesis (vs a cytoplasmic and inactivated status in cholesterol-replete serum), thus elucidating a clear and direct role in cholesterol homoeostasis via gene regulation (Fig. 4.8).

When cholesterol is present in excess in the cells, mechanism of efflux exists through pumps like ATP-binding cassette transporters A1 and G1 (ABCA1 and ABCG1) that transport cholesterol from the cells to a waiting HDL for the molecule to be recycled [65] (Fig. 4.9). The exported cholesterol may be re-used for cell repair, steroid hormone synthesis or eliminated through bile or by transintestinal cholesterol elimination (TICE) [65].

Cholesterol content of the body can be considered as brain, intestinal, tissue, liver, and lipoprotein-associated pools. The amount of cholesterol is closely regulated in all pools except for a flux in the lipoprotein pool which can vary depending on the metabolic status and nutritional intake of cholesterol (Fig. 4.10).

In a vegan who ingests no cholesterol, the entire daily requirement of cholesterol of about 1–1.5 g is through de novo synthesis. In individuals on a standard American diet, who ingest about 300 mg of cholesterol, the de novo synthesis is adjusted to account for cholesterol absorption. However, only about 26% of dietary cholesterol is

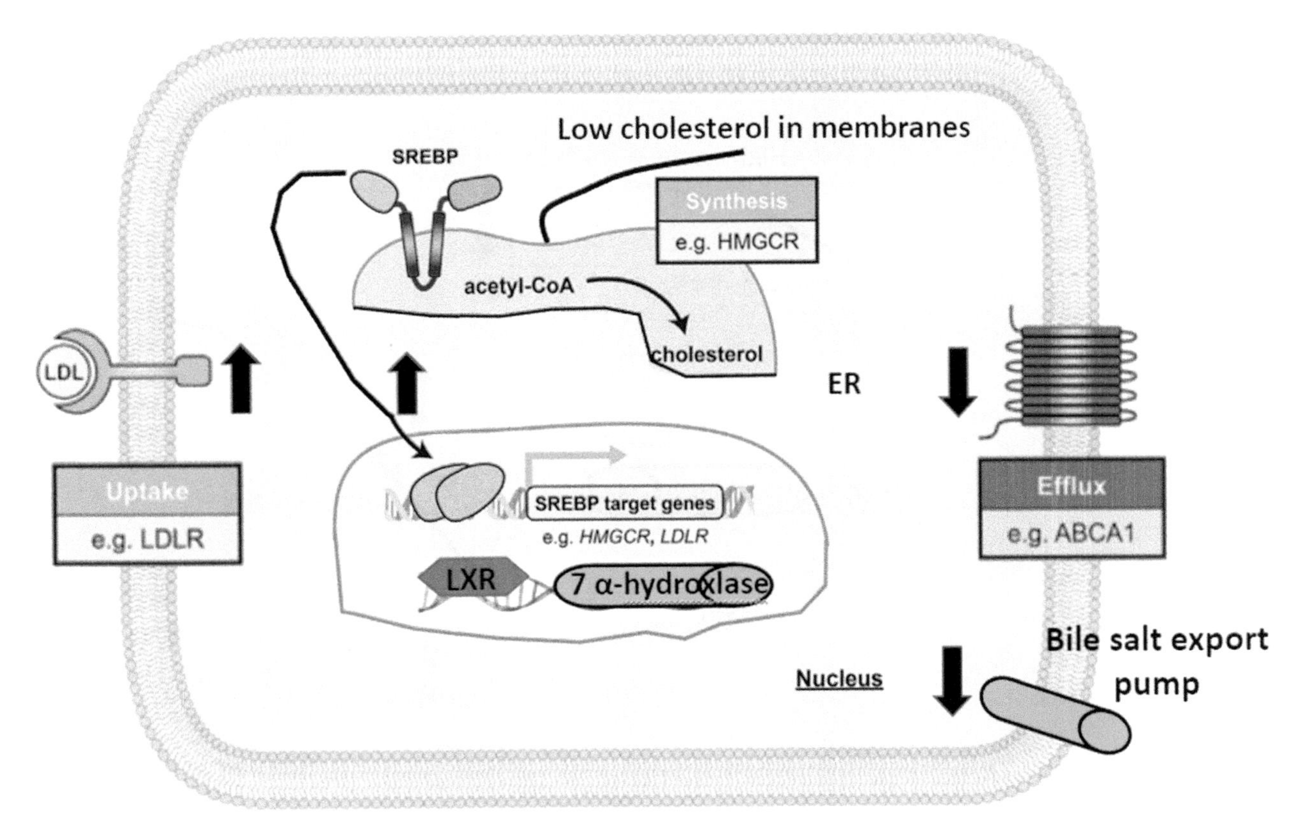

FIGURE 4.7 **Cholesterol regulation in deprived conditions.** When cholesterol levels are low, the sterol regulatory element binding proteins (SREBP) translocate to the nucleus. The SREBP is a transcription regulator that augments the synthesis of cholesterol synthetic enzymes and LDL receptors. In addition, cholesterol efflux and elimination via bile salts is downregulated [70]. *ABCA1*, ATP-binding cassette transporter; *HMGCR*, 3-hydroxy-3-methylglutaryl-CoA reductase; *LDLR*, low density lipoprotein receptor; *LXR*, liver X receptor.

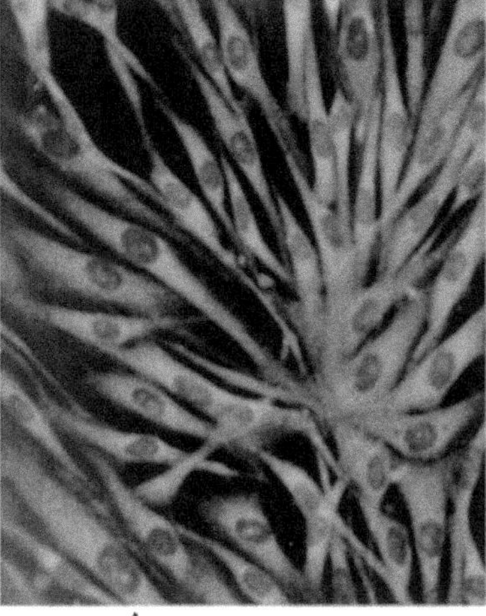

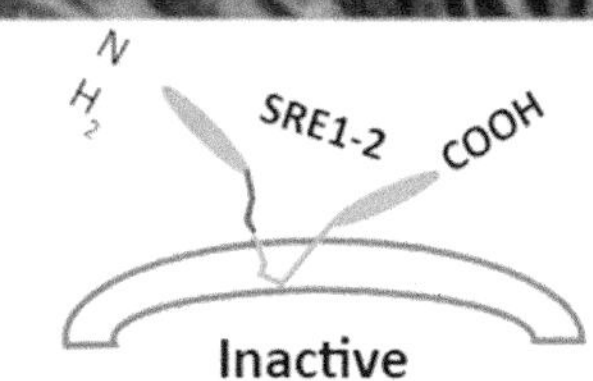

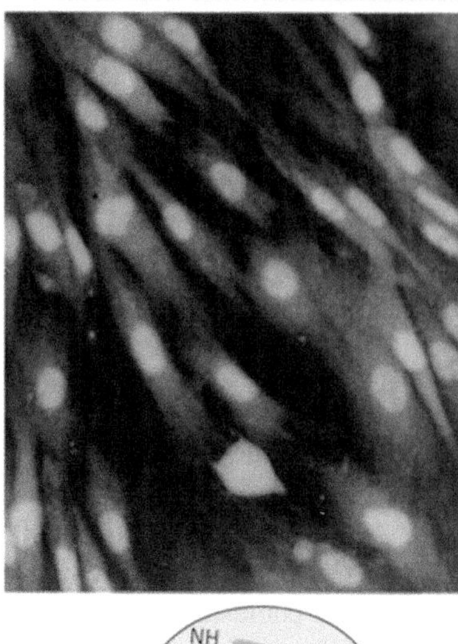

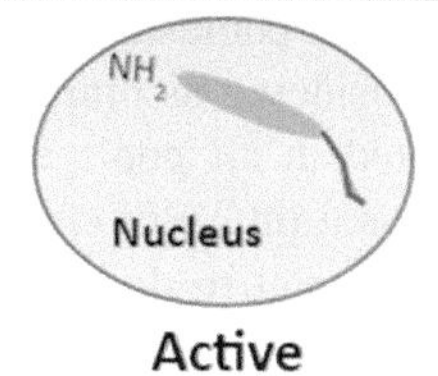

FIGURE 4.8 **SREBP-2 activity and location in human fibroblasts in the presence or absence of external cholesterol.** When these cells were incubated in whole serum containing cholesterol, the sterol regulatory element binding proteins (SREBPs) remained in the endoplasmic reticulum membrane and were thus not active in promoting the expression of cholesterol synthesis. The staining for these is exclusively in the cytoplasm (right panel). However, when the same cells were incubated in cholesterol depleted serum, there is bright staining for SREBPs in the nucleus, indicating that the need for cholesterol, translocated this transcription promoter to activate the enzymes for cholesterol synthesis (left panel). *SRE*, Sterol regulatory element-binding protein; *COOH*, carboxyl group. *Figure extracted and modified from Brown MS, Goldstein JL. The SREBP pathway: regulation of cholesterol metabolism by proteolysis of a membrane-bound transcription factor. Cell. 1997;89(3):331–340.*

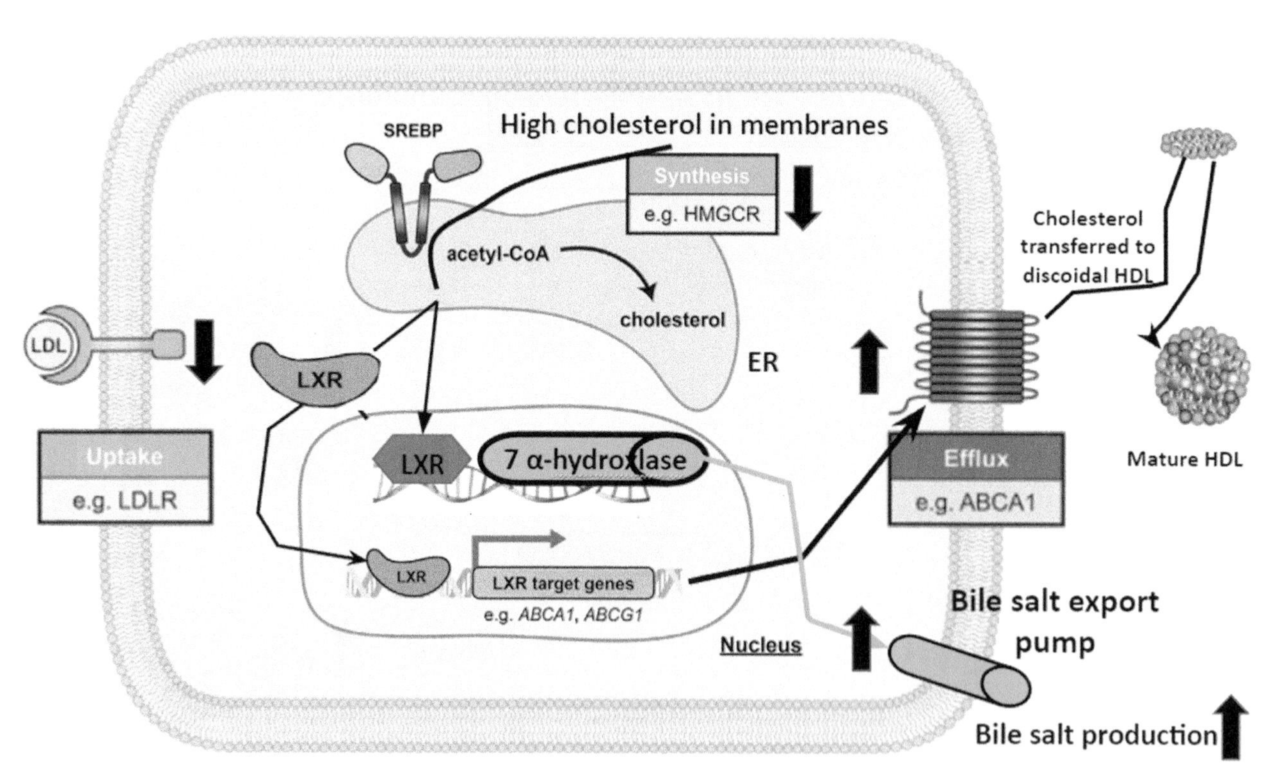

FIGURE 4.9 **Cholesterol regulation in replete conditions.** When cholesterol is present in excess in the cells, mechanism of efflux exists through pumps like ATP-binding cassette transporters A1 and G1 (ABCA1 and ABCG1) that transport cholesterol from the cells to a waiting HDL for the molecule to be recycled. It is also eliminated as bile in hepatic cells as well as through transintestinal cholesterol elimination (TICE). *ABCA1*, ATP-binding cassette transporter; HMGCR, 3-hydroxy-3-methylglutaryl-CoA reductase; *LDLR*, low density lipoprotein receptor; *LXR*, liver X receptor; SREBP, sterol regulatory element binding proteins.

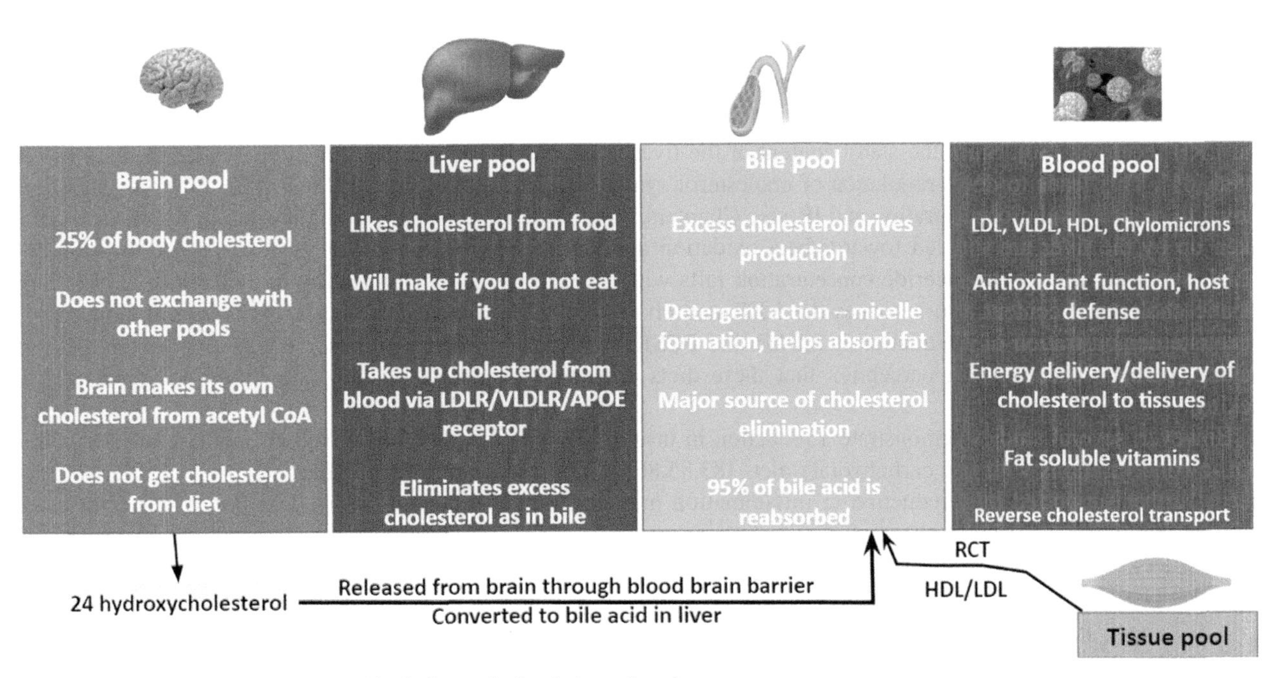

FIGURE 4.10 Distribution of cholesterol in the human body: cholesterol pools.

absorbed. The rest of the daily requirement for cellular processes is internally synthesised. In an individual on a low carbohydrate animal-sourced diet, the amount of cholesterol ingested can be over a gram. Even though there is an increase in the absolute amount of exogenous cholesterol absorbed, there is a reduction in the percentage of ingested cholesterol absorbed and cholesterol balance is maintained by a combination of reduction in synthesis and an increase in elimination of cholesterol as bile acid and neutral sterols [65]. It should be noted that there is a paucity of studies on alteration of de novo synthesis and cholesterol excretion in humans as intake increases from vegans (negligible intake) to standard American diet (over 300 mg), and culminates in the high intake of a carnivore diet (over 1 g).

4.3.2.1 Fasting and cholesterol regulation

In a fasted state, cholesterol and bile are not secreted into the gastrointestinal tract, resulting in almost zero cholesterol elimination. In addition, fasting induces autophagy and lipolysis (Chapter 10: Therapeutic fasting), both processes resulting in release of cholesterol from cells and adipose tissue into lipoproteins, specifically HDL [72]. The process of reverse cholesterol transport is activated, and cholesterol is brought back to the liver by means of both LDLR and SR-B1 [73]. The hepatic content of cholesterol is increased and thus there is downregulation of cholesterol synthesis in the liver [74]. This leads to inactivation of SREBP-2, which in turn not only reduces the transcription of cholesterol synthesis enzymes, but also reduces PCSK9 as well as LDLR transcription [75]. The reduction in LDLR leads to an increase in LDL-c concentration in serum. The reason for the mild increase in HDL-c concentration with fasting is most likely mediated by autophagy induced sterol sensor LXR which activates the cholesterol efflux pump, the ABCA1 transporter [76].

Fatty acids released from triglycerides are used as fuel to drive beta oxidation, and the glycerol moiety is used for gluconeogenesis. Consequently, there is limited to no re-esterification of fatty acids and glycerol into triglycerides. This manifests as reduced VLDL synthesis and reduced triglyceride concentration in serum [77]. Elegant demonstration of reduction in triglycerides, lathosterol, and PCSK9 with fasting, along with an increase in LDL-c has been previously demonstrated [78,79].

To summarise, fasting reduces cholesterol synthesis, PCSK9 concentrations, LDLR expression, while promoting cholesterol efflux through ABCA1 transporters, resulting in significantly increased LDL-c and a small rise in HDL-c concentration in serum.

It should be noted that while there is change in distribution of cholesterol in different pools, the cholesterol balance is maintained by reduction in synthesis since elimination is virtually eliminated.

4.3.2.2 *Therapeutic carbohydrate restriction and cholesterol regulation*

Individuals on TCR diets ingest relatively high quantities of both saturated fat and cholesterol. This increases the cholesterol content of the liver since there is hepatic uptake of chylomicron remnant particles through the action of Apo E and LRH receptors [80]. Since the sterol content of the liver is increased, the sterol sensing element, SREBP, is inactivated [81]. This leads to down-regulation of cholesterol synthesis, LDLR, as well as PCSK9 [82]. TCR has also been shown to reduce insulin concentration and IR (see Chapters 1 and 2). This creates a metabolic state in which fatty acids taken up by the liver are shuttled towards beta oxidation and ketone body formation rather than re-esterification and VLDL synthesis. Hence, triglyceride concentration falls with TCR in metabolically healthy individuals [83]. The high hepatic cholesterol content also activates the LXR and cholesterol efflux into HDL via the ABCA1 transporter [84]. Adequate demonstration of a reduction in LDLR and PCSK9 with high cholesterol diets, such as a carnivore diet, are lacking, perhaps because of a perception that these diets are atherogenic and funding into this type of research is lacking.

However, several studies demonstrate a reduction in insulin, triglyceride, and VLDL and an increase in HDL-c and LDL-c concentrations with low carbohydrate diets [83,85,86]. The presence of a favourable metabolic profile with this diet is further supported by a reduction in inflammation markers, weight reduction, as well as improvement in blood pressure [86–88].

4.3.2.3 *Lean mass hyper responder*

This term refers to a specific lipoprotein profile in physically active individuals with a normal body mass index (BMI) who consume a carbohydrate restricted diet [89–91]. Typically, these individuals have triglyceride concentrations below or equal to 0.79 mmol/L (70 mg/dL), and HDL concentrations equal or higher than 2.07 mmol/L (80 mg/dL) [91] with a ratio of triglycerides/HDL less than 1.5. Their LDL concentrations are generally above 5.17 mmol/L (200 mg/dL) [91] and not uncommonly in the 7.76–10.34 mmol/L (300–400 mg/dL) range. The consumption of a predominantly animal sourced food as well as intermittent fasting or time restricted feeding are factors that increase the LDL concentrations into 7.76–10.34 mmol/L (300–400 mg/dL) range in these individuals.

There is universal agreement that a low triglyceride with higher HDL is a favourable antiatherogenic profile. The extremely high LDL concentrations present in these individuals were previously observed only in individuals with genetic variants of familial hypercholesterolaemia. The reason for the high LDL concentrations is perhaps related to:

- Low insulin concentrations and insulin sensitivity
- Reduction in the number of LDLR on the liver
- The synthesis and export of predominantly LDL rather than VLDL by the liver

The mechanisms by which these factors lead to high LDL concentrations is explained elsewhere in this chapter.

4.3.2.4 *Bile acids - role in cholesterol elimination and control of lipid and glucose metabolism*

The catabolism of cholesterol into bile acids is regulated by cholesterol and oxysterol content of the liver [92]. The oxysterols bind to Liver X receptor (LXR) and cause feed forward induction of the rate limiting enzyme cholesterol 7 alpha-hydroxylase in bile acid synthesis [93]. The bile acids form micelles of phospholipid and cholesterol and are essential for solubilisation and absorption of fat, cholesterol, and fat-soluble vitamins in the gut. The pool of bile acid is about 2 g. After they aid in absorption of hydrophobic fats, cholesterol, and fat-soluble vitamins the bile acids are actively reabsorbed in the distal part of the small intestines, ileum by active transport mechanisms. This is called the enterohepatic circulation of bile acids and about 12–20 g of bile acids go through this process each day. While 95% of the bile acid are re-absorbed, the 5% that escapes this process is designed as a mechanism for cholesterol excretion. The bile acids are actively secreted at the canalicular side of the hepatic cell by bile salt export pump. This process not only stimulates bile acid secretion but also the excretion of excess hepatic cholesterol into the bile [94].

The bile acid pool serves to control its own synthesis through activation of the farnesoid X receptor (FXR), which is responsible for repression of transcription of rate limiting enzymes cholesterol 7 alpha-hydroxylase [95]. FXR belongs to the superfamily of ligand-activated nuclear receptor transcription factors. FXR not only reduces bile acid synthesis but is also involved in the repression of hepatic SREBP-1c expression, a nuclear transcription factor that promotes de novo lipogenesis. In addition, the role of bile acid in glucose regulation is also emerging. The role of bile acid in control of lipid and glucose metabolism is beyond the scope of this review and the reader is directed to the work of Bart Staels and co-workers [96].

In summary, bile acids serve several important roles:

1. Micelle formation for solubilisation of fat, fat-soluble vitamins, and cholesterol for absorption in the gut.
2. The catabolic end-products of cholesterol metabolism and their synthesis is driven by the hepatic content of cholesterol and cholesterol products like oxysterols.
3. Their secretion also stimulates the excretion of excess hepatic cholesterol in bile.
4. Control not only their own synthesis through FXR but also modulate de novo lipogenesis by repressing SREB-1c and regulate glucose metabolism.

4.3.2.5 Trans intestinal cholesterol elimination

While bile and biliary cholesterol orchestrate the elimination of cholesterol in faeces, an important role of intestines in sterol homoeostasis has recently been highlighted. The process named trans intestinal cholesterol elimination (TICE) is an active process that is estimated to contribute to about 35% of sterol excretion to maintain cholesterol balance [97]. The cholesterol elimination via TICE occurs in the proximal intestines. The augmentation of TICE is through activation of LXR which is involved in sterol sensing not only in hepatic cells but also in the intestines. In addition, the role of peroxisome proliferator-activated receptor-d and FXR in augmenting TICE has also been illustrated. The mechanisms underlying TICE are not completely understood. The source of cholesterol for TICE is most likely the liver but an intestinal source is not excluded. The transport of cholesterol from the liver to intestines for TICE may involve both PCSK9 and LDL, but definitive evidence is lacking. HDL is not involved in TICE [98]. The excretion of cholesterol from the apical luminal side of intestinal cells is most likely accomplished by ABCG5/G8 transporters, but other transporters are perhaps also involved. There is also evidence that TICE can be augmented in the context of hepatobiliary disease.

In summary, cholesterol balance is regulated not only by controlling its synthesis, but by precisely manipulating its elimination via bile and TICE.

4.3.2.6 Cholesterol modulating medications

4.3.2.6.1 Statins

The Selling of Statins as 'Miracle Drugs'

David M. Diamond

In the first half of the 20th century, the finding of cholesterol in the arteries of people who had died from coronary heart disease (CHD) led clinicians to postulate that cholesterol had infiltrated and then thickened the walls of the coronary arteries, thereby choking off blood flow to the heart [99]. In 1938, Muller suggested that a reduction of serum cholesterol may serve as a prophylactic treatment against premature CHD [100]. Hence, the search for a strategy to reduce cholesterol to improve CHD outcomes began decades before the statin era.

In the 1950s, investigators discovered that consumption of corn oil reduced cholesterol concentrations, which, in theory, would protect people from CHD [101]. An unequivocal test of this hypothesis was provided by Rose et al. [102] men at high risk of CHD that consumed corn oil each day had lower cholesterol concentrations, but they died or had heart attacks at a greater rate than those in the untreated group. Clinical trials over the next two decades with different cholesterol lowering approaches were also unsuccessful at prolonging the lives of people with high cholesterol. In 1992, Professor Michael Oliver summarised the decades of failed trials on heart disease protection by declaring '... we are now learning to live with the fact that lowering cholesterol concentrations in men at high risk does not reduce total mortality and may actually increase non-cardiac mortality' [103]. The failure of LDL cholesterol (LDL-c) reduction to have beneficial effects may be because high concentrations of LDL-c, particularly in the elderly, are associated with greater longevity compared to people with low LDL-c [104].

Astonishingly, built on this background of decades of failed attempts at showing cholesterol reduction protects people from CHD mortality, statins, a class of drugs that reduces LDL-c via inhibition of HMG-CoA reductase, have become the treatment of choice for CHD. William Roberts, M.D., editor of the American Journal of Cardiology refers to statins as 'miracle drugs', which 'are to atherosclerosis what penicillin was to infectious diseases' (Roberts, 1996). Praise for statins has been so strong that anyone that dares to criticise them has been labelled a member of the 'statin denial cult' [105].

One representative clinical trial illustrates why statins have been promoted as 'miracle drugs', when, in fact, statin benefits are quite meagre. CHD benefits from treatment with the statin, Crestor, were greeted with great enthusiasm [106]. Dr. John Kastelein presented the JUPITER trial findings in the media with the following statement: 'It's spectacular... We finally have strong data' that a statin prevents a first heart attack. Kastelein reported that Crestor cut the rate of heart attacks and strokes by 50%.

The finding that a drug can reduce the likelihood of a coronary event by 50% does sound like a miracle treatment, as it would appear as if half of all statin-treated people would be protected from ever having a heart attack. However, this is not

(Continued)

(Continued)

what the 50% figure represents. In the Crestor study (as in all statin studies), coronary events (myocardial infarction, stroke or death from CVD) rarely occurred; only 1.8% of the placebo-treated and 0.9% of the statin-treated subjects experienced a major coronary event over the course of the 1.9-year trial. These findings are illustrated in the left side of Fig. 4.11.

How does less than a 1% difference in event rate between the groups transform into a 50% reduction in events? Because 0.9% is 50% of 1.8%. The 50% value is called the hazard ratio or relative risk reduction (RRR). The benefit to the patient, in terms of the difference in the rate of events between groups (1.8%–0.9%) is 0.9%, which is the absolute risk reduction (ARR).

The 0.9% ARR is transformed into a clinically relevant value, the number needed to treat (NNT), which is the reciprocal of the ARR, extrapolated to 2 years. As reported in the publication, the NNT for Crestor was 95. This means that 95 patients would need to be treated with Crestor for 2 years for just 1 of the 95 patients to have 1 less heart attack, stroke, or cardiovascular-related death. The remaining 94 patients would derive no benefit from statin treatment.

The emphasis on the RRR (50%) and exclusion of any mention of the ARR (0.9%) by clinical trial directors has been denounced by experts in biostatistics. For example, Gigerenzer et al., (2010) declared that the portrayal of the RRR without including the ARR provides 'incomplete and misleading risk information', and that 'Conveying relative risks without baseline risk is the first "sin" against transparent reporting'. The exaggeration of the appearance of the benefits of statins with the isolated presentation of the RRR is a form of deception which is routinely employed by statin trial directors [107].

Although the 0.9% ARR benefit of statin treatment is much smaller than the advertised values of 50%, a 0.9% benefit would be better than no benefit at all, that is if statins did not have any adverse effects. However, the adverse effects of statins are more extensive than statin trial directors have led the public and practitioners to believe, including cognitive deficits, diabetes mellitus, and muscle injury [108].

Finally, is there evidence of a benefit of statin treatment in people who are on a low carbohydrate diet (LCD)? Although a trial to address this question has not been conducted, indirect evidence provides an answer. A re-analysis of the 4S trial addressed whether statins benefited subjects with high LDL-c, high triglycerides and low HDL-c (an unhealthy lipid triad), compared to subjects with high LDL-c, low triglycerides and high HDL-c (a lipid triad commonly found in people on LCD) [109]. This analysis revealed that subjects with the unhealthy lipid triad had a modest benefit from statin treatment, which was likely produced by the drug's pleiotropic effects, such as its mild anti-inflammatory and anticoagulant effects, which are independent of LDL reduction [110]. More importantly, those subjects with a lipid triad that would match someone on an LCD exhibited no benefit from statin treatment.

In summary, nearly a century of research has unjustly implicated cholesterol as a causal factor in CHD, when other factors, such as hyperglycaemia, hypercoagulation and inflammation, are the culprits that promote atherosclerosis [111,112]. Despite the fanfare about statins being 'miracle drugs', statin treatment provides only a small benefit to a subset of individuals, and the benefits are more than offset by the adverse effects. Ultimately, the shift from a carbohydrate-rich diet to an LCD is likely to provide greater benefits than statin treatment, without the adverse side effects.

4.3.2.6.2 Statins and cholesterol regulation – the untold story of phytosterols

The paradigm that LDL-c is atherogenic has led to widespread use of statins for most adult populations of the world. There is a small but inconsistent benefit of statins in certain populations at risk. Statins reduce cholesterol production by competitively inhibiting the rate-limiting enzyme, HMG-CoA reductase, early in the cascade of enzymes involved in

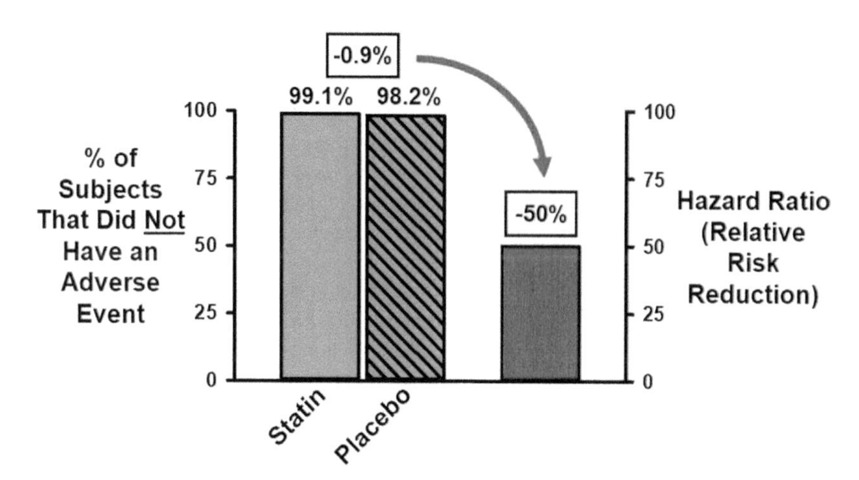

FIGURE 4.11 Crestor study results. The left side of the graph depicts the per cent of subjects in the statin and placebo groups that did not have a myocardial infarction, stroke or death from cardiovascular causes in the JUPITER study [106]. Data above each bar indicate the numerical value for each group. The −0.9% value is the numerical difference in major coronary event rates between the treated and placebo groups (absolute risk reduction; ARR). The red arrow provides a visual connection between the ARR and the hazard ratio (also referred to as the relative risk reduction; RRR), in which the −0.9% group difference is transformed into a 50% reduction in the rate of events.

cholesterol synthesis [113]. The ensuing reduction in sterols in the membranes of the cell is sensed by SREBP-2 which is activated and transported to the nucleus to increase the synthesis of cholesterol synthetic enzymes, LDLR and PCSK9 [114]. The increase in LDLR increases LDL uptake by the liver and a reduction of this lipoprotein in the serum by about 30%–60% depending on the potency and dose of statin utilised [115]. It should be noted that in certain individuals the synthesis of PCSK9 is robust and reduces the effectiveness of LDL lowering by statins [116]. The increased PCSK9 concentrations binds LDLR and takes it down the path of internalisation and lysosomal destruction reducing the ability of statins to lower LDL concentrations.

In a study done by Gylling and co-workers, high dose statin increased relative and total cholesterol absorption from 26% to 53% and 65 mg/d to 153 mg/d respectively [117]. It is clear from this study that inhibition of synthesis is associated with the body trying to absorb more cholesterol from dietary intake. One should not be careful to dismiss this as a compensatory homoeostatic response since it creates a situation where absorption of sterols becomes indiscriminate. The cholesterol absorption by the Niemann-Pick type C1-like 1 (NPC1L1) receptor is designed to reject plant sterols or phytosterols [118]. What little plant sterol gets into the intestinal cell is actively extruded by the ABCG5/8 transporters [118]. With high dose statin use, this is no longer the case and the concentrations of phytosterols increase in blood as evidenced by an increase in sitosterol in serum in patients on high dose atorvastatin [119]. Phytosterols get incorporated into cell membranes with detrimental alteration in its fluidity and membrane integrity [120]. In addition, data on phytosterol incorporation adversely modulating specialised cholesterol-rich domains in cell membranes such as caveolae and lipid rafts has not been investigated. Given the widespread use of statins and their association with IR, it is quite likely that alteration in insulin receptor function may be mediated by such a mechanism and deserve further study [121].

4.3.2.6.3 PCSK9 and PCSK9 inhibitors

The PCSK9 has a function of regulating the lipid and cholesterol content of the liver and pancreas by regulating the presence of cell surface LDLR, VLDLR, ApoER, and CD36. A deficiency of these receptors, as can happen with loss of function mutations of PCSK9 or with monoclonal antibody inhibitors of PCSK9, leads to an abundance of these lipoprotein receptors on the cell surface of hepatic cells and islets. This leads to unregulated lipid accumulation in these cells resulting in fatty liver and its attendant consequence as well as β-cell apoptosis.

The PCSK9 not only internalises the LDLR receptor and commits it to lysosomal degradation, but it also mediates a similar process for other lipoprotein receptors such as VLDLR, ApoE receptor, LDLR-related protein (LRP1), and cluster of differentiation 36 receptor (CD36). These receptors are involved in the uptake of VLDL, IDL, and chylomicron remnants. The PCSK9 inhibitor trials have shown that not only is there a robust reduction in LDL, but there is modest reduction in triglyceride rich lipoproteins such as VLDL, IDL and chylomicron remnants, accompanied by a small increase in HDL. While this may appear to be the most beneficial lipoprotein phenotype, that is low LDL, accompanied by high HDL and low triglycerides, it is occurring at the expense of lipid accumulation in the liver, pancreas and heart and associated perhaps with functionally deficient HDL.

Human demographic studies in individuals with PCSK9 mutations have demonstrated complex relationships with an increased risk of diabetes and visceral obesity in some variants [122], notably those with a loss-of-function variant [123]. This confirms the observations from animal and cell culture studies, which demonstrate that PCSK9 regulates not only lipoprotein pool of cholesterol but also controls intracellular triglyceride and cholesterol concentrations. However, it was too enticing given the LDL hypothesis of atherosclerosis to test the role of PCSK9 inhibitors in reducing coronary ischaemic events. There is a robust and potent reduction in LDL concentrations with the administration of monoclonal antibody inhibitors of PCSK9. The reservation one should have about their negative impact on visceral obesity, β-cell apoptosis, and fatty liver disease were largely ignored or explained by preliminary observations that PCSK9 inhibitors only target soluble PSCK9 of hepatic origin and that cellular PCSK9 present in β-cells, intestines, or VSMCs is not inhibited [124].

The results of a representative phase III clinical trial with the PCSK9 inhibitor Evolocumab nicely illustrates the abject failure of this intervention in reducing cardiac and overall mortality in individuals who were at high risk of cardiac ischaemic events such as myocardial infarction and coronary death (Fig. 4.12) [125].

One should also question the validity of the LDL hypothesis since, the LDL concentrations in the treatment group were approximately 30 mg/dL which is a lower concentration compared to other previous clinical trials [126]. At the very least, one should question the hypothesis that lower is better for LDL, a prevailing concept that is used to justify potent therapy with high dose statins and PCSK9 inhibitors. In addition, there are data from meta-analysis that both the duration and potency of PCSK9 inhibitor therapy are associated with the risk of arising HbA1c as well as the occurrence of new-onset diabetes [127].

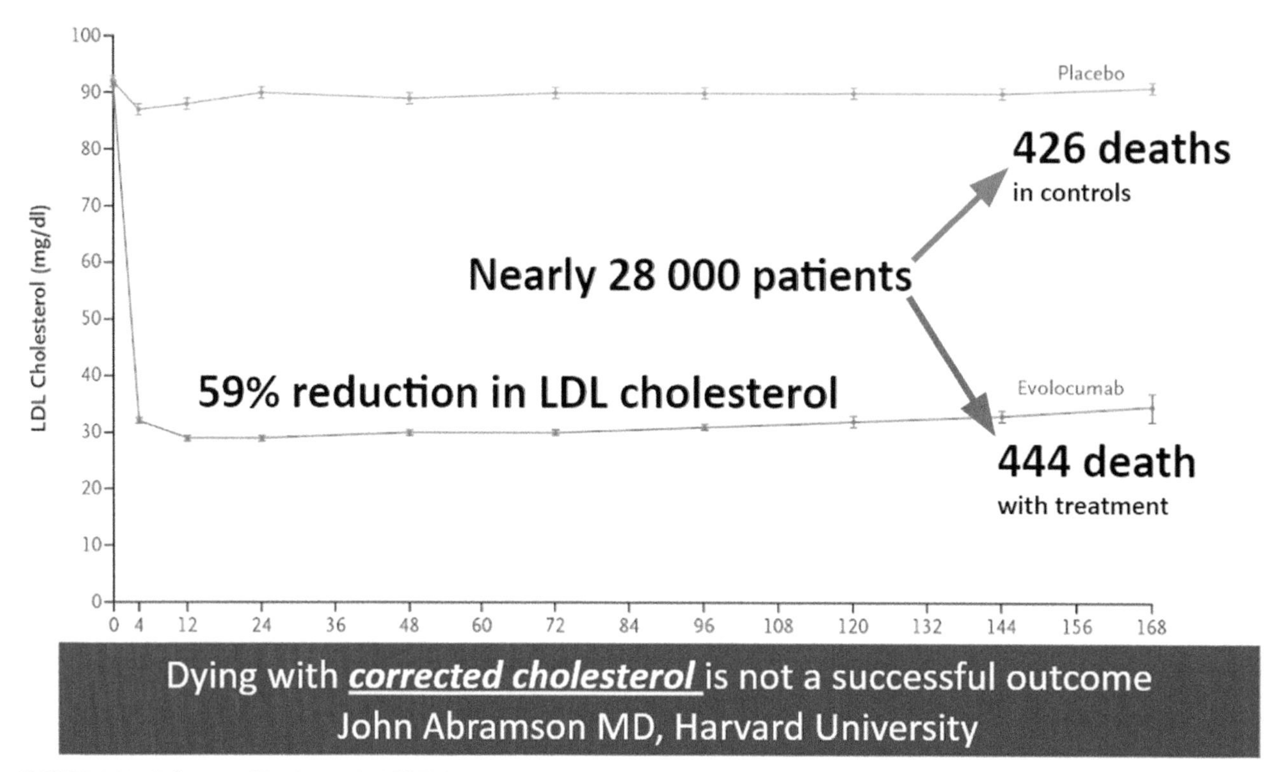

FIGURE 4.12 Influence of Evolocumab (PCSK9 inhibitor) on cardiac and overall mortality in patients with cardiovascular disease. *Figure extracted and modified from Sabatine et al. (2017).*

4.4 Lipoproteins

4.4.1 Lipoprotein structure and physiology

There are two major classes of lipoproteins based on their identifying protein, apolipoprotein B (apo B) and apolipoprotein A1 (apo A1). The apo B is the identifying lipoprotein of VLDL, LDL and chylomicrons. It is longer in VLDL and LDL and is called apo B100 and is truncated in chylomicrons to apo B48. The apo A1 is the defining apoprotein of HDL. As mentioned, the central hydrophobic core of these multifunctional molecules is composed of neutral lipid and CE. Their surface however is rich in amphipathic proteins, phospholipids, and free cholesterol. The cholesterol is oriented with its hydrophilic tail pointed internally and the polar 3β OH moiety oriented externally. This is similar to the free cholesterol orientation observed in cell membranes [128].

In addition to their unique identifying proteins, these molecules are rich in other functional proteins. Some of these are involved in lipid metabolism such as apo E, apolipoprotein C-11, C-III, phospholipid transfer protein (PLTP), CETP and lecithin cholesterol acyltransferase (LCAT). There are other proteins associated with HDL, LDL and VLDL that are involved in other biological functions like inflammation, immune modulation and host defence.

The enterocyte is the site of production of the chylomicron from ingested fat, phospholipids, and cholesterol. These dietary components are assembled along with apo B48 and secreted into the lymphatic system, gaining entry to blood through the thoracic duct. It is interesting that long chain fatty acids and cholesterol are directly escorted into blood in chylomicrons, bypassing the portal circulation. Shorter chain fatty acids (less than 14 carbons in length), amino acids, and monosaccharides, which are digestion products of protein and carbohydrates, on the other hand, are first processed by the liver before entering systemic circulation [129].

The chylomicron is the largest lipoprotein in humans and along with VLDL, are triglyceride-rich and synthesised by the liver. These molecules undergo lipolysis in the muscles and adipose tissue in order to deliver their lipid cargo for energy use or storage. The process of lipolysis is aided by the enzyme LPL present in muscle and adipose tissue along with a cofactor protein, apo C-II, present on both VLDL and chylomicrons. After delipidation they are much smaller and are referred to as chylomicron and VLDL remnants [130].

These remnants which are cholesterol-rich are cleared by the liver through several different receptors. A factor that aids remnant particle clearance is apo E. The apo E is genetically polymorphic. It is inherited from each parent. The possible variations in apo E are E2/2, E2/3, E2/4, E3/3, E3/4, and E4/4. For simplicity is better to conceptualise them as apo E2, E3 and E4 phenotypes. The apo E4 has the highest affinity for the liver receptors responsible for clearance of chylomicron/VLDL remnants and is rapidly taken up by the liver. The apo E2 has the slowest clearance while apo E3 is middle range for receptor affinity. There is association of apo E4 with early onset dementia and CAD (CAD) but this is largely modulated by IR [131].

After delivery of its lipid cargo VLDL is relatively cholesterol-rich and is now referred to as LDL. The majority of LDL is derived from VLDL, except in situations of fasting and TCR, where LDL is directly synthesised and exported by the liver [132]. Apo B100 is the structural protein for LDL and is recognised by the LDLR on the liver and peripheral tissues for endocytosis and cholesterol delivery and uptake [133].

The other cholesterol-rich lipoprotein, HDL, begins its journey as a nascent protein apo A1, without cargo, after its synthesis by the hepatocytes and enterocytes. Apo A1 is a ligand for lipid transfer proteins on the membranes of peripheral cells and macrophages called ABCA1 [134]. The function of this interaction between these two proteins is to transfer cholesterol and phospholipids into the nascent HDL molecule. HDL is protein rich and smaller in size compared to other lipoproteins. It contains many other proteins such as apo E, PLTP, and CETP in order to collaborate with LDL/VLDL to exchange lipids between lipoprotein particles. Cholesterol, unlike fat, protein and carbohydrate cannot be used as an energy source. Cholesterol released by cell injury and death needs to be cleared. In addition, the number of enzymatic steps required to synthesise cholesterol is energy expensive and consumes approximately 100 ATP molecules [135]. Thus, it would make sense for human biology to recycle cholesterol rather than make it anew.

4.4.1.1 Lipid transport and lipoproteins

Lipoproteins are the primary mechanism for lipid transport and were originally called large lipid transport proteins. As a courier for dietary and endogenous triglycerides, they transport fat energy from the intestines and liver to the muscles for energy and adipose tissue for storage. Their second major role is to function as bidirectional transport vehicles for cholesterol between liver and peripheral cells. Cellular growth requires cholesterol in large quantities that cannot be provided by de novo synthesis in the cells themselves and most tissues depend on the liver for supply. The brain is an exception to this rule. RCT occurs in cells undergoing injury and autophagy. In addition, cholesterol is taken up by the macrophages in the process of vessel wall injury from oxLDL.

4.4.1.2 Lipoproteins' antioxidant function

The inner core of lipoprotein particles VLDL, LDL, and HDL contains antioxidants such as vitamin E, beta carotene, and ubiquinol CoQ10. In addition, the phospholipid bilayer can undergo oxidation in the setting of free radical injury associated with inflammation.

In an elegant experiment in ten healthy humans, the group of Alleva et al. (1995) were able to demonstrate that CoQ10 concentrations were reduced in the small dense sub-fractions of the LDL, which have been implicated in the atherosclerotic process [136]. In the small dense LDL, not only was the CoQ10 concentration low in the small dense LDL particle, but it was accompanied by greater oxidative injury to the lipoprotein particle [136]. Alleva et al. (1995) were able to demonstrate an increase in CoQ10 concentrations in the LDL lipoprotein with oral supplementation. Furthermore, when these supplement-enhanced LDL particles were subjected to free radical damage a reduced susceptibility to oxidation was observed. The antioxidant function of the resident tocopherol in the LDL molecule is similar to that of CoQ10 and confirmed by a number of different researchers [23,24].

In addition to resident antioxidants of the lipoprotein core and its structural protein, there are several other antioxidant proteins embedded in low abundance on the surface [137]. Many of them are still being characterised by lipoproteomic analysis. The HDL is associated with LPS- binding protein, paraoxonase, and clusterin, an incomplete list that participates in inflammation modulation. The lysozyme C and LPS binding protein have been identified in LDL and can neutralise invading pathogens and their cellular components, hence reducing inflammation and injury. These observations give credence to the role of LDL and HDL in particular, and lipoproteins in general, as host defence mechanisms against invading pathogens, as well as modulators of inflammation. A detailed description of these pathways are beyond the scope of this chapter and can be found in this review [138].

4.4.1.3 Fat as energy

Chylomicrons and VLDL are couriers of triglycerides for energy supply to various cells like the muscle and for storage in adipose tissue. As such, some consider VLDL as the predominant source of endogenous fat energy supply to peripheral cells. However, this may not be the case. In fact, the increased synthesis and export of VLDL may be considered as dysfunctional lipid metabolism.

Consider the case of prolonged fasting or TCR. Both scenarios are associated with low insulin concentrations and hence a decrease in the synthesis of VLDL by the hepatocytes. The fatty acids entering the liver do not undergo re-esterification to triglycerides for export in newly synthesised VLDL particles. Instead, the fatty acids are diverted in the liver for β-oxidation and conversion to ketones. Ketones are small molecules derived from fat but function as an energy substrate for the brain in lieu of glucose. Both fasting and TCR induce a hormonal state of low insulin and high glucagon. Consequently, not only is β-oxidation of fatty acids promoted but so is the conversion of the glycerol moiety of triglycerides and certain amino acids to glucose via the process of gluconeogenesis. Thus, the predominant source of fat energy supply in TCR or a fasted state comes from free fatty acids (FFA) derived from adipose tissue lipolysis rather than fat energy exported as VLDL by the liver. The FFA are carried in the circulation bound to albumin. While the liver is picking up more FFA in a carbohydrate-restricted and -fasted state, it uses them for the synthesis of ketone bodies and not for re-esterification into triglycerides.

Now let us examine a situation of high carbohydrate intake with an element of IR. The high insulin state is not conducive for beta-oxidation of fatty acids. Hence, fatty acids are re-esterified to triglycerides. Humans have limited ability to store carbohydrates as glycogen. The carbohydrate consumed that cannot be utilised for energy or stored as glycogen is converted in the liver to triglyceride in a process termed de novo lipogenesis (DNL). Thus, in this metabolic state, the liver has a surplus of triglycerides, which are attached to apo B100 and exported as VLDL. One would expect this VLDL to serve as a source of fat energy for muscle. However, muscle is in the same metabolic situation as the liver: there is plenty of carbohydrate energy to utilise first. The fat energy from VLDL is therefore not used by the muscles. The fate of VLDL now depends on the health of the adipose tissue. If the adipose tissue has room to accommodate the lipid energy carried by VLDL, then VLDL residence time in the bloodstream will be short. The delipidated VLDL will get converted to LDL. In the setting of MetS however, the adipose tissue is already full and/or insulin resistant. Then triglyceride-rich lipoproteins, like VLDL and chylomicrons, cannot unload their cargo, and their residence time in blood increases. This is manifested as high triglyceride concentration on a lipid panel.

Thus, optimal energy homoeostasis is one of minimal VLDL production since its synthesis requires an oversupply of carbohydrate energy, leading to insulin concentrations not conducive to β-oxidation in the liver or peripheral cells. The fate of VLDL in the setting of dietary carbohydrate excess depends on the ability of adipose tissue to take triglycerides. Early work by Cahill and others [139,140] demonstrated these seminal observations which have unfortunately gone unnoticed by health professionals setting nutritional intake guidelines (see Chapter 1.3: The adoption and evolution of dietary guidelines). This perhaps stems from the universal view that fat and cholesterol intake is somehow toxic and causal in atherosclerosis and CAD, a paradigm that needs re-examination.

4.4.2 Lipoproteins as surrogate marker of insulin resistance

IR can be characterised as the pathophysiological condition of reduced insulin responsiveness in target tissues like liver, muscle, and adipose tissue. While IR is predominantly considered in the context of carbohydrate metabolism, there are major alterations in lipoprotein metabolism that predispose to a concomitantly higher risk of CAD. The dyslipidaemia of IR is characterised by a triad of lipoprotein abnormalities:

1. Increase in triglyceride rich lipoprotein particles (TRLP)
2. A reduction in HDL-c
3. Unchanged LDL-c concentration but a preponderant increase in small dense LDL-c

The increase in TRLP is from the action of CETP, which mediates the exchange of core lipids (triglyceride and CE) between VLDL and HDL. It is important to recognise the pathophysiological mechanism for increased VLDL assembly and export by the liver in the setting of IR, as well as the presence of hepatic steatosis in IR, which occurs despite increased VLDL secretion by the liver.

There are three sources for triglycerides required for VLDL assembly in the liver:

1. FFAs bound to albumin in plasma
2. uptake of VLDL and chylomicron remnants after the delipidation of core triglycerides of these TRLP by Lpl in adipose tissue
3. hepatic de novo triglyceride synthesis (DNL).

The assembly and secretion of VLDL is substrate driven. Impaired insulin signalling at the level of adipose tissues results in a failure of insulin-mediated suppression of lipolysis. There is an unregulated release of fatty acids (FA) from adipose tissue, more so from visceral depots that are relatively more insulin resistant [141]. This increases the availability of FA to the liver, which are a substrate for VLDL.

IR also impairs the metabolism of LPL-mediated lipolysis of VLDL and chylomicrons. There is an increase in both fasting, but more predominantly postprandial, TRLP concentration. IR is characterised by an increased secretion of ApoCIII, which is an inhibitor of LPL, further impairing the clearance of TRLP. However, the increase in chylomicrons and VLDL is not just from defective clearance but also from augmented hepatic and intestinal secretion [142].

If this were not enough, there is a mechanism of 'spillover effect' of dietary chylomicron triglyceride-FA. Spillover reflects the fraction of fatty acids that cannot be taken up into local tissues and become part of the plasma FFA content which is a feature of dysfunctional storage mechanisms common in insulin resistance [143]. As this TRLP is undergoing lipolysis, significant quantities of FA escape local re-esterification in adipose tissue. This adds to the pool of FA available to the liver to drive VLDL assembly and secretion [143].

The third factor contributing to increased VLDL secretion is increased hepatic de novo lipogenesis (DNL) in IR. This has been well documented not only in rat studies [144], but DNL also contributes to triglycerides in humans with obesity and IR [144]. Nearly all genes involved in FA and triglyceride synthesis are upregulated in IR [145]. The regulation of hepatic DNL is mediated through sterol response element binding protein-1c (SREBP-1c), a transcription factor that has been described in great detail [146]. Insulin plays a central role in the upregulation of hepatic SREBP-1c gene regulation either directly or via LXR [147].

Studies in mice that are fasted for 24 hours and then re-fed a high carbohydrate chow have significant insulin release [148]. This insulin release illustrates its role in the marked stimulation of key genes and proteins that are involved in DNL. It should be pointed out that hepatic IR is selectively directed at increasing VLDL secretion as well as hepatic steatosis [144]. There is differential regulation of hepatic glucose and lipid metabolism. The pathophysiological basis of IR to persistently stimulate DNL, while at the same time, the inability of the hormone to suppress hepatic glucose output has been well described [149].

The disposition of hepatic triglycerides in the setting of IR is via three pathways. It can store the triglyceride in lipid droplets, utilise it for beta-oxidation or export it as VLDL. Studies have shown that IR does not reduce beta-oxidation to a significant degree [150]. The secretion of VLDL involves the lipidation of apo B, a process that is mediated by a chaperone protein called microsomal lipid transfer protein (MTP) [151]. In insulin-sensitive individuals, there is inhibition of MTP synthesis as well as targeting of apo B towards proteolytic degradation [152]. However, in the presence of IR, both the inhibition of MTP and the degradation of apo B are impaired [144]. There is unopposed countervailing stimulation of VLDL secretion by hepatic triglyceride content, which is markedly increased in IR [153].

The remaining dilemma is the accumulation of triglyceride leading to steatosis despite IR mediated increase in VLDL secretion [154]. It is estimated that there is a three to fivefold increase in hepatic VLDL output by IR livers compared to metabolically healthy individuals [144]. This range of VLDL secretion contributes to the development of fatty liver [144]. A factor that is causal is endoplasmic reticulum stress due to the high turnover of FA derived from all three sources, namely increased uptake of both FA and TRLP remnants by the liver as well as the upregulation of DNL [155]. Despite the ER stress, VLDL secretion is at an elevated level compared to metabolically healthy individuals and is parabolic [144]. If the level of ER stress is moderate, then VLDL secretion is increased. However, it is not adequate to maintain normal hepatic triglyceride balance. Additionally, with ongoing IR, there will be a point at which the milder nonalcoholic steatohepatitis is replaced by hepatic steatosis. At this juncture, ER stress is increased, the VLDL assembly and secretion drops, with worsening of liver pathology. However, if calorie restriction and/or intermittent fasting is practised, there is a reduction in substrate driven formation of triglycerides, and a reduced need for VLDL secretion. This leads to improved insulin sensitivity, inhibition of MTP and apo B degradation with improvement in liver pathology.

4.5 Carbohydrate restricted diets and specific cardiac disorders

4.5.1 Congestive heart failure

TCR is useful for the management of congestive heart failure [156]. In these individuals with reduced cardiac output due to a reduction in the contractility of the left ventricle have hormonal changes that lead to fluid retention. There is activation of the RAAS mediating sodium and fluid retention. The presence of IR exacerbates this process. TCR diets most likely work through reducing insulin concentrations and promoting insulin sensitivity. There is also an improvement in blood pressure accompanying a low insulin state which can improve cardiac contractility and cardiac output. Finally, not to be discounted is the improvement in functioning most individuals experience from weight loss associated with TCR diets. There is considerable clinical experience amongst low carbohydrate practitioners about the utility of TCR diets in the treatment of CHF. However, well-designed observational studies are lacking, and there are no randomised studies to clarify its use.

Heart failure and the role of ketones

Sarah M. Rice

Emerging evidence suggests a therapeutic role for ketones in heart disease and the failing heart.

The healthy heart uses fatty acids, metabolised to fatty acyl-CoA, to produce ATP as the major fuel source. Glucose is a minor contributor and the contribution of ketone bodies is influenced by availability [4,157]. Heart disease is accompanied by a loss of metabolic flexibility where the inability to use fatty acids for fuel drives a move to glucose utilisation and the potential for myocardial energy deficit, which affects contractile function [4,157,158]. Under conditions of heart failure, circulating ketones and ketone use in the heart increase, which improves contractile function [4,157]. This is thought to be an adaptive response to physiological stress and there appears to be a dose-response relationship between the level of circulating ketones and ketone uptake and use by the heart [157,158].

Beyond the direct fuelling effects, ketones also act indirectly: reducing inflammation by inhibiting NLRP3 inflammasome; acting on the endothelium by increasing the expression of nitric oxide synthase and promoting vasodilation; reducing oxidative stress by inhibiting class I histone deacetylases; providing an alternative energy source for mitochondria thereby protecting function [4,157]. CVD risk factors may also be addressed contributing to therapeutic effects which include blood pressure, glycaemic control, weight, and lipid profile [4]. This may also be achieved using nutritional ketosis [159].

Studies where ketone bodies are elevated have shown increased uptake and oxidation of ketones by the myocardium and improvements in cardiac function [4,158].

This emerging area of therapeutic application for ketone bodies and carbohydrate restriction in heart failure shows promise and warrants further investigation.

4.5.2 Coronary artery disease

The presence of CAD is synonymous with LDL-c in mainstream medicine. Since low carbohydrate diets increase LDL-c concentrations, their use is discouraged strongly by conventional medical practitioners. In the majority of individuals with healthy fat cells and normal triglyceride concentrations, a TCR diet is associated with an increase in HDL-c concentrations and a reduction in TRLP, a profile associated with anti-atherogenic potential [160]. The reduction in IR is also a beneficial aspect of TCR diets in the setting of CAD. There is also associated reduction in high blood pressure, weight loss, and reduction in systemic inflammation further augmenting the benefits of TCR diets. To date there are no well-designed studies to address this paradigm. The clinical experience of low carbohydrate practitioners attests to the lack of progression of CAD with TCR use when implemented with an emphasis on intermittent fasting and exercise. However, it should be noted that there is near universal disagreement about their safety and utility by mainstream medicine.

4.5.3 Cardiac rhythm disturbances

The practice of TCR is commonly accompanied by some form of intermittent fasting or time restricted feeding. To separate the contributions of these two lifestyle changes on the occurrence of cardiac rhythm disturbances is not possible. It is the opinion of most practitioners who have clinical experience with TCR diets that there is a small increase in the risk of premature beats as well as atrial fibrillation (AF). AF is an arrhythmia that is initiated in the upper chambers of the heart, the heart rhythm is irregular, and the heart rate is over a 100 beats per minute at rest. This is usually observed in individuals who already have a diathesis for this rhythm disturbance. An increase in magnesium supplementation reduces the risk of developing AF [161]. A retrospective evaluation through a dietary questionnaire in the ARIC study (1987–89), when TCR diets were not popular or well defined, observed an increased risk of AF when carbohydrate intake was restricted [162]. Well-designed observational and randomised studies are needed to make firm conclusions.

4.6 Conclusion

Lipoproteins are a surrogate marker of metabolic health. Perhaps, the presence of high triglycerides accompanied by low HDL-c concentrations along with small dense LDL is a marker of metabolic ill health with far reaching adverse consequences than any LDL concentration. There are no reliable pharmaceutical means to lower triglycerides. The manipulation of HDL is feasible but not with assurances of HDL functionality. TCR with intermittent fasting and exercise is the best method to improve lipoprotein quality, namely low triglycerides, high HDL as well as large buoyant LDL. This lifestyle is associated with higher LDL concentrations, many times in ranges that are not previously seen by mainstream medicine. This creates a level of anxiety given our dogma that high LDL-c is the proximate cause of CAD. This chapter has presented evidence to dispel this hypothesis and show LDL, in the setting of insulin sensitivity, low inflammation markers, low triglycerides, and high HDL, as a marker of metabolic health. We can increase our confidence by evaluating the absence of CAD by CAC scoring or showing its stability.

A word of caution: based on clinical experience, metabolic health in individuals with severe IR, inflamed adipose tissue and high triglycerides cannot be achieved through the practice of TCR alone, as this may lead to lipotoxicity in the short run with the possibility of ischaemic vascular events as observed in some clinical cases [163]. As such our recommendations may have to be modified by greater emphasis on intermittent and long-term fasting (which prioritises adipose tissue fat oxidation as the primary fuel source) along with exercise guided by recovery, rather than TCR alone.

References

[1] Alkhalil M, Choudhury RP. Current concepts in atherosclerosis. Indian J Thorac Cardiovasc Surg 2018;34(Suppl 3):198–205.

[2] Li Z, Wu N, Wang J, Zhang Q. Roles of endovascular calyx related enzymes in endothelial dysfunction and diabetic vascular complications. Front Pharmacol 2020; [cited 2022 Jul 25];11. Available from: https://www.frontiersin.org/articles/10.3389/fphar.2020.590614.

[3] Cleasby ME, Jamieson PM, Atherton PJ. Insulin resistance and sarcopenia: mechanistic links between common co-morbidities. J Endocrinol 2016;229(2):R67–81.

[4] Yurista SR, Chong CR, Badimon JJ, Kelly DP, de Boer RA, Westenbrink BD. Therapeutic potential of ketone bodies for patients with cardiovascular disease: JACC state-of-the-art review. J Am Coll Cardiol 2021;77(13):1660–9.

[5] Galkina E, Ley K. Immune and inflammatory mechanisms of atherosclerosis. Annu Rev Immunol 2009;27:165–97.

[6] Tabas I, Williams KJ, Borén J. Subendothelial lipoprotein retention as the initiating process in atherosclerosis: update and therapeutic implications. Circulation. 2007;116(16):1832–44.

[7] Normal and oxidized low density lipoproteins accumulate deep in physiologically thickened intima of human coronary arteries | Laboratory Investigation [Internet]. [cited 2022 Aug 3]. Available from: https://www.nature.com/articles/3780550.

[8] Jimi S, Sakata N, Matunaga A, Takebayashi S. Low density lipoproteins bind more to type I and III collagens by negative charge-dependent mechanisms than to type IV and V collagens. Atherosclerosis 1994;107(1):109–16.

[9] Oxidized low-density lipoprotein downregulates endothelial basic fibroblast growth factor through a Pertussis toxin-sensitive G-protein pathway | Circulation [Internet]. [cited 2022 Aug 3]. Available from: https://www.ahajournals.org/doi/10.1161/hc3101.092213.

[10] Yano Y, Shimokawa K, Okada Y, Noma A. Immunolocalization of lipoprotein(a) in wounded tissues. J Histochem Cytochem 1997;45 (4):559–68.

[11] A D, C H, L S, Jl M. Small concentrations of oxLDL induce capillary tube formation from endothelial cells via LOX-1-dependent redox-sensitive pathway. Arterioscler Thromb Vasc Biol [Internet]. 2007 Nov [cited 2022 Aug 6];27(11). Available from: https://pubmed.ncbi.nlm.nih.gov/17717293/.

[12] Paraoxonase and atherosclerosis | Arterioscler Thromb Vasc Biol [Internet]. [cited 2022 Aug 9]. Available from: https://www.ahajournals.org/doi/10.1161/01.ATV.21.4.473.

[13] Regulation of cell growth by oxidized LDL - PubMed [Internet]. [cited 2022 Aug 3]. Available from: https://pubmed.ncbi.nlm.nih.gov/10946211/.

[14] Li M, Yu J, Li Y, Li D, Yan D, Qu Z, et al. CXCR4 positive bone mesenchymal stem cells migrate to human endothelial cell stimulated by ox-LDL via SDF-1alpha/CXCR4 signaling axis. Exp Mol Pathol 2010;88(2):250–5.

[15] Reduced antioxidant potential of LDL is associated with increased susceptibility to LDL peroxidation in type II diabetic patients - PMC [Internet]. [cited 2022 Aug 9]. Available from: https://www.ncbi.nlm.nih.gov/pmc/articles/PMC3693637/.

[16] Young IS, Woodside JV. Antioxidants in health and disease. J Clin Pathol 2001;54(3):176–86.

[17] Stocker R, Bowry VW, Frei B. Ubiquinol-10 protects human low density lipoprotein more efficiently against lipid peroxidation than does alpha-tocopherol. Proc Natl Acad Sci 1991;88(5):1646–50.

[18] Ferri N, Tibolla G, Pirillo A, Cipollone F, Mezzetti A, Pacia S, et al. Proprotein convertase subtilisin kexin type 9 (PCSK9) secreted by cultured smooth muscle cells reduces macrophages LDLR levels. Atherosclerosis. 2012;220(2):381–6.

[19] Ding Z, Liu S, Wang X, Theus S, Deng X, Fan Y, et al. PCSK9 regulates expression of scavenger receptors and ox-LDL uptake in macrophages. Cardiovasc Res 2018;114(8):1145–53.

[20] Ishiyama J, Taguchi R, Yamamoto A, Murakami K. Palmitic acid enhances lectin-like oxidized LDL receptor (LOX-1) expression and promotes uptake of oxidized LDL in macrophage cells. Atherosclerosis 2010;209(1):118–24.

[21] Autophagy regulates cholesterol efflux from macrophage foam cells via lysosomal acid lipase - ScienceDirect [Internet]. [cited 2022 Aug 3]. Available from: https://www.sciencedirect.com/science/article/pii/S1550413111001811.

[22] Di Pietro N, Formoso G, Pandolfi A. Physiology and pathophysiology of oxLDL uptake by vascular wall cells in atherosclerosis. Vasc Pharmacol 2016;84:1–7.

[23] Patsch JR, Miesenböck G, Hopferwieser T, Mühlberger V, Knapp E, Dunn JK, et al. Relation of triglyceride metabolism and coronary artery disease. Studies in the postprandial state. Arterioscler Thromb 1992;12(11):1336–45.

[24] Lagos KG, Filippatos TD, Tsimihodimos V, Gazi IF, Rizos C, Tselepis AD, et al. Alterations in the high density lipoprotein phenotype and HDL-associated enzymes in subjects with metabolic syndrome. Lipids. 2009;44(1):9.

[25] Barter PJ, Caulfield M, Eriksson M, Grundy SM, Kastelein JJP, Komajda M, et al. Effects of torcetrapib in patients at high risk for coronary events. N Engl J Med 2007;357(21):2109–22.

[26] Chaudhary R, Garg J, Shah N, Sumner A. PCSK9 inhibitors: a new era of lipid lowering therapy. World J Cardiol 2017;9(2):76–91.

[27] HDL cholesterol efflux capacity and incident cardiovascular events | NEJM [Internet]. [cited 2022 Aug 3]. Available from: https://www.nejm.org/doi/full/10.1056/NEJMoa1409065.

[28] Insulin resistance affects the regulation of lipoprotein lipase in the postprandial period and in an adipose tissue-specific manner - Panarotto - 2002 - European Journal of Clinical Investigation - Wiley Online Library [Internet]. [cited 2022 Aug 31]. Available from: https://onlinelibrary.wiley.com/doi/full/10.1046/j.1365-2362.2002.00945.x?casa_token = d75uk9G7yx0AAAAA%3Au-WCHBn7rlzHa-AYrJCMJ4J885BMmCcPnyMwXNA_Rw0CliH3AJF0jSaRlhP92JzrP8iI4gr3-aMm-IXD.

[29] Chapman MJ, Ginsberg HN, Amarenco P, Andreotti F, Borén J, Catapano AL, et al. Triglyceride-rich lipoproteins and high-density lipoprotein cholesterol in patients at high risk of cardiovascular disease: evidence and guidance for management. Eur Heart J 2011;32(11):1345–61.

[30] Aronson D, Rayfield EJ. How hyperglycemia promotes atherosclerosis: molecular mechanisms. Cardiovasc Diabetol 2002;1:1 Apr 8.

[31] Dharmashankar K, Widlansky ME. Vascular endothelial function and hypertension: insights and directions. Curr Hypertens Rep 2010;12(6):448–55.

[32] Horita S, Seki G, Yamada H, Suzuki M, Koike K, Fujita T. Insulin resistance, obesity, hypertension, and renal sodium transport. Int J Hypertens 2011;391762 Apr 12;2011.

[33] Mahmoud AM, Ali MM, Miranda ER, Mey JT, Blackburn BK, Haus JM, et al. Nox2 contributes to hyperinsulinemia-induced redox imbalance and impaired vascular function. Redox Biol 2017;13:288–300 Jun 3.

[34] Sonal Sekhar M, Marupuru S, Reddy BS, Kurian SJ, Rao M. Chapter 21 - physiological role of cholesterol in human body In: Preuss HG, Bagchi D, editors. Dietary sugar, salt and fat in human health [Internet]. Academic Press; 2020[cited 2022 Jul 25]. p. 453–81. Available from. Available from: https://www.sciencedirect.com/science/article/pii/B9780128169186000214.

[35] Bickel PE. Lipid rafts and insulin signaling. Am J Physiol Endocrinol Metab 2002;282(1):E1–10.

[36] Inhibition of cholesterol biosynthesis disrupts lipid raft/caveolae and affects insulin receptor activation in 3T3-L1 preadipocytes - PubMed [Internet]. [cited 2022 Aug 2]. Available from: https://pubmed.ncbi.nlm.nih.gov/19433058/.

[37] Bile salts in control of lipid metabolism - PubMed [Internet]. [cited 2022 Aug 2]. Available from: https://pubmed.ncbi.nlm.nih.gov/27031274/.

[38] Genaro-Mattos TC, Anderson A, Allen LB, Korade Z, Mirnics K. Cholesterol biosynthesis and uptake in developing neurons. ACS Chem Neurosci 2019;10(8):3671–81.

[39] Cholesterol: a novel regulatory role in myelin formation - PubMed [Internet]. [cited 2022 Aug 2]. Available from: https://pubmed.ncbi.nlm.nih.gov/21343408/.

[40] Dai L, Zou L, Meng L, Qiang G, Yan M, Zhang Z. Cholesterol metabolism in neurodegenerative diseases: molecular mechanisms and therapeutic targets. Mol Neurobiol 2021;58(5):2183–201.

[41] Lütjohann D. Cholesterol metabolism in the brain: importance of 24S-hydroxylation. Acta Neurol Scand 2006;114(s185):33–42.

[42] Smolič T, Zorec R, Vardjan N. Pathophysiology of lipid droplets in neuroglia. Antioxidants. 2022;11(1):22.

[43] Wollmer MA, Streffer JR, Lütjohann D, Tsolaki M, Iakovidou V, Hegi T, et al. ABCA1 modulates CSF cholesterol levels and influences the age at onset of Alzheimer's disease. Neurobiol Aging 2003;24(3):421–6.

[44] Kirsch C, Eckert GP, Mueller WE. Statin effects on cholesterol micro-domains in brain plasma membranes. Biochem Pharmacol 2003;65(5):843–56.

[45] Sierra S, Ramos MC, Molina P, Esteo C, Vázquez JA, Burgos JS. Statins as neuroprotectants: a comparative in vitro study of lipophilicity, blood-brain-barrier penetration, lowering of brain cholesterol, and decrease of neuron cell death. J Alzheimer's Dis 2011;23(2):307–18.

[46] Dahlgren K, Gibas KJ. Ketogenic diet, high intensity interval training (HIIT) and memory training in the treatment of mild cognitive impairment: a case study. Diabetes Metab Syndrome Clin Res & Rev 2018;12(5):819–22.

[47] Phillips MCL, Deprez LM, Mortimer GMN, Murtagh DKJ, McCoy S, Mylchreest R, et al. Randomized crossover trial of a modified ketogenic diet in Alzheimer's disease. Alzheimer's Res & Ther 2021;13(1):51.

[48] Frontiers | The role of intermittent fasting in Parkinson's disease [Internet]. [cited 2022 Aug 5]. Available from: https://www.frontiersin.org/articles/10.3389/fneur.2021.682184/full.

[49] Gudden J, Vasquez AA, Bloemendaal M. The effects of intermittent fasting on brain and cognitive function. 2021 Aug 27 [cited 2022 Aug 5]; Available from: https://www.preprints.org/manuscript/202108.0528/v1.

[50] Vitamin D and the immune system | J Investig Med [Internet]. [cited 2022 Aug 2]. Available from: https://jim.bmj.com/content/59/6/881.abstract.

[51] Davies G, Garami AR, Byers J. Evidence supports a causal role for vitamin D status in global COVID-19 outcomes. medRxiv. 2020 Jun 13;2020.05.01.20087965.

[52] Vitamin D production after UVB exposure depends on baseline vitamin D and total cholesterol but not on skin pigmentation - PubMed [Internet]. [cited 2022 Aug 2]. Available from: https://pubmed.ncbi.nlm.nih.gov/19812604/.

[53] Carbone LD, Rosenberg EW, Tolley EA, Holick MF, Hughes TA, Watsky MA, et al. 25-Hydroxyvitamin D, cholesterol, and ultraviolet irradiation. Metabolism 2008;57(6):741–8.

[54] Grimes DS. Statins and vitamin D. Cardiovasc Drugs Ther 2009;23(4):261–2.
[55] Ravnskov U. High cholesterol may protect against infections and atherosclerosis. QJM: Int J Med 2003;96(12):927–34.
[56] Manifold-Wheeler BC, Elmore BO, Triplett KD, Castleman MJ, Otto M, Hall PR. Serum lipoproteins are critical for pulmonary innate defense against Staphylococcus aureus quorum sensing. J Immunol 2016;196(1):328–35.
[57] Herz J, Hamann U, Rogne S, Myklebost O, Gausepohl H, Stanley KK. Surface location and high affinity for calcium of a 500-kd liver membrane protein closely related to the LDL-receptor suggest a physiological role as lipoprotein receptor. EMBO J 1988;7(13):4119–27.
[58] Chen HW. Role of cholesterol metabolism in cell growth. Fed Proc 1984;43(1):126–30.
[59] LDL cholesterol recycles to the plasma membrane via a Rab8a-Myosin5b-Actin-dependent membrane transport route - ScienceDirect [Internet]. [cited 2022 Aug 3]. https://www.sciencedirect.com/science/article/pii/S153458071300542X.
[60] Yang ST, Kreutzberger AJB, Lee J, Kiessling V, Tamm LK. The role of cholesterol in membrane fusion. Chem Phys Lipids 2016;199:136–43.
[61] Mbuyane LL, Bauer FF, Divol B. The metabolism of lipids in yeasts and applications in oenology. Food Res Int 2021;141:110142.
[62] Cohen DE. Balancing cholesterol synthesis and absorption in the gastrointestinal tract. J Clin Lipidol 2008;2(2):S1–3.
[63] Brown AJ, Coates HW, Sharpe LJ. Chapter 10 - cholesterol synthesis. In: Ridgway ND, McLeod RS, editors. Biochemistry of lipids, lipoproteins and membranes. Seventh Edition Elsevier; 2021 [cited 2022 Aug 4]. p. 317–55. https://www.sciencedirect.com/science/article/pii/B9780128240489000055.
[64] Mitsche MA, McDonald JG, Hobbs HH, Cohen JC. Flux analysis of cholesterol biosynthesis in vivo reveals multiple tissue and cell-type specific pathways. eLife. 4:e07999.
[65] Afonso MS, Machado RM, Lavrador MS, Quintao ECR, Moore KJ, Lottenberg AM. Molecular pathways underlying cholesterol homeostasis. Nutrients. 2018;10(6):760.
[66] Field FJ, Kam NTP, Mathur SN. Regulation of cholesterol metabolism in the intestine. Gastroenterology 1990;99(2):539–51.
[67] Hu J, Zhang Z, Shen WJ, Azhar S. Cellular cholesterol delivery, intracellular processing and utilization for biosynthesis of steroid hormones. Nutr Metab (Lond) 2010;7:47.
[68] Zhang J, Liu Q. Cholesterol metabolism and homeostasis in the brain. Protein Cell 2015;6(4):254–64.
[69] Maxfield FR, van Meer G. Cholesterol, the central lipid of mammalian cells. Curr Opin Cell Biol 2010;22(4):422–9.
[70] Jensen MD, Haymond MW, Gerich JE, Cryer PE, Miles JM. Lipolysis during fasting. Decreased suppression by insulin and increased stimulation by epinephrine. J Clin Invest 1987;79(1):207–13.
[71] Brown MS, Goldstein JL. The SREBP pathway: regulation of cholesterol metabolism by proteolysis of a membrane-bound transcription factor. Cell 1997;89(3):331–40.
[72] Jaishy B, Abel ED. Lipids, lysosomes, and autophagy. J Lipid Res. 2016;57(9):1619–35.
[73] Abnormal reverse cholesterol transport in controlled type II diabetic patients | Arterioscler Thromb Vasc Biol [Internet]. [cited 2022 Aug 1]. Available from: https://www.ahajournals.org/doi/full/10.1161/01.ATV.15.12.2130.
[74] Dietschy JM, Gamel WG. Cholesterol synthesis in the intestine of man: regional differences and control mechanisms. J Clin Invest 1971;50 (4):872–80.
[75] Lagace TA. PCSK9 and LDLR degradation: regulatory mechanisms in circulation and in cells. Curr Opin Lipidol 2014;25(5):387–93.
[76] Hammer SS, Vieira CP, McFarland D, Sandler M, Levitsky Y, Dorweiler TF, et al. Fasting and fasting-mimicking treatment activate SIRT1/LXRα and alleviate diabetes-induced systemic and microvascular dysfunction. Diabetologia 2021;64(7):1674–89.
[77] Wirth A, Ritthaler F, Roth A, Schlierf G. Reduced uptake and esterification of free fatty acids during prolonged fasting. Int J Obes 1983;7(4):353–9.
[78] Browning JD, Horton JD. Fasting reduces plasma proprotein convertase, subtilisin/kexin type 9 and cholesterol biosynthesis in humans. J Lipid Res 2010;51(11):3359–63.
[79] Persson L, Cao G, Ståhle L, Sjöberg BG, Troutt JS, Konrad RJ, et al. Circulating proprotein convertase subtilisin kexin type 9 has a diurnal rhythm synchronous with cholesterol synthesis and is reduced by fasting in humans. Arterioscler Thromb Vasc Biol 2010;30(12):2666–72.
[80] Lambert MS, Avella MA, Botham KM, Mayes PA. The type of dietary fat alters the hepatic uptake and biliary excretion of cholesterol from chylomicron remnants. Br J Nutr 2000;83(4):431–8.
[81] Regulation of cholesterol and fatty acid synthesis - PubMed [Internet]. [cited 2022 Aug 15]. Available from: https://pubmed.ncbi.nlm.nih.gov/21504873/.
[82] Hernández-Rodas MC, Valenzuela R, Echeverría F, Rincón-Cervera MÁ, Espinosa A, Illesca P, et al. Supplementation with Docosahexaenoic acid and extra virgin olive oil prevents liver steatosis induced by a high-fat diet in mice through PPAR-α and Nrf2 upregulation with concomitant SREBP-1c and NF-kB downregulation. Mol Nutr Food Res 2017;61(12):1700479.
[83] Astrup A, Larsen TM, Harper A. Atkins and other low-carbohydrate diets: hoax or an effective tool for weight loss? Lancet 2004;364(9437):897–9.
[84] Jacobo-Albavera L, Posadas-Romero C, Vargas-Alarcón G, Romero-Hidalgo S, Posadas-Sánchez R, González-Salazar Mdel C, et al. Dietary fat and carbohydrate modulate the effect of the ATP-binding cassette A1 (ABCA1) R230C variant on metabolic risk parameters in premenopausal women from the Genetics of Atherosclerotic Disease (GEA) Study. Nutr Metab (Lond) 2015;12(1):45.
[85] Westman EC, Yancy WS, Olsen MK, Dudley T, Guyton JR. Effect of a low-carbohydrate, ketogenic diet program compared to a low-fat diet on fasting lipoprotein subclasses. Int J Cardiology 2006;110(2):212–16.
[86] Partsalaki Ioanna, Karvela A, Spiliotis BE. Metabolic impact of a ketogenic diet compared to a hypocaloric diet in obese children and adolescents. J Pediatr Endocrinol Metab 2012;25(7–8):697–704.
[87] Meckling KA, Gauthier M, Grubb R, Sanford J. Effects of a hypocaloric, low-carbohydrate diet on weight loss, blood lipids, blood pressure, glucose tolerance, and body composition in free-living overweight women. Can J Physiol Pharmacol 2002;80(11):1095–105.

[88] Ketogenic diet exhibits anti-inflammatory properties - Dupuis - 2015 - Epilepsia - Wiley Online Library [Internet]. [cited 2022 Aug 2]. Available from: https://onlinelibrary.wiley.com/doi/full/10.1111/epi.13038.

[89] Norwitz NG, Soto-Mota A, Kaplan B, Ludwig DS, Budoff M, Kontush A, et al. The lipid energy model: reimagining lipoprotein function in the context of carbohydrate-restricted diets. Metabolites. 2022;12(5):460.

[90] Norwitz NG, Soto-Mota A, Feldman D, Parpos S, Budoff M. Case report: hypercholesterolemia 'lean mass hyper-responder' phenotype presents in the context of a low saturated fat carbohydrate-restricted diet. Front Endocrinol (Lausanne) 2022;13:830325.

[91] Norwitz NG, Feldman D, Soto-Mota A, Kalayjian T, Ludwig DS. Elevated LDL cholesterol with a carbohydrate-restricted diet: evidence for a "lean mass hyper-responder" phenotype. Curr Dev Nutr 2021;6(1):nzab144.

[92] Björkhem I. Do oxysterols control cholesterol homeostasis? J Clin Invest 2002;110(6):725–30.

[93] Wolf G. The role of oxysterols in cholesterol homeostasis. Nutr Rev 1999;57(6):196–8.

[94] Overexpression of cholesterol 7α-hydroxylase promotes hepatic bile acid synthesis and secretion and maintains cholesterol homeostasis - Li - 2011 - Hepatology - Wiley Online Library [Internet]. [cited 2022 Aug 2]. Available from: https://aasldpubs.onlinelibrary.wiley.com/doi/full/10.1002/hep.24107.

[95] Tu H, Okamoto AY, Shan B. FXR, a bile acid receptor and biological sensor. Trends Cardiovascular Med 2000;10(1):30–5.

[96] Role of bile acids and bile acid receptors in metabolic regulation | Physiological Reviews [Internet]. [cited 2022 Aug 2]. Available from: https://journals.physiology.org/doi/full/10.1152/physrev.00010.2008.

[97] Reeskamp LF, Meessen ECE, Groen AK. Transintestinal cholesterol excretion in humans. Curr OpLipidol 2018;29(1):10–17.

[98] Trans-intestinal cholesterol efflux is not mediated through high density lipoprotein - Journal of Lipid Research [Internet]. [cited 2022 Aug 2]. Available from: https://www.jlr.org/article/S0022-2275(20)43179-7/fulltext.

[99] Tuberous Xanthomatosis - PMC [Internet]. [cited 2022 Aug 27]. Available from: https://www.ncbi.nlm.nih.gov/pmc/articles/PMC503662/.

[100] Müller C. Xanthomata, hypercholesterolemia, angina pectoris. Acta Medica Scand 1938;95(S89):75–84.

[101] 'Essential' fatty acids, degree of unsaturation, and effect of corn (maize) oil on the serumcholesterol level in man. [Internet]. [cited 2022 Aug 27]. Available from: https://www.cabdirect.org/cabdirect/abstract/19571403743.

[102] Rose GA, Thomson WB, Williams RT. Corn Oil in treatment of ischaemic heart disease. Br Med J 1965;1(5449):1531–3.

[103] Oliver MF. Doubts about preventing coronary heart disease. BMJ. 1992;304(6824):393–4.

[104] Ravnskov U, Diamond DM, Hama R, Hamazaki T, Hammarskjöld B, Hynes N, et al. Lack of an association or an inverse association between low-density-lipoprotein cholesterol and mortality in the elderly: a systematic review. BMJ Open 2016;6(6):e010401.

[105] Nissen SE. Statin denial: an internet-driven cult with deadly consequences. Ann Intern Med 2017;167(4):281–2.

[106] Rosuvastatin to prevent vascular events in men and women with elevated C-reactive protein | NEJM [Internet]. [cited 2022 Aug 27]. Available from: https://www.nejm.org/doi/full/10.1056/NEJMoa0807646.

[107] How statistical deception created the appearance that statins are safe and effective in primary and secondary prevention of cardiovascular disease: Expert Review of Clinical Pharmacology: Vol 8, No 2 [Internet]. [cited 2022 Aug 27]. Available from: https://www.tandfonline.com/doi/abs/10.1586/17512433.2015.1012494.

[108] Systematic review of the predictors of statin adherence for the primary prevention of cardiovascular disease | PLoS ONE [Internet]. [cited 2022 Aug 27]. Available from: https://journals.plos.org/plosone/article?id = 10.1371/journal.pone.0201196.

[109] Influence of low high-density lipoprotein cholesterol and elevated triglyceride on coronary heart disease events and response to simvastatin therapy in 4S | Circulation [Internet]. [cited 2022 Aug 27]. Available from: https://www.ahajournals.org/doi/full/10.1161/hc5001.100624.

[110] Davignon J, Laaksonen R. Low-density lipoprotein-independent effects of statins. Curr Opin Lipidol 1999;10(6):543–59.

[111] Noakes TD. The 2012 University of Cape Town Faculty of Health Sciences centenary debate "Cholesterol is not an important risk factor for heart disease, and the current dietary recommendations do more harm than good.". South Afr J Clin Nutr 2015;28(1):19–33.

[112] Ravnskov U, de Lorgeril M, Kendrick M, Diamond DM. Inborn coagulation factors are more important cardiovascular risk factors than high LDL-cholesterol in familial hypercholesterolemia. Med Hypotheses 2018;121:60–3.

[113] Istvan ES, Deisenhofer J. Structural mechanism for statin inhibition of HMG-CoA reductase. Science 2001;292(5519):1160–4.

[114] Dong B, Wu M, Li H, Kraemer FB, Adeli K, Seidah NG, et al. Strong induction of PCSK9 gene expression through HNF1α and SREBP2: mechanism for the resistance to LDL-cholesterol lowering effect of statins in dyslipidemic hamsters. J Lipid Res 2010;51(6):1486–95.

[115] Ridker PM, Mora S, Rose L, the JUPITER Trial Study Group. Percent reduction in LDL cholesterol following high-intensity statin therapy: potential implications for guidelines and for the prescription of emerging lipid-lowering agents. Eur Heart J 2016;37(17):1373–9.

[116] Melendez QM, Krishnaji ST, Wooten CJ, Lopez D. Hypercholesterolemia: the role of PCSK9. Arch Biochem Biophysics 2017;625–626:39–53.

[117] Synthesis and absorption markers of cholesterol in serum and lipoproteins during a large dose of statin treatment - Miettinen - 2003 - Eur J Clin Investig - Wiley Online Library [Internet]. [cited 2022 Aug 2]. Available from: https://onlinelibrary.wiley.com/doi/full/10.1046/j.1365-2362.2003.01229.x?casa_token = 2FXTQPwoq-EAAAAA%3Alk3G-Extbz5YXVxkST3eNIABOM8q_4Lq2IGjwHY8jVhBo4vMAfDevrIhqjd5qQMCt2tM7vtDFI4yLAY.

[118] Melenotte C, Carrié A, Serratrice J, Weiller PJ. Sitosterolemia: a new mutation in a Mediterranean patient. J Clin Lipidol 2014;8(4):451–4.

[119] Miettinen TA, Gylling H. The effects of statins and sitosterols: benefit or not? Curr Atheroscler Rep 2009;11(1):23–7.

[120] Clayton PT, Whitfield P, Iyer K. The role of phytosterols in the pathogenesis of liver complications of pediatric parenteral nutrition. Nutrition. 1998;14(1):158–64.

[121] Abbasi F, Lamendola C, Harris CS, Harris V, Tsai MS, Tripathi P, et al. statins are associated with increased insulin resistance and secretion. Arterioscler Thromb Vasc Biol 2021;41(11):2786–97.

[122] Gai MT, Adi D, Chen XC, Liu F, Xie X, Yang YN, et al. Polymorphisms of rs2483205 and rs562556 in the PCSK9 gene are associated with coronary artery disease and cardiovascular risk factors. Sci Rep 2021;11(1):11450.

[123] Schmidt AF, Swerdlow DI, Holmes MV, Patel RS, Fairhurst-Hunter Z, Lyall DM, et al. PCSK9 genetic variants and risk of type 2 diabetes: a mendelian randomisation study. Lancet Diabetes Endocrinol 2017;5(2):97–105.

[124] PCSK9 deficiency reduces insulin secretion and promotes glucose intolerance: the role of the low-density lipoprotein receptor - PubMed [Internet]. [cited 2022 Aug 27]. Available from: https://pubmed.ncbi.nlm.nih.gov/29982592/.

[125] Evolocumab and clinical outcomes in patients with cardiovascular disease | NEJM [Internet]. [cited 2022 Aug 5]. Available from: https://www.nejm.org/doi/full/10.1056/nejmoa1615664.

[126] Katzmann JL, Gouni-Berthold I, Laufs U. PCSK9 inhibition: insights from clinical trials and future prospects Front Physiol [Internet] 2020; [cited 2022 Aug 31];11. Available from: https://www.frontiersin.org/articles/10.3389/fphys.2020.595819.

[127] de Carvalho LSF, Campos AM, Sposito AC. Proprotein convertase subtilisin/kexin type 9 (PCSK9) inhibitors and incident type 2 diabetes: a systematic review and meta-analysis with over 96,000 patient-years. Diabetes Care 2017;41(2):364–7.

[128] Song Y, Kenworthy AK, Sanders CR. Cholesterol as a co-solvent and a ligand for membrane proteins. Protein Sci 2014;23(1):1–22.

[129] Oliphant K, Allen-Vercoe E. Macronutrient metabolism by the human gut microbiome: major fermentation by-products and their impact on host health. Microbiome. 2019;7(1):91.

[130] Nakajima K, Nakano T, Tokita Y, Nagamine T, Inazu A, Kobayashi J, et al. Postprandial lipoprotein metabolism; VLDL vs chylomicrons. Clin Chim Acta 2011;412(15–16):1306–18.

[131] Starks EJ, Patrick O'Grady J, Hoscheidt SM, Racine AM, Carlsson CM, Zetterberg H, et al. Insulin resistance is associated with higher cerebrospinal fluid tau levels in asymptomatic APOEε4 carriers. J Alzheimers Dis 2015;46(2):525–33.

[132] (1) (PDF) Metabolic origins and clinical significance of LDLC heterogeneity [Internet]. [cited 2022 Aug 27]. Available from: https://www.researchgate.net/publication/11155851_Metabolic_origins_and_clinical_significance_of_LDLC_heterogeneity.

[133] Beglova N, Blacklow SC. The LDL receptor: how acid pulls the trigger. Trends Biochemical Sci 2005;30(6):309–17.

[134] Tall AR, Yvan-Charvet L. Cholesterol, inflammation and innate immunity. Nat Rev Immunol 2015;15(2):104–16.

[135] Biochemistry of lipids, lipoproteins and membranes, sixth edition [PDF] [286j0fbr6eb0] [Internet]. [cited 2022 Aug 3]. Available from: https://vdoc.pub/documents/biochemistry-of-lipids-lipoproteins-and-membranes-sixth-edition-286j0fbr6eb0.

[136] Alleva R, Tomasetti M, Battino M, Curatola G, Littarru GP, Folkers K. The roles of coenzyme Q10 and vitamin E on the peroxidation of human low density lipoprotein subfractions. Proc Natl Acad Sci USA 1995;92(20):9388–91.

[137] Hoofnagle AN, Heinecke JW. Lipoproteomics: using mass spectrometry-based proteomics to explore the assembly, structure, and function of lipoproteins: Thematic Review Series: Proteomics. J Lipid Res 2009;50(10):1967–75.

[138] Zhu X, Parks JS. New roles of HDL in inflammation and hematopoiesis. Annu Rev Nutr 2012;32. Available from: https://doi.org/10.1146/annurev-nutr-071811-150709 Aug 21.

[139] Cahill GF. Ketosis. Kidney Int 1981;20(3):416–25.

[140] Ruderman NB, Jones AL, Krauss RM, Shafrir E. A biochemical and morphologic study of very low density lipoproteins in carbohydrate-induced hypertriglyceridemia. J Clin Invest 1971;50(6):1355–68.

[141] Bickerton AST, Roberts R, Fielding BA, Tornqvist H, Blaak EE, Wagenmakers AJM, et al. Adipose tissue fatty acid metabolism in insulin-resistant men. Diabetologia. 2008;51(8):1466.

[142] Avramoglu RK, Qiu W, Adeli K. Mechanisms of metabolic dyslipidemia in insulin resistant states: deregulation of hepatic and intestinal lipoprotein secretion. Front Biosci 2003;8:d464–76.

[143] Almandoz JP, Singh E, Howell LA, Grothe K, Vlazny DT, Smailovic A, et al. Spillover of fatty acids during dietary fat storage in type 2 diabetes. Diabetes. 2013;62(6):1897–903.

[144] Choi SH, Ginsberg HN. Increased very low density lipoprotein (VLDL) secretion, hepatic steatosis, and insulin resistance. Trends Endocrinol Metab 2011;22(9):353–63.

[145] JCI - Insulin resistance and cardiovascular disease [Internet]. [cited 2022 Aug 3]. Available from: https://www.jci.org/articles/view/10762.

[146] Ferré P, Foufelle F. SREBP-1c transcription factor and lipid homeostasis: clinical perspective. HRP 2007;68(2):72–82.

[147] Dif N, Euthine V, Gonnet E, Laville M, Vidal H, Lefai E. Insulin activates human sterol-regulatory-element-binding protein-1c (SREBP-1c) promoter through SRE motifs. Biochem J 2006;400(1):179–88.

[148] Horton JD, Bashmakov Y, Shimomura I, Shimano H. Regulation of sterol regulatory element binding proteins in livers of fasted and refed mice. Proc Natl Acad Sci 1998;95(11):5987–92.

[149] Zang M. The molecular basis of hepatic de novo lipogenesis in insulin resistance In: Ntambi JM, editor. Hepatic de novo lipogenesis and regulation of metabolism [Internet]. Cham: Springer International Publishing; 2016[cited 2022 Aug 6]. p. 33–58. Available from. Available from: https://doi.org/10.1007/978-3-319-25065-6_2.

[150] Nonalcoholic steatohepatitis: association of insulin resistance and mitochondrial abnormalities - ScienceDirect [Internet]. [cited 2022 Aug 3]. Available from: https://www.sciencedirect.com/science/article/abs/pii/S0016508501007491.

[151] Shelness GS, Sellers JA. Very-low-density lipoprotein assembly and secretion. Curr OpLipidol 2001;12(2):151–7.

[152] Mason TM. The role of factors that regulate the synthesis and secretion of very-low-density lipoprotein by hepatocytes. Crit Rev Clin Lab Sci 1998;35(6):461–87.

[153] Adiels M, Westerbacka J, Soro-Paavonen A, Häkkinen AM, Vehkavaara S, Caslake MJ, et al. Acute suppression of VLDL1 secretion rate by insulin is associated with hepatic fat content and insulin resistance. Diabetologia. 2007;50(11):2356–65.

[154] Ferré P, Foufelle F. Hepatic steatosis: a role for de novo lipogenesis and the transcription factor SREBP-1c. Diabetes Obes Metab 2010;12(s2):83–92.

[155] Differing endoplasmic reticulum stress response to excess lipogenesis versus lipid oversupply in relation to hepatic steatosis and insulin resistance. PLoS ONE [Internet]. [cited 2022 Aug 3]. Available from: https://journals.plos.org/plosone/article?id = 10.1371/journal.pone.0030816.

[156] Takahara S, Soni S, Maayah ZH, Ferdaoussi M, Dyck JRB. Ketone therapy for heart failure: current evidence for clinical use. Cardiovasc Res 2022;118(4):977–87.

[157] Takahara S, Soni S, Maayah ZH, Ferdaoussi M, Dyck JRB. Ketone therapy for heart failure: current evidence for clinical use. Cardiovasc Res 2021; Mar 10.

[158] Nielsen R, Møller N, Gormsen LC, Tolbod LP, Hansson NH, Sorensen J, et al. Cardiovascular effects of treatment with the ketone body 3-hydroxybutyrate in chronic heart failure patients. Circulation 2019;139(18):2129–41.

[159] Athinarayanan SJ, Hallberg SJ, McKenzie AL, Lechner K, King S, McCarter JP, et al. Impact of a 2-year trial of nutritional ketosis on indices of cardiovascular disease risk in patients with type 2 diabetes. Cardiovasc Diabetol 2020;19(1):208.

[160] Gershuni VM, Yan SL, Medici V. Nutritional ketosis for weight management and reversal of metabolic syndrome. Curr Nutr Rep 2018;7(3):97–106.

[161] Gums JG. Magnesium in cardiovascular and other disorders. Am J Health-Syst Pharm 2004;61(15):1569–76.

[162] Zhang S, Zhuang X, Lin X, Zhong X, Zhou H, Sun X, et al. Low-carbohydrate diets and risk of incident atrial fibrillation: a prospective cohort study. J Am Heart Assoc 2019;8(9):e011955.

[163] Lipotoxicity in the heart - ScienceDirect [Internet]. [cited 2022 Aug 27]. Available from: https://www.sciencedirect.com/science/article/pii/S1388198109002364?casa_token = C8PITXinPOAAAAAA:n16rzex922J_qr_nfcCQxkolJ4sMinK-QAz47lqTUr0f6GuTgJBQJcEGmwsYdUlDq4fzql4R1A.

Chapter 5

Neurology

Michael Hoffmann[1,2], Robert Cywes[3], Ann M. Childers[4], Meredith M. Kossoff[5], Eric H. Kossoff[6], David Perlmutter[7,8], Mathew C.L. Phillips[9], Georgia Edes[10], Amy Berger[11], Angela A. Stanton[12], Laurie Rauch[13], Julienne Fenwick[14], Joshua Rossi[15], Elisa Marie Rossi[15], Elizabeth Gonzalez[15] and Fabian Rossi[15,16]

[1]*University of Central Florida, Orlando, FL, United States,* [2]*Orlando VA Medical Center, Orlando, FL, United States,* [3]*JSAPA Metabolic Centre, Jupiter, FL, United States,* [4]*Oregon City, OR, United States,* [5]*Cornell University, Ithaca, NY, United States,* [6]*Departments of Neurology and Paediatrics, Johns Hopkins Hospital, Baltimore, MD, United States,* [7]*American Nutrition Association, Hinsdale, IL, United States,* [8]*University of Miami Miller School of Medicine, Miami, FL, United States,* [9]*Waikato Hospital, Hamilton, New Zealand,* [10]*Psychiatrist in Private Practice,* [11]*Nutritionist in Private Practice,* [12]*Stanton Migraine Protocol, Anaheim, CA, United States,* [13]*Physiological Sciences, Faculty of Health Sciences, University of Cape Town, Cape Town, South Africa,* [14]*Best of both Wellness, Hermanus, Western Cape, South Africa,* [15]*UCF Medical School, Orlando, FL, United States,* [16]*Clinical Neurophysiology Lab, Orlando VA Medical Center, Orlando, FL, United States*

5.1 A ketogenic diet addresses the pathophysiology underlying diverse neurological disorders

Michael Hoffmann

5.1.1 Introduction

The basic sciences have long informed the clinical sciences, but a recent surge of interest in evolutionary medicine supports this to be even more fundamental in understanding and guiding human biology. A renowned biologist, Theodosius Dobzhansky, cautioned us almost 50 years ago, 'Nothing in biology makes sense except in the light of evolution'. Such insights are not only useful to understand the present-day structure and function of the human brain but also what nutrients are essential for optimum brain and body health. The monumental expansion of the cerebral circuitry came at a price. The increasing connectomic complexity is limited by energetic constraints and the risk of psychosis. The human connectome (maps of connections within the nervous system) has vulnerable hubs and is prone to failure in most neurological diseases [1]. The prefrontal cortex is the most vulnerable of all [2] and is also implicated in the dysconnectivity of schizophrenia [3]. The fragility of our extensive white matter circuitry also predisposes us to mild cognitive impairment, mild behavioural impairment, dementia and stroke if metabolism is disrupted, principally by suboptimal nutrition [4]. Connectopathies, synaptopathies, autoimmune encephalitis and neuropsychiatric disease are all manifestations of the white matter tract, synaptic and immunocompetence vulnerability, with nutrition a fundamental pillar of brain health.

5.1.2 Pathophysiology

5.1.2.1 Modulating inflammation

The KD has been advocated for over 100 years, initially for refractory epilepsy. Accruing evidence from animal models, as well as small and uncontrolled human clinical trials for neurodegenerative (Alzheimer's disease [AD], PD, and frontotemporal syndromes) disorders in general, has advocated implementing a KD. Because neurodegenerative conditions have underlying neuroinflammation, the ketogenic-type diet has been investigated both for symptom relief and potential disease modifying effects. Ketone bodies (β-hydroxybutyrate, acetoacetate, and acetone) are neuroprotective, with antioxidant and anti-inflammatory effects and regarded as a disease modifying type therapy, especially in the case of epilepsy where anticonvulsant therapy alone is not regarded as disease modifying [5,6].

Additionally, the elevated fatty acids associated with a KD activate anti-inflammatory mechanisms such as peroxisome proliferator-activated receptor alpha, which inhibits proinflammatory transcription factors, such as nuclear factor kappa-light-chain-enhancer of activated B cells (NF-kappa B) [7].

Inflammation is a natural and beneficial host response to infections that requires tight control to avoid excessive or prolonged activity. NF-kappa B is a transcription factor that has a central role in regulating other genes that in turn

Ketogenic. DOI: https://doi.org/10.1016/B978-0-12-821617-0.00006-1

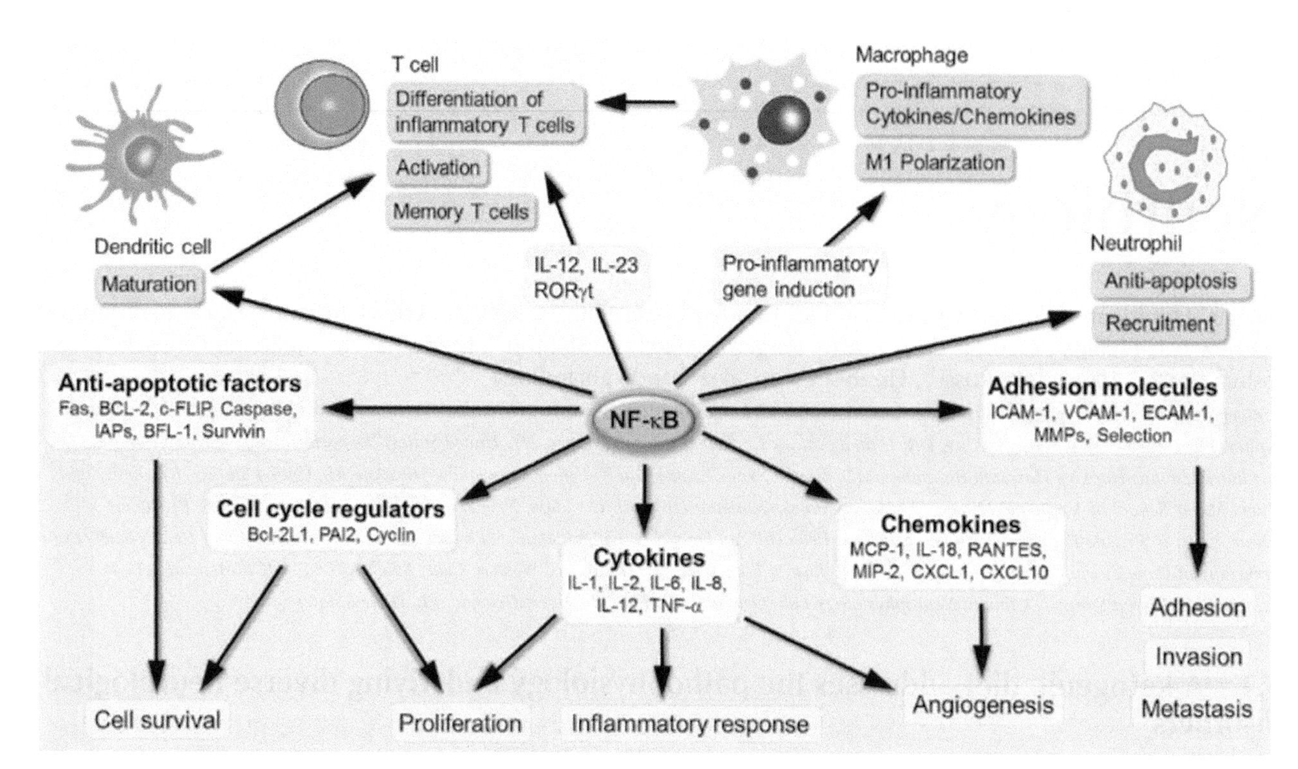

FIGURE 5.1 **Vital statistics of the brain.** Non-conscious activity uses most of the energy and is the dominant brain activity. Even willed movement is initially non-conscious.

control inflammatory and immune responses [8]. Ubiquitous in animal cells, it provides a mechanism of countering microbial antigens, stress, free radicals, ultraviolet light radiation, and heavy metals (Fig. 5.1).

Activation of NF-κB can regulate inflammation directly via cytokine/adhesion molecules/chemokine upregulation, but also indirectly via regulating the cell cycle and genes regulating inflammation as an inducible transcription factor. Nuclear factor kappa B (NF-κB); B-cell lymphoma 2 (BCL-2); cellular FLICE-like inhibitory protein (c-FLIP); inhibitor of apoptosis (IAP); Bcl-2-related protein A1 (BFL-1); Bcl-2-like protein 1 (BCL-2L1); Plasminogen activator inhibitor type-2 (PAI-2); interleukin (IL); Retineic-acid-receptor-related orphan nuclear receptor gamma (RORγt); Tumour necrosis factor alpha (TNF-α); Monocyte Chemoattractant Protein-1 (MCP-1); Regulated upon Activation, Normal T Cell Expressed and Presumably Secreted (RANTES); Macrophage Inflammatory Protein 2 (MIP-2); C-X-C Motif Chemokine Ligand (CXCL); Intercellular adhesion molecule-1 (ICAM-1); vascular cell adhesion molecule 1 (VCAM-1); epithelial cell adhesion molecule-1 (ECAM1); Matrix metalloproteinases (MMPs) (figure obtained from ref. [8]).

With dysregulation of NF-kappa B, autoimmune disease, inflammatory disease and cancer develop [9]. From the point of view of nutrition as a method of combating a chronic autoimmune and or inflammatory disease such as multiple sclerosis (Ms) (Section 5.7), NF-kappa B represents a key target as a central genetic switch that amplifies the inflammatory response. An anti-inflammatory diet such as a KD may be viewed as a method of gene silencing and upstream intervention. Pharmacological agents have a downstream intervention, so the ketogenic diet is a more elegant method to impact NF-kappaB, the primary molecular inflammatory target [8].

Diet and inflammation are tightly linked with the innate immune system and the sensitivity to nutrients dates back several hundred million years [10]. Certain nutrients (arachidonic acid) may activate the inflammatory cascade and some can inhibit it (docosahexaenoic acid (DHA), eicosapentaenoic acid (EPA), polyphenols). Reported neurophysiological mechanisms mediating the relationship of omega 3 fatty acids and other brain-specific nutrients with depression, bipolar disease, and other neuropsychiatric and neurodegenerative conditions, include cytokine expression (IL-1, IL-6, IL8, and TNF alpha), neurotransmitter augmentation (serotonin, dopamine) BDNF release, and augmentation of cerebral blood flow and eicosanoid production [11,12].

5.1.2.2 Ameliorates glutamate-mediated toxicity

Countering glutamate-mediated toxicity attenuation of glutamate-induced formation of reactive oxygen species (ROS) is one of the many mechanisms whereby the KD confers neuroprotection [13].

5.1.2.3 *Effects on γ-aminobutyric acid systems*

KD-induced neuroprotection may also be attained by augmenting γ-aminobutyric acid (GABA) concentrations, with a consequent increase in GABA- mediated inhibition [14].

5.1.2.4 *Antioxidant mechanisms*

Ketone bodies reduce coenzyme Q semiquinone with consequent reduction of free radical production [15]. Glutathione peroxidase is another important enzyme in reactive oxygen species (ROS) regulation that prevents lipid peroxidation by reducing lipid hydroperoxides due to glutathione peroxidase activity, which was first reported in the rat hippocampus [16]. Another KD effect is to augment the production of mitochondrial uncoupling proteins (UCPs) namely, UCP2, UCP4, and UCP5, which function to dispel the mitochondrial membrane potential, thereby reducing ROS [17].

5.1.2.5 *Energy metabolism*

Ketone bodies are a more efficient source of cerebral energy per unit oxygen as opposed to glucose ([18]) with rodent studies revealing an increase in hippocampal mitochondrial profiles (mitochondrial biogenesis) by electron micrographic analysis in rats fed the KD.

5.1.2.6 *Gut microbiome*

Diet and exposure to the natural environment is critical to microbial diversity. Research on ancestral diets reveals much greater microbial diversity than in people who have T2D and obesity, termed gastrointestinal microbial deprivation with predominantly inflammatory gut microbiota in those pursuing a Westernised type diet [19]. A ketogenic diet can modulate the microbiome, playing a role in the therapeutic effect [20].

5.1.3 Conclusion

A ketogenic diet can address many aspects of the pathophysiology underlying neurological disorders, which include reducing inflammation, mediating the glutamate and GABA pathways, supporting antioxidant mechanisms, and improving energy metabolism. These are just some of the mechanisms involved. A well-formulated ketogenic diet is nutritionally dense and can provide DHA and other essential fats while improving aspects of the microbiome, an emerging therapeutic target of interest.

5.2 Neurophysiology and energy metabolism

Michael Hoffmann

5.2.1 Anatomy and physiology of the neuron and neuronal signalling

Diverse cellular components make up the central nervous system (CNS) These include neurons (~100 billion), astrocytes (approximately 1 trillion), oligodendroglia (make CNS myelin), microglia (brain macrophages), ependymal cells (line the ventricles, part of blood cerebrospinal fluid barrier – BCSFB) and endothelial cells (components of brain blood vessels and part of the BBB). A classic image of a neuron comprises the cell body called perikaryon, an axon that sends electrical signals out and many dendrites that receive signals. Whereas proteins are key components for general body growth, lipids comprise approximately 60% of the brain's structural components. The primary functions of lipids (cholesterol, complex lipids) are as components of neuronal membranes, signal transduction, synthesis of myelin and formation of neuro-steroids. The dietary essential long chain polyunsaturated fatty acids (LC-PUFA) are the major limiting nutrients for the construction of brain lipids and neuronal membranes and yet are not that readily available in foods [21].

Neurons are electrically excitable cells due to a negative membrane potential enabled by the sodium-potassium (Na/K) pump. This in turn allows the neurons to signal to each other via action potentials. The currents from positively charged sodium (Na^+) and potassium (K^+) ion channels account for the majority of the current need to generate an axon potential. The initial opening of the Na^+ channel is followed by the K^+ opening, briefly reversing the resting positive charge on the outside and negative charge on the inside, and then due to the nodes of Ranvier, which have a ten-fold increase in Na^+ channels that enable much faster propagation of the electrical impulse. This jumping from node to node is termed saltatory conduction [22]. An action potential is propagated down the axon, which is myelinated to allow fifty-fold faster conduction compared to unmyelinated axons. The increased conduction speed allows for increased information processing in response to stimuli (e.g., a predatory attack), increased temporal precision and spatial localisation of stimuli and faster communication between the brain and distant body parts. This also provides several hundred-fold more metabolic efficiency for the cost of neuronal traffic. However, on the downside, because lipids are required to synthesise myelin, myelin, and consequently efficacy of neural conduction, is dependent on good food quality [23]. The frequency of spiking may vary widely, and several examples include single spiking, slow and rapid spike trains and chattering spiking [24]. These electrical signals connect one neuron to another through chemical synapses, allowing one neuron to influence another. Electrical synapses are gap junctions between neurons and have a much simpler design. This characteristic translates into speed and efficiency of conduction and hence is able to excite, inhibit, conduct bidirectionally and synchronise neuronal chatter [25].

5.2.2 Brain energy metabolism

Human neural processing of information has been determined to be metabolically expensive. Considering that the human brain is approximately 2% of the body's weight, it nevertheless accounts for around 20% of its basal metabolic rate. Overall, the action potentials use 47% and the subsequent glutamate postsynaptic signalling uses 34%, consuming the most energy. Maintaining the resting potential gradient consumes about 13%, whereas glutamate recycling consumes around 3% [26].

The brain's energy is derived predominantly from glucose oxidation with synaptic transmission, maintenance of ion gradients, axonal transport, and phospholipid synthesis being the main energy hungry processes. A continuous and reliable energy supply is vital for brain cellular performance as glycogen storage is minimal. With fasting, increasing amounts of ketone bodies are utilised. This is underscored by the neurodegenerative diseases, all of which are characterised by metabolic impairment, as well as neuroinflammation, mitochondrial dysfunction, and protein aggregation, induced by energy failure. Recent clinical studies support the use of ketone bodies for the treatment of neurodegenerative diseases, which improve neuronal metabolism. Interestingly, sodium glucose co-transporter 2 inhibitors, which increase ketone body concentrations similar to ketogenic type diets, correlated with a lower risk of developing dementia [27].

The function of cerebral insulin includes nutrient homoeostasis, cognition, memory function, neuromodulatory, and neuroprotective properties. When these processes malfunction, there may be impairment of central insulin resistance, T2D or AD. The well-known relationship between AD and T2D is particularly notable with AD being twice as likely in people with T2D and referred to as type 3 diabetes [28].

5.2.3 The high-energy-demanding human brain

The most extensively connected hub nodes of the cerebral networks have the highest metabolic demands because of their long-distance connections. These high demands, at the same time, render them more prone to the consequences of vascular, metabolic, and neurodegenerative diseases [26]. The dependency of our brain's energy demands also makes us susceptible to human-specific conditions such as degenerative (AD, frontotemporal dementias) and developmental (schizophrenia, autism) diseases [26]. Larger brains also feature more synapses per neuron and disproportionately more fibre tracts, with exorbitant energy demands. The majority of the energetic costs are incurred by synaptic signalling and maintaining neuronal electrochemical gradients and subsequent oxidative stress [26]. Whether due to metabolic deficiency or injury, these are preferentially affected and seen as vulnerable areas of the human connectome [29,30]. Energy consumption attributions are noted in Table 5.1. Non-conscious activity is the dominant brain activity and hence, uses most of the energy. Willed movement has an initial non-conscious component, with a 'readiness potential' preceding awareness of the movement by approximately 1 s and as much as 8 s prior, in the frontopolar cortex [31,32].

TABLE 5.1 Neurochemistry, energy consumption %.

1	Action potentials energy	47
2	Postsynaptic processing	34
3	Resting neuronal potential	13
4	Glutamate recycling	3

5.2.4 The big human brain

The threefold increase in human brain volume in comparison to extant great apes (over the last seven to eight million years since our divergence from the common ancestor) is eclipsed by the even more dramatic expansion in the white matter tracts and the respective cerebral networks [33]. In addition, glial cell proliferation, the expansion of the cortical granular layer, and synaptic complexity escalation, together, enabled humans to have a much higher processing speed. The constituent human brain comprises approximately 100 billion neurons, 700 km of blood vessels, and sixfold more glial cells (approximately 1 trillion) than neurons (Fig. 5.2). Perhaps the most mind-boggling statistic is the 150,000 km (the same distance as four times around the Earth) of nerve fibres, the basis of the human connectome. Neuronal complex networks also interact with the complex networks at the metabolic, immune, genetic, and social networks.

5.2.5 Glial cells augment complex human brain processing

Other brain processing dimensions in three-dimensional space and time, include astroglial networks (gliotransmission) and epigenetic mechanisms. Glial cells enable mammals to attain more swiftness in motion, more complex brain functions, and vastly increased speed of reaction and information processing. Overall, with increasing complexity amongst animals, there occurs an increase in glial cell to neuron ratio with the human ratio approximately 6:1. Astrocytic processes are intimately associated with blood vessels and neural synapses (forming the tripartite synapse) and are integral to the BBB, control potassium homoeostasis, and mediate uptake of cellular waste [34]. Notably, astrocytes, also have receptors for the principal neurotransmitters (glutamate and GABA). In the prefrontal cortex and other parts of tertiary association areas, such as the inferior parietal cortex, there are more glial cells in humans than in any other animal, except for cetaceans. Einstein's brain revealed a twofold increase in glial to neuron cell ratio, in the inferior parietal lobule, as compared to the human norm of 11 male controls [35,36].

Glial cells eavesdrop on neuronal signalling and have their own neurotransmitter receptors, which allows for additional dimensions into information processing. A single astrocyte can envelop and influence approximately two million synapses and incorporate large groups of neurons and their synapses into functional units [37]. The expansive glial domains and their chemical cellular transmission diffuses widely and allows transgression of the hardwired tracts of neuronal connections, enabling a more global scale of information processing compared to the point-to-point synapse-based neuronal systems. Global glial communication networks also coordinate immunological, hormonal, and vascular networks.

Astrocytic complexity and the glio-neuronal functional unit augment the human brain's processing power to surpass most if not all other species [38]. Burgeoning connectivity has occurred at a molecular level, at a cellular level, as well

Neuroanatomy (hardware)

- All our cells 10^{13} (10 trillion)
- Neurons 10^{11} (100 billion)
- Glial cells 10^{12} (1 trillion)
- Synapses 10^{15} (1 quadrillion)
- Connectome 150 000 km of axons
- Blood vessels 700 km
- Microbiome 1.5 kg
- Microbes $2x10^{14}$ (200 trillion)

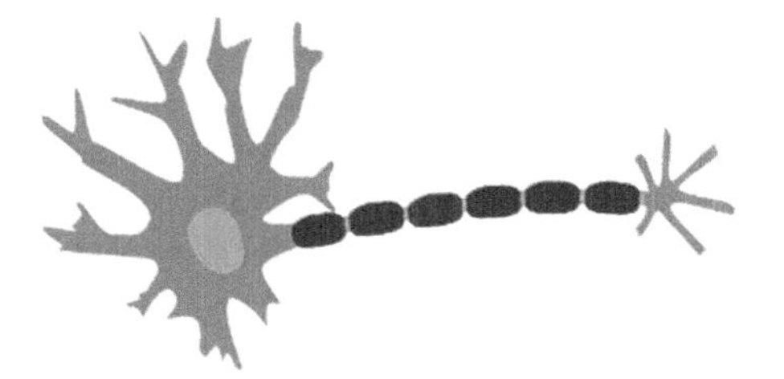

Neurophysiology (software)

- Human sensory systems receive ~ 11 million bits of information/sec
- Conscious mind processing ~16-50 bits per second
- Conscious activity ~ 5% of all cognition
- Non-conscious activity ~ 95% of processing

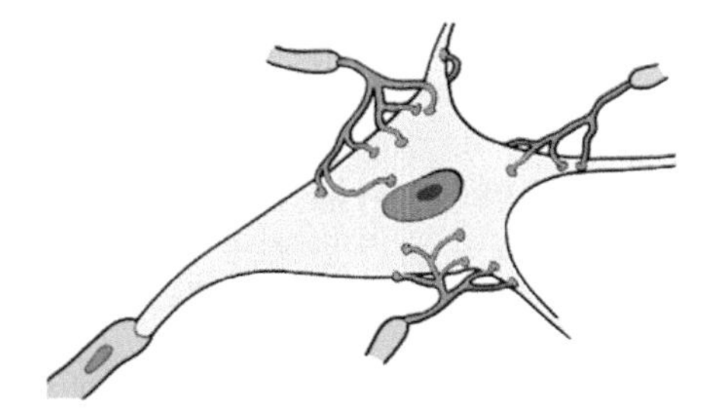

FIGURE 5.2 The pivotal role of NF-κB, which increases cytokines, adhesion molecules, chemokines and anti apoptotic factors.

as at a connectomal level. Glial cells are increasingly being implicated in almost all neurological disorders including, stroke, dementia, and migraine epilepsy through their ability to influence blood flow regulation, cell signalling, oxidative stress, inflammation, and apoptosis [39].

5.2.6 Higher processing-speed synapses evolved in humans

Information processing and storage in the human brain is dependent on pyramidal cell firing, synaptic transmission, and the plasticity of neuronal circuitry. Pyramidal cells make up approximately 70% of the cortical neurons and compared to rodent brains, human pyramidal cell information transfer is greater by a factor of four to ninefold, with frequencies measured in the beta and gamma range. Sensory synaptic features that process temporal data were also conveyed at higherprocessing-speed in humans compared to rodents. A human feature of 'fast recovering synapses' augments the information transfer during spike trains. Human pyramidal cells also have the capability of encoding higher quantities of synaptic. Together, these and probably other features have enabled human cerebral microcircuits to transmit information at overall higher processing-speeds in comparison to rodent micro-circuitry [40].

5.2.7 Epigenetics shape the human mind

In addition to genetic drivers, various epigenetic-based mechanisms shape the human mind. DNA differences between modern humans and Neanderthals, our closest extinct relative are miniscule, with our genome 99.8% the same. Our genome even differs very little from chimpanzees, our closest extant relative, only by about 1%. Epigenetic mechanisms, the switching of genes on and off, explain more of our differences. These epigenetic 'switches' affect gene regulation and behaviour and may be reversible. Epigenetics involves a change in gene expression without altering DNA sequences and may also be transgenerational, extending beyond a person's lifetime, being passed from parent to child [41]. Epigenetic mechanisms allow the interjection of additional sources of variation among biological systems in response to environmental influences. Epigenetic variation also occurs at a much higher rate than genomic changes, and is therefore more responsive to environmental factors, such as climate and nutrition [42]. The neurobiological mechanisms involved include DNA methylation, histone acetylation, and micro RNA interference [41].

5.2.8 Information acquisition: the ultimate purpose of the brain

The ultimate purpose of the brain is information acquisition and application as rapidly as possible in demanding environments or circumstances. It has been conjectured that we may be at both the physical and physiological limits of brain size and processing speed ability, with the fundamental impediments including basic physics laws and inter-neuronal communication capacity. Intellectual performance and functional brain network efficiency are correlated. Resting state connectivity (default mode network) and efficiency are predictive of cognitive potential [43]. Our overall intellectual performance is correlated with how efficiently our brains integrate and assimilate information from several different brain regions, which has important evolutionary- based consequences [44]. The more rapidly a specific type of environmental information can be processed as a function of time, the more likely is the chance of survival or success of a chosen course of action. This is also dependent on how rapidly information processing can occur with respect to consulting the repository's long-term memory stores, which may influence decision making with regards to a particular challenge.

5.2.9 Food and reward

Ultimately our neurophysiology allows us to have an inherent drive for knowledge acquisition, which is linked to our hedonic reward circuitry. A good example is reading, which is a widespread leisure activity and may be reflective of this drive within us [45]. Acquiring information may be through perusing novelty information, termed 'diversive curiosity', as seen, for example, in activities like surfing the web. However, when a specific focus exists, such that there is an integration of knowledge with that which is already present in the brain, this is termed epistemic knowledge. By involving/engaging more expansive brain circuitry, more information is trans-modally available [46,47]. The more knowledgeable and informed we are, pertaining to our environment, the more likely we are to make more favourable decisions.

Healthy living requires the intake of six major food components aided by six different taste senses. Intake of macronutrients (fats, proteins, carbohydrates), micronutrients (minerals, fat soluble and water-soluble vitamins) and water are guided by the currently known six different known taste senses, augmented by our sense of smell (olfaction). The different taste senses include salt, umami (savoury, amino acid detection), fat detection, sweet, bitter, and sour. The first four are linked to our hedonic dopaminergic system and underlie the concept of hyperpalatable foods with sugar, salt, fat excesses seen in many foods available today (particularly those termed ultra-processed food, UPF). Sour taste allows for detection of acids or spoiled foods and bitter helps discriminate potentially toxic substances from beneficial ones [48]. Highly processed (UPF) and high sugar foods impact the food/reward system of our brains because these are typically made hyperpalatable by the mixture of salty, sweet, and fatty components, which, in combination, are linked to our brain's hedonic reward systems.

5.2.10 The gut-brain connection

Dietary quantity, type, and food combinations can lead to improved memory, cognition, stave off dementia and cardiovascular disease, improve athletic prowess, have antidepressant effects, and diminish infections [49]. This is accomplished by an extensive anatomical and neurochemical communication network between our brain, the enteric (gastrointestinal) nervous system, and the microbiome; all are interdependent on each other [50]. The microbiome constitutes a complex system with approximately 200 trillion (2×10^{14}) organisms resident, and contributes to the psychobiome, or the microbial contribution to our brain's functioning, processing, and mental health [51].

Nowadays, we are confronted with a mass marketing of UPF, which generally are nutrient poor, calorie rich. This is widely considered an important factor in the approximately 700% increase in T2D, vascular disease, obesity, and a range of mental disorders. Microbiome analysis also points to a reduction in the beneficial versus harmful gut bacteria associated with such diets, termed dysbiosis. The biochemical consequences of dysbiosis include increased intestinal mucosal permeability, which in turn triggers an augmented immune response, cytokine production, and chronic neuroinflammation, a significant cause of mental illness [52].

5.2.11 Human brain evolution: shore vs land

The quality of food is most important. Docosahexaenoic acid (DHA) and eicosapentaenoic acid (EPA) are not only necessary but also critical for brain health. DHA has been conserved as the principal lipid molecular component of visual and neural signalling membranes from cephalopods to fish, amphibians, reptiles, birds, and all mammals [53]. The extreme conservation as well as the preservation of DHA for over 600 million years for neural signalling systems, despite multiple genomic changes over 600 million years insinuates that DHA is directed to DNA rather than the other way around [53]. It is possible that a shore-based environment may have been necessary for human brain development due to the provision of other vital brain-selective nutrients found in higher quantities in that habitat, in addition to DHA and EPA, namely iodine, iron, copper, selenium, and zinc. Brain selective nutrients co-occur with fat. Hence, a relatively high protein and lower fat diet would have been insufficient to sustain human brain evolution. All of these nutrients are richly sourced from shellfish, and other seafoods, eggs, meat, organ meats, and marrow. Approximately 1 kg of shellfish is required to obtain all five of these essential brain-specific nutrients, which may constitute the best overall dietary source of brain-specific nutrients. Eggs are virtually as good except for their lower relative copper content. Fish generally have optimal iodine and selenium concentrations but have relatively lower copper, zinc, and iron. Of the fish, cold water 'SMASH' (S – salmon, M – mackerel, A – anchovies, S – sardines, H – herring) fish have the highest DHA content. Hence, a combination of shellfish, fish, eggs, and meat comprises optimal nutrition to support adult brain health, maintain healthy infant body fat stores, and curtailing chronic diseases [54].

5.2.12 Summary/conclusion

The human brain is a very large and complicated organ with unfathomable levels of processing, neural connections, and structural integrity. As a consequence, the brain is the most metabolically sensitive and demanding organ in the body. Current research is elucidating the ever-expansive connections of the brain to the gut, and thus the importance of fuel types on its function and its development, particularly the well documented essentiality of DHA and EPA in both human evolution and modern neurological health, which are only adequately obtainable on a high-fat, animal-based diet. Diet has the capacity to prevent most modern neurological diseases and hence should be a major clinical consideration in the treatment, management, and/or prevention of mental illness, neuroinflammation, neurodegeneration, and beyond.

5.3 Cerebrovascular disease and stroke

Michael Hoffmann

5.3.1 Introduction

Stroke is the fifth leading cause of death and the leading cause of long-term disability in the United States [55,56]. Cerebrovascular diseases are particularly amenable to intervention, as most of the risk factors can be controlled, with 90% of strokes all being potentially treatable (Table 5.2).

The WHO has calculated that 80% of all cases of cardiovascular disease (CVD) and type 2 diabetes (T2D) and 40% of cancers can be prevented through the three pillars of healthy diet, physical activity and avoiding tobacco [59]. Possible stroke risk factors continue to be identified in epidemiological research, such as periodontal disease, vitamin D deficiency, air pollution, sleep apnoea and low fruit intake [57,58,60,61].

The original TOAST (The Trial of Org 10172 in Acute Stroke Treatment (TOAST)) classification of stroke causes has been expanded to be more inclusive of an increasing number of aetiologies, each with differing treatments (Table 5.3). Five subtypes of ischaemic stroke were defined, including, large-artery atherosclerosis, cardioembolism, small-vessel occlusion, stroke of other determined aetiology, and stroke of undetermined aetiology [62,63].

5.3.1.1 Clinical presentation and investigations

It is important to distinguish between stroke risk factors and stroke triggering events to ensure appropriate treatment. For example, alcohol binge drinking, infection, psychological stress, and cardiac dysrhythmias are triggering events, some of which cause platelet activation [64]. Any occurrence of a relatively sudden neurological deficit, especially in the setting of one or more stroke risk factors, should prompt immediate triage to an emergency room, preferably one attached to a primary or comprehensive stroke centre. With a typical infarct, as every minute passes, approximately 1.9 million neurons, 14 billion synapses, and 12 km (7.5 miles) of fibre tracts are destroyed [65].

Stroke presentation may be dramatic (hemiplegia or aphasia) or subtle, as in transient ischaemic attacks (TIA), with symptoms lasting usually less than 1 h. The risk of recurrent stroke after TIA can be objectivised by using the $ABCD^2$ score (A-age, B-blood pressure, C-clinical features such as unilateral weakness aphasia, D-duration, D-Diabetes). With

TABLE 5.2 Stroke risk factors and odds ratio in brackets [57,58].

1	Hypertension	(2.64)
2	Cardiac causes	(2.38)
3	Smoking current	(2.09)
4	Apolipoprotein B/A1	(1.89)
5	Waist to hip ratio	(1.65)
6	Alcohol intake	(1.51)
7	Diabetes mellitus	(1.36)
8	Diet risk score	(1.35)
9	Depression	(1.35)
10	Psychosocial stress	(1.30)
11	Sleep apnoea	(4.31)
12	Periodontal disease	(2.60)
13	Air pollution	(1.24)
14	Physical exercise	(0.69)
15	Mediterranean type diet	(0.65)
16	Vitamin D >440 IU/day	(0.70)

TABLE 5.3 Ischaemic stroke expanded aetiological TOAST classification (A) and cerebral haemorrhage causes (B).

A. Ischaemic stroke causes
- prothrombotic states
- dissection
- cerebral venous thrombosis
- vasculitis
- migraine related
- miscellaneous vasculopathy
- aortic arch atheroma
- vessel redundancy syndrome
- vertebrobasilar hypoplasia
- arterial fenestrations
- vessel dolichoectasia
- eclampsia
- Call Fleming syndrome
- fibromuscular dysplasia
- Moya Moya syndrome
- substance abuse related

B. Cerebral haemorrhage causes

More common causes of cerebral haemorrhage
- Hypertensive related ICH
- Amyloid haemorrhage
- Anticoagulation
- Illicit drugs
- Bleeding diatheses

Less common causes of cerebral haemorrhage
- Aneurysms
- Cerebral neoplasms
- Arteriovenous malformations
- Cavernous malformations
- Moya moya syndrome
- Vasculitis
- Post stroke arterial infarction
- Post stroke venous infarction/occlusion
- Post operative, carotid hyperperfusion syndrome
- Delayed post traumatic
- ICH due vasculopathies include
- Liver cirrhosis
- Cold exposure
- Low cholesterol (<160 mg/dL) in Japanese and Hawaiian men

more accurate Magnetic Resonance Imaging (MRI) imaging, so-called TIAs are increasingly being recognised as minor strokes, called sneak attacks or cerebral infarct with transient symptoms (CITS). Acute stroke is subject to potential treatment with clot-busting agents, tissue plasminogen activator (tPA), within the so-called golden first hour of stroke onset.

Sudden neurological events may not always signify a stroke. Both stroke mimics and stroke chameleons need to be considered (Table 5.4). Stroke chameleons are atypical stroke presentations that may be misinterpreted as due to conditions other than stroke [66].

5.3.1.2 *Acute stroke assessment*

Clinical scoring is performed by emergency personnel using the Cincinnati Prehospital scale (FAS) and clinical stroke severity by the National Institutes of Health (NIH) stroke scale (0–42) and outcome of treatments by the modified Rankin Disability scale (0–6). Neuroimaging evaluation with stat computerised tomography (CT) brain scanning and calculation of the ASPECTS score of the anterior circulation with a score of less than 7 predicting a worse functional outcome at three months and symptomatic haemorrhage. A modified ASPECTS score is also used when the posterior circulation is involved [67]. Diffusion weighted MRI and perfusion CT measurements define ischaemic brain tissue that

TABLE 5.4 Stroke mimic and stroke chameleons.

Stroke mimics
• Partial seizure, Todd's paresis
• Encephalitis/meningitis
• Subdural/epidural haematoma
• Brain tumour, metastasis
• Multiple sclerosis
• Plexus/root/peripheral nerve lesions
• Migraine
• Metabolic (hyper/hypoglycaemia)
• Fat embolism
• Re-emergent (unmasking) symptoms post stroke
Stroke chameleons - most common examples
• Acute confusional state
• Limb shaking TIA
• Alien hand syndrome
• Acute vestibular syndrome
• Acute monoparesis; cortical hand and cortical foot syndrome
• Isolated sensory symptoms
• Isolated dysarthria
• Cerebral venous thrombosis

is irreversibly damaged (core). Magnetic resonance angiography (MRA) or computed tomography angiography (CTA) are both emergent scans for the location of intracranial arterial occlusions.

5.3.2 Managing the patient

Stroke is an eminently treatable disorder from the perspective of primary or secondary prevention (see Chapter 4), as well as in the acute phase when it constitutes one of the most critical medical emergencies.

5.3.2.1 Treatment

5.3.2.1.1 Thrombolysis

If a haemorrhagic stroke has been excluded, thrombolysis with alteplase has been shown beneficial if administered within 4.5. h of stroke onset [68–70]. Mechanical thrombectomy may be considered in certain cases [71,72]. Antiplatelet agents (e.g., aspirin and clopidogrel) administered within 48 h of stroke onset decreases stroke recurrence [73,74].

5.3.2.1.2 Cerebral haemorrhage

Approximatetly 15% of strokes are haemorrhagic, of which two thirds constitute intracerebral haemorrhage (ICH) and one third subarachnoid haemorrhage (SAH). The leading causes of haemorrhagic stroke are hypertension and cerebral amyloid angiopathy (in which amyloid beta peptide deposits are not sufficiently cleared from in brain blood vessels) [75]. It is estimated that one third of haemorrhagic strokes could be avoided by effective treatment of hypertension [76]. See Section 3.1 and Chapter 4, for more information regarding the use of TCR to manage hypertension.

5.3.2.1.3 Surgical treatment

If cerebellar haemorrhages are larger than 3 cm in diameter or presence of brainstem compression or hydrocephalus is present, these subgroups do better with surgery [77].

5.3.2.2 Secondary prevention of stroke

Treating an individual's risk factors is paramount and addresses the underlying cause of stroke. Up to 90% of first strokes can be prevented with the appropriate risk factor amelioration [58]. In particular CVD risk factors, namely hypertension and atherosclerosis (see Chapter 4), and physical inactivity should be addressed [78].

As such, lifestyle therapy is imperative post discharge, and can be combined with the following therapies:

5.3.2.2.1 Antiplatelet therapy, single and dual indications

Current options include aspirin, clopidogrel, aspirin-dipyridamole, cilostazol, dipyridamole, ticagrelor. The aspirin–dipyridamole combination (Aggrenox) has been shown to be twice as effective as either ASA or clopidogrel alone in preventing recurrent stroke. Cilostazol causes less haemorrhage than ASA and is a safer choice for those subgroups at risk of haemorrhage such as CAA. Cilostazol also has an endothelial protective effect, mediating the blood–brain barrier and microvasculature protection via MMP9 and decreasing cerebral arterial pulsatility. Dipyridamole is a phosphodiesterase inhibitor with neuroprotective and anti-inflammatory effects and inhibitory effects on the proliferation of smooth muscle cells. Dipyridamole also induces the release of tissue plasminogen activator from brain microvascular endothelial cells [77,79].

5.3.2.2.2 Antihypertensive agents

Hypertension is the most prevalent risk factor for stroke. Those with less than 130 mmHg systolic blood pressure have 19% less risk (HR 0.81) of lacunar stroke than those with blood pressure of 130–140 mmHg [80]. The SPS3 study group reported a 63% reduction in the risk of haemorrhagic stroke in secondary prevention. First-line hypertension treatment is lifestyle and diet, as described in Section 3.1 and Chapter 4. Both ACE Inhibitors and angiotensin receptor blockers (ARBs) can be considered for the treatment of hypertension and for their stroke-protective effects [81].

5.3.2.2.3 Anticoagulation

With atrial fibrillation and other cardiac indications such as cardiomyopathy or cardiac failure, treatment with the newer oral anticoagulant agents (NOAC) is very effective [82]. The indication for anticoagulation is guided by the CHA_2DS_2VASc score and if anticoagulation is instituted, the bleeding risk may be calculated using the HAS-BLED score [83]. These can now all be reversed, if necessary, by Andexxa (coagulation factor Xa recombinant) for Apixaban, Rivaroxaban, Edoxaban and Idarucizumab (monoclonal antibody fragment) for Dabigatran reversal [84].

5.3.2.2.4 Lipid profile

Hyperlipidaemia is independently associated with lower severity of white matter hyperintensities or leukoaraiosis and hyperlipidaemia is also related to a lower intracerebral haemorrhage risk suggesting a protective role in small vessel disease [85]. Although statins have so-called pleiotropic stroke-protective properties, their use in stroke remains controversial [86]. Ezetimimibe or proprotein convertase subtilisin/kexin 9 inhibitors in selected patients also remain controversial [87]. The relationship between lipids and ischaemic stroke is complex where atherosclerotic subtypes carry the strongest association [88] which may be mediated by insulin resistance [89].

5.3.2.2.5 Glycaemic control

First line treatment should be lifestyle and dietary interventions (see Chapter 3.2). In patients with insulin resistance but not with diabetes mellitus, Rosiglitazone may be of benefit [90].

5.3.2.2.6 Surgery

Other surgical options are considered for all other aetiologies of stroke, for example, left atrial appendage closure, revascularization of the carotid arteries by endarterectomy and stenting, intracranial revascularisation, patent foramen oval (PFO) closure in cryptogenic stroke, aneurysm surgery, and arteriovenous malformation surgery.

5.3.2.3 Nutrition and physical exercise in stroke primary and secondary prevention

Evidence for atherosclerosis has been documented in Ancient Egyptian Mummies dating back to over 3000 years ago. In the Horus study, 34% of mummies had probable or definite atherosclerosis [91] (Fig. 5.3). A significant grain-based diet is regarded as causative and their reputation as Artophagoi, 'eaters of bread'.

Increased triglycerides, but not other lipid fractions were associated with MRI markers of small vessel disease in the brain [93]. C-reactive protein (CRP) is a stronger predictor of cardiovascular events than LDL cholesterol concentrations. The Mediterranean diet is associated with a 30% lower risk of major cardiovascular events (myocardial infarction, stroke, and death) in high-risk patients, compared to a low fat diet [94]. The cerebral white matter disease (leukoaraiosis) volume reduction associated with cognitive decline was also decreased by following this diet [95,96]. The pivotal

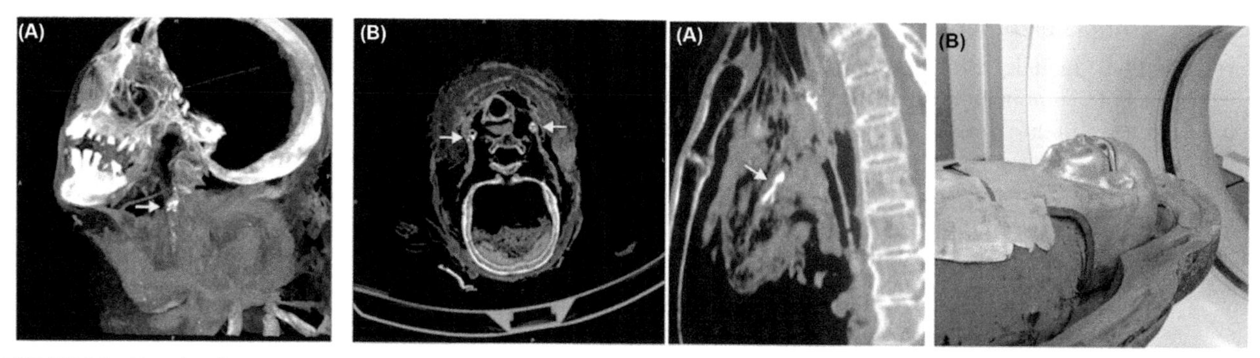

FIGURE 5.3 Egyptian diets and vascular disease. The A and B subfigures to the left depict carotid calcification, the right A subfigure depicts cardiac calcification, and the right B subfigure shows the methodological CT scanning of the mummies [92].

Finnish FINGER study demonstrated that multidomain intervention with physical exercise, cognitive stimulation, and high-fat, low-carbohydrate nutrition significantly curbs cognitive decline [97]. A groundswell of similar studies have followed suit in many countries including North America (POINTER study) [98], Singapore (SINGER study) [99], Australia (MYB study) [100], and China (MIND-CHINA) [101].

Ketogenic and similar diets have support from both animal and clinical studies in a wide range of neurological disorders including epilepsy, AD, migraine, motor neuron disease (MND), glioma, and stroke [102,103]. The pleiotropic mechanisms of the ketogenic diet (KD) are mediated by neurotransmitter and synaptic effects, antioxidant, and anti-inflammatory effects [103]. Clinical studies have already shown efficacy in some acute neurological disorders such as traumatic brain injury and animal studies of ischaemic stroke [102,103].

Overall, at least four-fifths of recurrent vascular events in patients with cerebrovascular disease might be prevented using a comprehensive, multifactorial approach [104]. Thirty-year data from the prospective Caerphilly study revealed major reductions in several important chronic diseases in middle aged men who followed four of five healthy living behaviours (vigorous exercise, healthy diet, normal body mass index, low alcohol use, and no smoking). These included a 50% reduction in diabetes, 50% in vascular disease, 60% in cognitive impairment, and dementia and 60% all-cause mortality [105]. Physical exercise was found to be the most important. Unsurprisingly, in 2016, the AHA Scientific Statement of 2016 recommended that cardiorespiratory fitness be measured and monitored as a vital sign [106].

5.4 Epilepsy

Meredith M. Kossoff and Eric H. Kossoff

5.4.1 Part 1: Epilepsy and where ketogenic diet (KD) therapy plays a role

5.4.1.1 Definition and epidemiology

A seizure is a convulsion or alteration in awareness caused by synchronous brain activity; however, experiencing one seizure does not necessarily indicate the presence of epilepsy. It is not uncommon to have a single seizure and then never have one again. A seizure can be symptomatic and can occur due to many factors including trauma, syncope, brain tumour, fever (in young children), alcohol use, Alzheimer disease, and metabolic derangement (e.g., hypoglycaemia or hyponatremia) [107]. After one seizure, the chances of experiencing a second episode are 50%, although abnormalities on an electroencephalogram (EEG) will increase the risk. After two seizures without a clear trigger, patients are then formally diagnosed with epilepsy, at times referred to as idiopathic [108]. At this point, the chances of having a third seizure rise to 70%, and treatment is often recommended. Epilepsy is currently defined as more than one seizure not due to a symptomatic cause (e.g., alcohol, fever, low blood glucose), or one seizure with an EEG strongly suggestive of an underlying epilepsy [108]. Approximately 1 in 26 Americans develops epilepsy, it affects 65,000,000 people in the world today, and epilepsy is particularly common in young children and the elderly (http://www.epilepsy.com.statistics).

5.4.1.2 *Clinical presentation*

Clinical presentation of epilepsy is variable as seizures can be focal or generalised, aware, or unaware [109]. Focal seizures begin in one area of one hemisphere or region of the brain while generalised seizures affect both hemispheres simultaneously, theorized to come from deep brain structures. Focal seizures can then spread throughout the brain, even becoming secondarily generalised seizures. In focal aware seizures, the patient can maintain awareness of their surroundings during a seizure [109].

In the majority of cases, people with epilepsy have focal unaware seizures, which typically last 30–60 s and then self-resolve. Contrary to the presentation of seizures in television and film, patients do not usually bite their tongues or require aggressive intervention during an event (other than being laid on their side). Afterwards the patient may have a headache or be tired, called a postictal period. Patients with epilepsy otherwise look normal in between events. Some patients have an aura or warning, but most do not, making epilepsy often frightening and unpredictable for patients trying to work, drive, and/or attend school. Mortality can occur from a prolonged seizure in patients with epilepsy. There is a risk of death during sleep called SUDEP (sudden unexpected death in epilepsy patients), which occurs in 1 in 1000 patients [110]. Some children outgrow their epilepsy in puberty with approximately 60% eventually achieving complete remission [111].

5.4.1.3 *Investigations*

Patients with epilepsy will generally first have an EEG performed to look at brain waves. EEGs are used to ascertain the source of seizures and determine if an epilepsy syndrome is present. Other tests include an MRI of the brain, basic laboratory studies, and occasionally genetic panels. There are dozens of epilepsy syndromes, with hundreds of genes identified as the cause of epilepsy, however in many cases, no aetiology is found, and these cases are referred to as idiopathic. Epilepsy is not caused by stress or nutritional imbalance in most cases, although these can be triggers for seizures in those with underlying epilepsy. Additionally, no two patients are alike. So, unlike with cancer, asthma, or diabetes, treatment is neither protocolized nor the same for every patient.

5.4.2 Managing the patient

There are four major treatment categories used for epilepsy: antiseizure drugs (ASDs), diet (ketogenic and others), neurostimulation (vagus or direct brain stimulation devices), and epilepsy surgery. Treatment is initiated when the seizures become frequent or epilepsy is officially diagnosed. Not all patients start or need treatment, and the decision to treat is made by the patient/parent in combination with their neurologist.

Nearly universally started first, ASDs are highly effective and there are over 20 on the market today [112]. Many have unique mechanisms of action that target excitability in the brain (or enhance inhibition) through channels or neurotransmitters. These drugs come in tablets, liquids, and intravenous preparations, and many are generic and affordable. Even medical marijuana, previously perceived as an alternative therapy, now has a drug version (cannabidiol) that was FDA approved in 2018. These drugs do not change the underlying epilepsy or lead to quicker resolution in those who may outgrow it. Rather, they act to raise the threshold for seizures to happen [113].

As mentioned previously, there is no universally-accepted protocol for treatment with ASDs. No medication is preferred; neurologists typically choose one medication, start low and increase the dose slowly as needed for seizure control. This is a highly successful strategy, with 70% of patients responding with seizure freedom to either the first or second medication chosen [114]. Side effects certainly exist for all ASDs and may include sedation, dizziness, weight change, rash, or haematologic or hepatic abnormalities. However, they tend to be manageable and if not, ASDs can be switched. Sometimes a patient's epilepsy will not respond to trials of multiple ASDs. After two drugs have failed to bring seizures under control, a patient is considered to have refractory epilepsy, a difficult to treat form of epilepsy that may require one of the other major epilepsy treatments [114].

Epilepsy surgery is considered when the following three conditions are met: several ASDs have failed, there is only one area of the brain where seizures are originating, and the area is safe to remove surgically [115]. If correct and successful, epilepsy surgery can be permanently curative. Neurostimulation is used mostly if two to three ASDs have failed and epilepsy surgery is not a viable option [115]. Devices are implanted and stimulate nerves (e.g., vagus or trigeminal) or even directly to the cortex or thalamus of the brain. Seizure freedom is rare, but side effects are minimal.

Finally, diet therapy is an option. It is utilised mostly in children but also increasingly in adults with epilepsy, typically when two to three drugs have been tried and failed. In Part 2 and the remainder of this chapter, we will focus on this helpful treatment.

5.4.3 Part 2: Ketogenic diets for epilepsy

5.4.3.1 History

The classic KD was first published in the medical literature as a treatment for epilepsy in 1921 by the Mayo Clinic as a high fat, low carbohydrate diet (LCD) initially theorized to mimic fasting and starvation, which had been described for centuries as helpful for seizure control [116]. The KD was traditionally initiated in the hospital following a 48-h fasting period. The KD remained popular for the following two decades but its use waned as new ASDs became more prevalent in the mid-twentieth century. By the 1980s, the KD was not widely used. Articles and chapters would refer to it as alternative and even nontraditional medicine, despite over 60 years of research. That changed dramatically in 1994 when media attention related to a young boy named Charlie Abrahams and the creation of the Charlie Foundation (http://www.charliefoundation.org) brought about a resurgence of the KD [117]. Now at just over 100 years after its initial description by the Mayo Clinic, the KD is a mainstream treatment for paediatric epilepsy, offered in approximately 75 countries, and the presence of a KD centre is one of the criteria judged for inclusion in the annual US News and World Report hospital rankings. The neurological community using diet therapy has recently formed a society entitled the International Neurologic Ketogenic Society (INKS) to continue to advocate for expanded use and organise biannual scientific conferences (http://www.neuroketo.org).

5.4.3.2 Mechanisms of action

Currently, there is evidence of multiple mechanisms of action of diet therapy in both humans and animal models. Research indicates that the KD impacts metabolism, and the mitochondria specifically, in a variety of complex manners [118]. Although for many years it was believed that ketone bodies directly worked as ASDs do, it is less clear today that ketones are the major factor involved in seizure control. Rather, they may represent evidence that the patient has made the metabolic shift to burn fat over carbohydrates, and serve as a method of assessing compliance, in a way similar to ASD blood concentrations [118]. Recent evidence in mice also suggests that alteration of the gut microbiota by the KD may play a role in seizure control by increasing bacteria that create gamma aminobutyric acid (GABA) [119]. Many pharmaceutical companies are very interested today in diet therapy as a pathway to a new class of ASDs, at times referred to as 'metabolism-based treatments'.

5.4.3.3 Versions of the ketogenic diet

In addition to the classic KD which uses long-chain triglycerides (LCT) as the primary fat source, there are four other major ketogenic diet therapies (KDTs): the medium-chain triglyceride (MCT) diet, the Modified Atkins Diet (MAD), the modified ketogenic diet (MKD), and the Low Glycemic Index Treatment (LGIT) [120]. Typical foods for these diets are similar and include high-fat foods such as oils, butter, bacon, eggs, heavy whipping cream, and mayonnaise while restricting carbohydrates. Studies have shown similar efficacy between these diets; details about their compositions are listed below.

5.4.3.3.1 The classic ketogenic diet

The classic KD is offered by most paediatric epilepsy centres and has been extensively researched for 100 years. It is a high-fat, low-carbohydrate diet in which 90% of calories are from fat, which is much higher than the 'keto diet' used for weight loss by many people today. The KD is implemented by maintaining a 4:1 ratio in which 4 g of fat are consumed for every 1 g of protein and carbohydrate. Sometimes a 3:1 ratio can be used, especially when the KD is used for infants [120]. Since it maintains a weight-based ratio, parents measure foods on a scale and follow dietitian-prescribed recipes. Although historically the KD involved calorie restriction to 80%–90% of the daily recommended intake, fluid restriction to 90%, and a universal 24–48 h fasting period, these practices were found to be largely unnecessary and are not currently the norm [120]. The classic KD is initiated in the hospital over a 2–3-day period, with the help of a neurologist and dietitian.

5.4.3.3.2 The MCT ketogenic diet

The traditional MCT diet was created in the 1970s and similar to the classic KD, it is usually started in the hospital [121]. However, the traditional MCT diet derives 60% of its calories from MCTs, which are often provided by MCT oil supplements. Further research has shown that 60% may be too high for some children, so patients often now consume 40%–50% of calories from MCTs [122]. The remaining percentage of calories comes from protein, carbohydrates, and fats that are naturally in foods. Advantages include higher percentages of carbohydrates and protein and possibly improved lipid profiles. It is used primarily in the UK and Canada today.

5.4.3.3.2.1 The modified Atkins diet In 2003, the MAD was created at Johns Hopkins Hospital. It is similar to the classic KD except instead of setting a 4:1 ratio, daily carbohydrate intake is monitored using food labels and usually restricted to 20 glycaemic (net) grams (of carbohydrate) per day [123]. Patients are instructed to increase their fat intake but no specific amounts of fat or protein are provided. The MAD simplifies meal planning since overall calories are not limited and exact calculations of a ratio or percentage are not needed [120]. Unlike the KD and MCT, the MAD is initiated in an outpatient setting, often in group teaching sessions. Studies have demonstrated that the MAD and KD have similar efficacy in children with refractory epilepsy (Kim et al., 2016) [124].

5.4.3.3.3 The low glycemic index treatment

The LGIT was developed in 2002 at Massachusetts General Hospital and like the MAD, it is initiated as outpatient. The LGIT is more flexible than the other three major KDs as it allows 40–60 g of carbohydrates per day. These carbohydrates are largely supposed to have low glycaemic indices of <50 [125]. Calories and fat amounts are loosely monitored. This diet has relatively fewer publications describing efficacy, but one recent comparison study suggested similar efficacy to the MAD and classic KD, but fewer side effects [124].

5.4.3.3.4 Modified ketogenic diet

There is a fifth, newest form of the KD entitled the MKD [126]. Created in the UK, the MKD uses a 1:1 ratio of carbohydrates to fat but is otherwise similar to the classic KD. Foods are weighed and measured, but fat and carbohydrate choice lists (ranging from 1 to 10 g/portion) are provided for meals in order to approximate 75% fat, 20% protein, and 5% carbohydrate daily.

The choice of diet therapy is a combination of neurologist and parent/patient choice, but in the case of infants and enterally fed patients, the KD can be provided in an all-liquid, formula-based diet as therefore the classic KD is chosen. When given as a liquid-based diet, the KD has high compliance rates and efficacy, making it an excellent option for these specific patients [127]. Adolescents and adults are universally started on either the MAD or LGIT due to their less restrictive nature [120,128].

5.4.3.4 Overall outcomes

Over the past century, there have been several randomised controlled trials and hundreds of prospective single- and multi-centre trials demonstrating efficacy [120]. There is no longer any debate in the medical community about whether the diet is effective. On average, approximately 50%–60% of those on any diet therapy will have a >50% seizure reduction within 2–3 months [120]. Diet therapy works quickly when it is effective; 75% of children have seizure reduction within 14 days, but experts agree that treatment should continue for about 3 months on average in order to determine if the KDT is effective [129]. If the KDT is working, it is generally continued for 2 years before stopping (in children). Children, even those with refractory epilepsy, may outgrow their epilepsy and thus do not require lifelong therapy, KDT or otherwise.

5.4.3.5 Indications for use

Some types of epilepsy have a >50% chance of 50% reduction in seizures (Table 5.5), and these patients are considered to be ideal candidates. For patients with Glut1 deficiency syndrome (GLUT1DS) and pyruvate dehydrogenase deficiency (PDHD), the KD is the treatment of choice [120] and for infantile spasms, it has been reported as beneficial as a first-line therapy [130]. For other forms of epilepsy, diet therapy is generally considered after two medications have failed. This is due to the lack of any other data suggesting the superiority (or even equivalency) of KDT as a first-line therapy.

Certain contraindications must be ruled out before beginning diet therapy (Table 5.6). Since KDTs make lipids the primary energy source, absolute contraindications are those disorders that prevent the normal metabolism of fats [120].

TABLE 5.5 Epilepsy syndromes and conditions (listed alphabetically) in which KD has been consistently reported as more beneficial (>70%) than the average 50% KD response (defined as >50% seizure reduction).

Angelman syndrome
Complex 1 mitochondrial disorders
Dravet syndrome
Epilepsy with myoclonic-atonic seizures (Doose syndrome)
Febrile infection-related epilepsy syndrome (FIRES)
Formula-fed (solely) children or infants
Glucose transporter protein 1 (Glut-1) deficiency syndrome (Glut1DS)
Infantile spasms
Ohtahara syndrome
Pyruvate dehydrogenase deficiency (PDHD)
Super-refractory status epilepticus
Tuberous sclerosis complex

TABLE 5.6 Contraindications to the use of KDT.

Absolute
Carnitine deficiency (primary)
Carnitine palmitoyltransferase (CPT) I or II deficiency
Carnitine translocase deficiency
β-oxidation defects
Pyruvate carboxylase deficiency
Porphyria
Relative
Inability to maintain adequate nutrition
Surgical focus identified by neuroimaging and video-EEG monitoring
Parent or caregiver noncompliance
Propofol concurrent use (risk of propofol infusion syndrome may be higher)

Laboratory tests (e.g., comprehensive metabolic profile, urine organic acids, plasma amino acids, and genetic testing) are usually obtained for a patient with epilepsy due to an unknown cause before starting any diet therapy to rule out any contraindication.

5.4.3.6 *Adverse effects*

Some adverse effects of diet therapy as used for epilepsy do exist and include constipation, weight loss, growth slowing, kidney stones, hypercholesterolaemia, bone density changes, cardiac abnormalities (prolonged QT syndrome), and pancreatitis [120,131]. Possible side effects are carefully monitored during the course of treatment and can often be prevented with supplements such as standard multivitamins, calcium, Vitamin D, laxatives, salt, and oral citrates (e.g., sodium or potassium citrates). They rarely lead to KD discontinuation; the primary reason for stopping diet therapy is a lack of sufficient seizure control.

5.4.3.7 *Discontinuation*

Diet therapy is typically discontinued if there is no seizure reduction after 3 months of treatment. When the KDT is effectively decreasing seizures in children, it is maintained for 2 years and then gradually discontinued, as many cases of even refractory paediatric epilepsy can be outgrown and no longer require treatment. However, sometimes families and many adults choose to continue the KDT for more than 2 years if they are experiencing nearly complete seizure reduction and no adverse effects [120]. There is no upper limit to KDT and the time period to continue KDT is often a mutual decision between patients and the neurologist. When a decision is made to discontinue KDT, it is usually weaned over 3–4 weeks with careful monitoring [132].

5.5 Alzheimer's disease

A. Berger, G. Ede

5.5.1 Introduction

Worldwide, approximately 35 million people are living with AD [133] and this number is expected to more than double by 2050 [134]. Despite more than 200 clinical trials conducted over nearly three decades and costing billions of dollars, not a single medicine has yet emerged that can provide meaningful relief of symptoms, let alone alter the course of the illness [135].

Fortunately, multiple lines of robust scientific evidence conducted over the past twenty years or so now point compellingly to insulin resistance as a key driving force behind most cases of late-onset AD. The growing understanding that AD is largely the result of long-term systemic metabolic dysfunction opens up promising new avenues for intervention and potential prevention.

5.5.1.1 Clinical presentation

In acknowledgement of the fact that AD develops silently over decades, diagnostic criteria were revised in 2011 to include a symptom-free preclinical stage detectable only with brain imaging or lumbar puncture, a phase marked by subtle symptoms called mild cognitive impairment (MCI) which may or may not progress to Alzheimer's dementia, and Alzheimer's dementia itself, characterised by memory, language, and orientation difficulties that interfere with independent function [136].

5.5.1.2 Investigations

As there is no reliable test for AD, the diagnosis is essentially a clinical one, and much of the evaluation is geared towards ruling out other oetiologies. A thorough investigation consists of a complete history and physical examination, medication review, laboratory and brain imaging studies, third-party interviews of close contacts, and cognitive measures ranging from simple office-based assessments to formal neuropsychological testing. Diagnostic certainty is only possible after death using neuropathological techniques [137].

5.5.2 Pathophysiology

5.5.2.1 Alzheimer's disease as type 3 diabetes

Brown University neuroscientist Dr. Suzanne de la Monte [138], a leading researcher in the field, has called AD 'a brain form of diabetes' owing to the significant overlap between the biochemical and physiological abnormalities in T2D and AD. The phrases type 3 diabetes (T3D) and 'brain insulin resistance' are now regularly used to describe AD [139,140]. An important pathological feature of AD is reduced brain uptake and metabolism of glucose, resulting in a neuronal fuel shortage. This 'chronic starvation' due to brain glucose hypometabolism may contribute to the neurodegenerative changes and functional decline observed in AD [141].

At just 2% of body weight, the brain demands approximately 20% of the body's glucose. Therefore, a reduction in fuel metabolism can prove catastrophic for brain cell function, particularly for neurons involved in memory and cognition, which are the first to suffer when energy availability is compromised [142].

In individuals who eventually develop AD, baseline cerebral glucose utilisation declines more quickly than in those who remain cognitively healthy [143]. This eventually results in up to a 45% reduction in glucose metabolism, a phenomenon described as 'the predominant abnormality' in late-onset AD [144].

This steady decline in glucose utilisation likely represents the earliest detectable harbinger of future AD, preceding symptoms and brain atrophy by years and possibly even decades [145–147]. Indeed, evidence of sluggish brain glucose metabolism has been detected in genetically susceptible, cognitively normal individuals in their 20s and 30s [148].

5.5.2.2 The role of chronic hyperinsulinemia

While it is well established that chronically elevated blood glucose increases the risk for memory problems and dementia [149,150], chronically elevated insulin, even in the context of normal blood glucose concentrations, has emerged as a strong independent risk factor for cognitive decline. One study determined that the risk for AD nearly doubled in subjects with hyperinsulinemia, even in the absence of T2D [151]. Hyperinsulinemia 'is usually at or near the top of the list of known lifestyle-related factors heightening the risk of declining cognition in the elderly' [141].

Insulin crosses the blood-brain barrier via a saturable transporter, the actions of which are altered by hyperglycaemia, and resistance to insulin action in the CNS is associated with peripheral insulin resistance, as abnormal systemic insulin metabolism impairs cerebral insulin transport and function [152,153]. Paradoxically, while many AD patients have high insulin concentrations in the blood, they have lower concentrations of insulin in the brain and central nervous system compared to age-matched controls, possibly resulting from downregulation of insulin receptors at the blood-brain barrier in response to overexposure to insulin [154,155]. This cerebral insulin deficit is particularly problematic for regions of the brain key to learning and memory, such as the hippocampus, which depends on robust insulin supply and is therefore especially rich in insulin receptors [156].

5.5.2.3 Reconciling conflicting theories of the origin of Alzheimer's disease

It is becoming clear that conventional theories about dementia development and pharmaceutical research have largely focused on the anatomical consequences of the disease process rather than its root causes. An excellent example of this is the amyloid hypothesis.

5.5.2.3.1 The amyloid hypothesis

Decades of research have focused on amyloid as the key driving force behind AD, yet the amyloid hypothesis is not supported by the majority of experimental evidence [157]. Many inconsistencies surround the amyloid hypothesis [158], including the fact that a substantial number of individuals with AD are free of significant plaque buildup while many without AD have a substantial plaque burden [157].

Rather than being a cause of neuronal injury, amyloid beta (Aβ) is secreted in response to neuronal injury to help defend the brain against oxidative stress and may even play a role in promoting neurite outgrowth and tissue regeneration [159]. This may explain not only the repeated failure of anti-amyloid therapies to favourably impact disease progression [160], but also the accelerated deterioration of patients in one Phase III anti-amyloid drug trial, forcing its early discontinuation [161].

In fact, it is impaired clearance, not overproduction, which leads to Aβ accumulation; Aβ clearance rate may be as much as 30% lower in AD patients compared to cognitively normal individuals [162]. One possible explanation for this is lower concentrations of an enzyme that helps to clear Aβ from the brain: insulin-degrading enzyme (IDE), which, as its name implies, is also responsible for breaking down insulin molecules. In APOE ε4 + AD patients, brain IDE expression is greatly reduced. Since the production of IDE is stimulated by insulin itself, in a low-insulin environment such as the AD brain, reduced availability of IDE would make it easier for amyloid to accumulate and clump into plaques [163].

In addition to setting the stage for excess amyloid accumulation, cerebral insulin deficiency also directly contributes to many other abnormalities seen in the Alzheimer's brain, including:

- *Neurofibrillary tangles.* Insulin prevents the clumping of individual tau molecules into toxic tangles that can disrupt cell architecture and lead to cell death [164].
- *Cholinergic cell dysfunction.* Insulin supports the synthesis of acetylcholine, a neurotransmitter central to learning and memory [165,166]. AD medications such as donepezil attempt to support dwindling acetylcholine activity [167].
- *Glutamate dysregulation.* Insulin resistance interferes with healthy glutamate metabolism and function. The AD drug memantine targets glutamate imbalances [168].

5.5.2.3.2 The ApoE4 'Alzheimer's susceptibility gene'

ApoE4 is often called the Alzheimer's 'susceptibility gene' [148] because in some populations, carriers of this gene have up to a fivefold increased risk of developing AD compared to non-carriers, with the risk appearing dose-dependent: homozygotes have a greater risk compared to heterozygotes [169]. Despite this seemingly predictive genetic heritage, the ApoE4 allele is neither required nor sufficient for the development of AD, as 50% of people with AD are not carriers, and some E4 homozygotes never develop the disease [170]. It may be that the ApoE4 genotype is not inherently damaging, but may only be deleterious in the context of the modern industrialised diet, as E4 may be mismatched to an evolutionarily novel preponderance of refined carbohydrates and seed oils [171]. It is critical to note, however, that hyperinsulinemia elevates risk for AD independently of ApoE status [171].

5.5.3 Managing the patient

5.5.3.1 Pharmacotherapy

Pharmacologic treatments for AD are limited to prescription medications of three types: cholinesterase inhibitors such as donepezil, memantine (a glutamate regulator), and the new anti-amyloid agent aducanumab.

5.5.3.2 Lifestyle related considerations

Nonpharmacologic approaches to the management of AD include blood pressure management, cognitive training, and lifestyle changes such as physical exercise and dietary strategies (most commonly the Mediterranean–DASH intervention for neurodegenerative delay [MIND] diet, which has yet to be tested in interventional studies) [172].

5.5.3.3 Diet: ketogenic therapies for cognitive dysfunction

Research regarding ketogenic interventions for AD and mild cognitive impairment (MCI) is admittedly in its infancy. Studies typically use small sample sizes and subjects with early or mild disease, but findings are promising. A 2020 systematic review of ketogenic therapies for AD and MCI, which included ten randomised controlled trials that employed either a KD or various MCT preparations, concluded that while this research is in its early stages and is highly heterogeneous, ketogenic interventions are promising for improving acute and long-term cognition [173]. The most rigorous study to date was a six-week randomised crossover trial of 21 patients with mild AD in which a KD was compared to a low-fat diet. When following a KD that produced average beta-hydroxybutyrate (BHB) blood concentrations of 0.95 mmol/L, subjects scored higher on measures of quality of life and activities of daily living, but they did not score higher on cognitive tests [174].

The primary goal of ketogenic interventions is to deliver energy to neurons that can no longer metabolise glucose properly. Although cells in the Alzheimer's brain do not take up or metabolise glucose effectively, it's been shown that brain ketone uptake and metabolism remain just as robust in those with MCI and early AD as in cognitively healthy older subjects [175]. The brain energy deficit in MCI and AD is specific to glucose, so elevating serum ketone concentrations generally results in acute cognitive improvements [147].

Under typical dietary circumstances, in which carbohydrates comprise a significant percentage of calories, the brain requires approximately 120 g of glucose per day. However, in a ketogenic state, some of this energy can be supplied by ketones, helping to close the fuel gap faced by the low-insulin Alzheimer's brain.

Outside of pathological ketoacidosis, ketones are typically only produced endogenously under conditions of either fasting or carbohydrate restriction. Under conditions of fasting, a serum BHB concentration of 0.3–0.5 mmol/L can provide 3%–5% of the brain's energy, 1.5 mmol/L (8.7 mg/dL) can provide up to 18% of the brain's energy, and a concentration of 5 mmol/L (29.04 mg/dL) can provide as much as 60% of the brain's energy [142]. The latter concentration would be difficult to achieve through diet alone, but a range of 1.0–3.0 mmol/L (5.8–17.4 mg/dL) is not uncommon in those following strict KDs.

Non-dietary methods may also be used to increase serum ketone concentration. Most of the research studies regarding ketogenic therapies for AD and MCI have employed exogenous ketones in the form of βOHB salts or esters, or medium-chain triglyceride (MCT) formulas, as MCTs are more readily converted into ketones than other types of fatty acids. MCTs offer potential benefit to the MCI or AD patient because they are metabolised to ketones even in the fed state and when dietary carbohydrate is not reduced.

5.5.3.3.1 Medium-chain triglyceride formulas

MCT preparations have shown promise in the limited research conducted to date, although it should be noted that non-E4 carriers appear to respond more favourably compared to E4 + individuals [176]. Chronic administration of doses of various MCT formulations providing up to 20 g/day of MCT has been shown to improve memory and processing speed in subjects with mild-to-moderate AD [177], improve cognition as assessed by the AD Assessment Scale-Cognitive Subscale (ADAS-Cog) in non-E4 carriers with mild-to-moderate AD [178], and increase total brain energy metabolism (in direct proportion to the plasma ketone concentration achieved) in subjects with mild-to-moderate AD [179]. Among subjects with MCI, a dose of 30 g/day of an MCT formula taken for six months was shown to improve several measures of cognition. Brain ketone metabolism was increased by 230% while brain glucose uptake was unchanged [180].

Owing to gastrointestinal upset that may be induced by high doses of MCTs, it may be difficult to administer MCT formulas in high enough concentrations to result in truly substantial improvements in cognition. βOHB esters typically induce a much larger rise in serum ketones, which could potentially have a greater impact on cognition. Research is very limited, but one case report documents remarkable improvements in cognition and quality of life in a sexagenarian male ApoE4 carrier in whom the ketone ester elevated serum βOHB to as much as 3–7 mmol/L (17.4–40 mg/dL) depending on the dose [181].

5.5.3.3.2 Ketogenic diets

An important limitation to exogenous ketogenic therapies is that they raise ketone concentrations without lowering blood glucose and insulin concentrations, and therefore do not address the underlying metabolic dysfunction that may continue to drive the disease process forward.

KDs, which are typically very low in carbohydrate, moderate in protein, and higher in fat than standard diets, not only facilitate endogenous ketone synthesis to support brain metabolism, but also reduce blood glucose and insulin concentrations, directly addressing these important likely root causes of neurodegeneration.

At the time of this writing, research using KDs in patients with MCI or AD is limited to small, uncontrolled clinical trials and several case reports. Two six-week studies of subjects with MCI [182] showed that dietary carbohydrate restriction resulted in small but statistically significant improvements on long-term memory tests and other cognitive tests (the latter also included MCT oil supplementation).

Case Studies

Limited but intriguing case reports have documented significant metabolic, cognitive, and quality of life improvements when low-carbohydrate diets were used in conjunction with other lifestyle interventions:

- A 68 year old male, heterozygous for ApoE4, with mild AD and diagnosed with T2D, followed a KD (with an 8-h time-restricted eating window), plus moderate intensity exercise for ten weeks [183]. The following improvements were observed:
  - Montreal Cognitive Assessment (MoCA) score: 23/30 to 29/30 (mild AD to normal)
  - Fasting blood glucose: 7.2 mmol/L to 5.4 mmol/L (129 mg/dL to 98 mg/dL) (−24%)
  - Fasting insulin: 97.2 mIU/L to 14.3 mIU/L (675 pmol/L to 99.31 pmol/L) (−85.3%)
  - HOMA-IR: 31.0 to 3.5 (−88%)
  - Haemoglobin A1c: 7.8% to 5.5% (−29.5%; diabetic to normal)
  - HDL-C: 0.72 mmol/L to 0.98 mmol/L (28 mg/dL to 38 mg/dL) (+35.7%)
  - Triglycerides: 1.55 mmol/L to 0.92 mmol/L (137 mg/dL to 83 mg/dL) (−39.4%)
- A 38-year-old male ApoE4 carrier with metabolic syndrome (MetS) and self-reported memory problems followed a KD plus intense exercise for 10 weeks [184]. The following improvements were documented:
  - MoCA score: 22/30 to 30/30 (MCI to normal)
  - Fasting insulin: 15.6 mUI/L to 7.1 mUI/L (108.33 pmol/L to 49.31 pmol/L) (−54%)
  - HOMA-IR: 4.3 to 1.8 (-58%)
  - Triglycerides: 6.47 mmol/L to 1.89 mmol/L (573 mg/dL to 167 mg/dL) (−71%)
  - Triglyceride-to-HDL-C ratio: 14.7 to 3.4 (−77%)
- A 57-year-old female with MCI and MetS followed a KD plus high-intensity exercise and use of an electronic memory training app for 12 weeks with the following results [185]:
  - MoCA score: 22/30 to 30/30 (MCI to normal)
  - HDL-C: 26% increase
  - Triglycerides: 56% decrease

  The below case comes from the practice of Deborah Gordon, MD, founder of the Northwest Memory and Wellness Center in Ashland, Oregon, US, which specialises in healthy ageing.

I first saw Harriet in 2018. She cheerily said she noticed no memory problems; her sister had urged her to come in and accompanied her to the appointment. Their paternal grandparents had been diagnosed with dementia at a late age, but the 'A' word was never used.

(Continued)

(Continued)

Harriet was involved in her community, liked to walk with friends, slept well, and read books for mental stimulation. She had a preference for sweet, grain-rich breakfasts and tended to snack constantly throughout her day. She had quit smoking cigarettes in 2016 and drank a glass or two of wine about twice a week. She was taking vitamin C, vitamin E, probiotics, and fish oil; her only medication was atorvastatin, prescribed by a physician who had told her to throw out her egg yolks. At 5'5" (165 cm) tall, she was overweight at 152 pounds (69 kg), with a waist circumference of 38 inches (96 cm). Her medical history was notable for GERD (gastroesophageal reflux disease) and osteopenia.

Initial metrics of note:

- MoCA score 18/30
- Haemoglobin A1C 5.5%, fasting insulin 7.1 mIU/L (49.31 pmol/L), hsCRP 1.35 mg/L.
- ApoE status: ApoE3/4
- MRI: 25th percentile for brain volume with marked asymmetry

At her initial visit, we increased her dosage of fish oil, added a multivitamin, ashwagandha, gotu kola, pyrroloquinoline quinone (PQQ), pregnenolone, resveratrol, zinc, alpha-lipoic acid, berberine, cinnamon, and a mixed-nutrient brain supplement containing acetyl-l-carnitine. We prescribed oestradiol, progesterone, and testosterone for documented hormone deficiencies. She wanted to continue the statin, as her PCP had recommended it, so we changed the atorvastatin to rosuvastatin, as it is less likely to cross the blood-brain barrier.

We counselled Harriet on the 'KetoFlex' diet as described by Dr. Dale Bredesen. Rather than specific macronutrient targets, we suggested she fill 2/3 to 3/4 of every plate with non-starchy vegetables and the rest with whole eggs, wild-caught fish, and/or pasture-raised meat/poultry. 'Forbidden foods' included sweets, breads, granola, bananas, and tropical fruits, and alcohol was limited to half a glass once or twice a week.

With her highly motivated sister in the role of chef, Harriet has been compliant with the dietary changes and supplements, with home ketone concentrations ranging between 0.7 and 1.4 mmol/L (4.1 mg/dL to 8.1 mg/dL).

By month 12, her MoCA score had improved to 24/30, and at 24 months, it remains stable at 24/30. Now 73 years old, she has lost 4 inches around her waist and is free of GERD symptoms. Her fasting insulin has decreased to 5.3 mIU/L.

I've learned from Harriet that the 'A' word just sets her back, as it's inextricably linked to serious decline. Instead, we talk generally about the memory issues she has had, as we compliment her for her brain's improvement and her increasing taste for eggs, meat, and vegetables!

5.5.3.3.3 Implementing ketogenic diets in patients with cognitive disorders

The case examples help illustrate several clinical principles important to bear in mind when using dietary interventions in the treatment of people with cognitive disorders:

1. Poor insight into the diagnosis of AD is common and can interfere with thorough assessment, therapeutic alliance, and treatment planning. Shifting the focus of the conversation to metabolic health is often a more welcome and productive strategy.
2. Dietary interventions in those with cognitive impairment often require dedicated caregiver support for proper implementation.
3. While maintaining at least moderate ketosis may be more beneficial, KDs need not involve complicated macronutrient ratios, special foods, carbohydrate counting, or ketone monitoring to be helpful.
4. For those unable or unwilling to make dietary changes, exogenous ketogenic therapies may improve cognition and quality of life despite not altering the course of the disease.
5. Given that AD is a serious neurodegenerative disease with no known cure, patients, families, clinicians, and even researchers rarely feel comfortable employing the KD as a sole therapy, opting instead to implement a variety of lifestyle interventions and supplements in hopes of optimising outcomes. This makes it impossible to determine the proportional contribution of each element and understand which elements of treatment may be most responsible for improvements. It seems reasonable, however, to propose that anything that improves insulin sensitivity, whether from MetS or T2D (dietary changes, lifestyle changes, or a combination of these) has the potential to benefit cognition.

5.5.3.4 Conclusion: a new way forward

Given the dismal track record of other approaches, it is noteworthy that any improvement in cognition at all has been observed among subjects with MCI or AD, and that it has been observed in association with elevation of serum ketones. Researchers note, 'A core element of this interpretation is that brain cells and/or networks that were previously dysfunctional can start to function more normally again once they are provided with more fuel, i.e., they were starving or exhausting but not dead; otherwise this cognitive improvement would not be possible' [147].

By the time the diagnosis of AD is made, the process of neurodegeneration is already well underway, so we propose that ketogenic therapies be implemented as early in the disease course as possible. Since most of the research has been conducted with subjects with MCI or mild-to-moderate AD, it is unknown whether individuals with more advanced disease might also improve with ketogenic therapies. There may be a point of no return after which the damage is so severe and widespread that the potential for improvement in those with advanced disease is unknown [186].

The current pharmaceutical treatment paradigm for AD is of minimal clinical value and does not address metabolic aberrations that appear to contribute directly to disease pathology.

Unlike age, genetics, and family history, insulin resistance is a powerful risk factor for AD that clinicians and patients can actually do something about, making ketogenic interventions uniquely empowering therapeutic strategies. Ketogenic interventions, including exogenous ketones and MCT preparations, but particularly the KD, have the potential to restore some degree of cognitive function and improve overall health, thereby enhancing not only the patient's quality of life but also that of their loved ones and caregivers.

5.6 The ketogenic diet in mood disorders

Ann M. Childers

5.6.1 Introduction

The field of nutritional psychiatry is in its nascent era. While some psychiatrists declare a special interest in nutritional psychiatry, the definition of nutritional psychiatry is unstandardised, and opinions diverge as to which nutritional approach is optimal for treating patients with mental illness. Most studies on the effects of nutrition and diet can be problematic and controversial. What little research has been conducted is promising, but sample sizes tend to be small and study time frames short. This section provides an overview of the KD as it pertains to mood disorders, major depressive disorder, and bipolar spectrum disorders in particular.

The most common mood disorders encountered by mental health practitioners are divided into five types: major depression, persistent depressive disorder (dysthymia), bipolar disorder, mood disorder due to a general medical condition, and substance-induced mood disorder. Despite the criteria set by the DSM-5 to define each category and subcategory of diagnosis, there is still little evidence that each category has a natural boundary. Further complicating matters is that physical and psychiatric comorbidities are the rule rather than the exception, so while psychiatric diagnostic categories and criteria appear distinct at first glance, nothing could be further from the truth. The vast majority of patients with depression, for example, have anxiety as well, andhaving metabolic conditions such as insulin resistance doubles the odds of having depression [187,188].

5.6.1.1 Depression

Depression is a mood disorder that causes a persistent feeling of sadness and loss of interest. Features common to all depressive disorders are sadness, emptiness, or irritable mood, accompanied by somatic and cognitive changes significantly impacting the individual's capacity to function [189]. Biological and environmental factors can promote depression. There are genetic components to depression that impact some families, or depression may occur de novo [190]. Conditions that increase with age, such as diabetes and dementia, are often preceded by, or accompanied by depression. In addition, anxiety is recognised as a common cause of, and/or comorbidity with, depression. In the US, a national survey of adults found 10.4% had a one-year prevalence of moderate to severe depression (associated with comorbidity and impairment), and this increased to a lifetime prevalence of 20.6%. A national survey of 36,309 US adults found the 12-month and lifetime prevalences of major depressive disorder were 10.4% and 20.6%, respectively, with most being of moderate or severe intensity, and associated with comorbidity and impairment [191]. Major depressive disorders (MDD) impose a significant economic burden as well. In 2021 Greenberg, et al. reported that, between 2005 and 2010, the incremental economic burden of major depressive disorders (MDDs) in the United States increased by 21.5%, from $173.2 billion to $210.5 billion inflation-related dollars, with direct medical costs accounting for 47% of dollars spent

[192]. Depressive disorders can be life threatening. A Danish longitudinal study of 176,347 persons found that in men, the absolute risk of suicide in men with unipolar depression was second only to the absolute risk of suicide from bipolar disorder [193].

5.6.1.2 Bipolar disorder

Bipolar disorder is a chronic, usually lifelong illness characterised by recurrent manic, hypomanic, mixed, and depressive episodes, with the most common phase being depression. Bipolar 1 disorder has the highest genetic linkage of all psychiatric disorders with heritability estimated at 85% (19% concordance in dizygotic twins and 67% in monozygotic twins) [194]. Lifetime prevalence for bipolar disorder ranges from 1% for bipolar I to 3.5% for bipolar II disorder and subthreshold or soft-spectrum bipolar disorder [195]. The economic burden of bipolar I and II disorders is substantial. Based on 56 studies included in their 2020 systematic review of US economic impacts of Bipolar 1 and Bipolar II disorders, Bessonova et al. [196] estimated the total annual national economic burden was more than $195 billion in 2018 US dollars, with approximately 25% attributed to direct medical costs [196]. Bipolar disorder is a life-threatening condition, with suicide death rates among patients estimated to be 20–30 times higher than the corresponding rate in the general population [197]. Existing research worldwide shows 20%–60% of persons with bipolar disorder attempt suicide at least once in their lifetime, with up to 20% (many untreated) ending life by suicide [198].

5.6.2 Pathophysiology

For patients with mood disorders, no laboratory results or imaging study currently establishes a psychiatric diagnosis [199]. Charlton [200] postulates that malaise, with sickness behaviour, similar to that observed in animals, is at the core of depression. This model presents depression as a physical illness [200]. Indeed, appetite disturbance may lead to observable increases or decreases in weight, and psychiatric patients may present with measurable biomarkers of physical illness proposed to be mediated by cytokines [200]. Mental illnesses, including depression and bipolar disorder, share a number of metabolic features in common with other neurological disorders. Norwitz et al. [201] propose four categories: inflammation, glucose hypometabolism, neurotransmitter imbalances, and oxidative stress, and that these metabolic states can be modified by a KD [201].

5.6.2.1 Inflammation

Inflammation is not only a common feature of physical illness, but is evident in mental illness as well. As many as 30% of depressed patients are unresponsive to standard treatments, and they have been shown to demonstrate significantly elevated cytokines [202]. Inflammatory cytokines could play a significant role in depression [202,203]. Depression is a side effect of the cytokine treatment interferon-alpha in 30%–50% of patients receiving it [202,203].

In their review and meta-analysis of 69 studies, Enache et al. [204] found significant elevations in pro-inflammatory Interleukin-6 and tumour necrosis factor-alpha in both cerebrospinal fluid and the brains of individuals known to suffer from depression, suggesting a physical contribution to depression in the individuals studied. While it is more difficult to determine inflammation in a live brain, microglia activation, measured with positron emission tomography (PET), indicates that brain inflammation is present in the brains of individuals with depression and bipolar disorder [204]. Microglial brain cells exhibit pro-inflammatory and anti-inflammatory (neuroprotective) states.

5.6.2.2 Glucose hypometabolism

Functional brain imaging studies demonstrate abnormalities in regional cerebral glucose metabolism in the prefrontal cortex in patients with mood disorders, depression, and bipolar disorder [205]. Other brain regions appear to be involved as well. While, in some areas glucose is taken up by brain tissue at a higher rate, in most affected areas glucose uptake is reduced.

5.6.2.3 Neurotransmitter imbalances: glutamate and gamma amino butyric acid

In patients with major depressive disorder or bipolar disorder, abnormalities in excitatory and/or inhibitory neurotransmission may lead to dysfunctional connectivity between brain cells [206]. Glutamate is an excitatory neurotransmitter, and gamma amino butyric acid (GABA) is an inhibitory neurotransmitter. Glutamate promotes neuron firing and

GABA inhibits it. Both must be in balance for the intricate network of neurons in the brain to work in a coordinated manner; too much of either causes problems. Increased glutamate signalling can cause excitotoxicity and may result in neuronal death. If GABA inhibits neurons too much, it becomes sedating.

5.6.2.4 Oxidative stress

Oxidative stress is a component of both bipolar disorder and major depressive disorder representing a potentially harmful imbalance between reactive oxygen species [207].

5.6.3 Managing the patient

5.6.3.1 Pharmacotherapy

Psychotropic drugs combined with psychotherapy are the most common approach to the treatment of bipolar and depressive disorders. There are risks and benefits to each, and the relationship with the mental health provider exerts a primary influence on a patient's treatment compliance. This said, the role of medication side effects in medication non-compliance cannot be overlooked. It is not uncommon for a previously treated patient to show reluctance to enter further treatment after experiencing noxious side effects from one or more medications. Both depression and bipolar patients complain that medications make them feel less like themselves. Other side effects patients complain of include, but are not limited to, nausea, dizziness, fatigue, and skin rashes. Metabolic changes trending toward pre-diabetes and T2D, as evidenced by features such as weight gain (for women in particular), increased waist size, hyperlipidaemia, hypertension, and hyperglycaemia influence treatment satisfaction as well [208]. This is particularly true of second-generation antipsychotic medications, most frequently prescribed for bipolar disorders but also used in the treatment of depressive disorders. Most second-generation antipsychotics, clozapine, and olanzapine in particular, require metabolic monitoring. Even when they appear to be well tolerated and effective, metabolic changes can limit their use, or necessitate the addition of one or more antidiabetic drugs. These are among the reasons patients may prefer to remain untreated, putting them at greater risk of early mortality [208–212].

5.6.3.2 Diet

5.6.3.2.1 Evidence for the role of carbohydrates in mental illness

Effects of high glycaemic index (GI) carbohydrates on mood have been studied. In 2015, a report based on the Women's Health Initiative study found that in post-menopausal women, a high GI diet was associated with depression. Participants in the fourth and fifth quintiles for dietary GI were significantly more likely to experience incident depression, and those in the fifth quintile were more likely to be depressed at time of follow up three years later [213]. A 2019 systematic review and meta-analysis found no significant association between dietary GI or glycaemic load (GL) and odds of depression in cross-sectional studies. However, the authors found a significant association between a high GI diet and risk of depression in cohort studies. When they combined results from two clinical trials, a significant increase in depression score after consumption of a high-GL diet was found. The authors concluded that the findings together suggest a possible causal relationship between dietary GI, GL, and depression [214]. Due to its macronutrient composition (high fat, moderate protein, and very low carbohydrate content), TCR or KD is the lowest GI/GL diet.

At a blood glucose of equal to, or greater than 15 mmol/L (270 mg/dL), a study series of Type 1 and Type 2 diabetics showed temporary mild cognitive dysfunction, including difficulties with calculations and slowed processing speed [215]. Data from the cross-sectional Maastritch Study (2017) showed that, compared to those with normal glucose metabolism, individuals with T2D performed worse in all cognitive domains measured (memory, processing speed, executive function, and attention), whereas individuals with prediabetes did not. Hyperglycaemia and hypertension (not insulin resistance) modulated some of these differences, but neither accounted for differences in memory [216]. While hyperglycaemia is a known occurrence in diabetics, a 2018 Stanford continuous glucose monitor (CGM) study found hyperglycaemia to occur in healthy subjects as well [217]. Contrary to what researchers expected, 80% of healthy subjects showed pre-diabetic or diabetic-like glucose spikes after eating unsweetened cornflakes and milk [217].

Given the high GI of ultra-processed foods, and of corn flakes in particular, such a result would be expected in persons with insulin resistance. However, 80% of subjects considered healthy would not be expected to exhibit insulin resistance. A 2019 study from the University of North Carolina at Chapel Hill based on data from 8721 participants in the US National Health and Nutrition Examination Survey (NHANES) years 2009–16, may help explain this unexpected result. Measurements from this population were used to determine how many adults are at low versus high risk for chronic disease. According to researchers, just 12% of American adults were found to be in optimal metabolic health; that is to say, their metabolic measurements met recommended targets for cardiovascular risk factors management. Not only does this place 88% of the US population at higher risk for hyperglycaemia, but for hypoglycaemia as well.

When insulin is overproduced, if the liver fails to deliver glucose via glycogenolysis, or both, symptoms of hypoglycaemia may occur. Hypoglycaemic symptoms may occur in the presence or absence of abnormally low glucose. While symptoms rarely occur above 3.3 mmol/L (60 mg/dL), a rapid fall in glucose may result in symptomatic hypoglycaemia at higher glucose concentrations [218]. Symptoms of hypoglycaemia include, but are not limited to, one or more of the following: anxiety, headache, fast heartbeat, palpitations, irritability, tremors, sweating, hunger, dizziness, blurred vision, cognitive difficulty, feeling faint, and disrupted sleep. Mood swings, irritability, apathy, and other changes in mental status during hypoglycaemia can be mistaken for psychiatric disorders such as depression and anxiety [219]. Anger and aggressive behaviours, or lack thereof, are also reported to be related to glucose status [220,221].

5.6.3.3 *Mechanism of action*

Evidence indicates that a KD improves many of the pathophysiological processes underlying mood disorders:

5.6.3.3.1 Inflammation

Morris et al. (2020) reviewed mechanisms by which the KD may play a role in converting microglia from a pro-inflammatory state to an anti-inflammatory state and suppressed the microglial gene activity responsible for the inflammatory state [222].

5.6.3.3.2 Glucose hypermetabolism

In 1972, Drenick demonstrated the ability of the ketone BHB to protect the brain, allowing the men in his study to tolerate exceedingly low blood glucose without seizures or other adverse effects [223]. It is currently recognised that ketones can provide an alternative fuel for the brain when glucose, or glucose uptake, is low [27].

5.6.3.3.3 Neurotransmitter imbalances

Evidence suggests the KD may restore balance in these neurotransmitters, as evidenced in the treatment of seizure disorders [224]. While this characteristic of the KD looks promising, whether its influence on GABA and glutamate as demonstrated in persons with epilepsy generalises to mood disorders is not established.

5.6.3.3.4 Oxidative stress

The KD reduces oxidative stress [225]. Compared to glucose, BHB produced fewer reactive oxygen species when catabolized. Through other mechanisms, BHB also inhibits pro-oxidant factors and promotes antioxidant factors [201]. In this way, it shows promise in its ability to control the role of ROS in mood disorders [226].

Additionally, the KD may be employed as a means of controlling the metabolic side effects of many psychotropic medications used to stabilise mood, such as the second-generation antipsychotics. Routine monitoring of lipids and glucose is still recommended as, for some patients, the metabolic effects of these medications may not be controlled by diet alone.

5.6.4 Conclusion

Research on the KD as a treatment, or an adjunct to treatment, of mood disorders is encouraging [227–232], and side effects of a well-formulated KD are minimal [233]. Under medical supervision in a clinical setting, the KD can be utilised as a low-risk approach to mood disorders, with the understanding that it is currently an investigational treatment and its effectiveness, while promising, is not established. Given the personal and societal impacts of mood disorders, studies of treatments acceptable to patients that have minimal side effects are urgently needed. As the scientific literature on the use of the KD in psychiatry expands and its impact on the mechanisms of mood disorders becomes clearer the KD may find its role as a standard treatment of mood disorders (Boxes 9.5 and 9.6).

BOX 5.1 Case 1.

Angie is a married caucasian non-diabetic woman in her mid-thirties. She was referred by a mental health professional for a psychiatric evaluation to rule out bipolar disorder. Angie's complaint was, 'I get angry for no reason'. Her symptoms became intolerable when she was faced with legal charges when she assaulted her husband in public 'after a couple of drinks'. She described her typical drinking habits as between zero and one drink daily. She took no medications. A thyroid stimulating hormone test drawn five days prior to her visit was within normal limits. Angie did not describe symptoms meeting criteria for mania or hypomania, but complained of sudden 'mood swings'. She described experiencing two or more episodes of labile mood with severe irritability daily. Angie reported irritability typically occurring one to 3 h after eating. A continuous glucose monitor confirmed episodes of hypoglycaemia during the day. She was sent to a laboratory to undergo an oral glucose tolerance test with insulin. Fasting insulin and glucose were drawn together at 9am. She finished drinking 75 g glucose at approximately 9:05am, after which samples of glucose and insulin were drawn at intervals. Thirty-five minutes after glucose ingestion Angie's blood glucose reached a peak of 6.7 mmol/L (120 mg/dL), after which it began its descent, reaching a nadir of 1.2 mmol/L (21 mg/dL) 2 h and 9 min after glucose ingestion (Fig. 5.4).

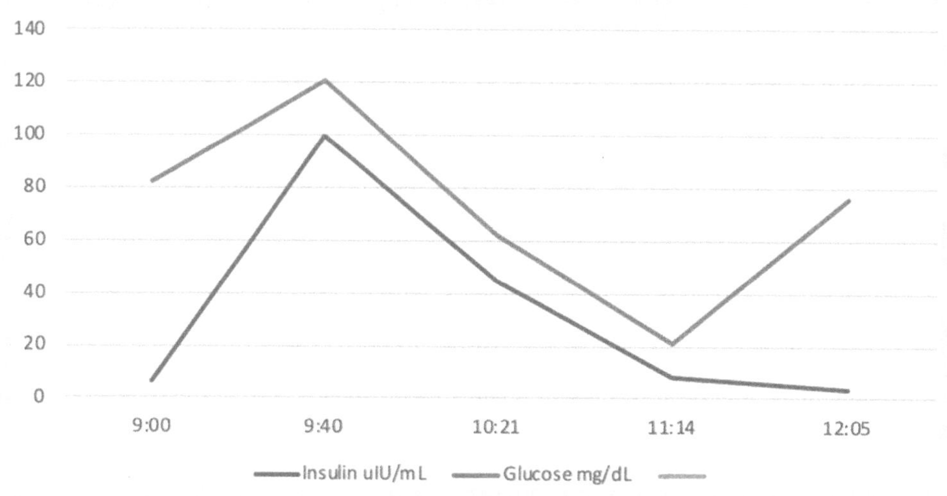

FIGURE 5.4 Graph of Angie's OGTT. Insulin and glucose were drawn at 9:00 AM, 9:40 AM, 10:21 AM, 11:14 AM and 12:05 PM. Her lowest glucose result was 1.2 mmol/L (21 mg/dL) at 11:14 AM.

Angie did not meet the criteria for bipolar disorder. Given what appeared to be severe reactive hypoglycaemia, it was suspected her 'couple of drinks' promoted a marked decline in blood glucose the night of the assault. When this data was presented in court, assault charges were dropped. A consulting endocrinologist advised her to adopt a low carbohydrate diet, and to make arrangements with the endocrine department of a local university medical centre for further evaluation.

BOX 5.2 Case 2.

Greg is a married caucasian male in his forties with untreated T2D. He was employed in an industry that demanded concentration and a strong cognitive capacity. While he reported mild symptoms of depression, his chief concern was 'brain fog' so disabling he worried he would have to stop work in the near future. Questionnaires revealed moderate depression and mild anxiety. During the course of his initial psychiatric evaluation, he agreed to wear a continuous glucose monitor for two weeks. At his one-week appointment his psychiatrist interpreted and shared his first week of continuous glucose monitor data, and suggested hyperglycaemia was a likely source of anxiety, depression, and cognitive issues ('brain fog') he complained of. A copy of his report is below (Fig. 5.5). He was educated about carbohydrate sources and encouraged to adopt a high fat, moderate protein, low carbohydrate diet, beginning with a ketogenic breakfast. At his two-week follow-up he reported improved mood, less anxiety, and resolution of 'brain fog' [234].

(Continued)

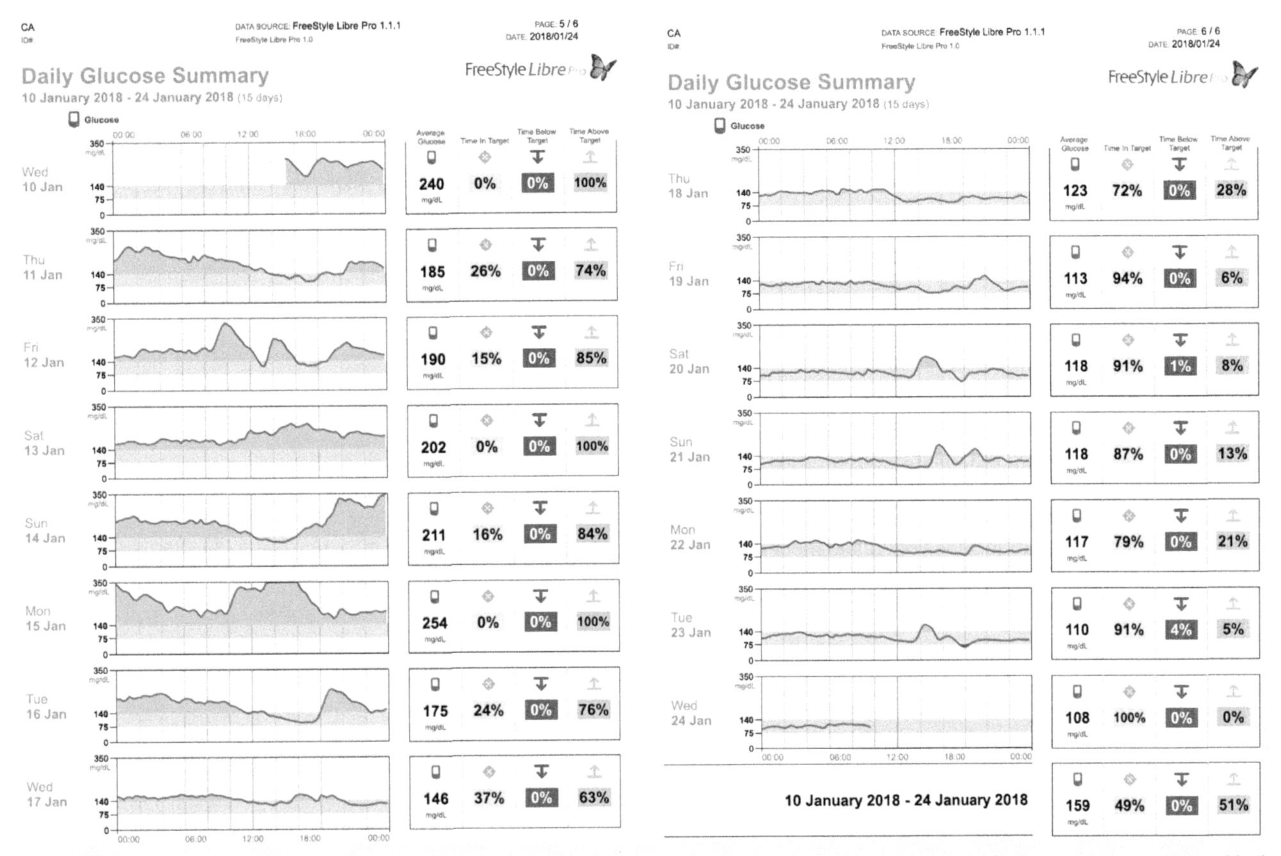

FIGURE 5.5 Abbott Freestyle Libre Pro continuous glucose monitor data. Left, Week 1. Yellow under the curve signifies hyperglycaemia. His psychiatric appointment with discussion of results and dietary recommendations took place the morning of January 17. Right, Week 2. Hyperglycaemia is largely resolved.

Mood disorder case study

G. Ede

On December 23, 2019, WW suddenly awoke from a sound sleep at one o'clock in the morning with severe physical agitation, 'I felt like a deer in the headlights'. Unable to shake the discomfort with his usual relaxation and breathing techniques, he left his house in the middle of the night and walked... for eight miles... but to no avail. 'It was like a startle response that wouldn't go away'. Over the ensuing three months, this profound restlessness continued to come and go seemingly randomly; leaving him in peace for a day or two only to repeatedly revisit him for as long as 24 h, and prompting him to walk for up to 25 miles a day with little to no relief.

WW is a 65-year-old married salesman with a lifelong history of anxiety, depression, and attention deficit disorder, which he had learned to manage with cognitive therapy and physical exercise. An avid cyclist, he typically rode about 100 miles per week. Despite these strategies, his depression had been slowly worsening in the years leading up to this acute period of unrest, which he thought may have been related to an increase in stress at work that month.

In early February 2020, he attended a weeklong family reunion which he looks forward to as the highlight of his year, expecting it would help him relax and feel better; but to his dismay, the agitation was much worse despite his loving family and positive environment.

In late February, he went to his primary care doctor for a physical exam and was told his blood tests were all normal, although his fasting glucose was 5.6 mmol/L (101 mg/dL). Melatonin was recommended, which helped him fall asleep at night but the intermittent agitation then simply waited until dawn to overtake him.

He told me he was determined to avoid psychiatric medications, because about 15 years prior, he'd undergone extensive psychiatric evaluation at a private ADHD specialty clinic and had been prescribed venlafaxine, clonazepam, and mixed amphetamine salts. He soon started to feel 'super-human', 'highly focused', 'full of energy' and became uncharacteristically arrogant and extraverted. To

(Continued)

(Continued)

temper these manic symptoms, he added marijuana to the medications, was eventually diagnosed with bipolar disorder type II, and urged to take a mood stabiliser. To his great credit, he brought himself back from the brink of divorce and homelessness by stopping all medications and joining Marijuana Anonymous.

In early March, when he first consulted with me, he embarked on a LCD, switching to a plant-free carnivore diet after a few days, of his own accord, in hopes that it might bring the fastest possible relief. His score on the GAD-7, a validated measure of anxiety symptoms, was 17 on a scale of 0–21 (with 21 being the most severe), and his score on the PHQ-9, a validated measure of depression symptoms, was 15 on a scale of 0–27 (with 27 being the most severe).

Almost 40 days after adopting the low carbohydrate carnivore diet, both his GAD-7 and PHQ-9 scores had fallen to *zero*.

Just another awesome week. That now makes six weeks without any symptoms of anxiety, agitation, or depression. Nada, zilch, none-...yeah!! Overall I am consistently feeling better than I have for my entire life.

After a lifetime of eating a standard American diet, a food plan consisting entirely of beef, pork, eggs, and cheese appears to have completely reversed his mood disorder, and normalised his fasting glucose, which now typically runs between 4.4 and 4.8 mmol/L (80 and 87 mg/dL). He reported mild ketosis by urine testing (0.9–2.6 mmol/L or 5–15 mg/dL) every day.

The only problem we encountered was that, despite eating 1.5–1.8 kg of fatty animal food per day, he was not able to regain the ten pounds he'd lost since the acute agitation had begun; at 180 cm tall, he weighed 69 kg. Therefore, we recently began relaxing his diet to include yogurt and modest amounts of select fruits and root vegetables to promote healthy weight restoration, support athletic performance, and add variety. He is thriving on his low-carbohydrate whole food diet and remains symptom-free at the time of this writing, a full seven months later.

5.7 Multiple sclerosis and nutrition

Michael Hoffmann.

5.7.1 Introduction

5.7.1.1 Definition/description

From a pathophysiological point of view, Ms is an inflammatory and demyelinating condition of the human nervous system, which causes recurrent neurological deficits. These occur mostly in a subacute time frame and cause both white and grey matter damage. Importantly, it is an autoimmune disease with autoreactive lymphocytes proliferating and gaining access to the CNS. Both T lymphocytes and B cells are involved in the pathogenetic neuroinflammatory process. These mechanisms have been realised by the use of efficacious B -depleting antibody treatments. Demyelination is a characteristic part of the pathology but axonal, subcortical grey matter as well as cortical grey matter involvement is increasingly appreciated, especially with higher Tesla magnetic resonance imaging (MRI) scanners.

5.7.1.2 Clinical presentation

Ms has a number of initial common clinical presentations that may prompt an immediate clinical possibility of the disorder. Thereafter, a number of different trajectories may occur (Table 5.7). Initial clinical presentations include the

TABLE 5.7 Demyelinating syndrome classification.

A. Multiple sclerosis
- Relapsing remitting
- Secondary progressive
- Primary progressive
- Acute multiple sclerosis (Marburg disease, tumefactive Ms)
- Diffuse cerebral sclerosis (Schilders and concentric sclerosis of Balo)

B. Neuromyelitis optica (Devic disease)
C. Acute disseminated encephalomyelitis (ADEM)
D. Acute haemorrhagic encephalitis (Weston Hurst disease)
E. Demyelination associated with autoimmune disease
F. Sarcoid related demyelination
G. Graft versus host disease

originally described Charcot triad of staccato speech, intention tremor, and nystagmus (characterised by repetitive uncontrolled eye movements). Other frequent clinical presentations include optic neuritis, occurring in about 25% of people with Ms, other cerebellar syndromes, spinal presentations, particularly the transverse myelitis syndrome (spinal cord inflammation), brainstem presentations such as internuclear ophthalmoplegias (extraocular muscle palsies), diplopia (double vision), trigeminal neuralgia (electric type facial shock sensations) and a number of cognitive impairment syndromes. Swelling of the optic nerve head (papillitis) occurs in about one third of people with optic neuritis, with retrobulbar neuritis found more commonly with a normal appearing optic nerve head. More subtle forms of optic nerve involvement may be diagnosed by the afferent pupillary defect (RAPD) sign. Paraclinical tests such as visual evoked responses, and optical coherence tomography (OCT) are sensitive tests aiding diagnosis. Vision recovers in at least half of people with optic neuritis within weeks of presentation. Residual visual impairment taking the form of dyschromatopsia, contrast sensitivity deficits and the Pulfrich phenomenon may persist (lateral motion two-dimensional objects are perceived in three dimensions due to differential signal timing of the two eyes). Other common clinical presentations include sensory deficits and/or motor deficits in approximately one third of people, an electric type sensation, at times with tingling radiating to the shoulders and down the spine with flexion of the neck (Lhermitte's sign). Lhermitte's sign is not specific to Ms, occurring also with cervical spondylosis. Less common clinical accompaniments may be seen more commonly with established disease including bladder dysfunction, spastic ataxia, cognitive disorders such as involuntary emotional expression disorder (IEED), inappropriate euphoria ('la belle indifference'), executive dysfunction, marked fatigue, vertigo, paroxysmal attacks of neurological deficit in the order of seconds to minutes duration, tic douloureux, and algesic dysesthesias.

5.7.1.3 Diagnostic criteria

All diagnostic criteria (from the earliest Schumacher to the most recent McDonald and Polman criteria) are variations of five principles domains including [235,236]:

1. a typical Ms syndrome,
2. objective evidence of nervous system involvement (examples are clinical spinal fluid or MRI brain imaging),
3. evidence of dissemination over time,
4. evidence of dissemination in space (systemic spread of symptoms), and
5. no competing or more likely alternative diagnosis (a formidable list of differential diagnostic entities requires specific exclusion).

Pseudo relapses may complicate presentations with conditions such as fever, anxiety, stress or drugs precipitating a transient recurrence resembling a previous attack of Ms that turns out on investigation not to be a new Ms-related lesion.

5.7.2 Pathophysiology

Although genetic and environmental factors are generally regarded as contributing to the pathophysiological process, no Mendelian Ms examples have been reported, with the concordance rate for monozygotic twins of approximately 25% and dizygotic twins, only around 5% [237]. To date, human leucocyte antigen (HLA)-related genes have shown the strongest association with HLA-DRB1* 15:01 with an approximately threefold odds ratio and HLA-A*02 associated with a reduced risk of developing Ms [238]. Epigenetic and environmental risk factors appear to play a much more influential factor than mendelian genetics in the development of Ms [239]. Known risk factors include [240–244]:

1. Epstein–Barr virus (EBV) seropositivity

   EBV infection involves both antibody dependent processes, as well as cytotoxic T cells. This virus has evolved to evade both
2. Infectious mononucleosis (IM)

   Approximately, 90% of IM is due to EBV infection with other causes including cytomegalovirus, adenovirus, Rubella, hepatitis, and human immunodeficiency virus. Both antibody dependent processes and cytotoxic T cells are implicated.
3. Obesity

   Obesity impacts the cellular immune responses posed by infections resulting in chronic immune-related inflammation. There is also a correlation between obesity and previous IM, which may contribute to explain our finding of an interaction between adolescent BMI and past IM.

4. Tobacco smoking

   Cigarette smoke exposure impairs all immune system components; innate immunity, B- and T-lymphocytes, natural killer cells as well as nitric oxide perturbation that leads to demyelination and axonal damage.
5. Shift work

   Both sleep deprivation and circadian disruption are common in shift workers and have well known immune disruptive effects.
6. Higher latitudes

   The most comprehensive meta-analysis to date supported a much greater role for environmental factors that whereby latitude and its relation to ultraviolet light and vitamin D status mediated various immune impairments.
7. Vitamin D deficiency

   Vitamin D is also a steroid hormone regulating over 200 genes for growth, enzymes and proteins with sunlight being the best source. Those in low sunlight environments are prone to low concentrations and at risk of hyperactive immune responses and cytokine storm seen with COVID-19 infections.
8. Low sunlight exposure particularly lack of ultraviolet light B [240–244]

With Ms termed a sunlight deficiency disease, sun exposure has protective properties, aside from vitamin D concentrations. Other mechanistic processes include a role for the type I IFN and MC1R pathway and immune related T cell divergence

The microbiome may also play a role in Ms risk. Individuals with Ms have altered gut microbiota compared to control patients [245,246], with immunomodulatory and neurotransmitter related effects on the host immune system [247]. Genetic susceptibility in addition to a combination of the environmental risk factors appears to be the most likely scenario for triggering the disease.

5.7.3 Managing the patient

5.7.3.1 Aims of care

Management of Ms involves both emergency care and long-term disability care. In addition, lifelong patient education with regards to important lifestyle adherence and understanding the nature of Ms. Accurate clinical assessments are key and should include Ms-specific clinical scales. Treatments may be divided into:

- Symptomatic treatment
- Acute attack treatment
- Treatment aimed at preventing attacks with disease modifying treatments
- Neural repair and treatments aimed at remyelination (investigational at this time)

5.7.3.2 Investigations

The combination of magnetic resonance imaging (MRI) multimodality imaging (to establish the requirement of dissemination in time and space of lesions) and cerebrospinal fluid (CSF) analysis (for specific intrathecal antibody synthesis) is commonly employed to substantiate a typical clinical Ms diagnosis [248]. Electrophysiological and other paraclinical tests such as optical coherence tomography (OCT) (which tests optical and retinal nerve fibre thickness) may also be conducted.

5.7.3.3 Educating the patient

It is important to educate patients about the Ms disease process as it may encompass wide ranging symptomatology and treatment options.

5.7.3.4 Lifestyle related considerations

A strong recommendation for Ms, as well as for all neurological illnesses in general, is to adhere to five basic brain fitness rules that stress the concept that a fit mind and brain requires a fit body. Diet and its importance for Ms is the specific focus of this brief overview. The four other components integral to maintaining a healthy mind, brain, and body are physical exercise, cognitive exercise, sleep hygiene, and socialisation [249].

5.7.3.5 *Monitoring*

This includes a general clinical neurological examination for typical Ms-related syndromes and recurrences. Overall elementary neurological deficit and disability-related measurements may be objectively graded with the Kurtzke Expanded Disability Status Score (EDSS) and Functional Status Score (pyramidal, cerebellar, brain stem, sensory, bowel and bladder, visual, and cerebral cognitive functions). The scoring system ranges from 0 (normal neurological examination) and 10 (death from Ms) [250]. Cognitive and behavioural neurological impairment may be conveniently and rapidly evaluated by the computerised CNS-VS subscales with one specifically designed for Ms monitoring [251].

5.7.3.6 *Pharmacotherapy*

5.7.3.6.1 Acute attacks

Intravenous methylprednisolone, variously using regimens of 500–1000 mg for three to five days, has been used since 1951 and has remained the mainstay of treatment since. Evidence indicates that intravenous and oral delivery of steroid therapies are equally effective [252,253]. Only three other options have been investigated to date: corticosteroids, adrenocorticotropic hormone (ACTH), and plasma exchange for Ms relapses. None have been found more efficacious to date and hence are considered second line agents.

5.7.3.6.2 Disease modifying therapies

These agents are deployed in the hopes of ameliorating exacerbations of relapsing remitting, secondary progressive, primary progressive and aggressive forms of Ms (Table 5.8) [255,256].

A recommendation of Ms medication according to time and severity of the disease is given in Fig. 5.6.

5.7.3.7 *Figure obtained from Gross RH, Corboy JR. Monitoring, switching, and stopping multiple sclerosis disease- modifying therapies.* Continuum (Minneap Minn) *2019;25(3):715-735. Diet*

Important clues for newer potential treatment strategies for Ms may be deduced from known risk factors. Of particular interest is the risk imposed by obesity, lack of sunlight exposure, vitamin D deficiency and other inflammatory neurological conditions such as autoimmune diseases and migraine. In addition, Ms itself is a neuroinflammatory disease. Furthermore, cerebrovascular reactivity has been shown to be deficient in people with Ms underscoring the critical role of vascular health that is heavily dependent on a healthy lifestyle [257]. There appear to be correlations between lack of

TABLE 5.8 Immunomodulatory and immunosuppressive medications approved for the treatment of Ms (listed in order of increasing efficacy and relative toxicity).

Mildly effective (in general reduce relapse rates in 30%–35% range)
Interferon beta 1a, Interferon 1b: principle side effects are flu like symptoms, hepatotoxicity Glatiramer acetate: regarded as safe in pregnancy, no flu like side effects
Moderately effective
Fingolimod: first- and second-degree heart block risk Dimethyl fumarate: gastrointestinal side effects, occasional progressive multifocal leukoencephalopathy (PML) risk Teriflunomide: Stevens Johnson side effect risk, teratogenicity
Most effective (in general reduce relapse rates in 60% range)
Mitoxantrone hydrochloride: potentially cardiotoxic Natalizumab: ~30% autoimmune disorder risk, progressive multifocal leukoencephalopathy due JC virus infection Ocrelizumab: elevated risk of malignancies, decreases new MRI lesions by ~95% Alemtuzumab: autoimmune disorder and malignancy risk side effect, especially thyroid
Promising investigative therapies
Sphingosine 1 phosphate receptor antagonists Remyelination strategies Bone marrow transplantation High dose biotin [254]

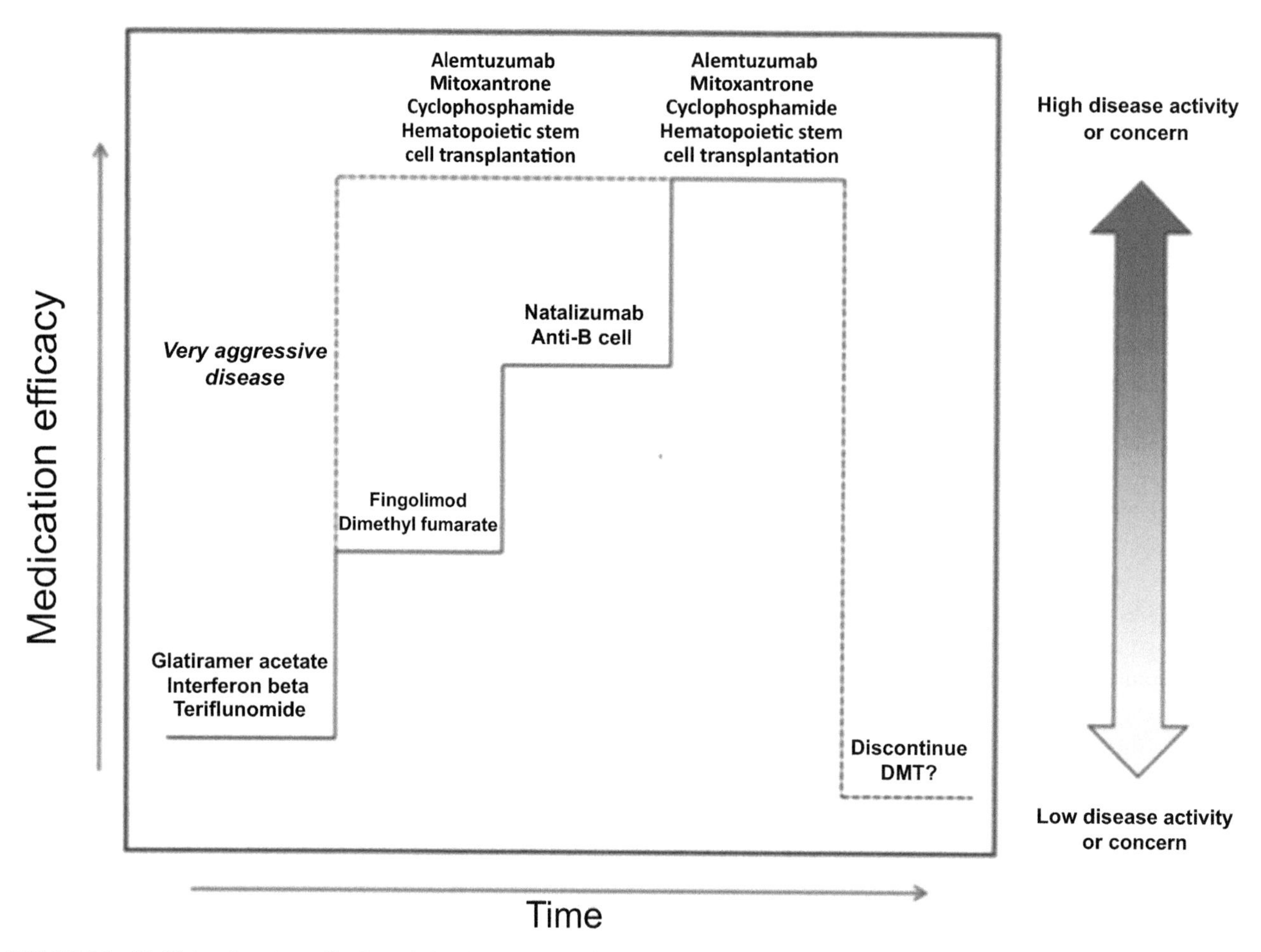

FIGURE 5.6 **Multiple sclerosis medications: balancing disease activity with medication efficacy over time.** Medications change in accordance with the severity of the disease upon identifying treatment failure in a patient over a brief period of time. This treatment is contingent upon frequent follow-ups for success.

vitamin D and Ms, Ms and obesity and obesity and autoimmune syndromes. Current recommendations for heliotherapy (sunlight exposure), which may mitigate a number of these risks, includes 30–60 min sun exposure daily, with approximately half the skin surface area exposed, preferably around midday, to maximise UV-B light absorption. Importantly, any diet that counters obesity will also be expected to lessen Ms incidence and severity.

5.7.3.7.1 Pathophysiological insights: the neuroprotective effect of the ketogenic diet

The KD's neuroprotective effects and potential benefits for Ms are likely multimodal, and are reviewed in Section 5.3. A ketogenic diet addresses the pathophysiology underlying diverse neurological disorders, and summarised below:

5.7.3.7.1.1 Modulating inflammation Any modality that may reduce or mitigate inflammation in the body may be assumed to be of benefit. An anti-inflammatory diet such as ketogenic type diet or similar have already been tested in a number of trials which have shown benefit [11,258]. Physical exercise is one of the most potent anti-inflammatory methods and has also been shown to improve working memory clinically and lessen hippocampal atrophy in people with Ms [259,260].

A recent pilot study in Ms patients, with one of the many KD formats, the modified Atkins diet, noted improvement in fatigue, depression, reduction in pro-inflammatory adipokines and weight loss [261]. The diet was well tolerated in the 20 subjects with relapsing Ms. Data from these subjects has been expanded with the number of participants increased to 65 for a phase two study [262]. Over six months improvements in inflammation, neurological function, quality of life, and body composition were reported. The ketogenic diet was well tolerated and found to be safe. A review of the potential application of this diet with regards to progressive form of Ms, highlighted the importance of mitochondrial dysfunction and its relation to the neurodegeneration in Ms as opposed to the inflammatory process [263].

In view of pro-inflammatory eicosanoids being involved in the pathogenesis of Ms, which increase vascular permeability and allow leucocyte migration into the cerebrum, KDs were investigated in 60 adult patients in a prospective randomised controlled trial. The expression of the pro-inflammatory ALOX5 in the treatment group was significantly reduced compared to the control group [264].

5.7.3.7.1.2 ***Gut microbiome*** A small study of ten people adhering to a KD for six months revealed much greater biofermentive bacteria, compared to counts prior to commencing the KD, resembling the study healthy control group [265]. This may be expected to confer neuroprotective benefits in Ms, based on the inter-relationship between the microbiome and the central nervous system, or the 'psychobiome'

In addition to a KD's anti-inflammatory and microbiome-modulating effects it may also benefit Ms by the following mechanisms (reviewed in Section 5.3. Ketogenic diet addresses the pathophysiology underlying diverse neurological disorders):

- Ameliorates glutamate-mediated toxicity and consequent ROS formation
- Effects on γ-aminobutyric acid systems
- Antioxidant mechanisms
- Energy metabolism

5.7.4 Conclusion

Given the risks associated with Ms, such as vitamin D deficiency and obesity, a dietary intervention may provide significant neuroprotection. The KD as a potent anti-inflammatory diet may provide multiple effects on Ms prevention and treatment. With relatively no contraindications and benefits observed in studies, the KD is worth both further investigation and clinical application.

5.8 Parkinson's disease

David Perlmutter and Mathew C.L. Phillips

5.8.1 Introduction

PD is a slow progressive, CNS disorder that affects movement, resulting in unintended and uncontrolled movements, loss of coordination, and tremors. Affecting approximately 10 million people worldwide, PD is a devastating neurodegenerative disorder second only to AD in terms of prevalence [266].

5.8.2 Pathophysiology

One of the fundamental neuropathological hallmarks of the disease is loss of pigmented melanin-containing neurons in the midbrain reflecting degeneration of dopaminergic neurons in the substantia nigra, a consequence of which is a marked decline in the availability of the neurotransmitter, dopamine, in the striatum [267].

A pivotal event in our mechanistic understanding of what underlies this disease occurred in 1982. Dr. William Langston, working as the Director of Neurology at the Santa Clara Valley Medical Center in California was called to evaluate a patient who had experienced a rapid onset of parkinsonian features. Within a short time, he and his team identified six other similar cases and discovered that all had been exposed to 'synthetic heroin' that had recently become available. Moreover, seven patients showed dramatic improvement when given standard L-DOPA therapy.

Dr. Langston and his team were able to obtain the illicit drug and found that it was almost pure 1-methyl-4-phenyl-1,2,3,6-propionoxypiperidine (MPTP). Researchers began animal research in rodents and primates using MPTP and soon learned that its administration did indeed induce PD like disease in these models and further, was aggressively toxic, specifically to dopaminergic neurons in the substantia nigra.

Further research revealed that MPTP itself wasn't specifically toxic, but once it entered the brain, MPTP, through the action of the enzyme, monoamine oxidase-B, was rapidly biotransformed into the toxic metabolite, 1-methyl-4-phenylpyridinium, or MPP+. MPP+ is then rapidly accumulated into dopaminergic neurons in the substantia nigra and reaches toxic concentrations within the mitochondria. Damage to mitochondrial function then ensues with compromise of electron transport function, specifically involving complex I [268].

While this human event and the animal research that followed were intriguing, questions were appropriately raised concerning the broader application of these discoveries to the population of patients with idiopathic PD. Researchers subsequently discovered that, similar to the mitochondrial dysfunction seen in the MPTP animal model, humans diagnosed with idiopathic PD likewise showed mitochondrial dysfunction, specifically involving complex I, as measured in platelets' mitochondria [269]. Other researchers have shown deficiencies of not just complex I, but also complex II and IV in muscle tissue of PD patients [270].

More recently, the herbicide paraquat has gained interest due to similarities in its chemical structure with MPTP and likewise has the ability to affect mitochondrial function [271] and influence gene expression [272]. Another herbicide, rotenone has also been shown to inhibit complex I of the mitochondrial electron transport chain [273]. Observations that exposure to these herbicides may be associated with increased risk for PD are debated [273–276]. However their use in producing animal models of disease suggests exposure may be a contributing factor [277].

A small proportion of PD patients appear to have genetic polymorphism (PINK1, DJ1, and triplication of the alpha-synuclein gene) that may increase their vulnerability to environmental exposures [275,277,278]. There is evidence that alpha-synuclein, a small protein that aggregates in the PD brain, inhibits complex-I and can drive mitochondrial abnormalities [278].

The profound effects of these environmental toxins on mitochondrial function coupled with the manifestation of parkinsonian features have led to the consideration of the central role of mitochondrial dysfunction in the genesis of PD.

5.8.2.1 Clinical presentation

Beyond the classic motor issues that characterise PD, the majority of these patients suffer from non-motor symptoms which contribute to their morbidity and mortality [279]. These include mood and affect disorders, fatigue, compulsive behaviours, autonomic dysfunction including orthostatic hypotension and constipation, psychosis, dementia, and sleep disorders. Over time, these issues become more obvious and significantly impact quality of life, the progression of disability, and the need for assisted care [280].

5.8.2.2 Investigations

The medical assessment (which is ideally performed alongside the nutritional assessment (see Diet below) in a combined clinic) involves a description of the patient's baseline medical status. The PD motor and nonmotor symptoms must be documented - this can be qualitative, although quantitative measurements using validated assessment tools, such as the Unified PD Rating Scale, [281] may be more useful for comparison with subsequent clinical reviews. Comorbidities, particularly those related to metabolic syndrome, should be recorded as these may also be affected by the diet. Medications must be documented, particularly L-DOPA and insulin. The former must be timed properly to avoid protein interference, the dose of the latter will likely need to be gradually lowered over time. A baseline neurological examination and standard blood investigations should be performed, including complete blood count, electrolytes, liver and kidney function tests, glycosylated haemoglobin, and a lipid profile.

5.8.3 Managing the patient

5.8.3.1 Aims of care

The functional decline in striatal dopamine represents a central player in the characteristic symptomatic manifestations of PD and has served as a major focal point for the development of therapeutic intervention.

5.8.3.2 Pharmacotherapy

In 1960, considering the likelihood of the central role of dopamine deficiency in the disease, Birkmayer and Hornykiewicz administered L-DOPA (levodopa), the blood-brain barrier penetrating precursor to dopamine, intravenously to PD patients and achieved 'miraculous' improvement of motor symptoms [282].

To this day, dopaminergic enhancement remains the gold standard in the treatment of the myriad motor manifestations of PD. Over time, strategies for achieving this goal have become nuanced with the use of agents that enhance the central availability of orally administered L-DOPA by inhibiting its peripheral degrading enzyme, L-DOPA-decarboxylase (benserazide, carbidopa) or its centrally active degrading enzyme, monoamine oxidase B (selegiline, rasagiline). Dopamine agonists have been developed and have gained widespread acceptance. They include pramipexole, ropinirole, and piribedil given orally with rotigotine administered transdermally [283,284].

As is the case with motor complications of PD, the various non-motor manifestations are managed using multiple modalities with the goal of reducing symptoms. Indeed almost all therapeutic protocols described for the treatment of PD are specifically designed around the goal of symptom amelioration. The extensive array of interventions now available to practitioners has had a dramatic impact on symptom management for these patients. However, while symptom management interventions are efficacious, it is important to explore the mechanisms underlying the process of neuronal dysfunction and degeneration that are characteristic of this disorder. Understanding these mechanisms may facilitate strategies that may slow disease progression and as such, help reduce the need for symptom-relieving medications, as well as allow the consideration of disease prevention.

5.8.3.3 Non-pharmacological medical interventions

Non-pharmaceutical approaches targeting the neurotransmitter imbalance in the motor circuitry of the basal ganglia have also gained significant attention. Deep brain stimulation (DBS) involves the stereotactic placement of stimulating electrodes into either the subthalamic nucleus or internal parts of the globus pallidus [285]. And this procedure has demonstrated clear effectiveness in reducing motor symptoms not only in patients with advanced disease, but in PD patients very early in their disease process [286].

5.8.3.4 Lifestyle considerations

5.8.3.4.1 Exercise

The role of exercise in the management of PD is well described. It may attenuate progression by supporting neuroplasticity, reducing oxidative stress, and promoting release of dopamine. Exercise therapy may lead to improvement or protection of function such as balance, bradykinesia, and gait. Other benefits such as improved sleep, cognition, and quality of life can also be experienced when exercise is included as an adjunct therapy [287]. A variety of exercise options can be considered including dance, walking, Tai Chi, personalised, or self-directed community based [288]. Various assisted exercise strategies can also be considered such as robot-assisted gait training [287]. Some studies suggest exercise may enhance medication effects and attenuate side effects [289].

5.8.3.5 Diet

5.8.3.5.1 Fasting

With evidence supporting the central role of mitochondrial bioenergetics (See Pathophysiology above) in PD, strategies designed to enhance and protect mitochondrial function are warranted. One such approach is fasting, defined as a voluntary abstinence from food and drink for specified, recurring periods of time [290,291]. Following 12–36 h of fasting, the human body enters a physiological state of ketosis characterised by the hepatic production of fat-derived ketones, which serve as a major energy source for the brain [292]. Compared to glucose, ketones produce more energy per unit oxygen, [293] and they may also circumvent the PD complex I defect via a complex II-dependent mechanism, enhancing mitochondrial respiration [294]. Fasting also invokes a number of additional metabolic mechanisms that collectively enhance mitochondrial biogenesis and function [295]. While fasting has been explored as a therapy in animal models of PD, despite it's sound theoretical advantages, it has only recently begun being investigated in human studies [296].

5.8.3.5.2 Ketogenic diet

One other strategy that may enhance and protect mitochondrial function in PD is a KD, which is a high-fat, adequate-protein, low-carbohydrate diet that forces the body to burn fat rather than carbohydrate as the primary energy source. KDs mimic a fasted metabolic state by generating ketones and inducing many of the metabolic mechanisms induced by fasting. Historically, KDs have been classified on the basis of their macronutrient ratio into four main KD therapies, [297] but the long-term viability of these therapeutic KDs is hampered by their imposed culinary and social restrictions, [298] making them less attractive in PD. Fortunately, recent years have seen the emergence of modified ketogenic diets (MKDs), which are more relaxed with respect to the macronutrient ratio. Practically speaking, an MKD is any diet that provides adequate nutritional intake while sustaining physiological ketosis (blood BHB concentrations of 0.5 mmol/L or higher) [299]. Importantly, MKDs can be tailored to the individual and are more flexible in social settings, which is highly appealing in PD.

To date, very few interventional studies have examined the impact of a KD in people with PD. One, a single-arm study, examined the effect of a four week 'hyperketogenic' diet (containing extremely low levels of carbohydrate and protein) in seven PD patients [300]. The five completers improved their motor symptom scores, but the study was limited by the low protein content of the diet, which likely enhanced levodopa bioavailability, and the lack of a control group. Another, a randomised controlled study, examined the effects of an eight-week MKD in 47 PD patients [301]. Patients on the KD experienced a 41% improvement in non-motor symptoms (compared to 11% in the low-fat control group), with the largest between group improvements seen in urinary problems, pain, fatigue, daytime sleepiness, and cognitive impairment. Given that these particular nonmotor symptoms represent some of the most disabling, least levodopa-responsive aspects of PD, the latter study's findings suggested that an MKD could play a complementary role alongside levodopa.

Since these findings are preliminary, KDs cannot yet be routinely recommended to people with PD. However, given the positive results of the few pilot studies, [232,302–304] MKDs can be considered in educated and enthusiastic patients. An outline of one suggested approach is described in Table 5.9.

5.8.3.5.3 Assessment

Patient selection should take place at an introductory visit (this can occur at a regular clinical appointment), during which the patient's suitability for an MKD is ascertained. Patients with very severe PD (Hoehn and Yahr score of 4–5), a very low body-mass index (less than 20), or lacking sufficient ability or support to institute a diet change may not be suitable. Patient education is paramount, as a KD involves a significant lifestyle change, it is vital to convey that an MKD is a comprehensive metabolic therapy (as opposed to a mere dietary change). Following this discussion, the patient's level of motivation for the diet should be reevaluated; if they remain enthusiastic, further information should be provided so that the patient can return home and self-research the approach before the next visit.

The nutritional assessment involves collaborating with the patient to create an individualised MKD that maximises their chances of long-term adherence. Culinary and social restrictions should be minimised so that the patient feels empowered by their diet, rather than confined by it. A list of acceptable recipe options in accordance with their tastes will retain their ability to eat a variety of enjoyable meals at home, whereas a list of acceptable ketogenic (or at least,

TABLE 5.9 A suggested approach for instituting a modified ketogenic diet (MKD) in Parkinson's disease (PD).

Stage	Steps
Introductory visit	Assess contraindications
	Educate patient
	Assess patient motivation
	Provide additional information
Medical assessment	Describe PD symptoms
	Record comorbidities
	Document medications
	Perform baseline neurological examination
	Order baseline blood investigations
Nutritional assessment	Create individualised MKD
	Provide list of recipe options
	Provide list of foods for social settings
	Consider need for supplementation
	Record physical parameters
	Show how to obtain and use monitor
Regular ongoing follow-up	Provide guidance
	Manage adverse effects
	Repeat blood investigations at 2–3 months
	Arrange further clinical review

low-carbohydrate) food options to eat at restaurants or events will maintain their ability to attend social activities. Calcium and vitamin D supplementation may be worthwhile in a patient with osteopenia or osteoporosis and a multivitamin can be considered. Physical parameters, such as weight and body-mass index, should be recorded. Lastly, the patient must be shown how to obtain and use a blood glucose and BHB monitor, which provides feedback as to whether they are achieving a sustained BHB concentration of 0.5 mmol/L or higher. BHB concentrations are ideally monitored daily for the first several weeks or months. The frequency can be decreased over time as the patient becomes more adept at sustaining physiological ketosis.

5.8.3.5.4 Monitoring

Regular ongoing follow-up (via phone or email) is critical, particularly during the first month as this is the period when patients will require the most guidance and when most potential adverse effects will occur. Some PD patients on an MKD may experience an intermittent exacerbation of the tremor or rigidity as they commence the diet. As long as these are tolerable, they can be reassured that the exacerbations will probably decrease in frequency and severity within weeks. Increased irritability, hunger, and sugar cravings represent transient effects related to a significant reduction in carbohydrate intake, and should also improve within weeks. Patients experiencing thirst, presyncope, headache, or cramps are usually low in water or salt intake, which can be rectified by increasing both water and salt. Cramps may also be mitigated with high-dose magnesium supplementation. Weight loss can also occur as a result of reduced appetite. If this is not desired, the patient can be reassured that the loss slows with time, and can be mitigated by increasing food intake. A repeat blood test should be performed two to three months after initiating the diet, prior to the next clinical review.

5.8.4 Conclusion

In conclusion, current therapy for PD focuses on symptom management. Symptom-based approaches will doubtless remain useful in the foreseeable future. However, it is also vital that we discover disease-modifying therapies aimed at alleviating the mitochondrial dysfunction that lies at the heart of this disorder. Although the evidence supporting KDs as a therapy in Parkinson's is only in its preliminary stages, MKDs represent one potentially promising strategy for treating this disorder at its most fundamental level.

5.9 Neurodevelopment and autism spectrum disorder

Robert Cywes

5.9.1 Introduction

5.9.1.1 Definition/description

ASD is defined as a range of pervasive developmental, communication, and behavioural disorders starting in early childhood characterised by impaired communication and social interaction, excessive rigidity, and emotional detachment with restricted or repetitive patterns of thought, behaviour, and interests limiting or impairing daily functioning associated with variable forms of anatomical derangement of brain white matter. ASD is a pervasive developmental disorder. To meet diagnostic criteria for ASD according to DSM-V, a child must have persistent deficits in each of the three areas of social communication and interaction plus at least two of four types of restricted, repetitive behaviours. Severity is based on social communication impairments and restricted, repetitive patterns of behaviour. Previously, under DSM-IV ASD required three levels of severity and consisting of five distinct disorders: (1) autistic disorder, (2) childhood disintegrative disorder, (3) pervasive developmental disorder – not otherwise specified (NOS), (4) Asperger Syndrome, (5) and Rett Syndrome [305]. Diagnosis is based on behavioural assessment independent of correlation with brain and white matter anatomy. However, predictability scores for at-risk babies can be made as early as three months of age by brain magnetic resonance imaging (MRI) criteria [306].

5.9.1.2 Epidemiology

Originally described in 1938 by Hans Asberger and in 1943 by Leo Kanner, the incidence has increased from 1:15,000 in 1970 to 1:44 (2.3%) in 2018 in the United States [307]. The global prevalence (median) of autism is 100/10,000 with a 4:1 male preponderance [308]. Understanding the reason behind this rising prevalence is essential to prevent its continuance in coming generations.

5.9.2 Pathophysiology

5.9.2.1 Spontaneous genetic mutation theory

While some cases have specific aetiology (<10%), assigning cause is problematic because of misinformed conspiratorial popularism (e.g., The Vaccination Theory) that has been comprehensively debunked yet remains a common belief [309], assumptions of genetic spontaneous mutations despite lack of genetic or statistical evidence, wishful thinking and cognitive dissonance. While altered gene expression remains an unresolved factor, despite vast spending on defining new genetic mutation aetiology, little concrete evidence exists to support the pervasively stated factual claim to this effect [310], including the low incidence of autism risk across generations. There is little evidence that children of autistic parents have autism, while parents of autistic children do have a higher percentage of autism traits, there is no direct genetic lineage even in autosomal recessive patterns [311]. No specific genetic mutation or cluster of mutations has been identified to adequately account for ASD on a genetic basis.

Observed behavioural diagnostic criteria correlate directly with white matter structural (and thereby functional) disturbance [312] but assumes spontaneous genetic mutations in white matter development rather than considering post-genetic substrate and assembly disturbances because of the cognitive dissonance that low fat, low cholesterol, plant-based high carbohydrate diets are ideal for foetal and early childhood brain development [310,313,314].

Statistically, a 277-fold increase in incidence over 50 years and an astonishing 556% increase in prevalence between 1991 and 1997 [314] defy the new mutation theory particularly for a condition that was extremely rare before the 1970s. Current conventional understanding of the aetiology of autism is based on 'multiple interacting genetic factors' interacting with 'environmental factors', leading to a neurodevelopmental process that results in the expression of ASD in the child [314]. A firm foundation for this theory despite a lack of genetic proof is the 2%–8% recurrence rate [315] in siblings of affected children and twin studies reporting 60% concordance for classic autism in monozygotic twins versus less than 10% in dizygotic twins [314,316].

A more plausible understanding of aetiology correlates ASD with structural developmental abnormalities of the nervous system that can be seen on imaging or pathological sectioning [312], in particular the supportive white matter, leading to abnormal brain function and intercellular communication between grey matter cells, which affects emotion, learning ability, self-control, and memory. Based upon brain imaging studies, comparisons of white matter fibre density and bundle morphology and global white matter volume find that individuals with ASD have reduced fibre density, suggestive of decreased axonal count in several major white matter tracts, including the corpus callosum, bilateral inferior frontal-occipital fasciculus, right arcuate fasciculus, and right uncinate fasciculus, as well as a global white matter reduction [317]. Social impairment severity correlates with splenium of the corpus callosum fibre density [318]. Thus, primary microstructural white matter abnormality is the anatomical basis for ASD.

Structural brain development begins in the third week of gestation through the first five to six years of life [319,320], with ongoing modification beyond 50 years of life [321]. The effects of neurodevelopmental disorders last for a person's lifetime [322]. Expansion of prefrontal white matter, associated with development of higher-order cognitive functions, defines human brain evolution. While aberrant trajectories of prefrontal white matter development are implicated in psychiatric disorders such as ASD.

APOE4 influences brain development early in life. Infants with APOE4 have slower myelination and reduced cortical area and volume [323]. White-matter MRI analyses showed that myelination begins a few weeks earlier in APOE4 carriers than noncarriers. However, by one year of age, the noncarriers have caught up, and at two-and-a-half years they have more myelin than APOE4 carriers in all white-matter areas. This impact of APOE on myelination rate is explained by the fact that APOE mediates the metabolism of two key components of myelin: cholesterol and lipids. Carrying the APOE4 allele results in an anatomic vulnerability that is present very early in life and may affect behavioural ASD early but does not impact cognitive function until neurodegenerative processes associated with ageing come into play. However, the entirety of the expression of any APOE4 effect is substrate-driven [323].

White matter microstructural development, under genetic control, is the anatomical defect that causes the behavioural aberrations clinically called ASD [324,325]. However, this is where root cause theory is divergent. The majority of structural abnormality theories consider de novo genetic mutations in lipid membrane formation to be responsible for maldevelopment [326,327].

5.9.2.2 Substrate availability theory

Cognitive dissonance regarding a shift in dietary recommendations over the past 70 years has influenced neurodevelopmental substrate provision and assembly, particularly in pregnancy, early formula-fed infants, toddler beverages, and plant/grain-based low-fat dietary recommendations.

Humans are evolutionarily defined by brain development. Unquestionably evolved to nourish infants, human breast milk reveals the nature and proportion of substrates necessary for healthy human development. The structure, ratio, and function of different components, including fat, define the relative importance of essential newborn requirements (Table 5.10). Foetal substrate provision and the ratio of essential nutrients in the maternal diet, as well as maternal nutritional hormonal state, directly influence foetal development. Post-partum, despite maternal dietary and conditioning diversity, breast milk remains superior in quality and relatively consistent [328]. Studies on the evolution and composition of mammalian milk indicate that 50% of the total fatty acids (FA) contained are saturated fatty acids (SFA) [329]. These lipid components have an important role acting as structural building blocks, providing fuel, and participating in other metabolic processes. The genome responsible for lipid production has been preserved over time, suggesting a primary function of mammalian milk is to deliver lipids potentially providing unique metabolic benefits [329,330].

5.9.2.2.1 The lipophilic brain

Over the past 70 years, due to societal lipophobia, inadequate substrate provision, particularly saturated fat, essential omega-3 long chain polyunsaturated fatty acids (LC-PUFA) and micronutrients, primarily in the maternal diet during pregnancy and in formula-fed and weaned infants, have influenced the development of the foetus and newborn child, in particular the brain. These substrate deficiencies have led to a combination of structural inadequacy (particularly in the white matter of the brain) as well as a substitution of membrane components [331]. Membrane structure reflects a decrease in essential LC-PUFA, cholesterol, and ultra-long chain saturated FAs with a significantly higher proportion of non-essential PUFAs, pro-inflammatory omega-6 PUFAs, 16 palmitic acid (a fatty acid derivative of glucose de novo lipogenesis in the liver and brain) and a deficiency in particular of ketone bodies and vitamin D (a steroid hormone) [332,333]. In addition, foetal and maternal insulin resistance and loss of hormonal and substrate cycling, due to increased frequency of snacking on refined carbohydrates devoid of fat, has flattened hormonal diurnal variation [334]. This leads to abnormal structural cellular development (particularly prominent in the high essential fatty acid-requiring white matter of the brain) [335–338], which in turn would be expected to result in a dramatic rise in ASD incidence concomitant with the adoption of a high carbohydrate, low fat, low cholesterol, and low salt diet.

The brain is one of the fastest growing organs in the foetal body with the head comprising one third of a newborn's mass. Hyperplastic neuronal and support cell mitosis only occurs in the early foetal and childhood developing brain to any significant extent. As such, substrate demands are vastly greater during this period than at any other time of life. The growing brain has to incorporate whole structural FAs into cell and organelle phospholipid membranes. However, the rate of transport of whole FAs across the placenta and blood-brain barrier is too slow, which means that the manufacture of FAs by dividing cells is a critical part of growth [339]. Ideally, substrate for such FA creation comes from ketones [340], but in the modern era of chronic excessive carbohydrate consumption, insulin resistance, and reduction in saturated and essential FA consumption, glucose has become a primary substrate for lipogenesis. Glucose-based lipogenesis generates predominantly C-16 and C-18 palmitic and oleic acids (energy storage fats) rather than phospholipid structural fat [341]. These compete with and displace cholesterol, docosahexaenoic acid (DHA) and ecosapentanoic

TABLE 5.10 Macronutrient composition breast milk versus infant formulas.

Breast milk	Infant formula
FAT 4g (2g saturated) 36 Cal	FAT 4g (1.4g saturated) 36 Cal
All animal origin	All plant origin
Carbohydrate 7g 28 Cal	Carbohydrate 7g 28 Cal
Protein 1g 4 Cal	Protein 1.5g 6 Cal (whey)
Cholesterol 15 mg	Cholesterol 0 mg
DHA 0.5% of total fat PUFA	DHA 0.4% of total fat PUFA
EPA (AA) 0.7% of total fat PUFA	EPA (AA) 0.2% of total fat PUFA
Total 70 Cal	Total 70 Cal
Salt 25–30 mg	Salt 15 mg
40% cell membrane SFA	28% cell membrane SFA
30% cholesterol	0% cholesterol
DHA:EPA ratio 1:2 to 1:3	DHA:EPA ratio 2:1 to 3:2
3:6 OFA ratio 1:1–4	3:6 OFA ratio 1:10–17
Fibre 0g	Fibre 0–1g

acid (EPA) in the cell membrane yielding less flexible less functional membranes with fewer protein and receptor attachments, more prone to inflammatory cascading, particularly in the white matter, where the type and ratio of FAs and cholesterol matter for membrane rigidity, protein attachment, and inflammation [342–344]. Healthy cell membranes require a preponderance of longer carbon chain (C-20 and greater, whether saturated or polyunsaturated) structural FAs [345,346] that are the predominant lipids in insulin-sensitive maternal states and breast milk, whereas shorter C-16 and C-18 energy FAs predominate in insulin resistant states [345] and when plant-based lipids are used in infant formulas [347]. In particular, shorter (< C-18) chain PUFAs, found in hydrogenated oils, displace essential LC-PUFAs (and SFAs) affecting particularly myelin sheath white matter function [348,349].

5.9.2.2.2 Essential long chain polyunsaturated fatty acids

Approximately 65% of the human brain is fat, while 75% of the white matter myelin is fat. Of that, approximately 35%–40% is made up of essential long chain PUFA (EFAs). Only two FAs are essential for humans: alpha-linolenic acid (ALA, an omega-3 fatty acid) and linoleic acid (LA, an omega-6 fatty acid), t. However, fatty acid derivatives of these two EFAs are conditionally essential in the developing brain because of their high volume requirement during early brain growth, meaning that they are essential under developmental conditions including docosahexaenoic acid and eicosapentaenoic acid (DHA and EPA omega-3 FA), and arachidonic acid, gamma-linolenic acid and dihomo gamma-linoleic acid (AA, GLA and DGLA omega-6 FA). During pregnancy under the influence of oestrogen, there is an 8%–21% increase in maternal conversion of LA and ALA to DHA, EPA and AA, but if the maternal diet is deficient in these essential EFAs, there is reduction in conditionally essential PUFAs for the foetus. The omega-3 to omega-6 ratio, in high carbohydrate low fat diets, promotes pathogenic membrane structural development due to opposing effects of omega-3 and omega-6 FA on the brain via molecular mechanisms. Increased dietary intake of LA leads to oxidation and alters the ratio of other EFA in cell membrane phospholipids. Both omega-6 and omega-3 FA influence gene expression by directly competing for transcription factors, binding to modulate the expression of different sets of target genes. So the de novo spontaneous mutation theory of ASD may be related to altered post-translational gene expression rather than de novo gene mutation because of the EFA ratio influence. Omega 3 and 6 fatty acids also compete for the same set of enzymes to produce signalling molecules that have opposing inflammatory physiological functions: anti-inflammatory and pro-inflammatory, respectively. They compete to be incorporated into cell membranes, directly impacting the function of the membrane. While endocannabinoid:arachidonic acid ratio simultaneously affects mood and behaviour. The optimal omega-3/omega-6 ratio is 1:1–1:3. On a high carbohydrate low fat diet, the ratio is more often in the 1:15 range, which profoundly affects membrane function and inflammation [350].

The ratio and cascades of these EFAs are critically important for neuronal cell growth but also cross over into inflammatory cascades that may be implicated in ASD. Two competing EFA cascades, AA and EPA, balance inflammation in the growing brain so that both absolute substrate provision and the ratio of substrates are critical to healthy structural brain growth. Maternal diets and baby formulas have become increasingly deficient in these EFAs and the ratio of omega -3 and -6 FA has shifted greatly towards LA derivatives because of the increased use of plant-derived LC-PUFAs and a decrease in fish oils [351]. DHA and AA are essential components of oligodendrocyte membranes in a 1:2 ratio. which form the myelin sheaths of axons. Particular characteristics such as membrane fluidity and membrane cohesion [352] are important for myelin formation as well as myelin membrane stabilisation and function. Over the past 70 years, a dramatic decrease in maternal and early childhood EFA consumption correlates directly with the rising ASD incidence, particularly in formula-fed babies. While compensation of 3 and 6 omega LCFAs has been made by the addition to baby formulas, the ratios are often incorrect, closer to 1:10–15 and there is no EFA compensation in toddler high carbohydrate low fat diets.

Approximately 50% of developing brain cell membranes comprises SFA that should include an array of long chain (more than 16 carbons in length) SFA that ideally come from a combination of maternal diet (although transport into the brain across the placenta and blood-brain barrier is a limiting factor), as well as ketone-sourced lipogenesis. However under lipophobic, hyperinsulinaemic dietary conditions, the majority come from de novo lipogenesis of glucose to palmitic (c16) FAs that are not ideally suited to membrane phospholipids.

5.9.2.2.3 Cholesterol

The brain contains 25%–30% of the entire body's cholesterol, 70% of the brain cholesterol is found in myelin sheaths. Cholesterol facilitates membrane fluidity and anchors proteins, provides insulation for nerve conduction, and is the common precursor for all steroid hormones critical in pregnancy, including vitamin D3. Importantly, cholesterol is an indispensable component of myelin membranes, and cholesterol availability in oligodendrocytes is a rate-limiting factor for brain maturation [353]. Cholesterol comprises 40% of the brain outer lipid membrane and about 3% of the inner membrane. The rate of early childhood brain growth is so rapid that at least two thirds of the required cholesterol comes from the diet or hepatic generation, while one third is made in the brain from ketones. Due to increases in high carbohydrate low fat dietary recommendations, maternal diets are inadequate in cholesterol consumption, and maternal insulin resistance precluding hepatic ketone production is increasingly prevalent, so that there is both a reduction in dietary as well as de novo cholesterol availability for the developing brain [354]. Insulin resistance reduces de novo neuronal cholesterol synthesis [355,356].

5.9.2.2.4 Ketones, brain energy and structural growth

Cellular hyperplasia requires enormous amounts of energy, and ketones are essential to brain fuel security. Seventy five percent of all newborn energy is used by the infant brain, and ketone uptake is five times faster than in adults. Ketones are also essential as structural fat substrates in the developing brain. The early embryo uses maternal glucose until eight weeks of gestation when the foetal liver begins ketone production. At the same time, 70% of brain energy is from FAs, mostly ketones, while 30% is from glucose. All newborns are born in ketosis, using brown fat stored in the third trimester as a source for ketone production. Ketone supply is negatively affected by insulin resistance and maternal high carbohydrate low fat diets. Additionally, high glucose baby formulas block ketosis.

In a meta-analysis of seven publications, children with ASD are significantly less likely to have been breastfed than children without ASD (OR = 0.61, 95% CI = 0.45–0.83, P = 0.002) [357]. Formula-fed babies have reduced intake of Vitamin D, saturated fat, salt, DHA, and higher intake of simple carbohydrates and non-essential PUFA. Soybean oil (the most commonly used oil source for infant formula) contains 7%–10% palmitic acid, 2%–5% stearic acid, 1%–3% arachidic acid, 22%–30% oleic acid, 50%–60% linoleic acid, and 5%–9% linolenic acid. The FA composition of soybean oil includes a high level of PUFA that significantly lowers serum cholesterol concentrations (considered by many to be healthy in the modern anti-cholesterol era).

In a comparative ultrasound study, exclusive breastfeeding was associated with statistically significant optimal brain development, particularly specific aspects of white matter structures, compared with babies who were bottle-fed or never breastfed [347].

Primary nutritional factors associated with both behavioural ASD and structural brain white matter abnormalities include a high carbohydrate low saturated fat, low cholesterol, low essential omega-3 DHA and omega-6 AA LC-PUFA, low vitamin D diet [358,359]. These factors are also associated with a statistically significantly higher incidence of maternal insulin resistance and development of insulin resistance in toddlers on high carbohydrate weaning diets [336,360,361].

5.9.2.2.5 The development of foetal insulin resistance and link to Autism Spectrum Disorder

Further confirmatory evidence implicating high carbohydrate, low-fat diets, insulin resistance, and nutrient availability is the high correlation of maternal diabetes of any kind with ASD [362]. Embryologically, the liver and pancreas form, starting on gestational day 16 (in the third week), at the confluence of the umbilical veins. These veins carry all of the nutrient-rich, oxygenated blood from the placenta directly to the liver for processing, including fat and fat-soluble vitamins but not maternal hormones (insulin does not cross the placenta) [363]. Thus, unlike post-partum, the early foetus is exposed to preformed proteins, FA, phospholipids and glucose, at concentrations similar to that of the maternal blood that enter the foetal circulation and can directly be used for cellular development and growth. However, lack of foetal regulation of concentrations such as glucose, and diseases such as gestational diabetes have devastating consequences on the foetus (e.g., gestational diabetes increases a foetus' mortality risk sevenfold).

The islets of Langerhans that produce insulin, glucagon, and somatostatin begin to secrete in the 15th week [364]. The portal vein carries hormone-rich blood from the foetal intestine and pancreas directly to the sinusoidal system of capillaries in the liver where foetal hormones regulate maternal nutrient supply and liver metabolism. These hormones are endogenously produced by the foetus and do not cross the placenta from the mother [365]. Therefore, maternal insulin resistance, gestational diabetes and hyperglycaemia causes unregulatable foetal hyperglycaemia very early in embryology that affects foetal organogenesis, particularly foetal brain or neurodevelopment, sometimes fatally [366]. Once insulin is produced in the second half of foetal life, insulin overproduction leads to foetal insulin resistance and chronically elevated insulin concentrations, which affects insulin-sensitive carbohydrate, lipid and protein metabolism and organogenesis as well as steroid hormone production. Maternal hyperglycaemia directly affects foetal brain development particularly in the first trimester when organogenesis is most active.

Pregnant mother diabetes incidence was 17.6% in 2014, up from 11% a decade previously [367]. There is a 42% increased absolute risk of ASD in mothers diagnosed with gestational or T2D by 26 weeks of gestation [368]. In a large study of 419, 425 children from 1995 to 2012, 5827 (1.4%) had ASD diagnosed by seven years of age and 11% of pregnant mothers were found to have type 1, type 2 or gestational diabetes but had 2.3% incidence of ASD (a 61% increase over non-diabetic mothers). Unadjusted average annual ASD incidence rates per 1000 children were 4.4 for exposure to type 1 diabetes; 3.6 for T2D; 2.9 for gestational diabetes by 26 weeks; 2.1 for gestational diabetes after 26 weeks; and 1.8 for no diabetes. Relative to no diabetes exposure, the adjusted hazard ratios for exposure to maternal diabetes were 2.36 (95% CI, 1.36–4.12) for type 1 diabetes, 1.45 (95% CI, 1.24–1.70) for T2D, 1.30 (95% CI, 1.12–1.51) for gestational diabetes by 26 weeks' gestation, and 0.99 (95% CI, 0.88–1.12) for GDM after 26 weeks [369].

5.9.2.2.6 Summary

ASD is the behavioural expression of a diversity of predominantly white matter brain structural maldevelopment with a wide spectrum of behavioural expression due to the diversity of white matter injury from radiologically undetectable to obvious, although always detectable upon anatomical dissection [312]. While there are multiple specific causes of white matter damage, less than 10% are specifically diagnosable, and the vast remainder are a direct consequence of maternal and early childhood nutritional substrate deficits resulting in metabolic hormonal disruption in the foetus and young child. The most common being deficiency of saturated fat, cholesterol and essential FA in the maternal and early childhood diet together with an excess of non-essential PUFAs and dominance of carbohydrate consumption causing insulin resistance as the primary energy substrate.

5.9.2.3 Dietary guidelines

Current 2020 US Dietary Guidelines for the first time include recommendations from birth to age 24 months, the critical period in brain growth [370].

5.9.2.3.1 Birth to 6 months

The 2020 Dietary Guidelines Committee recommends breastfeeding for the first six months, acknowledging that evidence suggests that human breast milk feeding and brain growth may correlate beneficially with higher infant saturated fatty acid status, which is in turn influenced by maternal diet [370]. Despite this, they were unable to separate themselves from the belief that saturated fat consumption exacerbates cardiovascular disease (CVD) risk. Their concern around saturated fat and CVD in adults (including lactating mothers) conflicts with the admitted benefits of this FA to the growing infant brain. Their recommendations support lactating women to consume food sources of long-chain PUFA, such as fish, but not saturated fat. While recommending avoiding sugar-sweetened beverages in children under two, adults (including lactating mothers) are told that all beverages (including milk and 100% fruit juice) contribute to hydration needs and can help meet nutrient goals, further promoting an anti-fat pro-carbohydrate ideology. Across the post-partum lifecycle, the guidelines promote plant-based PUFAs in place of saturated fat and cholesterol-rich animal fats, which conflict with the biology of the growing human brain and alter the lipid content of the nutritional gold standard for infant health: breast milk. Adults (including lactating mothers) are encouraged to eat plant-based foods over bioavailable, nutrient-rich animal foods, further exacerbating this evolutionary inconsistency in infant nutrition.

5.9.2.3.2 Six to twelve months

Despite accepting that nutrient needs are high relative to energy requirements for children ages six to 24 months, the Committee was unable to establish a recommended food pattern for infants aged 6 to 12 months.

5.9.2.3.3 Twelve to twenty-four months

For toddlers aged 12–24 months who are not fed cow's milk or formula, the Committee recommends a food pattern that 'allows for a variety of nutrient-rich animal-source foods, including meat, poultry, seafood, eggs, and dairy products, as well as nuts and seeds, fruits, vegetables, and grain products', prepared according to developmental stage.

5.9.2.3.4 Childhood

While acknowledging excess sugar causes obesity, they found insufficient evidence to condemn sugar-sweetened beverages compared to low- or no-calorie sweetened beverages in children, despite the significant increase in early childhood insulin resistance [371] that directly affects behaviour and brain development.

5.9.2.3.5 Summary

While the Committee strongly recommends breast milk for infants, their entire dietary recommendation exactly opposes the formulation of breast milk. The non-evidence-based concern over dietary saturated fat and cholesterol may have particularly deleterious consequences for the delivery of essential fat substrate to the developing brain. Logic, human biology, and embryologic scientific evidence suggests that this macronutrient dietary shift is the root cause of the structural defects seen in the brains of children with ASD and should be primarily addressed until there is evidence to the contrary.

5.9.3 Managing the patient

5.9.3.1 Clinical presentation

The DSM classification is discussed at the start of this section. Concomitant psychiatric disorders are common in ASD from schizophrenia to depression-anxiety disorders. Concomitant seizure disorders occur in 5%–40% of ASD patients, and there is a high incidence of attention deficit, learning, and hyperactivity disorders, while sensory hypersensitivity to food texture makes diet a significant challenge for ASD patients. Concomitant diseases of CECC and Insulin Resistance such as obesity, MetS and T2D are also more widespread in ASD and add requirement for TCR dietary interventions, but increase the challenges associated with initiating and sustaining such dietary changes.

5.9.3.2 Therapeutic intervention

5.9.3.2.1 Aims of care

ASD is a permanent anatomical brain disorder that cannot be structurally ameliorated beyond the age of 5–6 years of age. However, treatment aimed at stabilising and improving, even possibly to remission, ancillary psychiatric, psychologic and IR-related diseases with stabilisation and even improvement of behavioural elements including seizure control is becoming a larger part of ASD management specifically utilising ketogenic TCR while reducing the risk of comorbid carbohydrate-associated diseases [372–375]. Brain deterioration with dementia and Alzheimer's is also accelerated in the untreated ASD patient and early strategies to stabilise and reduce post-natal structural brain decay are also available. Cognitive behavioural modification programmes as well as regular intentional physical activity and improved sleep strategies also add value in the minimisation of ASD symptoms and reduction in comorbid disease [337,339–341,371,376–380].

5.9.3.2.2 Diet and lifestyle interventions

In our practice we have a particular therapeutic algorithm as outlined below:

1. Progressive migration toward TCR prioritising high protein-fat animal products for comprehensive dietary-sourced micro- and -macronutrient supply, taking into account food sensory needs of the patient such as smoothness, crunch and spices. Ideally BG and blood ketones are measured in the early ketogenic adaptive phase until fat-adapted by bloodwork
2. Intermittent fasting with no more than two to three calorie-consuming meals per day and no snacking in between
3. Developing a relationship with a non-calorie containing hydrating drink as an ever-present source of comfort and soothing distraction to sip on throughout the day
4. Prioritising marine sources of food including fish and seafood with the addition of at minimum 1000 mg DHA fish oil supplement
5. 15 mL of MCT oil or coconut oil twice a day
6. Sunlight and nature for anxiety management
7. Salt and electrolyte replenishment daily. Typically, 3–5 g iodised salt daily
8. Other minerals, vitamins, supplements, and additives only as required because of measurable deficiencies. Minimalism is better
9. Regular intentional exercise daily, daily engagement in a creative art of choice, intentional meditative time with at least 7 h of sleep. Routines offset the anxiety of chaos and assist in handling unexpected stresses
10. Daily conversational human interaction focussed on understanding and implementing the concept of empathy at first with a trained therapist then
11. Group therapy and group engagement that offers enormous therapeutic benefit particularly in higher functioning ASD

5.9.3.2.3 Pharmacotherapy

The following pharmacotherapeutic guidelines have been found helpful in clinical practice:

1. Never statin therapy - deprescribe
2. Preferably enrol the heavily medicated patient in an in-patient or intensive out-patient detoxification deprescription programme that utilises TCR as a foundational diet
3. Possible addition of 81 mg aspirin alternate days if signs of MetS or IR
4. Insulin resistance medication whether with the biguanide Metformin or a GLP-1 agonist/GIP receptor antagonist in combination or alone. Incretin medication is not used in underweight patients, but has profound value if MetS, IR, T2D or obesity is present.
5. If the patient is on psychiatric or anti seizure medication, referral to a psychiatrist comfortable with progressive medication deprescription is warranted or may be performed within our metabolic practice. Many patients can significantly reduce sedative medications and lift the dysfunctional brain fog that suppresses mental functioning in ASD patients.
6. ADHD medications such as methylphenidate-based psychostimulants or amphetamine-based psychostimulants may be carefully used early on to gain focus and suppress appetite particularly in IR but great caution is required to avoid abuse.
7. Aggressive management of migraines and headaches to remission (see migraine section)

5.9.3.2.4 Preventive strategies

Autism prevention strategies are generally lacking in the literature because of the ideology that it is due to spontaneous genetic mutation. A substrate deficiency theory as proposed in this section, however, lends itself to a readily preventable strategy in four parts:

1. Maternal diet prior to conception

   Establishing a fat-adapted insulin sensitive maternal biology using TCR increases the likelihood of conception and provides an ideal nutrient environment for the early developing embryo that is entirely and directly dependent on intact maternal substrate and hormonal provision prior to foetal organogenesis. This includes essential TCR strategies inclusive of adequate protein (preferably animal source) and saturated, essential, and mono-unsaturated fatty acid intake. Hydration is less dependent on large amounts of fluid intake than adequate salt, electrolyte and mineral intake, since salt regulates blood volume and pressure. Supplementation recommendations are for prenatal multivitamin with adequate folate, 3- and 6-omega PUFA supplementation and sunlight. Supplementation ideally takes the form of frequent small fish consumption, liver, eggs, nuts, fish roe, high-fat dairy or may be taken in pill form. Avoidance of processed and high-carbohydrate foods is essential as well as avoidance of foods that may contain high levels of heavy metals and environmental toxins, including nicotine and high alcohol consumption. Teratogenic effects of medications also need to be considered. Eating no more than two meals a day is ideal unless underweight or exercising heavily to restore nutritional hormonal cycling and a steady supply-demand nutritional cycle [381,382].
2. Maternal diet during pregnancy

   Dietary recommendations preconception apply during pregnancy. Folate-rich prenatal multivitamin including vitamins A, D, E, K, and 1000–3000 mg of DHA fish oil (providing 3-omega EFA) supplementation each day, particularly if there is a family history of dementia or Alzheimer's disease or either parent carries the APOE4 gene allele. High-fat dairy, pasteurised or safely raw is recommended if possible. Expect hyperemesis gravidarum (morning sickness) in the first trimester related to hormonal surges. Plan for this by eating when less symptomatic without resorting to high carbohydrate intake.
3. Infants up to 6 months of age

   3a. Breast Feeding: Same as above for the mother. Breast milk is a pure carnivore diet. Recommend exclusive breastfeeding for the first four to six months. Breastfeeding on demand or at least eight feeds per day for the first 12 weeks then wean to six to eight feeds until four to six months of age. Track on growth charts. Babies may be slightly lower on weight charts. Safe to supplement with infant Vitamin D, iron and iodine enriched drops. Liquid DHA fish oil supplementation daily is strongly recommended.

   3b. Formula Feeding: Exclusively only for four to six months of a term (37 week gestation) baby. Ketogenic formula rather than standard commercial plant-based formula. Add liquid DHA-enriched fish oil to any formula daily. Excess EPA and DHA is readily converted to other fats including ketones. Add 20–30 mg iodised salt or electrolytes. Add goat ghee or butter if possible. Avoid cow dairy, but may use small amounts of raw goat's milk and butter for cholesterol supplementation. Supplement with infant Vitamin D, iron and iodine enriched drops.

4. Infants six to 12 months of age

After 4 to 6 months of age, start complementary feeding with a high fat animal-based diet, including any meat, poultry, fish, cheese (preferably goat's milk), eggs, pureed, three times a day supplemented with breast or formula feedings, and sucking on strips of high fat meat until the first teeth come in. Include avocado and vegetable purees with animal products as foundation. Butter, Ghee, tallow, and cheese can be added to each meal. Vitamin D and fish oil drops may be supplemented. No fruit, grains, or fluids other than breast milk or formula and water is recommended. Allow baby-led weaning. Raw goat's milk is a reasonable substitute for formula after eight months if available. Allow the baby to gum, chew, or suck on solid juicy pieces of meat but watch for choking. If the parents are following a real food TCR diet, there should be no reason to ever purchase 'baby' food.

5. Over 1 year of age

Breastfeeding should continue for at least the first six months of life, and preferably up to two years and beyond. After 12–18 months of age weaning to full fat dairy and water as fluids is optional. Continue animal-based diet to provide optimal fat and protein. Include fish if tolerated. Provide food that requires chewing. Avoid fruit if possible. Avoid high carbohydrate and grain products. Avoid all commercial toddler beverages.

A diet adequate in 3- and 6-omega fatty acids in the correct ratio with the addition of LCHF TCR, adequate cholesterol, saturated fat, food-based micronutrients, and salt consumption creating a biological environment of insulin sensitivity, ketosis, and fluctuating hormonal feedback pathways is most likely to allow intact microstructural white matter development and prevent ASD.

5.9.4 Summary

In an era of enormous societal cognitive dissonance regarding diet in general, the likelihood of redirection away from a spontaneous genetic mutation towards a substrate provision theory of ASD development and treatment is a long way away. Influencing individual prospective parents to understand the importance of prevention of the ever-increasing rate of diet-related maternal-foetal complications including ASD is a priority for readers since societal correction is a long distance from addressing the root cause of ASD as a lifelong challenging yet possibly preventable disorder.

5.10 Migraine

Angela A. Stanton

5.10.1 Introduction

Migraine is the third most prevalent neurological condition with 15% of the population afflicted [383]. Migraine causes the highest rate of disability is the age group under 50 [384]. Nearly 3% of all disabilities globally are attributed to migraines [385]. The pathophysiology of migraine is known [386].

Normal neuronal signalling happens when electrical signals travel through the neuron's axon via spike train, facilitated by voltage-gated sodium and potassium channels down the axon. A critical function of neurons is the movement of sodium and potassium ions to create chemical and electrical gradients across the neuronal membrane to generate alternating action potentials (firing) and resting potential (-70 mV, the potential difference across the neuronal membrane when it is at rest), as well as refractory periods. generation of alternating action and resting potentials, as well as refractory periods. During the refractory period, the neuron rests and the channels cannot operate to create another action potential. During this time, the sodium-potassium pumps repolarize the membrane by actively moving sodium back out of the neuron and potassium back in, using the ATPase sodium/potassium pump.

5.10.2 Pathophysiology

Having insufficient sodium ions prevents the sodium and potassium pumps from creating a large enough action potential to open the gates [387], causing an extended refractory state. If neurons cannot create action potential, blocking neurotransmitter release, they may stay in an extended refractory period. Following this, a slow-moving wave of energy, cortical spreading depression (CSD), starts, which is a flow of sodium (depolarisation) [388], with its goal of resetting the neurons to an operational state [389]. If there is no recovery, the CSD reaches the nociceptors in the dura, which start the pain [390]. CSD is the initiating phase of migraine, which is called the prodrome phase. It is followed by two additional phases: migraine and postdrome.

5.10.2.1 Migraine and hyponatremia

Sodium shortage is associated with migraine, and mechanistic data indicates that the relationship may be causal [391]. Migraineurs experience significant diuresis and natriuresis during migraines [392] and eliminate 50% more urinary sodium [393] than non-migraineurs, resulting in electrolyte disturbance [394]. Reduced sodium increases renin and aldosterone (responsible for the maintenance of electrolyte homoeostasis), which then wastes water and potassium to re-establish electrolyte homoeostasis [395].

Additionally, a migraine brain is associated with sodium imbalance and problems with glucose metabolism and insulin resistance [396] in more than one ways. Nearly all migraineurs' sodium coupled glucose transporters (SGLT) are variants [397]. SGLT facilitates glucose uptake into cells by actively transporting sodium across the cell membrane alongside glucose. The movement of sodium ions from inside the cell to extracellular space provides the driving force for secondary active transporters such as membrane transport proteins, which import glucose and other nutrients into the cell by use of the sodium ion gradient. High blood glucose levels from carbohydrate consumption or a hypersensitive stress response exacerbate the problem because with higher concentrations of glucose entering the neurons, more sodium also leaves these cells via the active transport, causing an electrolyte imbalance. In addition, since these sodium-potassium-ATPase pumps also manage cell volume [398], failure of these pumps causes swelling in the neuron. The swelling itself causes these pumps to try to reset the proper osmolality (ion concentrations inside and outside of the neuron). But these pumps are variants in the migraine-brain and don't operate the expected way. Neurons use the Na, K ATPase pump to reverse postsynaptic sodium flux to re-establish the potassium and sodium gradients which are necessary to fire action potentials [399]. In addition, studies show that reduced dietary sodium is associated with metabolic disease, and migraineurs are salt-wasters by excreting more sodium in their urine than non-migraineurs [393], suggesting that the remaining cerebral hyponatremia [400] also predisposes them to metabolic disease [401].

5.10.2.2 Migraines, stress hyperreactivity, hyperglycaemia

Migraine starts with an excitatory stimulus [383], followed by three phases: prodromes, migraine, and postdrome (Fig. 5.7). Stress hormones release and the fight-or-flight response starts [402], increasing glucose [403], oxygen, and heart rate [404], stopping digestion, causing vomiting, diarrhoea, excess urination, restless legs, irritability, and yawning. Migraineurs see better in the dark [405] and have vivid dreams [406]. Everything so far described is an integral part of 'getting away from danger' [407].

Fight-or-flight is an evolutionary response to danger and for a migraineur's hypersensitive sensory organs [408], which perceives loud sound, strong odour, or bright light as danger that is not different from a predator appearing in terms of stress hormones. Migraineurs, particularly those with aura, may have superior responsiveness to brain stimuli and increased brain connectivity related to visuospatial ability, perception, and sensory integration [405] as well as vivid dreams [409]. Migraineurs also have different pupil size and pupil responses from the general population [410].

Migraineurs' hypersensitivity to stress may also result in hyperglycaemia and a predisposition to insulin resistance. During stress, insulin levels fall, glucagon, adrenaline and cortisol rise, gluconeogenesis is initiated and glucose is released from the liver [411]. At the same time, growth hormone and cortisol increase, causing body tissues (muscle and fat) to be less sensitive to insulin [412]. As a result, more glucose is available in the bloodstream to support the fight-or-flight response. All this leads to 'stress hyperglycaemia', which long term may cause insulin resistance [413,414].

5.10.3 Managing the patient

5.10.3.1 Dietary intervention

Various low-carbohydrate diets with increased salt prevent migraines. Therapeutic carbohydrate restriction (TCR), carnivore (CD), and ketogenic (KD) diets have been reported to prevent migraines. This may be because sodium is not displaced by glucose. Migraineurs also need to increase sodium in their diet. Adding 300 mg sodium (750 mg salt or an eighth of a teaspoon of fine salt) to every cup of water and eating food containing a close to 1:1 ratio of potassium to sodium prevents migraine. Drinking water with salt, ensuring adequate hydration, may have the additional benefits of increasing oxytocin, a neurotransmitter known to initiate comfort and reduce anxiety and stress while increasing trust and comfort [415,416].

It is not necessary to be in ketosis for migraine prevention. The carbohydrate level found to be effective for migraine prevention is below 70 carbs gr for women and below 85 gr for men, with the very low carbohydrate CD the most beneficial. In addition, the ideal migraine-preventing diet is high in protein, with a minimum of 25% of energy coming from

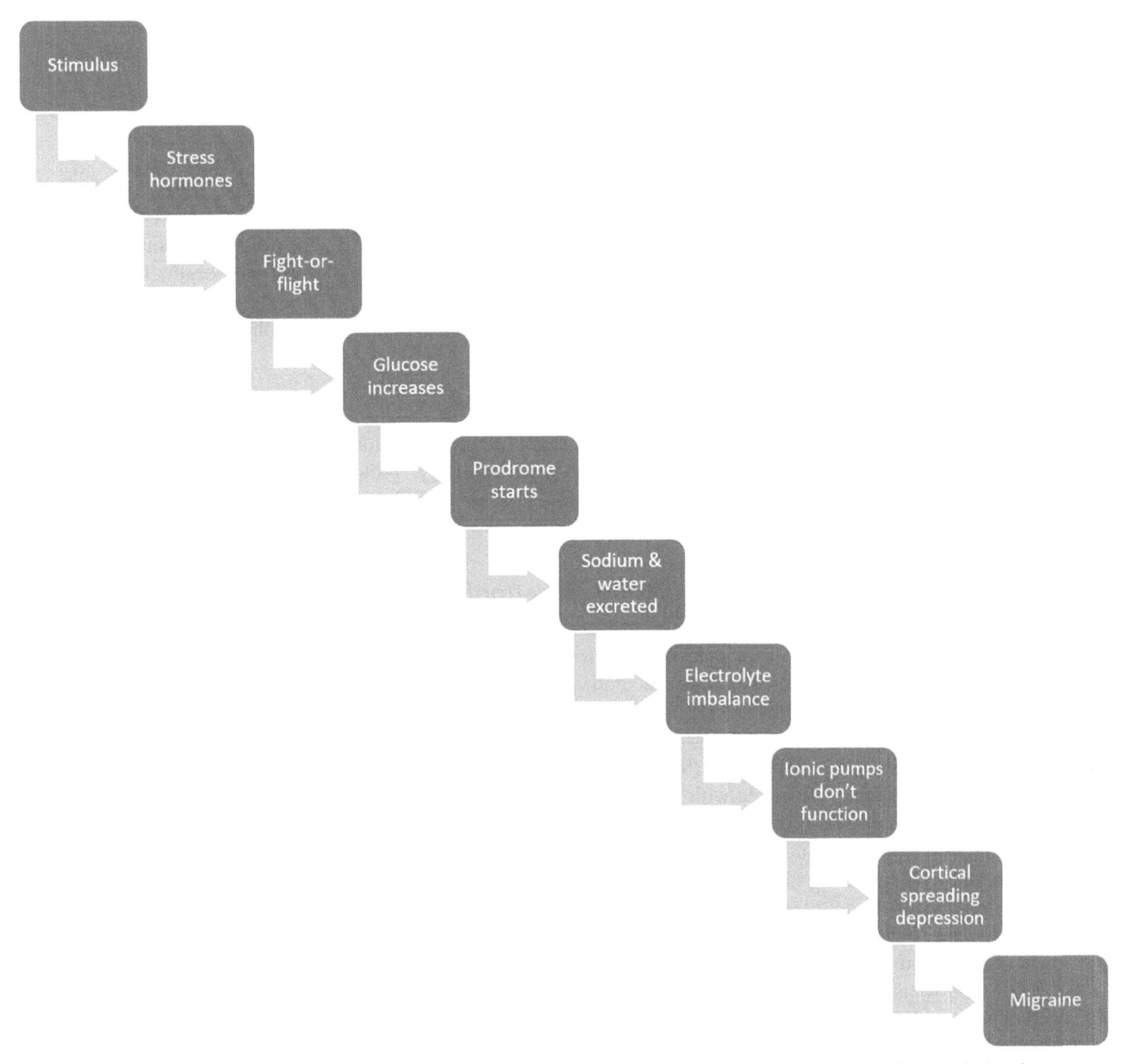

FIGURE 5.7 **Migraine sequelae.** A stimulus promotes stress hormone secretion, activating fight or flight responses. Hypercortisolaemia encourages hyperglycaemia, initiating prodrome, leading to sodium and water excretion. This creates an electrolyte imbalance, eventually leading to ionic pump dysfunction, creating the cortical spreading depression behind a migraine.

animal proteins on TCR and KD, and about 50% on the CD. The ideal sodium level appears to be dependent on water amount: ideally starting with 300 mg sodium per every second cup of water and increasing to every cup as the minimum water levels are reached. In addition, starting every morning with salt and water and ending every day with salt and water appears to be the most important part of migraine prevention in practice.

While migraineurs appear to be carbohydrate intolerant, making sudden changes can exacerbate symptoms. Regular monitoring of blood glucose and ketones concentrations is recommended to ensure there is no hypoglycaemia (<3.9 mmol/L or 70 mg/dL) and blood ketone concentrations don't increase above 3 mmol/L, since both scenarios have been reported to result in migraines. In addition, there are anecdotal reports of many migraine medications interacting with ketosis, especially heart medications and psychotropics. Interaction with heart medications may present as palpitations, tachycardia, heart arrhythmia, and similar symptoms while interactions with psychotropics may present as anxiety or mood and eating disorders. These medications should be used with caution and only under close medical supervision.

5.11 Amyotrophic lateral sclerosis

Joshua Rossi, Elisa Marie Rossi, Elisa Marie Rossi, Fabian Rossi

5.11.1 Introduction

ALS is a fatal neurodegenerative disorder with a progressive degeneration of both upper and lower motor neurons [417,418]. Degeneration of the upper motor neuron leads to increased muscle tone and spastic paresis. Degeneration of lower motor neurons causes fasciculations, atrophy, and muscle weakness [419,420]. The progressive muscle weakness is virtually inevitable and finally leads to tetraplegia, anarthria, aphagia, respiratory failure, and death. The prevalence of ALS has been reported to be five to eight in 100,000 in industrialised countries, with a peak of disease manifestation between 50 and 70 years of age. About 90% of ALS cases are spontaneous while 10% are inherited [419–421].

5.11.2 Pathophysiology

Different pathophysiological mechanisms had been implicated in the degeneration of the motor neuron, including loss of oxidative control, excessive production of free radicals, excitotoxicity, protein misfolding/aggregation, defective autophagy, glutamate toxicity, and mitochondrial dysfunction. Mitochondrial dysfunction is a key step in the pathogenesis of ALS [420–422].

5.11.2.1 Hypermetabolism, mitochondria and Amyotrophic Lateral Sclerosis

Animals and individuals with ALS experience a reduction in food intake and energy consumption resulting from progressive dysphagia and weakness in the masticatory and respiratory muscles. However, despite this reduction in energy intake, an increase in energy expenditure (hypermetabolism) has been reported in familial and sporadic cases of ALS, especially at rest. This suggests an abnormality in the energy haemostasis as an essential aspect of ALS pathophysiology [423].

Mutations in the superoxide dismutase-1 (SOD1) and TDP-43 genes are linked to ALS. In these transgenic mice, there is a hypermetabolic state associated with loss of body weight, reduced fat mass, and reduced blood lipid concentrations compared with the wild-type mice [424,425]. The possible causes of this hypermetabolic state are increased oxygen consumption by raised mitochondrial activity, uncontrolled fasciculations, increased respiratory muscle work, and mitochondrial abnormalities [424,426]. These animal models reveal abnormalities in mitochondria, not only in the nervous system, but also in muscles and other organs [424,426,427]. The decrement in muscle mitochondrial function was associated with reduction in ATP production, overexpression of uncoupling proteins, and increased concentration of markers of lipids and carbohydrate use, which worsen as the disease advances [424,426,427].

In G37R SOD1 transgenic mice, membrane-bound vacuoles derived from mitochondrial degeneration were found in axons and dendrites [428]. G93A SOD1 transgenic mice showed severe mitochondrial degeneration at the motor neuron that occurred even before the onset of the disease [429]. Mitochondrial impairments in the electron transfer chain activity and ATP production were seen in animal models [430]. These mitochondrial abnormalities are localised especially in close proximity to the neuromuscular junction. In SOD1-ALS transgenic mice it is speculated that the muscle hypermetabolic state is responsible for the muscle atrophy, the detachment between muscle and nerve (denervation) and then the motor neuron damage that follows [424,431]. It is important to note that the altered metabolic rate was identified in ALS mice before the onset of clinical features [424].

A total of 25%–68% of humans with ALS also present with a phenotype of hypermetabolic state, most likely secondary to muscle hypermetabolism despite muscle hypomobility [432]. This muscle hyperactivity and degeneration also precedes the motor neuron degeneration [433,434]. Mitochondrial abnormalities are also seen in patients with ALS showing mitochondria fragmentation and aggregation [435]. Therefore, improving mitochondrial function seems a potential strategy that could benefit patients with ALS and should be considered early.

5.11.3 Managing the patient

5.11.3.1 Aims of care

In view of the lack of effective treatments, therapeutic interventions facilitating the improvement of the mitochondria function, such as TCR, should be considered.

5.11.3.2 *Pharmacotherapy*

Only two compounds have been approved for the treatment of ALS: riluzole (possibly protecting motor neurons from glutamate excitotoxicity) and endaravone which has been postulated to scavenge free oxygen radicals [419]. However, both medications can only be considered as disease-modifying as they do not actually halt its progression.

5.11.3.3 *Diet*

5.11.3.3.1 High fat diets

There is evidence for high-fat diets benefiting ALS in animal models and human studies. In SOD1-ALS mice, a high-fat diet corrected the energy deficiency and postponed the onset of the disease, reduced muscle denervation, improved motor neuron survival, and increased life span [424]. In mouse ALS models, a high-calorie, high-fat diet lengthens life-span [436] while a calorie restricted diet shortens it [437].

Increased body mass index (BMI) and pre-diagnosis body fat improve survival, while lower BMI worsens prognosis [438], implying that high energy intake and associated body weight may also be beneficial in humans with ALS. In a small, randomised, double-blinded placebo- controlled phase two trial including 24 patients with late stage ALS disease, there was some improvement in survival in the groups that received a high calorie diet (though there was no difference between high-carbohydrate and high-fat diet groups) [439]. High dietary fat intake may facilitate increased energy intake though. A Japanese study showed that diets rich in total, saturated, monounsaturated and long-chain polyunsaturated fatty acids appeared to have a neuroprotective effect, reducing the risk of developing ALS. Conversely, low-fat and high- carbohydrate diets were associated with higher risk of developing ALS [440]. Elevation of 5'adenosine monophosphate-activated protein kinase (AMPK) occurs during disease progression. AMPK is a sensor and regulator of energy concentrations. When ATP production is reduced AMPK is activated to restore energy and keep energy homoeostasis [441,442]. A high-fat diet modulates the high-energy state demonstrated by delayed AMPK activation and prolonged survival of TDP-43 [442] and SOD1 mice [424,443].

Diets rich in omega-3 long-chain polyunsaturated fatty acids (PUFA) may be particularly neuroprotective. In one large prospective study, 995 of the approximately one million participants developed ALS. Diets rich in omega-3 PUFA were associated with a 34% reduction in the risk of developing ALS [444]. In another study, 132 patients with definite, probable or possible ALS, a 50%–60% reduced risk of developing ALS was observed in those who consumed a high intake of omega-3 PUFA and vitamin E [445]. Omega-3 PUFA (eicosatetraenoic acid (EPA), docosahexaenoic acid (DHA) and alpha linolenic acid (ALA)) commonly found in fish also appear to have neuro-protective effects in other neurodegenerative disorders [446]. EPA and DHA compete with arachidonic acid (a derivative of omega-6 PUFA) for the cyclooxygenase enzyme for conversion into prostaglandins, which have anti-inflammatory effects [420]. Inflammation and cyclooxygenase upregulation is implicated in the pathogenesis of ALS [447]. Omega-3 PUFA also share a neuroprotective benefit via an anti-glutaminergic effect [445,447].

5.11.3.3.2 Ketogenic diet in amyotrophic lateral sclerosis

The main source of energy for the brain is glucose. The brain cannot utilise fatty acids as they cannot cross the blood-brain-barrier. After fasting for a few days, there is a drastic loss in glucose reserves leading the brain to use an alternative source of energy: ketone bodies (KB). KB are produced by the liver in a process called ketosis. When KB concentrations reach 4 mmol/L (23 mg/dL) (non-fasted individuals on standard diets usually see KB concentrations below 0.3 mmol/L (1.7 mg/dL)), the brain starts to utilise them as a source of energy. The KB in the mitochondria are able to produce higher amounts of ATP than from glucose [448].

A state of ketosis could also be reached by the ketogenic diet (KD), which is high in fats, normal in protein, and low in carbohydrates. A KD leads the body to burn fats rather than carbohydrates, having a similar effect to calorie restriction, undernutrition, or fasting. A KD has the same activating effect on AMPK as low caloric restriction diets [448,449]. There are different versions of KD based on the ratio of fat *to* protein *to* carbohydrates and based on the type of fat being used (usually long-chain and/or medium chain triglycerides). KD could have 90% fats and 8.4% carbohydrates as in the classical KD, or 60% fats and 5% carbohydrates as in the Atkins diet, whereas the typical American diet contains 35% fats and 50% carbohydrates with protein making up the remainder [450].

In G93A SOD1 transgenic mice, a KD was associated with delayed loss in motor function, better preserved body weight, and more motor neurons in their spinal cord at autopsy compared with mice not eating a KD [451]. Another study in mice showed that a diet supplemented with caprylic acid (a medium chain triglyceride and KB precursor), was associated with an improvement in motor function compared to controls and was protective against motor neuron loss [452].

KD could potentially benefit ALS patients through the following mechanisms:

1. improving brain mitochondrial energy production [450]
2. decreasing excitotoxicity via reduction in brain glutamate concentrations [450]
3. reducing neuroinflammation via inhibition caspase-1 activation and blocking the release of proinflammatory cytokines [450]
4. reducing oxidative stress via boosting endogenous antioxidants [450]
5. Providing cholesterol and phospholipids which have a key role in the axonal membrane injury repair process (also see discussions earlier in this chapter) [453,454]

5.11.4 Conclusion

In summary, early data from animal and human studies suggests that high-fat and high-fat low-carbohydrate diets could be considered as a potential nutritional intervention to treat ALS.

5.12 Traumatic brain injury

Julienne Fenwick, Laurie Rauch

5.12.1 Introduction

A person who suffers a traumatic brain injury (TBI) sustains both primary and secondary injuries. Primary injuries, such as skull fracture, contusions (bleeding), shearing of nerve fibres, and compression of the surrounding brain tissue, occur during the initial traumatic insult to the brain. Secondary injuries such as ischaemia, hypoxaemia, cerebral oedema, hyper- or hypo- glycaemia, hyper- or hypo- capnia, hyper-or hypo- tension, hyperthermia and dysautonomia, occur as an indirect result of the primary injuries. Preventing and treating secondary injuries are thus of crucial importance to optimise the chances of a good outcome.

5.12.1.1 Clinical presentation

5.12.1.1.1 Initial presentation

The mild TBI patient is initially stunned or dazed for a few seconds or minutes. Following this, the patient remains alert with little or no post-traumatic amnesia. Complete recovery is usual. In more serious injuries, the duration of unconsciousness and particularly of post-traumatic amnesia helps grade the severity [455]. Consciousness should be examined over 24 h as grading can go up or down during this time. In terms of TBI, the Glasgow coma scale (GCS) is used to record the degree of coma and is used for its prognostic value. A severe GCS is in the range of 3–8, and the early score relates to expected outcomes, a lower score predicting increased mortality risk [456].

5.12.1.1.2 Recovery of severe traumatic brain injury

Recovery from severe TBI takes many weeks or months [455,457]. During the first couple of weeks patients are intermittently restless or lethargic and have focal deficits such as hemiparesis or aphasia. Gradually, they become more aware or may remain in posttraumatic amnesia, being unable to recall any continuous memory despite being awake. This amnesia may last weeks or more, though it may not be as clinically obvious. Post-traumatic amnesia is a predictor of outcome that is used very often. Usually, if it lasts longer than 2 weeks, it implies persistent organic cognitive deficits, although it can return to baseline but this takes a lot of work [458,459].

5.12.1.1.3 Late sequelae of traumatic brain injury

The late sequelae of TBI depend on the cause but do have important social and medico-legal consequences. About 65% of patients who sustain a moderate or severe TBI complain of cognitive impairment. Physical impairments may also be present [460]. Additionally, post-traumatic epilepsy can be quite disruptive, and post-traumatic (post-concussional) syndrome results in headaches, dizziness, malaise, and often being out of work for a long time due to depression and handicaps [458,461,462]. Other late sequelae include benign paroxysmal positional vertigo, chronic subdural haematoma, hydrocephalus, and chronic traumatic encephalopathy (confused patient) [461].

5.12.2 Pathophysiology of secondary brain injury following traumatic brain injury

TBI causes a hypermetabolic state with increased energy requirements necessitating adequate supplies of oxygen and glucose and optimisation of nutrition to meet the increased demands of the recovery processes ([463,464]). What complicates matters are the cellular perturbations that may occur as a result of the primary injury, such as disruptions to cellular membranes and to the blood–brain barrier (BBB) that lead to increased cytokine concentrations in the brain, increased endogenous catecholamine concentrations, and mitochondrial dysfunction, amongst other things [465,466]. These perturbations, in combination with the earlier-mentioned late sequelae, can play havoc with energy metabolism [463], and lead to increased oxidative stress [467] and apoptosis [468]. In addition, TBI causes haemodynamic perturbations [469] and often lengthy delays in normalisation of autonomic dysfunction ([470]; Kahlid 2019).

Autonomic nervous system (ANS) dysfunction typically manifests as a decrease in vagal nerve activity (the main nerve of the parasympathetic nervous system (PNS) that supports rest and digest and gut-to-brain processes) and increased sympathetic nervous system (SNS) activity (stress or fight-and-flight response) [465,471]. A healthy ANS is thus critical for maintenance of a healthy gut-brain axis. These far-reaching health effects emphasise the importance of addressing ANS dysfunction to improve short- and long-term health in TBI.

5.12.3 Managing the patient/therapeutic intervention

5.12.3.1 Aims of care

Following the immediate management of the patient, the next priority is to minimise oxidative stress of the injured brain tissue, to take steps to limit bodily inflammatory processes and cytokine production that can cross the disrupted BBB, and to ensure adequate energy supply to the injured brain tissue as well as to take steps to restore a healthy gastrointestinal tract.

5.12.3.2 Immediate management

Follow the Advanced Trauma Life Skills (ATLS) principles: Airways, bleeding, circulation (ABC), coma, stress fracture and if there is suspicion of intracranial haematoma, a computerised tomography (CT) image must be done and immediately get the neurosurgeon involved [457,472–474]. Stabilise from that point of view. In South Africa the approach is usually to immediately do a CT scan if GCS is less than 8 or on its way to 8, intubate and sedate the patient responsibly and give oxygen if the patient is restless. It is rare that TBI is an isolated injury [472,474]. So once ABC is taken, a careful neurological examination is of paramount importance.

5.12.3.3 Rehabilitation

Rehabilitation is usually prolonged, and it takes an energetic team of many different specialties (preferably including a specific functional nutritionist or dietitian for management of the gut). In the days following a TBI the gut microbiome becomes dysbiotic resulting in significant indirect effects via the vagus nerve and production of serotonin and dopamine (70% to 90% of which is formed in the gut). Stress on the gut is generally paid little attention, which often impacts neuroendocrine hormones, sleep, mood, and it can also completely disrupt the reward centres. If no attention is paid to this, it can prolong the recovery [475,476]. Refer to Chapter 8 for guidance regarding promoting a healthy gut and microbiome. You can activate your vagus nerve by engaging in rhythmic deep slow '10 s breathing', consisting of 4 s in-breaths and 6 s out-breaths [477]. A further crucial element necessary for vagal nerve activation is to quieten your thoughts. A good way to quieten your thoughts is by focussing your mind on your breathing rhythm. Alternatively, if you find your mind is too overwhelmed to keep a single-minded focus on your breath, a more practical way to quieten your thoughts and activate your vagus nerve is by engaging in slow rhythmic movements around the T7 spine such as occurs during natural movement, qigong, Tai Chi, etc [478].

5.12.3.4 Diet

5.12.3.4.1 Therapeutic carbohydrate restriction

The brain normally requires 100–150 g of glucose a day and uses about 20% of the total bodily oxygen [479]. TBI frequently leads to mitochondrial disruptions that impair oxidative phosphorylation of glucose ([480]) and enhances the rate of anaerobic glycolysis [480,481]. Unlike muscle and liver cells, brain cells have limited glycogen storage capacity [482], thus the injured and hypermetabolic brain tissue requires an immediate and steady supply of blood glucose from the periphery.

Meier and co-workers [483] suggested that blood glucose concentrations be kept between 5 and 8 mmol/L (90 and 144 mg/dL) during the first week of brain injury to prevent possible hypoglycaemic damage, and then from the second week onwards, at slightly lower concentrations (3.5–6.5 mmol/L or 63–117 mg/dL) to prevent hyperglycaemic complications such as cellular swelling, tissue acidosis, oxidative stress, microcirculatory damage/blood brain barrier disruptions [483,484].

The difficulty with keeping blood glucose concentrations set is that it requires constant monitoring and tweaking. Hyperglycaemia is common in critical illness via multiple mechanisms that include stress response, elevated cytokines during inflammatory response driving insulin resistance, existing conditions of dysglycaemia, and medications [485]. Low-carbohydrate, high-fat formulas may reduce hyperglycaemia and can be considered especially if there is pre-existing dysglycaemia [485]. Ketogenic nutrition (4:1) has been shown to be feasible and safe in an early study in adults with TBI [486]. Another feasibility study in patients with post-concussion syndrome using a ketogenic diet (5%−10% carbohydrate, 70%−75% fat, and 20%−25% protein, plus MCT oil) showed a potential for benefit that warrants further investigation [487]. Using a different approach, ketone bodies such as BHB can be used both enterally and intravenously as an alternate fuel source for the brain [293,488,489], with research indicating improved blood glucose control once a hyperketotic state is reached [490]. Ketone bodies also have the ability to decrease oxidative damage to injured brain tissue via coenzyme Q and glutathione peroxidase [293,491].

5.12.3.4.2 Dietary considerations

The nutrients outlined in Table 5.11 may support recovery in TBI.

TABLE 5.11 Nutrients that may support recovery from traumatic brain injury.

Nutrients that may support recovery from TBI [492,493]	Mechanism of action	Food (if patient is able to eat)	Supplements (if patient is unable to chew, swallow or has gut motility dysfunction post TBI)
Flavonoids rich in antioxidants [493−495]	Anti-oxidant action counters effects of free radical damage to brain cells; reduces inflammation.	Blueberries, cranberries, green tea, cacao, baby spinach	Curcumin extract daily [496] Vitamin C daily [497] Vitamin E daily [498]
Omega-3 Fatty Acids [499]	Enhanced neuronal cell survival, decreased Neuro-inflammation	Fatty fish (sardines, mackerel, salmon, tuna); flaxseeds, chia seeds, walnuts	Omega 3 (DHA and EPA) daily
Methylcobalamin (B12) [500]	Enhanced nerve repair	Meat and dairy	Vitamin B12 (methylcobalamin)
Trace elements: magnesium [501], zinc [502], selenium [503]	Enhanced synaptic transmission between brain cells (zinc). Protection against secondary effects of trauma (magnesium, selenium)	Unprocessed red meat, 70% dark chocolate (dairy and sugar free), nuts, legumes, seeds, seafood.	Magnesium, selenium and zinc daily
Vitamin D3 [504,505]	Modulates immune and ROS response	Oily fish, liver, egg yolk	Vitamin D3 daily (adjust to blood concentrations)
Prebiotics and probiotics for microbiome support [506]	Gut-brain axis optimisation, immune-modulation	Wide variety of vegetables with each meal. Fermented foods and beverages (kimchi, sauerkraut, kefir, kombucha)	Probiotic capsule daily before meals
Ketogenic foods (high fat (70%); moderate protein (20%); carbohydrates (10%)) per day depending on patient's needs [492,507,508]		Full fat dairy, unprocessed meat, fish, eggs, bone broth, free-range chicken, healthy oils, avocado, seeds, nuts, low-carb green vegetables, cacao, dark chocolate, tea and coffee (unsweetened)	
Foods to avoid in ketogenic diet		Sugar, honey, syrup, fruit (except berries), grains, starchy vegetables, sweetened foods and beverages	

5.12.3.5 Monitoring

Heart rate variability and the baroreflex index can be used as non-invasive markers of autonomic control, representing practical and cost-effective ways to track recovery from brain injury.

Blood tests of the various organ systems should be done. Kidney and liver function tests, full blood count with ferritin concentrations and differential white cell count should be done. Additional tests should include a full lipogram, hs-CRP, vitamins B12, and D3 concentrations, thyroid hormones (T3, T4, and TSH), as well as fasting blood glucose parameters (HbA1c, and fasting glucose and insulin). This should form part of the initial work-up, and tests can be repeated every one to three months to monitor the patient's response to the appropriate treatments.

5.12.4 Conclusion/summary

A person who suffers a TBI sustains both primary and secondary injuries that cause a hypermetabolic state with increased energy requirements. Steps must be taken to restore a healthy gastrointestinal tract and to minimise oxidative stress of the injured brain tissue by limiting bodily inflammatory processes and cytokine production able to cross the disrupted BBB. Adequate supplies of oxygen and glucose and optimisation of nutrition are needed to meet the increased demands of the recovery processes. Ketone bodies such as BHB, provided by nutritional ketosis and/or exogenous ketone supplementation, can be used as an alternate fuel source for the brain and have also been shown to decrease oxidative damage to injured brain tissue.

Useful websites

http://www.epilepsy.com/ketonews
http://www.neuroketo.org
http://www.epilepsy.com/learn/about-epilepsy-basics
http://www.charliefoundation.org
http://www.matthewsfriends.org
http://www.ncbi.nlm.nih.gov/pmc/articles/PMC5983110/pdf/EPI4-3-175.pdf (2018 Ketogenic Diet Consensus Guideline)

References

[1] Crossley NA, Mechelli A, Scott J et al. The hubs of the human connectome are generally implicated in the anatomy of brain disorders. Brain 2014;137:2382–95.

[2] Arnsten AF. Stress weakens prefrontal networks: molecular insults to higher cognition. Nat Neurosci 2015;18:1376–85.

[3] Vertes PE, Seidlitz J. Towards a natural history of schizophrenia. Brain 2019;142:3669–71.

[4] Stam CJ. Modern network science of neurological disorders. Nat Rev Neurosci 2014;15:683–95.

[5] Gasior M, Rogawski MA, Hartman AL. Neuroprotective and disease-modifying effects of the ketogenic diet. Behav Pharmacol 2006;17 (5–6):431–9.

[6] Schachter SC. Current evidence indicates that antiepileptic drugs are anti-ictal, not antiepileptic. Epilepsy Res 2002;50:67–70.

[7] Pinto A, Bonucci A, Maggi E, Corsi M, Businaro R. Anti-oxidant and anti-inflammatory activity of ketogenic diet: new perspectives for neuroprotection in Alzheimer's disease. Antioxidants (Basel) 2018;7(5):63. Available from: https://doi.org/10.3390/antiox7050063; PMID: 29710809.

[8] Liu T, Zhang L, Joo D, Sun S-C. NF-κB signaling in inflammation. Signal Transduct Target Ther 2017;2:e17023. Available from: https://doi.org/10.1038/sigtrans.2017.23.

[9] Barnabei L, Laplantine E, Mbongo W, Rieux-Laucat F, Weil R. NF-κB: at the borders of autoimmunity and inflammation. Front Immunol 2021;12:716469. Available from: https://doi.org/10.3389/fimmu.2021.716469; PMID: 34434197.

[10] Alcock J, Franklin ML, Kuzawa CW. Nutrient signaling: evolutionary origins of the immune-modulating effects of dietary fat. Q Rev Biol 2012;87(3):187–223. Available from: https://doi.org/10.1086/666828.

[11] Di Majo D, Cacciabaudo F, Accardi G, Gambino G, Giglia G, Ferraro G, et al. Ketogenic and modified mediterranean diet as a tool to counteract neuroinflammation in multiple sclerosis: nutritional suggestions. Nutrients. 2022;14(12):2384. Available from: https://doi.org/10.3390/nu14122384; PMID: 35745113.

[12] Tolkien K, Bradburn S, Murgatroyd C. An anti-inflammatory diet as a potential intervention for depressive disorders: A systematic review and meta-analysis. Clin Nutr 2018. Available from: http://doi.prg/10.1016/j.clnu.2018.11.007.

[13] Noh HS, Hah YS, Nilufar R, Han J, Bong JH, Kang SS, et al. Acetoacetate protects neuronal cells from oxidative glutamate toxicity. J Neurosci Res 2006;83:702–9.

[14] Erecinska M, Nelson D, Daikhin Y, Yudkoff M. Regulation of GABA level in rat brain synaptosomes: fluxes through enzymes of the GABA shunt and effects of glutamate, calcium, and ketone bodies. J Neurochem 1996;67:2325–34.

[15] Veech RL. The therapeutic implications of ketone bodies: the effects of ketone bodies in pathological conditions: ketosis, ketogenic diet, redox states, insulin resistance, and mitochondrial metabolism. Prostaglandins Leukot Essent Fatty Acids 2004;70:309–19.

[16] Ziegler DR, Ribeiro LC, Hagenn M, Siqueira IR, Araujo E, Torres IL, et al. Ketogenic diet increases glutathione peroxidase activity in rat hippocampus. Neurochem Res 2003;28:1793–7.

[17] Sullivan PG, Rippy NA, Dorenbos K, Concepcion RC, Agarwal AK, Rho JM. The ketogenic diet increases mitochondrial uncoupling protein levels and activity. Ann Neurol 2004;55:576–80.

[18] Veech RL, Chance B, Kashiwaya Y, Lardy HA, Cahill Jr GF. Ketone bodies, potential therapeutic uses. IUBMB Life 2001;51(4):241–47.

[19] Seo YS, Lee HB, Kim Y, Park HY. Dietary carbohydrate constituents related to gut dysbiosis and health. Microorganisms 2020;8(3):427.

[20] Rawat K, Singh N, Kumari P, Saha L. A review on preventive role of ketogenic diet (KD) in CNS disorders from the gut microbiota perspective. Rev Neurosci 2020;32(2):143–57. Available from: https://doi.org/10.1515/revneuro-2020-0078; PMID: 33070123.

[21] Broadhurst CL, Wang Y, Crawford MA, Cunnane SC, Parkington JE, Schmidt WF. Brain specific lipids from marine, lacustrine or terrestrial resources: potential impact on early African Homo sapiens. Comp Biochem Physiol Part B 2002;131:653–73.

[22] Brady ST, Siegel J, Albers RW, Price DL, editors. Basic Neurochemistry. 8th ed. Oxford, United Kingdom: Academic Press, Elsevier; 2012.

[23] Hussain G, Wang J, Rasul A, et al. Role of cholesterol and sphingolipids in brain development and neurological diseases. Lipids Health Dis 2019;18:26. Available from: https://doi.org/10.1186/s12944-019-0965-z.

[24] Bucher D, Goaillard J-M. Beyond faithful conduction: short-term dynamics, neuromodulation, and long-term regulation of spike propagation in the axon. Prog Neurobiol 2011;94(4):307–46.

[25] Connors BW. Synchrony and so much more: diverse roles for electrical synapses in neural circuits. Dev Neurobiol 2017;77(5):610–24.

[26] Attwell D, Laughlin SB. An energy budget for signaling in the grey matter of the brain. J Cereb Blood Flow Metab 2001;21:1133–45.

[27] Jensen NJ, Wodschow HZ, Nilsson M, Rungby J. Effects of ketone bodies on brain metabolism and function in neurodegenerative diseases. Int. J. Mol. Sci. 2020;21:8767. Available from: https://doi.org/10.3390/ijms21228767.

[28] Blazquez E, Velazquez E, Hurtado-Cameiro, et al. Insulin in the brain: its pathophysiological implications for states related with central insulin resistance, type 2 diabetes and Alzheimer's disease. Front Endocrinol 2014. Available from: https://doi.org/10.3389/fendo.2014.00161.

[29] Liu X, Li G, Xiong S, Nan J, Li J, et al. Hierarchical alteration of brain structural and functional networks in female migraine sufferers. PLoS One 2012;7:e51250.

[30] Saxena S, Caroni P. Selective neuronal vulnerability in neurodegenerative disease: from stressor thresholds to degeneration. Neuron 2011;71:35–48.

[31] Hassin RR, Uleman JS, Bargh JA. The New Unconscious. Oxford: Oxford University Press; 2005.

[32] Libet B, Gleason CA, Wright EW, Pearl DK. Time of conscious intention to act in relation to onset of cerebral activity (readiness potential): the unconscious initiation of a freely voluntary act. Brain 1983;106:623–42.

[33] Stephan H, Baron G, Frahm H. Comparative Brain Research in Mammals, 1. New York: Insectivora, Springer; 1991.

[34] Oberheim NA, Takano T, Han X, et al. Uniquely hominid features of adult human astrocytes. J Neurosci 2009;29(10):3276. Available from: https://doi.org/10.1523/JNEUROSCI.4707-08.2009.

[35] Diamond MC, Scheibel AB, Murphy Jr GM, Harvey T. On the brain of a scientist: Albert Einstein. Exp Neurol 1985;88(1):198–204.

[36] Falk D. Glial cells may be a factor in superior intellectual ability [Falk D. New information about Albert Einstein's Brain]. Front Evol Neurosci 2009;1:3. Available from: https://doi.org/10.3389/neuro.18.003.2009.

[37] Verkhratsky A, Nedergaard M. The homeostatic astroglia emerges from evolutionary specialization of neural cells. Philos Trans R Soc Lond B Biol Sci 2016;371(1700):20150428. Available from: https://doi.org/10.1098/rstb.2015.0428; PMID: 27377722.

[38] Oberheim NA, Wang X, Goldman S, Nedergaard M. Astrocyte complexity distinguishes the human brain. Trends Neurosci 2006;29:547–53.

[39] Ricci G, Volpi L, Pasquali L, Petrozzi L, Siciliano G. Astrocyte–neuron interactions in neurological disorders. J Biol Phys 2009;35:317–36.

[40] Testa-Silva G, Verhoog MG, Linaro D, et al. High bandwidth synaptic communication and frequency tracking in human neocortex. PLoS Biol 2014;12(Issue 11):e1002007.

[41] Carey N. The Epigenetics Revolution. New York: Columbia University Press; 2012.

[42] Jablonka E, Lamb MJ. Evolution in four dimensions. Cambridge MA: MIT Press; 2014.

[43] Douglas Fox D. The Limits of Intelligence. Scientific American; 2011.

[44] Van den Heuvel MP, Stam CJ, Kahn RS, Hulshoff Pol HE. Efficiency of functional brain networks and intellectual performance. J Neurosci 2009;29:7619–24.

[45] Kringelbach MI, Vuust P, Geake J. The pleasure of reading. Interdiscip Sci Rev 2008;33:321–33.

[46] Leslie I. Curious. The desire to know and why your future depends on it. New York: Basic Books; 2014.

[47] Berlyne DE. Uncertainty and epistemic curiosity. Br J Psychol 1962;53:27–34.

[48] Gomez-Pinilla F. Brain Foods: the effects of nutrients on brain function. Nature Reviews Neurosci 2008;9:568–78.

[49] Vaynman S, Gomez-Pinilla F. Revenge of the "sit": how lifestyle impacts neuronal and cognitive health through molecular systems that interface energy metabolism with neuronal plascticity. J Neurosci Res 2006;84:699–715.

[50] Montiel-Castro AJ, González-Cervantes RM, Bravo-Ruiseco G, Pacheco-López G. The microbiota-gut-brain axis: neurobehavioral correlates, health and sociality. Front Integr Neurosci 2013;7:70.

[51] Catalioto RJ, Maggi CA, Giuliani S. Intestinal epithelial barrier dysfunction in disease and possible therapeutical interventions. Curr Med Chem 2011;18:398–426.

[52] Mörkl S, Wagner-Skacel J, Lahousen T, et al. The role of nutrition and the gut-brain axis in psychiatry: a review of the literature. Neuropyschobiology 2018. Available from: https://doi.org/10.1159/000492834.

[53] Crawford MA, Bloom M, Broadhurst CL, Schmidt WF, Cunnane SC, Galli C, et al. Evidence for the unique function of docosahexanoic acid during the evolution of the modern hominid brain. Lipids 1999;34:S39–47.
[54] Cunnane SC, Stewart KM. Human Brain Evolution: The Influence of Freshwater and Marine Food Resources. Hoboken NJ: Wiley-Blackwell; 2010.
[55] Benjamin EJ, Virani SS, Callaway CW, et al. Heart disease and stroke statistics – 2018 update: a report from the American Heart Association. Circulation 2018;137:e67–e492.
[56] Centers for Disease Control and Prevention. Prevalence of the most common causes of disability among adults: United Stats 2005. MMWR Morb Mortal Rep 2009;58:421–6.
[57] Arzt M, Young T, Finn L. Association of sleep-disordered breathing and the occurrence of stroke. Am J Respir Crit Care Med 2005;172:1447–51.
[58] Meschia JF, Bushnell C, Boden-Albala B, et al. Guidelines for the primary prevention of stroke: a statement for healthcare professionals from the American Heart Association/American Stroke Association. Stroke 2014;45:3754–832.
[59] Bulletin of the World Health Organization 2016;94:634-634A. Available from: https://doi.org/10.2471/BLT.16.181636
[60] Gottesman RF, Albert MS, Alonso A, et al. Associations between midlife vascular risk factors and 25-year incident dementia in the atherosclerosis risk in communities (ARIC) Cohort. JAMA Neurol 2017;74(10):1246–54.
[61] Johnson KG, Johnson DC. Frequency of sleep apnea in stroke and TIA patients: a meta-analysis. J Clin Sleep Med 2010;6:131–7.
[62] Adams HP, Bendixen BH, Kappelle LJ, Biller J, Love BB, Gordon DL, et al.EE and TOAST Investigators Classification of Subtype of Acute Ischaemic Stroke. Stroke 1993;24:35–41.
[63] Nakagawa E, Hoffmann M. Young women's stroke etiology differs from that in young men. An analysis of 511 patients Neurol Int 2013. 09-16 10:00:56. Available from: https://doi.org/10.4081/ni.2013.e12.
[64] Guiraud V, et al. Triggers of ischemic stroke. A Systematic Review Stroke 2010;41:2669–77.
[65] Saver JL. Neurostereology: time is brain quantified. Stroke 2006;37:263–6.
[66] Dupre CM, Libman R, Dupre SI, et al. Stroke chameleons. J Stroke Cerebrovasc Dis 2014;23:374–8.
[67] Barber PA, Demchuk AM, Zhang J, Buchan AM. Validity and reliability of a quantitative computed tomography score in predicting outcome of hyperacute stroke before thrombolytic therapy. Lancet 2000;355:1670 4.
[68] Emberson J, Lees KR, Lyden P, et al. Effect of treatment delay, age, and stroke severity on the effects of intravenous thrombolysis with alteplase for acute ischaemic stroke: a meta-analysis of individual patient data from randomised trials. Lancet 2014;384:1929–35.
[69] Hacke W, Donnan G, Fieschi C, et al.and the ATLANTIS Trials Investigators, and the ECASS Trials Investigators, and the NINDS rt-PA Study Group Investigators Association of outcome with early stroke treatment: pooled analysis of ATLANTIS, ECASS, and NINDS rt-PA stroke trials. Lancet 2004;363:768–74.
[70] Campbell BCV, Ma H, Ringleb PA, et al. Extending thrombolysis to 4.5–9 h and wake-up stroke using perfusion imaging: a systematic review and meta-analysis of individual patient data. Lancet 2019;394:139–47.
[71] Goyal M, Menon BK, van Zwam WH, et al. Endovascular thrombectomy after large-vessel ischaemic stroke: a meta- analysis of individual patient data from five randomised trials. Lancet 2016;387:1723–31.
[72] Thomalla G, Simonsen CZ, Boutitie F, et al. MRI-guided thrombolysis for stroke with unknown time of onset. N Engl J Med 2018;379:611–22.
[73] Wang Y, Pan Y, Zhao X, et al. Clopido- grel with aspirin in acute minor stroke or transient ischemic attack (CHANCE) trial: one-year outcomes. Circulation 2015;132:40–6.
[74] Chen ZM, Sandercock P, Pan HC, et al. Indications for early aspirin use in acute ischemic stroke: a combined analysis of 40 000 randomized patients from the Chinese Acute Stroke Trial and the Inter- national Stroke Trial. Stroke 2000;31:1240–9.
[75] Vasilevko V, Passos GF, Quiring D, Head E, Kim RC, Fisher M, et al. Aging and cerebrovascular dysfunction: contribution of hypertension, cerebral amyloid angiopathy, and immunotherapy. Ann N Y Acad Sci 2010;1207:58–70. Available from: https://doi.org/10.1111/j.1749-6632.2010.05786.x; PMID: 20955427.
[76] Woo D, Haverbusch M, Sekar P, Kissela B, Khoury J, Schneider A, et al. Effect of untreated hypertension on hemorrhagic stroke. Stroke 2004;35(7):1703–8.
[77] Hemphill JC, Greenberg SM, Anderson CS, et al. Guidelines for the management of spontaneous intracerebral hemorrhage. Stroke 2015;46:2032–60. Available from: https://doi.org/10.1161/STR.0000000000000069.
[78] Turan TN, Nizam A, Lynn MJ, Egan BM, Le NA, Lopes-Virella MF, et al. Relationship between risk factor control and vascular events in the SAMMPRIS trial. Neurology 2017;88(4):379–85. Available from: https://doi.org/10.1212/WNL.0000000000003534; Epub 2016 Dec 21. PMID: 28003500.
[79] Niu PP, Guo ZN, Jin H, et al. Antiplatelet regimens in the long term secondary prevention of transient ischemic attack and ischemic stroke: an updated network meta-analysis. BMJ Open 2016;6(3):e009013. Available from: https://doi.org/10.1136/bmjopen-2015-009013.
[80] Benavente OR, White CL, Pearce L, et al. The secondary prevention of small subcortical strokes (SPS3) study. Int J Stroke 2011;6(2):164–75. Available from: https://doi.org/10.1111/j.1747-4949.2010.00573.x.
[81] PROGRESS Collaborative Group. Randomised trial of a perindopril-based blood-pressure-lowering regimen among 6,105 individuals with previous stroke or transient ischaemic attack. Lancet 2001;358(9287):1033–41. Available from: https://doi.org/10.1016/S0140-6736(01)06178-5.
[82] Kerr Saraiva JF. Stroke prevention with oral anticoagulants: summary of the evidence and efficacy measures as an aid to treatment choices. Cardiol Ther 2018;7(1):15–24. Available from: https://doi.org/10.1007/s40119-018-0106-1.

[83] Zhu W, He W, Guo L, et al. The HAS-BLED score for predicting major bleeding risk in anticoagulated patients with atrial fibrillation: a systematic review and meta-analysis. Clin Cardiol 2015;38(9):555–61. Available from: https://doi.org/10.1002/clc.22435.

[84] Levy JH, Douketis J, Weitz JI. Reversal agents for non-vitamin K antagonist oral anticoagulants. Nat Rev Cardiol 2018;15(5):273–81. Available from: https://doi.org/10.1038/nrcardio.2017.223.

[85] Jimenez-Conde J, Biffi A, Rahman R, Kanakis A, Butler C, Sonni S, et al. Hyperlipidemia and reduced white matter hyperintensity volume in patients with ischemic stroke. Stroke 2010;41(3):437–42.

[86] Wang X, Dong Y, Qi X, et al. Cholesterol levels and risk of hemorrhagic stroke: as systematic review and meta-analysis. Stroke 2013;44:1833–9.

[87] Zhan S, Tang M, Liu F, et al. Ezetimibe for the prevention of cardiovascular disease and all-cause mortality events. Cochrane Database Syst Rev 2018;11(11):CD012502. Available from: https://doi.org/10.1002/14651858.CD012502.pub2.

[88] Yaghi S, Elkind MS. Lipids and cerebrovascular disease: research and practice. Stroke 2015;46(11):3322–8. Available from: https://doi.org/10.1161/STROKEAHA.115.011164; Epub 2015 Oct 8. PMID: 26451029.

[89] Deng XL, Liu Z, Wang C, Li Y, Cai Z. Insulin resistance in ischemic stroke. Metab Brain Dis 2017;32(5):1323–34.

[90] Han L, Cai W, Mao L, et al. Rosiglitazone promotes white matter integrity and long-term functional recover after focal cerebral ischemia. Stroke 2015;46:2628–36.

[91] Thompson RC, Allam AH, Lombardi GP, et al. Atherosclerosis across 4000 years of human history: the Horus study of four ancient populations. Lancet 2013;381:1211–22.

[92] Allam AH, Thompson RC, Wann LS, et al. Atherosclerosis in Ancient Egyptian Mummies. JACC Cardiovasc Imaging 2011;4:315–27.

[93] Schilling S, Tzourio C, Dufouil C, et al. Plasma lipids and cerebral small vessel disease. Neurology 2014;83:1844–52.

[94] Estruch R, Ros E, Salas-Salvadó J, et al. Primary prevention of cardiovascular disease with a Mediterranean diet. Collaborators (233). N Engl J Med 2013;368(14):1279–90.

[95] Gardener H, Scarmeas N, Gu Y, Boden Albala B, Elkind MSV, Sacco RL, et al. Mediterranean diet and white matter hyperintensity volume in the Northern Manhattan Stroke Study. Arch Neurol 2012;69:251–6.

[96] O'Donnell MJ, et al. Risk Factors for ischemic and intracerebral hemorrhagic stroke in 22 countries (Interstroke study): a case control study. Lancet 2010;376:112–23.

[97] Ngandu T, Lehtisalo J, Solomon A, et al. A 2-year multidomain intervention of diet, exercise, cognitive training, and vascular risk monitoring versus control to prevent cognitive decline in at-risk elderly people (FINGER): a randomised controlled trial. Lancet 2015;385:2255 226.

[98] Baker LD, Espeland MA, Kivipelto M, Whitmer RA, Snyder HM, Carrillo MC, et al. US POINTER (USA) World-Wide FINGERS network: The first global network of multidomain dementia prevention trials. Alzheimer's & Dementia 2020;16:e046951.

[99] Xu X, Chew KA, Wong ZX, Phua AK, Chong EJ, Teo CK, et al. The SINgapore GERiatric Intervention Study to Reduce Cognitive Decline and Physical Frailty (SINGER): Study Design and Protocol. J Prev Alzheimers Dis 2022;9(1):40–8.

[100] Heffernan M, Andrews G, Fiatarone Singh MA, Valenzuela M, Anstey KJ, Maeder AJ, et al. Maintain your brain: protocol of a 3-year randomized controlled trial of a personalized multi-modal digital health intervention to prevent cognitive decline among community dwelling 55 to 77 year olds. J Alzheimers Dis 2019;70(s1):S221–37.

[101] Wang Y, Han X, Zhang X, Zhang Z, Cong L, Tang S, et al. Health status and risk profiles for brain aging of rural-dwelling older adults: Data from the interdisciplinary baseline assessments in MIND-China. Alzheimer's Dement: Transl Res Clin Interv 2022;8(1):e12254.

[102] Arora NA, Mehta TR. Role of the ketogenic diet in acute neurological diseases. Clin Neurol Neurosurg 2020;192. Available from: https://doi.org/10.1016/j.clineuro.2020.105727.

[103] McDonald TJW, Cervanka MC. Ketogenic diets for adult neurological disorders. Neurotherapeutics 2018;15:1018–31.

[104] Daniel G, Hackam DG, Spence DJ. Combining Multiple approaches for the secondary prevention of vascular events after stroke. a quantitative modeling study. Stroke 2007;38:1881–5.

[105] Elwood P, Galante J, Pickering J, et al. Healthy lifestyles reduce the incidence of chronic diseases and dementia: evidence from the caerphilly cohort study. PLoS One 1877;8(12):e8. Available from: https://doi.org/10.1371/journal.pone.0081877.

[106] Ross R, Blair SN, Arena R, et al. Importance of assessing cardiorespiratory fitness in clinical practice: a case for fitness as a clinical vital sign. Circulation 2016;134:e653–99.

[107] Beghi E. The epidemiology of epilepsy. Neuroepidemiology 2020;54(2):185–91. Available from: https://doi.org/10.1159/000503831.

[108] Fisher RS, Acevedo C, Arzimanoglou A, Bogacz A, Cross JH, Elger CE, et al. ILAE official report: a practical clinical definition of epilepsy. Epilepsia 2014;55(4):475–82. Available from: https://doi.org/10.1111/epi.12550.

[109] Pack AM. Epilepsy overview and revised classification of seizures and epilepsies. Continuum 2019;25(2):306–21. Available from: https://doi.org/10.1212/CON.0000000000000707.

[110] Cooper K, Kirkpatrick P, Brand C, Rolfe A, Florida-James S. Discussing sudden unexpected death in epilepsy with children and young people with epilepsy and their parents/carers: A mixed methods systematic review. Seizure 2020;78:159–67. Available from: https://doi.org/10.1016/j.seizure.2019.10.002.

[111] Berg AT, Rychlik K. The course of childhood-onset epilepsy over the first two decades: a prospective, longitudinal study. Epilepsia 2015;56(1):40–8. Available from: https://doi.org/10.1111/epi.12862.

[112] Perucca E, Brodie MJ, Kwan P, Tomson T. 30 years of second-generation antiseizure medications: impact and future perspectives. Lancet Neurol 2020;19(6):544–56. Available from: https://doi.org/10.1016/S1474-4422(20)30035-1.

[113] Arts WF, Geerts AT. When to start drug treatment for childhood epilepsy: the clinical-epidemiological evidence. Eur J Pediatr Neurol 2009;13(2):93–101. Available from: https://doi.org/10.1016/j.ejpn.2008.02.010.

[114] Chen Z, Brodie MJ, Liew D, Kwan P. Treatment outcomes in patients with newly diagnosed epilepsy treated with established and new antiepileptic drugs: A 30-year longitudinal cohort study. JAMA Neurol 2018;75(3):279–86. Available from: https://doi.org/10.1001/jamaneurol.2017.3949.

[115] Hoffman CE, Parker WE, Rapoport BI, Zhao M, Ma H, Schwartz TH. Innovations in the Neurosurgical Management of Epilepsy. World Neurosurg 2020;139:775–88. Available from: https://doi.org/10.1016/j.wneu.2020.03.031.

[116] Wilder RM. The effect of ketonemia on the course of epilepsy. Mayo Clinic Bull 1921;2:307–8.

[117] Wheless JW. History of the ketogenic diet. Epilepsia 2008;49(Suppl 8):3–5. Available from: https://doi.org/10.1111/j.1528-1167.2008.01821.x.

[118] Masino SA, Rho JM. Metabolism and epilepsy: Ketogenic diets as a homeostatic link. Brain Res 2019;170:26–30. Available from: https://doi.org/10.1016/j.brainres.2018.05.049.

[119] Olson CA, Vuong HE, Yano JM, Liang QY, Nusbaum DJ, Hsiao EY. The gut microbiota mediates the anti-seizure effects of the ketogenic diet. Cell 2018;174(2):497. Available from: https://doi.org/10.1016/j.cell.2018.06.051.

[120] Kossoff EH, Zupec-Kania BA, Auvin S, Ballaban-Gil KR, Christina Bergqvist AG, Blackford R, et al. Optimal clinical management of children receiving dietary therapies for epilepsy: Updated recommendations of the International Ketogenic Diet Study Group. Epilepsia Open 2018;3(2):175–92. Available from: https://doi.org/10.1002/epi4.12225.

[121] Huttenlocher P. Ketonemia and seizures: Metabolic and anticonvulsant effects of two ketogenic diets in childhood epilepsy. Pediatr Res 1976;10(5):536–40. Available from: https://doi.org/10.1203/00006450-197605000-00006.

[122] Neal EG, Chaffe H, Schwartz RH, Lawson MS, Edwards N, Fitzsimmons G, et al. A randomized trial of classical and medium-chain triglyceride ketogenic diets in the treatment of childhood epilepsy. Epilepsia 2009;50(5):1109–17. Available from: https://doi.org/10.1111/j.1528-1167.2008.01870.x.

[123] Kossoff EH, McGrogan JR, Bluml RM, Pillas DJ, Rubenstein JE, Vining EP. A modified Atkins diet is effective for the treatment of intractable pediatric epilepsy. Epilepsia 2006;47(2):421–4. Available from: https://doi.org/10.1111/j.1528-1167.2006.00438.x.

[124] Sondhi V, Agarwala A, Pandey RM, Chakrabarty B, Jauhari P, Lodha R, et al. Efficacy of ketogenic diet, modified Atkins diet, and low glycemic index therapy diet among children with drug-resistant epilepsy: A randomized clinical trial. JAMA Pediatr 2020;e202282. Available from: https://doi.org/10.1001/jamapediatrics.2020.2282.

[125] Muzykewicz DA, Lyczkowski DA, Memon N, Conant KD, Pfeifer HH, Thiele EA. Efficacy, safety, and tolerability of the low glycemic index treatment in pediatric epilepsy. Epilepsia 2009;50(5):1118–26. Available from: https://doi.org/10.1111/j.1528-1167.2008.01959.x.

[126] Martin-McGill KJ, Lambert B, Whiteley VJ, Wood S, Neal EG, Simpson ZR, et al. Understanding the core principles of a 'modified ketogenic diet': a UK and Ireland perspective. J Hum Nutr Diet 2019;32(3):385–90. Available from: https://doi.org/10.1111/jhn.12637.

[127] Hosain SA, La Vega-Talbott M, Solomon GE. Ketogenic diet in pediatric epilepsy patients with gastrostomy feeding. Pediatr Neurol 2005;32(2):81–3. Available from: https://doi.org/10.1016/j.pediatrneurol.2004.09.006.

[128] Cervenka MC, Henry BJ, Felton EA, Patton K, Kossoff EH. Establishing an Adult Epilepsy Diet Center: Experience, efficacy and challenges. Epilep Behav 2016;58:61–8. Available from: https://doi.org/10.1016/j.yebeh.2016.02.038.

[129] Kossoff EH, Laux LC, Blackford R, Morrison PF, Pyzik PL, Hamdy RM, et al. When do seizures improve with the ketogenic diet? Epilepsia 2008;49(2):329–33. Available from: https://doi.org/10.1111/j.1528-1167.2007.01417.x.

[130] Dressler A, Benninger F, Trimmel-Schwahofer P, Gröppel G, Porsche B, Abraham K, et al. Efficacy and tolerability of the ketogenic diet versus high-dose adrenocorticotropic hormone for infantile spasms: A single-center parallel-cohort randomized controlled trial. Epilepsia 2019;60(3):441–51. Available from: https://doi.org/10.1111/epi.14679.

[131] Kang HC, Chung DE, Kim DW, Kim HD. Early and late-onset complications of the ketogenic diet for intractable epilepsy. Epilepsia 2004;45(9):1116–23. Available from: https://doi.org/10.1111/j.0013-9580.2004.10004.x.

[132] Worden LT, Turner Z, Pyzik PL, Rubenstein JE, Kossoff EH. Is there an ideal way to discontinue the ketogenic diet? Epilepsy Res 2011;95(3):232–6. Available from: https://doi.org/10.1016/j.eplepsyres.2011.04.003.

[133] World Health Organization (2019). Dementia Fact Sheet. Updated Sept 2019. Accessed from https://www.who.int/news-room/fact-sheets/detail/dementia

[134] Alzheimer's Association (2020). Facts and Figures. https://www.alz.org/alzheimers-dementia/facts-figures. Accessed Sept 12, 2020.

[135] Belluck, P. (2018, November 19). Will we ever cure Alzheimer's? The New York Times. https://www.nytimes.com/2018/11/19/health/dementia-alzheimers-cure-drugs.html. Accessed October 31, 2020.

[136] Sperling RA, Aisen PS, Beckett LA, Bennett DA, Craft S, Fagan AM, et al. Toward defining the preclinical stages of Alzheimer's disease: Recommendations from the National Institute on Aging-Alzheimer's Association workgroups on diagnostic guidelines for Alzheimer's disease. Alzheimers Dement 2011;7(3):280–92. Available from: https://doi.org/10.1016/j.jalz.2011.03.003.

[137] DeTure MA, Dickson DW. The neuropathological diagnosis of Alzheimer's disease. Mol Neurodegener 2019;14(1):32. Available from: https://doi.org/10.1186/s13024-019-0333-5.

[138] de la Monte SM. The full spectrum of Alzheimer's disease is rooted in metabolic derangements that drive type 3 diabetes. Adv Exp Med Biol 2019;1128:45–83. Available from: https://doi.org/10.1007/978-981-13-3540-2_4.

[139] Arnold SE, Arvanitakis Z, Macauley-Rambach SL, Koenig AM, Wang HY, Ahima RS, et al. Brain insulin resistance in type 2 diabetes and Alzheimer disease: concepts and conundrums. Nat Rev Neurol 2018;14(3):168–81. Available from: https://doi.org/10.1038/nrneurol.2017.185.

[140] Leszek J, Trypka E, Tarasov VV, Ashraf GM, Aliev G. Type 3 diabetes mellitus: a novel implication of Alzheimers disease. Curr Top Med Chem 2017;17(12):1331–5. Available from: https://doi.org/10.2174/1568026617666170103163403.

[141] Cunnane S, Nugent S, Roy M, Courchesne-Loyer A, Croteau E, Tremblay S, et al. Brain fuel metabolism, aging, and Alzheimer's disease. Nutrition 2011;27(1):3–20. Available from: https://doi.org/10.1016/j.nut.2010.07.021.

[142] Hashim SA, VanItallie TB. Ketone body therapy: From the ketogenic diet to the oral administration of ketone ester. J Lipid Res 2014;55 (9):1818–26. Available from: https://doi.org/10.1194/jlr.R046599.

[143] Mosconi L, De Santi S, Li J, Tsui WH, Li Y, Boppana M, et al. Hippocampal hypometabolism predicts cognitive decline from normal aging. Neurobiol Aging 2008;29(5):676–92. Available from: https://doi.org/10.1016/j.neurobiolaging.2006.12.008.

[144] Fukuyama H, Ogawa M, Yamauchi H, Yamaguchi S, Kimura J, Yonekura Y, et al. Altered cerebral energy metabolism in Alzheimer's disease: a PET study. J Nucl Med 1994;35(1):1–6.

[145] Baker LD, Cross DJ, Minoshima S, Belongia D, Watson GS, Craft S. Insulin resistance and Alzheimer-like reductions in regional cerebral glucose metabolism for cognitively normal adults with prediabetes or early type 2 diabetes. Arch Neurol 2011;68(1):51–7. Available from: https://doi.org/10.1001/archneurol.2010.225.

[146] Mosconi L, Sorbi S, de Leon MJ, Li Y, Nacmias B, Myoung PS, et al. Hypometabolism exceeds atrophy in presymptomatic early-onset familial Alzheimer's disease. J Nucl Med 2006;47(11):1778–86.

[147] Cunnane SC, Courchesne-Loyer A, Vandenberghe C, St-Pierre V, Fortier M, Hennebelle M, et al. Can ketones help rescue brain fuel supply in later life? Implications for cognitive health during aging and the treatment of Alzheimer's disease. Front Mol Neurosci 2016;9:53. Available from: https://doi.org/10.3389/fnmol.2016.00053.

[148] Reiman EM, Chen K, Alexander GE, Caselli RJ, Bandy D, Osborne D, et al. Functional brain abnormalities in young adults at genetic risk for late-onset Alzheimer's dementia. Proc Natl Acad Sci USA 2004;101(1):284–9. Available from: https://doi.org/10.1073/pnas.2635903100.

[149] Kerti L, Witte AV, Winkler A, Grittner U, Rujescu D, Flöel A. Higher glucose levels associated with lower memory and reduced hippocampal microstructure. Neurology 2013;81(20):1746–52. Available from: https://doi.org/10.1212/01.wnl.0000435561.00234.ee.

[150] Crane PK, Walker R, Hubbard RA, Li G, Nathan DM, Zheng H, et al. Glucose levels and risk of dementia. N Engl J Med 2013;369 (6):540–8. Available from: https://doi.org/10.1056/NEJMoa1215740.

[151] Young SE, Mainous 3rd AG, Carnemolla M. Hyperinsulinemia and cognitive decline in a middle-aged cohort. Diabetes Care 2006;29 (12):2688–93. Available from: https://doi.org/10.2337/dc06-0915.

[152] Banks WA, Owen JB, Erickson MA. Insulin in the brain: There and back again. Pharmacol Ther 2012;136(1):82–93. Available from: https://doi.org/10.1016/j.pharmthera.2012.07.006.

[153] Correia SC, Santos RX, Carvalho C, Cardoso S, Candeias E, Santos MS, et al. Insulin signaling, glucose metabolism and mitochondria: major players in Alzheimer's disease and diabetes interrelation. Brain Res 2012;1441:64–78. Available from: https://doi.org/10.1016/j.brainres.2011.12.063 Mar 2.

[154] Kellar D, Craft S. Brain insulin resistance in Alzheimer's disease and related disorders: mechanisms and therapeutic approaches. Lancet Neurol 2020;19(9):758–66. Available from: https://doi.org/10.1016/S1474-4422(20)30231-3.

[155] Cholerton B, Baker LD, Craft S. Insulin, cognition, and dementia. Eur J Pharmacol 2013;719(1-3):170–9. Available from: https://doi.org/10.1016/j.ejphar.2013.08.008.

[156] Cholerton B, Baker LD, Montine TJ, Craft S. Type 2 diabetes, cognition, and dementia in older adults: toward a precision health approach. Diab Spectrum 2016;29(4):210–19. Available from: https://doi.org/10.2337/ds16-0041.

[157] Castello MA, Jeppson JD, Soriano S. Moving beyond anti-amyloid therapy for the prevention and treatment of Alzheimer's disease. BMC Neurol 2014;14:169. Available from: https://doi.org/10.1186/s12883-014-0169-0.

[158] Morris GP, Clark IA, Vissel B. Inconsistencies and controversies surrounding the amyloid hypothesis of Alzheimer's disease. Acta Neuropathol Commun 2014;2:135. Available from: https://doi.org/10.1186/s40478-014-0135-5.

[159] Mamelak M. Alzheimer' s disease, oxidative stress and gammahydroxybutyrate. Neurobiol Aging 2007;28(9):1340–60. Available from: https://doi.org/10.1016/j.neurobiolaging.2006.06.008.

[160] Castello MA, Soriano S. On the origin of Alzheimer's disease: trials and tribulations of the amyloid hypothesis. Ageing Res Rev 2014;13:10–12. Available from: https://doi.org/10.1016/j.arr.2013.10.001.

[161] Eli Lilly and Company. (2010, August 17). Lilly halts development of semagacestat for Alzheimer's disease based on preliminary results of Phase III clinical trials. https://investor.lilly.com/news-releases/news-release-details/lilly-halts-development-semagacestat-alzheimers-disease-based?releaseid = 499794. Accessed Sept 12, 2020.

[162] Mawuenyega KG, Sigurdson W, Ovod V, Munsell L, Kasten T, Morris JC, et al. Decreased clearance of CNS beta-amyloid in Alzheimer's disease. Science 2010;330(6012):1774. Available from: https://doi.org/10.1126/science.1197623.

[163] Mullins RJ, Diehl TC, Chia CW, Kapogiannis D. Insulin resistance as a link between amyloid-beta and tau pathologies in Alzheimer's disease. Front Aging Neurosci 2017;9:118. Available from: https://doi.org/10.3389/fnagi.2017.00118.

[164] Orr ME, Sullivan AC, Frost B. A brief overview of tauopathy: causes, consequences, and therapeutic strategies. Trends Pharmacol Sci 2017;38(7):637–48. Available from: https://doi.org/10.1016/j.tips.2017.03.011.

[165] Fishwick KJ, Rylett RJ. Insulin regulates the activity of the high-affinity choline transporter CHT. PLoS One 2015;10(7):e0132934. Available from: https://doi.org/10.1371/journal.pone.0132934.

[166] Sposato V, Canu N, Fico E, Fusco S, Bolasco G, Ciotti MT, et al. The medial septum is insulin resistant in the AD presymptomatic phase: Rescue by nerve growth factor-driven IRS1 activation. Mol Neurobiol 2019;56(1):535–52. Available from: https://doi.org/10.1007/s12035-018-1038-4.

[167] Hampel H, Mesulam MM, Cuello AC, Farlow MR, Giacobini E, Grossberg GT, et al. The cholinergic system in the pathophysiology and treatment of Alzheimer's disease. Brain 2018;141(7):1917–33. Available from: https://doi.org/10.1093/brain/awy132.

[168] Fried PJ, Pascual-Leone A, Bolo NR. Diabetes and the link between neuroplasticity and glutamate in the aging human motor cortex. Clin Neurophysiol 2019;130(9):1502–10. Available from: https://doi.org/10.1016/j.clinph.2019.04.721.

[169] Kamboh MI. Apolipoprotein E polymorphism and susceptibility to Alzheimer's disease. Hum Biol 1995;67(2):195–215.

[170] Qiu WQ, Folstein MF. Insulin, insulin-degrading enzyme and amyloid-beta peptide in Alzheimer's disease: review and hypothesis. Neurobiol Aging 2006;27(2):190–8. Available from: https://doi.org/10.1016/j.neurobiolaging.2005.01.004.

[171] Henderson ST. High carbohydrate diets and Alzheimer's disease. Med Hypotheses 2004;62(5):689–700. Available from: https://doi.org/10.1016/j.mehy.2003.11.028.

[172] National Institute on Aging. (2019, September 27). What do we know about diet and prevention of Alzheimer's Disease? https://www.nia.nih.gov/health/what-do-we-know-about-diet-and-prevention-alzheimers-disease

[173] Grammatikopoulou MG, Goulis DG, Gkiouras K, Theodoridis X, Gkouskou KK, Evangeliou A, et al. To keto or not to keto? A systematic review of randomized controlled trials assessing the effects of ketogenic therapy on Alzheimer disease Adv Nutr 2020;nmaa073. Advance online publication. Available from: https://doi.org/10.1093/advances/nmaa073.

[174] Phillips M, Deprez LM, Mortimer G, Murtagh D, McCoy S, Mylchreest R, et al. Randomized crossover trial of a modified ketogenic diet in Alzheimer's disease. Alzheimer's Res Ther 2021;13(1):51. Available from: https://doi.org/10.1186/s13195-021-00783-x.

[175] Croteau E, Castellano CA, Fortier M, Bocti C, Fulop T, Paquet N, et al. A cross-sectional comparison of brain glucose and ketone metabolism in cognitively healthy older adults, mild cognitive impairment and early Alzheimer's disease. Exp Gerontol 2018;107:18–26. Available from: https://doi.org/10.1016/j.exger.2017.07.004.

[176] Henderson ST, Vogel JL, Barr LJ, Garvin F, Jones JJ, Costantini LC. Study of the ketogenic agent AC-1202 in mild to moderate Alzheimer's disease: a randomized, double-blind, placebo-controlled, multicenter trial. Nutr Metab (Lond.) 2009;6:31. Available from: https://doi.org/10.1186/1743-7075-6-31.

[177] Ota M, Matsuo J, Ishida I, Takano H, Yokoi Y, Hori H, et al. Effects of a medium-chain triglyceride-based ketogenic formula on cognitive function in patients with mild-to-moderate Alzheimer's disease. Neurosci Lett 2019;690:232–6. Available from: https://doi.org/10.1016/j.neulet.2018.10.048.

[178] Xu Q, Zhang Y, Zhang X, Liu L, Zhou B, Mo R, et al. Medium-chain triglycerides improved cognition and lipid metabolomics in mild to moderate Alzheimer's disease patients with APOE4$^{-/-}$: a double-blind, randomized, placebo-controlled crossover trial. Clinical Nutrition (Edinburgh, Scotland) 2020;39(7):2092–105. Available from: https://doi.org/10.1016/j.clnu.2019.10.017.

[179] Croteau E, Castellano CA, Richard MA, Fortier M, Nugent S, Lepage M, et al. Ketogenic medium chain triglycerides increase brain energy metabolism in Alzheimer's disease. Journal of Alzheimer's Disease: JAD 2018;64(2):551–61. Available from: https://doi.org/10.3233/JAD-180202.

[180] Fortier M, Castellano CA, Croteau E, Langlois F, Bocti C, St-Pierre V, et al. A ketogenic drink improves brain energy and some measures of cognition in mild cognitive impairment. Alzheimer's & Dementia: The Journal of the Alzheimer's Association 2019;15(5):625–34. Available from: https://doi.org/10.1016/j.jalz.2018.12.017.

[181] Newport MT, VanItallie TB, Kashiwaya Y, King MT, Veech RL. A new way to produce hyperketonemia: use of ketone ester in a case of Alzheimer's disease. Alzheimer's & Dementia: The Journal of the Alzheimer's Association 2015;11(1):99–103. Available from: https://doi.org/10.1016/j.jalz.2014.01.006.

[182] Krikorian R, Shidler MD, Dangelo K, Couch SC, Benoit SC, Clegg DJ. Dietary ketosis enhances memory in mild cognitive impairment Neurobiol Aging 2012;33(2):425. e19–425.e4.25E27. Available from: https://doi.org/10.1016/j.neurobiolaging.2010.10.006.

[183] Stoykovich S, Gibas K. *APOE* ε4, the door to insulin-resistant dyslipidemia and brain fog? A case study. Alzheimer's & Dementia (Amsterdam, Netherlands) 2019;11:264–9. Available from: https://doi.org/10.1016/j.dadm.2019.01.009.

[184] Brown D, Gibas KJ. Metabolic syndrome marks early risk for cognitive decline with APOE4 gene variation: A case study. Diabetes & Metabolic Syndrome 2018;12(5):823–7. Available from: https://doi.org/10.1016/j.dsx.2018.04.030.

[185] Dahlgren K, Gibas KJ. Ketogenic diet, high intensity interval training (HIIT) and memory training in the treatment of mild cognitive impairment: a case study. Diabetes & Metabolic Syndrome 2018;12(5):819–22. Available from: https://doi.org/10.1016/j.dsx.2018.04.031.

[186] Stafstrom CE, Rho JM. The ketogenic diet as a treatment paradigm for diverse neurological disorders. Frontiers in Pharmacology 2012;3:59. Available from: https://doi.org/10.3389/fphar.2012.00059.

[187] Anderson RJ, Freedland KE, Clouse RE, Lustman PJ. The prevalence of comorbid depression in adults with diabetes: a meta-analysis. Diabetes Care 2001;24(6):1069–78.

[188] Watson KT, Simard JF, Henderson VW, Nutkiewicz L, Lamers F, Nasca C, et al. Incident Major Depressive Disorder Predicted by Three Measures of Insulin Resistance: A Dutch Cohort Study. AJP 2021;178(10):914–20.

[189] Chand SP, Arif H. Depression StatPearls [Internet]. Treasure Island (FL): StatPearls Publishing; 2020 [cited 2020 Nov 1]. Available from. Available from: http://www.ncbi.nlm.nih.gov/books/NBK430847/.

[190] Deleted in review.

[191] Hasin DS, Sarvet AL, Meyers JL, Saha TD, Ruan WJ, Stohl M, et al. Epidemiology of Adult DSM-5 Major Depressive Disorder and Its Specifiers in the United States. JAMA Psychiatry 2018;75(4):336–46.

[192] Greenberg PE, Fournier A-A, Sisitsky T, Simes M, Berman R, Koenigsberg SH, et al. The Economic Burden of Adults with Major Depressive Disorder in the United States (2010 and 2018). Pharmacoeconomics 2021;39(6):653 65.1.

[193] Nordentoft M, Mortensen PB, Pedersen CB. Absolute Risk of Suicide After First Hospital Contact in Mental Disorder. Arch Gen Psychiatry 2011;68(10):1058–64.

[194] McGuffin P, Rijsdijk F, Andrew M, Sham P, Katz R, Cardno A. The heritability of bipolar affective disorder and the genetic relationship to unipolar depression. Arch Gen Psychiatry 2003;60(5):497–502.

[195] Merikangas KR, Akiskal HS, Angst J, Greenberg PE, Hirschfeld RMA, Petukhova M, et al. Lifetime and 12-Month Prevalence of Bipolar Spectrum Disorder in the National Comorbidity Survey Replication. Arch Gen Psychiatry 2007;64(5):543–52.

[196] Bessonova L, Ogden K, Doane MJ, O'Sullivan AK, Tohen M. The Economic Burden of Bipolar Disorder in the United States: A Systematic Literature Review. Clinicoecon Outcomes Res 2020;12:481–97.

[197] Monson ET, Shabalin AA, Docherty AR, DiBlasi E, Bakian AV, Li QS, et al. Assessment of suicide attempt and death in bipolar affective disorder: a combined clinical and genetic approach. Transl Psychiatry 2021;11(1):1–8.

[198] Dome P, Rihmer Z, Gonda X. Suicide Risk in Bipolar Disorder: A Brief Review. Medicina (Kaunas) 2019;55(8):E403.

[199] First MB, Drevets WC, Carter C, et al. Clinical Applications of Neuroimaging in Psychiatric Disorders. Am J Psychiatry 2018;175(9):915–16. Available from: https://doi.org/10.1176/appi.ajp.2018.1750701.

[200] Charlton BG. The malaise theory of depression: major depressive disorder is sickness behavior and antidepressants are analgesic. Med Hypotheses 2000;54(1):126–30.

[201] Norwitz NG, Dalai SS, Palmer CM. Ketogenic diet as a metabolic treatment for mental illness. Curr Opin Endocrinol Diabetes Obes 2020;27 (5):269–74.

[202] Osimo EF, Pillinger T, Rodriguez IM, Khandaker GM, Pariante CM, Howes OD. Inflammatory markers in depression: A meta-analysis of mean differences and variability in 5,166 patients and 5,083 controls. Brain Behav Immun 2020;87:901–9. 2020/02/27 ed.

[203] Felger JC, Lotrich FE. Inflammatory Cytokines in Depression: Neurobiological Mechanisms and Therapeutic Implications. Neuroscience 2013;246:199–229.

[204] Enache D, Pariante CM, Mondelli V. Markers of central inflammation in major depressive disorder: A systematic review and meta-analysis of studies examining cerebrospinal fluid, positron emission tomography and post-mortem brain tissue. Brain Behav Immun 2019;81:24–40.

[205] Morris G, Puri BK, Carvalho A, Maes M, Berk M, Ruusunen A, et al. Induced Ketosis as a Treatment for Neuroprogressive Disorders: Food for Thought? Int J Neuropsychopharmacol 2020;23(6):366–84.

[206] Duman RS, Sanacora G, Krystal JH. Altered Connectivity in Depression: GABA and Glutamate Neurotransmitter Deficits and Reversal by Novel Treatments. Neuron 2019;102(1):75–90.

[207] Salim S. Oxidative stress and psychological disorders. Curr Neuropharmacol 2014;12(2):140–7.

[208] Fakhoury WKH, Wright D, Wallace M. Prevalence and extent of distress of adverse effects of antipsychotics among callers to a United Kingdom National Mental Health Helpline. Int Clin Psychopharmacol 2001;16(3):153–62.

[209] Himmerich H, Minkwitz J, Kirkby KC. Weight Gain and Metabolic Changes During Treatment with Antipsychotics and Antidepressants. Endocr Metab Immune Disord Drug Targets 2015;15(4):252–60. Available from: https://doi.org/10.2174/1871530315666150623092031; PMID: 26100432.

[210] Marvanova M. Strategies for prevention and management of second generation antipsychotic-induced metabolic side effects. Mental Health Clinician 2013;3(3):154–61.

[211] Miller JN, Black DW. Bipolar Disorder and Suicide: a Review. Curr Psychiatry Rep 2020;22(2):6.

[212] Semahegn A, Torpey K, Manu A, Assefa N, Tesfaye G, Ankomah A. Psychotropic medication non-adherence and its associated factors among patients with major psychiatric disorders: a systematic review and meta-analysis. Systematic Reviews 2020;9(1):17.

[213] Gangwisch JE, Hale L, Garcia L, Malaspina D, Opler MG, Payne ME, et al. High glycemic index diet as a risk factor for depression: analyses from the Women's Health Initiative. Am J Clin Nutr 2015;102(2):454–63. Available from: https://doi.org/10.3945/ajcn.114.103846; Epub 2015 Jun 24. PMID: 26109579.

[214] Salari-Moghaddam A, Saneei P, Larijani B, Esmaillzadeh A. Glycemic index, glycemic load, and depression: a systematic review and meta-analysis. Eur J Clin Nutr 2019;73(3):356–65.

[215] Cox DJ, Kovatchev BP, Gonder-Frederick LA, Summers KH, McCall A, Grimm KJ, et al. Relationships Between Hyperglycemia and Cognitive Performance Among Adults With Type 1 and Type 2 Diabetes. Diabetes Care 2005;28(1):71.

[216] Geijselaers SLC, Sep SJS, Claessens D, Schram MT, van Boxtel MPJ, Henry RMA, et al. The Role of Hyperglycemia, Insulin Resistance, and Blood Pressure in Diabetes-Associated Differences in Cognitive Performance-The Maastricht Study. Diabetes Care 2017;40(11):1537–47.

[217] Hall H, Perelman D, Breschi A, Limcaoco P, Kellogg R, McLaughlin T, et al. Glucotypes reveal new patterns of glucose dysregulation. PLoS Biol 2018;16(7):e2005143. Available from: https://doi.org/10.1371/journal.pbio.2005143.

[218] Hypoglycemia - Hormonal and Metabolic Disorders [Internet]. Merck Manuals Consumer Version. [cited 2022 Jan 9]. Available from: https://www.merckmanuals.com/home/hormonal-and-metabolic-disorders/diabetes-mellitus-dm-and-disorders-of-blood-sugar-metabolism/hypoglycemia.

[219] Low Blood Glucose (Hypoglycemia) | American Diabetes Association [Internet]. Available from: https://professional.diabetes.org/pel/low-blood-glucose-hypoglycemia-english.

[220] DeWall CN, Deckman T, Gailliot MT, Bushman BJ. Sweetened blood cools hot tempers: physiological self-control and aggression. Aggress Behav 2011;37(1):73–80.

[221] Bushman B, Dewall C, Pond JR, Hanus M. Low glucose relates to greater aggression in married couples. Proceedings of the National Academy of Sciences of the United States of America 2014;111.

[222] Morris G, Puri BK, Maes M, Olive L, Berk M, Carvalho AF. The role of microglia in neuroprogressive disorders: mechanisms and possible neurotherapeutic effects of induced ketosis. Progress in Neuro-Psychopharmacology and Biological Psychiatry 2020;99:109858.

[223] Drenick EJ, Alvarez LC, Tamasi GC, Brickman AS. Resistance to Symptomatic Insulin Reactions after Fasting. J Clin Invest 1972;51(10):2757–62.

[224] Brietzke E, Mansur RB, Subramaniapillai M, Balanzá-Martínez V, Vinberg M, González-Pinto A, et al. Ketogenic diet as a metabolic therapy for mood disorders: Evidence and developments. Neurosci Biobehav Rev 2018;94:11–16.

[225] Rojas-Morales P, Pedraza-Chaverri J, Tapia E. Ketone bodies, stress response, and redox homeostasis. Redox Biol 2019;29:101395.

[226] Umare MD, Wankhede NL, Bajaj KK, Trivedi RV, Taksande BG, Umekar MJ, et al. Interweaving of reactive oxygen species and major neurological and psychiatric disorders. Annales Pharmaceutiques Françaises. Elsevier Masson; 2021.

[227] Adams RN, et al. Depressive symptoms improve over 2 years of type 2 diabetes treatment via a digital continuous remote care intervention focused on carbohydrate restriction. Journal of Behavioral Medicine [Preprint] 2022. Available from: https://doi.org/10.1007/s10865-021-00272-4.

[228] Ortí JE, de la R, et al. Can ketogenic diet improve Alzheimer's disease? Association with anxiety, depression, and glutamate system. Frontiers in Nutrition 2021;8. Available from: https://doi.org/10.3389/fnut.2021.744398.

[229] Palmer CM. Ketogenic diet in the treatment of schizoaffective disorder: Two case studies. Schizophr Res 2017;189:208–9. Available from: https://doi.org/10.1016/j.schres.2017.01.053.

[230] Palmer CM, Gilbert-Jaramillo J, Westman EC. The ketogenic diet and remission of psychotic symptoms in schizophrenia: Two case studies. Schizophrenia Research [Preprint] 2019. Available from: https://doi.org/10.1016/j.schres.2019.03.019.

[231] Pieklik A, et al. The ketogenic diet: a co-therapy in the treatment of mood disorders and obesity - a case report Current Problems of Psychiatry 2021. 0(0), p. 000010247820210002. Available from: https://doi.org/10.2478/cpp-2021-0002.

[232] Tidman MM, White D, White T. Effects of an low carbohydrate/healthy fat/ketogenic diet on biomarkers of health and symptoms, anxiety and depression in Parkinson's disease: a pilot study. Neurodegenerative Disease Management [Preprint] 2022. Available from: https://doi.org/10.2217/nmt-2021-0033.

[233] Ludwig DS. The ketogenic diet: evidence for optimism but high-quality research needed. J Nutr 2020;150(6):1354–9. Available from: https://doi.org/10.1093/jn/nxz308; PMID: 31825066.

[234] Deleted in review.

[235] Schumacher GA, Beebe G, Kibler RF, et al. Problems of experimental trials of therapy in multiple sclerosis: report by the panel on the evaluation of experimental trials of therapy in multiple sclerosis. Ann N Y Acad Sci 1965;122:552–68. Available from: https://doi.org/10.1111/j.1749-6632.1965.tb20235.x.

[236] Thompson AJ, Banwell BL, Barkhof F, et al. Diagnosis of multiple sclerosis: 2017 revisions of the McDonald criteria. Lancet Neurol 2018;17(2):162–73. Available from: https://doi.org/10.1016/S1474-4422(17)30470-2.

[237] Willer CJ, Dyment DA, Risch NJ, et al. Twin concordance and sibling recurrence rates in multiple sclerosis. Proc Natl Acad Sci U S A 2003;100(22):12877–82. Available from: https://doi.org/10.1073/pnas.1932604100.

[238] Moutsianas L, Jostins L, Beecham AH, et al. Class II HLA interactions modulate genetic risk for multiple sclerosis. Nat Genet 2015;47(10):1107–13. Available from: https://doi.org/10.1038/ng.3395.

[239] Hedström AK, Bomfim IL, Barcellos L, et al. Interaction between adolescent obesity and HLA risk genes in the etiology of multiple sclerosis. Neurology 2014;82(10):865–72. Available from: https://doi.org/10.1212/WNL.0000000000000203.

[240] Hedström AK, Åkerstedt T, Olsson T, Alfredsson L. Shift work influences multiple sclerosis risk. Mult Scler 2015;21(9):1195–9. Available from: https://doi.org/10.1177/1352458514563592.

[241] Huseby ES, Liggitt D, Brabb T, et al. A pathogenic role for myelin-specific CD8(+) T cells in a model for multiple sclerosis. J Exp Med 2001;194(5):669–76. Available from: https://doi.org/10.1084/jem.194.5.669.

[242] Bäärnhielm M, Hedström AK, Kockum I, et al. Sunlight is associated with decreased multiple sclerosis risk: no interaction with human leukocyte antigen-DRB1*15. Eur J Neurol 2012;19(7):955–62. Available from: https://doi.org/10.1111/j.1468-1331.2011.03650.x.

[243] Lucas RM, Ponsonby AL, Dear K, et al. Sun exposure and vitamin D are independent risk factors for CNS demyelination. Neurology 2011;76(6):540–8. Available from: https://doi.org/10.1212/WNL.0b013e31820af93d.

[244] Alfredsson L, Olsson T. Lifestyle and environmental factors in multiple sclerosis. Cold Spring Harb Perspect Med. 2019;9(4):a028944. Available from: https://doi.org/10.1101/cshperspect.a028944 PMID: 29735578; PMCID: PMC6444694.

[245] Tremlett H, Fadrosh DW, Faruqi AA, et al. Gut microbiota in early pediatric multiple sclerosis: a case-control study. Eur J Neurol 2016;23(8):1308–21. Available from: https://doi.org/10.1111/ene.13026.

[246] Chen J, Chia N, Kalari KR, et al. Multiple sclerosis patients have a distinct gut microbiota compared to healthy controls. Sci Rep 2016;6:28484. Available from: https://doi.org/10.1038/srep28484.

[247] Baranzini SE, Oksenberg JR. The genetics of multiple sclerosis: from 0 to 200 in 50 years. Trends Genet 2017;33(12):960–70. Available from: https://doi.org/10.1016/j.tig.2017.09.004.

[248] Rovira A, et al. MAGNIMS consensus guidelines on the use of MRI in multiple sclerosis—clinical implementation in the diagnostic process. Nat. Rev. Neurol. 2015;11:471–82.

[249] Hoffmann M. Clinical Mentation Evaluation. A Connectomal Approach to Rapid and Comprehensive Assessment. New York: Springer; 2020. p. 147. Available from: https://doi.org/10.1007/978-3-030-46324-3.

[250] Kurtzke JF. Rating neurologic impairment in multiple sclerosis: An expanded disability status scale EDSS. Neurology 1983;33:1444–52. Available from: https://doi.org/10.1212/wnl.33.11.1444.

[251] CNS Vital Signs - Computerized Neurocognitive Assessment Software [Internet]. [cited 2022 Aug 24]. Available from: https://www.cnsvs.com/

[252] Le Page E, Veillard D, Laplaud DA, et al. Oral versus intravenous high-dose methylprednisolone for treatment of relapses in patients with multiple sclerosis (COPOUSEP): a randomised, controlled, double-blind, non-inferiority trial. Lancet 2015;386(9997):974–81. Available from: https://doi.org/10.1016/S0140-6736(15)61137-0.

[253] Morrow SA, Alexander J, Day FC, et al. Effect of treating acute optic neuritis with bioequivalent oral vs intravenous corticosteroids. a randomized clinical trial. JAMA Neurol. 2018;75(6):690–6. Available from: https://doi.org/10.1001/jamaneurol.2018.0024.

[254] Sedel F, Bernard D, Mock DM, Tourbah A. Targeting demyelination and virtual hypoxia with high-dose biotin as a treatment for progressive multiple sclerosis. Neuropharmacology 2016;110:644–53.

[255] Gross RH, Corboy JR. Monitoring, switching, and stopping multiple sclerosis disease- modifying therapies. Continuum (Minneap Minn) 2019;25(3):715–35.

[256] Rae-Grant A, Day GS, Marrie RA, et al. Practice guideline recommendations summary: disease-modifying therapies for adults with multiple sclerosis: report of the Guideline Development, Dissemination, and Implementation Subcommittee of the American Academy of Neurology. Neurology 2018;90(17):777–88. Available from: https://doi.org/10.1212/WNL.0000000000005347.

[257] Marshall O, Lu H, Brisset J-C, Xu F, Liu P, Herbert J, et al. Impaired cerebrovascular reactivity in multiple sclerosis. JAMA Neurology 2014;71:1275–81.

[258] Benlloch M, López-Rodríguez MM, Cuerda-Ballester M, Drehmer E, Carrera S, Ceron JJ, et al. Satiating effect of a ketogenic diet and its impact on muscle improvement and oxidation state in multiple sclerosis patients. Nutrients. 2019;11(5):1156.

[259] Leavitt VM, et al. Aerobic exercise increases hippocampal volume and improves memory in multiple sclerosis: preliminary findings. Neurocase 2014;20:695–7.

[260] Shobeiri P, Karimi A, Momtazmanesh S, et al. Exercise-induced increase in blood-based brain-derived neurotrophic factor (BDNF) in people with multiple sclerosis: A systematic review and meta-analysis of exercise intervention trials. PLoS One 2022. Available from: https://doi.org/10.1371/journal.pone.0264557.

[261] Brenton JN, Banwell B, Bergqvist AGC, et al. Pilot study of a ketogenic diet in relapsing- remitting MS. Neurol Neuroimmunol Neuroinflamm 2019;6:e565. Available from: https://doi.org/10.1212/NXI.0000000000000565.

[262] Brenton JN, Lehner-Gulotta D, Woolbright E, Banwell B, Bergqvist AGC, Chen S, et al. Phase II study of ketogenic diets in relapsing multiple sclerosis: safety, tolerability and potential clinical benefits J Neurol Neurosurg Psychiatry [Internet] 2022; Apr 13 [cited 2022 Apr 24]; Available from. Available from: https://jnnp.bmj.com/content/early/2022/04/13/jnnp-2022-329074.

[263] Storoni M, Plant GT. The therapeutic potential of the ketogenic diet in treating progressive multiple sclerosis. Multiple Sclerosis International 2015;Volume:9. Available from: https://doi.org/10.1016/j.ebiom.2018.08.057; Article ID 681289.

[264] Bock M, Karber M, Kuhn H. Ketogenic diets attenuate cyclooxygenase and lipoxygenase gene expression in multiple sclerosis. EBioMedicine 2018;36:293–303.

[265] Swidsinski A., Dörffel Y., Loening Baucke V. et al. Reduced mass and diversity of the colonic microbiome in patients with multiple sclerosis and their improvement with ketogenic diet. Front. Microbiol, 28. Available from: https://doi.org/10.3389/fmicb.2017.01141

[266] Parkinson's News Today. Accessed June 5, 2020. Parkinson's Disease Statistics. {https://parkinsonsnewstoday.com/parkinsons-disease-statistics/}

[267] Haining R, Achat-Mendes C. Neuromelanin, one of the most overlooked molecules in modern medicine, is not a spectator. Neural Regen Res 2017;12(3):372–5.

[268] Langston W. The MPTP Story. Journal of Parkinson's Disease 2017;7(s1):S11–19.

[269] Parker W, Boyson S. Abnormalities of the electron transport chain in idiopathic Parkinson's disease. Ann Neurol 1989;26(6):719–23.

[270] Bindoff L, Birch-Machin M, Cartlidge N, et al. Respiratory chain abnormalities in skeletal muscle from patients with Parkinson's disease. J Neurol Sci 1991;104:203–8.

[271] Franco-Iborra S, Vila M, Perier C. Mitochondrial quality control in neurodegenerative diseases: focus on Parkinson's Disease and Huntington's disease. Frontiers in Neuroscience 2018;12. https://www.frontiersin.org/article/10.3389/fnins.2018.00342.

[272] Wang Q, Ren N, Cai Z, et al. Paraquat and MPTP induce neurodegeneration and alteration in the expression profile of microRNAs: the role of transcription factor Nrf2. NPJ Parkinsons Dis 2017;3:31. Available from: https://doi.org/10.1038/s41531-017-0033-1; Published 2017 Oct 20.

[273] Tanner CM, Kamel F, Ross GW, et al. Rotenone, paraquat, and Parkinson's disease. Environ Health Perspect 2011;119(6):866–72. Available from: https://doi.org/10.1289/ehp.1002839.

[274] Tangamornsuksan W, Lohitnavy O, Sruamsiri R, Chaiyakunapruk N, Norman Scholfield C, Reisfeld B, et al. Paraquat exposure and Parkinson's disease: A systematic review and meta-analysis. Arch Environ Occup Health. 2019;74(5):225–38. Available from: https://doi.org/10.1080/19338244.2018.1492894 Epub 2018 Nov 25. Erratum in: Arch Environ Occup Health. 2019;74(5):292-293. PMID: 30474499.

[275] Vaccari C, El Dib R, Gomaa H, Lopes LC, de Camargo JL. Paraquat and Parkinson's disease: a systematic review and meta-analysis of observational studies. J Toxicol Environ Health B Crit Rev 2019;22(5-6):172–202. Available from: https://doi.org/10.1080/10937404.2019.1659197.

[276] Weed DL. Does paraquat cause Parkinson's disease? A review of reviews. Neurotoxicology 2021;86:180–4.

[277] Wen S, Aki T, Unuma K, Uemura K. Chemically induced models of Parkinson's disease: history and perspectives for the involvement of ferroptosis Frontiers in Cellular Neuroscience [Internet] 2020;14[cited 2022 Mar 9]. Available from: https://www.frontiersin.org/article/10.3389/fncel.2020.581191.

[278] Devi L, Raghavendran V, Prabhu BM, Avadhani NG, Anandatheerthavarada H. Mitochondrial import and accumulation of alpha-synuclein impair complex I in human dopaminergic neuronal cultures and Parkinson disease brain. J Biol Chem 2008;283:9089–100.

[279] Lim S, Lang A. The nonmotor symptoms of Parkinson's disease—an overview. Mov Disord 2010;25(Suppl 1):S123–30.

[280] Seppi K, Weintraub D, et al. The *movement* disorder society evidence-based medicine review update: treatments for the non-motor symptoms of Parkinson's disease. Mov Disord 2011;26(03):S42–80.

[281] Fahn S, Elton RL, UPDRS Program Members. Unified Parkinson's disease rating scale. In: Fahn S, Marsden CD, Goldstein M, Calne DB, editors. Recent developments in Parkinson's disease, 2. Florham Park, NJ: Macmillan Healthcare Information; 1987.

[282] Birkmayer W, Hornykiewicz O. [The L-3,4-dioxyphenylalanine (DOPA)-effect in Parkinson-akinesia]. Wien Klin Wochenschr 1961;73:787–8.

[283] Dong J, Cui Y, Li S, Le W. Current pharmaceutical treatments and alternative therapies of Parkinson's disease. Curr Neuropharmacol 2016;14(4):339.

[284] Armstrong MJ, Okun MS. Diagnosis and treatment of parkinson disease: a review. JAMA 2020;323(6):548–60.

[285] Deuschl G, Schade-Brittinger C, Krack P, et al. A randomized trial of deep-brain stimulation for Parkinson's disease. N Engl J Med 2006;355 (9):896–908.

[286] Schuepbach WM, Rau J, Knudsen K, et al. Neurostimulation for Parkinson's disease with early motor complications. N Engl J Med 2013;368 (7):610–22.

[287] Feng YS, Yang SD, Tan ZX, Wang MM, Xing Y, Dong F, et al. The benefits and mechanisms of exercise training for Parkinson's disease. Life Sci 2020;245:117345. Available from: https://doi.org/10.1016/j.lfs.2020.117345; Epub 2020 Jan 22. PMID: 31981631.

[288] Kulisevsky J, Oliveira L, Fox SH. Update in therapeutic strategies for Parkinson's disease. Curr Opin Neurol 2018;31(4):439–47. Available from: https://doi.org/10.1097/WCO.0000000000000579; PMID: 29746402.

[289] Xu X, Fu Z, Le W. Exercise and Parkinson's disease. Int Rev Neurobiol 2019;147:45–74. Available from: https://doi.org/10.1016/bs.irn.2019.06.003; Epub 2019 Jun 20. PMID: 31607362.

[290] Longo VD, Mattson MP. Fasting: Molecular mechanisms and clinical applications. Cell Metab 2014;19:181–92.

[291] Patterson RE, Sears DD. Metabolic effects of intermittent fasting. Annu Rev Nutr 2017;37:371–93.

[292] Puchalska P, Crawford PA. Multi-dimensional roles of ketone bodies in fuel metabolism, signaling, and therapeutics. Cell Metab 2017;25:262–84.

[293] Veech RL, Chance B, Kashiwaya Y, et al. Ketone bodies, potential therapeutic uses. IUBMB Life 2001;51:241–7.

[294] Tieu K, Perier C, Caspersen C, et al. D-beta-hydroxybutyrate rescues mitochondrial respiration and mitigates features of Parkinson disease. J Clin Investig 2003;112:892–901.

[295] Phillips MCL. Fasting as a therapy in neurological disease. Nutrients 2019;11(10):E2501.

[296] Neth BJ, Bauer BA, Benarroch EE, Savica R. The role of intermittent fasting in parkinson's disease. Front Neurol 2021;12:682184. Available from: https://doi.org/10.3389/fneur.2021.682184; Published 2021 Jun 1.

[297] Schoeler NE, Cross JH. Ketogenic dietary therapies in adults with epilepsy: A practical guide. Pract Neurol 2016;16:208–14.

[298] Klein P, Tyrlikova I, Mathews GC. Dietary treatment in adults with refractory epilepsy: A review. Neurology 2014;83:1978–85.

[299] Volek J, Phinney SD. The art and science of low carbohydrate living: an expert guide to making the life-saving benefits of carbohydrate restriction sustainable and enjoyable. 1st edition Beyond Obesity LLC; 2011.

[300] Vanitallie TB, Nonas C, Di Rocco A, et al. Treatment of Parkinson disease with diet-induced hyperketonemia: a feasibility study. Neurology 2005;64:728–30.

[301] Phillips MCL, Murtagh DK, Gilbertson LJ, et al. Low-fat versus ketogenic diet in Parkinson's disease: A pilot randomized controlled trial. Mov Disord 2018;33:1306–14.

[302] Koyuncu H, et al. Effect of ketogenic diet versus regular diet on voice quality of patients with Parkinson's disease. Acta Neurologica Belgica [Preprint] 2020. Available from: https://doi.org/10.1007/s13760-020-01486-0.

[303] Krikorian R, et al. Nutritional ketosis for mild cognitive impairment in Parkinson's disease: A controlled pilot trial. Clinical Parkinsonism & Related Disorders [Preprint] 2019. Available from: https://doi.org/10.1016/j.prdoa.2019.07.006.

[304] Tidman M. Effects of a ketogenic diet on symptoms, biomarkers, depression, and anxiety in parkinson's disease: a case study. Cureus [Internet] 2022;(3):14. https://www.cureus.com/articles/90565-effects-of-a-ketogenic-diet-on-symptoms-biomarkers-depression-and-anxiety-in-parkinsons-disease-a-case-study.

[305] DSM-5 [Internet]. [cited 2022 Mar 24]. Available from: https://www.psychiatry.org/psychiatrists/practice/dsm

[306] Rashid B, Calhoun V. Towards a brain-based predictome of mental illness. Hum Brain Mapp 2020;41(12):3468–535.

[307] Maenner MJ, Shaw KA, Bakian AV, Bilder DA, Durkin MS, Esler A, et al. Prevalence and characteristics of autism spectrum disorder among children aged 8 years—autism and developmental disabilities monitoring network, 11 sites, United States, 2018. MMWR Surveill Summ 2021;70(11):1–16.

[308] Zeidan J, Fombonne E, Scorah J, Ibrahim A, Durkin MS, Saxena S, et al. Global prevalence of autism: A systematic review update. Autism Research 2022;15(5):778–90.

[309] Doja A, Roberts W. Immunizations and autism: a review of the literature. Can J Neurol Sci 2006;33(4):341–6.

[310] Turner TN, Coe BP, Dickel DE, Hoekzema K, Nelson BJ, Zody MC, et al. Genomic Patterns of De Novo Mutation in Simplex Autism. Cell. 2017;171(3):710–22 e12.

[311] Frans EM, Sandin S, Reichenberg A, Långström N, Lichtenstein P, McGrath JJ, et al. Autism risk across generations: a population-based study of advancing grandpaternal and paternal age. JAMA Psychiatry 2013;70(5):516–21.

[312] Wegiel J, Kaczmarski W, Flory M, Martinez-Cerdeno V, Wisniewski T, Nowicki K, et al. Deficit of corpus callosum axons, reduced axon diameter and decreased area are markers of abnormal development of interhemispheric connections in autistic subjects. Acta Neuropathol Commun 2018;6(1):143.

[313] Martinat M, Rossitto M, Di Miceli M, Layé S. Perinatal dietary polyunsaturated fatty acids in brain development, role in neurodevelopmental disorders. Nutrients. 2021;13(4):1185.

[314] Muhle R, Trentacoste SV, Rapin I. The genetics of autism. Pediatrics 2004;113(5):e472–86.

[315] Sandin S, Lichtenstein P, Kuja-Halkola R, Larsson H, Hultman CM, Reichenberg A. The familial risk of autism. JAMA 2014;311(17):1770–7.

[316] Castelbaum L, Sylvester CM, Zhang Y, Yu Q, Constantino JN. On the nature of monozygotic twin concordance and discordance for autistic trait severity: a quantitative analysis. Behav Genet 2020;50(4):263–72.

[317] Jou RJ, Reed HE, Kaiser MD, Voos AC, Volkmar FR, Pelphrey KA. White matter abnormalities in autism and unaffected siblings. JNP 2016;28(1):49–55.

[318] Dimond D, Schuetze M, Smith RE, Dhollander T, Cho I, Vinette S, et al. Reduced White Matter Fiber Density in Autism Spectrum Disorder. Cereb Cortex 2019;29(4):1778–88.

[319] Huang H, Vasung L. Gaining insight of fetal brain development with diffusion MRI and histology. Int J Dev Neurosci 2014;32:11–22.

[320] Stiles J, Jernigan TL. The basics of brain development. Neuropsychol Rev 2010;20(4):327–48.

[321] Fjell AM, Walhovd KB. Structural brain changes in aging: courses, causes and cognitive consequences. Rev Neurosci 2010;21(3):187–221. Available from: https://doi.org/10.1515/revneuro.2010.21.3.187; PMID: 20879692.

[322] Thapar A, Cooper M, Rutter M. Neurodevelopmental disorders. Lancet Psychiatry 2017;4(4):339–46.

[323] Remer J, Dean DC, Chen K, Reiman RA, Huentelman MJ, Reiman EM, et al. Longitudinal white matter and cognitive development in pediatric carriers of the apolipoprotein ε4 allele. Neuroimage 2020;222:117243.

[324] Gilmore JH, Santelli RK, Gao W. Imaging structural and functional brain development in early childhood. Nat Rev Neurosci 2018;19(3):123–37.

[325] Sun C, Zou M, Wang X, Xia W, Ma Y, Liang S, et al. FADS1-FADS2 and ELOVL2 gene polymorphisms in susceptibility to autism spectrum disorders in Chinese children. BMC Psychiatry 2018;18:283.

[326] Grant PE, Im K, Ahtam B, Laurentys CT, Chan WM, Brainard M, et al. Altered White Matter Organization in the TUBB3 E410K Syndrome. Cerebral Cortex (New York, NY) 2019;29(8):3561.

[327] Guo H, Wang T, Wu H, Long M, Coe BP, Li H, et al. Inherited and multiple de novo mutations in autism/developmental delay risk genes suggest a multifactorial model. Molecular Autism 2018;9(1):64.

[328] Kim SY, Yi DY. Components of human breast milk: from macronutrient to microbiome and microRNA. Clin Exp Pediatr 2020;63(8):301–9.

[329] German JB, Dillard CJ. Saturated fats: a perspective from lactation and milk composition. Lipids 2010;45(10):915–23.

[330] Lemay D.G., Lynn D.J., Martin W.F., Neville M.C., Casey T.M., Rincon G., et al. The bovine lactation genome: insights into the evolution of mammalian milk. Genome Biol;10(4):R43.

[331] van Elst K, Bruining H, Birtoli B, Terreaux C, Buitelaar JK, Kas MJ. Food for thought: dietary changes in essential fatty acid ratios and the increase in autism spectrum disorders. Neurosci Biobehav Rev 2014;45:369–78.

[332] Hirokawa K, Kimura T, Ikehara S, Honjo K, Ueda K, Sato T, et al. Associations between broader autism phenotype and dietary intake: a cross-sectional study (Japan Environment & Children's Study). J Autism Dev Disord 2020;50(8):2698–709.

[333] Kinney DK, Barch DH, Chayka B, Napoleon S, Munir KM. Environmental risk factors for autism: do they help cause de novo genetic mutations that contribute to the disorder? Med Hypotheses 2010;74(1):102–6.

[334] Stenvers DJ, Scheer FAJL, Schrauwen P, la Fleur SE, Kalsbeek A. Circadian clocks and insulin resistance. Nat Rev Endocrinol 2019;15 (2):75–89.

[335] Giona F, Pagano J, Verpelli C, Sala C. Another step toward understanding brain functional connectivity alterations in autism. J Neurochem 2021;159(1):12–14.

[336] Krakowiak P, Walker CK, Bremer AA, Baker AS, Ozonoff S, Hansen RL, et al. Maternal metabolic conditions and risk for autism and other neurodevelopmental disorders. Pediatrics 2012;129(5):e1121–8. Available from: https://doi.org/10.1542/peds.2011-2583; Epub 2012 Apr 9. PMID: 22492772.

[337] Martins BP, Bandarra NM, Figueiredo-Braga M. The role of marine omega-3 in human neurodevelopment, including autism spectrum disorders and attention-deficit/hyperactivity disorder—a review. Crit Rev Food Sci Nutr 2020;60(9):1431–46.

[338] Bhattamisra SK, Shin LY, Saad HIBM, Rao V, Candasamy M, Pandey M, et al. Interlink between insulin resistance and neurodegeneration with an update on current therapeutic approaches. CNS Neurol Disord Drug Targets 2020;19(3):174–83.

[339] Murru E, Manca C, Carta G, Banni S. Impact of dietary palmitic acid on lipid metabolism Front Nutr [Internet] 2022;9 cited 2022 Jul 5. Available from: https://www.frontiersin.org/articles/10.3389/fnut.2022.861664.

[340] Yeh YY, Sheehan PM. Preferential utilization of ketone bodies in the brain and lung of newborn rats. Fed Proc 1985;44(7):2352–8.

[341] Kingsbury KJ, Paul S, Crossley A, Morgan DM. The fatty acid composition of human depot fat. Biochem J 1961;78(3):541–50.

[342] Dietschy JM, Turley SD. Cholesterol metabolism in the brain. Curr Opin Lipidol 2001;12(2):105–12.

[343] Dietschy JM, Turley SD. Thematic review series: brain lipids. Cholesterol metabolism in the central nervous system during early development and in the mature animal. J Lipid Res 2004;45(8):1375–97.

[344] Zeisel SH. The supply of choline is important for fetal progenitor cells. Semin Cell Dev Biol 2011;22(6):624–8.

[345] Jo D, Yoon G, Song J. Role of EXENDIN-4 IN BRAIN INSULIN RESISTANCE, MITOCHONDRIAL FUNCTION, AND NEURITE OUTGROWTH IN NEURONS UNDER PALMITIC ACID-INDUCED OXIDATIVE STress. Antioxidants (Basel) 2021;10(1):78.

[346] Kihara A. Very long-chain fatty acids: elongation, physiology and related disorders. The Journal of Biochemistry 2012;152(5):387–95.

[347] Herba CM, Roza S, Govaert P, Hofman A, Jaddoe V, Verhulst FC, et al. Breastfeeding and early brain development: the generation R study. Matern Child Nutr 2013;9(3):332–49.

[348] Amine H, Benomar Y, Taouis M. Palmitic acid promotes resistin-induced insulin resistance and inflammation in SH-SY5Y human neuroblastoma. Sci Rep 2021;11:5427.

[349] Almaguel FG, Liu JW, Pacheco FJ, De Leon D, Casiano CA, De Leon M. Lipotoxicity mediated cell dysfunction and death involves lysosomal membrane permeabilization and cathepsin L activity. Brain Res 2010;1318 C:133–43.

[350] Simopoulos AP. The importance of the ratio of omega-6/omega-3 essential fatty acids. Biomed Pharmacother 2002;56(8):365–79.

[351] Sanders TAB. DHA status of vegetarians. Prostaglandins Leukot Essent Fatty Acids 2009;81(2–3):137–41.

[352] Kinsella JE. Lipids, membrane receptors, and enzymes: effects of dietary fatty acids. Journal of Parenteral and Enteral Nutrition 1990;14(5 S): 200S−17S.

[353] Saher G, Brügger B, Lappe-Siefke C, Möbius W, Tozawa Richi, Wehr MC, et al. High cholesterol level is essential for myelin membrane growth. Nat Neurosci 2005;8(4):468−75.

[354] Genaro-Mattos TC, Anderson A, Allen LB, Korade Z, Mirnics K. Cholesterol biosynthesis and uptake in developing neurons. ACS Chem Neurosci 2019;10(8):3671−81.

[355] Kleinridders A, Ferris HA, Cai W, Kahn CR. Insulin Action in brain regulates systemic metabolism and brain function. Diabetes 2014;63 (7):2232−43.

[356] Schell M, Chudoba C, Leboucher A, Alfine E, Flore T, Ritter K, et al. Interplay of dietary fatty acids and cholesterol impacts brain mitochondria and insulin action. Nutrients 2020;12(5):1518.

[357] Tseng PT, Chen YW, Stubbs B, Carvalho AF, Whiteley P, Tang CH, et al. Maternal breastfeeding and autism spectrum disorder in children: A systematic review and meta-analysis. Nutr Neurosci 2019;22(5):354−62.

[358] Katz J, Reichenberg A, Kolevzon A. Prenatal and perinatal metabolic risk factors for autism: a review and integration of findings from population-based studies. Curr Opin Psychiatry 2021;34(2):94−104.

[359] Zhong C, Tessing J, Lee BK, Lyall K. Maternal dietary factors and the risk of autism spectrum disorders: a systematic review of existing evidence. Autism Res 2020;13(10):1634−58.

[360] Patel BP, McLellan SS, Hanley AJ, Retnakaran R, Hamilton JK. Greater nutritional risk scores in 2-year-old children exposed to gestational diabetes mellitus in utero and their relationship to homeostasis model assessment for insulin resistance at age 5 years. Can J Diabetes 2021;45 (5):390−4.

[361] Rivell A, Mattson MP. Intergenerational Metabolic Syndrome and Neuronal Network Hyperexcitability in Autism. Trends Neurosci 2019;42 (10):709−26.

[362] Xu G, Jing J, Bowers K, Liu B, Bao W. Maternal diabetes and the risk of autism spectrum disorders in the offspring: a systematic review and meta-analysis. J Autism Dev Disord 2014;44(4):766−75.

[363] Herrera E, Desoye G. Maternal and fetal lipid metabolism under normal and gestational diabetic conditions. Horm Mol Biol Clin Investig 2016;26(2):109−27.

[364] Grasso S, Palumbo G, Rugolo S, Cianci A, Tumino G, Reitano G. Human fetal insulin secretion in response to maternal glucose and leucine administration. Pediatr Res 1980;14(5):782−3.

[365] Coltart TM, Beard RW, Turner RC, Oakley NW. Blood glucose and insulin relationships in the human mother and fetus before onset of labour. Br Med J 1969;4(5674):17−19.

[366] Tennant PWG, Glinianaia SV, Bilous RW, Rankin J, Bell R. Pre-existing diabetes, maternal glycated haemoglobin, and the risks of fetal and infant death: a population-based study. Diabetologia 2014;57(2):285−94.

[367] Pouliot A, Elmahboubi R, Adam C. Incidence and outcomes of gestational diabetes mellitus using the new international association of diabetes in pregnancy study group criteria in hôpital Maisonneuve-Rosemont. Can J Diabetes 2019;43(8):594−9.

[368] Xiang AH, Wang X, Martinez MP, Walthall JC, Curry ES, Page K, et al. Association of maternal diabetes with autism in offspring. JAMA 2015;313(14):1425−34.

[369] Xiang AH, Wang X, Martinez MP, Page K, Buchanan TA, Feldman RK. Maternal Type 1 Diabetes and Risk of Autism in Offspring. JAMA 2018;320(1):89−91.

[370] Dietary Guidelines for Americans, 2020-2025: 164.

[371] Isganaitis E, Lustig RH. Fast food, central nervous system insulin resistance, and obesity. Arterioscler Thromb Vasc Biol 2005;25 (12):2451−62.

[372] Garcia-Penas JJ. [Autism spectrum disorder and epilepsy: the role of ketogenic diet]. Rev Neurol 2016;62(Suppl 1):S73−8.

[373] Li H, Liu H, Chen X, Zhang J, Tong G, Sun Y. Association of food hypersensitivity in children with the risk of autism spectrum disorder: a meta-analysis. Eur J Pediatr 2021;180(4):999−1008.

[374] Peretti S, Mariano M, Mazzocchetti C, Mazza M, Pino MC, Verrotti Di Pianella A, et al. Diet: the keystone of autism spectrum disorder? Nutr Neurosci 2019;22(12):825−39.

[375] Verrotti A, Iapadre G, Pisano S, Coppola G. Ketogenic diet and childhood neurological disorders other than epilepsy: an overview. Expert Rev Neurother 2017;17(5):461−73.

[376] Evangeliou A, et al. Application of a ketogenic diet in children with autistic behavior: pilot study. J Child Neurol 2003;18(2):113−18. Available from: https://doi.org/10.1177/08830738030180020501.

[377] Herbert MR, Buckley JA. Autism and dietary therapy: case report and review of the literature. J Child Neurol 2013;28(8):975−82. Available from: https://doi.org/10.1177/0883073813488668.

[378] Lee RWY, et al. A modified ketogenic gluten-free diet with MCT improves behavior in children with autism spectrum disorder. Physiol Behav 2018;188:205−11. Available from: https://doi.org/10.1016/j.physbeh.2018.02.006.

[379] Żarnowska I, et al. Therapeutic use of carbohydrate-restricted diets in an autistic child; a case report of clinical and 18FDG PET findings. Metab Brain Dis 2018;33(4):1187−92. Available from: https://doi.org/10.1007/s11011-018-0219-1.

[380] Al Qassimi A, Al Otiabi M, Al Rabeeah F. A case report: an approach to recognize a role in ketogenic diet response in autism with positive CHD8. Recent Developments in Medicine and Medical Research 2021;9:17−22. Available from: https://doi.org/10.9734/bpi/rdmmr/v9/4654F.

[381] Lyall K, Schmidt RJ, Hertz-Picciotto I. Maternal lifestyle and environmental risk factors for autism spectrum disorders. Int J Epidemiol 2014;43(2):443–64.
[382] Cheng J, Eskenazi B, Widjaja F, Cordero JF, Hendren RL. Improving autism perinatal risk factors: A systematic review. Med Hypotheses 2019;127:26–33.
[383] Burstein R, Noseda R, Borsook D. Migraine: multiple processes, complex pathophysiology. J Neurosci 2015;35(17):6619–29.
[384] Steiner TJ, Stovner LJ, Vos T, Jensen R, Katsarava Z. Migraine is first cause of disability in under 50 s: will health politicians now take notice? J Headache Pain 2018;19(1):17.
[385] Leonardi M, Raggi A. Burden of migraine: international perspectives. Neurol Sci 2013;34(Suppl 1):S117–18.
[386] Schwedt TJ, Dodick DW. Advanced neuroimaging of migraine. Lancet Neurol 2009;8(6):560–8.
[387] Covey E. editor Chapter 4 Structure and Cell Biology of The Neuron. Washington: Washington Uo; 1980.
[388] Zukin RS, Jover T, Yokota H, Calderone A, Simionescu M, Lau CG. Chapter 42 - Molecular and cellular mechanisms of ischemia-induced neuronal death. In: Mohr JP, Choi DW, Grotta JC, Weir B, Wolf PA, editors. Stroke. Fourth Edition Philadelphia: Churchill Livingstone; 2004. p. 829–54.
[389] Lambert G, Michalicek J. Cortical spreading depression reduces dural blood flow—a possible mechanism for migraine pain? Cephalalgia 1994;14(6):430–6.
[390] Levy D. Endogenous mechanisms underlying the activation and sensitization of meningeal nociceptors: the role of immuno-vascular interactions and cortical spreading depression. Curr Pain Headache Rep 2012;16.
[391] Pogoda JM, Gross NB, Arakaki X, Fonteh AN, Cowan RP, Harrington MG. Severe headache or migraine history is inversely correlated with dietary sodium intake: NHANES 1999–2004. Headache 2016; n/a-n/a.
[392] Poole CJ, Lightman SL. Inhibition of vasopressin secretion during migraine. J Neurol Neurosurg Psychiatry 1988;51:4.
[393] Campbell DA, Tonks EM, Hay KM. An investigation of the salt and water balance in migraine. Br Med J 1951;1424–9.
[394] Longo DL, Fauci AS, Kasper DL, Hauser SL, Jameson JL, Loscalzo J. Harrison's Manual of Medicine. 18th Edition New York: McGraw Hill Medical; 2013.
[395] Laragh JH, Sealey JE. Renin–Angiotensin–Aldosterone System and the Renal Regulation of Sodium, Potassium, and Blood Pressure Homeostasis. Comprehensive Physiology: John Wiley & Sons, Inc; 2010.
[396] Guldiken B, Guldiken S, Taskiran B, Koc G, Turgut N, Kabayel L. Migraine in metabolic syndrome. Neurologist 2009;15.
[397] Science WIo. The Human Gene Database Internet: Weizmann Institute of Science; 2017 [cited 2017 1/28/2017]. The Human Genome Database. Available from: http://www.genecards.org.
[398] Armstrong CM. The Na/K pump, Cl ion, and osmotic stabilization of cells. Proc Natl Acad Sci 2003;100(10):6257–62.
[399] Pirahanchi Y, Jessu R, Aeddula NR. Physiology, Sodium Potassium Pump. StatPearls [Internet] 2021.
[400] Tenny ST, William. Cerebral Salt Wasting Syndrome. StatPearls [Internet]. NCBI: StatPearls Publishing; 2021.
[401] Reaven G, Hoffman BA. Role for insulin in the aetiology and course of hypertension? Lancet 1987;330(8556):435–7.
[402] Augustyn A. Fight-or-flight response. Physiology. Encyclopaedia Britannica: Encyclopaedia Britannica; 2019.
[403] McCowen KC, Malhotra A, Bistrian BR. Stress-induced hyperglycemia. Crit Care Clin 2001;17(1):107–24.
[404] Fuller MD, Emrick MA, Sadilek M, Scheuer T, Catterall WA. Molecular mechanism of calcium channel regulation in the fight-or-flight response. Sci Signal 2010;3(141) ra70-ra.
[405] Tedeschi G, Russo A, Conte F, Corbo D, Caiazzo G, Giordano A, et al. Increased interictal visual network connectivity in patients with migraine with aura. Cephalalgia 2015;.
[406] Lin Y-K, Lin G-Y, Lee J-T, Lee M-S, Tsai C-K, Hsu Y-W, et al. Associations between sleep quality and migraine frequency: a cross-sectional case-control study. Medicine 2016;95(17):e3554.
[407] Adeniyi PO. Stress, a major determinant of nutritional and health status. American Journal of Public Health Research 2015;3(1):15–20.
[408] Schwedt TJ. Multisensory integration in migraine. Curr Opin Neurol 2013;248–53.
[409] Lin G-Y, Lin Y-K, Lee J-T, Lee M-S, Lin C-C, Tsai C-K, et al. Prevalence of restless legs syndrome in migraine patients with and without aura: a cross-sectional, case-controlled study. J Headache Pain 2016;17(1):97.
[410] Cortez MM, Rea NA, Hunter LA, Digre KB, Brennan K. Altered pupillary light response scales with disease severity in migrainous photophobia. Cephalalgia 2017;37(8):801–11.
[411] UCSF. Blood Sugar & Stress [Website]. Diabetes Teaching Center at the University of California, San Francisco; [cited 2021 11/21/2021]. [Educational Article]. Available from: https://dtc.ucsf.edu/types-of-diabetes/type2/understanding-type-2-diabetes/how-the-body-processes-sugar/blood-sugar-stress/.
[412] Ferris H.A., Kahn C.R. New mechanisms of glucocorticoid-induced insulin resistance: make no bones about it. J Clin Invest 122(11):3854-3857.
[413] Li L, Li X, Zhou W, Messina JL. Acute psychological stress results in the rapid development of insulin resistance. J Endocrinol 2013;217(2):175–84.
[414] Marik PE, Bellomo R. Stress hyperglycemia: an essential survival response!. Crit Care 2013;17(2):305.
[415] Krause EG, de Kloet AD, Flak JN, Smeltzer MD, Solomon MB, Evanson NK, et al. Hydration state controls stress responsiveness and social behavior. J Neurosci 2011;31(14):5470–6.
[416] Zak PJ, Stanton AA, Ahmadi S. Oxytocin increases generosity in humans. PLoS One 2007;2(11):e1128.
[417] Goyal NA, Berry JD, Windebank A, Staff NP, Maragakis NJ, Berg LH, et al. Addressing heterogeneity in amyotrophic lateral sclerosis clinical trials. Muscle Nerve 2020;. Available from: https://doi.org/10.1002/mus.26801.

[418] Nicolle MW. Sleep and Neuromuscular Disease. Semin Neurol 2009;29:429–37. Available from: https://doi.org/10.1055/s-0029-1237119.
[419] Fujisawa A, Yamamoto Y. Edaravone, a potent free radical scavenger, reacts with peroxynitrite to produce predominantly 4-NO-edaravone. Redox Rep 2016;21(3):98–103. Available from: https://doi.org/10.1179/1351000215Y.0000000025; Epub 2016 Feb 18. PMID: 26196041.
[420] Bagga D, Wang L, Farias-Eisner R, Glaspy JA, Reddy ST. Differential effects of prostaglandin derived from ω-6 and ω-3 polyunsaturated fatty acids on COX-2 expression and IL-6 secretion. Proc Natl Acad Sci 2003;100(4):1751–6.
[421] Deleted in review.
[422] Morgan S, Orrell RW. Pathogenesis of amyotrophic lateral sclerosis. Br Med Bull 2016;119(1):87–98. Available from: https://doi.org/10.1093/bmb/ldw026.
[423] Ferri A, Coccurello R. What is 'hyper' in the ALS hypermtabolism? Hindawi 2017; article ID 7821672.
[424] Dupuis L, Oudart H, Rene F, Gonzalez de Aguilar JL, Loeffler JP. Evidence for defective energy homeostasis in amyotrophic lateral sclerosis: benefit of a high-energy diet in transgenic mouse model. Proc Natl Acad Sci 2004;101(30):11159–64.
[425] Chiang PM, Ling J, Jeong YH, Price DLAja SM, Wong PC. Deletion of TDP-43 down regulate Tbc1d1 a gene link to obesity, and alter body fat metabolism. Proc Natl Acad Sci USA 2010;107:16320–4.
[426] Dupuis L, Pradat PF, Ludolph AC, Loeffler JP. Energy metabolism and amyotrophic lateral sclerosis. Lancet Neurol 2011;10:75–82.
[427] Muydermann H, Chen T. Mitochondrial dysfunction in amyotrophic lateral sclerosis – a valid pharmacological target? Br J Pharmacol 2014;171:2191–205.
[428] Wong PC, Pardo CA, Borchelt DR, Lee MK, Copeland NG, Jenkins NA, et al. An adverse property of a familial ALS-linked SOD1 mutation causes motor neuron disease characterized by vacuolar degeneration of mitochondria. Neuron 1995;14(6):1105–16.
[429] Kong J, Xu ZJ. Familial amyotrophic lateral sclerosis mutants of copper. Neurosci 1998;18:3241–50.
[430] Mattiazzi M, D'Aurelio M, Gajewski CD, Matushova K, Kiaei M, Beal MF, et al. Mutated human SOD1 causes dysfunction of oxidative phosphorylation in mitochondria of transgenic mice. Biol Chem 2002;277:29626–33.
[431] Monks DA, Johansen JA, Mo K. Overexpression of wild-type androgen receptor in muscle recapitulates polyglutamine. Proc Natl Acad Sci USA 2007;104:18259–64.
[432] Steyn FJ, Ioannides ZA, Van Eijk RP, Heggie S, Thorpe KA, Ceslis A, et al. Hypermetabolism in ALS is associated with greater functional decline and shorter survival. J Neurol Neurosurg Psychiatry 2018;89(10):1016–23.
[433] Dadon-Nachum M, Melamed E, Offen D. The "dying-back" phenomenon of motor neurons in ALS. J Mol Neurosci 2011;43(3):470–7. Available from: https://doi.org/10.1007/s12031-010-9467-1; Epub 2010/11/09. PubMed PMID: 21057983.
[434] Marcuzzo S, Zucca I, Mastropietro A, de Rosbo NK, Cavalcante P, Tartari S. Hind limb muscle atrophy precedes cerebral neuronal degeneration in G93A-SOD1 mouse model of amyotrophic lateral sclerosis: a longitudinal MRI study. Exp Neurol 2011;231(1):30–7. Available from: https://doi.org/10.1016/j.expneurol.2011.05.007; Epub 2011/05/31. PubMed PMID: 21620832.
[435] Ferri A, Coccurello R. What is "Hyper" in the ALS Hypermetabolism? Mediators Inflamm 2017;2017:7821672. Available from: https://doi.org/10.1155/2017/7821672; Epub 2017/10/31. PubMed PMID: 29081604.
[436] Gallo V, Wark PA, Jenab M, Pearce N, Brayne C, Vermeulen R. Pre-diagnostic body fat and risk of death from amyotrophic lateral sclerosis: the EPIC cohort. Neurology 2013;80(9):829–38. Available from: https://doi.org/10.1212/WNL.0b013e3182840689; Epub 2013/02/08. PubMed PMID: 23390184.
[437] Patel BP, Safdar A, Raha S, Tarnopolsky MA, Hamadeh MJ. Caloric restriction shortens lifespan through an increased in peroxidation, inflammation and apoptosis in the G93 A mouse, and animal model in ALS. PLoS One 2010;5:e9386.
[438] Ahmed RM, Mioshi E, Caga J, Shibata M, Zoing M, Bartley L, et al. Body mass index delineates ALS from FTD: implications for metabolic health. J Neurol 2014;261(9):1774–80.
[439] Wills A.M., Hubbard J., Macklin E.A., Glass J., Tandan R., Simpson E.P., et al. Hypercaloric enteral nutrition in patient with amyotrophic lateral sclerosis: a randomized, double-blind, placebo controlled phase 2 trial. Lancet 383, 2065-2072.
[440] Okamoto K, Kihira T, Kondo T. Nutritional status and risk of amyotrophic lateral sclerosis in Japan. Amyotroph Lateral Scler 2007;8 (5):300–4.
[441] Long YC, Zierath. AMP-activated protein kinase signaling in etaboliuc regulation. J Clin Invest 2006;116:1776–83.
[442] Coughlan KS, Halang L, Woodss I, Prehn JH. A high-fat jelly diet restores bioenergetics balance and extends lifespan in the presence of motor dysfunction and lumbar spinal cord motor neuron loss in TDP-43 mutant C57BL6/J mice. Dis Model Mech 2016;9(9):1029–37.
[443] Zhao Z, Sui Y, Gao W, Cai B, Fan D. Effects of diet on adenosine monophosphate-activated protein kinase activity and disease progression in an amyotrophic lateral sclerosis model. J Int Med Res 2015;43(1):67–79.
[444] Fitzgerald KC, O'Reilly EJ, Falcone G J, McCullough ML, Park Y, Kolonel LN, et al. Dietary omega 3 polyunsaturated fatty acids intake and risk for amyotrophic lateral sclerosis. JAMA Neurol 2014;71(9):1102–10.
[445] Veldink JH, Kalmijn S, Groeneveld GJ, Wunderink W, Koster A, de Vries JH, et al. Intake of polyunsaturated fatty acids and vitamin E reduces the risk of developing amyotrophic lateral sclerosis. J Neurol Neurosurg Psychiatry 2007;78(4):367–71.
[446] Kalmijn S, Launer LJ, Ott A. Dietary Fat intake and the risk of incident dementia in the Rotternda Study. Ann Neurol 1997;42:776–82.
[447] Yasojima K, Tourtellote WW, McGeer EG. Marked increased in cyclooxygenase-2 in ALS spinal cord. Neurology 2005;57:952–6.
[448] Paoli A, Bianco A, Damiani E, Bosco G. Ketogenic diet in neuromuscular and neurodegenerative diseases. BioMed Res Int 2014;. Available from: https://doi.org/10.1155/2014/474296; Article ID 474296.
[449] Newman JC, Verdin E. "ketones bodies as signaling metabolites". Trend Endocrinol Metab 2014;25:42–52.

[450] Bedlack R, Barkhaus PE, Barnes B, Beauchamp M, Bertorini T, Bromber MB, et al. ALS untangled #63 ketogenic diet. Amyotroph Lateral Scler Frontotemporal Degener 2021;. Available from: https://doi.org/10.1080/21678421.2021.1990346.

[451] Zhao Z, Lange DJ, Voustianiouk A, MacGrogan D, Ho L, Suh J, et al. A ketogenic diet as potential novel therapeutics intervention in amyotrophic lateral sclerosis. BMC Neurosci 2006;7(29). Available from: https://doi.org/10.1186/1471-2202-7-29.

[452] Zhao W, Varghese M, Vempati P. Caprylic triglyceride as a novel therapeutic approach to effectively improve the performance and attenuate the symptoms due to motor neuron loss in ALS disease. PLoS One 2012;7(11) Ide 49191.

[453] Dupuis L, Corcia P, Fergani J, Gonzalez de Aguilar L, Bonnefront-Rousselot D, Bittar R, et al. Dyslipidemia is a protective factor in amyotrophic lateral sclerosis. Neurology 2008;70(3). Available from: https://doi.org/10.1212/01.wnl.000285080./70324.27.

[454] Posse de la Chaves EI, Rusinol AE, Vance DE, Campenot RB, Vance JE. Role of lipoproteins in the delivery if lipids to axons during axonal regeneration. J Biol Chem 1997;272(49):30766–73.

[455] Halliday J, Absalom AR. Traumatic brain injury: from impact to rehabilitation. Br J Hosp Med (Lond) 2008;69(5):284–9. Available from: https://doi.org/10.12968/hmed.2008.69.5.29362; PMID: 18557556.

[456] Jain S, Iverson LM. Glasgow coma scale StatPearls [Internet]. Treasure Island (FL): StatPearls Publishing; 2022 cited 2022 Aug 3]. Available from. Available from: http://www.ncbi.nlm.nih.gov/books/NBK513298/.

[457] Najem D, Rennie K, Ribecco-Lutkiewicz M, Ly D, Haukenfrers J, Liu Q, et al. Traumatic brain injury: classification, models, and markers. Biochem Cell Biol 2018;96(4):391–406. Available from: https://doi.org/10.1139/bcb-2016-0160; Epub 2018 Jan 25. PMID: 29370536.

[458] Fordington S, Manford M. A review of seizures and epilepsy following traumatic brain injury. J Neurol 2020;267(10):3105–11. Available from: https://doi.org/10.1007/s00415-020-09926-w; Epub 2020 May 22. PMID: 32444981.

[459] McGinn MJ, Povlishock JT. Pathophysiology of traumatic brain injury. Neurosurg Clin N Am 2016;27(4):397–407. Available from: https://doi.org/10.1016/j.nec.2016.06.002; Epub 2016 Aug 10. PMID: 27637392.

[460] Rabinowitz AR, Levin HS. Cognitive sequelae of traumatic brain injury. Psychiatr Clin North Am 2014;37(1):1–11.

[461] Dwyer B, Katz DI. Postconcussion syndrome. Handb Clin Neurol 2018;158:163–78. Available from: https://doi.org/10.1016/B978-0-444-63954-7.00017-3; PMID: 30482344.

[462] Capizzi A, Woo J, Verduzco-Gutierrez M. Traumatic brain injury: an overview of epidemiology, pathophysiology, and medical management. Med Clin North Am 2020;104(2):213–38. Available from: https://doi.org/10.1016/j.mcna.2019.11.001; PMID: 32035565.

[463] Giza C, Hovda DA. The new neurometabolic cascade of concussion. Neurosurgery 2014;75:S24–33. Available from: https://doi.org/10.1227/NEU.0000000000000505.

[464] Lazzarino G, Amorini AM, Signoretti S, Musumeci G, Lazzarino G, Caruso G, et al. Pyruvate dehydrogenase and tricarboxylic acid cycle enzymes are sensitive targets of traumatic brain injury induced metabolic derangement. Int J Mol Sci. 2019;20(22):5774. Available from: https://doi.org/10.3390/ijms20225774; PMID: 31744143.

[465] Lemke DM. Sympathetic storming after severe traumatic brain injury. Crit Care Nurse 2007;27(1):30–7 quiz 38. PMID: 17244857.

[466] Chen Y-H, Huang EY-K, Kuo T-T, Miller J, Chiang Y-H, Hoffer BJ. Impact of traumatic brain injury on dopaminergic transmission. Cell Transplant 2017;1156–68. Available from: https://doi.org/10.1177/0963689717714105.

[467] Lewén A, Fujimura M, Sugawara T, Matz P, Copin JC, Chan PH. Oxidative stress-dependent release of mitochondrial cytochrome c after traumatic brain injury. J Cereb Blood Flow Metab 2001;21(8):914–20. Available from: https://doi.org/10.1097/00004647-200108000-00003; PMID: 11487726.

[468] Herrero-Mendez A, Almeida A, Fernández E, Maestre C, Moncada S, Bolaños JP. The bioenergetic and antioxidant status of neurons is controlled by continuous degradation of a key glycolytic enzyme by APC/C-Cdh1. Nat Cell Biol 2009;11(6):747–52. Available from: https://doi.org/10.1038/ncb1881; Epub 2009 May 17. PMID: 19448625.

[469] Honda M, Sase S, Yokota K, Ichibayashi R, Yoshihara K, Masuda H, et al. Early cerebral circulation disturbance in patients suffering from different types of severe traumatic brain injury: a xenon CT and perfusion CT study. Acta Neurochir Suppl 2013;118:259–63. Available from: https://doi.org/10.1007/978-3-7091-1434-6_49; PMID: 23564144.

[470] Chan KH, et al. "Intracranial blood flow velocity after head injury: relationship to severity of injury, time, neurological status and outcome.". J Neurol Neurosurg Psychiatry 1992;55(9):787–91. Available from: https://doi.org/10.1136/jnnp.55.9.787.

[471] Baguley IJ, Perkes IE, Fernandez-Ortega JF, Rabinstein AA, Dolce G, Hendricks HTConsensus Working Group. Paroxysmal sympathetic hyperactivity after acquired brain injury: consensus on conceptual definition, nomenclature, and diagnostic criteria. J Neurotrauma 2014;31(17):1515–20. Available from: https://doi.org/10.1089/neu.2013.3301; Epub 2014 Jul 28. PMID: 24731076.

[472] Hackenberg K, Unterberg A. Schädel-Hirn-Trauma [traumatic brain injury]. Nervenarzt. 2016;87(2):203–14. Available from: https://doi.org/10.1007/s00115-015-0051-3; quiz 215-6. German. PMID: 26810405.

[473] Meyfroidt G, Bouzat P, Casaer MP, Chesnut R, Hamada SR, Helbok R, et al. Management of moderate to severe traumatic brain injury: an update for the intensivist. Intensive Care Med. 2022;48(6):649–66. Available from: https://doi.org/10.1007/s00134-022-06702-4; Epub 2022 May 20. Erratum in: Intensive Care Med. 2022 Jun 20; PMID: 35595999.

[474] Vella MA, Crandall ML, Patel MB. Acute management of traumatic brain injury. Surg Clin North Am 2017;97(5):1015–30. Available from: https://doi.org/10.1016/j.suc.2017.06.003; PMID: 28958355.

[475] George AK, Behera J, Homme RP, Tyagi N, Tyagi SC, Singh M. Rebuilding microbiome for mitigating traumatic brain injury: importance of restructuring the gut-microbiome-brain axis. Mol Neurobiol 2021;58(8):3614–27. Available from: https://doi.org/10.1007/s12035-021-02357-2; Epub 2021 Mar 27. PMID: 33774742.

[476] Panther EJ, Dodd W, Clark A, Lucke-Wold B. Gastrointestinal microbiome and neurologic injury. Biomedicines. 2022;10(2):500. Available from: https://doi.org/10.3390/biomedicines10020500; PMID: 35203709.

[477] Prinsloo GE, Derman WE, Lambert MI, Rauch HGL. The effect of biofeedback induced deep breathing on measures of heart rate variability during laboratory induced cognitive stress: *a pilot study*. Appl Psychophysiol Biofeedback 2013;38(2):81–90.

[478] Rauch H.G.L., S. Smit, D. Karpul, T.D. Noakes, Effect of Taijiquan training on autonomic re-activity and body position and postures during mock boxing, Book of Abstracts, 18th Congress of European College of Sport Science Barcelona, Spain, 25-28 June 2013.

[479] Cahill Jr GF, Herrera MG, Morgan AP, Soeldner JS, Steinke J, Levy PL. Reichard GA Jr, Kipnis DM. Hormone-fuel interrelationships during fasting. J Clin Invest 1966;45(11):1751–69. Available from: https://doi.org/10.1172/JCI105481; PMID: 5926444.

[480] Cheng G, Kong RH, Zhang LM, Zhang JN. Mitochondria in traumatic brain injury and mitochondrial-targeted multipotential therapeutic strategies. Br J Pharmacol 2012;167(4):699–719.

[481] Bergsneider M, Hovda DA, Shalmon E, Kelly DF, Vespa PM, Martin NA, et al. Cerebral hyperglycolysis following severe traumatic brain injury in humans: a positron emission tomography study. J Neurosurg 1997;86(2):241–51. Available from: https://doi.org/10.3171/jns.1997.86.2.0241; PMID: 9010426.

[482] Oz G, Seaquist ER, Kumar A, Criego AB, Benedict LE, Rao JP, et al. Human brain glycogen content and metabolism: implications on its role in brain energy metabolism. Am J Physiol Endocrinol Metab 2007;292(3):E946–51. Available from: https://doi.org/10.1152/ajpendo.00424.2006; Epub 2006 Nov 28. PMID: 17132822.

[483] Meier R, Béchir M, Ludwig S, Sommerfeld J, Keel M, Steiger P, et al. Differential temporal profile of lowered blood glucose levels (3.5 to 6.5 mmol/l versus 5 to 8 mmol/l) in patients with severe traumatic brain injury. Crit Care 2008;12(4):R98. Available from: https://doi.org/10.1186/cc6974; Epub 2008 Aug 4. PMID: 18680584.

[484] Shi J, Dong B, Mao Y, Guan W, Cao J, Zhu R, et al. Review: traumatic brain injury and hyperglycemia, a potentially modifiable risk factor. Oncotarget. 2016;7(43):71052–61.

[485] Burslem R, Rigassio Radler D, Parker A, Zelig R. Low-carbohydrate, high-fat enteral formulas for managing glycemic control in patients who are critically ill: A review of the evidence. Nut in Clin Prac 2022;37(1):68–80.

[486] Arora N, Litofsky NS, Golzy M, Aneja R, Staudenmyer D, Qualls K, et al. Phase I single center trial of ketogenic diet for adults with traumatic brain injury. Clin Nutr 2022;47:339–45.

[487] Rippee MA, Chen J, Taylor MK. The ketogenic diet in the treatment of post-concussion syndrome—a feasibility study. Front Nutr [Internet]. 2020; Sep 10 [cited 2020 Oct 6];7. https://www.ncbi.nlm.nih.gov/pmc/articles/PMC7511571/.

[488] Prins ML, Lee SM, Fujima LS, Hovda DA. Increased cerebral uptake and oxidation of exogenous betaHB improves ATP following traumatic brain injury in adult rats. J Neurochem 2004;90(3):666–72. Available from: https://doi.org/10.1111/j.1471-4159.2004.02542.x; PMID: 15255945.

[489] Ritter AM, Robertson CS, Goodman JC, Contant CF, Grossman RG. Evaluation of a carbohydrate-free diet for patients with severe head injury. J Neurotrauma 1996;13(8):473–85. Available from: https://doi.org/10.1089/neu.1996.13.473; PMID: 8880611.

[490] White H, Venkatesh B. Clinical review: Ketones and brain injury. Crit Care 2011;1519.

[491] Krebs HA, Veech RL. Equilibrium relations between pyridine nucleotides and adenine nucleotides and their roles in the regulation of metabolic processes. Adv Enzyme Regul 1969;7:397–413. Available from: https://doi.org/10.1016/0065-2571(69)90030-2; PMID: 4391643.

[492] Prins ML, Matsumoto JH. The collective therapeutic potential of cerebral ketone metabolism in traumatic brain injury. J Lipid Res 2014;55(12):2450–7. Available from: https://doi.org/10.1194/jlr.R046706; Epub 2014 Apr 10. PMID: 24721741.

[493] Vonder Haar C, Peterson TC, Martens KM, Hoane MR. Vitamins and nutrients as primary treatments in experimental brain injury: Clinical implications for nutraceutical therapies. Brain Res 2016;1640(Pt A):114–29. Available from: https://doi.org/10.1016/j.brainres.2015.12.030; Epub 2015 Dec 23. PMID: 26723564.

[494] Hall ED, Vaishnav RA, Mustafa AG. Antioxidant therapies for traumatic brain injury. Neurotherapeutics 2010;7(1):51–61. Available from: https://doi.org/10.1016/j.nurt.2009.10.021; PMID: 20129497.

[495] Shen Q, Hiebert JB, Hartwell J, Thimmesch AR, Pierce JD. Systematic review of traumatic brain injury and the impact of antioxidant therapy on clinical outcomes. Worldviews Evid Based Nurs 2016;13(5):380–9. Available from: https://doi.org/10.1111/wvn.12167; Epub 2016 May 31. PMID: 27243770.

[496] Farkhondeh T, Samarghandian S, Roshanravan B, Peivasteh-Roudsari L. Impact of curcumin on traumatic brain injury and involved molecular signaling pathways. Recent Pat Food Nutr Agric 2020;11(2):137–44. Available from: https://doi.org/10.2174/2212798410666190617161523; PMID: 31288732.

[497] Grünewald RA. Ascorbic acid in the brain. Brain Res Brain Res Rev 1993;18(1):123–33. Available from: https://doi.org/10.1016/0165-0173(93)90010-w; PMID: 8467348.

[498] Brigelius-Flohé R, Traber MG. Vitamin E: function and metabolism. FASEB J 1999;13(10):1145–55 PMID: 10385606.

[499] Kumar PR, Essa MM, Al-Adawi S, Dradekh G, Memon MA, Akbar M, et al. Omega-3 fatty acids could alleviate the risks of traumatic brain injury - a mini review. J Tradit Complement Med. 2014;4(2):89–92. Available from: https://doi.org/10.4103/2225-4110.130374; PMID: 24860731.

[500] Wu F, Xu K, Liu L, Zhang K, Xia L, Zhang M, et al. Corrigendum: vitamin B12 enhances nerve repair and improves functional recovery after traumatic brain injury by inhibiting ER stress-induced neuron injury. Front Pharmacol. 2021;12:598335. Available from: https://doi.org/10.3389/fphar.2021.598335; Erratum for: Front Pharmacol. 2019 Apr 24;10:406. PMID: 33912034.

[501] Zhao L, Wang W, Zhong J, Li Y, Cheng Y, Su Z, et al. The effects of magnesium sulfate therapy after severe diffuse axonal injury. TCRM 2016;12:1481–6.

[502] Levenson CW. Zinc and traumatic brain injury: from chelation to supplementation. Med Sci (Basel). 2020;8(3):36. Available from: https://doi.org/10.3390/medsci8030036; PMID: 32824524.

[503] Khalili H, Ahl R, Cao Y, Paydar S, Sjölin G, Niakan A, et al. Early selenium treatment for traumatic brain injury: Does it improve survival and functional outcome? Injury 2017;48(9):1922–6.

[504] Lee JM, Jeong SW, Kim MY, Park JB, Kim MS. The effect of vitamin D supplementation in patients with acute traumatic brain injury. World Neurosurg. 2019;126:e1421–6. Available from: https://doi.org/10.1016/j.wneu.2019.02.244; Epub 2019 Mar 20. PMID: 30904798.

[505] Lee SY, Amatya B, Judson R, Truesdale M, Reinhardt JD, Uddin T, et al. Clinical practice guidelines for rehabilitation in traumatic brain injury: a critical appraisal. Brain Inj 2019;33(10):1263–71. Available from: https://doi.org/10.1080/02699052.2019.1641747; Epub 2019 Jul 17. PMID: 31314607.

[506] Hanscom M, Loane DJ, Shea-Donohue T. Brain-gut axis dysfunction in the pathogenesis of traumatic brain injury. J Clin Invest 2021;131(12): e143777. Available from: https://doi.org/10.1172/JCI143777; PMID: 34128471.

[507] McDougall A, Bayley M, Munce SE. The ketogenic diet as a treatment for traumatic brain injury: a scoping review. Brain Inj 2018;32 (4):416–22. Available from: https://doi.org/10.1080/02699052.2018.1429025; Epub 2018 Jan 23. PMID: 29359959.

[508] Shilpa J, Mohan V. Ketogenic diets: Boon or bane? Indian J Med Res 2018;148(3):251–3. Available from: https://doi.org/10.4103/ijmr. IJMR_1666_18; PMID: 30425213.

Chapter 6

Cancer

Timothy David Noakes[1,2], Miriam Kalamian[3], Thomas N. Seyfried[4], Purna Mukherjee[4], Dominic P. D'Agostino[5], Gabriel Arismendi-Morillo[6], Christos Chinopoulos[7], Martha Tettenborn[8] and Nasha Winters[9]

[1]*Department of Health and Wellness Sciences, Cape Peninsula University of Technology, Cape Town, South Africa,* [2]*Nutrition Network, Cape Town, South Africa,* [3]*Dietary Therapies LLC, Hamilton, MT, United States,* [4]*Biology Department, Boston College, Boston, MA, United States,* [5]*Department of Molecular Pharmacology and Physiology, University of South Florida, Tampa, FL, United States,* [6]*Instituto de Investigaciones Biológicas, Facultad de Medicina, Universidad del Zulia, Maracaibo, Venezuela,* [7]*Department of Medical Biochemistry, Semmelweis University, Budapest, Hungary,* [8]*Kemble, Ontario, Canada,* [9]*Metabolic Terrain Institute of Health, Wilmington, DE, United States*

6.1 Cancer as a modern disease

Timothy David Noakes

M. Tanchou is of opinion that cancer, like insanity, increases in direct ratio to the civilization of the country and of the people.

Viljhalmur Steffanson ([1], p. 28)

Upon such a basis of theory and facts I have come to the essential conclusion that there has been a decided increase in the cancer death rate and progressively so during the last century ending with 1930. From this I reflect that the profound changes in dietary habits and nutritional condition of the population taking place during the intervening years have been world wide and due to the rapid and almost universal introduction of modified food products, conserved or preserved, refrigerated, or sterilized, colored or modified, aside from positive adulteration by the addition of injurious mineral substances close to being of a poisonous nature. To a diminishing extent food is being consumed in its natural state, at least by urban populations everywhere, and to a lesser degree also among people in rural communities.

Frederick Hoffman ([2], p. 196).

6.1.1 Introduction

This book begins by describing the phases through which human nutrition has evolved over the millennia. It began three to four million years ago when our ancient ancestors began to source animal foods and so embarked on the long hard road to *Homo sapiens*. All went well until about 12,000 years ago when, perhaps driven by a scarcity of the large fat mammals that humans had recently hunted to extinction, an alternate food source was required.

The solution was the cultivation of cereals and grains and the domestication of animals (the Agricultural Revolution) beginning in the Fertile Crescent in Western Asia. Next in the late 1800s, the industrial Revolution produced what Weston Price [3] labelled the 'the displacing nutrition [foods] of [modern] commerce' including 'largely white-flour products, sugar, polished rice, jams, canned goods, and vegetable fats'. In other words, foods that are long-lived, nutrient-poor but energy-dense and which can be transported over great distances without the risk of spoiling. More recently in the past few decades, modern commerce has created an even more damaging dietary concoction: highly addictive ultra-processed foods (UPFs).

A key argument advanced in this textbook is that a carbohydrate- and sugar-restricted, animal-based diet, higher in fat and protein is the original diet to which modern humans, because of our evolutionary history, are best adapted. It is the natural species-specific human diet [4]. We argue that deviation from this diet has caused the pandemic growth of chronic human diseases especially obesity, type 2 diabetes (T2D) and the other conditions linked to insulin resistance.

In this chapter, we consider whether cancer is another disease triggered by this diet change.

Ketogenic. DOI: https://doi.org/10.1016/B978-0-12-821617-0.00012-7

6.1.2 Is cancer a disease of civilisation?

To theorise that the modern diet induces human cancers, requires convincing evidence that cancer did not exist in populations eating the natural human diet. Clearly, it is more difficult to prove that something does not exist than that it does. For the absence of proof is not proof of absence. The existing 'proof of absence' of cancer is also based mainly on the recorded observations of individual witnesses. Fortunately, these witnesses were free of obvious conflicts of interest that might have skewed their conclusions. In particular, they received no financial or other benefit for their opinions. They simply recorded those of their observations that had surprised them.

Accepting that personal observations cannot prove any theory, it is nevertheless clear that all those who expressed an opinion over the past 100 years were unanimous in their opinion that the common cancers were encountered infrequently, if at all, in populations eating the natural human diet. Whereas this apparent rarity of cancer mysteriously disappeared when those same peoples adopted Weston Price's 'displacing nutrition of [modern] commerce'.

6.1.2.1 Cancer is uncommon in mid-Victorian England

As reported in Section 1.1, an important observation is that the mid-Victorian English who ate a wholesome diet of farm-produced real foods, available in such surplus that even the working-class poor were eating highly nutritious foods in abundance, were very healthy. As a result, the life expectancy of those who reached adulthood was equal to, or even better, than it is in modern Britain, especially for men (by about three years) [5–8].

The profile of the common causes of death was also quite different from the causes of deaths of their descendants, a century later (Fig. 6.1; [8]).

These reliable data clearly establish that cancer was an extremely uncommon cause of death in England and Wales in 1880 accounting for less than 3% of deaths compared to more than 40% in 1997. This supports the hypothesis that cancer is a more modern disease.

6.1.2.2 Reports that cancer was uncommon in African populations eating their traditional diets

In 1904 Dr. R. U. Moffat who was then working for the British government in East Africa wrote that: 'There is a general unanimity of opinion in favour of the idea that cancer is a rare disease among the aboriginal tribes' [9]. During a decade working there he had observed only 'one undoubted case of cancer' [9].

The North American physician and one-time president of the American Medical Association, Nicholas Senn, travelled to Africa in 1906; the previous year he had accompanied Robert Perry on one of his expeditions to the Arctic. On both continents he found no evidence of cancer: 'After closely observing the conditions of health' in both regions Senn became 'convinced that cancer is purely a disease of civilization' [10].

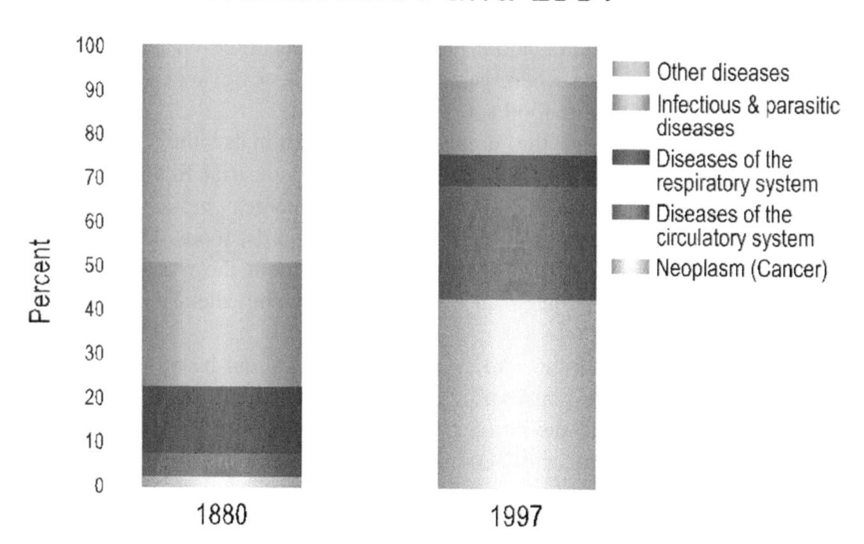

FIGURE 6.1 Comparison of causes of death in mid-Victorians living in England and Wales in 1880 compared with modern data from 1997. Note the large recent increases in deaths from cancers and diseases of the circulatory system, with reductions in deaths from infections, and parasitic and 'other' diseases. *Redrawn from Clayton P, Rowbotham J. How the mid-Victorians worked, ate and died. Int J Env Res Public Health 2009;6:1235–1253.*

The world-renowned physician and Nobel Peace Prize winner Albert Schweitzer, who worked as a physician in Gabon, Central Africa, for 41 years wrote: 'On my arrival in Gabon in 1913, I was astonished to encounter no case of cancer... I cannot, of course, say positively that there was no cancer at all, but like other frontier doctors. I can only say that if such cases existed they must have been quite rare. In the course of the years, we have seen cases of cancer in growing number in our region. My observation inclines me to attribute this to the fact that the natives were living more and more after the manner of the whites' [11]. Thus, Schweitzer reports an apparent increase in observed cancers after the adoption of the 'displacing foods of [modern] commerce'.

In 1923 the South African surgeon F. P. Fouche who spent six and a half years caring for 14,000 black (first nation) South Africans stated that he had not diagnosed a single case of cancer in that population. Whereas cancer '[was] frequently seen among the white or European population' [12].

Dr. Denis Burkitt, the grandfather of the dietary-fibre hypothesis [13] and who also discovered a specific cancer that now bears his name [14], spent 24 years in Uganda during and after the Second World War. He wrote that 44 hospitals he surveyed had never seen a single case of colon cancer or of heart disease, diverticulitis or appendicitis [15,16]. But he attributed this immunity to eating a diet high in fibre [13] rather than the avoidance of all the 'displacing nutrition of [modern] commerce'.

Others have drawn attention to the apparent rarity of cancer in other African populations eating their traditional diets [17,18]. A report in the British Medical Journal in April 1906 concluded: 'There can be no doubt that cancer in natives of British Central Africa is of the utmost rarity. Repeated efforts made by Government medical officers throughout the country for some time past have so far resulted in the discovery of but a single case' [19].

This rarity continued at least into the 1950s when the American physician John Higginson [20–22] reported that the prevalence of cancer in native African population yet untouched by the 'displacing nutrition of [modern] commerce' was remarkably low compared to reported cancer rates in Europe and the United States.

If these observations were true, the logical conclusion was that appropriate modifications of diet and lifestyle could prevent a proportion of cancers. Higginson suggested that the proportion could be as high as 70%–80%; Doll and Petro [23] agreed that at least 75%–80% of cancers in the United States might be preventable with appropriate modifications in diet and lifestyle.

But this suggestion has largely been ignored in favour of the theory that carcinogenic chemicals in the environment are the primary cancer-causing agents ([24], p. 210).

6.1.2.3 *Reports that cancer was uncommon in Arctic Inuit eating their traditional diets*

In the early 1900s, Vilhjamur Stefansson went to live for an extended period with the Inuit of the Canadian Arctic, describing his experiences in three classic books [24–26]. Three decades later, he dedicated his final book to an analysis of whether cancer is a modern disease [1].

Stefansson noted that when indoors the adult Inuit were naked above the waist and below the knees; children were completely naked. During his 10 years living with the Inuit and eating their traditional foods, Stefansson saw no visual evidence of cancer. Trained medical personnel who cared for the Inuit told him that 'cancer was not to be found amongst Eskimos who still lived native style' ([1], p. 16).

Stefansson also recorded the opinion of Dr. George Leavitt who had cared for up to 50,000 Inuit over a 15-year period. Encouraged by his physician brother to search for cases of cancer in the Inuit, Leavitt concluded that the search was futile because 'he was so sure by then that, except among civilized Eskimos, no native cancers would be found in the Arctic' ([1], p. 20). In the end it took him 50 years, from 1884 to 1933, to find a single case of cancer [1,18]. Another ship's surgeon with a similar experience, Dr. George Plummer Howe, concurred: 'It has been said that cancer does not exist among the Eskimos [Inuit]. So far as I can find out, this is true...' ([1], p. 16).

The Moravian Missionary doctor, Dr. Samuel King Hutton, who worked for 11 years in Labrador from 1902 to 1913 summarised his experience: 'Some diseases common in Europe have not come under my notice during a prolonged and careful survey of the health of the Eskimos [Inuit]. Of these diseases the most striking is cancer. I have not seen or heard of a case of malignant new growth in an Eskimo' ([1], p. 56; [27]).

In the autumn (fall) of 1931, F. S. Fellows was appointed Director of the Alaska Medical Services. Realising that there were no adequate statistics regarding death rates and causes of death in the four Alaskan judicial territories, he decided to instigate such a system. In 1934, he published a retrospective analysis of death rates and causes of death for the years 1926–1930 in the four territories [28]. Guyenet [29] has produced Fig. 6.2 from a table in that article [29]. The figure compares the cancer mortality rates amongst 'white' and Inuit persons in those four territories. Importantly the degree of 'Westernisation' of diet varies in the four territories; from most in Region 1 to least in

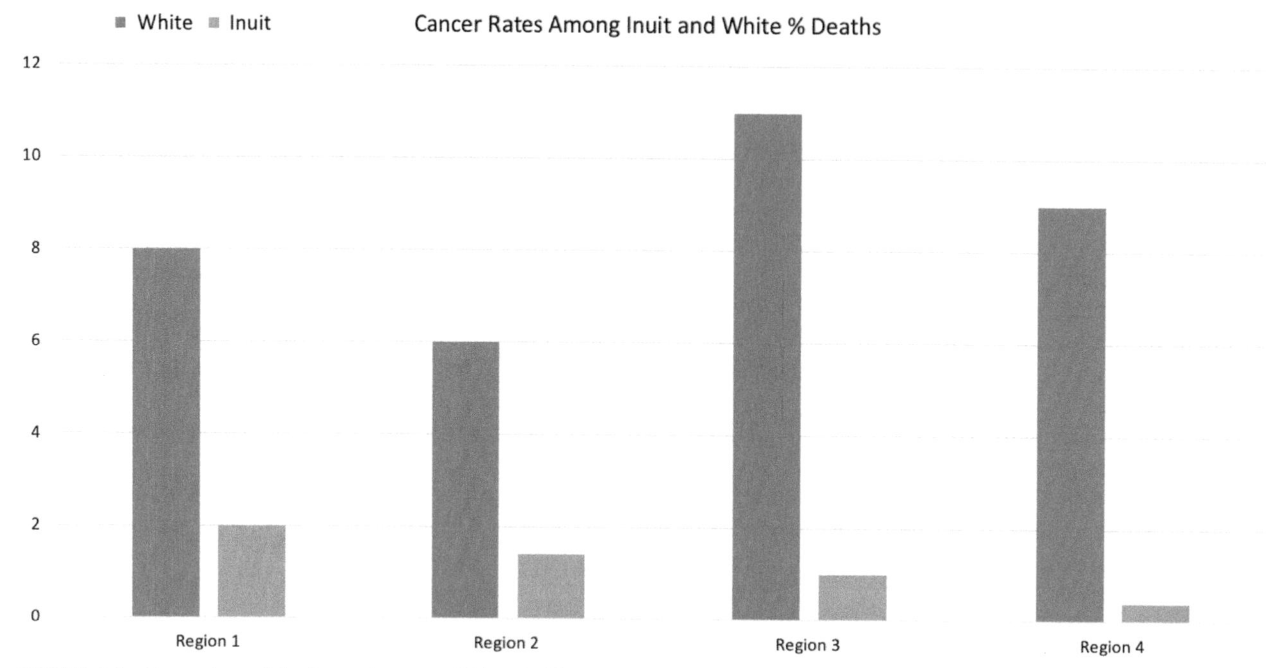

FIGURE 6.2 Comparison of death rates between 1926 and 1930 in four judicial territories in Alaska compared to 'white' and Inuit inhabitants of those territories. The degree of dietary 'Westernisation' fell progressively from Region 1 to Region 4.

Region 4. The degree of dietary 'Westernisation' was measured by the extent to which the 'displacing nutrition of [modern] commerce' especially wheat, flour, sugar canned goods and vegetable oils, had been adopted in the different regions.

Fig. 6.2 [29] shows that in all four territories (regions), cancer rates were substantially higher in the 'whites' than in the Inuit. The degree of dietary 'Westernisation' fell progressively from Region 1 to Region 4. Note that cancer deaths in the Inuit also fell from Regions 1 to 4 and were least and almost absent, amongst the Inuit living in Region 4 with the least dietary 'Westernisation'. This is to be predicted if cancer is a disease of dietary 'civilisation' or 'Westernisation'.

In conversation with Weston Price [3] in 1933, the Moravian Missionary Dr. Joseph Herman Romig reported that in his 36 years of contact with Eskimos (Inuit) and North American Indians who followed their traditional ways of life, he had never seen a case of malignant disease. But cancer had become more frequent when the Inuit became 'modernised' ([1], p. 47–48). Romig wrote: 'The women brought the biggest meal of the day.... mostly game and fish...Dried smoke salmon was much used, and other dried fish. Seal and fish oil was much in demand, and was a necessity; no one could be well without fats.... On this diet the people were strong and did not get scurvy... they did not have gastric ulcer, cancer, diabetes, malaria, or typhoid fever, or the common diseases of childhood known so well among the whites. For the most part they were a happy, carefree people...' ([1], p. 50).

A report in the Canadian Medical Journal in 1935 describes the experience of Dr. Urquhart from the Canadian/Alaskan border: '...as regards cancer... I have not in my seven years' experience ...seen a single case of malignancy in either Eskimo or Indian' [30].

A second article in the same journal in 1956 reported:

> *It has been said that 'cancer of the breast appears to have world-wide distribution and is in truth an arrant world citizen whose cellular turmoil shows no special predilection for race, climate, or geographical distribution [31]'.*
>
> *It would appear that the Canadian Eskimo may be an exception. For the past 10 years we have been aware of the relative freedom of Eskimos from breast cancer and cystic disease. In spite of strenuous efforts, we have so far been unable to discover one authenticated case of Eskimo breast malignancy. Dahl-Iversen has confirmed this observation in Greenland Eskimos ([32], p. 486).*

That cancer must have been encountered infrequently by doctors working in the Arctic is further suggested by single case reports of cancer in a Greenlander [33] and a Canadian [34] Inuit in the 1950s. The usual practise is to publish case reports of rare and unusual medical observations. Subsequently, the incidence of cancer has increased quite steeply in the Inuit [15,35–43].

In his publication documenting a rising incidence of cancers in Canadian Inuit from 1950 to 1973 [42], Schaefer noted that the change in cancer incidence occurred simultaneously with increases in all the chronic diseases:

> *Changes that have taken place in their (Inuit) dietary habits and their way of living have occurred with frightening speed. The fact that they are now growing faster, reaching puberty earlier, suffering from diabetes, cardiovascular disease, just about every disease prevalent among people who have been civilized for centuries, suggest that the metabolic turbulence created by a shift in diet is largely responsible for the less than pleasant outlook. The Eskimos' experience presents further evidence that behind many medical phenomena with which every practitioner in the Western world is now confronted lies a nutritional factor. How important we do not know. But important it certainly is ([42], p. 16).*

This changing pattern of neoplastic disease was associated with a reduction in daily protein intake from about 318 g/day in nomadic Inuit hunters to about 100 g/day in those living in urban areas. Carbohydrates provided approximately half of the total calories in urban Inuit compared to about 30% in traditional Inuit hunters (at that time) ([42], p. 10). The nature of the carbohydrates eaten had also changed in character with an increased consumption of refined, rapidly absorbed carbohydrates. Most importantly, sugar consumption had increased fourfold 'with almost a jolting abruptness in the last *twenty years* for the Canadian Eskimos' ([42], p. 11).

A more recent analysis has confirmed the rapidity and extent of these dietary changes. Between 1855 and 1970, the intake of sugar by the Greenland Inuit increased thirty-fold, and that of refined carbohydrates increased five- to sevenfold [44]. As a result, carbohydrate intake increased from 2%–8% to 40% of daily calories in the Greenland Inuit in the same period.

Today cancer is the leading cause of death amongst the Inuit in Alaska [15,43].

6.1.2.4 *Absence of cancer in traditional North and South American populations eating their usual diets*

A 460-page report based on interviews with physicians caring for First Nation native Americans of the southwestern United States and northern Mexico concluded that none had reported a 'clear case' of cancer [45]. A search of the remains of Native Americans also failed to find 'unequivocal signs of a malignant growth on an Indian bone' [45]. Hrdlicka concluded that if cancer existed at all among those peoples, it 'must be extremely rare'.

In his epic monograph, 'Mortality from Cancer' [46], Hoffman reported that he had found only two reports of cancer deaths among 63,000 Native Americans from different tribes ([46], p. 26).

Others reported that the North American Indians were free of the diseases that afflicted European settlers, including T2D, cancer, heart disease and most infectious diseases [15,47–50]: 'It is rare to see a sick body amongst them' [50]; they are 'unacquainted with a great many diseases that afflict the Europeans such as gout, gravel and dropsy, etc' [49]. 'While cancer is occasionally met with in primitive [*sic*] races, it occurs so seldom among the American Indians for instance, that this race may be considered practically immune from this disease' [48]; and 'In bodily proportions, color, gesture, dignity of bearing, the race is incomparable. It was free from our infectious scourges, tuberculosis and syphilis ... probably free from leprosy, scrofula and cancer, and it is safe to say that nervous prostration was unknown to the [American] Indian' [47].

The health of a population of hunter-gatherers, the Ache in Paraguay, South America, was extensively studied by Hill and Hurtado over 14 years in the 1970s. They published their findings in 1996 [51]. The data found that a significant percentage of the population reached the ages of 60 (30%) and 70 (20%) years; the main causes of death in Western populations (coronary heart disease, hypertension and T2D etc.) did not occur even in the elderly [52]. Moreover 'cases of death by cancer are not reported' [52].

Libertini suggests that the finding that old age can be reached without the development of cancer in the vast majority of a population (of hunter-gatherers), disproves the 'non-adaptive' hypothesis which posits that human ageing is caused by a reduction in the duplication capacities of stem cells, specifically to protect against the growth of cancers with increasing age.

6.1.2.5 *Absence of cancer in Torres Strait Islanders (Australian Aborigines)*

Of all the traditional populations that he and his wife studied, Weston Price [3] developed a special respect for the Australian Aborigines: '...their ability to build superb bodies and maintain them in excellent condition in so difficult an environment commands our genuine respect. It is a supreme test of human efficiency' (p. 152).

But he also wrote of the catastrophic effects of the lifestyle change produced by 'civilisation': 'It is doubtful if many places in the world can demonstrate so great a contrast in physical development and perfection of body as that which exists between the primitive (sic) Aborigines of Australia who have been the sole arbiters of their fate, and those Aborigines who have been under the influence of the white man' ([3], p. 152). For Price, 'the Aborigines represented the paradigm of moral and physical perfection' [53].

Although Price makes no mention of cancer rates amongst the Aborigines that he encountered, he did record the observation of Dr. J. R. Nimmo, the government physician caring for the health of the Torres Strait Islanders, a group considered indigenous Australians but who are ethnically distinct from the Australian Aborigines: 'In his thirteen years with them he (Nimmo) had not seen a single case of malignancy, and seen only one that he had suspected might be malignancy among the entire four thousand native populations. He stated that during this same period he had operated on several dozen malignancies for the white populations, which numbers about three hundred' ([3], p. 179).

Today lung and liver cancer rates are higher in Australian Aborigines and Torres Strait Islanders than in other Australians [54]. In addition Aborigines are more likely to die from their cancers than are other Australians [54].

6.1.2.6 Absence of cancer in the Hunzas living in the Himalayas

Major General Sir Robert McCarrison who died in 1960, is remembered as one of the first to understand the essential role of proper nutrition in human health [55].

In one of his iconic monographs, he wrote: 'the greatest single factor in the acquisition and maintenance of good health is perfectly constituted food...I know of nothing so potent in maintaining good health in a laboratory animal as perfectly constituted food; I know of nothing so potent in producing ill health as improperly constituted food. This, too, is the experience of stockbreeders. Is man an exception to a rule so universally applied to the higher animals?' [55]; '.. the fundamental fact (is) that a diet composed of natural foodstuffs, in proper proportions one to another, is the paramount influence in the maintenance of health' [56].

McCarrison spent most of his career studying the different dietary patterns and the health of the peoples living on the Indian continent. He documented the less-good health of those Indian populations existing almost exclusively on grains, particularly rice or wheat [55,56]. But he was particularly impressed by the health of Hunzas who lived in the Himalayas isolated far from the 'displacing nutrition of [modern] commerce' subsisting on an exclusive plant-based diet: 'During the period of my association with these people, I never saw a case of asthenic dyspepsia, of gastritis, or duodenal ulcer, or appendicitis, or mucous colitis, or cancer. Appendicitis, so common in Europe, was unknown' [56].

6.1.2.7 The twin monographs of Dr. Frederick Hoffman

Frederick Hoffman published two monumental texts – Mortality from Cancer throughout the World (1915) [46] and Cancer and Diet (1937) [2]. In the first, he acknowledged that the relative absence of reports of cancer in traditional population could not be ignored or easily explained away: 'There are no known reasons why cancer should not occasionally occur among any race or people...It is nevertheless a safe assumption that the large number of medical missionaries and other trained medical observers, living for years among native races throughout the world, would long ago have provided a more substantial basis of fact regarding the frequency of occurrence of malignant disease among the so-called 'uncivilised' races, if cancer were met with among them to anything like the degree common to practically all civilized countries' [46].

In his second monograph, Hoffman performed an exhaustive review of all the studies relevant to diet and cancer that had been published before 1937 [2]. He concluded that 'overabundant food consumption' is the root cause of all cancers ([2], p. 664).

6.1.2.8 Conclusion

On the basis of all this evidence, circumstantial as it may be, it seems reasonable to conclude that cancer is indeed a disease of 'civilisation' [57] that first appears in populations when they replace the natural human diet [4] with the 'displacing nutrition of [modern] commerce' [3].

This conclusion poses the question of what component(s) of this 'displacing nutrition' might be responsible.

6.1.3 Biological underpinnings linking diet and cancer

Proposed biological explanations for the apparent increase in cancer rates in populations following their adoption of diets that include the 'displacing nutrition of modern commerce'.

6.1.3.1 The Warburg Hypothesis

Nobel Laureate and acknowledged but flawed genius, Otto Warburg [58], was the first to suggest that a particular abnormality in glucose metabolism is the defining biochemical abnormality in all cancer cells. He showed that the cancer cells he studied in the 1930s preferred to 'ferment' glucose via the glycolytic pathway to lactic acid, rather than generate energy from mitochondrial respiration [59,60]. He postulated that this was due to hypoxic damage to the mitochondria of rapidly dividing cancer cells. The result, he proposed, was that all cancer cells were forced to rely purely on 'anaerobic' glucose fermentation into lactic acid for their energy and growth requirements.

Warburg's hypothesis flourished until others showed that mitochondrial function in the cells of many different forms of cancer is normal [61]. The discovery of the structure of DNA by Watson and Crick in 1953 [62] essentially killed the 'Warburg Hypothesis' and redirected the focus of cancer studies to the search for a genetic (DNA) cause for cancer.

In his exceptional book Ravenous [58], author Sam Apple brings Warburg's decades-long search for the cancer-diet connection into the modern era. He describes the modern evidence that Warburg was closer to the truth than is generally realised.

6.1.3.2 Overnutrition and cancer

In 1908 W. Roger Williams had written that 'Probably no single factor is more potent in determining the outbreak of cancer in the predisposed, than excessive feeding' [63]. Hoffman ends his exhaustive 767-page monograph 'Cancer and Diet' with the following conclusion: 'I consider my own duty discharged in presenting the facts as I have found them, which lead to the conclusion that overnutrition is common in the case of cancer patients to a remarkable degree, and that overabundant food consumption unquestionably is the underlying cause of the root condition of cancer in modern life' ([2], p. 664).

In their monograph 'The Causes of Cancer' [23] published 73 years later, Doll and Petro also concluded that 'overnutrition' was perhaps the most important but under-appreciated risk factor that could account for as many as 35% of all cancer deaths in the United States.

6.1.3.3 Type 2 diabetes, sugar consumption and cancer

Cancer is linked to rising rates of T2D and to increased global rates of sugar consumption. The increasing cancer rates that began in the late nineteenth century in the industrialised countries occurred simultaneously with rising rates of T2D; both followed increased global rates of sugar consumption.

The popular nutrition guide 'Food and Health' published in 1925 reported that: 'Not so long ago sugar was a rare luxury kept under lock and key in the tea caddy'. But with the rise of sugar beet production in Germany, the price of sugar fell in Europe so that consumption 'increased enormously.... Incidentally, cancer and diabetes, two scourges of civilization, have increased proportionately to the (rising) sugar consumption' [64].

In the United States Emerson and Larimore [65] noted that the incidence of T2D had increased more rapidly than any other disease; at the same time that sugar consumption had begun to increase exponentially in the mid to late 19th century. They asked: 'Do we need to eat three times as much sugar each year as our grandparents did?'.

They also noted, as would Cleave [66] a few decades later, that sugar consumption fell during the First (and Second) World Wars (Fig. 6.3) as did rates of T2D.

Note that sugar consumption dropped during both World Wars. This was reportedly associated with a reduced incidence of T2D during both Wars. Note also the exponential increase in sugar consumption from 1840 to 1895 (Fig. 6.3).

Others who linked increased rates of sugar consumption to rising rates of T2D (but without reference to cancer) were South African physician G. D. Campbell whose observational epidemiological studies in the 1960s established a link between the appearance of T2D in urbanised Zulu-speaking South Africans and their increased sugar consumption [67]. Cohen also reported rising T2D incidence rates in Yemenite immigrants to Israel associated with markedly increased rates of sugar consumption [68].

Interestingly, two of the most famous books identifying sugar as the key driver of a group of specific diseases – The Saccharine Diseases – make little, if any, reference to sugar as a direct cause of cancer [66,69].

However, the third iconic book in this collection, 'Pure, White and Deadly' by John Yudkin writes the following: 'The evidence at present comes chiefly from a study of international statistics and takes the form of an association between the average sugar consumption in different countries, and the incidence of two or three particular forms of cancer. The cancers that seem most likely to be related to sugar consumption are cancer of the large intestine in men and in women, and cancer of the breast in women. The death-rate for these three cancers in different countries is quite

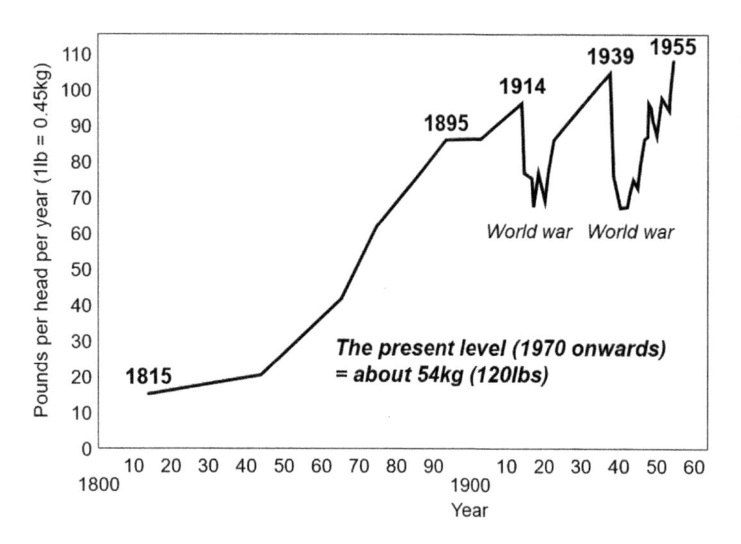

FIGURE 6.3 The rise in sugar consumption in the United Kingdom from 1800 to 1960. *Reproduced from fig. 6.1 in Cleave TL.* The Saccharine Disease. Conditions Caused by the Taking of Refined Carbohydrates, such as Sugar and White Flour. *John Wright and Sons Limited, Bristol, UK. 1974.*

closely associated with average sugar consumption, to about the same extent in fact as the association between sugar consumption or fat consumption with the death-rate due to coronary disease' [70].

Yudkin also noted that these cancers were most prevalent in the five countries with the highest rates of sugar consumption, specifically the United Kingdom, the Netherlands, Ireland, Denmark, and Canada. Whereas the countries with the lowest mortality from these cancers (Japan, Yugoslavia, Portugal, Spain, and Italy) also had the lowest rates of sugar consumption.

Doll and Armstrong also found epidemiological evidence linking sugar consumption with both the incidence of, and mortality from colon, rectal, breast, ovarian, prostate, kidney, nervous system, and testicular cancer [71,72].

Dr. Lewis Cantley whose research identified one molecular pathway through which insulin might favour cancer growth (by activating the phosphoinositide 3-kinase (PI3K) pathway [73,74]) has little doubt about the role of sugar in the causation of cancer [73]:

> *The high consumption of sugar over the past 40 years and the connection between obesity, elevated serum insulin and oncogenesis is almost certainly responsible for the increased rates of a variety of cancers in the developed world. It is far better to prevent cancers than to attempt to cure them after they are established. So I avoid sugar whenever possible. Someday, we will view this era of massive addiction to sugar in America in the same way that we now view the period of massive addiction to tobacco. In fact, sugar might be the more dangerous addiction because obesity, diabetes, cardiovascular disease and cancers probably have a greater negative impact on our health and the US economy than smoking-related diseases*

He goes even further: 'The evidence really suggests that if you have cancer, the sugar you're eating may be making it grow faster' ([58], p. 315).

Without suggesting any link to sugar consumption, a joint consensus statement issued by the American Diabetes Association and the American Cancer Association in 2010 concluded that: 'Epidemiological evidence suggests that people with diabetes are at significantly increased risk for many forms of cancer' [75].

It is also clear that those persons with T2D who develop cancer are less likely to survive than are those without that disease [75,76].

6.1.3.4 Insulin and cancer

Since persons with T2D are insulin resistant, inevitably the next advance would be the search for a linkage between hyperinsulinaemia and cancer. Already by 1990 it had been found that breast cancer cells overexpress insulin receptors [77]; numerous publications have since appeared linking cancer to elevated circulating blood insulin concentrations [75,78–91].

As recently reviewed in detail by Zhang et al. [91], hyperinsulinaemia is associated with an increased risk of both cancer incidence and death, even in those with normal body weight. Zhang et al. propose that 'hyperinsulinemia may promote cancer cell growth and prevent cancer cell death through both PI3K/AKT/mTORC and MAPK/ERK signaling' ([91], p. 292), in line with the work of Vander Heiden, Cantley, and Thompson [74] and Elstrom et al. [92]. This implies that insulin may be involved in the causation of cancer.

6.1.3.5 Fructose and cancer

Apple continues his exploration of the diet-cancer link by posing the question of why many populations have eaten high-carbohydrate diets for thousands of years without developing high rates of cancer (or T2D). For example, what dietary change could have produced higher rates of cancer (and T2D) in Asian populations in whom rice is the most important source of calories? Something else was necessary. Could it be the fructose component of sucrose [93]?

Apple argues that because it raises blood glucose and insulin concentrations, the glucose component of the sucrose molecule has always been considered the toxic component of sucrose for those with T2D.

Yet fructose may be at least as harmful because fructose specifically increases liver fat storage leading to non-alcoholic fatty liver disease (NAFLD) [94,95], which in turn exacerbates insulin resistance. Fructose-induced NAFLD must then inevitably cause persistent hyperinsulinaemia [96]. This persistent hyperinsulinaemia would be expected in turn to play a role in cancer causation.

6.1.3.6 High carbohydrate diets, genetics and cancer

There are possible biological mechanisms whereby diets high in carbohydrate, which produce hyperinsulinaemia or NAFLD, might be more likely to induce cancers.

Oncogenes linked to carbohydrate metabolism:

1. The genes coding for the enzyme lactate dehydrogenase (LDH), the key enzyme in the fermentation pathway producing lactic acid, were discovered as oncogenes in 1997 by researchers from Johns Hopkins hospital in Baltimore [97]. This provides indirect support for Warburg's hypothesis.
2. The gene coding for the production of phosphatidylinositol-3-kinase (PI_3K) has also been identified as an oncogene [73,74]. Crucially PI_3K is itself activated by insulin, specifically to activate the Warburg effect.
3. Dr. Craig Thompson of the Memorial Sloan Kettering Cancer Center discovered that dysfunctional mitochondria direct the cells in which they are located to destroy themselves (the process known as apoptosis). But apoptosis is prevented by growth factors external to the cell, which instruct the mitochondria to keep respiring and so to avoid apoptosis. Thompson realised that cancer cells no longer require these factors. His goal became to identify 'those specific genes that allow a (cancer) cell to (over)eat without permission from growth factors' ([58], p. 257).

The AKT/protein kinase B (PKB) gene [92] is one such that directs the production of these growth factors. This enzyme specifically increases the glucose uptake and metabolism of cancer cells, thereby activating the Warburg Effect.

Thompson argues that the Warburg Effect 'makes the cell independent of the normal signal transduction that controls its biology...We believe that's a fundamental shift in the way we should be thinking about cancer'. He argues that the advantages of deregulated glycolysis (the Warburg Effect) to a cancer cell are obvious: 'If you put more fuel in, things will work more efficiently... The deregulation of the Akt pathway [is] simply upregulating your ability to take up nutrients, to conserve amino acids and lipids... to fuel cell growth' ([98], p. 1806).

According to Thompson, in this gluttonous state, the cancer cell 'really doesn't ever think about dying. Now it thinks, 'I've got a lot of fuel; I could do a lot of other things'' ([58], p. 261). So '.. when the food exceeds their need to survive, they (cancer cells) begin to make copies of themselves, as many as they can' ([58], p. 264).

6.1.4 Summary

In 1927 the Journal 'Cancer' carried an article by Dr. William Howard Hay of Buffalo, New York entitled 'Cancer as a Disease of Either Election or Ignorance' [99]. Dr. Hay wrote ([57], p. 35; [99]):

> *A study of the distribution of cancer, among the races of the entire earth, shows a cancer ratio in about the proportion to which civilized living predominates; so evidently something inherent in the habits of civilization is responsible for the difference of cancer incidence as compared with the uncivilized (sic) races and tribes. Climate has nothing to do with this difference, as witness the fact that tribes living naturally will show a complete absence of cancer till mixture with more civilized man corrupts the naturalness of habit; and just as these habits conform to those civilizations, even so does cancer begin to show its head...*

Is it possible the cause of cancer is our departure from natural foods? It would surely look to any man from Mars; but we have so long lived on processed foods.... that we are in a state of unbalanced nutrition from birth... we have come to regard these foods as the hallmark of civilization, when it is in fact that these very foods set the stage for every sort of ill, including cancer...

The evidence presented in this article and in this Textbook suggests that Dr. William Howard Hay's comments were prescient.

6.2 Cancer as a mitochondrial metabolic disease

Thomas N. Seyfried, Gabriel Arismendi-Morillo, Purna Mukherjee, and Christos Chinopoulos

6.2.1 Introduction

According to the mitochondrial metabolic theory (MMT), most cancers arise in a two-step process. The first process involves defects in the number, structure, and function of mitochondria that would reduce ATP synthesis through oxidative phosphorylation (OxPhos) [100–108]. The second process involves a gradual increase in ATP synthesis through substrate level phosphorylation that would compensate for the reduced efficiency of OxPhos. Warburg first proposed this two-step process to account for the origin of cancer [108–111]. Warburg's central theory has been supported in a broad range of human and animal cancers [100,103,105,109,112–130]. Aerobic fermentation (aerobic glycolysis or Warburg Effect) involves ATP synthesis through substrate-level phosphorylation at the pyruvate kinase step in the glycolytic pathway [131]. The evidence for aerobic fermentation in cancer comes from the excessive production of glucose-derived lactate even in the presence of 100% oxygen [108–110,132,133]. The Warburg effect is linked in part to an abnormality in the Pasteur effect, which is an oxygen-mediated increase in ATP synthesis through OxPhos with a corresponding reduction in lactate production [134,135]. Aerobic fermentation is now recognised as a hallmark of cancer [131,136,137].

Although aerobic fermentation is seen in many cancers, Warburg placed little emphasis on the role of aerobic fermentation in tumour cells. He felt that aerobic fermentation was '*too labile and too dependent on external conditions*' due to the complex interactions of respiration and fermentation [108,110]. Warburg also described how aerobic fermentation would confuse the issue of cancer cell metabolism and should not be used as a test for cancer cells [110]. Support for his position that aerobic fermentation (glycolysis) confuses the issue of cancer metabolism came from the studies of R. J. O'Connor who misinterpreted the linkage of oxygen consumption to cell division in the early chick embryo [108,110,138]. It is known that anaerobic fermentation, not aerobic fermentation, is largely responsible for cell division in the early embryo [108,110]. Consequently, Warburg preferred to focus more on respiration and anaerobic fermentation than on aerobic fermentation in cancer cell metabolism. While persistent anaerobic fermentation is a common property of cancer cells, the linkage of oxygen consumption to ATP synthesis was, and continues to be, a controversial subject in the field of cancer metabolism [61,139]. As mitochondrial function is closely linked to mitochondrial structure [122,140–143], it is unclear how OxPhos would be unaffected in cancer cells with documented defects in the number, structure, and function of their mitochondria.

6.2.2 The mitochondrial network

The mitochondrion is a highly dynamic network organelle that undergoes rapid changes in size, length, and shape [144]. These changes are linked to metabolic and Ca^{2+} buffering requirements and to different cellular abnormalities. The ultrastructure of the mitochondrion consists of an outer and inner membrane. The outer membrane encloses the content of the mitochondrion, while the inner membrane comprises a series of folds, called cristae. The cristae project towards the interior matrix of the organelle. The intermembrane space is the area between the outer and inner membranes. The inner membrane encloses the matrix. The outer membrane contains the antagonists and agonists of apoptosis and the proteins regulating mitochondrial fission/fusion. The inner membrane includes the enzyme complexes and electron transporters of the respiratory chain that are necessary for generating 80%–90% of ATP through OxPhos in most mammalian tissues [117,131,145,146]. The shape and dimensions of the cristae modulate the kinetics and the structure of protein complexes that underlie the efficiency of OxPhos [143,147].

The mitochondrial matrix contains the enzymes for beta-oxidation and the tricarboxylic acid (TCA) cycle. Mitochondria display large, elongated, and branched structures in living human cells. These structures define the mitochondrial network, which extends throughout the cytosol and are in close contact with the membranes of other structures including the nucleus, the endoplasmic reticulum, the Golgi complex, and the cytoskeleton. Fusion and fission events continuously remodel the mitochondrial network [148]. Mitochondria can exist as single and randomly dispersed organelles in some cell types, and as dynamic networks that change shape and subcellular distribution in other cell types. Mitochondria can also display intracellular heterogeneity in morphology and biochemistry depending on cell type, [149,150].

Mitochondrial-associated membranes (MAM) are also part of the mitochondrial network [151]. MAM include the endoplasmic reticulum, the outer mitochondrial membrane, and membrane tether proteins. These components participate in trafficking and signalling events. MAM regulate metabolic pathways and participate in Ca^{2+} signalling, and the synthesis and exchange of lipids. The formation of MAM is linked to cellular demands or to changes in the microenvironment [144,152–155]. Structural and functional integrity of the mitochondrial network is essential for metabolic homoeostasis.

The mitochondrial network exhibits heterogeneous ultrastructural pathology in many human cancers [104,148,151,164,166]. The heterogeneous pathology involves abnormalities in the number of mitochondria, structural abnormalities in mitochondrial cristae, alterations in mitochondrial lipids and enzymes of the electron transport chain, and abnormalities in MAM. As MAM are intimately associated with mitochondrial function, alterations in MAM structure will alter mitochondrial function and reduce the efficiency of OxPhos [151]. Examples of mitochondrial and MAM ultrastructural abnormalities in breast cancer and glioblastoma are illustrated in Fig. 6.4A and B. A high cristae surface area is predicted to favour ATP synthesis [222]. Perturbations of mitochondrial-shaping proteins disrupt cristae organisation making the electron transport chain less efficient thereby decreasing the efficiency of OxPhos [143]. Alterations in the density, length, and width of the MAM and MAM-resident mTORC2 would increase ROS production thus causing a metabolic shift from energy production through OxPhos to energy production through glycolysis and glutaminolysis. Abnormalities in MAM ultrastructure have been found in glioma tissue that involve the density, length, and width of the interfacing membranes of the mitochondrial and ER. The ultrastructural abnormalities in mitochondria and MAM represent the submicroscopic base for abnormal cancer metabolism leading to a greater reliance on substrate level phosphorylation than on OxPhos for energy production. The motochondrial and MAM morphological abnormalities are dependent on the tumour microenvironment and are not specific for any tumour type.

In addition to the abnormalities in mitochondria and MAM ultrastructure, no cancer cell has been found with a normal composition or content of cardiolipin, the cristae-enriched phospholipid that contributes to OxPhos function [117,143,223–234]. Proton leak and uncoupling, which diminish respiratory efficiency [235], is also greater in tumour cells than in normal cells [236–238]. Based on the foundational biological principle that *structure determines function* [122,131,141,143,239], abnormalities in mitochondrial structure would alter mitochondrial function and effective ATP synthesis through OxPhos.

Despite the massive evidence presented showing that mitochondria are abnormal in cancer cells (Table 6.1), many investigators have claimed that mitochondria are functional and not impaired in cancer. This view is based largely from analysis of oxygen consumption by cultured tumour cells. Most investigators have equated oxygen consumption rate with OxPhos function. This is similar to the error made by R. J. O'Connor who misinterpreted the linkage of oxygen consumption to cell division mentioned above. Although the rate of oxygen consumption can be similar or greater in cancer cells than in normal cells, oxygen consumption can be a poor indicator for OxPhos in cancer cells [199,240–244]. Indeed, Ramanathan et al., stated it was: 'intriguing that cells with the highest tumorigenic potential consumed more oxygen and yet exhibit diminished oxygen dependent (aerobic) ATP synthesis' [243]. The authors considered that such tumour cells used the mitochondrial etc for reasons other than ATP synthesis by allowing leakage of the membrane potential thus producing heat and reactive oxygen species (ROS). Hence, caution is necessary in considering that mitochondria and OxPhos are normal in cancer cells based on the measurement of oxygen consumption alone.

Besides the above-documented abnormalities in mitochondrial number, structure, and function, genetic abnormalities that alter mitochondrial function have also been recognised in many cancers. The *p53* mutation, which is found in many cancers, can disrupt mitochondrial OxPhos [245–247]. The retinoblastoma tumour suppressor protein, Rb, has been linked to abnormalities in mitochondrial mass and OxPhos function [248]. Abnormalities in mitochondrial structure or function have also been associated with other cancer-related genes including *BCR-ABL* [249], the *V600E-BRAF* oncogene [199], and *BRCA* mutations [250–253]. Huang and colleagues showed that *K-rasG12v* transformation caused mitochondrial dysfunction and a metabolic switch from OxPhos to aerobic fermentation in direct support of the two-step MMT [115]. It appears that few if any cancer types are free of mitochondrial abnormalities, whether structural or functional, suggesting that OxPhos inefficiency is the signature metabolic hallmark of cancer, as hypothesised by Warburg. Hence, a reliance on fermentation metabolism for the synthesis of ATP and metabolic building blocks would

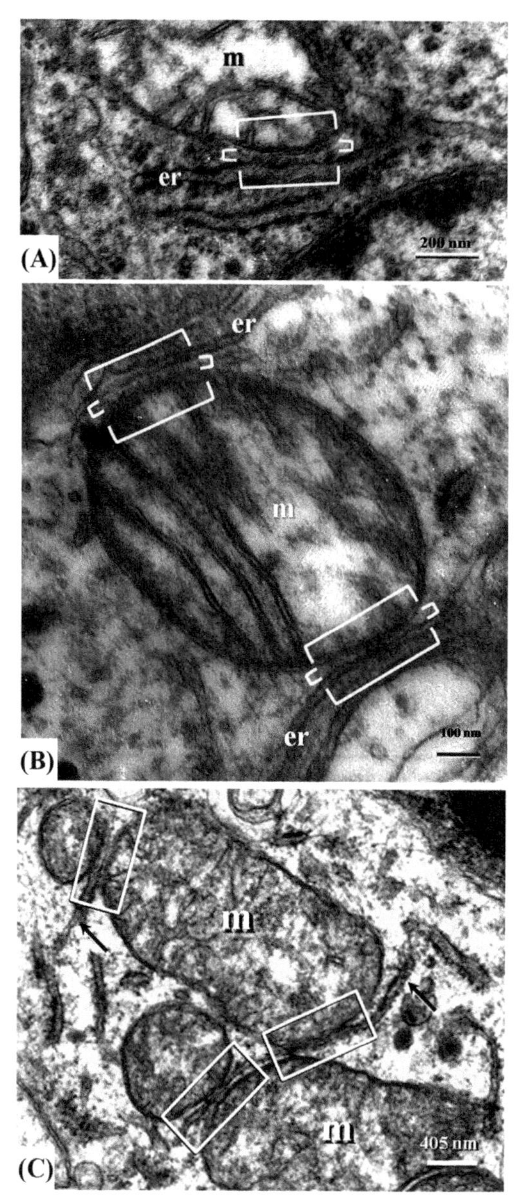

FIGURE 6.4 Ultrastructural mitochondrial and MAM abnormalities in human gliomas. Mitochondria with disarrangement of cristae and partial or total cristolysis, and MAM variations are seen. These structural abnormalities in the mitochondrial network would prevent sufficient ATP synthesis through OxPhos and thus requiring compensatory ATP synthesis through both substrate level phosphorylation in the cytoplasm using glucose as substrate (Warburg effect) and in mitochondria using glutamine as substrate (Q-Effect). Micrograph (A). MAM length 320 nm (long brackets). Mitochondria-Endoplasmic reticulum interface <30 nm (Directassociation) (short brackets). m: denotes electron-lucent mitochondria with partial cristolysis. er: nonexpanded endoplasmic reticulum profiles [159,162,168]. Reprinted with permission from [167]. Micrograph (B). MAM length 258,3–287,5 nm (long brackets). Mitochondria-Endoplasmic reticulum interface <30 nm (Direct association) (short brackets). m: denotes electron-lucent mitochondria with partial cristolysis. er: nonexpanded endoplasmic reticulum profiles. Micrograph (C). MAM length 96–652 nm, and Mitochondria-Endoplasmic reticulum interface <30 nm (Direct association) (rectangles). m: denotes electron-lucent mitochondria with total cristolysis. Arrows: nonexpanded endoplasmic reticulum profiles. Magnifications: ×5000–35,000. The mitochondria and MAM abnormalities found in gliomas have also been observed in other cancers and include abnormalities in calcium homeostasis, proliferation, metastasis, and chemotherapeutic resistance.

be the expected consequence of genetic abnormalities in the structure and function of mitochondria. As no cancer-associated gene has been found to be 100% penetrant, all cancer-associated gene abnormalities are considered secondary causes, rather than primary causes of cancer. Furthermore, the numerous somatic mutations present in cancer cells are considered downstream epiphenomena of dysfunctional OxPhos [107,245]. DNA repair is also dependent on ATP

TABLE 6.1 Evidence for abnormalities in mitochondrial number, structure, or function in various cancers.

Bladder cancer [156–158]
Breast/mammary cancers [105,122,159–170]
Colorectal cancers [105,171–173]
Gliomas [113,131,174–181]
Kidney/renal cancer [105,182–185]
Leukaemias/lymphoma including AML and ALL [105,164,186–190]
Liver/hepatic cancer [104,125,129,130,169,191–194]
Lung cancer [164,195–198]
Melanomas [193,199,200]
Neuroblastoma [201–203]
Osteosarcoma [204–207]
Ovarian cancer [208–210]
Pancreatic cancer [211–213]
Prostate cancer [105,214,215]
Rhabdomyosacromas [216,217]
Retinoblastoma [218,219]
Salivary gland/oral cancers [220,221]

synthesis through OxPhos [254]. ROS, arising largely from dysfunctional OxPhos, are carcinogenic and mutagenic [255]. Hence, most if not all somatic mutations seen in cancer cells arise as secondary effects of dysregulated cancer cell metabolism and are not the original cause of cancer.

6.2.3 Glutamine-driven mitochondrial substrate-level phosphorylation as a major energy source for cancer cells

Succinate-CoA ligase (SUCL, also known as succinyl-CoA synthetase) is a mitochondrial matrix enzyme that catalyses the conversion of succinyl-CoA and ADP (or GDP) to CoA-SH, succinate, and ATP (or GTP) [256]. SUCL is the only phosphorylation reaction occurring at the substrate level in the TCA cycle [257,258]. Notably, when SUCL proceeds towards ATP formation, it is termed mitochondrial substrate-level phosphorylation (mSLP); a process that can yield high-energy phosphates in the absence of oxygen. SUCL is a heterodimer composed of an invariant α-subunit encoded by the *SUCLG1* gene, and a substrate-specific β-subunit encoded by either the *SUCLA2* or *SUCLG2* genes. This dimer combination results in either of two reversible enzyme reactions, that is, a GTP-forming SUCL (EC 6.2.1.4) or an ATP-forming SUCL (EC 6.2.1.5) [259]. Chen recently suggested that mSLP could compensate for lost energy synthesis through either glycolysis or OxPhos [260]. Energy generation through mSLP is critically important in several metabolic pathways and could compensate for inefficient energy production through OxPhos in cancer cells [261,262].

It is our view that much of the confusion surrounding the issue of OxPhos impairment in cancer cell metabolism comes from the failure to recognise mSLP as a major source of ATP synthesis that can compensate for impaired ATP production through OxPhos. ATP synthesis through mSLP can be misinterpreted as energy through OxPhos unless experiments are designed to distinguish the two energy sources [263]. We recently described how the SUCL reaction in the TCA cycle could synthesise ATP (and/or GTP) thus 'bailing-in' cancer mitochondria from a reverse-operating F_0-F_1 ATP synthase when OxPhos function(s) are impaired [131]. The glutaminolysis pathway would support the production of high-energy phosphates through the sequential metabolism of glutamine -> glutamate -> alpha-ketoglutarate -> succinyl CoA -> succinate.

Glutamine has long been considered an essential metabolite for tumour cell growth [264–267]. We described how glutamine-derived *a*-ketoglutarate could branch out to become a substrate for both the reductive carboxylation and the oxidative decarboxylation pathways in the TCA cycle [131]. ATP synthesis through mSLP has been measured in cardiac and kidney tissues under conditions of hypoxia [268–270], and in cells with mtDNA mutations [260]. Indeed, OxPhos cannot be normal in cells containing numerous mtDNA mutations, as was recently found in most cancers [271]. Compensatory glutamine-dependent mSLP would therefore be the expected consequence of any defect, whether genetic or non-genetic, that would compromise OxPhos function. Recent studies also show that mitochondrial import of the ARHGAP11B protein facilitates proliferation of basal progenitor cells through mSLP and glutaminolysis during early brain development [272]. This is interesting, as emerging evidence shows that mSLP can also serve as a source of ATP synthesis in proliferating cancer cells [261,273]. Chen et al. also showed that glutamine utilisation is a common feature of cells with partial defects in OxPhos, irrespective of the specific OxPhos complex affected [260]. This finding could account in large part for the essential requirement for glutamine of cancers with partial defects in OxPhos [131]. It is our view that glutamine-supported mSLP can compensate for OxPhos deficiency in either hypoxic or normoxic growth environments.

Wallace McKeehan first described glutaminolysis as the second major energy pathway in cancer cells [266]. Although McKeehan recognised the SUCL reaction in the TCA cycle, he did not consider this reaction as a major source of ATP synthesis, but rather considered glutamine as a respiratory fuel for OxPhos, as have other investigators [264,266]. It is now known that the uncoupling action of glutamine in metastatic tumour cells would prevent ATP synthesis through OxPhos despite increased oxygen consumption [274], (and see below). While McKeehan considered malate-derived pyruvate as the end product of the glutaminolysis pathway, Moreadith and Lehninger showed that pyruvate was not the end product, as malate did not leave the mitochondria in five different tumour types [275]. We consider succinate, rather than pyruvate, as the end product of the glutaminolysis pathway [131,262,276]. This is important as succinate is known to stabilise HIF-1*a*, a transcription factor that together with c-Myc upregulates pathways necessary for the anaerobic metabolism of glucose and glutamine [277–282]. In addition to increasing glutaminolysis, c-Myc also enhances expression of the pyruvate kinase M2 isoform suggesting that succinic acid fermentation through glutaminolysis can enhance lactic acid fermentation through glycolysis (Warburg effect) [283,284]. These oncogenes facilitate tumour growth by upregulating glucose and glutamine fermentation pathways. Cells that cannot transition from OxPhos to fermentation will die, and rarely become tumorigenic [108]. Hence, oncogene activation becomes necessary for facilitating the transition from OxPhos to fermentation during tumorigenesis.

We recently proposed that mSLP was the missing link in Warburg's central theory that insufficient OxPhos coupled with compensatory fermentation is the origin of cancer [131]. In addition to cytoplasmic substrate level phosphorylation (Warburg effect), mSLP could also compensate for OxPhos deficiency. Direct evidence for this possibility comes from the data of Chen et al., showing that human cells with mitochondrial DNA mutations and OxPhos deficiency can rewire glutamine metabolism to obtain energy through mSLP [260]. As *Q* is the letter designation for glutamine, we have described this phenomenon as the *Q-Effect* to distinguish it from that involving the aerobic fermentation of glucose, that is, the *Warburg effect* [131]. Both the Warburg effect and the Q-effect arise from compromised OxPhos. Unfortunately, the role of glutaminolysis and mSLP in cellular energy metabolism was unknown to Warburg, as this information was discovered only after, or towards the end of his career [257,258,285,286]. Although we originally described this phenomenon as the Warburg Q-Effect, we removed the term *Warburg* from the effect, as Warburg did not envision amino acid fermentation as a second major compensatory energy source to OxPhos in his theory of cancer. Hence, mSLP and the Q-effect can be considered the missing metabolic link in the MMT of cancer.

Although many investigators have focused on aerobic fermentation (Warburg effect), none of the major review articles or previous studies on cancer energy metabolism have discussed or even recognised the role of SUCL activity and mSLP, as an energy mechanism that could compensate for deficient OxPhos in tumour cells [131,287]. The explanation for this oversight remains unexplained. Many investigators have also used the *Seahorse* instrument to link oxygen consumption to ATP synthesis through OxPhos. This instrument, however, can only infer that ATP flux is linked to oxygen consumption rate (OCR). As the *Seahorse* instrument is not yet capable of distinguishing ATP synthesis from mSLP or from OxPhos, caution is necessary in attempting to link oxygen consumption rate to ATP synthesis through OxPhos in cultured cancer cells using this instrument.

A reliance on mSLP for ATP synthesis would also be necessary for those tumours expressing the glycolytic pyruvate kinase M2 (PKM2) isoform, which predominates in many aggressive cancers and produces less ATP than the PKM1 isoform [137,283,284,288–290]. How could tumour cells with OxPhos deficiency and PKM2 expression synthesise ATP for growth? We consider mSLP as the dominant mechanism for ATP synthesis in tumour cells with deficient OxPhos, that overexpress PKM2, and that grow in hypoxic environments. Chen et al. showed recently that production of ATP through mSLP could compensate for deficiencies in either glycolysis or OxPhos [260]. mSLP would be the metabolic hallmark of tumour cell proliferation whether growth is in vivo or in vitro. The Crabtree effect might induce a similar process in non-tumorigenic cells that proliferate in vitro, but would not occur in normal cells that proliferate in vivo. Indeed, aerobic fermentation does not occur in proliferating non-transformed cells grown in vivo, for example, in regenerating liver cells and normal colon cells that use fatty acids and butyrate as respiratory fuels, respectively [131,291–293]. Confusion over the association of OxPhos with oxygen consumption and a general failure to appreciate the role of mSLP as a compensatory energy mechanism could explain in large part how some investigators might believe that OxPhos is functional and responsible for ATP synthesis in tumour cells.

6.2.4 Is it the mitochondrial metabolic theory or the somatic mutation theory that can best explain the origin of cancer?

A scientific theory is simply an attempt to explain the facts of nature. Reality is based on replicated facts, whereas interpretation of the facts is based on credible theories. The heliocentric theory was able to explain better the movements of celestial bodies than was the geocentric theory. The germ theory was able to explain better the origin of contagious diseases than was the miasma 'bad air' theory. The theory of evolution by natural selection was able to explain better the origin of species than was the theory of special creation. In none of these examples could a hybrid theory be envisioned. A theory that can best explain the facts of a phenomenon is more likely to advance knowledge than a theory that is less able to explain the facts. Can the MMT explain better the facts of cancer than can the somatic mutations theory (SMT)?

According to the SMT, cancer is a genetic disease that arises from inherited or spontaneous mutations in proto-oncogenes or tumour suppressor genes [136,294,295]. While many mutations have been found in various tumours, the so-called 'driver' gene mutations are thought to be most responsible for the disease [295]. Although the SMT is currently the dominant scientific explanation for the origin of cancer, numerous inconsistencies have emerged that seriously challenge the credibility of this theory. Major inconsistencies include:

1) The absence of gene mutations and chromosomal abnormalities in some cancers [296–300]. Specifically, Greenman et al., found no mutations following extensive sequencing in 73/210 cancers [294], whereas Parsons et al., found no mutations in the P53, the PI3K, or the RB1 pathways in the Br20P tissue sample of a glioblastoma patient [301]. These tissue samples should not exist according to the SMT.
2) The identification and clonal expansion of numerous driver gene mutations in a broad range of normal human tissues [302–306]. No clear explanation has been presented on how the SMT can account for malignant tumours that have no mutations or for normal cells and tissues that express driver mutations, but do not develop tumours.
3) The general absence of cancers in chimpanzees despite having about 98.5% gene and protein sequence identity with humans even at the BRCA1 locus [307–310]. Indeed, breast cancer has never been documented in a female chimpanzee suggesting that environmental factors (diet and lifestyle), rather than genetic mutations, are largely responsible for the disease [310,311]. As DNA replication would be similar in normal tissue stem cells in chimpanzees and humans, the rarity of cancer in all chimpanzee organs undermines the 'bad luck' hypothesis of Tomasetti and Vogelstein that cancer risk is due to random mutations arising during DNA replication in normal, noncancerous stem cells [312].
4) It is also interesting that Theodor Boveri, the person most recognised as the originator of the SMT [313,314], never directly studied cancer and was highly apologetic for his general lack of knowledge about the disease [315]. Despite these inconsistencies, the SMT is presented as if it were dogma in most current college textbooks of genetics, biochemistry, and cell biology, as well as in the National Cancer Institute in stating that, 'Cancer is a genetic disease—that is, it is caused by changes to genes that control the way our cells function, especially how they grow and divide' [316,317].

The most compelling evidence against the SMT comes from the nuclear/cytoplasm transfer experiments showing that normal cells and tissues can be produced from tumorigenic nuclei, as long as the tumorigenic nuclei are localised in cytoplasm containing normal mitochondria [317,318] (Fig. 6.5). Moreover, recent studies show that normal mitochondria can down-regulate multiple oncogenic pathways and growth behaviour in glioma, melanoma, and metastatic breast cancer cells [163,319–322]. These findings demonstrate that normal mitochondrial function can suppress tumorigenesis regardless of the gene or chromosomal abnormalities that might be present in the tumour nucleus. When viewed collectively, these findings suggest that the somatic mutations found in many cancers are not the primary cause of the disease and seriously challenge the SMT as a credible explanation for the origin of cancer.

It is our view that the MMT can explain better the hallmarks and facts of cancer than can the SMT (Fig. 6.6). The MMT is the only theory to provide a credible explanation for the 'oncogenic paradox' that has perplexed the cancer field for decades [323–325]. Albert Szent-Gyorgyi first described the oncogenic paradox as a specific process (malignant transformation) that could be initiated by a plethora of unspecific events (radiation, asbestos, viral infections, rare inherited mutations, irritation, inflammation, chemicals, etc.) [324]. Siddhartha Mukherjee also struggled to understand the paradox in stating on page 285 of his book: 'What, beyond abnormal, dysregulated cell division, was the common pathophysiological mechanism underlying cancer?' [323]. According to the MMT, the loss of OxPhos following mitochondrial damage is the common pathophysiological mechanism responsible for the origin of cancer. This damage

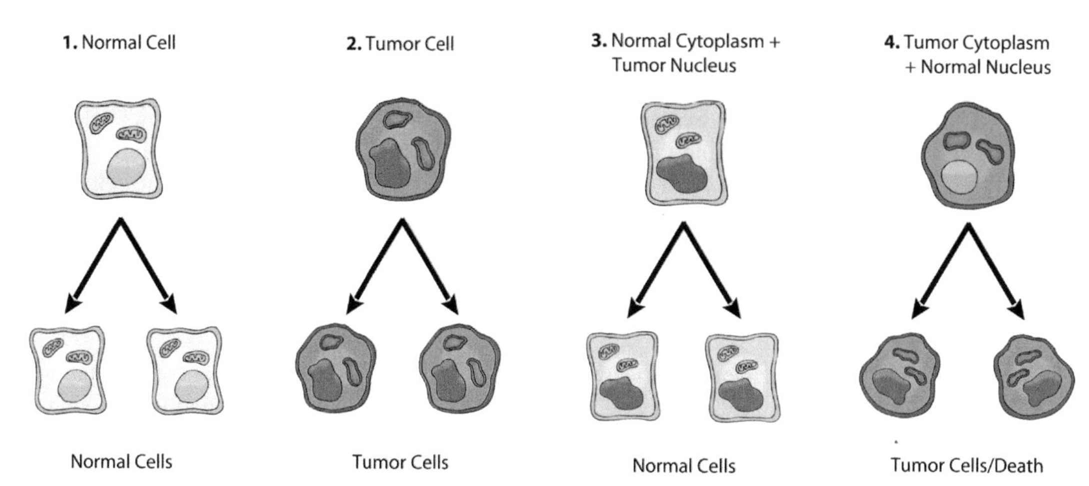

FIGURE 6.5 **Role of the nucleus and mitochondria in the origin of tumours.** This image summarises the broad range experimental evidence supporting a dominant role of the mitochondria in the origin of tumorigenesis as previously described [107,317,318]. Normal cells are depicted in green with mitochondrial and nuclear morphology indicative of normal respiration and nuclear gene expression, respectively. Tumour cells are depicted in red with abnormal mitochondrial and nuclear morphology indicative of abnormal respiration and genomic instability. (1) Normal cells beget normal cells. (2) Tumour cells beget tumour cells. (3) Delivery of a tumour cell nucleus into a normal cell cytoplasm begets normal cells despite the persistence of tumour-associated genomic abnormalities. (4) Delivery of a normal cell nucleus into a tumour cell cytoplasm begets tumour cells or dead cells, but not normal cells. The results provide the strongest evidence to date showing that tumours do not arise from nuclear genomic defects alone, and that normal mitochondria can suppress tumorigenesis. *Original diagram from Jeffrey Ling and Thomas N. Seyfried, with permission.*

could arise from any number of the unspecific processes. Such damage would induce compensatory energy production through the process of substrate level phosphorylation in both the cytoplasm and the mitochondria. As normal mitochondrial function maintains the differentiated state of cells, the rewiring of energy metabolism from respiration to fermentation would cause dedifferentiation and unbridled proliferation, [317]. How might these energy transitions explain the six major hallmarks of cancer as described by Hanahan and Weinberg?

Activation of oncogenes, for example, *Hif-1a* and c-*Myc*, become necessary for the upregulation of substrate level phosphorylation through the glycolysis and glutaminolysis pathways, respectively. This activation would be induced through the mitochondrial stress response or the retrograde signalling system [329–331]. The energy transition from OxPhos to substrate level phosphorylation will cause a cell to enter its default state of unbridled proliferation, that is, the metabolic state of existence for all cells during the dark and anaerobic period in the history of life [324]. The transition to this energetic state could explain the first three hallmarks of cancer (Fig. 6.6). Aerobic fermentation and sustained angiogenesis would be a consequence of Hif-1*a* stabilisation and could explain the fourth hallmark [279,280,336]. As mitochondria control apoptosis [337], evasion of apoptosis would be an expected outcome of dysfunctional mitochondria and could account for the fifth hallmark. While the rewiring of energy production from OxPhos to substrate level phosphorylation can explain the first five hallmarks of cancer, how might this energy rewiring be linked to metastasis?

Emerging evidence indicates that metastasis involves transformation of myeloid cells or fusion hybridisation between macrophages and transformed epithelial cells [334,338–343]. Macrophages and myeloid cells are mesenchymal cells that are programmed to intravasate blood vessels, to function in the circulation, and to extravasate for involvement in tissue repair. A macrophage/myeloid origin of metastasis is a compelling alternative to the epithelial mesenchymal transition (EMT) for the origin of metastasis [334]. Despite expressing aerobic fermentation (Warburg effect), it is the absence of macrophages and a cellular immune system in plant tumours that is considered the explanation for the absence of metastasis in crown-gall plant cancer [334,344]. Macrophages could acquire mitochondria with dysfunctional OxPhos through various fusion hybridisation events with neoplastic stem cells in an acidic and hypoxic microenvironment [339,345]. Radiation therapy can also facilitate tumour cell-macrophage/microglial fusion-hybridisation thus producing highly invasive metastatic cells [180,346]. It is also interesting that glutamine is a major energy metabolite for cells of the immune system including macrophages [347,348]. This fact could account in part for the glutamine dependency of metastatic cancer cells. As macrophages are immunosuppressive, metastatic cells with macrophage properties would be powerful

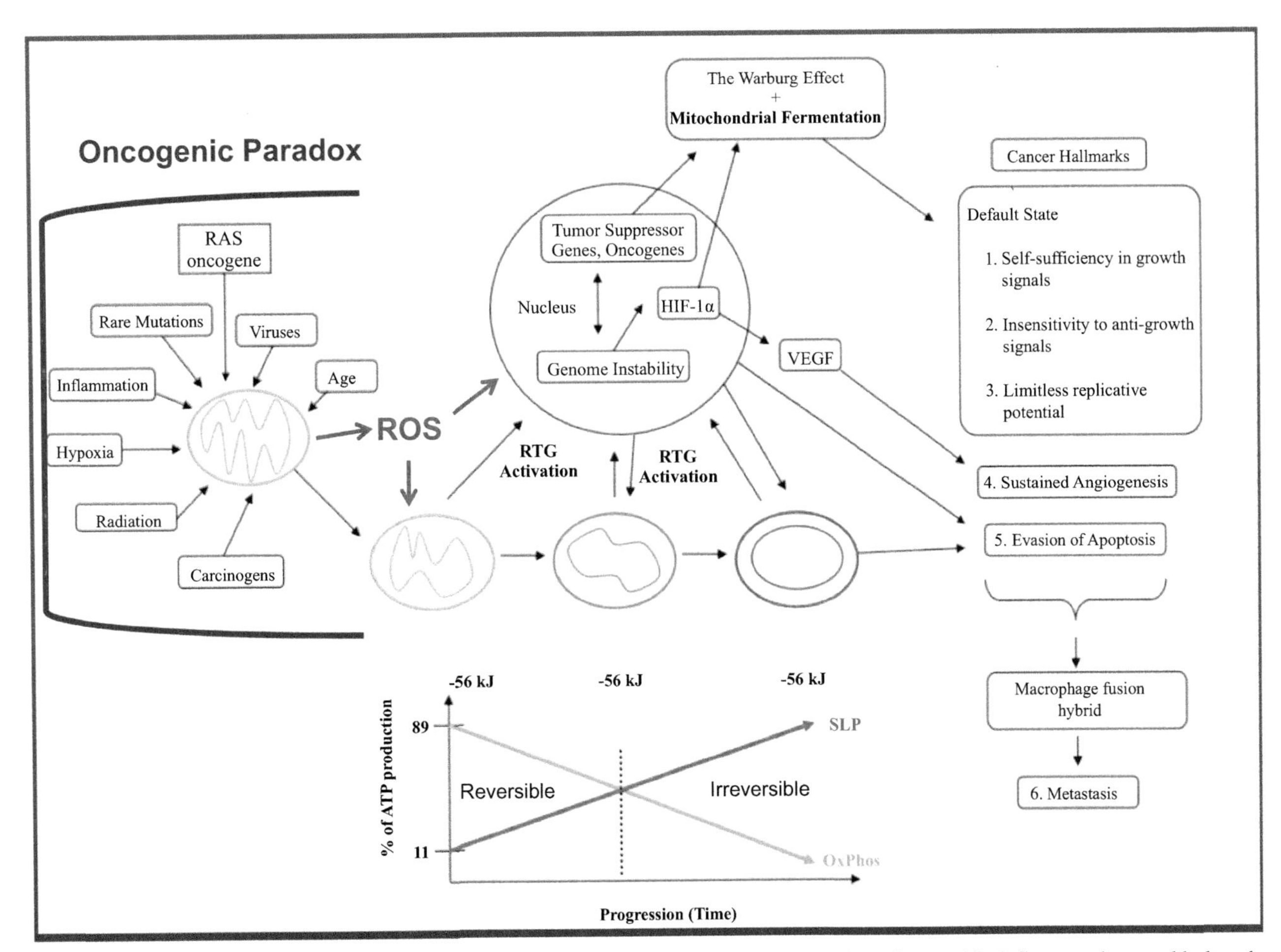

FIGURE 6.6 Cancer as a mitochondrial metabolic disease. Cancer can arise from any number of unspecific influences that would alter the number, structure, and function of mitochondria thus affecting energy production through OxPhos. The unspecific processes shown include, age, viral infections, the *Ras* oncogene, rare inherited mutations, chronic inflammation, intermittent hypoxia, radiation exposure, chemical carcinogens etc. The evidence supporting the carcinogenic properties of these unspecific processes was presented previously [106,107,115,237,326]. Any of these unspecific processes would increase the production of ROS within the mitochondria, which would ultimately link to the six major hallmarks of cancer [106,107,136]. Excessive ROS, mostly generated from OxPhos dysfunction, are carcinogenic and mutagenic and would cause significant damage to lipids, proteins, and nucleic acids in both the mitochondria and the nucleus [327]. Nuclear genomic instability including the vast array of somatic mutations and aneuploidy would arise as a consequence of ROS damage [107,255,328]. Indeed, mutations in the p53 tumour suppressor and genomic instability have been linked directly to mitochondrial ROS production in glioma stem cells [245]. Fermentation metabolism and ROS formation underlie the hyperproliferation of tumour cells. A gradual reduction in OxPhos efficiency would elicit a mitochondrial stress response through retrograde (RTG) signalling [329–331]. RTG activation would cause persistent expression of various oncogenes, for example, *Hif-1a* and c-*Myc*, that upregulate receptors and enzymes in both the glycolysis and the glutaminolysis pathways [279,331–333]. Oncogenes become facilitators of fermentation metabolism. ATP synthesis through mSLP will compensate for lost ATP synthesis from OxPhos or from PKM2 expression in glycolysis. The path to carcinogenesis will occur only in those cells capable of sustaining energy production through substrate level phosphorylation, (SLP). Cells unable to replace OxPhos with SLP, for example, CNS neurons or cardiomyocytes, would die and rarely become transformed. Despite the shift from respiration to SLP the delta G' of ATP hydrolysis remains fairly constant at approximately -56 kJ indicating that the energy from SLP compensates for the reduced energy from OxPhos. The mitochondrial stress response or retrograde signalling (RTG) will initiate oncogene up-regulation and tumour suppressor gene inactivation that are necessary to maintain the viability of incipient cancer cells when respiration becomes unable to maintain energy homoeostasis. Genomic instability will arise as a secondary consequence of protracted mitochondrial stress from disturbances in the intracellular and extracellular microenvironment. Metastasis arises from respiratory damage in cells of myeloid/macrophage origin either directly or after fusion hybridisation with epithelial-derived tumour cells [334]. Tumour progression and degree of malignancy are linked directly to ultrastructure abnormalities (cristolysis) and to the energy transition from OxPhos to substrate-level phosphorylation. The **T** signifies an arbitrary temporal threshold when the shift from OxPhos to SLP would become irreversible. This scenario links all major cancer hallmarks to extrachromosomal and epigenetic respiratory dysfunction and can explain the Oncogenic Paradox [335]. *Reprinted with modifications from Seyfried TN., and Shelton LM. Cancer as a metabolic disease.* Nutr Metab (Lond) *(2010) 7, 7.*

suppressors of the immune system. It is unlikely that random somatic mutations could be responsible for metastasis, as the metastatic cascade is a non-random phenomenon that is common to many cancer types [349]. Metastatic behaviour of cells can also occur in the absence of mutations [350,351]. Hence, the metastatic behaviour of tumour cells could arise from fusion hybridisation during tumour progression or following radiotherapy.

The origin of cancer has also been described under the tissue organisation field theory (TOFT), which is more compatible with the MMT than with the SMT [317]. Readers are referred to the excellent work of C. Sonnenschein and A. Soto for a comparative analysis of the TOFT and SMT of carcinogenesis [300,352–356].

6.2.5 Targeting glucose and glutamine for the metabolic management of cancer

Despite the billions of dollars spent on cancer therapies based on the SMT, over 1600 people die each day in the United States from cancer [357]. An accurate understanding of disease biology should lead to effective therapeutic strategies for management. The linkage of fermentation to malignancy is as solid as that of gravity to the redshift [110,180]. It is well recognised that most, if not all, tumour cells are dependent on glucose and glutamine for growth [267,281,358,359]. While amino acids other than glutamine can also provide energy through mSLP, glutamine is the only amino acid not requiring the expenditure of energy for the metabolic interconversions necessary to produce succinyl-CoA [131]. As the default state of metazoan cells is proliferation, not quiescence [300,353], unbridled proliferation becomes a consequence when SLP replaces OxPhos for ATP synthesis in cancer cells [100,180,317,324,360,361]. Indeed, unbridled proliferation was the dominant growth phenotype of all organisms before oxygen entered the atmosphere about 2.5 billion years ago [324,361]. The dependency of tumour cells on glycolysis and glutaminolysis will also make them resistant to apoptosis, ROS-induced damage, and chemotherapy drugs [362]. The activity of the p-glycoprotein, which protects cells from toxic chemotherapy, is driven by glycolysis [362,363]. The rewiring of ATP synthesis from OxPhos to fermentation involving SLP would cause a cell to enter its default state with consequent dedifferentiation, apoptotic resistance, and unbridled proliferation, that is, neoplasia [107,300,324].

Efforts to target glucose and glutamine simultaneously show promise as a therapeutic strategy for managing a broad range of cancers [360,364–367]. Leone et al. [364] showed that an analogue of the glutaminase inhibitor, 6-diazo-5-oxo-L-norleucine (DON), not only inhibited glutamine metabolism, but also inhibited glycolysis and related pathways, thus disabling the Warburg effect and significantly reducing tumour growth. Similar observations in reducing tumour growth were observed in combining glycolysis inhibitors (Glutor or lonidamine) with either DON or the glutaminase inhibitor CB-839 [366,367]. We also found a powerful therapeutic synergy in combining DON with a calorie-restricted ketogenic diet (KD-R) for managing late-stage growth in the VM-M3 and CT-2A syngeneic glioblastoma mouse tumours [365]. The KD-R not only reduced the ratio of glucose to non-fermentable ketone bodies in the blood, but also facilitated the delivery of DON to the tumours through the blood brain barrier. This therapeutic strategy simultaneously reduced the availability of glucose and glutamine to the glycolytic and glutaminolysis pathways in the tumour cells. Moreover, ketone bodies enhance the metabolic efficiency of the normal host cells, but are growth inhibitory or even toxic to many tumour cells [368–377]. Abnormalities in cardiolipin and other phospholipids in the inner mitochondrial membranes would prevent tumour cells from using ketone bodies for ATP synthesis [117,378,379]. Through their anti-angiogenic, anti-inflammatory, and pro-apoptotic actions, calorie restriction and KD-R can normalise the tumour microenvironment [336,380–384]. Maximal therapeutic benefit of glutamine-targeting drugs can be obtained for a broad range of cancers when administered to patients under reduced blood glucose and elevated ketone bodies, that is, nutritional ketosis [255,373,385–387]. Fig. 6.7 summarises how the simultaneous targeting of glucose and glutamine could help manage tumour growth. The simultaneous targeting of glucose and glutamine, while under nutritional ketosis, will selectively disrupt ATP synthesis in OxPhos-deficient cancer cells thus leading to their death and elimination. Based on the above information, we consider that the MMT can explain better the facts and origin of cancer than can the SMT.

6.2.6 Conclusions

Evidence is reviewed by comparing the facts of cancer in light of two competing theories that attempt to explain the origin of the disease, the MMT and the SMT. Overwhelming evidence now exists that undermines the SMT as a credible explanation for the origin of cancer. Most major cancers display abnormalities in the number, structure, and function of mitochondria that would compromise ATP synthesis through OxPhos. Glucose and glutamine drive cancer growth and metastasis through the glycolysis and glutaminolysis pathways, respectively. Compelling circumstantial evidence shows that mitochondrial substrate level phosphorylation at the succinate CoA ligase reaction in the TCA cycle can

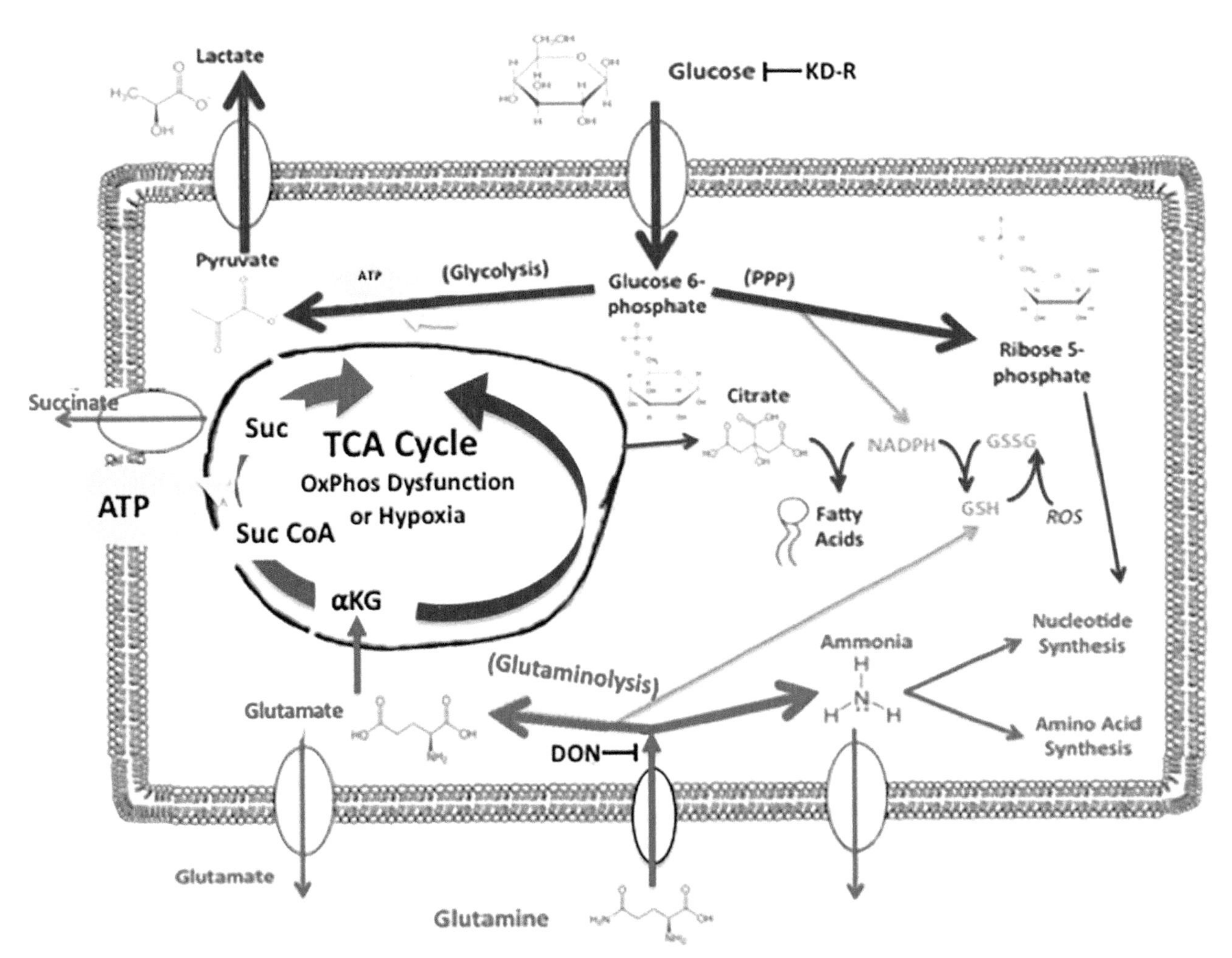

FIGURE 6.7 **Targeting glucose and glutamine for the metabolic management of cancer.** Most tumour cells, regardless of tissue origin, are largely dependent on glucose and glutamine for survival and growth. Energy through substrate-level phosphorylation (SLP) in the cytoplasm (glycolysis) and in the TCA cycle (glutaminolysis) will compensate for reduced energy through oxidative phosphorylation (OxPhos) or hypoxia that occurs in many solid tumours. The KD-R will reduce glucose carbons for both the glycolytic and pentose phosphate (PPP) pathways that supply ATP and precursors for synthesis of glutathione, lipids, and nucleotides. Glutaminase inhibitors, like DON, will deplete glutamate and the glutamine-derived amide nitrogen needed for ammonia and nucleotide synthesis. Depletion of glutamine-derived glutamate will reduce anapleurotic carbons to the TCA cycle through *a*-KG for protein synthesis, while also reducing ATP synthesis through the succinyl CoA ligase reaction in the TCA cycle. The glutamine-derived glutamate is also used for glutathione production that protects tumour cells from oxidative stress. The KD-R + DON will thus make tumour cells vulnerable to oxidative stress. The simultaneous targeting of glucose and glutamine using KD-R + DON will thus starve tumour cells of energy production while blocking their ability to synthesise proteins, lipids, and nucleotides. This metabolic starvation could also reduce extracellular acidification through the reduction of lactate and succinate. The elevation of non-fermentable ketone bodies will provide normal cells with an alternative energy source to glucose while also protecting them from oxidative stress. *Modified with permission from Seyfried TN, Yu G, Maroon JC, D'Agostino DP. Press-pulse: a novel therapeutic strategy for the metabolic management of cancer.* Nutr Metab (Lond) *(2017) 14, 19; and Mukherjee P, Augur ZM, Li M, Hill C, Greenwood B, Domin MA, et al. Therapeutic benefit of combining calorie-restricted ketogenic diet and glutamine targeting in late-stage experimental glioblastoma.* Commun Biol *(2019) 2, 200.*

provision ATP synthesis sufficient enough to compensate for reduced ATP synthesis through OxPhos in cancer cells. The simultaneous targeting of glucose and glutamine availability offers a parsimonious therapeutic strategy for managing most malignant cancers regardless of cell origin.

Acknowledgements

We thank the Foundation for Metabolic Cancer Therapies, CrossFit Inc., the Nelson and Claudia Peltz Foundation, Joseph C. Maroon, Mr. Edward Miller, Lewis Topper, the George Yu Foundation, Kenneth Rainin Foundation, Children with Cancer UK, and the Boston College Research Expense Fund for their support.

6.3 Cancer management using press-pulse ketogenic metabolic therapy

Thomas N. Seyfried, Purna Mukherjee, and Dominic P. D'Agostino

6.3.1 Introduction

Cancer is a systemic disease involving multiple time- and space-dependent changes in the health status of cells and tissues that ultimately lead to malignant tumours [107]. Neoplasia involving dysregulated cell growth is the biological endpoint of the disease [136,353]. Tumour cell invasion into surrounding tissues and their spread (metastasis) to distant organs is the primary cause of morbidity and mortality of most cancer patients [334,344,349,388]. Data from the American Cancer Society show that over 1600 people die each day in the United States from cancer with over 600,000 dying yearly [357]. Indeed, cancer is predicted to overtake heart disease as the leading cause of death in Western societies. The failure to clearly define the origin of cancer is responsible in large part for the failure to significantly reduce the cancer death rate from treatments and in developing cancer prevention strategies [237].

Cancer is generally considered a genetic disease where random somatic mutations underlie the origin and progression of the disease [136,295,302,317,389]. This general view is now under serious reconsideration in light of major inconsistencies with the gene theory [107,119,237,296,317,353,356,390–394]. In contrast to the extensive genetic heterogeneity seen in tumours, most if not all neoplastic cells within tumours share the common metabolic malady of substrate level phosphorylation arising from dysregulated oxidative phosphorylation [107,108,110,118,119,131,242]. It is more logical to target the common underlying metabolic malady then to target gene mutations, which are highly heterogeneous in cancer cells.

6.3.2 Tumour cell energy metabolites from cannibalism and phagocytosis

Emerging evidence indicates that macrophages, or their fusion hybrids with neoplastic stem cells, are the origin of metastatic cancer cells [334,341,395–398]. Cannibalism and phagocytosis of cellular debris are well-known characteristics of macrophages and of myeloid cancer cells with macrophage properties [395,399–404]. Shelton showed that glioblastoma cells with myeloid properties could survive in Matrigel (extracellular matrix material) in the absence of added glucose and glutamine [405]. The gradual accumulation of lactate in the media suggested that the glioblastoma cells survived through lysosomal digestion and aerobic fermentation of glycoconjugates present in the Matrigel. Glioblastoma cell death occurred immediately following the addition of chloroquine, which neutralises lysosomal acidity and digestion [405]. Shelton's findings are consistent with the more recent findings of Kamphorst et al. in showing that pancreatic ductal adenocarcinoma cells could obtain glutamine under nutrient poor conditions through lysosomal digestion of extracellular proteins [406]. It might therefore become necessary to also target lysosomal digestion under conditions of reduced glucose and glutamine availability by using chloroquine for the management of metastatic cancer.

6.3.3 Genome integrity and energy metabolism

The function of DNA repair enzymes and the integrity of the nuclear genome are dependent to a large extent on the energy derived from normal respiration [254,407–415]. Previous studies in yeast and mammalian cells show that disruption of aerobic respiration can cause mutations (loss of heterozygosity, chromosome instability, and epigenetic modifications etc.) in the nuclear genome [245,328,414,416]. A protracted reliance on fermentation causes oxidative stress leading to the production of ROS mostly through the mitochondrial coenzyme Q couple [376]. In addition to their role in oncogenic signalling, excess ROS production damages mitochondrial function, and are both carcinogenic and mutagenic [417,418]. The genomic instability seen in tumour cells thus arises from a protracted reliance on fermentation energy metabolism and a disruption of redox balance through excessive oxidative stress. A therapeutic strategy that can target the metabolic abnormality common to most tumour cells should be more effective in managing cancer than a strategy targeting genetic mutations that vary widely between tumours of the same histological grade and even within the same tumour.

6.3.4 Human evolution and adaptive versatility

Rick Potts, a palaeoanthropologist at the Smithsonian Institution, suggested that the evolutionary success of the human species has been due largely to the germline inheritance of traits that bestowed adaptive versatility [419–421]. Adaptability was determined based on three qualities: 'the ability of an organism to persist through major environmental shifts, to spread to new habitats, and to respond in novel ways to its surroundings' [421]. These characteristics were honed over millions of years and enabled humans to adapt rapidly to abrupt changes in the physical environment including changes in moisture, temperature, food resources etc. Adaptability to abrupt environmental change is a property of the genome, for which selection happened in order to ensure survival under environmental extremes [422,423].

Potts' hypothesis is an extension of Darwin's original theory (Chapter IV, Natural Selection) and can be applied to the individual cells of the organism, which exist as an integrated society of cells [422,423]. The success in dealing with environmental stress and disease is therefore dependent on the integrated action of all cells in the organism. Further, this integrated action depends on the flexibility of each cell's genome, which responds to both internal and external signals according to the needs of the organism. More specifically, only those cells possessing flexibility in nutrient utilisation will be able to survive under nutrient stress. Environmental forcing has therefore selected those genomes most capable of adapting to change in order to maintain metabolic homoeostasis [419,421,423,424]. This concept was first discussed in relation to the management of brain cancer [423].

The widely held notion that tumour cells have a growth advantage and are more fit than normal cells is not only inconsistent with Darwin's theory, but is also inconsistent with Potts' concept of adaptive versatility [421–423]. It is difficult to conceive how the non-uniform genomic instability seen in cancer cells could enhance their adaptability and fitness. It is important to recognise that mutations in *p53*, *K-Ras*, and *Raf* impact negatively on mitochondrial energy efficiency thus making cells with these mutations less metabolically flexible than are normal cells [115,199,245,246,408,425–427]. As long as the tumour cells have access to the metabolites needed for substrate level phosphorylation (glucose and glutamine), they will present the appearance of having a growth advantage over normal cells. According to Darwin and Potts, mutations that bestow a selective advantage are those that will enhance survival under environmental stress. If the multiple pathogenic point mutations, chromosomal rearrangements, and mitochondrial abnormalities confer a fitness or survival advantage to tumour cells, then survival under environmental stress and nutrient deprivation should be better in tumour cells than in normal cells [428]. However, when the hypothesis is tested, this is not what actually happens. An appreciation of evolutionary biology could help to develop therapeutic strategies that are more effective and less toxic than those in current use.

For example, when mice or persons with tumours are placed under energy stress using dietary energy restriction, many tumour cells die while normal cells survive. Indeed, the health and vitality of the normal cells improves with time under dietary energy reduction while hyper-glycolytic tumour cells experience an energetic crisis that triggers apoptotic death [429,430]. Support for this contention comes from studies in which brain tumours are provided with a dietary energy stress [336,370,380,381,383,431–436]. It is clear that adaptability to environmental stress is greater in normal cells than in tumour cells. This also explains why cell death is generally greater in tumour cells than in normal cells following exposure to toxic radiation and cancer drugs. Targeting glucose availability will therefore cause greater death in the tumour cells than in the normal cells, as the normal cells can transition to the metabolism of ketone bodies for survival. Mitochondrial defects will prevent tumour cells from using ketone bodies for energy. Consequently, glycolysis-dependent tumour cells are less adaptable to metabolic stress than are normal cells.

Therapeutic energy stress might also restore the morphogenetic field thus reversing abnormal energy metabolism and growth behaviour in tumour cells not containing genetic mutations [296,300]. In contrast to dietary energy reduction, radiation and toxic drugs can damage the microenvironment and transform normal cells into tumour cells while also creating tumour cells that become highly resistant to drugs and radiation. Drug-resistant tumour cells arise in large part from the damage to respiration in bystander pre-cancerous cells. These cells are often those that eventually become heavily dependent on fermentation for energy.

The greater adaptability of normal cells than tumour cells to energy stress is predicted by the theories of Darwin and Potts [422]. Metabolic flexibility allows the organism to respond in a coordinated way to environmental stress and limited substrate availability. Energy stress will force all normal cells to work together for the survival of the organism [422]. Pathogenic mutations and genomic instability will reduce adaptability and metabolic flexibility under energy stress. The greater the genomic instability in tumour cells, the less will be their capacity to adapt to stress. This concept is similar to that of Nowell's except it considers genomic instability as a liability rather than as an advantage to progression [422,437]. As energy generated through substrate level phosphorylation is greater in tumour cells than in normal cells, tumour cells are more dependent than normal cells on the availability of fermentable fuels (glucose and glutamine) [422]. Normal cells shift energy metabolism from glucose to ketone bodies and fats when placed under energy stress from glucose deprivation, insulin deficiency, and prolonged fasting. This shift is the result of adaptive versatility and genomic stability in cells and tissues with robust mitochondrial function, but the shift is lacking in most tumour cells due to the accumulation of random mutations. It is important to remember that 'nothing in cancer biology makes sense except in the light of evolution' [422].

Tumour cells will have difficulty surviving and growing if fermentable fuels become restricted in their microenvironment. Ketone bodies and fats are non-fermentable fuels [438]. Tumour cells have difficulty using ketone bodies and fats for fuel should the supply of glucose be reduced [372,374,439,440]. Although some tumour cells might appear to oxidise ketone bodies in the presence of ketolytic enzymes [441], ketone bodies and fats can provide sufficient energy for cell viability in the absence of glucose and glutamine. The studies in immunocompetent syngeneic mice and xenografts with brain tumours are proof of concept that tumour cells are less adaptable than normal cells when placed under energy stress [336,370,381–383,442,443]. Apoptosis under energy stress is greater in tumour cells than in normal cells [383]. The multiple genetic defects in tumour cells will reduce genomic flexibility thus increasing the likelihood of cell death under any environmental stresses that would lower glucose and ketone body availability. Regardless of when or how genomic defects become involved in the initiation or progression of tumours, these defects can be exploited for tumour management or resolution.

6.3.5 Press-pulse: a therapeutic strategy for the gradual elimination of cancer cells

The simultaneous occurrence of 'Press-pulse' disturbances is considered the mechanism responsible for the mass extinction of organisms during prior evolutionary epochs [444]. A 'press' disturbance is a chronic environmental stress on all organisms in an ecological community. The press disturbance promotes extinction through habitat loss, reduced reproduction, and restriction of range and resources. Press disturbances force biological communities into a new equilibrium where previously important species become non-viable. A press disturbance will shift the adaptive landscape to favour the fittest species while eliminating the weakest species. In contrast to the press disturbances, 'pulse' disturbances are acute events that disrupt biological communities and produce high mortality [444]. Through extensive mortality in the immediate aftermath of the event, a pulse disturbance can cause extinction. However, survival of some species could occur following a pulse disturbance, as the physical and biotic environments will eventually recover to their pre-disturbance equilibria [444]. It is only when both the press and the pulse disturbances coincide that mass extinction of species, without recovery, becomes probable. A modification of the press-pulse concept can be adopted for the eradication of tumour cells.

Mark Vincent suggested how a Press-pulse strategy could be used to stress tumour cells [445]. We have now expanded this concept to show how a press-pulse therapeutic strategy can be used for the non-toxic management and possible resolution of cancer. A calorie-restricted KD or dietary energy reduction creates chronic metabolic stress in the body. This energy stress acts as a press disturbance; the effects of which would be greater in the tumour cells than in the normal cells due to their dependency on fermentation energy metabolism, mitogens, anabolic signalling (IGF-1, mTOR, etc.), elevated redox stress, and mutational load.

Drugs that target the availability of glucose and glutamine would act as pulse disturbances by causing an acute reduction of these tumour-dependent fuels [367]. Hyperbaric oxygen therapy can also be considered another pulse disturbance in elevating ROS to a greater degree in tumour cells than in normal cells, thus promoting cancer cell death through redox stress [446]. Normal cells readily transition to ketone body metabolism for protection against ROS damage and oxidative stress. The goal therefore is to produce a therapeutic strategy that can more effectively manage cancer than can current toxic cancer therapies. The following examples illustrate the potential of press-pulse therapeutic strategies for cancer management.

6.3.6 Calorie restriction and restricted ketogenic diets: a press disturbance

Calorie restriction, water-only fasting, and restricted KDs reduce circulating glucose and insulin concentrations while elevating circulating concentrations of ketone bodies. KD are low-carbohydrate high-fat diets that are widely used to reduce refractory epileptic seizures in children [447,448]. The KD can more effectively reduce blood glucose and elevate blood ketone body concentrations than can CR alone making the KD potentially more therapeutic against tumours than CR [380,449,450]. The protein and fat composition of the KD differs from that of Atkins-type diets in having less protein and more fat than the Atkins diets. This is important as several amino acids found in proteins can be deaminated to form pyruvate, which can then be metabolised to form glucose through gluconeogenesis [451]. Campbell showed that tumour growth is greater under high protein (>20%) than under low protein content (<10%) in the diet [452]. Protein amino acids can be metabolised to glucose through the Cori cycle. The fats in KDs used clinically also contain more medium chain triglycerides than do Atkins diets. Consequently, blood glucose concentrations will be lower and ketone body concentrations will be higher with KDs than with Atkins-type diets. Calorie restriction, fasting, and restricted KDs are anti-angiogenic, anti-inflammatory, and pro-apoptotic and thus will target and eliminate tumour cells through multiple mechanisms [336,370,380–382,429,453,454]. KDs can also spare muscle protein and delay cancer cachexia, which is a major problem in the management of metastatic cancer [455–457]. This is important, as metastatic cancer cells are major consumers of muscle-derived glutamine due to their origin from macrophages [334]. Most metastatic cancers have the characteristics of macrophages. KD will therefore delay metastasis development and inhibit cachexia.

The therapeutic effects of KDs used alone or in combination with other therapies have been documented in preclinical studies for several cancer models including neuroblastoma [202,458], lung cancer [459], prostate cancer [460,461], breast and ovarian cancers [462,463], and, head & neck cancers [462], colon cancer [464], and glioblastoma [365]. These preclinical studies are also motivating case reports and pilot studies in humans with brain and other cancers [436,441,465–472]. It is clear from these studies, and from the original observation of Linda Nebeling and colleagues in children with gliomas [432], that treatment of cancer patients with KDs is generally safe and well tolerated, which is consistent with decades of research obtained from evaluation of children treated with KDs for the management of epilepsy [473]. Information on KDs can be obtained from Miriam Kalamian's book, *Keto For Cancer*, and from the Charlie Foundation web site (https://www.charliefoundation.org).

We developed the Glucose/Ketone Index calculator (GKIC) to assess the potential therapeutic effects of various low-carbohydrate and KDs for brain cancer management [449]. The GKIC is a simple tool that measures the ratio of blood glucose to blood ketone concentrations and can help monitor the efficacy of metabolic therapy in preclinical animal models and in clinical trials for malignant brain cancer or for any cancer that expresses aerobic fermentation. GKI values of 1.0 or below are considered therapeutic, though therapeutic benefit appears to be associated more with elevated ketone bodies and suppression of insulin than with reduced blood glucose concentrations [450,474]. However, the elevation of blood ketone concentrations is generally greater when blood glucose concentrations are lower than when blood glucose concentrations are higher [375,380,475]. The GKI can therefore serve as a biomarker to assess the therapeutic efficacy of various diets for the management of a broad range of cancers.

Reduced glucose availability and suppression of insulin signalling will produce chronic energy stress on those tumour cells that depend primarily on glucose for growth and survival. It is important to remember that insulin drives glycolysis through stimulation of the pyruvate dehydrogenase complex [476,477]. Reduced concentrations of glucose will also reduce substrates for both the glycolytic and the pentose phosphate pathways thus reducing cellular energy, as well as the synthesis of glutathione and nucleotide precursors (Fig. 6.7, in Section 6.2).

The water-soluble ketone bodies (D-β-hydroxybutyrate and acetoacetate) are produced largely in the liver from adipocyte-derived fatty acids and ketogenic dietary fat. Ketone bodies bypass glycolysis and directly enter the mitochondria for metabolism to acetyl-CoA [478]. In contrast to fatty acid metabolism, which generates both NADH and $FADH_2$, ketone body metabolism generates only NADH [376]. Moreover, ketone body metabolism does not induce mitochondrial uncoupling in contrast to metabolism of saturated fatty acids [376]. The metabolism of D-β-hydroxybutyrate in normal cells will therefore increase the redox span between Complexes I and III, thus increasing the delta G' of ATP hydrolysis while, at the same time, reducing ROS formation through the Complex II coenzyme Q couple [479,480]. Due to mitochondrial defects, tumour cells cannot exploit the therapeutic benefits of burning ketone bodies as normal cells would. Indeed, racemic mixtures of D-/L-ketone bodies can be toxic to tumour cells under both low and high glucose conditions [368–370,372,440,450]. Fine et al. found that uncoupling protein 2 is overexpressed in tumour cells, but not in normal control cells [368]. This finding provides a plausible molecular mechanism by which ketone bodies spare normal cells but suppress growth in cancer cell lines.

In contrast to D-β-hydroxybutyrate, L-β-hydroxybutyrate is beta-oxidised thus producing both NADH and $FADH_2$. $FADH_2$ will deliver electrons to Complex III, which can increase the semiquinone of Q, the half-reduced form. The Q semiquinone will react with molecular oxygen to form the superoxide $O_2^{\cdot -}$ free radical [376]. Therapeutic ketosis with racemic ketone esters can also make it feasible to safely sustain hypoglycaemia for inducing metabolic stress on cancer cells [481]. Hence, mixtures of L- and D-ketone esters have the potential to both enhance oxidative stress in tumour cells while reducing oxidative stress in normal cells, respectively [376,482]. There is also evidence showing that ketone bodies can inhibit histone deacetylases (HDAC) [483]. HDAC inhibitors play a role in targeting the cancer epigenome [484]. Deregulated inflammation is also considered to be one of the hallmarks of cancer. Therapeutic ketosis reduces circulating inflammatory markers, and ketones directly inhibit the NLRP3 inflammasome, an important proinflammatory pathway linked to carcinogenesis and an important target for cancer treatment response [485]. There are no adverse side effects of short-term therapeutic ketosis, but relatively mild adverse effects have been noted in some children with epilepsy after long-term use of KDs including constipation, kidney stones, electrolyte imbalances, and bone fracture [473]. These mild effects were easily managed with various supplements [486]. In general, there are no currently known cancer drugs that embody the therapeutic properties of ketone bodies.

6.3.7 Psychological stress reduction: a press disturbance

Chronic psychological stress is known to promote tumorigenesis through elevations of blood glucose, glucocorticoids, catecholamines, and Insulin-like growth factor (IGF-1) [487,488]. In addition to calorie-restricted KDs, psychological stress management involving exercise, yoga, music etc. also acts as press disturbances that can help reduce fatigue, depression, and anxiety in cancer patients and in animal models [489–492]. Ketone supplementation has also been shown to reduce anxiety behaviour in animal models [493]. The mechanism of action of psychological stress management for cancer control would largely involve reductions in blood glucose concentrations that contribute to tumour growth.

6.3.8 Restricted ketogenic diet used with 2-deoxyglucose

Calorie restriction or therapeutic fasting is anti-angiogenic, anti-inflammatory, and pro-apoptotic, and thus targets multiple cancer hallmarks [336,381–383,429,430,494–497]. This physiological state also enhances the efficacy of chemotherapy and radiation therapy, while reducing the side effects [498–500]. We showed a synergistic interaction between a calorie restricted ketogenic diet (KD-R) and the glycolysis inhibitor 2-deoxyglucose (2-DG) for the metabolic management of the syngeneic CT-2A malignant mouse glioma [501]. It was interesting to find that 2-DG (25 mg/kg) had no therapeutic effect on CT-2A tumour growth when administered alone to mice on a standard high carbohydrate diet, but produced a powerful therapeutic effect when administered with a KD-R. Indeed, this relatively low dose of 2-DG became somewhat toxic when used with the KD suggesting that lower dosing of some tumour-targeting drugs should also be effective when administered with KD-R. Besides 2-DG, a range of other glycolysis inhibitors might also produce similar therapeutic effects when combined with the KD-R including 3-bromopyruvate, oxaloacetate, and lonidamine [367,502–505]. In the example here the KD-R is the press making cancer cells selectively vulnerable to death and the 2-DG is the pulse, which could be used intermittently or cycled to avoid toxicity.

6.3.9 A ketogenic diet used with radiation therapy

Preclinical studies showed that the therapeutic efficacy of radiotherapy against the orthotopically grown GL261 mouse glioma could be greatly enhanced when combined with a commercially available KD [442]. Somewhat similar observations were obtained in patients with glioblastoma who received standard of care with a KD [433]. In these examples, the KD is the press and radiotherapy is the pulse. It is important to recognise, however, that the current standard of care (SOC) for glioblastoma, involving radiotherapy with temozolomide chemotherapy and dexamethasone, creates a tumour microenvironment rich in glucose and glutamine thus facilitating rapid tumour recurrence and patient death [180]. In this case, the KD can help delay the adverse effects of SOC.

6.3.10 A ketogenic diet used with hyperbaric oxygen therapy

Angela Poff and colleagues demonstrated that hyperbaric oxygen therapy (HBOT) enhanced the ability of the KD to reduce tumour growth and metastasis [446]. Evidence in animal models and in humans suggests that HBOT may have a modest anti-cancer effect when used alone [506], but appears most efficacious when it is used in combination with standard care [507]. Indeed, HBOT has proven effective when used prior to radiation therapy for GBM [508]. The mechanism of HBOT in tumour management is not yet clear, but saturating the tumour with oxygen could reverse hypoxia and suppress growth [506,509]. HBOT also increases oxidative stress and membrane lipid peroxidation of GBM cells *in vitro* [510]. The effects of the KD and HBOT can be enhanced with administration of exogenous ketones, which further suppressed tumour growth and metastasis [450]. Besides HBOT, intravenous vitamin C and dichloroacetate (DCA) can also be used with the KD to selectively increase oxidative stress in tumour cells [511,512]. Recent evidence also shows that ketone supplementation may enhance or preserve overall physical and mental health [513,514], which are often compromised due to disease progression and standard of care therapies. Under these conditions the KD with exogenous ketones serves as the press, while HBOT serves as the pulse. Although HBOT and radiotherapy both kill tumour cells through oxidative stress, HBOT is less toxic to normal cells than radiotherapy.

6.3.11 Calorie restriction and ketogenic diet used with glutamine targeting for metastatic cancer

While some tumours are more dependent on glucose than glutamine as a prime fuel for growth, other tumours are more dependent on glutamine than glucose, but most tumours are dependent on both glucose and glutamine for maximal growth [360,364–367,515]. Glutamine-dependent tumours are generally less detectable than glucose-dependent tumours under FDG-PET imaging, but could be detected under Glutamine-based PET imaging [516,517]. Glutamine targeting should have therapeutic benefit against those tumours that depend on glutamine for growth and survival.

We found that the highly metastatic VM-M3 tumour cells are dependent primarily on the availability of glutamine for growth and their ability to metastasise [518]. The glutaminase inhibitor DON (6-diazo-5-oxo-L-norleucine) has shown therapeutic benefit in the clinic, as long as the toxicity issue can be managed [367,519]. DON could work best when combined with inhibitors of glycolysis [365,367]. In addition to DON, other glutamine inhibitors (bis-2-(5-phenylacetamido-1,2, 4-thiadiazol-2-yl)ethyl sulphide (BPTES) or CB-839) could also be therapeutic in targeting glutamine-dependent tumours [520]. A greater attention to possible adverse effects will be needed for glutamine targeting than for glucose targeting, as glutamine is involved with several essential physiological functions especially for cells of the immune system [521,522]. Although glutamine is helpful for the gut and immune cell function, it is not yet clear if periodic glutamine supplementation would help or hinder glutamine targeting.

In the following study, spontaneously arising tumours (VM-M3) were observed in syngeneic immunocompetent VM/Dk inbred mice [523]. The tumour was classified as a glioblastoma (GBM) based on histological appearance, invasive growth behaviour in the brain, and systemic metastasis when given access to extra-neural sites [180,365,524–530]. The neoplastic VM-M3 tumour cells share several characteristics with mesenchymal microglia/macrophages, which are abundant in GBM and use glutamine as a major fuel [339,347]. Although calorie restriction could partially reduce the distal invasion of VM-M3 tumour cells in the brain and reduce primary tumour growth in flank, CR did not prevent systemic metastasis despite causing reduction in blood glucose and elevation of ketone body concentrations [384,518]. However, DON had a major effect in reducing both primary tumour size and systemic metastasis indicative of the importance of glutamine in driving this tumour [518]. A synergistic interaction was also seen when DON was combined with CR and the calorie restricted KD [180,365,531]. Indeed, KD-R not only reduced toxicity, but also facilitated DON delivery through the blood brain barrier [365]. Modifications of DON scheduling, timing, and dosing would be needed to improve efficacy and reduce toxicity. In this example, CR or KD is the press, and DON is the pulse. As glutamine is a major fuel of immune cells, glutamine targeting should be effective in reducing most metastatic cancers that have characteristics of macrophages and other immune cells [395]. While the mechanistic underpinnings of metastasis might remain elusive to many investigators, we know that metastatic cancer cells cannot survive under prolonged restriction of glucose and glutamine. We predict that the management of metastatic cancers will be improved significantly once oncology comes to understand this concept.

6.3.12 Optimisation of scheduling, timing, and dosing

The success of the press-pulse therapeutic strategy for the metabolic management of cancer will depend on optimisation of the scheduling, dosing, and timing of the various diets, drugs, and procedures used in order to achieve maximum synergistic interactions (Fig. 6.8). Scheduling will involve the order in which the chosen pulses are delivered to the subject while under dietary therapy. Timing will determine when and for how long the presses and pulses are given (e.g. number per day, week or month). Dosing will identify the optimal drug dosages needed to kill tumour cells while preventing or minimising systemic toxicity. Scheduling for each of these variables can be adjusted for the age, sex, and general health status of the subject. The strategy should degrade tumour cell populations gradually to prevent tumour lysis syndrome, which could cause excessive toxicity. Tumour imaging procedures involving FDG-PET, magnetic resonance imaging (MRI), and computed tomography perfusion (CTP), as well as the analysis of serum cancer biomarkers should be helpful in assessing therapeutic success. The goal of the press-pulse therapeutic strategy is to improve progression-free and overall survival from cancer without producing adverse effects from the treatment.

6.3.13 Conclusions

Many of the current treatments used for cancer management are based on the belief that cancer is a genetic disease. It is clear from the cancer death statistics that most current therapies are failing to reduce the yearly death rate or manage the disease without toxicity. Accumulating evidence indicates that cancer is a mitochondrial metabolic disease that depends on the availability of fermentable fuels for tumour cell growth and survival. Glucose and glutamine are the most abundant fermentable fuels present in the circulation and in the tumour microenvironment. Press-pulse ketogenic metabolic therapy is designed to target the availability of glucose and glutamine thus starving tumour cells of their most important fuels and increasing their vulnerability to oxidative stress and apoptotic death. Low-carbohydrate, high-fat KDs coupled with glycolysis inhibitors will reduce metabolic flux through the glycolytic and pentose phosphate pathways needed for synthesis of ATP, lipids, glutathione, and nucleotides. DON and other similar glutamine inhibitors will deprive proliferating tumour cells of the glutamine needed for TCA cycle anaplerosis, and the synthesis of glutathione, nucleotides, and proteins. Lysosomal targeting with chloroquine or similar drugs will reduce glucose and glutamine production following digestion of phagocytosed glycoconjugates and proteins. Glutamine targeting requires careful adjustments, as glutamine is a key

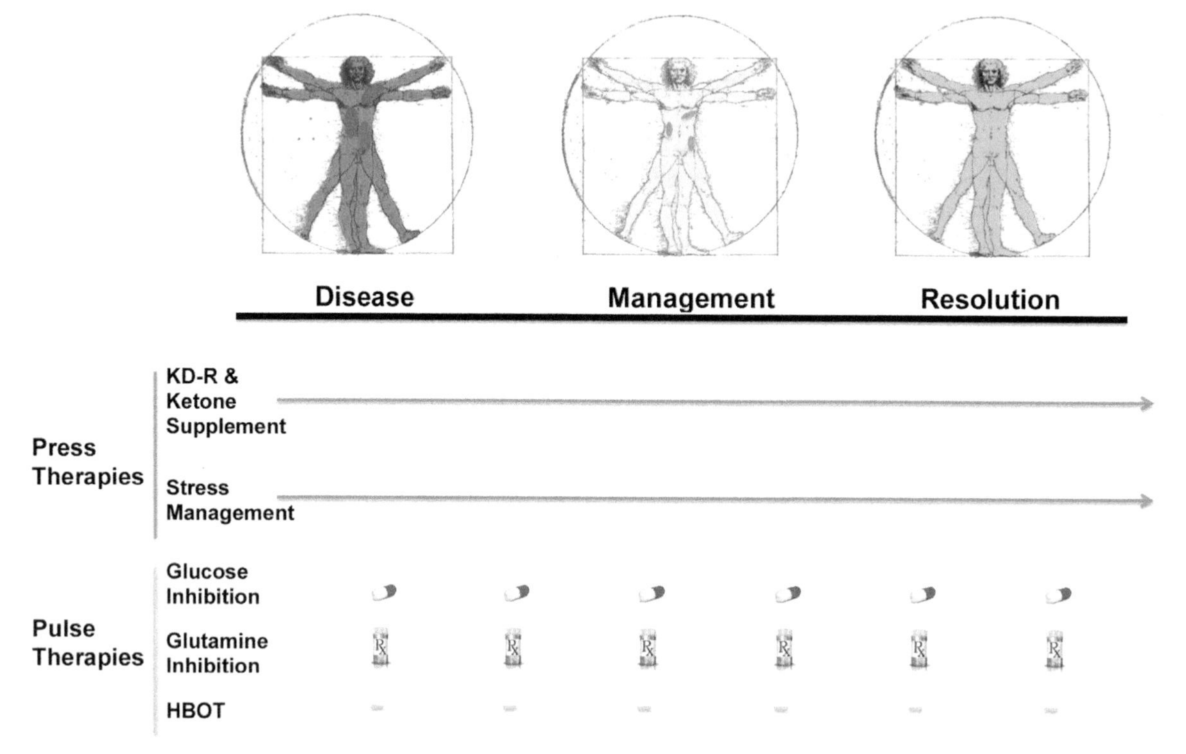

FIGURE 6.8 **Illustration of the press-pulse therapeutic strategy for cancer management.** Press-pulse ketogenic metabolic therapy considers cancer as a systemic disease regardless of the specific tissue or organ system containing invasive or metastatic tumour cells. This strategy is designed to target the glucose and glutamine dependency of tumour cells, while enhancing the metabolic efficiency in normal cells. Press therapies are designed to reduce systemic glucose availability while elevating blood concentrations of ketone bodies, which tumour cells cannot effectively use for energy generation. This approach pits the metabolic demands of normal cells against those of the mutated tumour cells, which are less capable than normal cells in adapting to metabolic stress from nutrient deprivation. Ketone body supplements could further reduce glucose concentration while enhancing the respiratory energy metabolism in normal cells. Stress management techniques together with exercise could further stress tumour cell metabolism while improving general health. The press therapies would be designed to work synergistically with acute pulse therapies to further target glucose and glutamine metabolism. HBOT will work together with the press therapies to selectively increase oxidative stress in tumour cells. The spacing between the various pulse therapies is designed to stress tumour cell metabolism while minimising toxicity to normal body cells. This therapeutic strategy will target the fermentation metabolism common to most tumour cells, thus gradually degrading tumour burden. The progressive colour change in the Vitruvian man drawing from red (diseased with darker red spots indicative of metastatic lesions), to yellow (reduced metastasis), to green (resolution) symbolises a gradual metabolic management and resolution of cancer. The pill symbol is indicative of glycolysis targeting that could be delivered orally. The Rx symbol is indicative of glutamine targeting that could be delivered intravenously or orally. Pulse therapies would terminate with evidence of management or resolution while press therapies could continue under modification or adjustment (arrow). Optimisation of dosing, timing, and scheduling of the therapeutic strategy will facilitate the eradication of tumour cells with minimal patient toxicity. This therapeutic strategy can be used as a framework for future clinical trials. HBOT, hyperbaric oxygen therapy; KD-R, calorie restricted ketogenic diet.

metabolite needed for the immune system and for other physiological functions. Hyperbaric oxygen therapy combined with the calorie-restricted KD will kill tumour cells through apoptotic and anti-angiogenic mechanisms while also reducing inflammation in the tumour microenvironment and systemically. It is our view that press-pulse ketogenic metabolic therapy is a compelling and parsimonious strategy for effectively managing the vast majority of malignant cancers with minimal toxicity. This therapeutic approach will target the major energy pathways responsible for tumour cell growth and survival while enhancing the energetic efficiency of normal body cells and tissues.

Acknowledgements

We would also like to thank Zachary Augur and Michael Pool for technical assistance, and Madam Trudy Dupont for providing us with valuable information and insight on the human experience of metabolic therapy for brain cancer management. We would also like to thank those that support our research: The Foundation for Metabolic Cancer Therapies, CrossFit Inc., the Nelson and Claudia Peltz Foundation, Dr. Joseph C. Maroon, Dr. Edward Miller, Lewis Topper, the George Yu Foundation, Kenneth Rainin Foundation, Children with Cancer UK, and the Boston College Research Expense Fund for their support.

6.4 Implementation of modifiable ketogenic diets in cancer

Miriam Kalamian

6.4.1 Purpose

'Better living through chemistry' sums up the current state of conventional cancer research and treatment: research identifies altered metabolic pathways then develops and tests pharmaceuticals that target these pathways. Conventional care then assembles these drugs into treatment plans with various toxicity profiles. In this model of cancer care, little to no attention is paid to the role of nutrition. Here, we present the steps needed to harness evolutionary adaptations to periods of food scarcity that favour the survival of normal cells at the expense of cancer cells.

The protocol presented here is intended to provide a framework for implementing a KD as an adjunct nutritional therapy in the treatment of cancer. KDs incorporate the first principles of therapeutic carbohydrate restriction (TCR) and therapeutic protein management (TPM) within the context of a nutritionally complete diet. At the cellular level, management of these macronutrients has been shown to inhibit activity in cancer-promoting pathways, lower inflammation in the tumour microenvironment, reduce availability of substrate for biomass synthesis, and limit angiogenesis in the network of blood vessels supplying tumour cells with nutrients [386].

6.4.2 Introduction

One in three women and nearly half of all men will receive a cancer diagnosis in their lifetime [532]. While some cancers can be adequately addressed through surgery alone, cancer treatment usually includes some combination of toxic drugs or radiation with adverse effects on normal cells that can significantly degrade quality of life. There is now a growing body of evidence suggesting that KDs implemented as adjunct treatments can slow the progression of many types of cancer, but to date, published reports lack the replicable protocols for implementation and data collection that are needed to move the science from the bench to the bedside [387,533]. This is one of the main obstacles to the use of ketogenic nutrition plans within conventional care settings.

6.4.3 Comparing ketogenic diet plans

6.4.3.1 Classic ketogenic diet

The classic KD for epilepsy was developed by Russell Wilder in the 1920s as a treatment for intractable paediatric epilepsy and is still used in some clinical and research settings. The patient's energy needs are calculated using standard formulas, such as Mifflin-St. Joer and macronutrients (carbohydrate, protein, and fat) are generally assigned in a 3:1 to 4:1 ratio of fat grams to the combination of carbohydrate-plus-protein grams. These diets are generally eucaloric to support the energetic needs of growing children. Given that the burden of cancer is much higher in adults than in children, it is essential to examine classic KDs in this light.

Pros:

- There is general consensus within the epilepsy community on how to initiate and support the plan [534].
- Absolute contraindications to use of the diet are clearly defined [534].
- The individual diet plan is developed by a registered dietician (RD) and potential side effects are prophylactically addressed and routinely monitored by the child's medical/neurological team.

Cons:

- Access to keto-trained RDs in medical settings is generally restricted to individuals with epilepsy.
- Adults require more protein than children in order to maintain their higher lean body mass (LBM); this lowers the diet ratio.
- High-ratio classic KDs are very high in dietary fat; this is often not well tolerated in adults, especially in those who are older, malnourished, and undergoing aggressive cancer treatments that interfere with digestion and uptake of nutrients.

6.4.3.2 Restricted ketogenic diet

As noted above, the classic KD is generally eucaloric given the needs of the paediatric population but there is evidence that eucaloric KDs may not result in a therapeutic response in cancer [535]. In contrast, the KD-R is consumed in restricted or reduced amounts. Research suggests that calorie restriction increases metabolic pressure on cancer cells by targeting angiogenesis and inhibiting activity in cancer-promoting pathways while simultaneously upregulating activities and signalling that maintain the status and function of metabolically healthy cells [535,536]. (It is highly recommended that researchers and clinicians read Dr. Thomas Seyfried's book, *Cancer as a Metabolic Disease*.) The protocol for using the KD-R must be individualised and monitored to ensure that calorie restriction does not result in malnutrition.

KD-R compared to classic eucaloric KDs has additional benefits in the clinical setting:

- Reducing total calories establishes an energy deficit that more closely mimics starvation-state cellular signalling, facilitating the metabolic shift to ketosis.
- The lower intake of dietary fat in KD-R compared to eucaloric KD improves tolerance, easing the adaptation to a high-fat diet.
- Lipolysis of fat stores generally results in higher concentrations of ketone bodies compared to what is achieved through dietary intake alone.
- KD-R is preferable for adults with overweight or obesity given that normalisation of weight is considered protective against recurrence in many cancers.

Caveat

Patients who are anorexic, cachexic, sarcopenic, malnourished or already at a low body weight should not be started on a KD-R. Instead, the nutrition plan should focus on reducing intake of sugars, grains, and highly refined starches while increasing intake of nutrient- and calorie-dense foods, including most above-ground vegetables, some berries and fruit, most legumes, specific nuts and seeds, and a variety of healthy fats and oils.

6.4.3.2.1 Macronutrient distribution

US government recommendations for macronutrient intake as a percentage of total calories are specified in a guideline known as the acceptable macronutrient distribution ranges (AMDR) [537]. As of 2022, the distribution ranges are 20%–35% fat, 10%–35% protein, and 45%–65% carbohydrate. Recently, advocates of TCR have proposed macronutrient distributions for use in KDs; these percentages are easier for the public to understand than diet ratio but there are some drawbacks. In a classic eucaloric KD and in mouse model research, the distribution is often presented as 90% fat with approximately 6% protein, and 4% carb [386,538]; that becomes the goalpost for many patients and practitioners. In KD-R, these percentages appear to fall short of the goal only because of the lower fat intake and higher protein intake relative to total calories.

Example of macronutrient distribution expressed as a percentage of total calories in a 1400 kcal restricted ketogenic diet.

- 80% fat provides 1120 kcals (124 g)
- 15% protein provides 210 kcals (52.5 g)
- 5% carb provides 64 kcals (16 g net carbs after deducting an estimated 8 g of fibre from total carbs)

6.4.3.3 *Modifiable ketogenic diet*

A high level of ketosis is generally seen as a primary goal of any ketogenic plan for cancer. However, given the potential of weight loss with a rigorous KD-R, the nutrition prescription for a malnourished and underweight client will be very different from the initial prescription for someone with excess weight. In the former, stabilising weight will require a more liberal plan supplemented with exogenous ketones. In the latter, a more rigorous plan will allow for deep ketosis without supplementation, most often with the beneficial 'side effect' of therapeutic weight loss.

The term 'modifiable ketogenic diet' (KD-M), suggested by Miriam Kalamian, incorporates the first principles of TCR and TPM but allows for a high degree of flexibility and customisation in the development of ketogenic macronutrient prescriptions. A KD-M can readily adapt to changes in patient status or protocols. A patient who may have been following a rigorous pre-surgery plan during neoadjuvant chemotherapy may be switched to a plan allowing for more protein during a postoperative recovery period. A patient who was sedentary at initiation may begin strength training, requiring more protein post-workout when muscle cells signal for more nutrients.

In a classic eucaloric KD, a 4:1 diet ratio specifies that for every combined carb + protein gram, the diet provides 4 g of fat. Mice can easily consume such high fat diets but this is more challenging in humans. For example, an 183-cm male who weighs 100 kg would require daily consumption of approximately 17 tbsp of fats or oils; an amount that is neither tolerable nor desirable especially given that ketosis is meant to mimic a semi-fasting state.

In place of ratios, KD-Ms assign gram targets to each macronutrient based on patient demographics, activity level, nutritional needs, the anticipated impact of treatments, and baseline health status. To simplify the calculations, investigators and clinicians are encouraged to use Cronometer, an online meal planning and tracking tool optimised for use with KDs. The process is simple:

- Enter patient demographics and current activity level to calculate estimated energy requirements.
- Set an initial carb limit; for example, 16–20 g net carbs ('rigorous'), 20–40 g net carbs ('moderate'), 40–80 g net carbs ('relaxed'). (Note that carb intake over 40 g may be necessary to prevent weight loss but may not be deeply ketogenic.)
- Estimate protein needs guided by an adequate assessment of the patient's lean body mass (LBM). The goal of TPM is to allow enough protein to maintain or even build LBM without providing excess nutrients that might be diverted to supply-driven gluconeogenesis or other activities that support cancer cell metabolism. To that end, consider an initial target of 1.2–1.5 g/kg LBM.
- Set a goal for fibre intake of at least 70% of the RDA.
- The amount of fat to include in the plan is based on estimated total energy needs and desired weight outcome (e.g., lose, maintain, gain). Caveats: Resting energy quotient of fit keto-adapted individuals may be lower due to heavier reliance on fatty acid oxidation [369,539,540] Patients with a long history of dieting may have a lower basal metabolic rate [386]. Patients with late-stage disease may need substantially more total calories to compensate for systemic alterations in whole body metabolism; this is especially true for those patients who develop cancer cachexia.

Additional guidance on protein intake

Cancer research has identified specific amino acids (primarily glutamine, methionine, and serine) that appear to aid cancer cell survival and drive progression in some cancers. What is less clear is how to distinguish what part of this progression may be due to dietary intake and what part is independent of intake; for example, resulting from metabolic rewiring of cellular activities that increase intracellular amino acid synthesis and recycling. Research here is ongoing and will likely result in future individualisation of the nutrition plan.

Despite the potential downside of too much protein, it is clear that some patients will benefit from a higher protein intake, perhaps approaching 2.0 g/kg LBM including those who:

- have low blood counts or nutrient deficiencies;
- regularly engage in strength training or sports;
- are recovering from surgery;
- are undergoing aggressive cancer treatment with chemo and/or radiation;
- struggle with GI issues that impair protein digestion;
- are at risk of sarcopenia or cachexia;
- are 'Older adults' (65 years old or older).

Protein and fat targets should be increased if weight loss continues in patients at or below a desirable weight. At all times with all patients, monitoring weight loss is a priority, especially if the patient is not tolerating the suggested amount of fat. This is more likely to happen in patients with low appetite or with compromised ability to digest fats and oils. Be prepared to discontinue the diet if these challenges are not resolved. That can be devastating to the morale of the patient: at that point, suggesting that they eat freely of all foods from the list of low-to-medium glycaemic index foods might be the best advice a clinician can offer.

For all patients, the goal is to liberalise the diet over time, making room for more variety in foods that still conform to the first principles. The lifetime plan for a cancer survivor should be more focused on metabolic flexibility; that is, maintaining energy homoeostasis in line with metabolic demands. The focus shifts to maintaining blood glucose concentrations in a low and tight range (e.g., 4–6 mmol/L, or 72–108 mg/dL) but with less emphasis on deep ketosis. Here, borderline ketosis may be enough to retain the evolutionary adaptations associated with metabolic health.

Feeding tubes

Chewing and swallowing often become major challenges in patients who receive radiation for head, neck, mouth, or lung cancer. In some cases, the temporary placement of a feeding tube can improve hydration and nutrition status. Although patients may baulk at the suggestion, encourage them to discuss this option with their medical team. They can continue to receive high-quality shakes, smoothies, or blenderised ketogenic meals through the tube.

6.4.3.4 *Medium-chain triglyceride diet*

Medium-chain triglyceride (MCT) oil has been safely used for decades to increase ketosis in children maintained on a KD for epilepsy. Their use has expanded into more general use, especially in KDs. C8 caprylic and C10 capric fatty acids do not undergo digestion by bile and pancreatic enzymes. Instead, soon after contact with the duodenum, they diffuse across the intestinal membrane into the hepatic capillary bed and are transported to the liver via the hepatic portal circulation. There, they can be readily converted into ketones and returned to the circulation for distribution throughout the body. Unfortunately, MCT oil is not universally well-tolerated in adults and some gastrointestinal issues (diarrhoea, bloating, GI pain, or pressure) limit its use although a gradual introduction may allow for at least minimal use.

MCT versions of the KD either specify a set amount of MCT (e.g., 2–8 tbsp) or a particular percentage (e.g., 10%–40% of total calories). Inclusion is intended to increase ketosis or liberalise the carbohydrate intake but occasionally it is suggested to lower the amount of other fats and oils in the plan. This is often due to continuing (and often misguided) concern over the potential adverse effects of 'high- fat diets' commonly promoted in conventional medical and nutrition settings. However, these misguided efforts to initiate protocols that call for high intake of MCT oil without considering compliance or tolerance issues have often backfired in clinical trial settings [541].

6.4.3.5 *Vegan and carnivore diets*

Best practice guidelines in KDs suffer from conflicting and often passionately charged opinions on whether or not to allow or even encourage the consumption of animal-sourced proteins and fat. Consequently, there exists a continuum spanning from resolute vegan (no animal products) to exclusively carnivore ('snout-to-tail'). Plans at either end of the continuum increase the challenges associated with implementing a well-formulated KD. Still, adaptations may need to be made for patients who engage in dietary practices that are integral to their social identity, such as vegetarianism in India or veganism in Seventh Day Adventists. Ideally, though, best practise sets aside personal beliefs and biases, utilising plans that include both plant and animal sources of all nutrients.

6.4.3.5.1 Clinical trial settings compared to private practice

It is important to note here that KD protocols in clinical trials typically do not allow for this degree of flexibility, either at initiation or at any point in the study time frame, as this obviously introduces confounders that detract from generalising the trial results. Therefore, the flexibility inherent in the KD-M is typically better suited to use in private medical practices. There are other critical differences between clinical trials and private practice. In conventional care, the intervention period ends, support is withdrawn, and the patient often returns to his or her former dietary pattern. In private practice, there is more emphasis on whole food nutrition and the patient is more likely to maintain new and healthier eating patterns over the long term.

6.4.4 Intake and assessment

In both private practise and clinical settings, the patient may arrive at that initial meeting having already started on a KD at home and without support. The nutritionist should review, revise, and build on this early start. At the initial meeting, the nutritionist should also outline the plan for continued contact and oversight by the nutrition team, setting parameters for what is the responsibility of the nutrition team versus what needs medical monitoring. The means and frequency of ongoing communication between the patient and the nutrition team should also be agreed upon.

Initial assessment should include (but is not limited to) the following:

- Absolute and relative contraindications to KDs
- Anthropometric data (age, gender, height, weight, body fat percentage)
- Medical history (comorbidities; other conditions that that affect appetite, oral intake, or digestion and uptake of nutrients)
- Nutrition (current dietary pattern; food preferences; allergies, aversions, and intolerances)
- Laboratory data (minimum: CBC, CMP, disease biomarkers including inflammatory markers)
- Medications and supplements (prescribed and self-selected)
- Challenges (physical, psychosocial, financial)
- Other considerations that impact food choices (cultural, religious, personally held beliefs)

6.4.4.1 *Absolute and relative contraindications*

There are very few absolute contraindications that make it unsafe to adopt a KD. For the most part, these are inborn errors that interfere with the ability to utilise fats for fuel and as such, they are generally diagnosed in early childhood.

The following list was adapted from the book *The KD and Modified Atkins Diets: Treatments for Epilepsy and Other Disorders* (6th ed. Demos Health. New York, NY, p. 33)

- Primary (i.e., inborn, not acquired) carnitine deficiencies
- Defects in pathways of fatty acid oxidation
- Pyruvate carboxylase deficiency
- Porphyria (certain forms of this can emerge in adulthood)

The list of relative contraindications is much broader and highly nuanced. Although none of these conditions rise to the level of absolute exclusion, they may require specialised medical or nutritional oversight.

6.4.4.1.1 Conditions that require interventions and/or intensive medical management

- Pregnancy or lactation
- Surgeries that affect GI structure or function (oesophageal surgery; Whipple procedure)
- Type 1 diabetes or poorly controlled T2D
- Diabetes medications that raise the risk for metabolic acidosis (e.g., SGLT2 inhibitors)
- History of gastric bypass surgery or current lap band
- Intractable constipation due to high dosages of opiate medications
- Impaired GI motility due to neuromuscular disorders or neurodegenerative disease
- Gallbladder obstruction
- History of pancreatitis
- Heart conditions (including elongated QT interval or rhythm disorders)
- Advanced renal disease
- Cancer cachexia

6.4.4.1.2 Conditions that require input and oversight from health care practitioners

- 'Red flags' in lab results (e.g., low blood counts, unbalanced electrolytes)
- Moderate-to-severe elevated liver enzymes
- Treatment-related side effects of anticancer drugs and/or radiation
- History of IBS, Crohn's disease, ulcerative colitis, short bowel syndrome
- Personal or family history of kidney stones or gallstones
- Hypo- or hyperthyroid (including Hashimoto's disease)
- Use of a feeding tube
- Impaired baseline nutrition or low body weight
- Cholecystectomy (gallbladder removal)
- Opiate medications
- Polypharmacy

6.4.4.1.3 Conditions that interfere with the ability to lower blood glucose concentrations

- Inflammation or injury caused by disease, surgery, radiation or drug therapies
- Concurrent use of steroid medications (most commonly, dexamethasone or prednisone)
- Persistent external or internal stressors that raise concentrations of stress hormones
- Tumour load (disrupts glucose homoeostasis)
- Excessive or vigorous exercise before keto-adaptation
- Epigenetic influence of certain single nucleotide polymorphisms (identified in direct-to-consumer genetic testing)

6.4.4.1.4 Conditions that complicate compliance with implementation guidelines

- Depression
- Fatigue
- Stress

- Constipation or diarrhoea
- Nausea or vomiting
- Illness or general malaise
- 'Keto Flu' in the first few weeks of the diet
- Difficulty tolerating fats and oils
- Comorbidities that impact gastrointestinal structure or function
- Self-imposed restrictive dietary patterns (e.g., Vegan, Gerson, Budwig)
- Impaired cognition and/or difficulty comprehending nutrition guidelines
- Physical limitations that interfere with activities of daily living
- Food choices which are consistently incompatible with the plan
- History of eating disorders
- Chronic and/or excessive intake of alcohol

6.4.4.1.5 Conditions that create obstacles in the social and emotional environment

- Resistance to change
- Feeling overwhelmed (commonly accompanies a cancer diagnosis)
- Orthorexia (here, additional food restrictions that extend beyond TCR/TPM)
- Feeling unsure about the safety of a KD
- Financial concerns over the cost of foods
- Competing demands on time or energy (shopping, meal planning, meal prep)
- Dissatisfaction with restrictions and limitations involved with following the diet
- Impact of unfavourable physical or social environments (e.g., chaos at home or work)
- Stress, both external and internal
- Reliance on food as comfort
- Interference or sabotage from family or friends
- Medical team opposition

6.4.5 Implementation

Implementation of KDs generally starts with one of these three approaches.

6.4.5.1 Water-only fasting

Patients with adequate body weight and in stable health might start with a two-to-three day medically monitored water-only fast (WOF). Therapeutic WOFs lower blood glucose and insulin concentrations and elevate blood ketone concentrations beyond what is typically seen in a KD-R, allowing most patients to quickly reach therapeutic ranges (as described by Seyfried and colleagues) as a glucose/ketone index of 1–2.5 [449]. While the degree of abstinence required for a WOF might sound draconian, fasting for several days, especially if the patient has transitioned to ketosis first, reduces the degree of lean tissue catabolism typically experienced in the first few days of fasting [455,542–544]. However, cancer patients often have comorbidities or situational limitations that make it unwise or less safe to conduct an initial multi-day WOF: for example, patients who live alone, are more medically fragile, or at a higher risk of sarcopenia.

Care should be taken to ensure that patients are educated on how to fast safely. This includes but is not limited to possibly reducing or discontinuing medications (under medical supervision), self-monitoring changes in blood pressure, and replenishing fluids and minerals (especially sodium and magnesium), which are depleted due to the diuretic effect of fasting. It is also crucial to have a ketogenic nutrition plan in place before ending the fast, or the benefits will be quickly lost.

Going hungry replenishes the body

Nasha Winters
Metabolic Terrain Institute of Health

Our food should be our medicine. Our medicine should be our food. But to eat when you are sick is to feed your sickness.

—Hippocrates

Fasting has been used as a therapeutic approach to wellness for a long time, even though it has fallen out of our conventional medicine toolbox. In 1909, Dr. Carlo Moreschi noted that caloric restriction led to decreased tumour growth, and since

(Continued)

(Continued)

then a large body of work has established that caloric restriction reduces the progression of tumours in animals [545]. By 1975, however, doctors recoiled at the idea of 'starving' their patients; the sentiment that fasting is antithetical to wellness still exists in both medical and public perceptions today.

One of the primary benefits to fasting is the activation of autophagy. Autophagy is our built-in self-cleaning process through which the body rids itself of all its broken down, old cellular parts. In the early stages of fasting, amino acid levels begin to increase, since autophagy has prompted the breakdown of cellular components [546]. Those amino acids are delivered to the liver for use in gluconeogenesis or incorporated into new proteins as they are generated. The autophagy process is unique to fasting since it is paused by the presence of glucose and insulin. In other words, the self-cleaning process stops the moment you begin to eat.

The process of cellular breakdown and protein synthesis has countless benefits for the body. In particular, it's key to combating two main conditions in which the accumulation of old, defective, or abnormal proteins results in disease: Alzheimer's disease and cancer [547,548].

As recently as 2014, Dr. Longo and his colleagues demonstrated that fasting in mice causes old and worn immune cells to die. Those immune cells were later replaced by stem cells, and the team concluded that a simple three-day fast could help regenerate the immune system in profound ways [549].

In addition to providing benefits to the immune system, Dr. Longo and his colleagues also demonstrated that a 48-h fast in mice slowed the growth and spread of five out of the eight cancers that they studied. They showed that the combination of fasting cycles with cycles of chemotherapy was more effective than chemotherapy alone in all cancers studied [550]. The team concluded that fasting reduces the concentrations of a number of anabolic hormones, growth factors, and inflammatory cytokines, reduces oxidative stress and cell proliferation, enhances autophagy, and leads to several DNA repair processes [551].

Only 2 years later, in 2016, a study published in the *Journal of American Medical Association* reported that women who fasted for 13 h overnight improved prognosis and lowered the recurrence rate of breast cancer as a result of improved glucoregulation [552]. Today, clinical studies continue to find that fasting and caloric restriction combat chronic illness by encouraging cellular repair.

6.4.5.1.1 Jumpstart a restricted ketogenic diet

If fasting is not an option, restricting carbohydrates to 20 net g/day and limiting protein to somewhere between 1.0 and 1.4 g/kg of LBM/day is usually sufficient to enter the therapeutic ranges for blood glucose and ketone concentrations within a period of time ranging from several days to several weeks. As in WOF, a KD-R is expected to have a diuretic effect so it is necessary to medically monitor any ongoing use of medications such as blood pressure medications. Electrolyte concentrations will also need to be monitored and/or replenished, especially during the transition to the KD. Proactively addressing transition side effects—such as hunger, cravings, and 'keto flu',—should reduce dropouts and minimise negative impacts on quality of life. Starting with a KD-R as opposed to a fast will also result in less degradation of muscle mass, which is crucial in protecting muscle in older adults as well as in those at high risk of sarcopenia and/or cachexia.

6.4.5.1.2 Gradual transition

Older patients as well as those with comorbidities, or where gastrointestinal structure or function has been compromised by disease or its treatment, may respond better to a more gradual transition to the diet. This is also the best option for those patients who are advised not to lose weight; for example, those at low or borderline weight at baseline, or have already undergone the process used to determine the radiotherapy treatment field. This transition period may range from several days to several weeks during which time fat intake is gradually increased at each meal as sugars and starches are withdrawn.

The more rigorous the initiation, the greater the impact on cancer pathways. However, ensuring the patient's safety is paramount, superseding any consideration of the potential benefits of a KD. Ultimately, the nutritionist in concert with the patient's wishes and medical team oversight should determine which implementation protocol is most appropriate. Be prepared to modify the plan to address the known and emerging side effects of the cancer treatment protocol.

6.4.5.2 Managing transition side effects

As noted, transition to ketosis often results in a predictable group of symptoms commonly referred to as 'keto flu' (Fig. 6.9). Nutrition education, ongoing communication, and psychosocial support for the patient and caregiver are crucial during the critical first few weeks of the transition. Materials such as the handout that follows are an important part of client education.

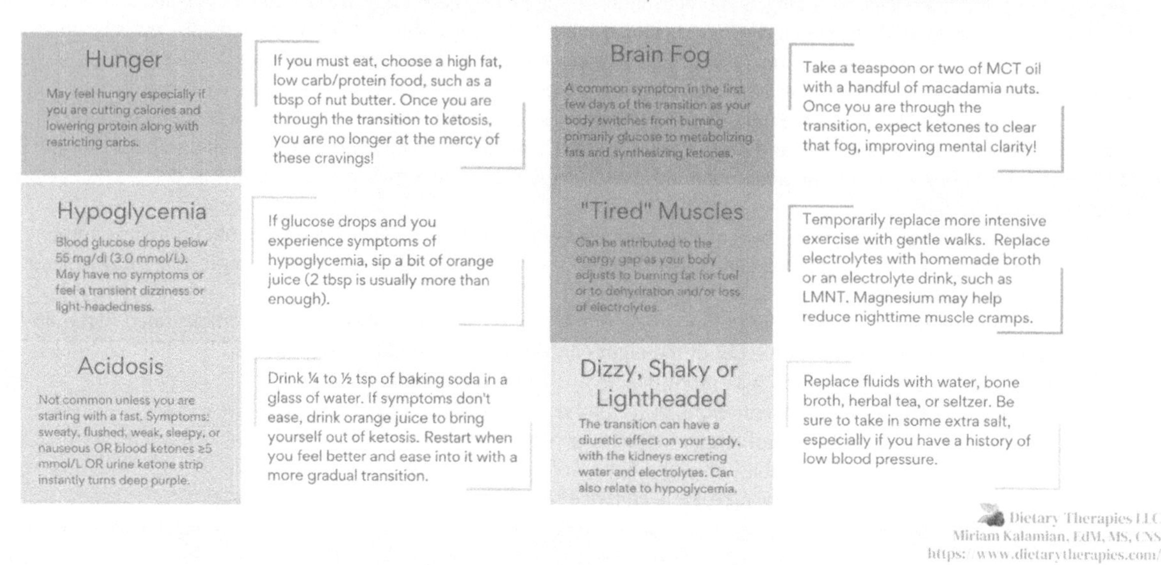

FIGURE 6.9 Common side effects of the patient undergoing transition to nutritional ketosis and their corresponding treatments.

Successful implementation of the KD often hinges on the education presented to patients prior to initiation as well as the ongoing support provided over an extended period of time as the patient and/or caregiver work through the obstacles and challenges commonly faced in the first few weeks. Unfortunately, nutrition education is often sparse and inadequate; for example, simply giving a patient a list of foods to include and foods to avoid does not ensure comprehension, competency or compliance. In contrast to experiences in some loosely designed KD clinical trials, the education and support given to patients with breast cancer in a recent German study is likely to have contributed to the low dropout rate in the KD group. The well-defined protocol allowed the researchers to offer valid conclusions on safety and feasibility for diets with similar parameters [553]. The following low-cost materials should be considered *minimum* education: keto-friendly food list, generic meal template (Fig. 6.10), sample meal plans, cookbooks, and a long list of reputable resources. The emphasis should be on whole food nutrition with packaged or processed food playing only a small supporting role. Equally important, the keto nutritionist should be available to answer patient/caregiver questions and to prophylactically address the anticipated negative impact of cancer treatment on appetite, intake, digestion, and uptake of nutrients.

The list of keto-friendly foods will vary from region to region based in part by what is locally available to the patient. It is important to note that this list is also likely to limit some foods that are usually included in low-carb and ketogenic nutrition plans for use in other applications, such as diabetes or weight loss. For example, a high intake of dairy proteins may stimulate the secretion of insulin, which might be desirable in diabetes. Given that cancer cells are programmed for growth, they often have more receptors for insulin: therefore, the nutritionist might want to set a limit on intake. Nuances aside, the basic plan can be represented by a simple graphic.

6.4.5.3 *Tracking blood glucose and ketone concentrations*

Tracking blood glucose and ketone concentration provides objective data on the patient's concentrations of ketosis. Along with food logs, this data also serves as a measure of dietary compliance. In the first few weeks (or months), patients should be encouraged to test concentration of blood glucose and ketones using a glucometer [554,555]. The nutrition team should work with the patient to establish an acceptable procedure for testing and recording these measurements. Testing protocols can be as basic as twice a day, fasting and at bedtime. Recording options include a log or spreadsheet, entries into a Cronometer or other platform, or even taking a picture of the metre measurement,

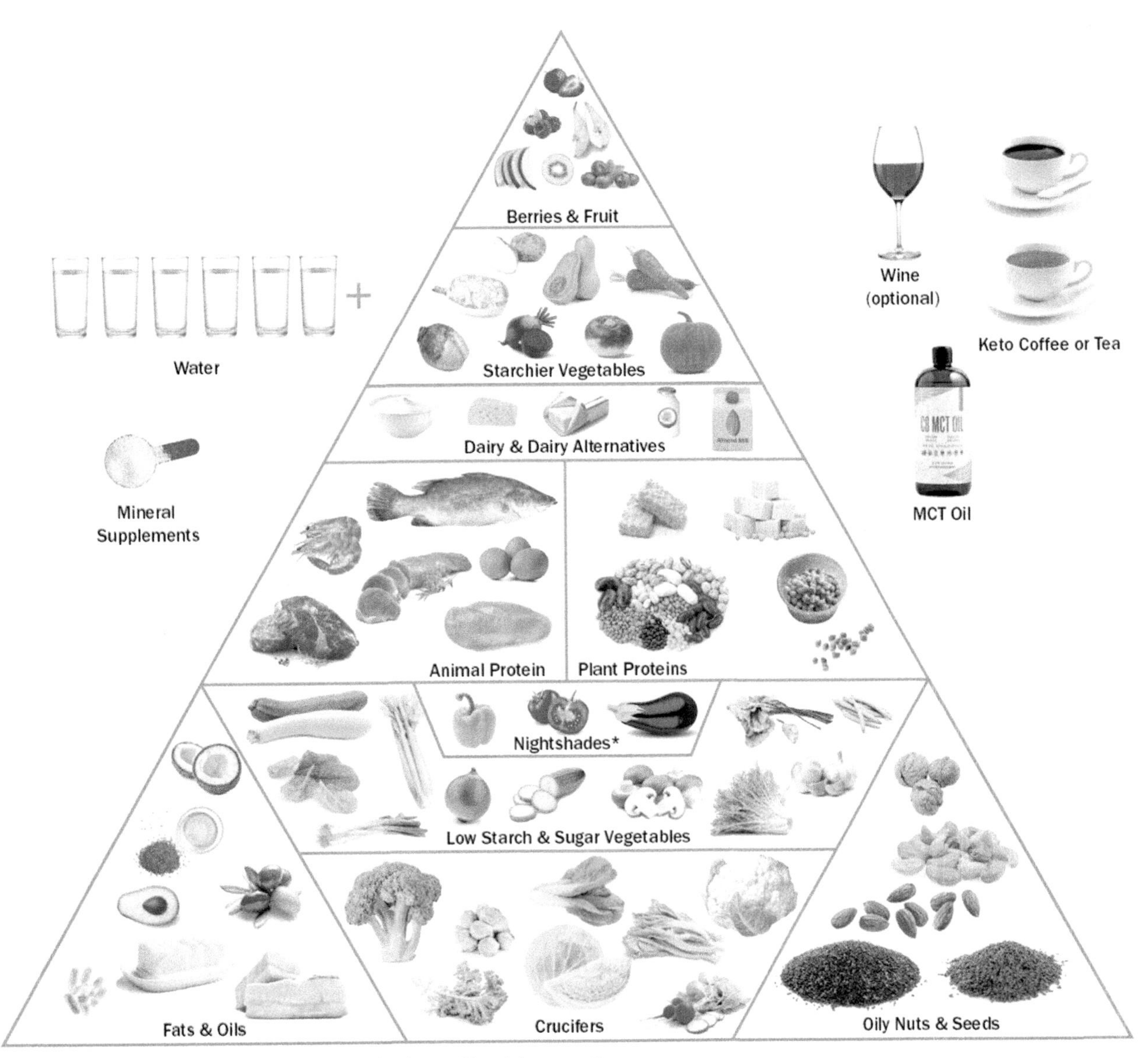

FIGURE 6.10 A ketogenic food pyramid consisting of ketogenic foods and their corresponding recommended proportions in the patient's diet. *Copyright retained. Graphic design by Suzi Smith.*

which is then shared with a nutrition team member. The nutrition team has leeway to expand on the testing schedule: for example, blood ketones may be measured once or twice a week before the evening meal, or glucose may be measured 1 or 2 h postprandial. Over time, the frequency of blood testing may be reduced to a few days per week.

6.4.5.3.1 Testing devices

The Abbott Precision Xtra glucose/ ketone metre has been the gold standard in research but other validated options (such as Keto-Mojo) may also be used. Patients need to be educated as to proper testing methods including finger sticking tips for getting a clean drop of blood.

Recently, there is growing interest in the use of continuous glucose monitors (CGMs) in place of or as adjuncts to glucometers. This reduces the burden of invasive finger stick testing for the patient but increases the cost. CGMs sample glucose from interstitial fluid rather than capillary blood. Glucose concentrations in interstitial fluid lag behind blood concentrations, which is reflected in the differences seen when CGM glucose readings are compared to measurements taken using a glucometer. Still, the information gained from continuous sampling allows practitioners to identify glucose trends associated with the patient's food choices, stressors, exercise, and sleep patterns. The data can also be used to reinforce food choices and lifestyle behaviours that are associated with desirably low and steady concentrations of glucose. Ideally, spot checks using the handheld glucose metre, either at home or with POC measurements taken during clinic visits, will help to identify any gross disparities between the two testing methods. At this time, Abbott's Freestyle Libre series are the easiest CGMs to obtain for this off-label use.

Breath analysers that sample acetone in the breath are an alternative to testing blood ketone concentrations. This method assesses the level of ketosis in units called ACEs (parts per million of breath acetone) [556]. In the past, breath acetone concentrations could not be easily correlated with blood concentrations of βHB but currently, at least one newer device, the Biosense breath analyser, has addressed this issue with a conversion algorithm, moving the device into position as a non-invasive alternative method for assessing ketosis. Similar to the CGM, the breath analyser reduces the burden of frequent finger stick testing. Although the accuracy of any single reading is questionable, the potential benefit of a breath analyser is in establishing the patient's daily ketone patterns from more frequent measurements. As with the CGM, it is still desirable to validate metre accuracy with spot checks of blood concentrations using a finger stick test.

Urine test strips are yet another non-invasive option for testing ketones. Their best use is a basic screening tool. Benefits include low cost, availability, and ease of use but there are many drawbacks. Urine strips test acetoacetate: over time and with keto-adaptation, less acetoacetate is excreted in the urine even in patients who are compliant to the diet. Urine strips are also highly sensitive to changes in water volume: they will falsely indicate high concentrations of ketones in a dehydrated state.

Initial weight loss is expected as patients transition to the diet. Early on, this is mostly water weight associated with the depletion of glycogen stores. Following the transition, it is suggested that the patient plan be recalculated to limit weight loss to no more than 1 kg/week in those with excess fat stores and to maintain weight in those already within an ideal weight range.

6.4.6 Accountability

A cancer diagnosis often creates a sense of overwhelming distress for both patients and caregivers who are now facing a multitude of new challenges, including family stress, constraints on time, increased fatigue, financial burdens, and a disconcerting array of conflicting recommendations coming from family, friends, and the internet. Diet accountability can add to the burden. For this reason, it may be best to approach the early days and weeks of the diet using only the food list, a simple meal template and examples of a weekly plan. Once the patient/caregiver is comfortable with the changes, they should be encouraged to keep accurate food records and to share this information with their team. Clinicians are encouraged to set up a Professional account with Cronometer or other online food tracking app that provides practitioner access to the patient's food diary, activity log, changes in weight, and glucose/ketone measurements. The collected data can then be assessed for nutritional adequacy and general health trends: feedback to the patient can assist them to improve these parameters over time. Video tutorials and/or the use of screenshare during a virtual meeting is often sufficient to ease patient concerns and impress upon them the value of the feedback on nutrition obtained through keeping accurate records. (In nutrition plans for children, clinicians should use the Charlie Foundation's KetoDietCalculator [557] as Cronometer is not designed to support KDs in the paediatric population.)

Rationale for the use of Cronometer:

- Provides a centralised platform for storing and sharing data
- High privacy setting, including a HIPPA compliant option
- Fosters patient accountability
- Identifies non-compliant foods or patterns (both intentional and inadvertent)
- Enhances communication between patient and nutrition team
- Integrates with fitness/sleep trackers providing data on sleep and exercise
- Syncs with devices such as Keto-Mojo and Biosense
- Graphs GKI from patient or team entries

6.4.7 Summary

It is clear from multiple case reports and the results of early clinical trials that well-formulated KDs undertaken with robust nutrition team support are both safe and feasible for those who meet baseline criteria. Private practise nutritionists and clinicians now have access to the tools and knowledge needed to develop safe and effective ketogenic nutrition plans.

6.4.8 Resources

Kalamian M. Keto for Cancer: Ketogenic Metabolic Therapy as a Targeted Nutritional Strategy. Chelsea Green, 2017.

Kalamian M. KetoMetabolic A Quickstart Guide to Integrative Cancer Care. Dietary Therapies, LLC. 2022. https://www.dietarytherapies.com/keto-for-cancer-book

American Nutrition Association. Ketogenic Nutrition Training Program. Includes a Module on Cancer. Available at: https://theana.org/trainings/ketogenic

6.5 Fasting and chemotherapy

Martha Tettenborn

Author of Hacking Chemo: Using Ketogenic Diet, Therapeutic Fasting and a Kickass Attitude to Power through Cancer

6.5.1 Benefits of combining fasting with chemotherapy

There are four main benefits of combining the use of fasting with chemotherapy in the management of cancer:

6.5.1.1 Improve chemotherapy's effectiveness

By fasting, the body is encouraged to enter a deeper state of ketosis whilst blood glucose concentrations are reduced, without major upward excursions when eating. Additionally, insulin production is minimised as a result of reduced stimulation by caloric or carbohydrate intake. This has the effect of stressing the cancer cells by reducing available fuel and by reducing the presence of growth factors such as insulin. These biological effects may potentiate the effectiveness of the chemotherapeutic drugs [550,558].

6.5.1.2 Reduce chemotherapy side effects

Normal physiological processes of cellular metabolism are down-regulated when the intake of food energy is reduced. Since most chemotherapy drugs are a 'blunt weapon', aimed at cells exhibiting an exaggerated rate of metabolism, the healthy cells escape notice by the chemotherapy drugs when they are in this suppressed state. This has the effect of reducing side effects such as mouth sores, nausea, vomiting, bowel issues, joint and muscular pains, peripheral neuropathy. Bone marrow suppression and hair loss, both more delayed effects of the chemo drugs, occur, but possibly to a reduced extent [559].

6.5.1.3 Reduce inflammation

Fasting reduces inflammation and some oncologists have begun to acknowledge this benefit by adjusting the dosage and/or timing of protocol steroid medications [560,561].

6.5.1.4 Improve quality of life

By allowing the cancer patient to manage one area of their cancer treatment, there is a sense of self-determination and control that is lacking in most cancer situations. This serves to reduce anxiety and allows the patient to feel that they are impacting positively on their cancer journey. By reducing side effects, there's a significant improvement in quality of life factors [500,559].

Fasting and weight loss

Miriam Kalamian

Weight loss is one of the often-cited concerns expressed in the conventional oncology setting. In anecdotal reports, unintended weight loss associated with short-term fasting has been minimal and mostly temporary. Fig. 6.11 is one example of improvements in baseline weight despite repeated cycles of fasting in a highly compliant patient.

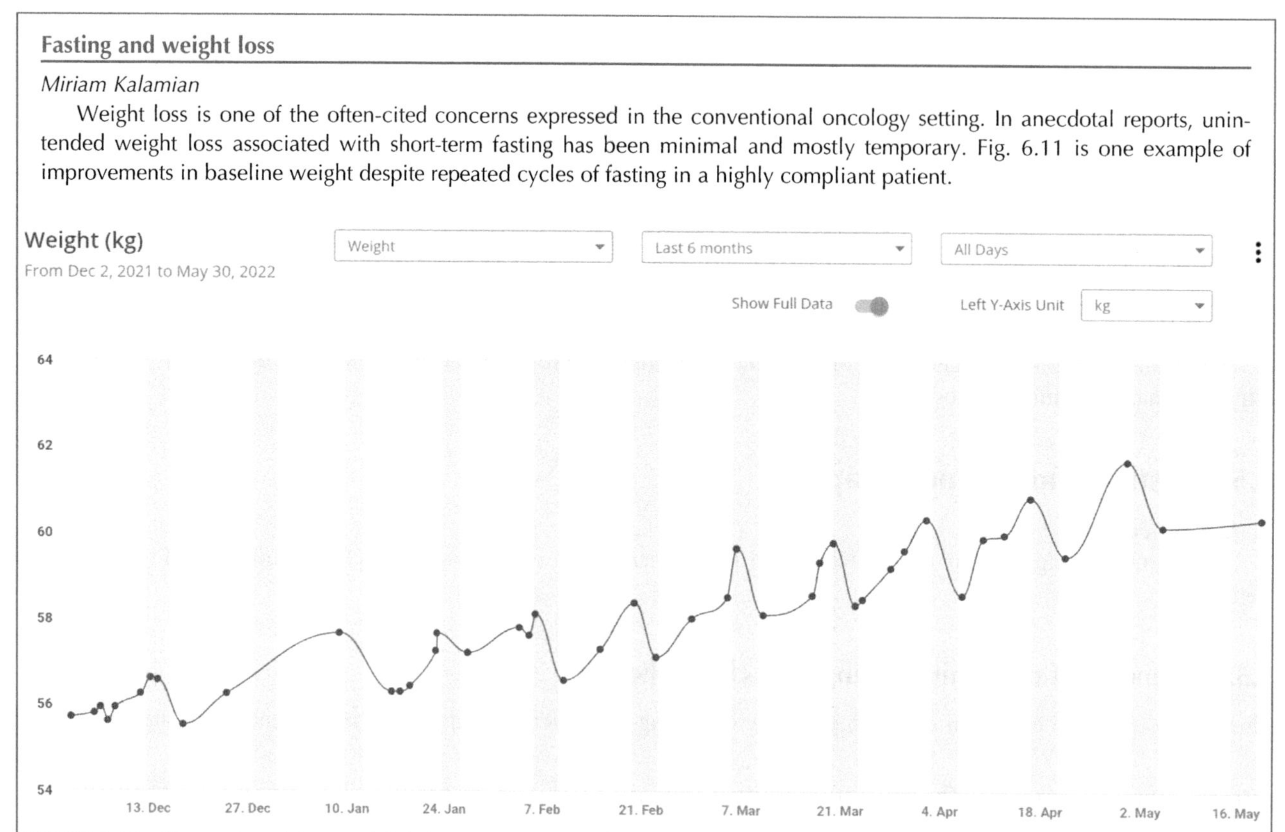

FIGURE 6.11 Changes in weight recorded during repeated cycles of chemotherapy (FOLFOXIRI plus bevacizumab) in the treatment of colorectal adenocarcinoma IV with metastases to the liver. The client is a 53-year-old white female, 168 cm, BMI at baseline was 19.7 kg/m^2, increasing to BMI of 21.4 kg/m^2 at 6 months. Modified fasting protocol of 3–5 days was maintained throughout each 2-week treatment cycle.

6.5.2 Managing the patient

These goals or benefits of fasting around chemo are maximised when the fasting is done in conjunction with maintaining a well-formulated KD between chemo treatments. The impact of a KD on lowering blood glucose and insulin, and elevating ketone concentrations makes for an inhospitable environment for promoting cancer growth. The ideal KD will be low enough in carbohydrate to promote at least mild ketosis (0.5–1.5 mmol/L), provide adequate caloric intake to maintain body weight, be sugar-free and low in non-nutritive sweeteners (due to their impact on insulin concentrations), and have little to no alcohol.

Although a water-only fast is possible, most patients will benefit from a fast that is supported with familiar and preferred calorie-free beverages (Table 6.2). Only fluids are used, as these do not stop in the stomach for digestion and stimulate gastric digestive hormonal and enzymatic responses. The goals of intake during fasting are adequate hydration and electrolytes (particularly sodium), provide satiety signals and simulate eating behaviours, thus meeting social, emotional and family requirements.

The timing of fasting around chemotherapy treatments has been studied, but not clearly defined. It appears that any fasting period prior to and post chemo is beneficial, but research has suggested a period of 24–72 h pre-chemo and 8–24 h post-chemo will have an impact on immediate side-effects, such as GI upset. An effective and relatively practical timing is 36–42 h before and 24 h after chemo administration (Table 6.3) [500].

6.5.3 Factors for success

Preparation is key to making this a successful intervention. Make bone broth ahead of time and have an adequate portion defrosted and ready before beginning the fast. Have adequate coffee, tea, soda, flavour enhancers, etc. Obtain a thermos for coffee, a separate one for tea or broth and a water bottle, so that appropriate fluids are always available.

TABLE 6.2 Allowed fluids during a chemotherapy-fast.

Fluid	Amount	Examples
Water	Ad libitum	Still, sparkling, club soda, flavour-infused waters with no sweeteners. Hot, room temperature, cold or iced.
Coffee	To tolerance of caffeine intake	Black or up to 1 tbsp coffee cream if needed (max one to two times/day). Hot or iced. Decaffeinated or regular.
Tea	Caffeinated teas: To tolerance of caffeine intake. Herbal teas: Ad libitum.	Black, green, white, herbal infusions with no added sugars or sweeteners. Hot or cold.
Bone broth	250–500 mL/day	Homemade or packaged bone broth. Not bouillon cubes or powder, not packaged chicken or beef soup base broth. Bone broth should be made using slow or pressure cooking methods from beef, pork, chicken, lamb or fish bones. Stovetop, crockpot or pressure cooker can be used. The resulting broth will provide a small amount of protein, mostly as collagen if joints are used, and minerals such as calcium and magnesium. Bone broth is also a good vehicle for providing salt (sea salt or pink salt preferred) and provides a sense of a 'meal' with good satiety.

Note: The goal is to drink 2–3 L per day.

TABLE 6.3 Timing and guidelines to fasting around chemotherapy treatments.

Day 1	2 days before chemo	Eat a well-formulated ketogenic diet until dinner, then commence fast after supper.
Day 2	Day before chemo	Use allowed beverages throughout the day. No solids, no sweetened beverages.
Day 3	Chemo administration day	Allowed beverages only throughout the day. Suggestion is to avoid taking broth into the chemo suite, due to potential for odour to be slightly off-putting for other clients. Lighter beverages such as tea or water are preferable for the chemo suite.
Day 4	24 h after the end of chemo administration (could be lunch or supper)	Plan for a light meal of a preferred food and be prepared for appetite to be smaller than normal.

In the pre-chemo period, stay busy and away from the kitchen as much as possible. Find activities that take place over the usual meal-time to reduce timing-related hunger. Use bone broth as a 'meal', sitting at the table and using a spoon to consume it if other family members or workmates are present.

Enlist support of others with whom one eats (e.g., family, workmates, friends). Share the rationale for the KD and the fasting protocol. Share the optimism and sense of control that dietary manipulation allows.

6.5.4 Monitoring

Clinicians working with patients, particularly those with the goal of publishing case series or reports, may choose to document outcomes, including changes in weight, body composition, GKI, blood counts, chemistries, insulin, IGF-1, cancer biomarkers and more general markers of inflammation.

6.5.5 Conclusion

Evidence indicates that fasting should be considered as an adjunct to chemotherapy to improve chemotherapy efficacy, reduce side effects and improve quality of life. A liquid fast, consisting of unsweetened beverages, may stretch from the day before to the day after a chemotherapy treatment, and is best combined with a KD during the non-fasting period. This effective, non-invasive and easy-to-apply therapeutic modality should be presented as an option to patients.

References

[1] Stefansson V. Cancer: Disease of Civilization? An anthropological and historical study. New York, NY: Hill and Wang; 1960.
[2] Hoffman FL. Cancer and Diet. With Facts and Observations of Related Subjects. Baltimore, MD: The Williams and Wilkins Company; 1937.
[3] Price WA. Nutrition and Physical Degeneration: A Comparison of Primitive and Modern Diets and Their Effects. 8th edition Price-Pottenger Nutrition Foundation; 1939.
[4] Ben-Dor M., Noakes T.D. Understanding human diet and disease. Sci Evolut Evid. (This Textbook).
[5] Rowbotham J, Clayton P. An unsuitable and degraded diet? Part three: Victorian consumption patterns and their health benefits. J R Soc Med 2008;101:454–62.
[6] Clayton P, Rowbotham J. An unsuitable and degraded diet. Part one: Public health lessons from the mid-Victorian working class diet. J R Soc Med 2008;101:282–9.
[7] Clayton P, Rowbotham J. An unsuitable and degraded diet? Part two: Realities of the mid-Victorian diet. J R Soc Med 2008;101:350–7.
[8] Clayton P, Rowbotham J. How the mid-Victorians worked, ate and died. Int J Env Res Public Health 2009;6:1235–53.
[9] Moffatt RU. Principal Medical Officer, Nairobi, to his Majesty's Commissioner. Anon 1906;35–6.
[10] Traveller brings new cancer theory. Philadelphia Inquirer, August 5, 1906.
[11] Berglas A. Foreword by Dr. Albert Schweitzer. Cancer: Nature, Cause and Cure. Institute Pasteur, Paris, France. 1957:27-58.
[12] Fouche FP. Freedom of Negro races from cancer. Br Med J 1923;3261:1116.
[13] Cummings JH, Engineer A. Denis Burkitt and the origins of the dietary fibre hypothesis. Nutr Res Rev 2018;31:1–15.
[14] Burkitt D. A sarcoma involving the jaws in African children. Br J Surg 1958;46:218–23.
[15] Lipski E. Traditional non-Western diets. Nutr Clin Pract 2010;25:585–93.
[16] Burkitt DP. Relationship between diseases and their etiological significance. Am J Clin Nutr 1977;30:262–7.
[17] Hearsey H. The rarity of cancer among the aborigines of British Central Africa. Br Med J 1906;1:1562–3.
[18] Kopp W. Significant dietary changes during human evolution and the development of cancer: From cells in trouble to cells causing trouble. J Carcinog Mutagen 2017;8:4.
[19] Anon. Cancer in the colonies. Br Med J 1906;2362:812.
[20] Higginson J. Developing concepts on environmental cancer: The role of geographical pathology. Env Mutagen 1983;5:929–40.
[21] Higginson J. From geographical pathology to environmental carcinogenesis: A historical reminiscence. Cancer Lett 1997;117:133–42.
[22] Higginson J. Rethinking the environmental causation of human cancer. Food Cosmetic Toxicol 1981;19:539–48.
[23] Doll R, Petro R. The causes of cancer: quantitative estimates of avoidable risks of cancer in the United States today. J Natl Cancer Inst 1981;66:1191–308.
[24] Taubes G. Good Calories Bad Calories: Challenging the Conventional Wisdom on Diet, Weight Control, and Disease. New York, NY: Alfred A. Knopf; 2007.
[25] Stefansson V. My life with the Eskimos. London, UK: The Macmillan Company; 1928.
[26] Stefansson V. The Friendly Arctic. London, UK: The Macmillan Company; 1921.
[27] Hutton SK. Among the Eskimos of Labrador: A Record of Five Years' Close Intercourse With the Eskimo Tribes of Labrador. Philadelphia, PA: J. B. Lippincott Co; 1912.
[28] Fellows FS. Mortality in the native races of the territory of Alaska, with special reference to tuberculosis. Pub Health Rep 1934;49:298–308.
[29] Guyenet S. Cancer among the Inuit Whole Health Source: Nutr Health Sci 2008;July 4th. Available from: http://wholehealthsource.blogspot.com/2008/07/cancer-among-inuit.html.
[30] Urquhart JA. The most northerly practice in Canada. Can Med Assoc J 1935;33:193–6.
[31] Lewison, EF. Paper delivered before Section on Surgery, AMA. 1956.
[32] Lawson RN, Saunders AL, Cowen RD. Breast cancer and heptaldehyde; preliminary report. Can Med Assoc J 1956;75:486–8.
[33] Fog-Poulson M. [Phaeochromocytoma in Greenlanders of pure Eskimo type]. Nord Med 1949;41:416–18.
[34] Brown GM, Cronk LB, Boag TJ. Occurrence of cancer in an Eskimo. Cancer 1952;5:142–3.
[35] Fortune R. Characteristics of cancer in the Eskimos of southern Alaska. Cancer 1969;23:468.
[36] Friborg JT, Melbye M. Cancer patterns in Inuit populations. Lancet Oncol 2008;9:892–900.
[37] Gottman AW. Report of 103 autopsies of Alaskan natives. Arch Pathol 1960;70:117–24.
[38] Arthraub JB. Cause of death in 339 Alaskan natives as determined by autopsy. Arch Path 1970;90:433.
[39] Hurst EE. Malignant tumors in Alaskan Eskimos: unique predominance of carcinoma of the oesophagus in Alaskan Eskimo women. Cancer 1964;17:1178.
[40] Lederman JM, Wallace AC, Hildes JA. Arteriosclerosis and neo-plasms in Canadian Eskimos. In: Biological Aspects of Aging; Proceedings of the 5th Congress of the International Association of Gerontology. Shock NW Editor. Columbia University Press, New York, NY, 1962.
[41] Schaefer O, Hildes JA, Medd LM, et al. The changing pattern of neoplastic disease in Canadian Eskimos. Can Med Assoc J 1975;112:1399–404.
[42] Schaefer O. When the Eskimo comes to town. Nutr Today 1971;8–16 Nov/Dec.
[43] Young TK, Kelly JJ, Friborg J, et al. Cancer among circumpolar populations: an emerging public health concern. J Circumpol Health 2016;75:10.
[44] DiNicolantonio JJ. Increase in the intake of refined carbohydrates and sugar may have led to the health decline of the Greenland Eskimos. Open Heart 2016;3:0000444.

[45] Hrdlicka A. Physiological and Medical Observations among the Indians of Southwestern United States and Northern Mexico. US Government Printing Office; 1908.
[46] Hoffman FL. The Mortality from Cancer throughout the World. Newark, NJ: Prudential Press; 1915.
[47] Hewett EL. Ancient life in the American Southwest. Indianapolis, IN: Bobbs-Merrill; 1930.
[48] Levin I. The study of the etiology of cancer based on clinical statistics. Ann Surg 1919;51:768–81.
[49] Obomsawin R. Historical and Scientific Perspectives on the Health of Canada's First Peoples; 2007.
[50] The Essays of Michael Lord of Montaigne. Florio J, trans-ed. Vol 1. New York, NY: J.M. Dent and Co; 1867.
[51] Hill K, Hurtado AM. Ache Life History. New York, NY: Aldine De Gruyter; 1996.
[52] Libertini G. Evidence for aging theories from the study of a hunter-gatherer people (Ache of Paraguay). Biochem (Mosc) 2013;78:1023–32.
[53] Fallon S, Enig MG. Australian aborigines: living off the fat of the land. West Price Found 2000;. Available from: https://www.westonaprice.org/health-topics/traditional-diets/australian-aborigines-living-off-the-fat-of-the-land/.
[54] Cunningham J, Rumbold AR, Zhang X, et al. Incidence, aetiology, and outcomes of cancer in indigenous peoples in Australia. Lancet Oncol 2008;9:585–95.
[55] McCarrison R. Studies in Deficiency Disease. London, UK: Henry Frowde and Hodder & Stoughton; 1945.
[56] McCarrison R. Nutrition and Health. London, UK: The McCarrison Society; 1982.
[57] Stefansson V. The Fat of the Land. London, UK: The Macmillan Company; 1960.
[58] Apple S. Ravenous. Otto Warburg, the Nazis, and the search for the Cancer-Diet Connection. New York, NY: Liveright Publishing Corporation; 2021.
[59] Warburg O. The Metabolism of Tumours. Investigations from the Kaiser Wilhelm Institute for Biology, Berlin-Dahlem. London, UK: Constable; 1930.
[60] Warburg O. The prime cause and prevention of cancer Part 1 with two prefaces on prevention. Revised lecture at the meeting of the Nobel-Laureates on June 30, 1966 at Lindau, Lake Constance, Germany. http://www.altered-states.net/barry/newsletter395/The_Prime_Cause_and_Prevention_of_Cancer.pdf.
[61] Weinhouse S. On respiratory impairment in cancer cells. Science 1956;124:267–9.
[62] Watson JD, Crick FHC. Molecular structure of nucleic acids: A structure for deoxyribose nucleic acid. Nature 1953;171:737–8.
[63] Williams HR. The Natural History of Cancer, with Special Reference to its Causation and Prevention. New York, NY: William Wood and Co.; 1908.
[64] Plimmer R, Plimmer V. Food and Health. London, UK: Longmans Green; 1925.
[65] Emerson H, Larimore LD. Diabetes mellitus. a contribution to its epidemiology based chiefly on mortality statistics. Arch Intern Med 1924;34:585–630.
[66] Cleave TL. The Saccharine Disease. Conditions Caused by the Taking of Refined Carbohydrates, such as Sugar and White Flour. Bristol, UK: John Wright and Sons Limited; 1974.
[67] Campbell GD. Diabetes in Indians and Africans in and around Durban. S Afr Med J 1963;37:1195–207.
[68] Cohen AM, Bavly S, Poznanski R. Change of diet of Yemenite Jews in relation to diabetes and ischemic heart-disease. Lancet 1961;2:1399–401.
[69] Cleave TL, Campbell GD, Painter NS. Diabetes, Coronary Thrombosis, and the Saccharine Disease. Second Edition Bristol, UK: John Wright and Sons Limited; 1969.
[70] Yudkin J. Pure, White and Deadly. London, UK: Penguin Books; 1972.
[71] Doll R, Armstrong B. Cancer. In: Trowell HC, Burkitt DP, editors. Western diseases. Their emergence and prevention. London, UK: Edward Arnold; 1981. p. 93–112.
[72] Armstrong B, Doll R. Environmental factors and cancer incidence and mortality in different countries, with special reference to dietary practices. Int J Cancer 1975;15:617–31.
[73] Cantley L. Seeking out the sweet spot in cancer therapeutics: an interview with Lewis Cantley. Dis Model Mech 2016;9:911–16.
[74] Vander Heiden MG, Cantley LC, Thompson CB. Understanding the Warburg Effect: The metabolic requirements of cell proliferation. Science 2009;324:1029–33.
[75] Giovannucci E, Harlan DM, Archer MA, et al. Diabetes and Cancer: A consensus report. CA Cancer J Clin 2010;60:207–21.
[76] Moore LL, Chadid S, Singer MR, et al. Metabolic health reduces risk of obesity-related cancer in Framingham study adults. Cancer Epidemiol Biomarkers Prev 2014;23:2057–65.
[77] Papa V, Pezzino V, Constantino A, et al. Elevated insulin receptor content in human breast cancer. J Clin Invest 1990;86:1503–10.
[78] Dankner R, Cohen C, Shanik MH, et al. Effect of elevated basal insulin on cancer incidence and mortality on cancer incident patients. The Israel GOH 29-year follow-up study. Diabetes Care 2012;35:1538–43.
[79] Gallagher EJ, LeRoith D. The proliferating role of insulin and insulin-like growth factors in cancer. Trends Endocrinol Metab 2010;21:610–18.
[80] Giovannucci E. Insulin and colon cancer. Cancer Cause Control 1995;6:164–79.
[81] Giovannuci E. Insulin, insulin-like growth factor and colon cancer: a review of the literature. J Nutr 2001;131(suppl):3109S–20S.
[82] Kaaks R, Lukanova A. Energy balance and cancer: The role of insulin and insulin-like growth factor 1. Proc Nutr Soc 2001;60:91–106.
[83] Kaaks R. Nutrition, hormones, and breast cancer risk: Is insulin the missing link? Cancer Cause Control 1996;7:605–25.
[84] LeRoith D, Roberts CT. The insulin-like growth factor system and cancer. Cancer Lett 2003;195:127–37.
[85] Pollak MN, Schernhammer ES, Hankinson SE. Insulin-like growth factors and neoplasia. Nat Rev Cancer 2004;4:505–18.

[86] Poloz Y, Stambolic V. Obesity and cancer: A case for insulin signalling. Cell Death Dis 2015;6:e2037.

[87] Rose DP, Vona-Davis L. The cellular and molecular mechanisms by which insulin influences breast cancer risk and progression. Endocrin Rel Cancer 2012;19:R225–41.

[88] Burroughs KD, Dunn SE, Barrett JC, et al. Insulin-like growth factor 1: a key regulator of human cancer risk? J Nat Cancer Inst 1999;91:579–81.

[89] Ter Braak B, Siezen CL, Lee JS, et al. Insulin-like growth factor 1 receptor activation promotes mammary gland tumor development by increasing glycolysis and promoting biomass production. Breast Canc Res 2017;19:14.

[90] Tsujimoto T, Kajio H, Sugiyama T. Association between hyperinsulinemia and increased risk of cancer death in nonobese and obese people: A population-based observational study. Int J Cancer 2017;141:102–11.

[91] Zhang AMY, Wellberg EA, Kopp JL, et al. Hyperinsulinemia in obesity, inflammation, and cancer. Diabet Metabl J 2021;45:285–311.

[92] Elstrom RL, Bauer DE, Buzzal M, et al. Akt stimulates aerobic glycolysis in cancer cells. Cancer Res 2004;64:3892–9.

[93] Ang B, Yu G. The role of fructose in type 2 diabetes and other metabolic diseases. Nutr & Food Sci 2017;8:1–4 May 2.

[94] DiStefano JK. Fructose-mediated effects on gene expression and epigenetic mechanisms associated with NAFLD pathogenesis. Cell Mol Life Sci 2020;77:2079–90.

[95] Jensen T, Abdelmalek MF, Sullivan S, et al. Fructose and sugar: A major mediator of nonalcoholic Fatty Liver Disease. J Hepatol 2018;68:1063–75.

[96] Godoy-Matos AF, Silva Junior WS, Valerio CM. NAFLD as a continuum: from obesity to metabolic syndrome and diabetes. Diabetol Metab Syndr 2020;12:60.

[97] Shim H, Dolde C, Lewis BC, et al. c-Myc transactivation of LDH-A: Implications for tumor metabolism and growth. Proc Nat Acad Sci 1997;94:6658–63.

[98] Garber K. Energy boost: the warburg effect returns in a new theory of cancer. J Nat Canc Instit 2004;96:1805–6.

[99] Hay WH. Cancer: A disease of either election or ignorance. Cancer. 1927;4:296–300.

[100] Fosslien E. Cancer morphogenesis: role of mitochondrial failure. Ann Clin Lab Sci 2008;38:307–29.

[101] Galluzzi L, Morselli E, Kepp O, Vitale I, Rigoni A, Vacchelli E, et al. Mitochondrial gateways to cancer. Mol Asp Med 2010;31:1–20.

[102] John AP. Dysfunctional mitochondria, not oxygen insufficiency, cause cancer cells to produce inordinate amounts of lactic acid: the impact of this on the treatment of cancer. Med Hypotheses 2001;57:429–31.

[103] Mayer N. Studies in Cancer X. Oxidative capacity of tumors. Can Res 1944;4:345–8.

[104] Pedersen PL. Tumor mitochondria and the bioenergetics of cancer cells. Prog Exp Tumor Res 1978;22:190–274.

[105] Roskelley RC, Mayer N, Horwitt BN, Salter WT. Studies in Cancer. Vii. Enzyme Deficiency in Human and Experimental Cancer. J Clin Invest 1943;22:743–51.

[106] Seyfried TN, Shelton LM. Cancer as a metabolic disease. Nutr Metab (Lond) 2010;7:7.

[107] Seyfried TN, Flores RE, Poff AM, D'Agostino DP. Cancer as a metabolic disease: implications for novel therapeutics. Carcinogenesis 2014;35:515–27.

[108] Warburg O. On the origin of cancer cells. Science 1956;123:309–14.

[109] Warburg O. The Metabolism of Tumours. New York: Richard R. Smith Inc.; 1931.

[110] Warburg O. On the respiratory impairment in cancer cells. Science 1956;124:269–70.

[111] Warburg O. Revised Lindau Lectures: The prime cause of cancer and prevention—Parts 1 & 2. In: Burk D, editor. Meeting of the Nobel-Laureates. Germany: K.Triltsch, Lindau, Lake Constance; 1969.

[112] Feichtinger RG, Weis S, Mayr JA, Zimmermann FA, Bogner B, Sperl W, et al. Alterations of oxidative phosphorylation in meningiomas and peripheral nerve sheath tumors. Neuro Oncol 2015.

[113] Feichtinger RG, Weis S, Mayr JA, Zimmermann F, Geilberger R, Sperl W, et al. Alterations of oxidative phosphorylation complexes in astrocytomas. Glia 2014;62:514–25.

[114] Formentini L, Martinez-Reyes I, Cuezva JM. The mitochondrial bioenergetic capacity of carcinomas. IUBMB life 2010;62:554–60.

[115] Hu Y, Lu W, Chen G, Wang P, Chen Z, Zhou Y, et al. K-ras(G12V) transformation leads to mitochondrial dysfunction and a metabolic switch from oxidative phosphorylation to glycolysis. Cell Res 2012;22:399–412.

[116] Isidoro A, Casado E, Redondo A, Acebo P, Espinosa E, Alonso AM, et al. Breast carcinomas fulfill the Warburg hypothesis and provide metabolic markers of cancer prognosis. Carcinogenesis 2005;26:2095–104.

[117] Kiebish MA, Han X, Cheng H, Chuang JH, Seyfried TN. Cardiolipin and electron transport chain abnormalities in mouse brain tumor mitochondria: lipidomic evidence supporting the Warburg theory of cancer. J lipid Res 2008;49:2545–56.

[118] Kim A. Mitochondria in cancer energy metabolism: culprits or bystanders? Toxicol Res 2015;31:323–30.

[119] Mazzocca A, Ferraro G, Misciagna G, Carr BI. A systemic evolutionary approach to cancer: Hepatocarcinogenesis as a paradigm. Med Hypotheses 2016;93:132–7.

[120] Pelicano H, Xu RH, Du M, Feng L, Sasaki R, Carew JS, et al. Mitochondrial respiration defects in cancer cells cause activation of Akt survival pathway through a redox-mediated mechanism. J Cell Biol 2006;175:913–23.

[121] Aisenberg AC. The Glycolysis and Respiration of Tumors. New York: Academic Press; 1961.

[122] Putignani L, Raffa S, Pescosolido R, Rizza T, Del Chierico F, Leone L, et al. Preliminary evidences on mitochondrial injury and impaired oxidative metabolism in breast cancer. Mitochondrion 2012;12:363–9.

[123] Ristow M. Oxidative metabolism in cancer growth. Curr Opin Clin Nutr Metab Care 2006;9:339–45.

[124] Warburg O, Wind F, Negelein E. The metabolism of tumors in the body. J Gen Physiol 1927;8:519–30.
[125] Capuano F, Guerrieri F, Papa S. Oxidative phosphorylation enzymes in normal and neoplastic cell growth. J Bioenerg Biomembr 1997;29:379–84.
[126] Cavalli LR, Liang BC. Mutagenesis, tumorigenicity, and apoptosis: are the mitochondria involved? Mutat Res 1998;398:19–26.
[127] Colowick SP. The status of Warburg's theory of glycolysis and respiration in tumors. Quart Rev Biol 1961.
[128] Cori CF, Cori GT. The carbohydrate metabolism of tumors. II. Changes in the sugar, lactic acid, and co-combining power of blood passing through a tumor. J Biol Chem 1925;65:397–405.
[129] Cuezva JM, Krajewska M, de Heredia ML, Krajewski S, Santamaria G, Kim H, et al. The bioenergetic signature of cancer: a marker of tumor progression. Cancer Res 2002;62:6674–81.
[130] Cuezva JM, Ortega AD, Willers I, Sanchez-Cenizo L, Aldea M, Sanchez-Arago M. The tumor suppressor function of mitochondria: Translation into the clinics. Biochimica et biophysica acta 2009;1792:1145–58.
[131] Chinopoulos C, Seyfried TN. Mitochondrial Substrate-Level Phosphorylation as Energy Source for Glioblastoma: Review and Hypothesis. ASN neuro 2018;10 1759091418818261.
[132] Burk D, Schade AL. On respiratory impairment in cancer cells. Science 1956;124:270–2.
[133] Burk D, Woods M, Hunter J. On the significance of glucolysis for cancer growth, with special reference to Morris rat hepatomas. J Natl Cancer Inst 1967;38:839–63.
[134] Racker E. Bioenergetics and the problem of tumor growth. Am scientist 1972;60:56–63.
[135] Racker E. History of the Pasteur effect and its pathobiology. Mol Cell Biochem 1974;5:17–23.
[136] Hanahan D, Weinberg RA. Hallmarks of cancer: the next generation. Cell 2011;144:646–74.
[137] Yu M, Chen S, Hong W, Gu Y, Huang B, Lin Y, et al. Prognostic role of glycolysis for cancer outcome: evidence from 86 studies. J Cancer Res Clin Oncol 2019;145:967–99.
[138] O'Connor RJ. The effect on cell division of inhibiting aerobic glycolysis. Br J Exp Pathol 1950;31:449–53.
[139] Weinhouse S. The Warburg hypothesis fifty years later. Z Krebsforsch Klin Onkol Cancer Res Clin Oncol 1976;87:115–26.
[140] Hackenbrock CR. Ultrastructural bases for metabolically linked mechanical activity in mitochondria. II. Electron transport-linked ultrastructural transformations in mitochondria. J Cell Biol 1968;37:345–69.
[141] Lehninger AL. The Mitochondrion: Molecular Basis of Structure and Function. New York: W.A. Benjamin, INC.; 1964.
[142] Stroud DA, Ryan MT. Mitochondria: organization of respiratory chain complexes becomes cristae-lized. Curr Biol: CB 2013;23: R969–71.
[143] Cogliati S, Enriquez JA, Scorrano L. Mitochondrial cristae: where beauty meets functionality. Trends Biochem Sci 2016;41:261–73.
[144] Sassano ML, van Vliet AR, Agostinis P. Mitochondria-associated membranes as networking platforms and regulators of cancer cell fate. Front Oncol 2017;7:174.
[145] Gilkerson RW, Selker JM, Capaldi RA. The cristal membrane of mitochondria is the principal site of oxidative phosphorylation. FEBS Lett 2003;546:355–8.
[146] Szewczyk A, Wojtczak L. Mitochondria as a pharmacological target. Pharmacol Rev 2002;54:101–27.
[147] Cogliati S, Frezza C, Soriano ME, Varanita T, Quintana-Cabrera R, Corrado M, et al. Mitochondrial cristae shape determines respiratory chain supercomplexes assembly and respiratory efficiency. Cell 2013;155:160–71.
[148] Arismendi-Morillo G. Electron microscopy morphology of the mitochondrial network in human cancer. Int J Biochem Cell Biol 2009;41:2062–8.
[149] Kiebish MA, Han X, Cheng H, Lunceford A, Clarke CF, Moon H, et al. Lipidomic analysis and electron transport chain activities in C57BL/6J mouse brain mitochondria. J neurochemistry 2008;106:299–312.
[150] Kuznetsov AV, Hermann M, Saks V, Hengster P, Margreiter R. The cell-type specificity of mitochondrial dynamics. Int J Biochem Cell Biol 2009;41:1928–39.
[151] Arismendi-Morillo G, Castellano-Ramirez A, Seyfried TN. Ultrastructural characterization of the Mitochondria-associated membranes abnormalities in human astrocytomas: Functional and therapeutics implications. Ultrastruct Pathol 2017;41:234–44.
[152] Giorgi C, Missiroli S, Patergnani S, Duszynski J, Wieckowski MR, Pinton P. Mitochondria-associated membranes: composition, molecular mechanisms, and physiopathological implications. Antioxid Redox Signal 2015;22:995–1019.
[153] Poston CN, Krishnan SC, Bazemore-Walker CR. In-depth proteomic analysis of mammalian mitochondria-associated membranes (MAM). J Proteom 2013;79:219–30.
[154] Theurey P, Rieusset J. Mitochondria-Associated Membranes Response to Nutrient Availability and Role in Metabolic Diseases. Trends Endocrinol Metab 2017;28:32–45.
[155] Theurey P, Tubbs E, Vial G, Jacquemetton J, Bendridi N, Chauvin MA, et al. Mitochondria-associated endoplasmic reticulum membranes allow adaptation of mitochondrial metabolism to glucose availability in the liver. J Mol Cell Biol 2016;8:129–43.
[156] Massari F, Ciccarese C, Santoni M, Iacovelli R, Mazzucchelli R, Piva F, et al. Metabolic phenotype of bladder cancer. Cancer Treat Rev 2016;45:46–57.
[157] Moriyama N, Yokoyama M, Niijima T. A morphometric study on the ultrastructure of well-differentiated tumours and inflammatory mucosa of the human urinary bladder. Virchows Arch A Pathol Anat Histopathol 1984;405:25–39.
[158] Papadimitriou JC, Drachenberg CB. Giant mitochondria with paracrystalline inclusions in paraganglioma of the urinary bladder: correlation with mitochondrial abnormalities in paragangliomas of other sites. Ultrastruct Pathol 1994;18:559–64.

[159] Elliott RL, Jiang XP, Head JF. Mitochondria organelle transplantation: introduction of normal epithelial mitochondria into human cancer cells inhibits proliferation and increases drug sensitivity. Breast cancer Res Treat 2012;136:347–54.

[160] Gadaleanu V, Craciun C. Malignant oncocytoma of the breast. Zentralbl Allg Pathol 1987;133:279–83.

[161] Guha M, Srinivasan S, Raman P, Jiang Y, Kaufman BA, Taylor D, et al. Aggressive triple negative breast cancers have unique molecular signature on the basis of mitochondrial genetic and functional defects. Biochim Biophys Acta Mol Basis Dis 2018;1864:1060–71.

[162] Jogalekar MP, Serrano EE. Morphometric analysis of a triple negative breast cancer cell line in hydrogel and monolayer culture environments. PeerJ 2018;6:e4340.

[163] Ma Y, Bai RK, Trieu R, Wong LJ. Mitochondrial dysfunction in human breast cancer cells and their transmitochondrial cybrids. Biochimica et biophysica acta 2010;1797:29–37.

[164] Morciano G, Marchi S, Morganti C, Sbano L, Bittremieux M, Kerkhofs M, et al. Role of mitochondria-associated ER membranes in calcium regulation in cancer-specific settings. Neoplasia 2018;20:510–23.

[165] Owens KM, Kulawiec M, Desouki MM, Vanniarajan A, Singh KK. Impaired OXPHOS complex III in breast cancer. PLoS One 2011;6: e23846.

[166] Pagano G, Talamanca AA, Castello G, Cordero MD, d'Ischia M, Gadaleta MN, et al. Oxidative stress and mitochondrial dysfunction across broad-ranging pathologies: toward mitochondria-targeted clinical strategies. Oxid Med Cell Longev 2014;2014:541230.

[167] Putignani L, Raffa S, Pescosolido R, Aimati L, Signore F, Torrisi MR, et al. Alteration of expression levels of the oxidative phosphorylation system (OXPHOS) in breast cancer cell mitochondria. Breast Cancer Res Treat 2008;110:439–52.

[168] Roddy HJ, Silverberg SG. Ultrastructural analysis of apocrine carcinoma of the human breast. Ultrastruct Pathol 1980;1:385–93.

[169] Rouiller C. Physiological and pathological changes in mitochondrial morphology. Int Rev Cytol 1960;9:227–92.

[170] Santidrian AF, Matsuno-Yagi A, Ritland M, Seo BB, LeBoeuf SE, Gay LJ, et al. Mitochondrial complex I activity and NAD + /NADH balance regulate breast cancer progression. J Clin Invest 2013;123:1068–81.

[171] Modica-Napolitano JS, Steele Jr. GD, Chen LB. Aberrant mitochondria in two human colon carcinoma cell lines. Cancer Res 1989;49:3369–73.

[172] Piscitelli D, Ingravallo G, Resta L, Fiore MG, Maiorano E. Oncocytic adenocarcinoma of the rectum with diffuse intra-luminal microcalcifications: the first reported case. Virchows Arch 2003;443:579–82.

[173] Sun AS, Sepkowitz K, Geller SA. A study of some mitochondrial and peroxisomal enzymes in human colonic adenocarcinoma. Lab Invest 1981;44:13–17.

[174] Deighton RF, Le Bihan T, Martin SF, Barrios-Llerena ME, Gerth AM, Kerr LE, et al. The proteomic response in glioblastoma in young patients. J neuro-oncology 2014;.

[175] Deighton RF, Le Bihan T, Martin SF, Gerth AM, McCulloch M, Edgar JM, et al. Interactions among mitochondrial proteins altered in glioblastoma. J neuro-oncology 2014;118:247–56.

[176] Arismendi-Morillo GJ, Castellano-Ramirez AV. Ultrastructural mitochondrial pathology in human astrocytic tumors: potentials implications pro-therapeutics strategies. J Electron Microsc (Tokyo) 2008;57:33–9.

[177] Katsetos CD, Anni H, Draber P. Mitochondrial dysfunction in gliomas. Sempediatric Neurol 2013;20:216–27.

[178] Oudard S, Boitier E, Miccoli L, Rousset S, Dutrillaux B, Poupon MF. Gliomas are driven by glycolysis: putative roles of hexokinase, oxidative phosphorylation and mitochondrial ultrastructure. Anticancer Res 1997;17:1903–11.

[179] Scheithauer BW, Bruner JM. Central nervous system tumors. Cllaboratory Med 1987;7:157–79.

[180] Seyfried TN, Shelton L, Arismendi-Morillo G, Kalamian M, Elsakka A, Maroon J, et al. Provocative Question: Should Ketogenic Metabolic Therapy Become the Standard of Care for Glioblastoma? Neurochem Res 2019.

[181] Sipe JC, Herman MM, Rubinstein LJ. Electron microscopic observations on human glioblastomas and astrocytomas maintained in organ culture systems. Am J Pathol 1973;73:589–606.

[182] Moreno SM, Benitez IA, Martinez Gonzalez MA. Ultrastructural studies in a series of 18 cases of chromophobe renal cell carcinoma. Ultrastruct Pathol 2005;29:377–87.

[183] Sarto C, Marocchi A, Sanchez JC, Giannone D, Frutiger S, Golaz O, et al. Renal cell carcinoma and normal kidney protein expression. Electrophoresis 1997;18:599–604.

[184] Simonnet H, Demont J, Pfeiffer K, Guenaneche L, Bouvier R, Brandt U, et al. Mitochondrial complex I is deficient in renal oncocytomas. Carcinogenesis 2003;24:1461–6.

[185] Yusenko MV, Ruppert T, Kovacs G. Analysis of differentially expressed mitochondrial proteins in chromophobe renal cell carcinomas and renal oncocytomas by 2-D gel electrophoresis. Int J Biol Sci 2010;6:213–24.

[186] Huhn D. Morphology, cytochemistry, and ultrastructure of leukemic cells with regard to the classification of leukemias. Recent Results Cancer Res 1984;93:51–68.

[187] Huhn D, Wochinger G, Darsow M. Mitochondrial changes in malignant lymphoma cells. Acta Haematol 1984;72:368–71.

[188] Kluza J, Jendoubi M, Ballot C, Dammak A, Jonneaux A, Idziorek T, et al. Exploiting mitochondrial dysfunction for effective elimination of imatinib-resistant leukemic cells. PLoS one 2011;6:e21924.

[189] Schumacher HR, Szekely IE, Fisher DR. Leukemic mitochondria. III. Acute lymphoblastic leukemia. Am J Pathol 1975;78:49–58.

[190] Schumacher HR, Szekely IE, Patel SB, Fisher DR. Leukemic mitochondria. I. Acute myeloblastic leukemia. Am J Pathol 1974;74:71–82.

[191] Lo C, Cristofalo VJ, Morris HP, Weinhouse S. Studies on respiration and glycolysis in transplanted hepatic tumors of the rat. Cancer Res 1968;28:1–10.

[192] Volman H. A morphologic and morphometric study of the mitochondria in several hepatoma cell lines and in isolated hepatocytes. Virchows Arch B Cell Pathol 1978;26:249–59.

[193] White MT, Arya DV, Tewari KK. Biochemical properties of neoplastic cell mitochondria. J Natl Cancer Inst 1974;53:553–9.

[194] Cheuk W, Chan JK. Clear cell variant of fibrolamellar carcinoma of the liver. Arch Pathol Lab Med 2001;125:1235–8.

[195] Fernandez BB, Hernanzez FJ, Spindler W. Metastatic cystosarcoma phyllodes: a light and electron microscopic study. Cancer 1976;37:1737–46.

[196] Momcilovic M, Jones A, Bailey ST, Waldmann CM, Li R, Lee JT, et al. In vivo imaging of mitochondrial membrane potential in non-small-cell lung cancer. Nature 2019;575:380–4.

[197] Nicolescu PG, Eskenasy A. Ultrastructure of macrocellular (large cell) carcinomas of the lung. Morphol Embryol (Bucur) 1984;30:211–16.

[198] Nicolescu PG, Eskenasy A. Electronmicroscopic observations on epidermoid (squamous cell) carcinomas of the lung. Morphol Embryol (Bucur) 1984;30:131–5.

[199] Hall A, Meyle KD, Lange MK, Klima M, Sanderhoff M, Dahl C, et al. Dysfunctional oxidative phosphorylation makes malignant melanoma cells addicted to glycolysis driven by the V600EBRAF oncogene. Oncotarget 2013;4:584–99.

[200] Taddei ML, Giannoni E, Raugei G, Scacco S, Sardanelli AM, Papa S, et al. Mitochondrial Oxidative Stress due to Complex I Dysfunction Promotes Fibroblast Activation and Melanoma Cell Invasiveness. J Signal Transduct 2012;2012:684592.

[201] Feichtinger RG, Zimmermann F, Mayr JA, Neureiter D, Hauser-Kronberger C, Schilling FH, et al. Low aerobic mitochondrial energy metabolism in poorly- or undifferentiated neuroblastoma. BMC Cancer 2010;10:149.

[202] Morscher RJ, Aminzadeh-Gohari S, Feichtinger RG, Mayr JA, Lang R, Neureiter D, et al. Inhibition of Neuroblastoma Tumor Growth by Ketogenic Diet and/or Calorie Restriction in a CD1-Nu Mouse Model. PLoS one 2015;10:e0129802.

[203] Brawn PN, Mackay B. Intracristal crystalline inclusions in mitochondria of a neuroblastoma. Ultrastruct Pathol 1980;1:495–7.

[204] Friedman B, Gold H. Ultrastructure of Ewing's sarcoma of bone. Cancer 1968;22:307–22.

[205] Ghadially FN, Mehta PN. Ultrastructure of osteogenic sarcoma. Cancer 1970;25:1457–67.

[206] Hou-Jensen K, Priori E, Dmochowski L. Studies on ultrastructure of Ewing's sarcoma of bone. Cancer 1972;29:280–6.

[207] van Waveren C, Sun Y, Cheung HS, Moraes CT. Oxidative phosphorylation dysfunction modulates expression of extracellular matrix–remodeling genes and invasion. Carcinogenesis 2006;27:409–18.

[208] Ishioka S, Sagae S, Ito E, Kudo R. Ultrastructural study of benign, low-malignant potential (LMP), and malignant ovarian tumors. Med Electron Microsc 2004;37:37–44.

[209] Andrews PA, Albright KD. Mitochondrial defects in cis-diamminedichloroplatinum(II)-resistant human ovarian carcinoma cells. Cancer Res 1992;52:1895–901.

[210] Dai Z, Yin J, He H, Li W, Hou C, Qian X, et al. Mitochondrial comparative proteomics of human ovarian cancer cells and their platinum-resistant sublines. Proteomics 2010;10:3789–99.

[211] Huntrakoon M. Oncocytic carcinoma of the pancreas. Cancer 1983;51:332–6.

[212] Legrand M, Pariente R. Electron microscopy in the cytological examination of metastatic pleural effusions. Thorax 1976;31:443–9.

[213] Novotny R, Ehrmann J, Tozzi di Angelo I, Prochazka V, Klos D, Lovecek M, et al. Mitochondrial changes in adenocarcinoma of the pancreas. Ultrastruct Pathol 2013;37:227–31.

[214] Mao P, Nakao K, Angrist A. Human prostatic carcinoma: an electron microscope study. Cancer Res 1966;26:955–73.

[215] Vayalil PK, Landar A. Mitochondrial oncobioenergetic index: A potential biomarker to predict progression from indolent to aggressive prostate cancer. Oncotarget 2015;6:43065–80.

[216] Li A, Blandford A, Chundury RV, Traboulsi EI, Anderson P, Murphy E, et al. Orbital rhabdomyosarcoma in a child with Leigh syndrome. J AAPOS 2018;22:150–2 e151.

[217] Bundtzen JL, Norback DH. The ultrastructure of poorly differentiated rhabdomyosarcomas: a case report and literature review. Hum Pathol 1982;13:301–13.

[218] Singh L, Nag TC, Kashyap S. Ultrastructural changes of mitochondria in human retinoblastoma: correlation with tumor differentiation and invasiveness. Tumour Biol 2015.

[219] Sun CN. Abnormal mitochondria in retinoblastoma. Experientia 1976;32:630–2.

[220] Kataoka R, Hyo Y, Hoshiya T, Miyahara H, Matsunaga T. Ultrastructural study of mitochondria in oncocytes. Ultrastruct Pathol 1991;15:231–9.

[221] Kummoona R, Jabbar A, Kareem Al-Rahal D. Proliferative activity in oral carcinomas studied with Ag-NOR and electron microscopy. Ultrastruct Pathol 2008;32:139–46.

[222] Quintana-Cabrera R, Mehrotra A, Rigoni G, Soriano ME. Who and how in the regulation of mitochondrial cristae shape and function. Biochem Biophys Res Commun 2018;500:94–101.

[223] Diatlovitskaia EV, Ianchevskaia GV, Bergel'son LD. [Tumor lipids. A comparative study of the phospholipids of the rat kidneys and nephroma RA]. Biokhimiia 1973;38:1186–91.

[224] Diatlovitskaia EV, Ianchevskaia GV, Kolesova NP, Bergel'son LD. [Tumor lipids. The positional distribution of fatty acids in rat liver glycerophospholipids and in hepatoma-27]. Biokhimiia 1973;38:749–55.

[225] Fry M, Green DE. Cardiolipin requirement for electron transfer in complex I and III of the mitochondrial respiratory chain. J Biol Chem 1981;256:1874–80.

[226] Garcea R, Canuto RA, Gautero B, Biocca M, Feo F. Phospholipid composition of inner and outer mitochondrial membranes isolated from Yoshida hepatoma AH-130. Cancer Lett 1980;11:133–9.

[227] Gohil VM, Hayes P, Matsuyama S, Schagger H, Schlame M, Greenberg ML. Cardiolipin biosynthesis and mitochondrial respiratory chain function are interdependent. J Biol Chem 2004;279:42612–18.

[228] Hostetler KY, Zenner BD, Morris HP. Phospholipid content of mitochondrial and microsomal membranes from Morris hepatomas of varying growth rates. Cancer Res 1979;39:2978–83.

[229] Houtkooper RH, Vaz FM. Cardiolipin, the heart of mitochondrial metabolism. Cell Mol Life Sci 2008;65:2493–506.

[230] Acehan D, Malhotra A, Xu Y, Ren M, Stokes DL, Schlame M. Cardiolipin affects the supramolecular organization of ATP synthase in mitochondria. Biophysical J 2011;100:2184–92.

[231] Randall EC, Zadra G, Chetta P, Lopez BGC, Syamala S, Basu SS, et al. Molecular Characterization of Prostate Cancer with Associated Gleason Score Using Mass Spectrometry Imaging. Mol Cancer Res 2019;17:1155–65.

[232] Sapandowski A, Stope M, Evert K, Evert M, Zimmermann U, Peter D, et al. Cardiolipin composition correlates with prostate cancer cell proliferation. Mol Cell Biochem 2015;410:175–85.

[233] Chicco AJ, Sparagna GC. Role of cardiolipin alterations in mitochondrial dysfunction and disease. Am J Physiol Cell Physiol 2007;292: C33–44.

[234] Claypool SM, Oktay Y, Boontheung P, Loo JA, Koehler CM. Cardiolipin defines the interactome of the major ADP/ATP carrier protein of the mitochondrial inner membrane. J Cell Biol 2008;182:937–50.

[235] Brand MD, Nicholls DG. Assessing mitochondrial dysfunction in cells. Biochem J 2011;435:297–312.

[236] Lemarie A, Grimm S. Mitochondrial respiratory chain complexes: apoptosis sensors mutated in cancer? Oncogene 2011;30:3985–4003.

[237] Seyfried TN. Respiratory dysfunction in cancer cells. Cancer as a Metabolic Disease: On the Origin, *Management, and Prevention of Cancer*. Hoboken, NJ: John Wiley & Sons; 2012. p. 73–105.

[238] Villalobo A, Lehninger AL. The proton stoichiometry of electron transport in Ehrlich ascites tumor mitochondria. J Biol Chem 1979;254:4352–8.

[239] Mayer E. The Growth of Biological Thought; Diversity, Evolution, and Inheritance. Harvard, Cambridge, MA: Belknap; 1982.

[240] Arcos JC, Tison MJ, Gosch HH, Fabian JA. Sequential alterations in mitochondrial inner and outer membrane electron transport and in respiratory control during feeding of amino azo dyes; stability of phosphorylation. Correlation with swelling-contraction changes and tumorigenesis threshold. Cancer Res 1969;29:1298–305.

[241] Leznev EI, Popova II, Lavrovskaja VP, Evtodienko YV. Comparison of oxygen consumption rates in minimally transformed BALB/3T3 and virus-transformed 3T3B-SV40 cells. Biochem (Mosc) 2013;78:904–8.

[242] Pacini N, Borziani F. Oncostatic-cytoprotective effect of melatonin and other bioactive molecules: a common target in mitochondrial respiration. Int J Mol Sci 2016;17.

[243] Ramanathan A, Wang C, Schreiber SL. Perturbational profiling of a cell-line model of tumorigenesis by using metabolic measurements. Proc Natl Acad Sci U S Am 2005;102:5992–7.

[244] Velez J, Hail Jr. N, Konopleva M, Zeng Z, Kojima K, Samudio I, et al. Mitochondrial uncoupling and the reprograming of intermediary metabolism in leukemia cells. Front Oncol 2013;3:67.

[245] Bartesaghi S, Graziano V, Galavotti S, Henriquez NV, Betts J, Saxena J, et al. Inhibition of oxidative metabolism leads to p53 genetic inactivation and transformation in neural stem cells. Proc Natl Acad Sci U S A 2015;112:1059–64.

[246] Matoba S, Kang JG, Patino WD, Wragg A, Boehm M, Gavrilova O, et al. p53 regulates mitochondrial respiration. Science 2006;312:1650–3.

[247] Zhou S, Kachhap S, Singh KK. Mitochondrial impairment in p53-deficient human cancer cells. Mutagenesis 2003;18:287–92.

[248] Nicolay BN, Danielian PS, Kottakis F, Lapek Jr. JD, Sanidas I, Miles WO, et al. Proteomic analysis of pRb loss highlights a signature of decreased mitochondrial oxidative phosphorylation. Genes Dev 2015;29:1875–89.

[249] Capala ME, Pruis M, Vellenga E, Schuringa JJ. Depletion of SAM50 Specifically Targets BCR-ABL-Expressing Leukemic Stem and Progenitor Cells by Interfering with Mitochondrial Functions. Stem Cell Dev 2016;25:427–37.

[250] Henderson BR. The BRCA1 Breast Cancer Suppressor: Regulation of Transport, Dynamics, and Function at Multiple Subcellular Locations. Scientifica (Cairo) 2012;2012:796808.

[251] Maniccia AW, Lewis C, Begum N, Xu J, Cui J, Chipitsyna G, et al. Mitochondrial localization, ELK-1 transcriptional regulation and growth inhibitory functions of BRCA1, BRCA1a, and BRCA1b proteins. J Cell Physiol 2009;219:634–41.

[252] Privat M, Radosevic-Robin N, Aubel C, Cayre A, Penault-Llorca F, Marceau G, et al. BRCA1 induces major energetic metabolism reprogramming in breast cancer cells. PLoS one 2014;9:e102438.

[253] Chung HJ, Korm S, Lee SI, Phorl S, Noh S, Han M, et al. RAP80 binds p32 to preserve the functional integrity of mitochondria. Biochem Biophys Res Commun 2017;492:441–6.

[254] Desler C, Lykke A, Rasmussen LJ. The effect of mitochondrial dysfunction on cytosolic nucleotide metabolism. J Nucleic Acids 2010;2010.

[255] Seyfried TN, Yu G, Maroon JC, D'Agostino DP. Press-pulse: a novel therapeutic strategy for the metabolic management of cancer. Nutr Metab (Lond) 2017;14:19.

[256] Johnson JD, Mehus JG, Tews K, Milavetz BI, Lambeth DO. Genetic evidence for the expression of ATP- and GTP-specific succinyl-CoA synthetases in multicellular eucaryotes. J Biol Chem 1998;273:27580–6.

[257] Hunter Jr. FE, Hixon WS. Phosphorylation coupled with the oxidation of alpha-ketoglutaric acid. J Biol Chem 1949;181:73–9.

[258] Kaufman S, Gilvarg C, Cori O, Ochoa S. Enzymatic oxidation of alpha-ketoglutarate and coupled phosphorylation. J Biol Chem 1953;203:869–88.
[259] Li X, Wu F, Beard DA. Identification of the kinetic mechanism of succinyl-CoA synthetase. Biosci Rep 2013;33:145–63.
[260] Chen Q, Kirk K, Shurubor YI, Zhao D, Arreguin AJ, Shahi I, et al. Rewiring of glutamine metabolism is a bioenergetic adaptation of human cells with mitochondrial DNA mutations. Cell Metab 2018;27:1007–25. e1005.
[261] Flores RE, Brown AK, Taus L, Khoury J, Glover F, Kami K, et al. Mycoplasma infection and hypoxia initiate succinate accumulation and release in the VM-M3 cancer cells. Biochimica et biophysica acta 2018.
[262] Tretter L, Patocs A, Chinopoulos C. Succinate, an intermediate in metabolism, signal transduction, ROS, hypoxia, and tumorigenesis. Biochimica et biophysica acta 2016;1857:1086–101.
[263] Chinopoulos C, Batzios S, van den Heuvel LP, Rodenburg R, Smeets R, Waterham HR, et al. Mutated SUCLG1 causes mislocalization of SUCLG2 protein, morphological alterations of mitochondria and an early-onset severe neurometabolic disorder. Mol Genet Metab 2019;126:43–52.
[264] Dang CV. Glutaminolysis: supplying carbon or nitrogen or both for cancer cells? Cell Cycle 2010;9:3884–6.
[265] DeBerardinis RJ, Cheng T. Q's next: the diverse functions of glutamine in metabolism, cell biology and cancer. Oncogene 2010;29:313–24.
[266] McKeehan WL. Glycolysis, glutaminolysis and cell proliferation. Cell Biol Int Rep 1982;6:635–50.
[267] Still ER, Yuneva MO. Hopefully devoted to Q: targeting glutamine addiction in cancer. Br J Cancer 2017;116:1375–81.
[268] Gronow GH, Cohen JJ. Substrate support for renal functions during hypoxia in the perfused rat kidney. Am J Physiol 1984;247:F618–31.
[269] Pisarenko OI, Solomatina ES, Ivanov VE, Studneva IM, Kapelko VI, Smirnov VN. On the mechanism of enhanced ATP formation in hypoxic myocardium caused by glutamic acid. Basic Res Cardiol 1985;80:126–34.
[270] Weinberg JM, Venkatachalam MA, Roeser NF, Nissim I. Mitochondrial dysfunction during hypoxia/reoxygenation and its correction by anaerobic metabolism of citric acid cycle intermediates. Proc Natl Acad Sci U S A 2000;97:2826–31.
[271] Yuan Y, Ju YS, Kim Y, Li J, Wang Y, Yoon CJ, et al. Comprehensive molecular characterization of mitochondrial genomes in human cancers. Nat Genet 2020;.
[272] Namba T, Doczi J, Pinson A, Xing L, Kalebic N, Wilsch-Brauninger M, et al. Human-Specific ARHGAP11B Acts in Mitochondria to Expand Neocortical Progenitors by Glutaminolysis. Neuron 2019.
[273] Gao C, Shen Y, Jin F, Miao Y, Qiu X. Cancer Stem cells in small cell lung cancer cell line H446: higher dependency on oxidative phosphorylation and mitochondrial substrate-level phosphorylation than non-stem cancer cells. PLoS One 2016;11:e0154576.
[274] Hurtaud C, Gelly C, Chen Z, Levi-Meyrueis C, Bouillaud F. Glutamine stimulates translation of uncoupling protein 2mRNA. Cell Mol Life Sci 2007;64:1853–60.
[275] Moreadith RW, Lehninger AL. The pathways of glutamate and glutamine oxidation by tumor cell mitochondria. Role of mitochondrial NAD (P) + -dependent malic enzyme. J Biol Chem 1984;259:6215–21.
[276] Chinopoulos C. Succinate in ischemia: Where does it come from? Int J Biochem Cell Biol 2019;115:105580.
[277] Dang CV. Therapeutic targeting of Myc-reprogrammed cancer cell metabolism. Cold Spring Harb symposia Quant Biol 2011;76:369–74.
[278] Semenza GL. HIF-1: upstream and downstream of cancer metabolism. Curr Opin Genet Dev 2010;20:51–6.
[279] Semenza GL. Hypoxia-inducible factors: coupling glucose metabolism and redox regulation with induction of the breast cancer stem cell phenotype. EMBO J 2017;36:252–9.
[280] Tannahill GM, Curtis AM, Adamik J, Palsson-McDermott EM, McGettrick AF, Goel G, et al. Succinate is an inflammatory signal that induces IL-1beta through HIF-1alpha. Nature 2013;496:238–42.
[281] Tardito S, Oudin A, Ahmed SU, Fack F, Keunen O, Zheng L, et al. Glutamine synthetase activity fuels nucleotide biosynthesis and supports growth of glutamine-restricted glioblastoma. Nat Cell Biol 2015;17:1556–68.
[282] Tennant DA, Duran RV, Boulahbel H, Gottlieb E. Metabolic transformation in cancer. Carcinogenesis 2009;30:1269–80.
[283] David CJ, Chen M, Assanah M, Canoll P, Manley JL. HnRNP proteins controlled by c-Myc deregulate pyruvate kinase mRNA splicing in cancer. Nature 2010;463:364–8.
[284] Dong G, Mao Q, Xia W, Xu Y, Wang J, Xu L, et al. PKM2 and cancer: The function of PKM2 beyond glycolysis. Oncol Lett 2016;11:1980–6.
[285] Ottaway JH, McClellan JA, Saunderson CL. Succinic thiokinase and metabolic control. Int J Biochem 1981;13:401–10.
[286] Sanadi DR, Gibson DM, Ayengar P, Jacob M. Alpha-ketoglutaric dehydrogenase. V. Guanosine diphosphate in coupled phosphorylation. J Biol Chem 1956;218:505–20.
[287] Seyfried TN. Is mitochondrial glutamine fermentation a missing link in the metabolic theory of cancer? in. Cancer as a Metabolic Disease: On the Origin, Management, and Prevention of Cancer. Hoboken, NJ: John Wiley & Sons; 2012, p. 133–44.
[288] Israelsen WJ, Dayton TL, Davidson SM, Fiske BP, Hosios AM, Bellinger G, et al. PKM2 isoform-specific deletion reveals a differential requirement for pyruvate kinase in tumor cells. Cell 2013;155:397–409.
[289] Mazurek S, Boschek CB, Hugo F, Eigenbrodt E. Pyruvate kinase type M2 and its role in tumor growth and spreading. Semcancer Biol 2005;15:300–8.
[290] Vander Heiden MG. Targeting cell metabolism in cancer patients. Sci Transl Med 2010;2: 31ed31.
[291] Hague A, Singh B, Paraskeva C. Butyrate acts as a survival factor for colonic epithelial cells: further fuel for the in vivo versus in vitro debate. Gastroenterology 1997;112:1036–40.

[292] Simek J, Sedlacek J. Effect of glucose administered in vivo or in vitro on the respiratory quotient of rat liver tissue after partial hepatectomy. Nature 1965;207:761–2.

[293] Thevananther S. Adipose to the rescue: peripheral fat fuels liver regeneration. Hepatology 2010;52:1875–6.

[294] Greenman C, Stephens P, Smith R, Dalgliesh GL, Hunter C, Bignell G, et al. Patterns of somatic mutation in human cancer genomes. Nature 2007;446:153–8.

[295] Vogelstein B, Papadopoulos N, Velculescu VE, Zhou S, Diaz Jr. LA, Kinzler KW. Cancer genome landscapes. Science 2013;339:1546–58.

[296] Baker SG. A cancer theory kerfuffle can lead to new lines of research. J Natl Cancer Inst 2015;107.

[297] Bayreuther K. Chromosomes in primary neoplastic growth. Nature 1960;186:6–9.

[298] Braun AC. On the origin of the cancer cells. Am Sci 1970;58:307–20.

[299] Pitot HC. Some biochemical aspects of malignancy. Ann Rev Biochem 1966;35:335–68.

[300] Soto AM, Sonnenschein C. The somatic mutation theory of cancer: growing problems with the paradigm? Bioessays 2004;26:1097–107.

[301] Parsons DW, Jones S, Zhang X, Lin JC, Leary RJ, Angenendt P, et al. An integrated genomic analysis of human glioblastoma multiforme. Science 2008;321:1807–12.

[302] Martincorena I, Campbell PJ. Somatic mutation in cancer and normal cells. Science 2015;349:1483–9.

[303] Martincorena I, Fowler JC, Wabik A, Lawson ARJ, Abascal F, Hall MWJ, et al. Somatic mutant clones colonize the human esophagus with age. Science 2018;362:911–17.

[304] Yizhak K, Aguet F, Kim J, Hess JM, Kubler K, Grimsby J, et al. RNA sequence analysis reveals macroscopic somatic clonal expansion across normal tissues. Science 2019;364.

[305] Yokoyama A, Kakiuchi N, Yoshizato T, Nannya Y, Suzuki H, Takeuchi Y, et al. Age-related remodelling of oesophageal epithelia by mutated cancer drivers. Nature 2019;565:312–17.

[306] Chanock SJ. The paradox of mutations and cancer. Science 2018;362:893–4.

[307] Huttley GA, Easteal S, Southey MC, Tesoriero A, Giles GG, McCredie MR, et al. Adaptive evolution of the tumour suppressor BRCA1 in humans and chimpanzees. Australian Breast Cancer Family Study. Nat Genet 2000;25:410–13.

[308] Lowenstine LJ, McManamon R, Terio KA. Comparative pathology of aging great apes: bonobos, chimpanzees, gorillas, and orangutans. Vet Pathol 2016;53:250–76.

[309] Puente XS, Velasco G, Gutierrez-Fernandez A, Bertranpetit J, King MC, Lopez-Otin C. Comparative analysis of cancer genes in the human and chimpanzee genomes. BMC Genomics 2006;7:15.

[310] Varki NM, Varki A. On the apparent rarity of epithelial cancers in captive chimpanzees. Philos Trans R Soc Lond B Biol Sci 2015;370.

[311] Kopp W. How western diet and lifestyle drive the pandemic of obesity and civilization diseases. Diabetes Metab Syndr Obes 2019;12:2221–36.

[312] Tomasetti C, Vogelstein B. Cancer etiology. Variation in cancer risk among tissues can be explained by the number of stem cell divisions. Science 2015;347:78–81.

[313] Barrett JC. Mechanisms of multistep carcinogenesis and carcinogen risk assessment. Env Health Perspect 1993;100:9–20.

[314] Knudson AG. Cancer genetics. Am J Med Genet 2002;111:96–102.

[315] Boveri T. Concerning the origin of malignant tumours by Theodor Boveri. Translated and annotated by Henry Harris. J Cell Sci 2008;121 (Suppl 1):1–84.

[316] National Cancer Institute.What Is Cancer?May 5, 2021; https://www.cancer.gov/about-cancer/understanding/what-is-cancer.

[317] Seyfried TN. Cancer as a mitochondrial metabolic disease. Front Cell developmental Biol 2015;3:43.

[318] Seyfried TN. Mitochondria: The ultimate tumor suppressor. in. Cancer as a Metabolic Disease: On the Origin, Management, and Prevention of Cancer. Hoboken, NJ: John Wiley & Sons; 2012. p. 195–205.

[319] Fu A, Hou Y, Yu Z, Zhao Z, Liu Z. Healthy mitochondria inhibit the metastatic melanoma in lungs. Int J Biol Sci 2019;15:2707–18.

[320] Kaipparettu BA, Ma Y, Park JH, Lee TL, Zhang Y, Yotnda P, et al. Crosstalk from non-cancerous mitochondria can inhibit tumor properties of metastatic cells by suppressing oncogenic pathways. PLoS one 2013;8:e61747.

[321] Sun C, Liu X, Wang B, Wang Z, Liu Y, Di C, et al. Endocytosis-mediated mitochondrial transplantation: Transferring normal human astrocytic mitochondria into glioma cells rescues aerobic respiration and enhances radiosensitivity. Theranostics 2019;9:3595–607.

[322] Chang JC, Chang HS, Wu YC, Cheng WL, Lin TT, Chang HJ, et al. Mitochondrial transplantation regulates antitumour activity, chemoresistance and mitochondrial dynamics in breast cancer. J Exp Clin Cancer Res 2019;38:30.

[323] Mukherjee S. The Emperor of All Maladies: A Biography of Cancer (pages 285, 303, 333, 342). New York: Scribner; 2010.

[324] Szent-Gyorgyi A. The living state and cancer. Proc Natl Acad Sci U S Am 1977;74:2844–7.

[325] Cairns J. The origin of human cancers. Nature 1981;289:353–7.

[326] Seyfried TN. Genes, respiration, viruses, and cancer. Cancer as a Metabolic Disease: On the Origin, Management, and Prevention of Cancer. Hoboken, NJ: John Wiley & Sons; 2012, p. 145–76.

[327] Zhu Y, Dean AE, Horikoshi N, Heer C, Spitz DR, Gius D. Emerging evidence for targeting mitochondrial metabolic dysfunction in cancer therapy. J Clin Invest 2018;128:3682–91.

[328] Seoane M, Mosquera-Miguel A, Gonzalez T, Fraga M, Salas A, Costoya JA. The Mitochondrial Genome Is a "Genetic Sanctuary" during the Oncogenic Process. PLoS one 2011;6:e23327.

[329] Biswas G, Srinivasan S, Anandatheerthavarada HK, Avadhani NG. Dioxin-mediated tumor progression through activation of mitochondria-to-nucleus stress signaling. Proc Natl Acad Sci U S Am 2008;105:186–91.

[330] Ryan MT, Hoogenraad NJ. Mitochondrial-nuclear communications. Annu Rev Biochem 2007;76:701–22.
[331] Srinivasan S, Guha M, Dong DW, Whelan KA, Ruthel G, Uchikado Y, et al. Disruption of cytochrome c oxidase function induces the Warburg effect and metabolic reprogramming. Oncogene 2016;35:1585–95.
[332] Dang CV, Semenza GL. Oncogenic alterations of metabolism. Trends Biochem Sci 1999;24:68–72.
[333] Yang D, Kim J. Mitochondrial retrograde signalling and metabolic alterations in the tumour microenvironment. Cells 2019;8.
[334] Seyfried TN, Huysentruyt LC. On the origin of cancer metastasis. Crit Rev oncogenesis 2013;18:43–73.
[335] Seyfried TN. Mitochondrial respiratory dysfunction and the extrachromosomal origin of cancer. Cancer as a Metabolic Disease: On the Origin, Management, and Prevention of Cancer. Hoboken, NJ: John Wiley & Sons; 2012, p. 253–9.
[336] Marsh J, Mukherjee P, Seyfried TN. Akt-dependent proapoptotic effects of dietary restriction on late-stage management of a phosphatase and tensin homologue/tuberous sclerosis complex 2-deficient mouse astrocytoma. Clin Cancer Res 2008;14:7751–62.
[337] Kwong JQ, Henning MS, Starkov AA, Manfredi G. The mitochondrial respiratory chain is a modulator of apoptosis. J Cell Biol 2007;179:1163–77.
[338] Garvin S, Vikhe Patil E, Arnesson LG, Oda H, Hedayati E, Lindstrom A, et al. Differences in intra-tumoral macrophage infiltration and radiotherapy response among intrinsic subtypes in pT1-T2 breast cancers treated with breast-conserving surgery. Virchows Arch 2019;475:151–62.
[339] Huysentruyt LC, Akgoc Z, Seyfried TN. Hypothesis: are neoplastic macrophages/microglia present in glioblastoma multiforme? ASN neuro 2011;3.
[340] Pawelek JM, Chakraborty AK. Fusion of tumour cells with bone marrow-derived cells: a unifying explanation for metastasis. Nat Rev Cancer 2008;8:377–86.
[341] Powell AE, Anderson EC, Davies PS, Silk AD, Pelz C, Impey S, et al. Fusion between Intestinal epithelial cells and macrophages in a cancer context results in nuclear reprogramming. Cancer Res 2011;71:1497–505.
[342] Ruff MR, Pert CB. Origin of human small cell lung cancer. Science 1985;229:680.
[343] Shabo I, Midtbo K, Andersson H, Akerlund E, Olsson H, Wegman P, et al. Macrophage traits in cancer cells are induced by macrophage-cancer cell fusion and cannot be explained by cellular interaction. BMC Cancer 2015;15:922.
[344] Tarin D. Cell and tissue interactions in carcinogenesis and metastasis and their clinical significance. Semin Cancer Biol 2011;21:72–82.
[345] Duelli D, Lazebnik Y. Cell fusion: a hidden enemy? Cancer Cell 2003;3:445–8.
[346] Davies PS, Powell AE, Swain JR, Wong MH. Inflammation and proliferation act together to mediate intestinal cell fusion. PLoS one 2009;4:e6530.
[347] Newsholme P. Why is L-glutamine metabolism important to cells of the immune system in health, postinjury, surgery or infection? J Nutr 2001;131:2515S–22S discussion 2523S-2514S.
[348] Newsholme P, Curi R, Gordon S, Newsholme EA. Metabolism of glucose, glutamine, long-chain fatty acids and ketone bodies by murine macrophages. Biochem J 1986;239:121–5.
[349] Fidler IJ. The pathogenesis of cancer metastasis: the 'seed and soil' hypothesis revisited. Nat Rev Cancer 2003;3:453–8.
[350] Lobikin M, Chernet B, Lobo D, Levin M. Resting potential, oncogene-induced tumorigenesis, and metastasis: the bioelectric basis of cancer in vivo. Phys Biol 2012;9:065002.
[351] Chernet B, Levin M. Endogenous Voltage Potentials and the Microenvironment: Bioelectric Signals that Reveal, Induce and Normalize Cancer. J Clin & Exp Oncol 2013;(Suppl 1).
[352] Sonnenschein C, Soto AM. The Society of Cells: Cancer and the Control of Cell Proliferation. New York: Springer-Verlag; 1999.
[353] Sonnenschein C, Soto AM. Somatic mutation theory of carcinogenesis: why it should be dropped and replaced. Mol Carcinog 2000;29:205–11.
[354] Sonnenschein C, Soto AM. Theories of carcinogenesis: an emerging perspective. Semin Cancer Biol 2008;18:372–7.
[355] Sonnenschein C, Soto AM. An integrative approach toward biology, organisms, and cancer. Methods Mol Biol 2018;1702:15–26.
[356] Soto AM, Sonnenschein C. Is systems biology a promising approach to resolve controversies in cancer research? Cancer Cell Int 2012;12:12.
[357] Siegel RL, Miller KD, Jemal A. Cancer statistics, 2020. CA Cancer J Clin 2020;70:7–30.
[358] Zielinski DC, Jamshidi N, Corbett AJ, Bordbar A, Thomas A, Palsson BO. Systems biology analysis of drivers underlying hallmarks of cancer cell metabolism. Sci Rep 2017;7:41241.
[359] Choi YK, Park KG. Targeting glutamine metabolism for cancer treatment. Biomol Ther (Seoul) 2018;26:19–28.
[360] Oronsky BT, Oronsky N, Fanger GR, Parker CW, Caroen SZ, Lybeck M, et al. Follow the ATP: tumor energy production: a perspective. Anticancer Agents Med Chem 2014;14:1187–98.
[361] Poljsak B, Kovac V, Dahmane R, Levec T, Starc A. Cancer etiology: a metabolic disease originating from life's major evolutionary transition? Oxid Med Cell Longev 2019;2019:7831952.
[362] Xu RH, Pelicano H, Zhou Y, Carew JS, Feng L, Bhalla KN, et al. Inhibition of glycolysis in cancer cells: a novel strategy to overcome drug resistance associated with mitochondrial respiratory defect and hypoxia. Cancer Res 2005;65:613–21.
[363] Horio M, Gottesman MM, Pastan I. ATP-dependent transport of vinblastine in vesicles from human multidrug-resistant cells. Proc Natl Acad Sci U S Am 1988;85:3580–4.
[364] Leone RD, Zhao L, Englert JM, Sun IM, Oh MH, Sun IH, et al. Glutamine blockade induces divergent metabolic programs to overcome tumor immune evasion. Science 2019;366:1013–21.
[365] Mukherjee P, Augur ZM, Li M, Hill C, Greenwood B, Domin MA, et al. Therapeutic benefit of combining calorie-restricted ketogenic diet and glutamine targeting in late-stage experimental glioblastoma. Commun Biol 2019;2:200.

[366] Reckzeh ES, Karageorgis G, Schwalfenberg M, Ceballos J, Nowacki J, Stroet MCM, et al. Inhibition of glucose transporters and glutaminase synergistically impairs tumor cell growth. Cell Chem Biol 2019;26:1214–28 e1225.

[367] Cervantes-Madrid D, Romero Y, Duenas-Gonzalez A. Reviving lonidamine and 6-Diazo-5-oxo-L-norleucine to be used in combination for metabolic cancer therapy. Biomed Res Int 2015;2015:690492.

[368] Fine EJ, Miller A, Quadros EV, Sequeira JM, Feinman RD. Acetoacetate reduces growth and ATP concentration in cancer cell lines which over-express uncoupling protein 2. Cancer Cell Int 2009;9:14.

[369] Hagihara K, Kajimoto K, Osaga S, Nagai N, Shimosegawa E, Nakata H, et al. Promising effect of a new ketogenic diet regimen in patients with advanced cancer. Nutrients 2020;12(5):1473.

[370] Ji CC, Hu YY, Cheng G, Liang L, Gao B, Ren YP, et al. A ketogenic diet attenuates proliferation and stemness of glioma stemlike cells by altering metabolism resulting in increased ROS production. Int J Oncol 2020;56:606–17.

[371] Bartmann C, Janaki Raman SR, Floter J, Schulze A, Bahlke K, Willingstorfer J, et al. Beta-hydroxybutyrate (3-OHB) can influence the energetic phenotype of breast cancer cells, but does not impact their proliferation and the response to chemotherapy or radiation. Cancer & Metab 2018;6:8.

[372] Magee BA, Potezny N, Rofe AM, Conyers RA. The inhibition of malignant cell growth by ketone bodies. Aust J Exp Biol Med Sci 1979;57:529–39.

[373] Poff A, Koutnik AP, Egan KM, Sahebjam S, D'Agostino D, Kumar NB. Targeting the Warburg effect for cancer treatment: Ketogenic diets for management of glioma. Semin Cancer Biol 2017.

[374] Skinner R, Trujillo A, Ma X, Beierle EA. Ketone bodies inhibit the viability of human neuroblastoma cells. J Pediatr Surg 2009;44:212–16 discussion 216.

[375] Cahill Jr. GF, Veech RL. Ketoacids? Good medicine? Trans Am Clin Climatol Assoc 2003;114:149–61 discussion 162-143.

[376] Veech RL. The therapeutic implications of ketone bodies: the effects of ketone bodies in pathological conditions: ketosis, ketogenic diet, redox states, insulin resistance, and mitochondrial metabolism. Prostaglandins Leukot Essent Fat Acids 2004;70:309–19.

[377] Clarke K, Tchabanenko K, Pawlosky R, Carter E, Todd King M, Musa-Veloso K, et al. Kinetics, safety and tolerability of (R)-3-hydroxybutyl (R)-3-hydroxybutyrate in healthy adult subjects. Regulatory Toxicol Pharmacol 2012;63:401–8.

[378] El Kebbaj MS, Latruffe N, Monsigny M, Obrenovitch A. Interactions between apo-(D-beta-hydroxybutyrate dehydrogenase) and phospholipids studied by intrinsic and extrinsic fluorescence. Biochem J 1986;237:359–64.

[379] Kiebish MA, Han X, Cheng H, Seyfried TN. In vitro growth environment produces lipidomic and electron transport chain abnormalities in mitochondria from non-tumorigenic astrocytes and brain tumours. ASN Neuro 2009;1:e00011.

[380] Zhou W, Mukherjee P, Kiebish MA, Markis WT, Mantis JG, Seyfried TN. The calorically restricted ketogenic diet, an effective alternative therapy for malignant brain cancer. Nutr Metab (Lond) 2007;4:5.

[381] Mukherjee P, Abate LE, Seyfried TN. Antiangiogenic and proapoptotic effects of dietary restriction on experimental mouse and human brain tumors. Clin Cancer Res 2004;10:5622–9.

[382] Mulrooney TJ, Marsh J, Urits I, Seyfried TN, Mukherjee P. Influence of caloric restriction on constitutive expression of NF-kappaB in an experimental mouse astrocytoma. PLoS One 2011;6:e18085.

[383] Mukherjee P, El-Abbadi MM, Kasperzyk JL, Ranes MK, Seyfried TN. Dietary restriction reduces angiogenesis and growth in an orthotopic mouse brain tumour model. Br J Cancer 2002;86:1615–21.

[384] Shelton LM, Huysentruyt LC, Mukherjee P, Seyfried TN. Calorie restriction as an anti-invasive therapy for malignant brain cancer in the VM mouse. ASN neuro 2010;2:e00038.

[385] Klement RJ. Beneficial effects of ketogenic diets for cancer patients: a realist review with focus on evidence and confirmation. Med Oncol 2017;34:132.

[386] Weber DD, Aminzadeh-Gohari S, Tulipan J, Catalano L, Feichtinger RG, Kofler B. Ketogenic diet in the treatment of cancer – Where do we stand? Mol Metab 2019;33:102–21. Available from: http://www.sciencedirect.com/science/article/pii/S2212877819304272.

[387] Winter SF, Loebel F, Dietrich J. Role of ketogenic metabolic therapy in malignant glioma: A systematic review. Crit Rev Oncol Hematol 2017;112:41–58.

[388] Lazebnik Y. What are the hallmarks of cancer? Nat Rev Cancer 2010;10:232–3.

[389] Alexandrov LB, Nik-Zainal S, Wedge DC, Aparicio SA, Behjati S, Biankin AV, et al. Signatures of mutational processes in human cancer. Nature 2013;500:415–21.

[390] Baker SG, Kramer BS. Paradoxes in carcinogenesis: new opportunities for research directions. BMC Cancer 2007;7:151.

[391] Bizzarri M, Cucina A. SMT and TOFT: why and how they are opposite and incompatible paradigms. Acta Biotheor 2016.

[392] Burgio E, Migliore L. Towards a systemic paradigm in carcinogenesis: linking epigenetics and genetics. Mol Biol Rep 2015;42:777–90.

[393] Seyfried TN, Mukherjee P, Iyikesici MS, Slocum A, Kalamian M, Spinosa JP, et al. Consideration of ketogenic metabolic therapy as a complementary or alternative approach for managing breast cancer. Front Nutr 2020;7:21.

[394] Wishart DS. Is cancer a genetic disease or a metabolic disease? EBioMedicine 2015;2:478–9.

[395] Huysentruyt LC, Seyfried TN. Perspectives on the mesenchymal origin of metastatic cancer. Cancer Metastasis Rev 2010;29:695–707.

[396] Kloc M, Li XC, Ghobrial RM. Are macrophages responsible for cancer metastasis? J Immuno Biol 2016;1:1.

[397] Pawelek JM. Tumour-cell fusion as a source of myeloid traits in cancer. Lancet Oncol 2005;6:988–93.

[398] Ruff MR, Pert CB. Small cell carcinoma of the lung: macrophage-specific antigens suggest hemopoietic stem cell origin. Science 1984;225:1034–6.

[399] Fais S. Cannibalism: a way to feed on metastatic tumors. Cancer Lett 2007;258:155–64.

[400] Gupta K, Dey P. Cell cannibalism: diagnostic marker of malignancy. Diagnostic cytopathology 2003;28:86–7.

[401] Abodief WT, Dey P, Al-Hattab O. Cell cannibalism in ductal carcinoma of breast. Cytopathology 2006;17:304–5.

[402] Kojima S, Sekine H, Fukui I, Ohshima H. Clinical significance of "cannibalism" in urinary cytology of bladder cancer. Acta Cytol 1998;42:1365–9.

[403] Lugini L, Matarrese P, Tinari A, Lozupone F, Federici C, Iessi E, et al. Cannibalism of live lymphocytes by human metastatic but not primary melanoma cells. Cancer Res 2006;66:3629–38.

[404] Matarrese P, Ciarlo L, Tinari A, Piacentini M, Malorni W. Xeno-cannibalism as an exacerbation of self-cannibalism: a possible fruitful survival strategy for cancer cells. Curr Pharm Des 2008;14:245–52.

[405] Shelton, L.M. (2010) Targeting energy metabolism in brain cancer. Ph.D., Boston College.

[406] Kamphorst JJ, Nofal M, Commisso C, Hackett SR, Lu W, Grabocka E, et al. Human pancreatic cancer tumors are nutrient poor and tumor cells actively scavenge extracellular protein. Cancer research, 75. 2015. p. 544–53.

[407] Delsite RL, Rasmussen LJ, Rasmussen AK, Kalen A, Goswami PC, Singh KK. Mitochondrial impairment is accompanied by impaired oxidative DNA repair in the nucleus. Mutagenesis 2003;18:497–503.

[408] Han SJ, Yang I, Otero JJ, Ahn BJ, Tihan T, McDermott MW, et al. Secondary gliosarcoma after diagnosis of glioblastoma: clinical experience with 30 consecutive patients. J Neurosurg 2010;112:990–6.

[409] Kulawiec M, Safina A, Desouki MM, Still I, Matsui SI, Bakin A, et al. Tumorigenic transformation of human breast epithelial cells induced by mitochondrial DNA depletion. Cancer Biol Ther 2008;7.

[410] Lu J, Sharma LK, Bai Y. Implications of mitochondrial DNA mutations and mitochondrial dysfunction in tumorigenesis. Cell Res 2009;19:802–15.

[411] Rasmussen AK, Chatterjee A, Rasmussen LJ, Singh KK. Mitochondria-mediated nuclear mutator phenotype in Saccharomyces cerevisiae. Nucleic Acids Res 2003;31:3909–17.

[412] Samper E, Nicholls DG, Melov S. Mitochondrial oxidative stress causes chromosomal instability of mouse embryonic fibroblasts. Aging Cell 2003;2:277–85.

[413] Smiraglia DJ, Kulawiec M, Bistulfi GL, Gupta SG, Singh KK. A novel role for mitochondria in regulating epigenetic modification in the nucleus. Cancer Biol Ther 2008;7:1182–90.

[414] Veatch JR, McMurray MA, Nelson ZW, Gottschling DE. Mitochondrial dysfunction leads to nuclear genome instability via an iron-sulfur cluster defect. Cell 2009;137:1247–58.

[415] Chandra D, Singh KK. Genetic insights into OXPHOS defect and its role in cancer. Biochimica et biophysica acta 2011;1807:620–5.

[416] Minocherhomji S, Tollefsbol TO, Singh KK. Mitochondrial regulation of epigenetics and its role in human diseases. Epigenetics: Off J DNA Methylation Soc 2012;7:326–34.

[417] Klaunig JE, Kamendulis LM, Hocevar BA. Oxidative stress and oxidative damage in carcinogenesis. Toxicol Pathol 2010;38:96–109.

[418] Sabharwal SS, Schumacker PT. Mitochondrial ROS in cancer: initiators, amplifiers or an Achilles' heel? Nat Rev Cancer 2014;14:709–21.

[419] Potts R. Humanity's Descent: The Consequences of Ecological Instability. New York: William Morrow & Co., Inc.; 1996.

[420] Potts R. Environmental hypotheses of hominin evolution. Am J Phys Anthropol 1998;Suppl 27:93–136.

[421] Potts R. Complexity of adaptability in human evolution. In: Goodman M, Moffat AS, editors. Probing Human Origins. Cambridge, MA: American Academy of Arts & Sciences; 2002, p. 33–57.

[422] Seyfried TN. Nothing in cancer biology makes sense except in the light of evolution. Cancer as a Metabolic Disease: On the Origin, Management, and Prevention of Cancer. Hoboken, NJ: John Wiley & Sons; 2012, p. 261–75.

[423] Seyfried TN, Mukherjee P. Targeting energy metabolism in brain cancer: review and hypothesis. Nutr Metab (Lond), 2. 2005, p. 30.

[424] Darwin C. On the Origin of Species by Means of Natural Selection, or on the Preservation of Favored Races in the Struggle for Life. London: John Murry; 1859.

[425] de Groof AJ, Te Lindert MM, van Dommelen MM, Wu M, Willemse M, Smift AL, et al. Increased OXPHOS activity precedes rise in glycolytic rate in H-RasV12/E1A transformed fibroblasts that develop a Warburg phenotype. Mol cancer 2009;8:54.

[426] Galmiche A, Fueller J. RAF kinases and mitochondria. Biochimica et biophysica acta 2007;1773:1256–62.

[427] Moiseeva O, Bourdeau V, Roux A, Deschenes-Simard X, Ferbeyre G. Mitochondrial dysfunction contributes to oncogene-induced senescence. Mol Cell Biol 2009;29:4495–507.

[428] Rozhok AI, DeGregori J. Toward an evolutionary model of cancer: Considering the mechanisms that govern the fate of somatic mutations. Proc Natl Acad Sci U S Am 2015;112:8914–21.

[429] Mukherjee P, Mulrooney TJ, Marsh J, Blair D, Chiles TC, Seyfried TN. Differential effects of energy stress on AMPK phosphorylation and apoptosis in experimental brain tumor and normal brain. Mol Cancer 2008;7:37.

[430] Mukherjee P, Sotnikov AV, Mangian HJ, Zhou JR, Visek WJ, Clinton SK. Energy intake and prostate tumor growth, angiogenesis, and vascular endothelial growth factor expression. J Natl Cancer Inst 1999;91:512–23.

[431] Elsakka AMA, Bary MA, Abdelzaher E, Elnaggar M, Kalamian M, Mukherjee P, et al. Management of glioblastoma multiforme in a patient treated with ketogenic metabolic therapy and modified standard of care: a 24-month follow-up. Front Nutr 2018;5:20.

[432] Nebeling LC, Miraldi F, Shurin SB, Lerner E. Effects of a ketogenic diet on tumor metabolism and nutritional status in pediatric oncology patients: two case reports. J Am Coll Nutr 1995;14:202–8.

[433] Panhans CM, Gresham G, Amaral JL, Hu J. Exploring the feasibility and effects of a ketogenic diet in patients with CNS malignancies: a retrospective case series. Front Neurosci 2020;14:390.
[434] Seyfried TN, Mukherjee P. Anti-angiogenic and pro-apoptotic effects of dietary restriction in experimental brain cancer: role of glucose and ketone bodies. In: Meadows GG, editor. Integration/Interaction of Oncologic Growth. 2nd Ed. New York: Kluwer Academic; 2005, p. 259–70.
[435] Seyfried TN, Sanderson TM, El-Abbadi MM, McGowan R, Mukherjee P. Role of glucose and ketone bodies in the metabolic control of experimental brain cancer. Br J Cancer 2003;89:1375–82.
[436] Zuccoli G, Marcello N, Pisanello A, Servadei F, Vaccaro S, Mukherjee P, et al. Metabolic management of glioblastoma multiforme using standard therapy together with a restricted ketogenic diet: case report. Nutr Metab (Lond) 2010;7:33.
[437] Nowell PC. The clonal evolution of tumor cell populations. Science 1976;194:23–8.
[438] Cahill Jr. GF. Fuel metabolism in starvation. Annu Rev Nutr 2006;26:1–22.
[439] Maurer GD, Brucker DP, Baehr O, Harter PN, Hattingen E, Walenta S, et al. Differential utilization of ketone bodies by neurons and glioma cell lines: a rationale for ketogenic diet as experimental glioma therapy. BMC cancer 2011;11:315.
[440] Poff AM, Ari C, Arnold P, Seyfried TN, D'Agostino DP. Ketone supplementation decreases tumor cell viability and prolongs survival of mice with metastatic cancer. Int J cancer J Int du cancer 2014;135:1711–20.
[441] Chang HT, Olson LK, Schwartz KA. Ketolytic and glycolytic enzymatic expression profiles in malignant gliomas: implication for ketogenic diet therapy. Nutr & Metab 2013;10:47.
[442] Abdelwahab MG, Fenton KE, Preul MC, Rho JM, Lynch A, Stafford P, et al. The ketogenic diet is an effective adjuvant to radiation therapy for the treatment of malignant glioma. PLoS one 2012;7:e36197.
[443] Martuscello RT, Vedam-Mai V, McCarthy DJ, Schmoll ME, Jundi MA, Louviere CD, et al. A supplemented high-fat low-carbohydrate diet for the treatment of glioblastoma. Clin Cancer Res 2016;22:2482–95.
[444] Arens NC, West ID. Press-pulse: a general theory of mass extinction? Paleobiology 2008;34:456–71.
[445] Vincent M. Cancer: a de-repression of a default survival program common to all cells?: a life-history perspective on the nature of cancer. BioEssays 2012;34:72–82.
[446] Poff AM, Ari C, Seyfried TN, D'Agostino DP. The ketogenic diet and hyperbaric oxygen therapy prolong survival in mice with systemic metastatic cancer. PLoS One 2013;8:e65522.
[447] Freeman JM, Kossoff EH. Ketosis and the ketogenic diet, 2010: advances in treating epilepsy and other disorders. Adv Pediatr 2010;57:315–29.
[448] Kossoff EH, Hartman AL. Ketogenic diets: new advances for metabolism-based therapies. Curr Opin Neurol 2012;25(2):173–8.
[449] Meidenbauer JJ, Mukherjee P, Seyfried TN. The glucose ketone index calculator: a simple tool to monitor therapeutic efficacy for metabolic management of brain cancer. Nutr & Metab 2015;12(1):12.
[450] Poff AM, Ward N, Seyfried TN, Arnold P, D'Agostino DP. Non-toxic metabolic management of metastatic cancer in VM mice: novel combination of ketogenic diet, ketone supplementation, and hyperbaric oxygen therapy. PLoS One 2015;10:e0127407.
[451] Burt ME, Gorschboth CM, Brennan MF. A controlled, prospective, randomized trial evaluating the metabolic effects of enteral and parenteral nutrition in the cancer patient. Cancer 1982;49:1092–105.
[452] Campbell TC. Dietary protein, growth factors, and cancer. Am J Clin Nutr 2007;85:1667.
[453] Jiang YS, Wang FR. Caloric restriction reduces edema and prolongs survival in a mouse glioma model. J neuro-oncology 2013;114:25–32.
[454] Lu Z, Xie J, Wu G, Shen J, Collins R, Chen W, et al. Fasting selectively blocks development of acute lymphoblastic leukemia via leptin-receptor upregulation. Nat Med 2017;23:79–90.
[455] Koutnik AP, Poff AM, Ward NP, DeBlasi JM, Soliven MA, Romero MA, et al. Ketone Bodies Attenuate Wasting in Models of Atrophy. J Cachexia Sarcopenia Muscle 2020;11:973–96.
[456] Tisdale MJ, Brennan RA. A comparison of long-chain triglycerides and medium-chain triglycerides on weight loss and tumour size in a cachexia model. Br-J-Cancer 1988;58:580–3.
[457] Tisdale MJ, Brennan RA, Fearon KC. Reduction of weight loss and tumour size in a cachexia model by a high fat diet. Br J Cancer 1987;56:39–43.
[458] Morscher RJ, Aminzadeh-Gohari S, Hauser-Kronberger C, Feichtinger RG, Sperl W, Kofler B. Combination of metronomic cyclophosphamide and dietary intervention inhibits neuroblastoma growth in a CD1-nu mouse model. Oncotarget 2016;7:17060–73.
[459] Allen BG, Bhatia SK, Buatti JM, Brandt KE, Lindholm KE, Button AM, et al. Ketogenic diets enhance oxidative stress and radio-chemo-therapy responses in lung cancer xenografts. Clin cancer Res: an Off J Am Assoc Cancer Res 2013;19:3905–13.
[460] Kim HS, Masko EM, Poulton SL, Kennedy KM, Pizzo SV, Dewhirst MW, et al. Carbohydrate restriction and lactate transporter inhibition in a mouse xenograft model of human prostate cancer. BJU Int 2012;110:1062–9.
[461] Mavropoulos JC, Buschemeyer 3rd WC, Tewari AK, Rokhfeld D, Pollak M, Zhao Y, et al. The effects of varying dietary carbohydrate and fat content on survival in a murine LNCaP prostate cancer xenograft model. Cancer Prev Res (Phila Pa) 2009;2:557–65.
[462] Lv M, Zhu X, Wang H, Wang F, Guan W. Roles of caloric restriction, ketogenic diet and intermittent fasting during initiation, progression and metastasis of cancer in animal models: a systematic review and meta-analysis. PLoS One 2014;9:e115147.
[463] Zhuang Y, Chan DK, Haugrud AB, Miskimins WK. Mechanisms by which low glucose enhances the cytotoxicity of metformin to cancer cells both in vitro and in vivo. PLoS One 2014;9:e108444.

[464] Hao GW, Chen YS, He DM, Wang HY, Wu GH, Zhang B. Growth of human colon cancer cells in nude mice is delayed by ketogenic diet with or without omega-3 fatty acids and medium-chain triglycerides. Asian Pac J Cancer Prev 2015;16:2061–8.

[465] Klement RJ. Calorie or carbohydrate restriction? The ketogenic diet as another option for supportive cancer treatment. Oncologist 2013;18:1056.

[466] Klement RJ. Restricting carbohydrates to fight head and neck cancer-is this realistic? Cancer Biol & Med 2014;11:145–61.

[467] Maroon JC, Seyfried TN, Donohue JP, Bost J. The role of metabolic therapy in treating glioblastoma multiforme. Surgical Neurol Int 2015;6:61.

[468] Rieger J, Bahr O, Maurer GD, Hattingen E, Franz K, Brucker D, et al. ERGO: a pilot study of ketogenic diet in recurrent glioblastoma. Int J Oncol 2014;44:1843–52.

[469] Schmidt M, Pfetzer N, Schwab M, Strauss I, Kammerer U. Effects of a ketogenic diet on the quality of life in 16 patients with advanced cancer: A pilot trial. Nutr & Metab 2011;8:54.

[470] Tan-Shalaby JL, Carrick J, Edinger K, Genovese D, Liman AD, Passero VA, et al. Modified Atkins diet in advanced malignancies - final results of a safety and feasibility trial within the Veterans Affairs Pittsburgh Healthcare System. Nutr Metab (Lond) 2016;13:52.

[471] Champ CE, Mishra MV, Showalter TN, Ohri N, Dicker AP, Simone NL. Dietary recommendations during and after cancer treatment: consistently inconsistent? Nutr cancer 2013;65:430–9.

[472] Champ CE, Palmer JD, Volek JS, Werner-Wasik M, Andrews DW, Evans JJ, et al. Targeting metabolism with a ketogenic diet during the treatment of glioblastoma multiforme. J neuro-oncology 2014;117:125–31.

[473] Freeman JM, Kossoff EH, Freeman JB, Kelly MT. The Ketogenic Diet: A Treatment for Children and Others with Epilepsy. Fourth ed. New York: Demos; 2007.

[474] Fine EJ, Segal-Isaacson CJ, Feinman RD, Herszkopf S, Romano MC, Tomuta N, et al. Targeting insulin inhibition as a metabolic therapy in advanced cancer: a pilot safety and feasibility dietary trial in 10 patients. Nutrition 2012;28:1028–35.

[475] Mantis JG, Centeno NA, Todorova MT, McGowan R, Seyfried TN. Management of multifactorial idiopathic epilepsy in EL mice with caloric restriction and the ketogenic diet: role of glucose and ketone bodies. Nutr Metab (Lond) 2004;1:11.

[476] Fein EJ, Feinman RD. Insulin, carbohydrate restriction, metabolic syndrome and cancer. Expert Rev Endocrinol & Metab 2015;10:15–24.

[477] Sato K, Kashiwaya Y, Keon CA, Tsuchiya N, King MT, Radda GK, et al. Insulin, ketone bodies, and mitochondrial energy transduction. Faseb J 1995;9:651–8.

[478] VanItallie TB, Nufert TH. Ketones: metabolism's ugly duckling. Nutr Rev 2003;61:327–41.

[479] Veech RL, Chance B, Kashiwaya Y, Lardy HA, Cahill Jr. GF. Ketone bodies, potential therapeutic uses. IUBMB Life 2001;51:241–7.

[480] Chance B, Sies H, Boveris A. Hydroperoxide metabolism in mammalian organs. Physiol Rev 1979;59:527–605.

[481] Ciraolo ST, Previs SF, Fernandez CA, Agarwal KC, David F, Koshy J, et al. Model of extreme hypoglycemia in dogs made ketotic with (R, S)-1,3-butanediol acetoacetate esters. Am J Physiol 1995;269:E67–75.

[482] Chance B, editor. Energy-Linked Functions of Mitochondria. New York: Academic Press; 1963.

[483] Shimazu T, Hirschey MD, Newman J, He W, Shirakawa K, Le Moan N, et al. Suppression of oxidative stress by beta-hydroxybutyrate, an endogenous histone deacetylase inhibitor. Science, 339. 2013. p. 211–4.

[484] West AC, Johnstone RW. New and emerging HDAC inhibitors for cancer treatment. J Clin Invest 2014;124:30–9.

[485] Youm YH, Nguyen KY, Grant RW, Goldberg EL, Bodogai M, Kim D, et al. The ketone metabolite beta-hydroxybutyrate blocks NLRP3 inflammasome-mediated inflammatory disease. Nat Med 2015;21:263–9.

[486] Kossoff EH, Zupec-Kania BA, Amark PE, Ballaban-Gil KR, Christina Bergqvist AG, Blackford R, et al. Optimal clinical management of children receiving the ketogenic diet: recommendations of the International Ketogenic Diet Study Group. Epilepsia 2009;50:304–17.

[487] Feng Z, Liu L, Zhang C, Zheng T, Wang J, Lin M, et al. Chronic restraint stress attenuates p53 function and promotes tumorigenesis. Proc Natl Acad Sci U S A 2012;109:7013–18.

[488] Jang HJ, Boo HJ, Lee HJ, Min HY, Lee HY. Chronic stress facilitates lung tumorigenesis by promoting exocytosis of igf2 in lung epithelial cells. Cancer Res 2016;76(22):6607–19.

[489] Levin GT, Greenwood KM, Singh F, Tsoi D, Newton RU. Exercise improves physical function and mental health of brain cancer survivors: two exploratory case studies. Integr Cancer Ther 2016;15:190–6.

[490] Lopes-Junior LC, Bomfim EO, Nascimento LC, Nunes MD, Pereira-da-Silva G, Lima RA. Non-pharmacological interventions to manage fatigue and psychological stress in children and adolescents with cancer: an integrative review. Eur J Cancer Care (Engl) 2016;25:921–35.

[491] Bradt J, Dileo C, Magill L, Teague A. Music interventions for improving psychological and physical outcomes in cancer patients. Cochrane Database Syst Rev 2016; CD006911.

[492] Sharma M, Rush SE. Mindfulness-based stress reduction as a stress management intervention for healthy individuals: a systematic review. J Evid Based Complementary Altern Med 2014;19:271–86.

[493] Ari C, Kovacs Z, Juhasz G, Murdun C, Goldhagen CR, Koutnik AM, et al. Exogenous ketone supplements reduce anxiety-related behavior in Sprague-Dawley and Wistar Albino Glaxo/Rijswijk rats. Front Mol Neurosci 2016;9:137.

[494] De Lorenzo MS, Baljinnyam E, Vatner DE, Abarzua P, Vatner SF, Rabson AB. Caloric restriction reduces growth of mammary tumors and metastases. Carcinogenesis 2011;32:1381–7.

[495] Longo VD, Mattson MP. Fasting: molecular mechanisms and clinical applications. Cell Metab 2014;19:181–92.

[496] Meynet O, Ricci JE. Caloric restriction and cancer: molecular mechanisms and clinical implications. Trends Mol Med 2014;20:419–27.

[497] Al-Wahab Z, Tebbe C, Chhina J, Dar SA, Morris RT, Ali-Fehmi R, et al. Dietary energy balance modulates ovarian cancer progression and metastasis. Oncotarget 2014;5:6063–75.

[498] Raffaghello L, Lee C, Safdie FM, Wei M, Madia F, Bianchi G, et al. Starvation-dependent differential stress resistance protects normal but not cancer cells against high-dose chemotherapy. Proc Natl Acad Sci U S A 2008;105:8215–20.

[499] Raffaghello L, Safdie F, Bianchi G, Dorff T, Fontana L, Longo VD. Fasting and differential chemotherapy protection in patients. Cell Cycle 2010;9:4474–6.

[500] Safdie FM, Dorff T, Quinn D, Fontana L, Wei M, Lee C, et al. Fasting and cancer treatment in humans: A case series report. Aging 2009;1 (12):988–1007. Available from: https://doi.org/10.18632/aging.100114.

[501] Marsh J, Mukherjee P, Seyfried TN. Drug/diet synergy for managing malignant astrocytoma in mice: 2-deoxy-D-glucose and the restricted ketogenic diet. Nutr Metab (Lond) 2008;5:33.

[502] Farah IO. Differential modulation of intracellular energetics in A549 and MRC-5 cells. Biomed Sci Instrum 2007;43:110–15.

[503] Pedersen PL. Warburg, me and Hexokinase 2: Multiple discoveries of key molecular events underlying one of cancers' most common phenotypes, the "Warburg Effect," i.e., elevated glycolysis in the presence of oxygen. J Bioenerg Biomembr 2007;39:211–22.

[504] Pelicano H, Martin DS, Xu RH, Huang P. Glycolysis inhibition for anticancer treatment. Oncogene 2006;25:4633–46.

[505] Williams DS, Cash A, Hamadani L, Diemer T. Oxaloacetate supplementation increases lifespan in Caenorhabditis elegans through an AMPK/FOXO-dependent pathway. Aging Cell 2009;8:765–8.

[506] Moen I, Stuhr LE. Hyperbaric oxygen therapy and cancer—a review. Target Oncol 2012;7:233–42.

[507] Iyikesici MS. Feasibility study of metabolically supported chemotherapy with weekly carboplatin/paclitaxel combined with ketogenic diet, hyperthermia and hyperbaric oxygen therapy in metastatic non-small cell lung cancer. Int J Hyperth 2019;36:446–55.

[508] Kohshi K, Beppu T, Tanaka K, Ogawa K, Inoue O, Kukita I, et al. Potential roles of hyperbaric oxygenation in the treatments of brain tumors. UHM 2013;40:351–62.

[509] Poff AM, Kernagis D, D'Agostino DP. Hyperbaric environment: oxygen and cellular damage versus protection. Comp Physiol 2017;7:213–34.

[510] D'Agostino DP, Colomb Jr. DG, Dean JB. Effects of hyperbaric gases on membrane nanostructure and function in neurons. J Appl Physiol 2009;106:996–1003.

[511] Ma Y, Chapman J, Levine M, Polireddy K, Drisko J, Chen Q. High-dose parenteral ascorbate enhanced chemosensitivity of ovarian cancer and reduced toxicity of chemotherapy. Sci Transl Med 2014;6 222ra218.

[512] Michelakis ED, Sutendra G, Dromparis P, Webster L, Haromy A, Niven E, et al. Metabolic modulation of glioblastoma with dichloroacetate. Sci Transl Med 2010;2 31ra34.

[513] Murray AJ, Knight NS, Cole MA, Cochlin LE, Carter E, Tchabanenko K, et al. Novel ketone diet enhances physical and cognitive performance. FASEB J 2016;.

[514] Cox PJ, Kirk T, Ashmore T, Willerton K, Evans R, Smith A, et al. Nutritional ketosis alters fuel preference and thereby endurance performance in athletes. Cell Metab 2016;24:256–68.

[515] Reitzer LJ, Wice BM, Kennell D. Evidence that glutamine, not sugar, is the major energy source for cultured HeLa cells. J Biol Chem 1979;254:2669–76.

[516] Baguet T, Verhoeven J, Pauwelyn G, Hu J, Lambe P, De Lombaerde S, et al. Radiosynthesis, in vitro and preliminary in vivo evaluation of the novel glutamine derived PET tracers [(18)F]fluorophenylglutamine and [(18)F]fluorobiphenylglutamine. Nucl Med Biol 2020;86–87:20–9.

[517] Venneti S, Dunphy MP, Zhang H, Pitter KL, Zanzonico P, Campos C, et al. Glutamine-based PET imaging facilitates enhanced metabolic evaluation of gliomas in vivo. Sci Transl Med 2015;7 274ra217.

[518] Shelton LM, Huysentruyt LC, Seyfried TN. Glutamine targeting inhibits systemic metastasis in the VM-M3 murine tumor model. Inter J Cancer 2010;127:2478–85.

[519] Mueller C, Al-Batran S, Jaeger E, Schmidt B, Bausch M, Unger C, et al. A phase IIa study of PEGylated glutaminase (PEG-PGA) plus 6-diazo-5-oxo-L-norleucine (DON) in patients with advanced refractory solid tumors, in *ASCO Annual Meeting*. J Clin Oncol 2008;26.

[520] Chakrabarti G, Moore ZR, Luo X, Ilcheva M, Ali A, Padanad M, et al. Targeting glutamine metabolism sensitizes pancreatic cancer to PARP-driven metabolic catastrophe induced by ss-lapachone. Cancer & Metab 2015;3:12.

[521] Mates JM, Segura JA, Campos-Sandoval JA, Lobo C, Alonso L, Alonso FJ, et al. Glutamine homeostasis and mitochondrial dynamics. Int J Biochem Cell Biol 2009;41:2051–61.

[522] Michalak KP, Mackowska-Kedziora A, Sobolewski B, Wozniak P. Key roles of glutamine pathways in reprogramming the cancer metabolism. Oxid Med Cell Longev 2015;2015:964321.

[523] Huysentruyt LC, Mukherjee P, Banerjee D, Shelton LM, Seyfried TN. Metastatic cancer cells with macrophage properties: evidence from a new murine tumor model. Int J Cancer 2008;123:73–84.

[524] Hamilton JD, Rapp M, Schneiderhan T, Sabel M, Hayman A, Scherer A, et al. Glioblastoma multiforme metastasis outside the CNS: three case reports and possible mechanisms of escape. J Clin Oncol 2014;32:e80–4.

[525] Hoffman HJ, Duffner PK. Extraneural metastases of central nervous system tumors. Cancer 1985;56:1778–82.

[526] Huysentruyt LC, Shelton LM, Seyfried TN. Influence of methotrexate and cisplatin on tumor progression and survival in the VM mouse model of systemic metastatic cancer. Int J Cancer 2010;126:65–72.

[527] Kalokhe G, Grimm SA, Chandler JP, Helenowski I, Rademaker A, Raizer JJ. Metastatic glioblastoma: case presentations and a review of the literature. J Neurooncol 2012;107:21–7.
[528] Shelton LM, Mukherjee P, Huysentruyt LC, Urits I, Rosenberg JA, Seyfried TN. A novel pre-clinical in vivo mouse model for malignant brain tumor growth and invasion. J Neurooncol 2010;99:165–76.
[529] Xu M, Wang Y, Xu J, Yao Y, Yu WX, Zhong P. Extensive therapies for extraneural metastases from glioblastoma, as confirmed with the OncoScan assay. World Neurosurg 2016;90 698 e697–698 e611.
[530] Yasuhara T, Tamiya T, Meguro T, Ichikawa T, Sato Y, Date I, et al. Glioblastoma with metastasis to the spleen–case report. Neurol Med Chir (Tokyo) 2003;43:452–6.
[531] Seyfried TN. Metabolic management of cancer. in. Cancer as a Metabolic Disease: On the Origin, Management, and Prevention of Cancer. Hoboken, NJ: John Wiley & Sons; 2012. p. 291–354.
[532] Hayat MJ, Howlader N, Reichman ME, Edwards BK. Cancer statistics, trends, and multiple primary cancer analyses from the surveillance, epidemiology, and end results (SEER) program. Oncologist 2007;12(1):20–37.
[533] Lane J, Brown NI, Williams S, Plaisance EP, Fontaine KR. Ketogenic diet for cancer: critical assessment and research recommendations. Nutrients. 2021;13(10):3562.
[534] Kossoff EH, Zupec-Kania BA, Auvin S, Ballaban-Gil KR, Christina Bergqvist AG, Blackford R, et al. Optimal clinical management of children receiving dietary therapies for epilepsy: Updated recommendations of the International Ketogenic Diet Study Group. Epilepsia Open 2018;3(2):175–92.
[535] O'Flanagan CH, Smith LA, McDonell SB, Hursting SD. When less may be more: calorie restriction and response to cancer therapy. BMC Med 2017;15:106.
[536] Roda N, Gambino V, Giorgio M. Metabolic constrains rule metastasis progression. Cells. 2020;9(9):2081.
[537] Manore MM. Exercise and the Institute of Medicine recommendations for nutrition. Curr Sports Med Rep 2005;4(4):193–8. Available from: https://doi.org/10.1097/01.csmr.0000306206.72186.00; PMID: 16004827.
[538] Sharma S, Jain P. The modified Atkins diet in refractory epilepsy. Epilepsy Res Treat 2014;2014:404202.
[539] Paoli A, Grimaldi K, Bianco A, Lodi A, Cenci L, Parmagnani A. Medium term effects of a ketogenic diet and a Mediterranean diet on resting energy expenditure and respiratory ratio. BMC Proc 2012;6(3):P37.
[540] Paoli A, Rubini A, Volek JS, Grimaldi KA. Beyond weight loss: a review of the therapeutic uses of very-low-carbohydrate (ketogenic) diets. Eur J Clin Nutr 2013;67(8):789–96.
[541] Juby AG, Blackburn TE, Mager DR. Use of medium chain triglyceride (MCT) oil in subjects with Alzheimer's disease: A randomized, double-blind, placebo-controlled, crossover study, with an open-label extension. Alzheimer's & Dementia: Transl Res & Clin Interventions 2022;8(1):e12259.
[542] Manninen AH. Very-low-carbohydrate diets and preservation of muscle mass. Nutr Metab (Lond) 2006;3(9).
[543] Thomsen HH, Rittig N, Johannsen M, Møller AB, Jørgensen JO, Jessen N, et al. Effects of 3-hydroxybutyrate and free fatty acids on muscle protein kinetics and signaling during LPS-induced inflammation in humans: anticatabolic impact of ketone bodies. Am J Clin Nutr 2018;108 (4):857–67.
[544] Catenacci VA, Pan Z, Ostendorf D, Brannon S, Gozansky WS, Mattson MP, et al. A randomized pilot study comparing zero-calorie alternate-day fasting to daily caloric restriction in adults with obesity. Obes (Silver Spring) 2016;24(9):1874–83.
[545] Moreschi C. Beziehungen zwischen ernährung und tumorwachstum. Z Immunitätsforsch Orig 1909;2:651–75.
[546] Mizushima N. Autophagy: process and function. Genes & Dev 2007;21(22):2861–73. Available from: https://doi.org/10.1101/gad.1599207.
[547] Hippert MM, O'Toole PS, Thorburn A. Autophagy in cancer: good, bad, or both? Cancer Res 2006;66(19):9349–51. Available from: https://doi.org/10.1158/0008-5472.CAN-06-1597.
[548] Cataldo AM, Hamilton DJ, Barnett JL, Paskevich PA, Nixon RA. Properties of the endosomal-lysosomal system in the human central nervous system: disturbances mark most neurons in populations at risk to degenerate in Alzheimer's disease. J Neurosci 1996;16(1):186–99. Available from: https://doi.org/10.1523/JNEUROSCI.16-01-00186.1996.
[549] Cheng CW, Adams GB, Perin L, Wei M, Zhou X, Lam BS, et al. Prolonged fasting reduces IGF-1/PKA to promote hematopoietic-stem-cell-based regeneration and reverse immunosuppression. Cell stem Cell 2014;14(6):810–23. Available from: https://doi.org/10.1016/j.stem.2014.04.014.
[550] Lee C, Raffaghello L, Brandhorst S, Safdie FM, Bianchi G, Martin-Montalvo A, et al. Fasting cycles retard growth of tumors and sensitize a range of cancer cell types to chemotherapy. Sci Transl Med 2012;4(124):124ra27. Available from: https://doi.org/10.1126/scitranslmed.3003293.
[551] Longo VD, Fontana L. Calorie restriction and cancer prevention: metabolic and molecular mechanisms. Trends Pharmacol Sci 2010;31 (2):89–98. Available from: https://doi.org/10.1016/j.tips.2009.11.004.
[552] Marinac CR, Nelson SH, Breen CI, Hartman SJ, Natarajan L, Pierce JP, et al. Prolonged nightly fasting and breast cancer prognosis. JAMA Oncol 2016;2(8):1049. Available from: https://doi.org/10.1001/jamaoncol.2016.0164.
[553] Klement RJ, Champ CE, Kämmerer U, Koebrunner PS, Krage K, Schäfer G, et al. Impact of a ketogenic diet intervention during radiotherapy on body composition: III—final results of the KETOCOMP study for breast cancer patients. Breast Cancer Res 2020;22(1):94.
[554] Seyfried TN, Kiebish MA, Marsh J, Shelton LM, Huysentruyt LC, Mukherjee P. Metabolic management of brain cancer. Biochim Biophys Acta 2011;1807(6):577–94.

[555] Seyfried TN, Marsh J, Shelton LM, Huysentruyt LC, Mukherjee P. Is the restricted ketogenic diet a viable alternative to the standard of care for managing malignant brain cancer? Epilepsy Res 2012;100(3):310–26.

[556] Alkedeh O, Priefer R. The ketogenic diet: breath acetone sensing technology. Biosens (Basel) 2021;11(1):26.

[557] KetoDietCalculator Home Page - KetoDietCalculator [Internet]. [cited 2022 Apr 21]. Available from: https://www.ketodietcalculator.org/keto-web/KetoStart.

[558] de Groot S, Vreeswijk MP, Welters MJ, Gravesteijn G, Boei JJ, Jochems A, et al. The effects of short-term fasting on tolerance to (neo) adjuvant chemotherapy in HER2-negative breast cancer patients: a randomized pilot study. BMC cancer 2015;15:652. Available from: https://doi.org/10.1186/s12885-015-1663-5.

[559] Bauersfeld SP, Kessler CS, Wischnewsky M, Jaensch A, Steckhan N, Stange R, et al. The effects of short-term fasting on quality of life and tolerance to chemotherapy in patients with breast and ovarian cancer: a randomized cross-over pilot study. BMC cancer 2018;18(1):476. Available from: https://doi.org/10.1186/s12885-018-4353-2.

[560] Dorff TB, Groshen S, Garcia A, Shah M, Tsao-Wei D, Pham H, et al. Safety and feasibility of fasting in combination with platinum-based chemotherapy. BMC Cancer 2016;16:360. Available from: https://www.ncbi.nlm.nih.gov/pmc/articles/PMC4901417.

[561] Tiwari S, Sapkota N, Han Z. Effect of fasting on cancer: a narrative review of scientific evidence. Cancer Sci 2022;. Available from: https://onlinelibrary.wiley.com/doi/abs/10.1111/cas.15492.

Further Reading

Augustin K, Khabbush A, Williams S, Eaton S, Orford M, Cross JH, et al. Mechanisms of action for the medium-chain triglyceride ketogenic diet in neurological and metabolic disorders. Lancet Neurol 2018;17(1):84–93.

Cronometer: Track nutrition & count calories [Internet]. [cited 2022 Apr 19]. Available from: https://cronometer.com/.

Han FY, Conboy-Schmidt L, Rybachuk G, Volk HA, Zanghi B, Pan Y, et al. Dietary medium chain triglycerides for management of epilepsy: New data from human, dog, and rodent studies. Epilepsia. 2021;62(8):1790–806.

Huttenlocher PR, Wilbourn AJ, Signore JM. Medium-chain triglycerides as a therapy for intractable childhood epilepsy. Neurology. 1971;21(11):1097–103.

Jaworski DM, Namboodiri AM, Moffett JR. Acetate as a metabolic and epigenetic modifier of cancer therapy. J Cell Biochem 2016;117:574–88.

Johannsen DL, Knuth ND, Huizenga R, Rood JC, Ravussin E, Hall KD. Metabolic slowing with massive weight loss despite preservation of fat-free mass. J Clin Endocrinol Metab 2012;97(7):2489–96.

Redman LM, Heilbronn LK, Martin CK, de Jonge L, Williamson DA, Delany JP, et al. Metabolic and behavioral compensations in response to caloric restriction: implications for the maintenance of weight loss. PLoS One 2009;4(2):e4377.

Römer M, Dörfler J, Huebner J. The use of ketogenic diets in cancer patients: a systematic review Clin Exp Med [Internet] 2021;[cited 2021 Apr 8]; Available from. Available from: https://doi.org/10.1007/s10238-021-00710-2.

Sargaço B, Oliveira PA, Antunes ML, Moreira AC. Effects of the ketogenic diet in the treatment of gliomas: a systematic review. Nutrients. 2022;14(5):1007.

Sills MA, Forsythe WI, Haidukewych D, MacDonald A, Robinson M. The medium chain triglyceride diet and intractable epilepsy. Arch Dis Child 1986;61(12):1168–72.

Symersky T, Vu MK, Frölich M, Biemond I, Masclee AAM. The effect of equicaloric medium-chain and long-chain triglycerides on pancreas enzyme secretion. Clin Physiol Funct Imaging 2002;22(5):307–11.

Yang YF, Mattamel PB, Joseph T, Huang J, Chen Q, Akinwunmi BO, et al. Efficacy of low-carbohydrate ketogenic diet as an adjuvant cancer therapy: a systematic review and meta-analysis of randomized controlled trials. Nutrients. 2021;13(5):1388.

Chapter 7

Musculoskeletal and immunological considerations

Gary Fettke[1], Bob Kaplan[2], Shawn Baker[3] and Sarah M. Rice[4]
[1]Launceston, Tasmania, Australia, [2]Independent researcher, Wayland, MA, United States, [3]Revero, San Francisco, CA, United States, [4]Nutrition Network, Cape Town, South Africa

7.1 Introduction

Musculoskeletal conditions are primarily thought to be as age-related and unavoidable. While age is a factor for musculoskeletal functional decline, an association with age should be considered alongside lifestyle factors. Inflammation accompanies musculoskeletal conditions, and should be targeted when considering interventions for these conditions. Diet is a key modulator of inflammation. The Western diet, which is high in carbohydrate, polyunsaturated seed oil, and processed food, is known to contribute to inflammation and can negatively affect the microbiome, both of which are implicated in autoimmune disease. Therapeutic carbohydrate restriction (TCR), on the other hand, shows promise for improving inflammation and the microbiome, as well as rheumatic and autoimmune conditions. As it relates to age associated declines, a well formulated TCR protocol naturally is animal nutrient-centric, which means it supplies sufficient protein, minerals, and fat-soluble vitamins to prevent or delay chronic conditions and bone and joint issues, when supplemented with exercise (which itself demonstrates similar preventative effects). TCR, in addition to metabolic improvement, has well-documented effects of improvement in age associated physiology, such as visceral adiposity, decline of cognition, bone mass, density, and muscle mass, and increased risk for chronic disease associated mortality. In this chapter the role of TCR as a promising supportive treatment for many rheumatic and autoimmune conditions, as well as age-related conditions is discussed.

7.2 Musculoskeletal conditions

Gary Fettke

7.2.1 Introduction

Our mobility is our freedom, our ability to survive and to source food to nourish our bodies.

The musculoskeletal system has dual purposes. The obvious reason is for structural stability, dexterity, and locomotion but it also has a significant metabolic role where the overall integrity is dependent on sound nutrition, mineral, and vitamin intake.

A deterioration in our musculoskeletal system is often observed in the form of pain, stiffness, or reduced function. It is one of the first parts of the body to respond to inappropriate load, activity, and inflammation. Deeper organs will continue their metabolic functions without giving specific warning signs until critical deterioration has occurred. The musculoskeletal system could be considered an early warning system.

The musculoskeletal system is affected by the complications of metabolic syndrome, obesity, inflammation and diabetes. Low carbohydrate healthy fat lifestyles such as a ketogenic diet (KD) show improvement and reversal of these background conditions, and as a result, dietary change should be considered as a first-line adjunctive management option [1–3]. A well-formulated nutritionally dense diet can have far-reaching effects on our musculoskeletal health.

7.2.2 Pathophysiology

Inflammation sits underneath virtually all pathological conditions and current evidence points towards a central role of nutrition in the inflammatory cascade [4]. The insulin-resistant (IR) state and metabolic syndrome promote inflammation and

Ketogenic. DOI: https://doi.org/10.1016/B978-0-12-821617-0.00004-8

immune dysregulation [5]. The excessive intake of carbohydrate, fructose and processed food, particularly high in polyunsaturated oils is an inflammatory diet resulting in inflammation in every blood vessel wall via insulin-mediated renin-angiotensin system (RAS), growth factors, cytokines, sympathetic nervous system (SNS), and C-reactive protein activation [6]. Every cell and mitochondrial membrane, and as a result, affects every organ in the body depending on its susceptibility [1–3,5,7–14].

Inflammation within tissue therefore will affect all tissues including joints, muscles, tendons as well as the soft tissues and nerves that run with them. The problems of excessive weight and diabetes upon these inflamed joints only compound the issue. The further observation is now of a society trying to outrun its bad diet by exercising to the extreme. This creates a further load on an already stressed musculoskeletal system.

Musculoskeletal injury is well noted in those individuals with diabetes [15]. The damage of chronic hyperglycaemia effectively stiffens the tissues affected, resulting in increased wear and degradation over time [16].

The Maillard reaction, the browning reaction seen when cooking at high heat, describes the binding reaction between glucose and proteins (protein glycosylation) to form advanced glycation end products (AGEs). With hyperglycaemia (e.g. in diabetes) comes an elevation in both blood glucose and tissue glucose. Under the effect of body heat, protein glycosylation occurs, resulting in soft tissue damage and vascular and neurological impairment. AGEs also further compound the chronic inflammatory state, which over time, results in tissue stiffness, scarring and dysregulation. All tissues are affected. Glycosylation is indirectly measured in the bloodstream erythrocytes with the HbA1c, but the major issue over time is the damage done within the tissues [10,16,17].

7.2.3 Clinical conditions

7.2.3.1 Osteoarthritis

At the joint level we have historically considered osteoarthritis to be a load-related condition, but it is increasingly being considered as an inflammatory arthritis. Inflammatory joint diseases such as rheumatoid arthritis, psoriatic arthritis, and lupus have their basis in inflammation and autoimmune disease. Reducing inflammation can be done with a variety of medications but the central role of nutrition has been overlooked for many decades. The emergence of TCR has seen transformational results in improving inflammatory and arthritis states, and often before weight loss [18–30].

The food we eat has an inflammatory potential and the response to that is critical. Emerging evidence is that joint inflammation is centrally tied to insulin load [20,23]. The consumption of carbohydrate provokes an insulin secretion by the pancreas and subsequent cascade of events. This includes not only the storage of excess carbohydrate intake as fat, but also insulin has a direct effect on the inflammation cascade as evidenced by synovial changes within the knee [20]. Insulin has also been shown to decrease human chondrocyte autophagy, thereby inhibiting cartilage formation and endochondral ossification, and thereby acting as another contributing factor to the development of osteoarthritis [23].

Significant reduction of carbohydrate intake is associated with a reduction in insulin secretion and immediate anti-inflammatory effect on joints [19]. This has been observed to result in pain reduction before significant weight loss in patients with osteoarthritis of the knee [19].

Reducing weight and load over time has secondary benefits for the musculoskeletal system. The knee has been studied more than most other joints. Two to three times the body weight goes through the knee in normal gait and six to eight times through the patellofemoral joint when going up and down stairs and arising from a chair. Reducing weight by at least 5% is associated with a significant improvement in functional outcome in osteoarthritis. That is increased significantly with 10% weight loss independent of age or severity of arthritis [23,27,29].

AGEs, which are related to long-term hyperglycaemia, accumulate in the cartilage of joints as well as in tendons and soft tissues. Their accumulation affects the elasticity of all those tissues and is associated with increased fatigue, wear and tear phenomena and then, symptomatic deterioration [27,31]. Reducing the hyperglycaemic state and elevated insulin concentrations over the long-term has clear implications for reducing AGEs accumulating in cartilage and tendons. Decreasing carbohydrate intake has the most immediate and effective benefit.

7.2.3.2 Osteoporosis

Osteoporosis is defined as the progressive loss of bone mineral content from the skeleton. Once a certain threshold is reached, which varies for age, the risk of pathological fractures increases. Osteopenia is the transitional state from normal bone to osteoporosis. Osteoporosis can be particularly debilitating with insufficiency fractures most commonly seen in the spine, hip and wrist. Modern society is plagued with a significant rate of osteoporosis [32]. Nutritional and vitamin deficiencies along with reduced activity being hallmark causes for the condition [33].

Our dietary guideline natural-fat-depleted diet of the last 40 years may have inadvertently led us to low intake of the fat-soluble vitamins A, D, E, K1, and K2. Those cultures that eat diets naturally high in dairy have lower rates of osteoporosis [34]. This has been traditionally considered as related to the calcium intake when it may be the vitamin K2 and fat intake that may have been the protective aspect.

There is increasing evidence that vitamin K2 may be the stabilising hormone, which moves calcium out of arterial walls and into bone. Vitamin K2 is naturally sourced from pasture fed meat, dairy and eggs as well as found in the Asian fermented soy product, natto [35,36]. Vitamin K2 has an anabolic effect on bone. It protects osteoblasts from apoptosis, stimulates osteocyte production, and inhibits osteoclasts from resorbing bone calcium matrix [35–40]. Vitamin K2 supplementation appears to be effective in the management of osteoporosis, particularly in combination with vitamin D – both of which are more readily available from a diet that includes pasture fed meat, dairy and eggs [38,41].

The state of nutritional ketosis or TCR does not appear to be detrimental to bone integrity. Well-formulated KD have not been associated with a deterioration in bone mineral density in observational studies out to 2 years [41–44].

Load-bearing exercise forms a central part of on-going management of osteoporosis, as does supplementation. The standards of supplementation have included calcium and vitamin D over a prolonged period but with increasing concern that they are not particularly effective [38] and at high doses, are associated with increased risks of cardiovascular disease [38]. This appears to be related to the deposition of calcification within the arterial wall [38].

The role of natural dietary fats and essential amino acids from proteins, with adequate exercise and sunlight and an appropriate intake of calcium, vitamin D, and vitamin K2 are protective against osteoporosis.

7.2.3.3 Gout

Elevated tissue and blood uric acid concentrations are associated with a condition called gout. The painful condition is caused by a precipitation of monosodium urate crystals within joints and soft tissues. There is an increasing incidence of gout in society over the last 20 years despite a reduction of meat and alcohol consumption. Uric acid is a by-product of fructose metabolism and part of the mechanistic damage done by fructose and its by-products [45]. An education towards a significant reduction of fructose intake, particularly sugar sweetened beverages, should be a primary intervention in the management of gout. A lower carbohydrate lifestyle reduces sugar and fructose intake directly reducing uric acid production [39,40,46–50]. See Chapter 7.3.

7.2.3.4 Tendinopathy

Tendon degeneration is generally considered as an ageing and overload process. Recent literature has seen the initial thoughts of chronic stress damage being replaced with a low-grade inflammatory response centred around by-products of excessive carbohydrate consumption. Biochemical studies have revealed the source of inflammation being associated with AGEs, glycosylated proteins and disruption of matrix metalloprotineases (MMPs) balance. These are the same processes that are occurring in the damage seen in articular cartilage of osteoarthritis [31,51–53].

The benefits of a lower carbohydrate lifestyle in tendinopathy are yet to be fully explored. There is anecdotal evidence which is yet to make it into the literature.

7.2.3.5 Pain

There is emerging evidence in the pain management field on the positive role of KDs for both acute and chronic pain issues [54,55].

7.2.3.6 Surgery

There are risks associated with obese and metabolically unwell individuals undergoing surgery. There are significant anaesthetic risks from ventilation, drug metabolism, and positional concerns [56,57]. Surgical approaches and incisions often need to be larger and are associated with the risks of operating through layers of poorly vascularised adipose tissue [58]. Surgical times are generally longer, particularly abdominal, and musculoskeletal surgery, and are associated with greater complication rates in both the short- and long-term [56,57].

Joint replacement surgery has been studied repeatedly, and there is clearly an increased risk of complications with longer surgical times, higher infection rates, longer hospitalisation and greater revision rates of surgery in those patients who are morbidly obese, particularly those who undergo knee replacement [59,60]. The complications and poorer outcomes of joint replacement surgery are only compounded in patients with obesity, particularly when diabetes is a comorbidity [60–65].

Patients regularly state that they are going to lose weight when they can exercise more following the surgery. This is a rare occurrence with only 23% of patients losing any weight in the post-operative period following knee replacement. Preoperative weight loss is a preferable pathway with delay of surgical intervention for many [60,62].

Sugar and carbohydrate intake are associated with poorer neutrophil function as well as T lymphocyte capacity [61,66]. A reduction of carbohydrate resulting in a ketogenic state is implicated in better immunity and outcome results [55,61,66,67]. The state of fasting improves white cell function [55,61,66,67].

7.2.3.7 Rheumatology

Rheumatology is the study of the changes, generally inflammatory and autoimmune, within soft tissues and the joints of the musculoskeletal system. Both inflammation and autoimmune disease can affect varying tissues with varying degrees at varying sites, but underlying all of that is a process of inflammation.

The patterns of involvement generally determine both the diagnosis and the management. For example, rheumatoid arthritis affects smaller joints more than larger ones. The traditional mainstays of medication therapy for rheumatological conditions include anti-inflammatories, corticosteroids, and anti-metabolites such as methotrexate, gold, and other disease-modifying anti-rheumatic drugs. Specific immunotherapies are now looking to target the autoimmune component of rheumatological conditions. Physical therapy has long been considered a management option, but there is now emerging evidence of the central role of diet as an adjunctive and first-line management [67–71].

IR, metabolic syndrome, and diabetes are associated with higher rates and poorer outcomes in those with rheumatoid arthritis. The benefits of a KD may be a promising adjunctive therapy and worth considering as an adjunctive option. Anecdotal claims are supported by experimental data [67–71].

7.2.3.8 Therapeutic intervention

The mainstay of musculoskeletal management is individual education on the central role of low carbohydrate or ketogenic eating patterns. Reducing sugar and carbohydrate consumption is an option for those who wish to choose it. The benefits are generally experienced within a few weeks.

Most patients understand the concept of sugar and carbohydrate ingestion provoking insulin secretion and the subsequent storage of excess as fat. Explaining the inflammatory effect of insulin allows them to take back control of their inflammation without drug intervention.

Patients who are compliant generally see an improvement in their symptoms prior to weight loss. Encouraging sound nutrition with resistance exercise, where possible, is effective without having to outrun a bad diet.

Shifting the concept from "I cannot exercise to lose weight" towards "controlling what you eat or don't eat" is an empowering moment for many patients.

With TCR as a first-line therapy for musculoskeletal conditions, monitoring the patient's outcome does not require significant investigation. Symptom severity, complemented by waist circumference and weight measurements, usually suffice. Blood investigations are generally part of a more systemic assessment.

7.2.4 Conclusion

A computer's safe mode can be used as an analogy for a state of ketosis. Traditionally, when we have been unwell, we are unable to move around, forage and eat. Our bodies move into a state of ketosis which is not only the safe mode, but also the reparative one.

The diet that has moved us into IR, metabolic syndrome, obesity, and diabetes, has been high in sugar, carbohydrates, and polyunsaturated oils. Reversing that to a low carbohydrate and ketogenic intake effectively allows the safe mode to operate and optimise bone and soft tissue health.

7.3 Gout

Gary Fettke

7.3.1 Introduction and description

Gout is the most common inflammatory arthritis disorder [72]. It is a debilitating and painful condition most often affecting the great toe (podagra) but can affect all joints, both large and small as well as the spine [73]. The effects are not just in the musculoskeletal system, as gout also affects the circulatory and renal systems [47,74].

7.3.2 Pathophysiology

Hyperuricaemia can result from an increase in uric acid production (high cellular turnover of DNA/RNA in cancer [75], psoriasis [76], protein [77], and fructose consumption [78]) or a decrease in urinary excretion (renal disease [79], alcohol [80], hyperinsulinaemia [81]), or a combination of both. Local precipitation of the uric acid as monosodium urate (MSU) crystals accounts for an acute inflammatory tissue response.

Comorbidities associated with gout include hypertension, diabetes mellitus, renal disease and morbid obesity [77].

There is a clear association of dietary intake, with a traditional understanding, that gout could be precipitated by high meat [82] and alcohol intakes [83] (purine pathways). However association studies are limited and may not account for other factors such as diet quality and metabolic health [84]. There is an increasing incidence of gout, particularly in developed nations [78], despite a move away from meat consumption in similar time frames [85]. A systematic review and meta-analysis from 2008 further support that alcohol and fructose may be greater contributors to hyperuricemia than meat consumption [82]. This increasing incidence of gout may be pathologically related to higher fructose consumption (fructose pathway) [47].

Fructose has uric acid as a byproduct of its metabolism [86]. Fructose induced hyperuricemia has a pathogenetic role in metabolic syndrome [78,87]. Higher insulin concentrations, associated with metabolic syndrome, reduce the renal excretion of uric acid [47,80,88]. Uric acid is an inhibitor of nitric oxide synthase, [78] which is the catalyst for nitric oxide, critical for circulatory and immune homeostasis.

Reducing circulating uric acid concentrations is one of the mechanistic components of improved blood pressure control that is observed with a reduction in fructose intake [89].

Uric acid precipitates out in affected tissue and joints as monosodium urate (MSU) crystals creating the painful symptomatic clinical condition.

The precipitation of MSU crystals in tissue is under the influence of the NLRP3 inflammasome [90]. The NLRP3 inflammasome has a central role in the inflammation cascade [91]. NLRP3 is inhibited by colchicine, a historic treatment for acute gout episodes. The same inhibitory effect has been observed with the ketone bodies β-hydroxybutyrate and acetoacetate [67].

7.3.2.1 Clinical presentation

Gout often presents as an acutely painful joint, commonly in the great toe (podagra), but all joints may be affected. There may or may not be a history of recurrent problems or dietary provocation. The subclinical picture may be a contributing factor to general malaise, hypertension, diabetes, obesity, and metabolic syndrome.

7.3.3 Managing the patient

7.3.3.1 Aims of care

The primary consideration in the presentation of an individual with an acutely painful joint is to exclude infection and trauma. Local examination may be difficult to differentiate as the joint is often swollen, very tender, and immobile. Plain X-rays may show evidence of gout, particularly with soft tissue calcification and periarticular erosions. A routine blood examination may reveal an elevated white cell count as well as elevated inflammatory markers (ESR and CRP). Serum uric acid concentrations are not definitive. The definitive diagnosis is from aspiration of joint fluid and imaging uric acid crystals by polarised light microscopy. Once confirmed as gout, there are pharmacotherapy and diet options to consider.

7.3.3.2 Pharmacotherapy

The treatment of gout involves acute and long-term management. Acute care includes traditional medications such as colchicine and non-steroidal anti-inflammatories and local splinting, rest, and ice. In a confirmed case of gout, there may be a role for intra-articular steroid injections. Uric acid lowering agents such as allopurinol may be used in addition. Allopurinol administration in an acute episode may exacerbate the immediate problem [92].

7.3.3.3 Diet

The fasting state promotes the production of ketones that are now recognised to have a mechanistic inhibitory effect via the NLRP3 inflammasome [90].

Longer-term management involves the avoidance of precipitating factors. A significant reduction in fructose load, both directly and indirectly via glucose intake and the polyol pathway, needs to be advised. The simple advice given over the last few decades to avoid meat has not been effective. Consumption of fructose and carbohydrate appears to have been the 'missing link'. Alcohol consumption is part of a greater lifestyle issue as it also raises serum uric acid and is an inhibitor of renal uric acid excretion [93].

7.3.4 Conclusion

The avoidance of carbohydrates and advantages of a nutritional ketotic state have a double benefit in the management of gout by reducing the production of uric acid and inhibiting the inflammatory response.

7.4 Ageing and therapeutic carbohydrate restriction

Bob Kaplan

7.4.1 Introduction

Ageing is associated with a number of physiological changes that can have an impact on nutritional needs. In women, menopause marks the end of a woman's reproductive years and can also have nutritional implications. Likewise, in many men (and women), andropause, or age-related testosterone deficiency, may influence nutritional demands. On average, there is a decline in muscle mass (i.e. sarcopenia) of 3%–8% per decade after age 30, and the rate of decline increases after the age of 60 [94]. During the same time, body fat increases, bone mass and density declines (i.e. osteoporosis), and these tissue changes are associated with an increased incidence of insulin resistance (IR) [95]. Both sarcopenia and osteoporosis contribute to an increased risk of debilitating falls and fractures. Ageing is claimed to be the major risk factor for death from all adult chronic diseases. From the age of 65, the four leading causes of death (cardiovascular disease (CVD, heart disease, and stroke), cancer, chronic lower respiratory disease, and Alzheimer disease (AD)) account for nearly 70% of all deaths, and the mortality rate for all of these diseases increases exponentially with age [96].

Research suggests that poor health does not have to be an inevitable consequence of ageing. An essential component of keeping older adults healthy is preventing or delaying chronic conditions and reducing associated complications. Diet quality plays an important role in physical condition, metabolism, vascular function, cognition, bone health, and the immune system. Therefore, improving the diet may be one of the most effective strategies for living better, longer. TCR dietary-related interventions have been shown to effectively treat all of the features of metabolic syndrome (MetS) (i.e. IR) and type 2 diabetes (T2D), two conditions that may be the central features that increase the risk for chronic diseases with the highest morbidity and mortality rates for aging adults [97].

7.4.2 Pathophysiology

7.4.2.1 Menopause and andropause

Menopause is the time in a woman's life when her menstrual cycle ends, defined as the point in time 12 months after a woman's last period. During the transition to menopause, an estimated 85% of women report at least one symptom, such as hot flushes, sleep disruption, or depressed mood [98]. These symptoms are generally a result of a decline in the production of the sex hormones oestrogen, progesterone, and testosterone. Menopause is associated with a decrease in bone density [99], cognitive impairment [100], osteoporosis [99], IR [39,40], increased fat accumulation [101], sarcopenia [101,102], and increased visceral fat accumulation [103]. Andropause is a term used to describe hormonal changes that happen to men as they age, and the symptoms are generally due to particularly low testosterone concentrations [104]. While menopause occurs in all women at a particular age, not all men experience andropause, and the age of onset is more varied. Many of the symptoms and associated conditions in menopause are observed in andropause: decreased bone density, increased fat accumulation, decreased skeletal muscle mass, and increased visceral fat accumulation [105,106]. Importantly, women also experience a decline in testosterone concentrations with age. After completion of menopause, average concentrations of testosterone are approximately 15% of premenopause concentrations [106]. For many women and men, menopause and andropause may increase the risk of sarcopenia, osteoporosis, and IR.

7.4.2.2 Sarcopenia and osteoporosis

Sarcopenia is typically defined as a progressive and age-related loss of muscle mass and function. The estimated prevalence in 60–70-year-old individuals is 5%–13% and increases to 11%–50% in people over 80 years of age [107]. Sarcopenia is associated with obesity, inflammation, IR, a drop in testosterone and oestrogen concentrations, and chronic diseases like T2D and CVD [108]. Osteoporosis is characterised by decreased bone mass and increased risk of fractures [109]. The first 20–30 years of life are spent building up the bones in our skeleton, then bone mass and density decline at a gradual rate, as much as 1% per year [110]. The lifetime risk of osteoporosis is 40%–50% among women and 13%–22% among men, contributing to the risk of fractures and falls [111]. Osteoporosis and sarcopenia often coexist in older populations [112], which is associated with a higher risk of frailty [113] and mortality [114] compared to having one of the conditions alone.

7.4.2.3 Common causes of death, chronic conditions, and comorbidities

The most common causes of death among US adults aged 65 or older include CVD, cancer, chronic lower respiratory disease, AD, diabetes, and accidents (of which falls are the leading cause) [115]. Almost 90% of older adults have one chronic condition, and about 65% of all older adults have two or more conditions [116]. Common chronic conditions include the causes of death listed above in addition to inflammatory joint disorders, hypertension, obesity, and dyslipidaemia. Strikingly, nearly 98% of older American adults with T2D have at least one comorbid condition, and nearly 90% have two comorbidities [117].

7.4.3 Managing the patient

7.4.3.1 Preventing or delaying sarcopenia

TCR—Preventing sarcopenia involves eating enough protein and performing resistance exercises to maintain or build skeletal muscle, but there is also evidence suggesting TCR preserves more muscle mass compared to other diets, especially during weight loss [118], which may help counteract sarcopenia.

Protein—Nutritional interventions using protein supplementation, especially when combined with resistance training, have been shown to oppose the effects of sarcopenia in older adults [119,120]. Older adults are less sensitive to the stimulatory effects of protein on muscle protein synthesis [121]. In older adults, compared to consumption of 20 g of protein, eating 35 and 40 g protein stimulates muscle protein synthesis to a greater extent at rest [121] and following exercise [122], respectively, and protein intakes of 1–1.5 g/kg of body weight per day are recommended for this population [123].

Exercise—Evidence that muscle loss as we age can be reduced (or even reversed) is found in dozens of randomised-controlled trials and meta-analyses showing resistance training helps older individuals increase muscle mass and strength [124–126]. A relatively higher protein diet from high-quality sources (i.e. animal-based protein and supplemental whey protein) combined with consistent resistance training may be the most effective strategy to offset sarcopenia.

Vitamins and minerals—Vitamin D appears to play an important role in reducing the risk of sarcopenia. Supplementing with vitamin D is associated with an increase in testosterone production and improves sarcopenia outcomes, particularly in women [127,128]. Sunlight is the predominant source of vitamin D, and sunlight also stimulates nitric oxide production [129]. Low concentrations of nitric oxide, also influenced by IR, may contribute to sarcopenia by impairing muscle protein synthesis [130]. Minerals such as calcium, magnesium, and selenium may also play a role in the prevention of sarcopenia [131].

7.4.3.2 Preventing or delaying osteoporosis

TCR—Eating foods rich in protein, fat-soluble vitamins, and minerals including calcium and magnesium can help protect bones throughout the life cycle.

Protein—Higher consumption of protein is associated with higher bone mineral density and a reduced risk of fractures in older adults [132]. Observational studies find that the greater the consumption of animal protein, the greater the associated increase in bone mineral density in elderly women [133] and that older men with the lowest protein intakes are associated with the greatest bone loss [134].

Exercise—Weight-bearing and resistance exercise increases lean muscle mass and bone density [135,136]. Weight-bearing activities add more bone during youth and prevent bone-resorbing cells from removing bone during ageing [110]. Resistance exercise has been shown to improve bone density in older adults [137–140], including women with low to very low bone mass [141]. Therefore, weight-bearing exercise throughout the life cycle may help combat osteoporosis.

Vitamins and minerals—Adequate intake of calcium, magnesium, zinc, and vitamins A, B12, D, and K may reduce fracture risk and reduce the risk of osteoporosis [142,143].

7.4.3.3 *Preventing or delaying chronic conditions and promoting a healthy lifespan*

TCR may help reduce the risk of the many chronic diseases that disproportionately affect the elderly. MetS (or IR) may be at the root of many chronic diseases, associated with less healthy ageing [144], and the leading causes of death in older adults. It's associated with T2D [145], CVD and hypertension [146], cancer [147], stroke [148], and AD [149]. Studies have shown that TCR improves all the features of MetS [150–152] and results in the reversal and remission of T2D [41]. It stands to reason that a diet that can reverse the features of MetS and T2D may also reduce the risk of the many chronic diseases associated with them. In addition, TCR reduces insulin concentrations and somatotropic signalling [153], which delays ageing and extends health span and lifespan in many species including rodents [154], and is associated with increased longevity in humans [155]. Taken together, TCR, providing adequate high-quality protein, vitamin and minerals, in addition to consistent weight-bearing activity, may help slow the rate of loss of physiological integrity and function that accompanies ageing [156], prevent morbidity and mortality related to physical decline, and prevent or delay chronic diseases, thus promoting a healthy lifespan into old age.

7.5 Autoimmunity

7.5.1 Autoimmunity and therapeutic carbohydrate restriction

Sarah M. Rice

7.5.1.1 *Introduction*

Though it is difficult to determine the exact cause of autoimmune disorders [157], several lines of evidence suggest nutrition and metabolic health are important, potentially modifiable, components. In metabolic syndrome and obesity, adipose tissue can modulate the immune response and the gut microbiome [158,159]. A bidirectional relationship between adipocytes and the gut microbiome influences the homeostasis of the innate and adaptive immune systems [159]. Autoimmune inflammation in adipose tissue, via T-cell priming, may cause altered antigen recognition and creation of autoantibodies [160]. Microbiome dysbiosis, genetics, and environmental exposures can also play a role in the development of autoimmunity [161]. Although there are many contributing factors [157] the impact of the Western diet on the microbiome, inflammation, and autoimmune conditions is well established [162,163]. As such, the removal of processed foods and a reduced carbohydrate approach may be expected to show benefit [164–167].

7.5.1.2 *Gut dysbiosis and autoimmunity*

Gut dysbiosis occurs when local homeostasis is disrupted via disrupted host-commensal relationships that include a decrease in beneficial (commensal) bacteria, an increase in harmful (opportunistic) bacteria, and reduced diversity or combinations of these (see Chapter 8). Any number of factors may contribute to dysbiosis including diet, toxins, drugs, and pathogens including viruses, bacteria and fungi [161]. Dysbiosis has been linked to specific gut disorders including autoimmune conditions such as inflammatory bowel disease (IBD) and coeliac disease, as well as irritable bowel syndrome (IBS) [157]. Altered gut homeostasis that reduces levels of butyrate-producing bacteria contributes to the development of gut permeability whereby intestinal epithelial integrity is compromised [168,169]. This loss of gut barrier function promotes an inflammatory state (modulated T reg response), which further contributes to increased permeability and can allow bacterial products like lipopolysaccharide (LPS), antigens, and toxins in the gastrointestinal tract to enter the bloodstream, leading to inappropriate antigen presentation and immune activation [160,169]. This can influence innate and adaptive immune responses, which may lead to failure of tolerance and autoimmune conditions [157,160,161,170,171]. A TCR approach has been shown to modify the microbiome beneficially, and as such, may be expected to attenuate autoimmunity in this way [172–175].

7.5.1.3 *Metabolic health and autoimmunity*

Autoimmune diseases have features in common, which can include MetS [176–179] and vitamin D deficiency [180,181], reflecting a role for screening for these in this population. The existence of vitamin D receptor (VDR) polymorphisms present in a proportion of the autoimmune population [182,183] is of interest and the role of supplements has been explored [181], though there are confounding factors [182]. One factor may be that insulin resistance can contribute to vitamin D deficiency and attenuate VDR gene expression, exacerbating any genetic predisposition to hypovitaminosis D [184]. Association of MetS with vitamin D deficiency is well documented [185]. Evidence supports TCR as one intervention for treating MetS and the pre-diabetes spectrum [186–189] (See Chapter 3.1. Metabolic Syndrome), and has also been shown to improve vitamin D levels in a type 2 diabetes (T2D) study [190]. TCR thus may be expected to offer some health benefit in those at risk of or suffering from autoimmunity.

7.5.1.4 Studies involving autoimmune conditions where therapeutic carbohydrate restriction has shown promise

Interest in and evidence for the application of TCR to autoimmune diseases are emerging. Autoimmune and gastrointestinal conditions may benefit from exclusion protocols that include zero carbohydrates [191–193].

The following list reflects an example of autoimmune conditions (or autoimmune components) where a nutritional intervention on the TCR spectrum has shown promise (includes fasting-mimicking, ketogenic, specific carbohydrate, zero carbohydrate, and other exclusion diets). This area is in its infancy and more high-quality trials are needed.

- Type 1 diabetes—may prolong honeymoon period [194,195] and improved BG control [196–198]
- Coeliac disease [199,200]
- Crohn's disease [192,193,201] and other inflammatory bowel diseases [164,202,203]
- Rheumatoid arthritis [204–206], ankylosing spondylitis [207–209], and other arthritis [210]
- Psoriasis [211–213]
- Hashimoto thyroiditis [166,214]
- Multiple sclerosis [173,215,216]
- Inclusion body myositis [217]

These observations are supported by review papers that indicate potential benefits of TCR spectrum approach in autoimmune conditions [167,218]. TCR, via various mechanisms, has demonstrated potential in neurological [219,220] and inflammatory [205,210,221] conditions that also support the use of this approach in the autoimmune patient.

7.5.1.5 Other lifestyle interventions

Other considerations in the management of autoimmune conditions include fasting [167,204,222–226], exercise [227], circadian rhythm [228], and stress reduction [229].

7.5.2 Conclusion

While individual responses will vary and the interplay between environment, genetics and other factors will influence outcomes, TCR is emerging as a promising intervention for a range of chronic conditions that include autoimmune disorders.

7.6 Perspective: autoimmunity in the context of plant and animal nutrition

Shawn Baker

7.6.1 Introduction

The prevalence of autoimmune diseases, like almost all other modern chronic diseases, has risen significantly. There are hundreds of named diseases that fall into this class with more being recognised each year. Rheumatoid arthritis, psoriasis, ulcerative colitis, Hashimotos' thyroiditis are but a few of the better known ones. Many autoimmune diseases are now treated with corticosteroids or expensive, side effect-prone immune-modulating medications, which often provide little benefit and tend to lose efficacy with time, as the underlying issues are not addressed. The importance of determining and addressing the causes of autoimmune diseases and their increasing prevalence cannot be underestimated.

7.6.1.1 Hypothesis: an evolutionarily inconsistent diet

The name itself, autoimmune disease, indicates some sort of problem with our immune system. However their origins are usually unknown (idiopathic), or put down to a special genetic susceptibility, leaving sufferers with no hope of a cure. Perhaps we just haven't considered some potentially obvious possibilities. Do we really think that some drastic shift in the human genome has occurred within the last 50–100 years that could account for this new increase in autoimmune disease? How about an alternative hypothesis? What if a chronic mismatch between what we eat and what we are best designed to eat ultimately leads to the expression of these diseases?

While our skin acts to protect our inner workings by excluding most of what we come into contact with, our gastrointestinal tract is designed to absorb. Our gut is where a huge portion of our immune system resides, and it is the primary interface between the external environment and our inner anatomy. It is at this interface that we are perhaps most susceptible. Researchers such as Alessio Fasano from Massachusetts General have put forth some interesting data around the associations between compromised gut permeability and the subsequent development of autoimmune diseases [230].

Most plants in the environment are acutely toxic to humans if we attempt to ingest them, making us sick or causing significant gastrointestinal upset [231,232]. Some are deadly [233]. Now of course, humans have been eating a myriad of plants for thousands if not millions of years to some degree, but most of those plants had to be carefully cultivated and required special preparation to reduce toxicity to prevent acute illness [234].

Foods that have been accepted into the human diet have generally not undergone rigorous testing to ensure the safety of the substance on long term human health [235]. In 1990, researcher Bruce Ames showed that naturally occurring pesticides produced by plants represent greater than 99% of all pesticides we generally consume [236]. Additionally, most of them have been identified as carcinogenic in animal studies depending upon dosages.

7.6.1.2 *Early evidence*

If indeed disruptions in gut permeability are the primary event in leading to autoimmune disease progression, how would we go about testing this? Let us suppose a group of people diagnosed with autoimmune disease were to alter their diet in a significant way and then subsequently no longer have the symptoms of autoimmune disease? What if this pattern were to happen to hundreds of people? What if this dietary pattern was one in which plants were excluded? Yes, even healthy fruits, vegetables, and whole grains. Interestingly, it just so turns out that an ever- growing population of people doing just that are now seeing all sorts of autoimmune diseases going into remission. They are coming off all medications and seeing clinically verifiable reversal of their disease states. Think of someone with ulcerative colitis with endoscopy proven disappearance of their disease despite having thrown away all expensive biological medication.

These things are happening and they are being seen more and more frequently within a community of people that have adopted fully meat-based diets. An informal survey of 11,000 of these community members (500 of which had an autoimmune disease) showed that reduction in autoimmune symptoms (Fig. 7.1) and medication (Fig. 7.2) correlated closely with time and increasing adherence to a strict meat-based diet.

These positive results have also been reflected in published survey studies [237,238]. Could it be that for some reason individual tolerance to certain toxic compounds found in plants varies, having a slow but steady deleterious effect on gut health in the vulnerable? [230–232].

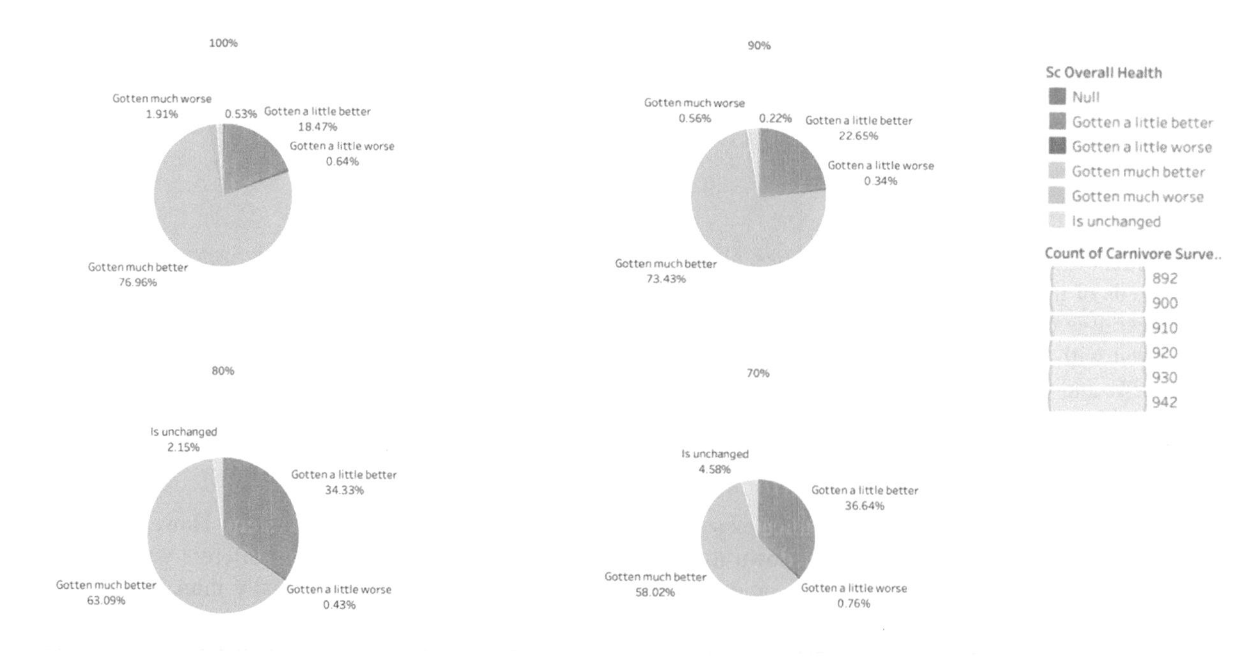

FIGURE 7.1 Autoimmune symptom relief (%) for various degrees of adherence (%) to a meat-based diet.

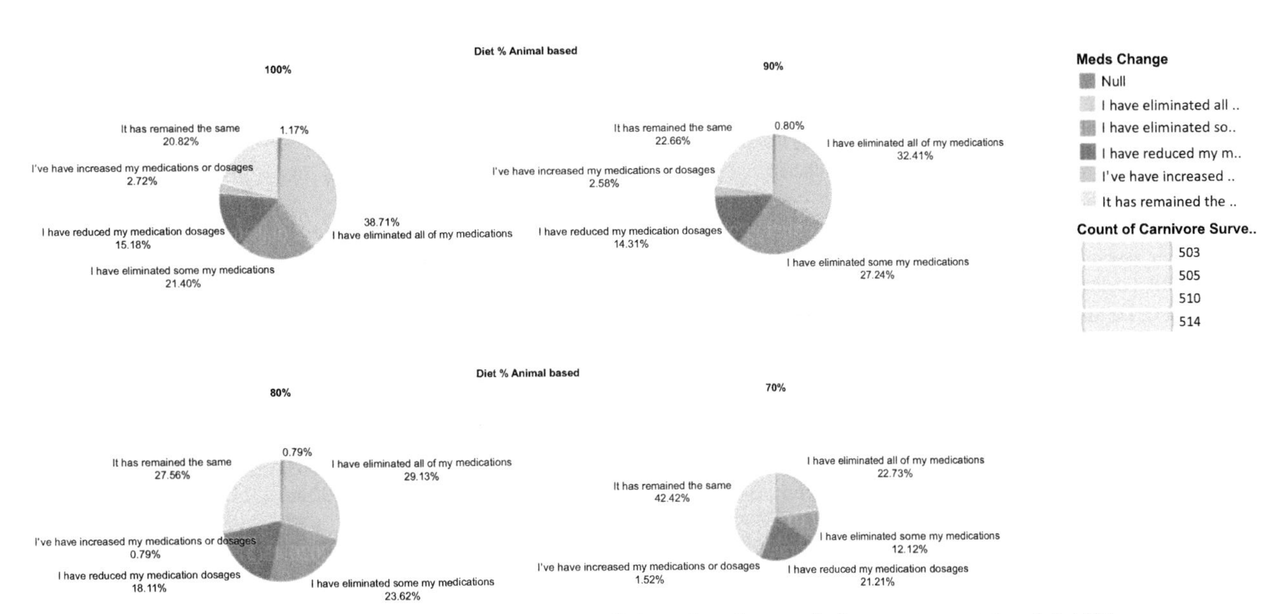

FIGURE 7.2 Reduction or elimination of autoimmune medications (%) for various degrees of adherence to a meat-based diet (%).

Hungarian researchers Csaba Tóth and Sofia Clemens have explored a meat-based dietary approach in their clinic, publishing a number of case studies [195,239,240]. Their data indicate a connection between the removal of plants from the diet, improvements in gut barrier function and subsequent reversal of clinical and laboratory signs of autoimmune disease.

7.6.2 Conclusion

Between Tóth and Clemens' case studies and unpublished community survey results, it appears that a population of hundreds with supposedly lifelong incurable autoimmune diseases, potentially related to compromised gut function, suddenly experienced a reversal of those diseases by eliminating foods that trigger a pathological response. This deserves rigorous study and further exploration. Conflicts of interest and dogmatic beliefs regarding nutrition need to be set aside, so that scientific questioning is encouraged and observations can be explored and verified.

References

[1] Choi YJ, Jeon SM, Shin S. Impact of a ketogenic diet on metabolic parameters in patients with obesity or overweight and with or without type 2 diabetes: a meta-analysis of randomized controlled trials. Nutrients 2020;12(7):2005. Available from: https://doi.org/10.3390/nu12072005.

[2] Myette-Côté É, Durrer C, Neudorf H, Bammert TD, Botezelli JD, Johnson JD, et al. The effect of a short-term low-carbohydrate, high-fat diet with or without postmeal walks on glycemic control and inflammation in type 2 diabetes: a randomized trial. Am J Physiol Regul Integr Comp Physiol 2018;315(6):R1210–19. Available from: https://doi.org/10.1152/ajpregu.00240.2018.

[3] Hallberg SJ, McKenzie AL, Williams PT, Bhanpuri NH, Peters AL, Campbell WW, et al. Effectiveness and safety of a novel care model for the management of type 2 diabetes at 1 year: an open-label, non-randomized, controlled study. Diabetes Therapy 2018;9(2):583–612. Available from: https://doi.org/10.1007/s13300-018-0373-9.

[4] Kiecolt-Glaser JK. Stress, food, and inflammation: psychoneuroimmunology and nutrition at the cutting edge. Psychosom Med 2010;72(4):365.

[5] Forsythe CE, Phinney SD, Fernandez ML, Quann EE, Wood RJ, Bibus DM, et al. Comparison of low fat and low carbohydrate diets on circulating fatty acid composition and markers of inflammation. Lipids 2008;43(1):65–77. Available from: https://doi.org/10.1007/s11745-007-3132-7.

[6] Kopp W. The atherogenic potential of dietary carbohydrate. Preventive Med 2006;42(5):336–42.

[7] Koletzko B. Human milk lipids. Ann Nutr & Metab 2016;69(Suppl 2):28–40. Available from: https://doi.org/10.1159/000452819.

[8] Lim JS, Mietus-Snyder M, Valente A, Schwarz JM, Lustig RH. The role of fructose in the pathogenesis of NAFLD and the metabolic syndrome. Nat Rev Gastroenterol Hepatol 2010;7(5):251–64. Available from: https://doi.org/10.1038/nrgastro.2010.41.

[9] Softic S, Cohen DE, Kahn CR. Role of dietary fructose and hepatic de novo lipogenesis in fatty liver disease. Digestive Dis Sci 2016;61(5):1282–93. Available from: https://doi.org/10.1007/s10620-016-4054-0.

[10] Thorpe SR, Baynes JW. Role of the Maillard reaction in diabetes mellitus and diseases of aging. Drugs Aging 1996;9(2):69–77. Available from: https://doi.org/10.2165/00002512-199609020-00001.

[11] Zhou L, Zhu DY. Neuronal nitric oxide synthase: structure, subcellular localization, regulation, and clinical implications. Nitric Oxide 2009;20 (4):223–30. Available from: https://doi.org/10.1016/j.niox.2009.03.001.

[12] DiNicolantonio JJ, O'Keefe JH. Omega-6 vegetable oils as a driver of coronary heart disease: the oxidized linoleic acid hypothesis. Open Heart 2018;5(2):e000898. Available from: https://doi.org/10.1136/openhrt-2018-000898.

[13] Giacco F, Brownlee M. Oxidative stress and diabetic complications. Circulation Res 2010;107(9):1058–70. Available from: https://doi.org/10.1161/CIRCRESAHA.110.223545.

[14] Gross LS, Li L, Ford ES, Liu S. Increased consumption of refined carbohydrates and the epidemic of type 2 diabetes in the United States: an ecologic assessment. Am J Clin Nutr 2004;79(5):774–9. Available from: https://doi.org/10.1093/ajcn/79.5.774.

[15] Kim RP, Edelman SV, Kim DD. Musculoskeletal complications of diabetes mellitus. Clin Diabetes 2001;19(3):132–5.

[16] Vistoli G, De Maddis D, Cipak A, Zarkovic N, Carini M, Aldini G. Advanced glycoxidation and lipoxidation end products (AGEs and ALEs): an overview of their mechanisms of formation. Free Radic Res 2013;47(Suppl 1):3–27. Available from: https://doi.org/10.3109/10715762.2013.815348.

[17] Vlassara H, Palace MR. Glycoxidation: the menace of diabetes and aging. Mt Sinai J Medicine, N Y 2003;70(4):232–41.

[18] Kluzek S, Newton JL, Arden NK. Is osteoarthritis a metabolic disorder? Br Med Bull 2015;115(1):111–21. Available from: https://doi.org/10.1093/bmb/ldv028.

[19] Monira Hussain S, Wang Y, Cicuttini FM, Simpson JA, Giles GG, Graves S, et al. Incidence of total knee and hip replacement for osteoarthritis in relation to the metabolic syndrome and its components: a prospective cohort study. Semin Arthritis Rheum 2014;43(4):429–36. Available from: https://doi.org/10.1016/j.semarthrit.2013.07.013.

[20] Qiao L, Li Y, Sun S. Insulin exacerbates inflammation in fibroblast-like synoviocytes. Inflammation 2020;43(3):916–36. Available from: https://doi.org/10.1007/s10753-020-01178-0.

[21] Rai MF, Sandell LJ. Inflammatory mediators: tracing links between obesity and osteoarthritis. Crit Rev Eukaryot Gene Expr 2011;21 (2):131–42. Available from: https://doi.org/10.1615/critreveukargeneexpr.v21.i2.30.

[22] Ribeiro M, López de Figueroa P, Blanco FJ, Mendes AF, Caramés B. Insulin decreases autophagy and leads to cartilage degradation. Osteoarthr Cartil 2016;24(4):731–9. Available from: https://doi.org/10.1016/j.joca.2015.10.017.

[23] Strath LJ, Jones CD, Philip George A, Lukens SL, Morrison SA, Soleymani T, et al. The effect of low-carbohydrate and low-fat diets on pain in individuals with knee osteoarthritis. Pain Med 2020;21(1):150–60. Available from: https://doi.org/10.1093/pm/pnz022.

[24] Berenbaum F, Eymard F, Houard X. Osteoarthritis, inflammation and obesity. Curr Opin Rheumatol 2013;25(1):114–18. Available from: https://doi.org/10.1097/BOR.0b013e32835a9414.

[25] Wang T, He C. Pro-inflammatory cytokines: the link between obesity and osteoarthritis. Cytokine Growth Factor Rev 2018;44:38–50. Available from: https://doi.org/10.1016/j.cytogfr.2018.10.002.

[26] Zhuo Q, Yang W, Chen J, Wang Y. Metabolic syndrome meets osteoarthritis. Nat Rev Rheumatol 2012;8(12):729–37. Available from: https://doi.org/10.1038/nrrheum.2012.135.

[27] Christensen R, Bartels EM, Astrup A, Bliddal H. Effect of weight reduction in obese patients diagnosed with knee osteoarthritis: a systematic review and meta-analysis. Ann Rheumatic Dis 2007;66(4):433–9. Available from: https://doi.org/10.1136/ard.2006.065904.

[28] Griffin TM, Scanzello CR. Innate inflammation and synovial macrophages in osteoarthritis pathophysiology. Clin Exp Rheumatol 2019;37 (5):57–63 *Suppl 120*.

[29] Gudbergsen H, Boesen M, Lohmander LS, Christensen R, Henriksen M, Bartels EM, et al. Weight loss is effective for symptomatic relief in obese subjects with knee osteoarthritis independently of joint damage severity assessed by high-field MRI and radiography. Osteoarthr Cartil 2012;20(6):495–502. Available from: https://doi.org/10.1016/j.joca.2012.02.639.

[30] Han D, Fang Y, Tan X, Jiang H, Gong X, Wang X, et al. The emerging role of fibroblast-like synoviocytes-mediated synovitis in osteoarthritis: an update. J Cell Mol Med 2020;. Available from: https://doi.org/10.1111/jcmm.15669 10.1111/jcmm.15669. Advance online publication.

[31] Rees JD, Stride M, Scott A. Tendons–time to revisit inflammation. Br J Sports Med 2014;48(21):1553–7. Available from: https://doi.org/10.1136/bjsports-2012-091957.

[32] Tatangelo G, et al. The cost of osteoporosis, osteopenia, and associated fractures in australia in 2017. J Bone Min Res 2019;34(4):616–25. Available from: https://doi.org/10.1002/jbmr.3640.

[33] NIH Consensus Development Panel on Osteoporosis Prevention, Diagnosis, and Therapy. Osteoporosis prevention, diagnosis, and therapy. JAMA 2001;285(6):785–95. Available from: https://doi.org/10.1001/jama.285.6.785.

[34] Hidayat K, et al. Systematic review and meta-analysis of the association between dairy consumption and the risk of hip fracture: critical interpretation of the currently available evidence. Osteoporos Int 2020;31(8):1411–25. Available from: https://doi.org/10.1007/s00198-020-05383-3.

[35] Myneni VD, Mezey E. Regulation of bone remodeling by vitamin K2. Oral Dis 2017;23(8):1021–8. Available from: https://doi.org/10.1111/odi.12624.

[36] Akbari S, Rasouli-Ghahroudi AA. Vitamin K and bone metabolism: a review of the latest evidence in preclinical studies. BioMed Res Int 2018;2018:4629383. Available from: https://doi.org/10.1155/2018/4629383.

[37] Saito E, Wachi H, Sato F, Sugitani H, Seyama Y. Treatment with vitamin k(2) combined with bisphosphonates synergistically inhibits calcification in cultured smooth muscle cells. J Atheroscler Thromb 2007;14(6):317–24. Available from: https://doi.org/10.5551/jat.e501.

[38] Villa J, Diaz M, Pizziolo VR, Martino H. Effect of vitamin K in bone metabolism and vascular calcification: A review of mechanisms of action and evidences. Crit Rev Food Sci Nutr 2017;57(18):3959–70. Available from: https://doi.org/10.1080/10408398.2016.1211616.

[39] Yan B, Liu D, Zhu J, Pang X. The effects of hyperuricemia on the differentiation and proliferation of osteoblasts and vascular smooth muscle cells are implicated in the elevated risk of osteopenia and vascular calcification in gout: An in vivo and in vitro analysis. J Cell Biochem 2019;120(12):19660–72. Available from: https://doi.org/10.1002/jcb.29272.

[40] Yan H, Yang W, Zhou F, Li X, Pan Q, Shen Z, et al. Estrogen improves insulin sensitivity and suppresses gluconeogenesis via the transcription factor Foxo1. Diabetes 2019;68:291–304.

[41] Athinarayanan SJ, Adams RN, Hallberg SJ, McKenzie AL, Bhanpuri NH, Campbell WW, et al. Long-term effects of a novel continuous remote care intervention including nutritional ketosis for the management of type 2 diabetes: a 2-year non-randomized clinical trial. Front Endocrinol (Lausanne) 2019;10:348. Available from: https://doi.org/10.3389/fendo.2019.00348.

[42] Krebs NF, Gao D, Gralla J, Collins JS, Johnson SL. Efficacy and safety of a high protein, low carbohydrate diet for weight loss in severely obese adolescents. J Pediatr 2010;157(2):252–8. Available from: https://doi.org/10.1016/j.jpeds.2010.02.010.

[43] Brinkworth GD, Wycherley TP, Noakes M, Buckley JD, Clifton PM. Long-term effects of a very-low-carbohydrate weight-loss diet and an iso-caloric low-fat diet on bone health in obese adults. Nutr (Burbank, Los Angeles County, Calif) 2016;32(9):1033–6. Available from: https://doi.org/10.1016/j.nut.2016.03.003.

[44] Foster GD, Wyatt HR, Hill JO, Makris AP, Rosenbaum DL, Brill C, et al. Weight and metabolic outcomes after 2 years on a low-carbohydrate versus low-fat diet: a randomized trial. Ann Intern Med 2010;153(3):147–57. Available from: https://doi.org/10.7326/0003-4819-153-3-201008030-00005.

[45] Caliceti C, et al. Fructose intake, serum uric acid, and cardiometabolic disorders: a critical review. Nutrients 2017;9(4):395. Available from: https://doi.org/10.3390/nu9040395.

[46] Ayoub-Charette S, Liu Q, Khan TA, Au-Yeung F, Blanco Mejia S, de Souza RJ, et al. Important food sources of fructose-containing sugars and incident gout: a systematic review and meta-analysis of prospective cohort studies. BMJ Open 2019;9(5):e024171. Available from: https://doi.org/10.1136/bmjopen-2018-024171.

[47] Rho YH, Zhu Y, Choi HK. The epidemiology of uric acid and fructose. Semnephrology 2011;31(5):410–19. Available from: https://doi.org/10.1016/j.semnephrol.2011.08.004.

[48] Choi HK, Curhan G. Soft drinks, fructose consumption, and the risk of gout in men: prospective cohort study. BMJ (Clin Res) 2008;336 (7639):309–12. Available from: https://doi.org/10.1136/bmj.39449.819271.BE.

[49] Ebrahimpour-Koujan S, Saneei P, Larijani B, Esmaillzadeh A. Consumption of sugar sweetened beverages and dietary fructose in relation to risk of gout and hyperuricemia: a systematic review and meta-analysis. Crit Rev Food Sci Nutr 2020;60(1):1–10. Available from: https://doi.org/10.1080/10408398.2018.1503155.

[50] Jamnik J, Rehman S, Blanco Mejia S, de Souza RJ, Khan TA, Leiter LA, et al. Fructose intake and risk of gout and hyperuricemia: a systematic review and meta-analysis of prospective cohort studies. BMJ Open 2016;6(10):e013191. Available from: https://doi.org/10.1136/bmjopen-2016-013191.

[51] Longo UG, Franceschi F, Ruzzini L, Spiezia F, Maffulli N, Denaro V. Higher fasting plasma glucose levels within the normoglycaemic range and rotator cuff tears. Br J Sports Med 2009;43(4):284–7. Available from: https://doi.org/10.1136/bjsm.2008.049320.

[52] Yang L, Zhang J, Ruan D, Zhao K, Chen X, Shen W. Clinical and structural outcomes after rotator cuff repair in patients with diabetes: a meta-analysis. Orthopaedic J Sports Med 2020;. Available from: https://doi.org/10.1177/2325967120948499.

[53] Fox AJ, Bedi A, Deng XH, Ying L, Harris PE, Warren RF, et al. Diabetes mellitus alters the mechanical properties of the native tendon in an experimental rat model. J Orthop Res 2011;29(6):880–5. Available from: https://doi.org/10.1002/jor.21327.

[54] Masino SA, Ruskin DN. Ketogenic diets and pain. J Child Neurol 2013;28(8):993–1001. Available from: https://doi.org/10.1177/0883073813487595.

[55] Goldberg EL, Molony RD, Kudo E, Sidorov S, Kong Y, Dixit VD, et al. Ketogenic diet activates protective γδ T cell responses against influenza virus infection. Sci Immunol 2019;4(41):eaav2026. Available from: https://doi.org/10.1126/sciimmunol.aav2026.

[56] Ball L, Hemmes S, Serpa Neto A, Bluth T, Canet J, Hiesmayr M, et al. Intraoperative ventilation settings and their associations with postoperative pulmonary complications in obese patients LAS VEGAS investigators, PROVE Network, & Clinical Trial Network of the European Society of AnaesthesiologyBr J Anaesth 2018;121(4):899–908. Available from: https://doi.org/10.1016/j.bja.2018.04.021.

[57] Bazurro S, Ball L, Pelosi P. Perioperative management of obese patient. Curr Opin Crit care 2018;24(6):560–7. Available from: https://doi.org/10.1097/MCC.0000000000000555.

[58] Pierpont YN, et al. Obesity and surgical wound healing: a current review. ISRN Obes 2014;2014:638936. Available from: https://doi.org/10.1155/2014/638936.

[59] Smith WA, Zucker-Levin A, Mihalko WM, Williams M, Loftin M, Gurney JG. A randomized study of exercise and fitness trackers in obese patients after total knee arthroplasty. Orthopedic Clin North Am 2019;50(1):35–45. Available from: https://doi.org/10.1016/j.ocl.2018.08.002.

[60] Smith WA, Zucker-Levin A, Mihalko WM, Williams M, Loftin M, Gurney JG. Physical function and physical activity in obese adults after total knee arthroplasty. Orthopedic Clin North Am 2017;48(2):117–25. Available from: https://doi.org/10.1016/j.ocl.2016.12.002.

[61] Phagocytosis and fasting - Sanchez A, Reeser JL, Lau HS, Yahiku PY, Willard RE, McMillan PJ, et al. Role of sugars in human neutrophilic phagocytosis. Am J Clin Nutr 1973;26(11):1180–4. Available from: https://doi.org/10.1093/ajcn/26.11.1180.

[62] Rodriguez-Merchan EC. Review article: outcome of total knee arthroplasty in obese patients. J Orthopaedic Surg (Hong Kong) 2015;23 (1):107–10. Available from: https://doi.org/10.1177/230949901502300124.

[63] Sun K, Li H. Body mass index as a predictor of outcome in total knee replace: a systemic review and meta-analysis. Knee 2017;24(5):917–24. Available from: https://doi.org/10.1016/j.knee.2017.05.022.

[64] Yeung E, Jackson M, Sexton S, Walter W, Zicat B, Walter W. The effect of obesity on the outcome of hip and knee arthroplasty. Int Orthop 2011;35(6):929–34. Available from: https://doi.org/10.1007/s00264-010-1051-3.

[65] Deakin AH, Iyayi-Igbinovia A, Love GJ. A comparison of outcomes in morbidly obese, obese and non-obese patients undergoing primary total knee and total hip arthroplasty. Surgeon 2018;16(1):40–5. Available from: https://doi.org/10.1016/j.surge.2016.10.005.

[66] Shodja MM, Knutsen R, Cao J, Oda K, Beeson LE, Fraser GE, et al. Effects of glycosylated hemoglobin levels on neutrophilic phagocytic functions. Jacobs J Diab Endocrinol 2017;8(2):9–16. Available from: https://doi.org/10.5897/JDE2017.0110.

[67] Youm YH, Nguyen KY, Grant RW, Goldberg EL, Bodogai M, Kim D, et al. The ketone metabolite β-hydroxybutyrate blocks NLRP3 inflammasome-mediated inflammatory disease. Nat Med 2015;21(3):263–9. Available from: https://doi.org/10.1038/nm.3804.

[68] Kornberg MD. The immunologic Warburg effect: evidence and therapeutic opportunities in autoimmunity. Wiley Interdiscip Rev Syst Biol Med 2020;12(5):e1486. Available from: https://doi.org/10.1002/wsbm.1486 Advance online publication.

[69] Nicolau J, Lequerré T, Bacquet H, Vittecoq O. Rheumatoid arthritis, insulin resistance, and diabetes. J Bone Spine 2017;84(4):411–16. Available from: https://doi.org/10.1016/j.jbspin.2016.09.001.

[70] Castañeda S, Remuzgo-Martínez S, López-Mejías R, Genre F, Calvo-Alén J, Llorente I, et al. Rapid beneficial effect of the IL-6 receptor blockade on insulin resistance and insulin sensitivity in non-diabetic patients with rheumatoid arthritis. Clin Exp Rheumatol 2019;37(3):465–73.

[71] Garcia-Carbonell R, Divakaruni AS, Lodi A, Vicente-Suarez I, Saha A, Cheroutre H, et al. Critical role of glucose metabolism in rheumatoid arthritis fibroblast-like synoviocytes. Arthritis Rheumatol 2016;68(7):1614–26. Available from: https://doi.org/10.1002/art.39608.

[72] Dehlin M, Jacobsson L, Roddy E. Global epidemiology of gout: prevalence, incidence, treatment patterns and risk factors. Nat Rev Rheumatol 2020;16:380–90. Available from: https://doi.org/10.1038/s41584-020-0441-1.

[73] Toprover M, Krasnokutsky S, Pillinger MH. Gout in the spine: imaging, diagnosis, and outcomes. Curr Rheumatol Rep 2015;17(12):70. Available from: https://doi.org/10.1007/s11926-015-0547-7.

[74] Gibson TJ. Hypertension, its treatment, hyperuricaemia and gout. Curr Opin Rheumatol 2013;25(2):217–22. Available from: https://doi.org/10.1097/BOR.0b013e32835cedd4.

[75] Ribeiro RC, Pui CH. Hyperuricemia in patients with cancer. Am J Cancer 2002;1:409–22. Available from: https://doi.org/10.2165/00024669-200201060-00004.

[76] Hu SC, Lin CL, Tu HP. Association between psoriasis, psoriatic arthritis and gout: a nationwide population-based study. J Eur Acad Dermatol Venereol 2019;33(3):560–7. Available from: https://doi.org/10.1111/jdv.15290.

[77] Li C, Hsieh MC, Chang SJ. Metabolic syndrome, diabetes, and hyperuricemia. Curr Opin Rheumatol 2013;25(2):210–16. Available from: https://doi.org/10.1097/BOR.0b013e32835d951e.

[78] Elfishawi MM, Zleik N, Kvrgic Z, Michet Jr CJ, Crowson CS, Matteson EL, et al. The rising incidence of gout and the increasing burden of comorbidities: a population-based study over 20 years. J Rheumatol 2018;45(4):574–9. Available from: https://doi.org/10.3899/jrheum.170806.

[79] Ter Maaten JC, Voorburg A, Heine RJ, Ter Wee PM, Donker AJ, Gans RO. Renal handling of urate and sodium during acute physiological hyperinsulinaemia in healthy subjects. Clin Sci 1997;92(1):51–8. Available from: https://doi.org/10.1042/cs0920051.

[80] de Oliveira EP, Burini RC. High plasma uric acid concentration: causes and consequences. Diabetol Metab Syndr 2012;4(1):12.

[81] Muscelli E, Natali A, Bianchi S, Bigazzi R, Galvan AQ, Sironi AM, et al. Effect of insulin on renal sodium and uric acid handling in essential hypertension. Am J Hypertens 1996;9(8):746–52. Available from: https://doi.org/10.1016/0895-7061(96)00098-2.

[82] Choi HK, Atkinson K, Karlson EW, Willett W, Curhan G. Purine-rich foods, dairy and protein intake, and the risk of gout in men. N Engl J Med 2004;350(11):1093–103. Available from: https://doi.org/10.1056/NEJMoa035700.

[83] Li R, Yu K, Li C. Dietary factors and risk of gout and hyperuricemia: a meta-analysis and systematic review. Asia Pac J Clin Nutr 2018;27(6):1344–56. Available from: https://doi.org/10.6133/apjcn.201811_27(6)0.0022.

[84] Yu KH, See LC, Huang YC, Yang CH, Sun JH. Dietary factors associated with hyperuricemia in adults. Semin Arthritis Rheum 2008;37(4):243–50. Available from: https://doi.org/10.1016/j.semarthrit.2007.04.007 Epub 2007 Jun 14. PMID: 17570471.

[85] United States Department of Agriculture. U.S. consumption of grains and protein foods were above recommendations in 2014. Economic Research Service. 2017. Retrieved 2022, from https://www.ers.usda.gov/webdocs/charts/84067/july17_finding_bentley_fig02.png?v = 42913

[86] Tappy L, Lê KA. Metabolic effects of fructose and the worldwide increase in obesity. Physiological Rev 2010;90(1):23–46. Available from: https://doi.org/10.1152/physrev.00019.2009.

[87] Nakagawa T, Hu H, Zharikov S, Tuttle KR, Short RA, Glushakova O, et al. A causal role for uric acid in fructose-induced metabolic syndrome. Am J Physiol Ren Physiol 2006;290(3):F625–31. Available from: https://doi.org/10.1152/ajprenal.00140.2005.

[88] Facchini F, Chen YD, Hollenbeck CB, Reaven GM. Relationship between resistance to insulin-mediated glucose uptake, urinary uric acid clearance, and plasma uric acid concentration. JAMA 1991;266(21):3008–11.

[89] Sanchez-Lozada LG, Rodriguez-Iturbe B, Kelley EE, Nakagawa T, Madero M, Feig DI, et al. Uric acid and hypertension: an update with recommendations. Am J Hypertens 2020;33(7):583–94. Available from: https://doi.org/10.1093/ajh/hpaa044.

[90] Kingsbury SR, Conaghan PG, McDermott MF. The role of the NLRP3 inflammasome in gout. J Inflamm Res 2011;4:39–49. Available from: https://doi.org/10.2147/JIR.S11330.

[91] Kelley N, Jeltema D, Duan Y, He Y. The NLRP3 inflammasome: an overview of mechanisms of activation and regulation. Int J Mol Sci 2019;20(13):3328. Available from: https://doi.org/10.3390/ijms20133328.

[92] Satpanich P, Pongsittisak W, Manavathongchai S. Early versus late allopurinol initiation in acute gout flare (ELAG): a randomized controlled trial. Clin Rheumatol 2022;41:213–21. Available from: https://doi.org/10.1007/s10067-021-05872-8.

[93] Yamamoto T, Moriwaki Y, Takahashi S. Effect of ethanol on metabolism of purine bases (hypoxanthine, xanthine, and uric acid). Clinica Chimica Acta 2005;356(1–2):35–57. Available from: https://doi.org/10.1016/j.cccn.2005.01.024.

[94] Holloszy JO. The biology of aging. Mayo Clin Proc 2000;75(Suppl):S3–8 discussion S8–9.

[95] Volpi E, Nazemi R, Fujita S. Muscle tissue changes with aging. Curr Opin Clin Nutr Metab Care 2004;7:405–10.

[96] Ferrucci L, Giallauria F, Guralnik JM. Epidemiology of aging. Radiol Clin North Am 2008;46 643–v.

[97] Facchini FS, Hua N, Abbasi F, Reaven GM. Insulin resistance as a predictor of age-related diseases. J Clin Endocrinol Metab 2001;86:3574–8.
[98] McKinlay SM, Brambilla DJ, Posner JG. The normal menopause transition. Maturitas 1992;14:103–15.
[99] Finkelstein JS, Brockwell SE, Mehta V, Greendale GA, Sowers MR, Ettinger B, et al. Bone mineral density changes during the menopause transition in a multiethnic cohort of women. J Clin Endocrinol Metab 2008;93:861–8.
[100] Kim SA, Jung H. Prevention of cognitive impairment in the midlife women. J Menopausal Med 2015;21:19–23.
[101] Greendale GA, Sternfeld B, Huang M, Han W, Karvonen-Gutierrez C, Ruppert K, et al. Changes in body composition and weight during the menopause transition. JCI Insight 2019;4.
[102] Sørensen MB. Changes in body composition at menopause–age, lifestyle or hormone deficiency? J Br Menopause Soc 2002;8:137–40.
[103] Davis SR, Castelo-Branco C, Chedraui P, Lumsden MA, Nappi RE, Shah D, et al. Understanding weight gain at menopause and Day 2012, as the W.G. of the I.M.S. for W.M. Climacteric 2012;15:419–29.
[104] Wu FCW, Tajar A, Pye SR, Silman AJ, Finn JD, O'Neill TW, et al. Hypothalamic-pituitary-testicular axis disruptions in older men are differentially linked to age and modifiable risk factors: the European male aging study. J Clin Endocrinol Metab 2008;93:2737–45.
[105] Allan CA, Strauss BJG, McLachlan RI. Body composition, metabolic syndrome and testosterone in ageing men. Int J Impot Res 2007;19:448–57.
[106] Horstman AM, Dillon EL, Urban RJ, Sheffield-Moore M. The Role of androgens and estrogens on healthy aging and longevity. J Gerontol A Biol Sci Med Sci 2012;67:1140–52.
[107] Cruz-Jentoft AJ, Baeyens JP, Bauer JM, Boirie Y, Cederholm T, Landi F, et al. Sarcopenia: European consensus on definition and diagnosis: report of the European working group on sarcopenia in older people. Age Ageing 2010;39:412–23.
[108] Hong S, Choi KM. Sarcopenic obesity, insulin resistance, and their implications in cardiovascular and metabolic consequences. Int J Mol Sci 2020;21.
[109] Golob AL, Laya MB. Osteoporosis: screening, prevention, and management. Med Clin North Am 2015;99:587–606.
[110] Pearson OM, Lieberman DE. The aging of Wolff's "law": Ontogeny and responses to mechanical loading in cortical bone. Am J Phys Anthropol 2004;125:63–99.
[111] Johnell O, Kanis J. Epidemiology of osteoporotic fractures. Osteoporos Int 2005;16(Suppl 2):S3–7.
[112] Nielsen BR, Abdulla J, Andersen HE, Schwarz P, Suetta C. Sarcopenia and osteoporosis in older people: a systematic review and meta-analysis. Eur Geriatr Med 2018;9:419–34.
[113] Wang Y-J, Wang Y, Zhan J-K, Tang Z-Y, He J-Y, Tan P, et al. Sarco-Osteoporosis: prevalence and association with frailty in chinese community-dwelling older adults. Int J Endocrinol 2015;2015.
[114] Yoo J-I, Kim H, Ha Y-C, Kwon H-B, Koo K-H. Osteosarcopenia in patients with hip fracture is related with high mortality. J Korean Med Sci 2018;33.
[115] Heron M.. Deaths: leading causes for 2018 (CDC), 2021.
[116] Boersma P. Prevalence of multiple chronic conditions among US adults, 2018. Prev Chronic Dis 2020;17.
[117] Iglay K, Hannachi H, Joseph Howie P, Xu J, Li X, Engel SS, et al. Prevalence and co-prevalence of comorbidities among patients with type 2 diabetes mellitus. Curr Med Res Opin 2016;32:1243–52.
[118] Manninen AH. Very-low-carbohydrate diets and preservation of muscle mass. Nutr Metab 2006;3:9.
[119] Phillips SM. Nutritional supplements in support of resistance exercise to counter age-related sarcopenia. Adv Nutr 2015;6:452–60.
[120] Devries MC, Phillips SM. Supplemental protein in support of muscle mass and health: advantage whey. J Food Sci 2015;80:A8–15.
[121] Pennings B, Groen B, de Lange A, Gijsen AP, Zorenc AH, Senden JMG, et al. Amino acid absorption and subsequent muscle protein accretion following graded intakes of whey protein in elderly men. Am J Physiol Endocrinol Metab 2012;302:E992–9.
[122] Yang Y, Breen L, Burd NA, Hector AJ, Churchward-Venne TA, Josse AR, et al. Resistance exercise enhances myofibrillar protein synthesis with graded intakes of whey protein in older men. Br J Nutr 2012;108:1780–8.
[123] Bauer J, Biolo G, Cederholm T, Cesari M, Cruz-Jentoft AJ, Morley JE, et al. Evidence-based recommendations for optimal dietary protein intake in older people: a position paper from the PROT-AGE study group. J Am Med Dir Assoc 2013;14:542–59.
[124] Lozano-Montoya I, Correa-Pérez A, Abraha I, Soiza RL, Cherubini A, O'Mahony D, et al. Nonpharmacological interventions to treat physical frailty and sarcopenia in older patients: a systematic overview – the SENATOR Project ONTOP Series. Clin Interv Aging 2017;12:721–40.
[125] Peterson MD, Sen A, Gordon PM. Influence of resistance exercise on lean body mass in aging adults: a meta-analysis. Med Sci Sports Exerc 2011;43:249–58.
[126] Beaudart C, Dawson A, Shaw SC, Harvey NC, Kanis JA, Binkley N, et al. Nutrition and physical activity in the prevention and treatment of sarcopenia: systematic review. Osteoporos Int 2017;28:1817–33.
[127] Oh C, Jeon BH, Reid Storm SN, Jho S, No J-K. The most effective factors to offset sarcopenia and obesity in the older Korean: Physical activity, vitamin D, and protein intake. Nutrition 2017;33:169–73.
[128] Park S, Ham J-O, Lee B-K. A positive association of vitamin D deficiency and sarcopenia in 50 year old women, but not men. Clin Nutr Edinb Scotl 2014;33:900–5.
[129] Weller RB. Sunlight has cardiovascular benefits independently of vitamin D. Blood Purif 2016;41:130–4.
[130] Marcell TJ. Review article: sarcopenia: causes, consequences, and preventions. J Gerontol Ser A 2003;58:M911–16.

[131] van Dronkelaar C, Velzen A, van, Abdelrazek M, Steen A, van der, Weijs PJM, Tieland M. Minerals and sarcopenia; the role of calcium, iron, magnesium, phosphorus, potassium, selenium, sodium, and zinc on muscle mass, muscle strength, and physical performance in older adults: a systematic review. J Am Med Dir Assoc 2018;19(6–11):e3.
[132] Weaver AA, Tooze JA, Cauley JA, Bauer DC, Tylavsky FA, Kritchevsky SB, et al. Effect of dietary protein intake on bone mineral density and fracture incidence in older adults in the health, aging, and body composition study. J Gerontol Ser A 2021;.
[133] Promislow JHE, Goodman-Gruen D, Slymen DJ, Barrett-Connor E. Protein consumption and bone mineral density in the elderly: the Rancho Bernardo Study. Am J Epidemiol 2002;155:636–44.
[134] Hannan MT, Tucker KL, Dawson-Hughes B, Cupples LA, Felson DT, Kiel DP. Effect of dietary protein on bone loss in elderly men and women: the Framingham osteoporosis study. J Bone Min Res J Am Soc Bone Min Res 2000;15:2504–12.
[135] Fiatarone MA, Marks EC, Ryan ND, Meredith CN, Lipsitz LA, Evans WJ. High-intensity strength training in nonagenarians. Eff Skelet muscle JAMA 1990;263:3029–34.
[136] American College of Sports Medicine, Chodzko-Zajko WJ, Proctor DN, Fiatarone Singh MA, Minson CT, Nigg CR, et al. American College of Sports Medicine position stand. Exercise and physical activity for older adults. Med Sci Sports Exerc 2009;41:1510–30.
[137] Nelson ME, Fiatarone MA, Morganti CM, Trice I, Greenberg RA, Evans WJ. Effects of high-intensity strength training on multiple risk factors for osteoporotic fractures: a randomized controlled trial. JAMA 1994;272:1909–14.
[138] Whiteford J, Ackland TR, Dhaliwal SS, James AP, Woodhouse JJ, Price R, et al. Effects of a 1-year randomized controlled trial of resistance training on lower limb bone and muscle structure and function in older men. Osteoporos Int 2010;21:1529–36.
[139] Bolam KA, van Uffelen JGZ, Taaffe DR. The effect of physical exercise on bone density in middle-aged and older men: A systematic review. Osteoporos Int 2013;24:2749–62.
[140] Huovinen V, Ivaska KK, Kiviranta R, Bucci M, Lipponen H, Sandboge S, et al. Bone mineral density is increased after a 16-week resistance training intervention in elderly women with decreased muscle strength. Eur J Endocrinol 2016;175:571–82.
[141] Watson SL, Weeks BK, Weis LJ, Horan SA, Beck BR. Heavy resistance training is safe and improves bone, function, and stature in postmenopausal women with low to very low bone mass: novel early findings from the LIFTMOR trial. Osteoporos Int 2015;26:2889–94.
[142] Kitchin B, Morgan SL. Not just calcium and vitamin D: other nutritional considerations in osteoporosis. Curr Rheumatol Rep 2007;9:85–92.
[143] Nieves JW. Calcium, vitamin D, and nutrition in elderly adults. Clin Geriatr Med 2003;19:321–35.
[144] Lin Y-H, Chiou J-M, Chen T-F, Lai L-C, Chen J-H, Chen Y-C. The association between metabolic syndrome and successful aging- using an extended definition of successful aging. PLoS One 2021;16:e0260550.
[145] Shin J, Lee J, Lim S, Ha H, Kwon H, Park Y, et al. Metabolic syndrome as a predictor of type 2 diabetes, and its clinical interpretations and usefulness. J Diabetes Investig 2013;4:334–43.
[146] Ginsberg HN. Insulin resistance and cardiovascular disease. J Clin Invest 2000;106:453–8.
[147] Arcidiacono B, Iiritano S, Nocera A, Possidente K, Nevolo MT, Ventura V, et al. Insulin resistance and cancer risk: an overview of the pathogenetic mechanisms. Exp Diabetes Res 2012;2012:e789174.
[148] Rundek T, Gardener H, Xu Q, Goldberg RB, Wright CB, Boden-Albala B, et al. Insulin resistance and risk of ischemic stroke among nondiabetic individuals from the northern Manhattan study. Arch Neurol 2010;67:1195–200.
[149] Watson GS, Craft S. The role of insulin resistance in the pathogenesis of Alzheimer's disease: implications for treatment. CNS Drugs 2003;17:27–45.
[150] Accurso A, Bernstein RK, Dahlqvist A, Draznin B, Feinman RD, Fine EJ, et al. Dietary carbohydrate restriction in type 2 diabetes mellitus and metabolic syndrome: time for a critical appraisal. Nutr Metab 2008;5:9.
[151] Volek JS, Feinman RD. Carbohydrate restriction improves the features of metabolic syndrome. Metabolic syndrome may be defined by the response to carbohydrate restriction. Nutr Metab 2005;2:31.
[152] Volek JS, Phinney SD, Forsythe CE, Quann EE, Wood RJ, Puglisi MJ, et al. Carbohydrate restriction has a more favorable impact on the metabolic syndrome than a low fat diet. Lipids 2009;44:297–309.
[153] Brown-Borg HM. Disentangling high fat, low carb, and healthy aging. Cell Metab 2017;26:458–9.
[154] Brown-Borg HM. The somatotropic axis and longevity in mice. Am J Physiol Endocrinol Metab 2015;309:E503–10.
[155] Milman S, Huffman DM, Barzilai N. The somatotropic axis in human aging: framework for the current state of knowledge and future research. Cell Metab 2016;23:980–9.
[156] López-Otín C, Blasco MA, Partridge L, Serrano M, Kroemer G. The hallmarks of aging. Cell 2013;153:1194–217.
[157] Forbes JD, Van Domselaar G, Bernstein CN. The gut microbiota in immune-mediated inflammatory diseases. Front Microbiol [Internet] 2016;7. Available from: https://www.frontiersin.org/article/10.3389/fmicb.2016.01081.
[158] Awan NM, Meurling IJ, O'Shea D. Understanding obesity: the role of adipose tissue microenvironment and the gut microbiome. Saudi J Med & Med Sci 2021;9(1):10.
[159] Khan S, Luck H, Winer S, Winer DA. Emerging concepts in intestinal immune control of obesity-related metabolic disease. Nat Commun 2021;12(1):2598.
[160] Petrelli A, Giovenzana A, Insalaco V, Phillips BE, Pietropaolo M, Giannoukakis N. Autoimmune inflammation and insulin resistance: hallmarks so far and yet so close to explain diabetes endotypes. Curr Diabetes Rep [Internet] 2021;21(12). Available from: https://www.ncbi.nlm.nih.gov/labs/pmc/articles/PMC8668851/.
[161] Luca FD, Shoenfeld Y. The microbiome in autoimmune diseases. Clin Exp Immunology 2019;195(1):74.

[162] Manzel A, Muller DN, Hafler DA, Erdman SE, Linker RA, Kleinewietfeld M. Role of "western diet" in inflammatory autoimmune diseases. Curr Allergy Asthma Rep 2013;14(1):404.

[163] Zinöcker MK, Lindseth IA. The western diet–microbiome-host interaction and its role in metabolic disease. Nutrients. 2018;10(3):365.

[164] Konijeti GG, Kim N, Lewis JD, Groven S, Chandrasekaran A, Grandhe S, et al. Efficacy of the autoimmune protocol diet for inflammatory bowel disease. Inflamm Bowel Dis 2017;23(11):2054.

[165] Kornberg MD. The immunologic Warburg effect: evidence and therapeutic opportunities in autoimmunity. WIREs Syst Biol Med 2020;e1486.

[166] Krysiak R, Szkróbka W, Okopień B. The effect of gluten-free diet on thyroid autoimmunity in drug-naïve women with Hashimoto's thyroiditis: a pilot study. Exp Clin Endocrinol Diabetes 2019;127(07):417–22.

[167] Choi IY, Lee C, Longo VD. Nutrition and fasting mimicking diets in the prevention and treatment of autoimmune diseases and immunosenescence. Mol Cell Endocrinol 2017;455:4–12 Nov 5.

[168] Saad MJA, Santos A, Prada PO. Linking gut microbiota and inflammation to obesity and insulin resistance. Physiology. 2016;31(4):283–93.

[169] Hills RD, Pontefract BA, Mishcon HR, Black CA, Sutton SC, Theberge CR. Gut microbiome: profound implications for diet and disease. Nutrients. 2019;11(7):1613.

[170] Clemente JC, Manasson J, Scher JU. State of the art review: the role of the gut microbiome in systemic inflammatory disease. BMJ [Internet] 2018;360. Available from: https://www.ncbi.nlm.nih.gov/labs/pmc/articles/PMC6889978/.

[171] Jiao Y, Wu L, Huntington ND, Zhang X. Crosstalk between gut microbiota and innate immunity and its implication in autoimmune diseases. Front Immunol [Internet] 2020;11. Available from: https://www.ncbi.nlm.nih.gov/labs/pmc/articles/PMC7047319/.

[172] Ren M, Zhang H, Qi J, Hu A, Jiang Q, Hou Y, et al. An almond-based low carbohydrate diet improves depression and glycometabolism in patients with type 2 diabetes through modulating gut microbiota and glp-1: a randomized controlled trial. Nutrients [Internet] 2020;12(10). Available from: https://www.ncbi.nlm.nih.gov/pmc/articles/PMC7601479/.

[173] Swidsinski A, Dörffel Y, Loening-Baucke V, Gille C, Göktas Ö, Reißhauer A, et al. Reduced mass and diversity of the colonic microbiome in patients with multiple sclerosis and their improvement with ketogenic diet. Front Microbiol [Internet] 2017;8. Available from: https://www.ncbi.nlm.nih.gov/pmc/articles/PMC5488402/.

[174] Xie G, Zhou Q, Qiu CZ, Dai WK, Wang HP, Li YH, et al. Ketogenic diet poses a significant effect on imbalanced gut microbiota in infants with refractory epilepsy. World J Gastroenterology 2017;23(33):6164.

[175] Yu D, Xie L, Chen W, Qin J, Zhang J, Lei M, et al. Dynamics of the gut bacteria and fungi accompanying low-carbohydrate diet-induced weight loss in overweight and obese adults. Front Nutr 2022;9:846378.

[176] Saroli Palumbo C, Restellini S, Chao CY, Aruljothy A, Lemieux C, Wild G, et al. Screening for nonalcoholic fatty liver disease in inflammatory bowel diseases: a cohort study using transient elastography. Inflamm Bowel Dis 2019;25(1):124–33.

[177] Ünlü B, Türsen Ü. Autoimmune skin diseases and the metabolic syndrome. Clin Dermatol 2018;36(1):67–71.

[178] Yamamoto EA, Jørgensen TN. Relationships between vitamin d, gut microbiome, and systemic autoimmunity. Front Immunology [Internet] 2019;10. Available from: https://www.ncbi.nlm.nih.gov/labs/pmc/articles/PMC6985452/.

[179] Caso F, Chimenti MS, Navarini L, Ruscitti P, Peluso R, Girolimetto N, et al. Metabolic syndrome and psoriatic arthritis: considerations for the clinician. Expert Rev Clin Immunol 2020; Mar 9.

[180] Murdaca G, Tonacci A, Negrini S, Greco M, Borro M, Puppo F, et al. Emerging role of vitamin D in autoimmune diseases: an update on evidence and therapeutic implications. Autoimmun Rev 2019;18(9):102350.

[181] Yang CY, Leung PSC, Adamopoulos IE, Gershwin ME. The implication of Vitamin D and autoimmunity: a comprehensive review. Clin Rev Allergy Immunol 2013;45(2):217–26.

[182] Bizzaro G, Antico A, Fortunato A, Bizzaro N. Vitamin D and autoimmune diseases: is vitamin D receptor (VDR) polymorphism the culprit? Isr Med Assoc J 2017;19:438–43.

[183] Dankers W, Colin EM, van Hamburg JP, Lubberts E. Vitamin D in autoimmunity: molecular mechanisms and therapeutic potential. Front Immunol 2017;7:697.

[184] Trimarco V, Manzi MV, Mancusi C, Strisciuglio T, Fucile I, Fiordelisi A, et al. Insulin resistance and vitamin D deficiency: a link beyond the appearances. Front Cardiovascular Med [Internet] 2022;9. Available from: https://www.frontiersin.org/articles/10.3389/fcvm.2022.859793.

[185] Strange RC, Shipman KE, Ramachandran S. Metabolic syndrome: a review of the role of vitamin D in mediating susceptibility and outcome. World J Diabetes 2015;6(7):896–911.

[186] McKenzie A, Athinarayanan S, Adams R, Hallberg S, Volek J, Phinney SD. Predictors of normalization of fasting glucose in patients with prediabetes using remote continuous care emphasizing low carbohydrate intake. J Endocr Soc 2021;5(Suppl 1):A323.

[187] McKenzie AL, Athinarayanan SJ, McCue JJ, Adams RN, Keyes M, McCarter JP, et al. Type 2 Diabetes prevention focused on normalization of glycemia: a two-year pilot study. Nutrients. 2021;13(3):749.

[188] Stentz FB, Brewer A, Wan J, Garber C, Daniels B, Sands C, et al. Remission of pre-diabetes to normal glucose tolerance in obese adults with high protein versus high carbohydrate diet: randomized control trial. BMJ Open Diabetes Res Care [Internet] 2016;4(1). Available from: https://www.ncbi.nlm.nih.gov/pmc/articles/PMC5093372/.

[189] Ismael SA. Effects of low carbohydrate diet compared to low fat diet on reversing the metabolic syndrome, using NCEP ATP III criteria: a randomized clinical trial. BMC Nutr 2021;7(1):62.

[190] Almsaid H, Muhsin H. The effect of ketogenic diet on vitamin D3 and testosterone hormone in patients with diabetes mellitus type 2. Curr Issues Pharm Med Sci 2021;33:202–5 Feb 19.

[191] Martin P, Johansson M, Ek A. A zero carbohydrate, carnivore diet can normalize hydrogen positive small intestinal bacterial overgrowth lactulose breath tests: a case report. Research Square 2021;. Available from: https://www.researchsquare.com/article/rs-148500/v1.

[192] Arjomand A, Suskind DL. Clinical and histologic remission in an adult Crohn's disease patient following the specific carbohydrate diet and its impact on healthcare costs. Cureus [Internet] 2022;14(2). Available from: https://www.cureus.com/articles/81257-clinical-and-histologic-remission-in-an-adult-crohns-disease-patient-following-the-specific-carbohydrate-diet-and-its-impact-on-healthcare-costs.

[193] Mehrtash F. Sustained Crohn's disease remission with an exclusive elemental and exclusion diet: a case report. Gastrointest Disord 2021;3 (3):129–37.

[194] Thewjitcharoen Y, Wanothayaroj E, Jaita H, Nakasatien S, Butadej S, Khurana I, et al. Prolonged honeymoon period in a thai patient with adult-onset type 1 diabetes mellitus. Case Rep Endocrinol 2021;2021:e3511281 Sep 2.

[195] Tóth C, Clemens Z. Type 1 diabetes mellitus successfully managed with the paleolithic ketogenic diet. Int J Case Rep Images 2014;5. Available from: https://doi.org/10.5348/ijcri-2014124-CR-10435.

[196] Krebs JD, Parry Strong A, Cresswell P, Reynolds AN, Hanna A, Haeusler S. A randomised trial of the feasibility of a low carbohydrate diet vs standard carbohydrate counting in adults with type 1 diabetes taking body weight into account. Asia Pac J Clin Nutr 2016;25(1):78–84.

[197] Lehmann V, Zueger T, Zeder A, Scott S, Bally L, Laimer M, et al. Lower daily carbohydrate intake is associated with improved glycemic control in adults with type 1 diabetes using a hybrid closed-loop system. Diabetes Care [Internet] 2020;. Available from: https://care.diabetesjournals.org/content/early/2020/09/29/dc20-1560.

[198] Nielsen JV, Gando C, Joensson E, Paulsson C. Low carbohydrate diet in type 1 diabetes, long-term improvement and adherence: a clinical audit. Diabetol Metab Syndr 2012;4(1):23.

[199] Reddel S, Putignani L, Del Chierico F. The impact of Low-FODMAPs, gluten-free, and ketogenic diets on gut microbiota modulation in pathological conditions. Nutrients. 2019;11(2).

[200] Roncoroni L, Bascuñán KA, Doneda L, Scricciolo A, Lombardo V, Branchi F, et al. A low FODMAP gluten-free diet improves functional gastrointestinal disorders and overall mental health of celiac disease patients: a randomized controlled trial. Nutrients [Internet] 2018;10(8). Available from: https://www.ncbi.nlm.nih.gov/pmc/articles/PMC6115770/.

[201] Suskind DL, Lee D, Kim YM, Wahbeh G, Singh N, Braly K, et al. The specific carbohydrate diet and diet modification as induction therapy for pediatric crohn's disease: a randomized diet controlled trial. Nutrients. 2020;12(12):3749.

[202] Norwitz NG, Loh V. A standard lipid panel is insufficient for the care of a patient on a high-fat, low-carbohydrate ketogenic diet. Front Med [Internet] 2020;7. Available from: https://www.frontiersin.org/articles/10.3389/fmed.2020.00097/full?&utm_source = Email_to_authors_&utm_medium = Email&utm_content = T1_11.5e1_author&utm_campaign = Email_publication&field&journalName = Frontiers_in_Medicine&id = 528189&fbclid = IwAR1JWAlCSjLv7GmrD_23h0fJOJ5mbqbQlYsRCEhWY-FTF0m1d-iAEr0tkeQ.

[203] Kakodkar S, Mutlu EA. Diet as a therapeutic option for adult inflammatory bowel disease. Gastroenterol Clin North Am 2017;46(4):745–67.

[204] Venetsanopoulou AI, Voulgari PV, Drosos AA. Fasting mimicking diets: a literature review of their impact on inflammatory arthritis. Mediterr J Rheumatol 2020;30(4):201–6.

[205] Ciaffi J, Mitselman D, Mancarella L, Brusi V, Lisi L, Ruscitti P, et al. The effect of ketogenic diet on inflammatory arthritis and cardiovascular health in rheumatic conditions: a mini review. Front Med [Internet] 2021;8. Available from: https://www.frontiersin.org/article/10.3389/fmed.2021.792846.

[206] Fioretti M, Gubinelli E, Pallotta S, Laurenti R. Diet in the management of psoriatic disease: ketogenic or Mediterranean diet? Preliminary data. Beyond Rheumatol [Internet] 2022;4(1). Available from: https://doi.org/10.53238/br_20223_383.

[207] Popa SL, Dumitrascu DI, Brata VD, Duse TA, Florea MD, Ismaiel A, et al. Nutrition in spondyloarthritis and related immune-mediated disorders. Nutrients. 2022;14(6):1278 Mar 17.

[208] Rashid T, Wilson C, Ebringer A. The link between ankylosing spondylitis, Crohn's disease, klebsiella, and starch consumption [Internet]. J Immunology Res 2013;. Available from: https://www.hindawi.com/journals/jir/2013/872632/.

[209] Ebringer A, Wilson C. The use of a low starch diet in the treatment of patients suffering from ankylosing spondylitis. Clin Rheumatol 1996;15(1):62–6.

[210] Strath LJ, Jones CD, Philip George A, Lukens SL, Morrison SA, Soleymani T, et al. The effect of low-carbohydrate and low-fat diets on pain in individuals with knee osteoarthritis. Pain Med 2019; Mar 13.

[211] Barrea L, Megna M, Cacciapuoti S, Frias-Toral E, Fabbrocini G, Savastano S, et al. Very low-calorie ketogenic diet (VLCKD) in patients with psoriasis and obesity: an update for dermatologists and nutritionists. Crit Rev Food Sci Nutr 2020;1–17 Sep 24.

[212] Castaldo G, Pagano I, Grimaldi M, Marino C, Molettieri P, Santoro A, et al. Effect of very-low-calorie ketogenic diet on psoriasis patients: a nuclear magnetic resonance-based metabolomic study. J Proteome Res 2020;.

[213] Castaldo G, Rastrelli L, Galdo G, Molettieri P, Aufiero FR, Cereda E. Aggressive weight loss program with a ketogenic induction phase for the treatment of chronic plaque psoriasis: a proof-of-concept, single-arm, open label clinical trial. Nutrition. 2020;110757.

[214] Esposito T, Lobaccaro JM, Esposito MG, Monda V, Messina A, Paolisso G, et al. Effects of low-carbohydrate diet therapy in overweight subject with autoimmune thyroiditis: possible synergism with ChREBP. DDDT. 2016;10:2939–46.

[215] Benlloch M, López-Rodríguez MM, Cuerda-Ballester M, Drehmer E, Carrera S, Ceron JJ, et al. Satiating effect of a ketogenic diet and its impact on muscle improvement and oxidation state in multiple sclerosis patients. Nutrients. 2019;11(5):1156.

[216] Brenton JN, Banwell B, Bergqvist AGC, Lehner-Gulotta D, Gampper L, Leytham E, et al. Pilot study of a ketogenic diet in relapsing-remitting MS. Neurol Neuroimmunol Neuroinflamm 2019;6(4):e565.

[217] Phillips MCL, Murtagh DKJ, Ziad F, Johnston SE, Moon BG. Impact of a ketogenic diet on sporadic inclusion body myositis: a case study. Front Neurol [Internet] 2020;11. Available from: https://www.frontiersin.org/articles/10.3389/fneur.2020.582402/full.

[218] Kornberg MD. The immunologic Warburg effect: evidence and therapeutic opportunities in autoimmunity. Wiley Interdiscip Rev Syst Biol Med 2020;12(5):e1486.

[219] Norwitz NG, Jaramillo JG, Clarke K, Soto A. Ketotherapeutics for neurodegenerative diseases. Int Rev Neurobiol 2020;155:141.

[220] Gasior M, Rogawski MA, Hartman AL. Neuroprotective and disease-modifying effects of the ketogenic diet. Behav Pharmacol 2006;17 (5−6):431−9.

[221] Masino SA, Ruskin DN. Nutritional recommendations to address pain: focus on ketogenic/low-carbohydrate diet. In: Pietramaggiori G, Scherer S, editors. Minimally Invasive Surgery for Chronic Pain Management: An Evidence-Based Approach [Internet]. Cham: Springer International Publishing; 2020. p. 69−71. Available from: https://doi.org/10.1007/978-3-030-50188-4_8.

[222] Michalsen A, Li C, Kaiser K, Lüdtke R, Meier L, Stange R, et al. In-patient treatment of fibromyalgia: a controlled nonrandomized comparison of conventional medicine versus integrative medicine including fasting therapy. Evid Based Complement Alternat Med 2013;2013. Available from: https://www.ncbi.nlm.nih.gov/pmc/articles/PMC3566607/.

[223] Adawi M, Damiani G, Bragazzi NL, Bridgewood C, Pacifico A, Conic RRZ, et al. The impact of intermittent fasting (ramadan fasting) on psoriatic arthritis disease activity, enthesitis, and dactylitis: a multicentre study. Nutrients. 2019;11(3).

[224] Adawi M, Watad A, Brown S, Aazza K, Aazza H, Zouhir M, et al. Ramadan fasting exerts immunomodulatory effects: insights from a systematic review. Front Immunol 2017;8. Available from: https://www.ncbi.nlm.nih.gov/pmc/articles/PMC5712070/.

[225] Fuhrman JM, Sarter B, Calabro DJ. Brief case reports of medically supervised, water-only fasting associated with remission of autoimmune disease. Alternative therapies health Med 2002;8(4):112 110−1.

[226] Hartmann AM, Dell'Oro M, Kessler CS, Schumann D, Steckhan N, Jeitler M, et al. Efficacy of therapeutic fasting and plant-based diet in patients with rheumatoid arthritis (NutriFast): study protocol for a randomised controlled clinical trial. BMJ Open 2021;11(8):e047758.

[227] Sharif K, Watad A, Bragazzi NL, Lichtbroun M, Amital H, Shoenfeld Y. Physical activity and autoimmune diseases: get moving and manage the disease. Autoimmun Rev 2018;17(1):53−72.

[228] Xiang K, Xu Z, Hu YQ, He YS, Wu GC, Li TY, et al. Circadian clock genes as promising therapeutic targets for autoimmune diseases. Autoimmunity Rev 2021;20(8):102866.

[229] Stojanovich L, Marisavljevich D. Stress as a trigger of autoimmune disease. Autoimmunity Rev 2008;7(3):209−13.

[230] Visser J, Rozing J, Sapone A, Lammers K, Fasano A. Tight junctions, intestinal permeability, and autoimmunity celiac disease and type 1 diabetes paradigms. Ann N Y Acad Sci 2009;1165:195−205. Available from: https://doi.org/10.1111/j.1749-6632.2009.04037.x May.

[231] Peumans WJ, Van Damme EJ. Lectins as plant defense proteins. Plant Physiol 1995;109(2):347.

[232] Thakur A, Sharma V, Thakur A. An overview of anti-nutritional factors in food. Int J Chem Stud 2019;7(1):2472−9.

[233] Bradberry SM, Dickers KJ, Rice P, Griffiths GD, Vale JA. Ricin poisoning. Toxicological Rev 2003;22(1):65−70.

[234] Petroski W, Minich DM. Is there such a thing as "anti-nutrients"? A narrative review of perceived problematic plant compounds. Nutrients. 2020;12(10):2929.

[235] Jackson LS. Chemical food safety issues in the United States: past, present, and future. J Agric Food Chem 2009;57(18):8161−70.

[236] Ames BN, Profet M, Swirsky Gold L. Dietary pesticides (99.99% all natural). Proc Natl Acad Sci 1990;87:7777−81. Available from: https://www.pnas.org/content/pnas/87/19/7777.full.pdf.

[237] Lennerz BS, et al. Behavioral characteristics and self-reported health status among 2029 adults consuming a "carnivore diet". Curr Dev Nutr [Prepr] 2021;nzab133. Available from: https://doi.org/10.1093/cdn/nzab133.

[238] Protogerou C, Leroy F, Hagger MS. Beliefs and experiences of individuals following a zero-carb diet. Behav Sci 2021;11(12):161. Available from: https://doi.org/10.3390/bs11120161.

[239] Tóth C, Clemens Z. A child with type 1 diabetes mellitus (T1DM) successfully treated with the paleolithic ketogenic diet: A 19-month insulin-freedom. Int J Case Rep Images 2015;6(12):752. Available from: https://doi.org/10.5348/ijcri-2015121-CR-10582.

[240] Tóth C, et al. Crohn's disease successfully treated with the paleolithic ketogenic diet. Int J Case Rep Images 2016;. Available from: https://doi.org/10.5348/ijcri-2016102-CR-10690.

Further reading

Kannus P, Uusi-Rasi K, Palvanen M, Parkkari J. Non-pharmacological means to prevent fractures among older adults. Ann Med 2005;37:303−10.

Ruskin DN, Suter TA, Ross JL, Masino SA. Ketogenic diets and thermal pain: dissociation of hypoalgesia, elevated ketones, and lowered glucose in rats. J Pain 2013;14(5):467−74. Available from: https://doi.org/10.1016/j.jpain.2012.12.015.

Chapter 8

Gastrointestinal health and therapeutic carbohydrate restriction

Natasha Campbell-McBride[1], Sarah M. Rice[2] and Tamzyn Murphy[2]
[1]GAPS Science Foundation, Cambridge, United Kingdom, [2]Nutrition Network, Cape Town, South Africa

8.1 Introduction

Natasha Campbell-McBride

All diseases begin in the gut!

Hippocrates (460–370 BC), the father of medicine.

The more we learn with our modern scientific tools, the more we have to agree with Hippocrates. From allergies to autoimmune diseases, from neurological to mental illness and learning disabilities, from endocrine dysfunction to chronic fatigue syndrome, all chronic health problems in children and adults seem to originate in the gut. Clinical experience shows that focusing on healing the gut lays the best foundation for treating and managing all chronic illnesses, no matter how far from the digestive system the disease may manifest.

Recent research in the human microbiome has laid a solid foundation for explaining this clinical observation. We learned that the human body is a microbial community: there are far more microbes in us than human cells. Our digestive system holds the majority of these microbes. Gut flora is a highly complex and sophisticated microbial community; it is the headquarters of the whole bodily microbiome, regulating it and affecting it in every conceivable way. Why was our digestive system put into such a central position? Because that is where food goes. Ask any microbiologist this question: what is the most powerful influence on any microbial community in nature? The answer will be simple and immediate: food. Change the food supply for a microbial community and the whole community will change. The food we consume on a daily basis has a profound effect on our microbiome and, through it, the health of the whole human organism (see Section 8.4). That is why understanding how the gut works and how to keep it healthy and functioning well is crucial for a clinician, no matter what speciality is practised (cardiology, rheumatology, neurology, psychiatry, endocrinology, dermatology etc.).

8.2 The human digestive system in health and disease

Natasha Campbell-McBride

Understanding the normal physiology of the digestive system is crucial to determining the root cause of gastrointestinal dysfunction and develop therapeutic interventions to restore health. The easiest way to examine the digestive system and its many functions is to travel through it with food.

8.2.1 Mouth

Our digestive system begins in the mouth, where chewing breaks up the food and mixes it with saliva, turning food into an easy-to-swallow bolus. The act of chewing and tasting food sends signals to the whole body through the autonomic nervous system, starting the digestive process and altering our mood and behaviour through hormonal changes [1].

Ketogenic. DOI: https://doi.org/10.1016/B978-0-12-821617-0.00001-2

8.2.1.1 *Saliva*

A very important element for keeping our mouths healthy is saliva. It is equipped with enzymes, antimicrobial elements, minerals, proteins, vitamins, lipids and other substances, which start digestion, keep normal pH, remineralise and heal our tooth enamel and maintain the right microbial community in the mouth [2]. In a healthy body, approximately 1.5 L of saliva is produced every day [2]. Saliva contains digestive enzymes: amylase (ptyalin) to digest carbohydrates and lipase to digest fats. When food is swallowed, salivary amylase gets inactivated by the stomach acid where digestion of carbohydrates stops. It will continue in the intestines, but thorough chewing is important to break down this group of nutrients [2].

Some 400 commonly prescribed pharmaceuticals reduce the production of saliva, making the mouth dry [3]. This makes the mouth environment abnormal and causes tooth decay, gum disease and other mouth problems. Normal saliva production is essential for the proper functioning of the whole digestive system. Clinicians need to be aware of this when prescribing medications. Chronic stress, food additives and artificial dental materials can also affect saliva production and its composition [3].

8.2.1.1.1 Teeth

Dental health has a profound effect on the health of the mouth [4]. Many dental materials change the environment in the mouth, promoting growth of pathogenic microbes via biofilms [5–7]. When we chew food with teeth that are chronically infected or contain toxic dental materials, these toxins are mixed with the food and swallowed [8]. The first place to suffer will be the gut itself. When these toxins are absorbed, they can cause systemic problems [8,9]. It is essential for a clinician to look at the teeth of any person with stomach and oesophagus problems, as toxins could leach from root canals, fillings, bridges, crowns, dental implants and other dental materials. This may contribute to indigestion, diarrhoea, constipation, abdominal pain, bloating and flatulence, leading to a common diagnosis of irritable bowel syndrome (IBS) [4,9].

8.2.1.1.2 Oral microflora

The mouth has a very rich microbial flora. Interestingly, the composition of this flora correlates with the flora found in the stool [10]. A healthy microbiome determines the health of all organs and tissues in the mouth and takes an active part in the digestive process. People with abnormal flora in the mouth often have mouth ulcers [11], tooth decay [12], breath odour [13] and digestive abnormalities [14].

8.2.1.2 *Tongue*

Looking at the tongue can give useful information to a clinician [15]. A white coating on the tongue is usually an overgrowth of fungi (*candida* in particular) [16]. A brown coating may indicate gastritis and liver congestion [17]. A swollen tongue, with indents on its sides left by the teeth, is a typical indication of low thyroid function [18]. A red and sore tongue is a symptom of B-vitamin deficiencies and is often accompanied by cracks in the corners of the mouth [19].

8.2.2 Oesophagus

The oesophagus passes food from the mouth and throat down into the stomach. It has powerful muscles to make sure that food can be swallowed in any position: vertical, horizontal and even upside down [20]. The lining of the oesophagus is well protected by extensive mucous production and has a similar microbial flora to the mouth [21]. A healthy microbiome promotes good oesophageal function. However, if the food and drink passing through the oesophagus contain toxins, this microbiome can become pathogenic [21]. Chemicals in processed foods and tap water, agricultural chemicals, pharmaceuticals and dental materials can cause damage, leading to chronic inflammation of the oesophagus (oesophagitis) [22]. Oesophagitis can make swallowing difficult and painful (dysphagia), causing nausea, vomiting and heartburn.

The oesophagus has two sphincters: upper and lower. The upper oesophageal sphincter (UOS) is positioned at the entry to the oesophagus (at the level of the larynx) to prevent food from going into the trachea. The lower oesophageal sphincter (LOS) is positioned at the entrance into the stomach to prevent stomach contents from going back up the oesophagus. When abnormal microbial flora develops in the oesophagus, pathogenic microbes can partially paralyse these sphincters, making them inefficient [23]. Usually both sphincters are affected, leading to regurgitation of food from the stomach (reflux), which can damage the oesophagus and cause chronic inflammation, ulcers and cancer of this organ [24].

When the LOS is not working properly, gastroesophageal reflux disease (*GORD or GERD*) develops. When the UOS is not working well, laryngopharyngeal reflux develops, which is more difficult to diagnose [25]. It can present with persistent sore throat and hoarseness of the voice, post-nasal drip, sleep apnoea, difficulty swallowing food and recurrent ear infections. Some people can develop allergic dysphagia of allergia eosiniphilic oesophagitis, when the UOS (or both sphincters) closes up on contact with a particular trigger substance [26]. Various artificial chemicals in food can trigger this reaction, most often in seafood (which may contain mercury) or smoked meats and fish (which were not smoked traditionally, but smeared with artificial chemicals to give them smoky flavour) [27]. When this happens, pain and discomfort in the throat and chest develops, as well as inability to swallow food, water or even saliva. This situation can last from a few minutes to a few hours. Clinical observation shows that patients with allergic dysphagia often had long-term amalgam fillings in their teeth.

8.2.3 Stomach

The stomach is our major food-digesting organ. It produces digestive enzymes and hydrochloric acid (HCl), as well as intrinsic factor (IF) to facilitate vitamin B12 absorption [28] The stomach is the place where protein digestion starts with the use of a proteolytic enzyme called *pepsin*. It is produced by the stomach wall in its inactive form of *pepsinogen*, which is converted into pepsin by the stomach acid. The pH in the stomach must go down to 1–2 to activate pepsinogen. Proteins are essential building blocks of the human body, and normal stomach acid production is crucial for supplying enough protein for the whole body to use. In infancy, another proteolytic enzyme is produced in the stomach—*rennin*—for digesting breast milk. After infancy, this enzyme disappears in the majority of people.

The stomach wall produces bicarbonate-rich mucous to protect itself from the HCl in the gastric juice. Painkillers (nonsteroidal antiinflammatory drugs, aspirin in particular) strip off this mucous protection and damage the stomach lining. These medications are by far the most common cause of stomach problems [29]. When the mucous protection is gone, stomach acid and pepsin deepen the damage, leading to gastritis. Modern food may contain agricultural chemicals and other toxins [30]. Dental care adds mercury, fluoride and other poisons leading to gastritis [31]. Smoking, drinking, chronic stress and negative mental attitudes can also be contributing factors [4].

When the stomach lining gets inflamed and sore, the body downregulates stomach acid production (to prevent further damage); this condition is called *hypochlorhydria* (low stomach acid) [32]. It presents devastating problems for the whole gastrointestinal tract (GIT), so let us discuss hypochlorhydria in detail.

8.2.3.1 Hypochlorhydria

An acidic environment is hostile to microbes. Normally, only a small resident microbiome lives on healthy stomach mucosa (largely *yeasts, lactobacilli* and *Helicobacter pylori*) [33]. In hypochlorhydria, these resident microbes can get out of control [34,35]. A good example is *H. pylori*, which is a normal inhabitant of a healthy stomach. Research shows that in countries with traditional ways of life, the majority of small children have this microbe in their stomachs, while in Western countries, very few children have it [36,37]. In regards to diet, our appetite and food consumption are regulated by hormones produced in the stomach and duodenum: ghrelin, leptin and other. *H. pylori* is involved in the normal production of these hormones; its absence leads to poor appetite control, abnormal metabolism and weight gain [37,38]. The absence of *H. pylori* is also linked to higher rates of asthma and allergies. This may be related to its action on ghrelin, which has an antiinflammatory role [37,38]. So, if *H. pylori* is detected, antibiotics need not be initiated to eliminate it, except in cases of stomach ulcers, stomach cancer or another serious stomach problem, and only as part of a holistic protocol which includes appropriate diet.

Stomach acid is the natural barrier for pathogenic microbes and parasites coming in with food and drink. In hypochlorhydria, these pathogens overgrow in the whole digestive system, including the stomach itself [39]. The most research in this area has been done in stomach cancer patients, the majority of whom show hypochlorhydria and microbial overgrowth in the stomach [36]. Proton pump inhibitors (PPIs) are a major cause of this situation [36] they are among the top 10 drugs most often prescribed in the developed world. They are commonly taken for indigestion, GORD and other stomach problems, leading to chronic hypochlorhydria.

Hypochlorhydria makes the whole digestive process abnormal, particularly digestion of protein. The most studied proteins in this situation are gluten and casein. In hypochlorhydria, these proteins are improperly digested and absorbed as opiate-like substances, called *gliadorphins* and *casomorphins*, which find their way to the nervous system and may affect mental health [40]. In hypochlorhydria, most proteins are absorbed in a partially digested state, causing problems in the body [41]. Stomach acidity is the major regulator of pancreatic and hepatic ability to respond to food; hence, hypochlorhydria leads to maldigestion, malabsorption and nutritional deficiencies [42]. It can lead to food allergies and intolerances [43], small intestinal bacterial overgrowth (SIBO) [43], IBS and cancer anywhere in the GIT [44]. Stomach acid is essential for production of IF, necessary for absorption of vitamin B12. Hypochlorhydria causes deficiency in this vitamin [45].

Microbes, overgrowing in a low-acid stomach, play an important role in causing stomach cancer, ulcers and gastritis [35–38,45,46]. Many of these microbes love to eat processed carbohydrates, producing toxins and gases (e.g. carbon dioxide and methane) [46]. Overproduction of gas causes excessive belching, while toxins make the inflammation in the stomach worse, increasing the severity of gastritis. Some of these microbial toxins cause a partial paralysis of the stomach muscle, called *gastroparesis*, which slows down stomach motility [47]. People with this condition complain that food stays in their stomach for long periods of time, not digesting or moving. Mechanical defects of the LOS are causally implicated in reflux [48]. Even with hypochlorhydria, there is some acid in the regurgitated food, which damages the walls of the oesophagus, leading to acid indigestion or heartburn and the development of *GORD* or *GERD*. Antacids and PPIs are usually prescribed for GORD, which may alleviate the immediate symptoms but, in the long run, make the whole situation worse, as they reduce stomach acid production even further and may also mask the presence of *H. pylori* [49].

Hypochlorhydria causes belching and bloating, because overgrowing yeasts, archaea and other microbes in the stomach produce excessive gas [46,50].

Another common symptom of chronic gastritis is *cyclic vomiting syndrome* [51]. Activity of worms, flukes and other residents of the digestive system can play an important role in this condition. The vomiting episodes happen in regular cycles coinciding with a particular stage in these creatures' life cycle (when they lay eggs or hatch into larvae) [52].

Healing the stomach must involve restoration of normal stomach acid production. It is an essential step in bringing health to the whole digestive system, normalising digestion and absorption of food and removing nutritional deficiencies [53].

8.2.4 Small intestine

The greatest part of digestion and absorption of food happens in the small intestine, which is made up of the duodenum (proximal), ileum and jejunum (distal) [54]. In the duodenum, bile and pancreatic enzymes are added to the food. For this process to go smoothly, the food has to arrive from the stomach with the right acidity (pH below 2) [55]. This acidity triggers production of hormones (*secretin, cholecystokinin* and other) in the walls of duodenum, which in turn regulate stomach, intestinal, pancreatic and liver functions [54]. If the food arriving from the stomach is not acidic enough, production of these hormones is impaired, leading to impaired digestion and absorption of food [56] (Fig. 8.1).

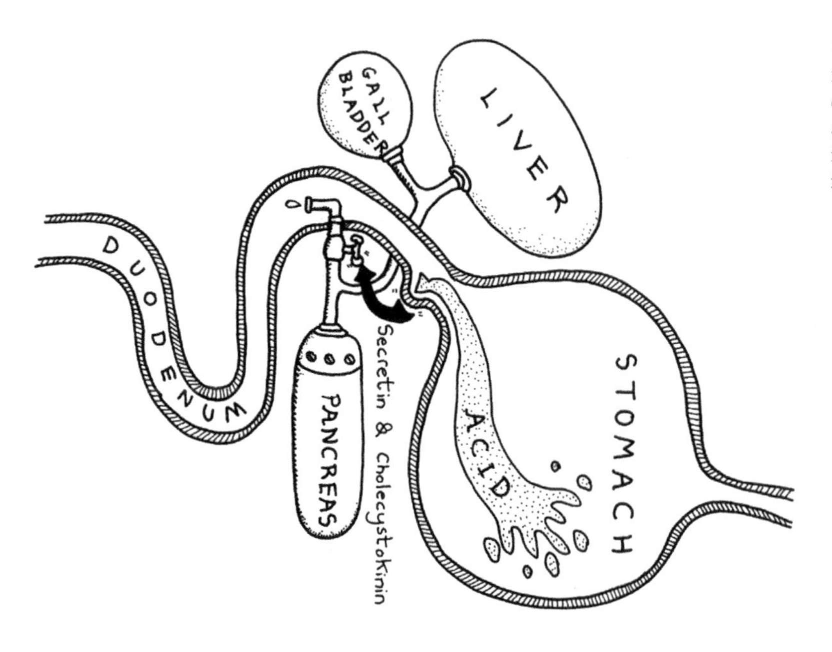

FIGURE 8.1 **Structure of the upper gastrointestinal tract.** Food processed with bile and pancreatic enzymes in the duodenum must enter from the stomach with an approximate pH of 2. Alkalinity can impair digestive hormone secretion as their function is pH-sensitive.

8.2.4.1 Enterocytes

The absorption of food happens in the small intestine, mainly in the duodenum and jejunum. Their walls form finger-like protrusions, called villi, lined by epithelial cells *enterocytes* [54] (Fig. 8.2).

The surface of enterocytes is covered by tiny hairs (microvilli or brush border) These hairs contain food-digesting brush border enzymes (peptidases, disaccharidases, lipases and other), which complete the digestive process before food is absorbed (Fig. 8.3).

Enterocytes live only a few days: born at the base of the villi, they travel to the top, slowly getting more mature on the way. When they reach the top, they are shed and replaced by new enterocytes moving up the villi (Fig. 8.4). This process of constant renewal of enterocytes is managed by the microbiome [55]. Animal experiments with sterilisation of the gut wall show that enterocytes mutate and become unable to perform their jobs of digestion and absorption of food [54,55].

The small intestine has more microbes living in it than the stomach, and the further from the stomach we get, the richer that flora becomes [55]. In a healthy duodenum, very few microbes are found ($0-10^5$ colonies/mL of intestinal content) and the species are similar to the stomach population. In a healthy ileum (the last third of the small intestine), the flora is the richest (10^3-10^6 colonies/mL of content), and at the lowest end, it becomes similar to the flora of the colon. Normal stomach acid production is essential for maintaining healthy intestinal microbiome [57]. In hypochlorhydria, upper intestines develop a much bigger population of microbes than normal, leading to IBS and SIBO [58]. Antibiotic therapy can make the whole situation worse, as fungi and other microbial species overgrow after antibiotics [59]. To help people with IBS and SIBO, stomach acid production needs to be improved.

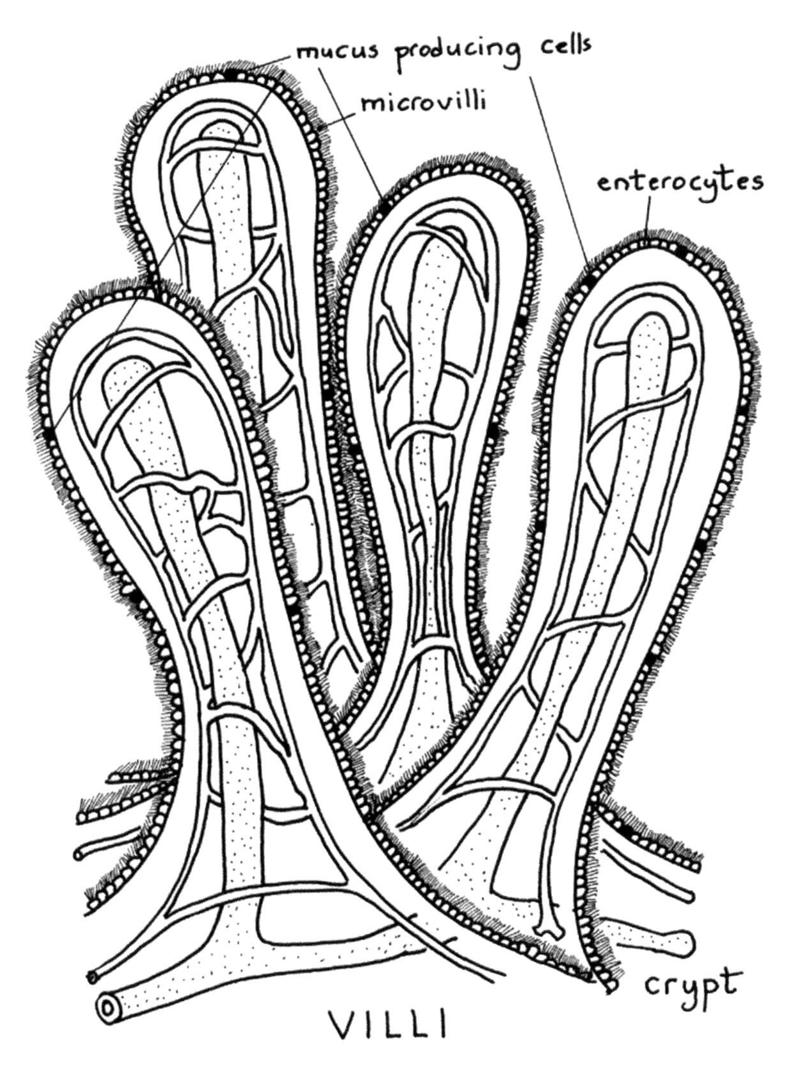

FIGURE 8.2 Simplified diagram of epithelial cells. Epithelial cells are lined by microvilli, which are the primary facilitators of digestion.

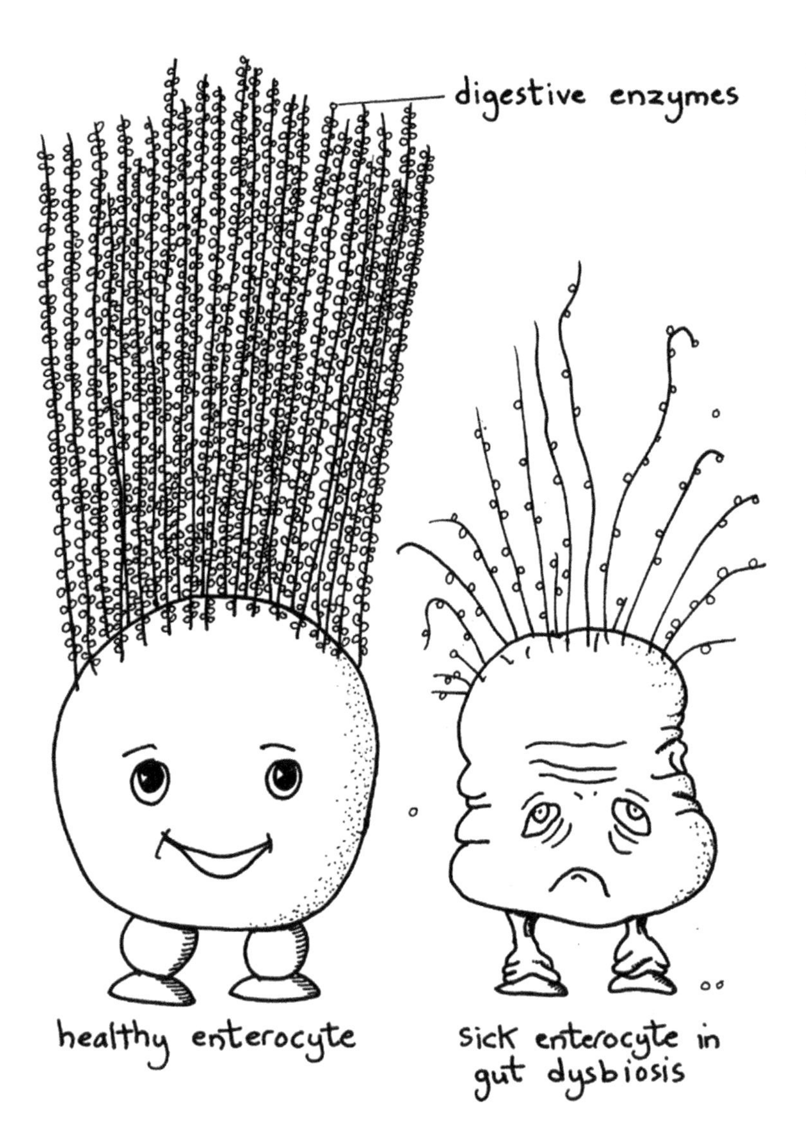

FIGURE 8.3 **A cartoon depiction of a healthy versus diseased enterocyte.** Healthy enterocytes are characterised by dense, active brush border enzymes, whereas a diseased enterocyte has dysfunctional brush border enzymes.

Unbalanced microbiome leads to *intestinal permeability (leaky gut)* [60]. The intestinal wall is covered by food-absorbing cells, called enterocytes. These cells form tight junctions between one another (Fig. 8.5).

When the intestinal microbiome is abnormal, tight junctions get damaged, making the gut wall permeable to compounds and microorganisms that would usually be prevented from entering the body (Fig. 8.6) [60].

Food does not get a chance to be digested properly before it gets absorbed through this damaged (leaky) wall. The immune system reacts to improperly digested food, clinically manifesting as food allergy or intolerance [61]. Symptoms of this condition are varied and multisystemic. Clinically they could manifest as an asthma attack or a panic attack, a skin rash or a migraine, a bout of cystitis or a drop in energy, lapses of memory or heart palpitations, emotional instability or arthritis. The reactions can be immediate or delayed, a reaction to one food or various foods, making identification of the offending substance difficult [62]. Following laboratory tests for food allergy (which may or may not identify an offending food), people often start removing foods until there is virtually nothing left to eat, but they are still reacting [63]. As long as the gut wall is like a sieve, they are likely to absorb all food in an improperly digested state and react to everything they eat. Instead of focusing on food, the focus should be on healing and sealing the intestinal wall. Once the tight junctions are restored, food gets absorbed in its properly digested state and food allergies/intolerances disappear. The following elimination diet usually proves effective in clinical practice: bone/meat broth, homemade whey, yoghurt or kefir, ginger tea and honey and water and well-cooked meat and vegetable soup or stew [64].

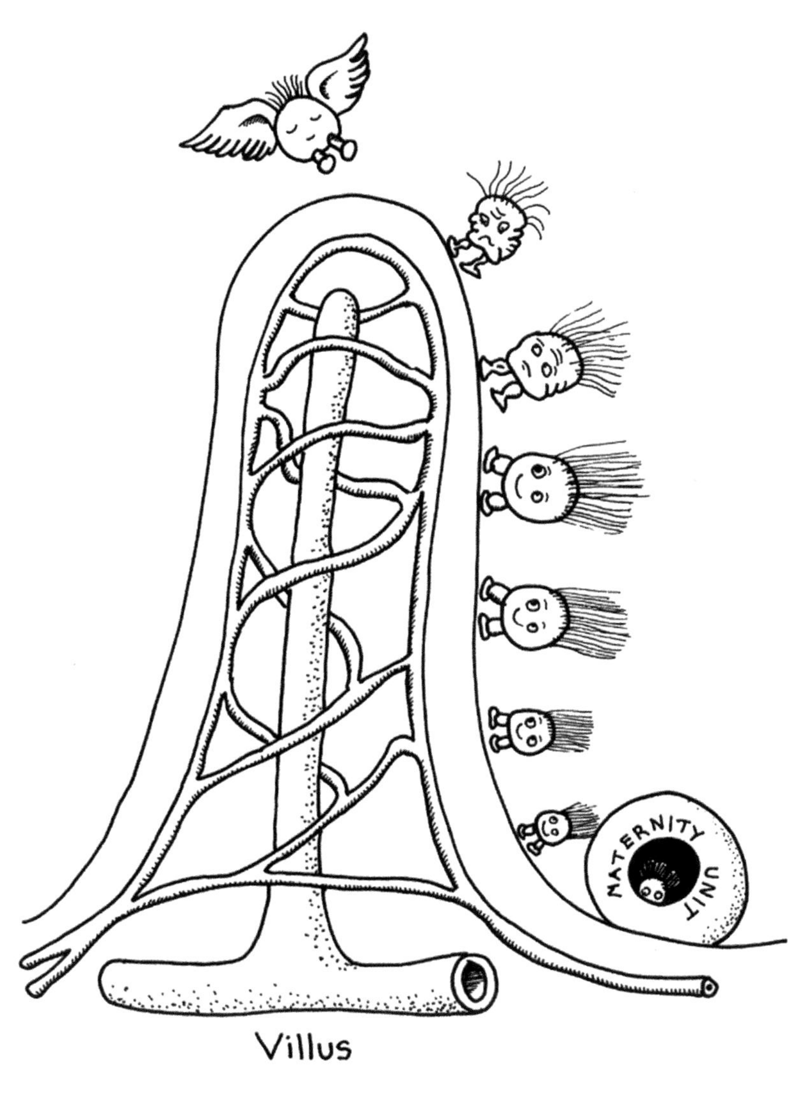

FIGURE 8.4 **Simplified depiction of the enterocyte life cycle.** Enterocytes are generated from the base of the villus, from which they age as they ascend the villus and are shed at the apex.

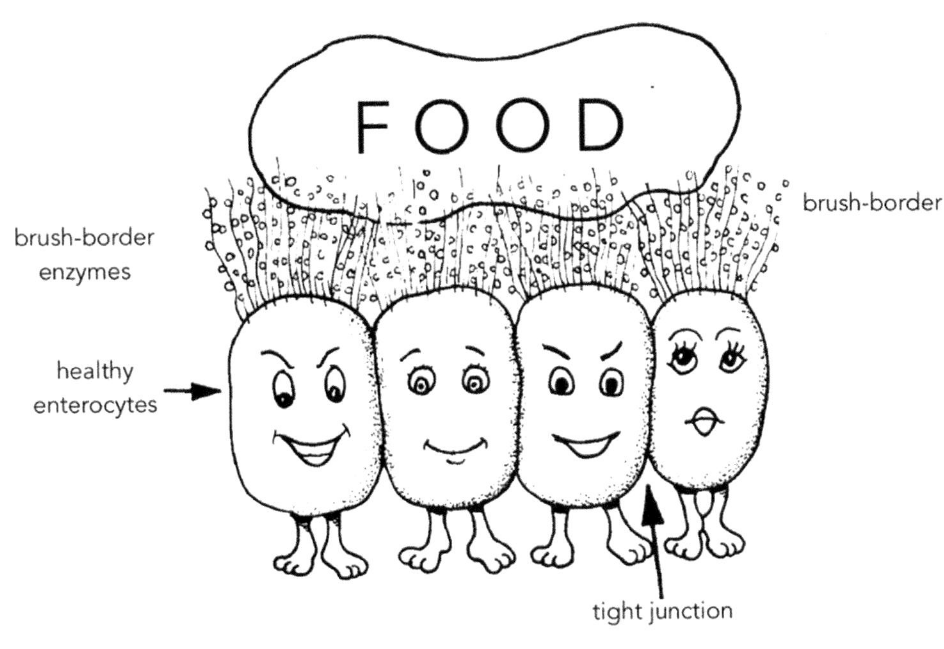

FIGURE 8.5 Simplified cartoon diagram of enterocytes, brush border enzymes and tight junctions.

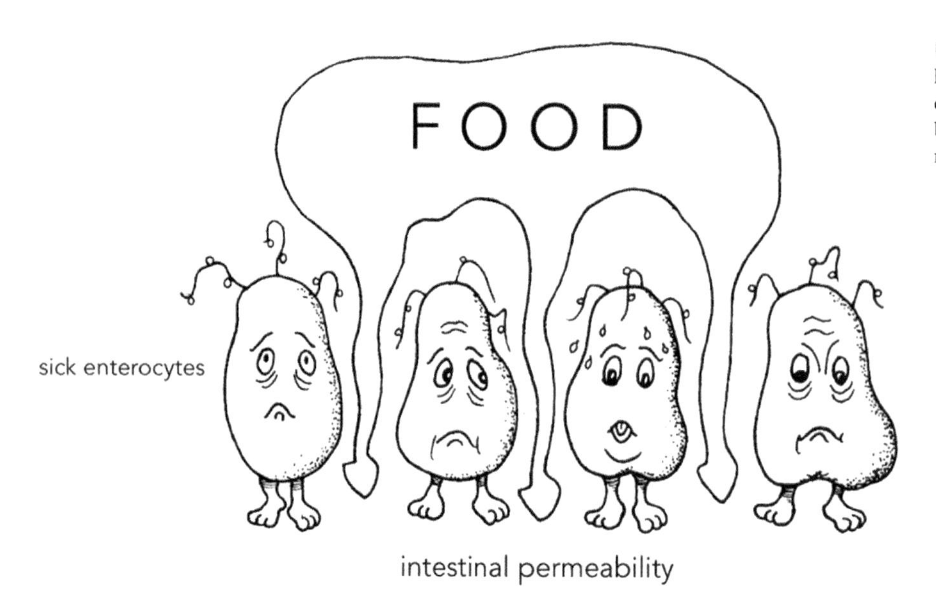

FIGURE 8.6 **Intestinal permeability: hallmark of digestive disease.** Diseased enterocytes have damaged tight junctions between them, allowing bypass of ingested molecules into the rest of the body.

8.2.5 Liver and gallbladder

Liver is an amazing organ fulfilling a myriad of functions: processing nutrients absorbed by the gut, manufacturing vital substances (blood proteins, cholesterol, enzymes, antioxidants and other), recycling enzymes, hormones and neurotransmitters, storing nutrients (glucose in the form of glycogen, for example) and many other jobs [65]. The liver is our major detoxification organ. It handles toxins from the gut and elsewhere in the body. Hepatic Kupffer cells phagocytose damaged white blood cells, microbes and debris. Toxins, which cannot be neutralised, get unloaded into the bile to be removed through the gut [66].

The liver produces approximately 600–1000 mL of bile every day [65,66]. Accumulating in the gallbladder, the bile becomes more concentrated and potent; when released into the duodenum, it neutralises stomach acid and emulsifies fats. Normal stomach acidity is essential for the bile to be released from the liver and gallbladder (through regulation by hormones secretin and cholecystokinin). Hypochlorhydria can impair bile production [67]. Without bile, dietary fats are lost in the stool, making it greasy and pale in colour (steatorrhea) [68]. This leads to deficiency in fats and fat-soluble vitamins (A, D, K and E), without which the body cannot assimilate proteins and minerals, cannot heal any damage or protect itself from infections. As a result, the person may develop poor immunity, lack of energy, poor memory and cognitive ability, endocrine problems, osteoporosis, dry skin and hair and many other problems [69].

People, who lack bile, find it difficult to digest fat and often limit its consumption; dietary fat makes them feel nauseous and unwell after a meal. In order for the liver to maintain the bile flow, we must consume natural fats with meals. When this stimulation does not happen for a long-enough time, the bile ducts can get blocked with bile stones [70].

Formation of bile stones is normal and occurs in everyone most of the time [71]. Once formed, these stones are tiny and soft and pass easily through the bile ducts. When we eat a meal with a good fat content, these tiny stones get flushed out into the gut and removed from the body in the stool. If a person is on a low-fat diet, there is no stimulation for the bile to flow and the stones stay in the bile ducts too long [71,72]. Calcium salts (e.g. calcium oxalate) accumulate in the outer parts of these stones, making them bigger, with a rough, hard surface. These stones are difficult to pass. They get stuck in the gallbladder or bile ducts. When enough biliary ducts are blocked with stones, fat digestion becomes problematic and the liver becomes congested, with reduced ability to detoxify, which can lead to nausea and slight jaundice [73,74]. Lack of bile flow is also a major cause of chronic constipation (discussed later) [75,76].

Haemorrhoids are the visible signs of high blood pressure in the portal system of veins, which bring the blood from the GIT to the liver [77]. If the liver is congested and cannot process the blood quickly enough, the pressure in the portal system increases and can become quite high (*portal hypertension*) [78]. They may also be associated with constipation [79].

Gallstones can also move to the pancreas, causing the pancreas's powerful proteolytic enzymes to build up behind the obstruction and damage the pancreas, which can lead to acute or chronic pancreatitis [80,81], pancreatic insufficiency [81] and pancreatic cancer [82] As the tissue of the pancreas gets damaged, the person may develop post-pancreatitis diabetes due to impaired insulin production in the pancreatic islets of Langerhans (beta cells) [83].

8.2.6 Pancreas

The pancreas is our major digestive-enzyme-producing organ [84]. It produces about 1.5 litres of alkaline pancreatic juice per day, full of enzymes necessary for us to break down food: protein-digesting trypsin and chymotrypsin, fat-digesting lipases and carbohydrate-digesting amylases. Pancreatic enzymes are released into the duodenum in an inactive form (called zymogens or proenzymes). The intestinal wall produces enterokinases, which activate these proenzymes and may also influence microbiota [85].

Production of pancreatic juice is regulated by cholecystokinin, secretin and other hormones [86]. These hormones are released by the duodenum if the stomach acidity is normal [87]. If the stomach acidity is low, reduced production of pancreatic juices can impair digestion.

The pancreas is hidden deep inside the abdomen close to the solar plexus (a complex formation of peripheral nerves). Perhaps for this reason, pancreatic problems are painful [88]. The pain can be severe and made worse by eating, and it can radiate into the back and spread to other parts of the abdomen. If the process is acute, the person may develop nausea and vomiting, have high fever and feel quite unwell. In chronic pancreatitis, loss of fat in the stool (steatorrhea) is common because the fats are not being digested properly, leading to deficiency in fatty acids and fat-soluble vitamins [89].

A healthy pancreas has its own microbial community living in its ducts [90]. When the pancreas is underproducing, this microbial community changes, encouraging growth of unhealthy microbes [91]. Poor pancreatic function leads to poor digestion of food, malabsorption and deficiencies in nutrients, weight loss, anaemia and failure to thrive. Undigested food, travelling through the intestines, feeds microbes, leading to an overgrowth of pathogenic microbes in the small and large intestines [92].

The good news is that the pancreas has a considerable ability to regenerate [93]. However, it is a team player: to heal the pancreas, it is essential to heal the whole digestive system. The microbiome and stomach acidity are important in this process [91,94]. When gut function improves, pancreatic exocrine function is supported, contributing to a normal microbiome in the pancreas and good health of this organ [91].

8.2.7 Large intestine (bowel or colon)

It normally takes approximately 24 hours for material to pass through the large intestine, where water and electrolytes are absorbed and stool is formed [95]. Colon has the richest population of microbes: this is where the bulk of gut microbiome resides to ferment undigested food components [96]. These microbes produce short-chain fatty acids (SCFAs; 95% of which are butyric, acetic and propionic acids), as well as vitamins, amino acids, neurotransmitters and other beneficial substances. Research has focused on bacteria in human stools; the predominant groups in healthy people include *Bacteroides* [97], *Bifidobacteria* [98] and *Clostridia* [99]. Maintaining the correct balance of the various bacterial subtypes is key for human health [100]. However, not only bacteria, but also a complex microbial community, including fungi, viruses, protozoa, archaea, worms and other creatures live in the gut, all of which are essential and important. A failure to account for this complexity makes the study of the gut microbiome clinically irrelevant so far. In a healthy person, this microbial community is balanced and works in harmony with the body. Modern lifestyles often damage our microbiome, leading to health problems in the gut and everywhere else in the body [101].

Part of the research has focussed on prebiotics (carbohydrates which feed bacteria) [102]. Prebiotics, starch, and fibre are considered to be good food for bacteria in the gut (again the focus is only on bacteria). However, clinical experience shows that these substances feed equally the 'good' and the 'bad' microbes in the gut (fungi in particular). If one's gut has a healthy, balanced microbiome, it will feast on the starch, fibre, and prebiotics, grow larger colonies and make one healthier as a result. However, if the gut is dominated by pathogenic microbes, then they will feed on these carbohydrates and make the person very sick [101,103–105]. In people with serious digestive disorders, prebiotics, starch and fibre may have to be removed for a long time to change the gut flora and heal the gut lining.

Well-functioning balanced gut flora is essential for forming normal stools and moving the bowel comfortably and regularly. People with abnormal microbiomes may suffer from diarrhoea, constipation and other abnormalities (see Section 8.4).

8.2.8 Beyond digestion

8.2.8.1 *Gut-associated lymphoid tissue*

Our digestive system is the biggest immune organ in the human body: Gut-associated lymphoid tissue (GALT) represents 70%–80% of the immune system by weight and cell content [106]. The gut can be seen as the headquarters of the immune system. It has a very complex and close relationship with the gut microbiome, which feeds it, informs it, balances it and keeps it healthy and well [107]. When the gut microbiome becomes abnormal, the immune system of the body may be affected, leading to inflammation and autoimmunity in any organ or system [108]. Allergies and autoimmune diseases such as asthma, hay fever, rheumatoid arthritis, multiple sclerosis, eczema, psoriasis, chronic fatigue syndrome, fibromyalgia, and more may have their roots in the gut, and addressing gut health is an important part of the treatment plan. Activities of GALT and microbiome are immensely complex. Both are largely dependent on what food is present in the GIT. The diet is of profound importance [109]. When things go wrong with the GALT and microbiome, many digestive disorders can develop, including inflammatory bowel diseases (IBD) (Crohn's disease and ulcerative colitis) [110]. Chronic inflammation and autoimmunity are both active in these disorders. So the mainstream approach, focusing on immune-suppression and symptom control, does not address the root cause. An appropriate diet and restoration of the gut microbiome must be the main steps in dealing with any digestive disorder, particularly with IBD (See Section 8.3).

Overexposure to oral antibiotics can play a role in IBD and other digestive disorders [111]. Antibiotics can negatively impact the delicate balance in the gut microbiome, which has a profound effect on the GALT and the rest of the immune system. It is also known that antibiotics weaken immune cells [112]. Antibiotics are life-saving medications and should only be used as such. Considering the phenomenal importance of gut microbiome and GALT for the health of the entire body, nonoral administration of antibiotics should be preferred in most situations.

8.2.8.2 Enteric nervous system

Our gut has an extensive nervous system (NS), called the enteric NS, connected to the brain through the gut–brain axis. Its complexity and functions are so monumental that the GIT has been called the second brain [113]. It influences the entire body through multiple channels: chemical, neuroendocrine, neuroimmune, sympathetic, parasympathetic, HPA axis and nutritional [113,114]. The gut microbiome works in partnership with the enteric NS and has a strong influence on its functions. Hormones, neurotransmitters, enzymes, peptides and many other powerful molecules are produced and modulated in the digestive system with the involvement of the gut flora [115]. For example, more than 90% of body's serotonin is produced in the GIT [116] and some 50% of dopamine [117]. A damaged gut and/or an abnormal microbiome impacts their secretion and activity, contributing to depression and other mood disorders [118].

In recent years, published research has been providing more evidence for a connection between the gut and the mind, connecting the GIT with autism [119], ADHD [120], Parkinson's disease [121], anxiety and mood disorders [122], Alzheimer's disease [123], schizophrenia [124] and other psychiatric and psychological problems [118–124]. This research brings hope to modern psychiatry, providing it with an explanation of the possible root cause or, at least, influential factor, in neuropsychiatric disorders and a path for an effective treatment.

8.2.8.3 Gut as an endocrine organ

The GIT is considered to be one of the biggest endocrine organs in the body [125]. It produces and modulates a plethora of hormones and microbial metabolites, regulating our hormonal balance [126]. Hormones are powerful molecules affecting functions of every cell in every organ, making the GIT immensely influential in the entire body. Bacteria in the gut have been found to produce hormones (serotonin, dopamine and somatostatin), convert glucocorticoids into androgens and regulate oestrogen balance in the body [127]. Gut dysbiosis could impact hormonal regulation [128]. Abnormal oestrogen metabolism alone has very serious implications: it drives cardiovascular disease (CVD), obesity, cancer and dementia, along with infertility, endometriosis, polycystic ovarian syndrome and cancers of reproductive organs [129].

8.2.9 Conclusion

Understanding the normal physiology of the GIT, from the mouth through to the colon, allows us to better identify the root of pathophysiological processes that result in gastrointestinal disorders and other further reaching systemic conditions. Understanding the pathophysiology in turn allows for effective targeted therapeutic intervention to restore gastrointestinal and systemic health.

8.3 Diet and gastrointestinal disorders

Natasha Campbell-McBride

8.3.1 Introduction

The digestive system is a long tube: what we fill this tube with has a direct effect on its well-being [130]. So, food should be the number one treatment for any digestive disorder. The gut microbiome, digestive wall and all its structures respond to dietary changes [131]. No matter what other methods of treatment we may consider, the diet must be changed first.

Before trying to change one's diet, it is important to address food addictions (see Section 11.3.2). Gut microbiome dictates our food preferences [131,132]. People with abnormal gut microbiome typically limit their diet to sweet and starchy foods [133]: bread, pasta, sugary drinks, biscuits, cakes, sweets, pizza, breakfast cereals, chocolates, chips, crisps and snacks. Common pathogens in their gut convert these processed carbohydrates into toxic substances, and the brain gets addicted to them [134]. As a result, foods that harm these patients become their favourite foods. In order to change the diet, food addictions must be dealt with and the patient may need help.

Accumulated clinical experience, the wisdom of traditional diets from all over the world combined with the scientific literature, has given us a successful dietary approach to begin healing from digestive disorders.

8.3.2 Nutritional components

8.3.2.1 Carbohydrates

Carbohydrates primarily are absorbed as the monosaccharides (single sugars) glucose, fructose and galactose [135]. Glucose and fructose are found in vegetables, ripe fruit and real honey. Honey is largely made of fructose and glucose and does not require much digestion. Galactose is found in soured (fermented) milk products, such as yoghurt, kefir, sour cream and cheese. *Monosaccharides do not require digestion to be absorbed* and thus do not pose a digestive challenge to people with digestive disorders. So monosaccharides should be the main form of carbohydrate consumed by these individuals.

The next size carbohydrates are disaccharides (made from two monosaccharides) [135]. The most common ones are sucrose (table sugar), made from one fructose and one glucose; lactose (the milk sugar), made from one galactose and one glucose; and maltose (from digestion of starch and other complex carbohydrates), made from two glucose molecules. Unhealthy enterocytes lose their ability to produce brush border enzymes and cannot digest disaccharides [136]. These sugars stay in the gut and provide food for pathogenic microbes, getting converted into toxic compounds such as lipopolysaccharides (LPS) [137], which damage the gut wall by disrupting tight junctions and leaching said toxins throughout the body inducing systemic inflammation [138]. Deficiencies in carbohydrate absorption accompany digestive disorders and other chronic illnesses (autoimmune diseases, allergies and other degenerative conditions) [138,139]. More complex carbohydrates, containing chains of mono- and disaccharides may be even harder to digest in gastrointestinal conditions [140].

So, double sugars and larger carbohydrates should be excluded from the diet for those with gastrointestinal disorders, including table sugar, unfermented dairy products and foods containing starch (and other complex sugars): all grains, most legumes and starchy root vegetables (potato, yams, sweet potato, Jerusalem artichoke, cassava and parsnips).

Clinical practice shows that when the gut has been given a long enough period without double sugars, starch, fibre and other complex carbohydrates, it has a good chance of recovery. Once this recovery takes place, many people find that they can start having grains and starchy vegetables again without ill effects.

8.3.2.1.1 Fibre

Consumption of fibre has been promoted for its purported health benefits such as good gut health [141] and even prevention of CVD [142], diabetes [143] and cancer [144]. However, the published evidence has failed to show that it is the fibre in the food, rather than other ingredients, that bestows benefits [145]. The hypothesis that fibre is responsible for this plethora of health benefits has been challenged from the beginning, particularly by clinicians. Clinical experience shows that fibre and starch can be deleterious for individuals with digestive disorders. Fibre is a complex carbohydrate indigestible (or partially indigestible) for humans (microbes can digest it to a degree). The problem is that both beneficial and pathogenic microbes can ferment fibre and other complex carbohydrates, converting them into many metabolites, some health-giving and some damaging [146,147]. If an individual's gut flora is dominated by a health-promoting balanced microbial community, it is possible that fibre, starch and other complex carbohydrates may bring some benefits. However, in a person with abnormal gut flora (which constitutes a growing proportion of the global population), these complex carbohydrates could be fermented by pathogenic microbes, causing diarrhoea, constipation, bloating, flatulence and other symptoms, often leading to a diagnosis of IBS [148,149].

Fibre proponents focus on the SCFAs, acetate, propionate and butyrate, produced by bacteria in the gut from complex carbohydrates. SCFAs, butyrate in particular, have been found to maintain the health of the gut wall [150], with systemic antiinflammatory effects [151]. From the growing research into ketogenic diet (KD), we now learn that in physiological ketosis, the liver can produce beta-hydroxybutyrate (a form of the SCFA butyrate), with resultant systemic benefits, including maintenance of the gut wall integrity [152] and health (see Section 2.3). More research like this may show that we do not need to consume fibre to produce SCFAs in the body. In the clinical setting, removing the bulk of fibre, starch and other complex carbohydrates (with or without physiological ketosis) reduces inflammation in the gut and allows it to heal.

The biggest claim made for fibre consumption is that it should resolve constipation. However, in some situations, consumption of fibre causes constipation or aggravates it, and reducing fibre ameliorates it [153]. It may depend on an individual's gut flora composition. The microbes in the gut that consume fibre are capable of causing constipation, diarrhoea or anything in between [154,155].

Dietary fibre has been divided into two groups: soluble (pectin, psyllium, beta-glucans and gums) and insoluble (cellulose, hemicellulose and lignin). Soluble fibre dissolves in water, and the health benefits of fibre consumption are largely assigned to this group. Insoluble fibre does not dissolve in water and is said to add bulk to the stool and stimulate peristalsis. Though grains, legumes and other seeds contain more insoluble fibre, all plant foods may contain both groups and, in a clinical setting, may have an equally damaging effect on a sensitive digestive system [156].

Fermentable oligo-, di-, monosaccharides and polyols (FODMAPs) are carbohydrates classified as dietary fibre [157]. They are actively fermented by unhealthy gut flora causing diarrhoea, constipation, flatulence, bloating, pain and other digestive symptoms. People with damaged gut microbiome find it helpful to avoid foods containing these substances, particularly people with IBS and IBD [158]. Common FODMAPs include fructose, lactose, fructans (particularly in wheat, spelt, rye and barley), galactans (found in large amounts in legumes), polyols (such as xylitol, sorbitol, maltitol and mannitol) and so forth. Many fruits, vegetables, grains, legumes, nuts and seeds contain FODMAPs. Avoiding them helps to control the symptoms, but may not bring sustainable benefits: when the person starts consuming them again, the symptoms return. Clinical experience indicates that healing the gut with an elimination diet protocol allows the patient to improve to the point when these highly fermentable carbohydrates can be consumed again without ill effects.

8.3.2.2 Protein

Enterocytes complete protein digestion by breaking peptides into amino acids with the use of brush border enzymes, called peptidases [142]. Damaged enterocytes may be unable to do this job. Pancreatic protein-digesting enzymes trypsin and chymotrypsin also need to be activated by enterokinases in the brush border. In a person with an abnormal gut microbiome, the intestinal wall deteriorates and may not be able to produce enterokinases, so pancreatic enzymes may not be fully activated. The two most researched proteins, which do not get broken down properly and get absorbed as peptides [159,160], are gluten from grains and casein from milk. These peptides have a structure similar to opiates and are called gluteomorphins and casomorphins [161]. They are absorbed and cross the blood brain barrier [162], causing depression [162], memory problems [163], inability to focus [163], sleep problems [163] and other mental symptoms [162]. Gluteomorphins and casomorphins were originally thought to play a role in autism and schizophrenia [162], but lately have been implicated in other mental health conditions [163]. Based on this research, a gluten and casein-free diet has been proposed for people with neuropsychiatric disorders [164]. Though it may bring some benefits, it does not heal the gut and delivers mixed results [165], as it only addresses two proteins.

The most difficult proteins for humans to digest are proteins from plants [166]. Grains, beans, pulses, nuts and other plant matter contain many proteins, which are indigestible for humans, and their amino acid composition is inappropriate for the human physiology [167]. The most researched plant protein is gluten, and we are rapidly coming to the conclusion that a growing proportion of humans cannot digest it [167,168]. Non-coeliac gluten sensitivity prevalence ranges considerably from 0.6% (US population) to 13% (UK population) depending on the country of analysis [169]. Gluten causes intestinal permeability (leaky gut), and non-coeliac gluten sensitivity can cause a plethora of health problems, from gastrointestinal to neurological and cognitive symptoms, to anaemia, neuropathy, headaches, fatigue, arthritis and autoimmune disease [167]. Depending on the person's general state of health and constitution, tolerance of gluten can vary dramatically, from full-blown coeliac disease to a few mild symptoms [167,168]. Bread (a major source of gluten) is a well-established staple in the world, and it may never occur to many people that their chronic headaches, arthritis, depression, allergies and other health problems could be caused by consuming bread day after day [167].

The best sources of easy-to-digest and very nourishing proteins for human beings are from animal sources: eggs, meats, seafood, poultry and well-fermented milk products, as the casein is largely digested during the fermentation process [170]. Proteins from these animal foods have the right amino acid composition for the human body to thrive on [171]. For people with digestive problems, it is important to eat easily digestible proteins to make work as easy as possible for their digestive systems.

8.3.2.3 Fats

Enterocytes do not have to do much work in absorbing fats [172]. That is likely why clinical practice shows that natural fats in the diet, animal fats in particular, are well tolerated by people with digestive disorders. However, many people with chronic illnesses find it difficult to digest fats due to poor bile flow. Clinical experience shows that when disaccharides, starches and other complex carbohydrates are out of the diet for a long-enough period, gallstones are naturally removed, bile flow improves and digestion of fats normalises [173].

8.3.2.4 Alcohol

Clinically, individuals with digestive disorders can tolerate small amounts of spirits and natural dry wine. Beer contains complex carbohydrates and should be avoided. It should be kept in mind that alcohol provides a burden for detoxification pathways in the liver, which can manifest with various symptoms, such as headaches, painful joints and fatigue [174–176]. For this reason, it is a good idea to avoid all alcoholic beverages until the digestive system heals to a large degree.

Some people with digestive disorders suffer from a so-called *auto brewery syndrome*, where pathogenic flora in the gut converts dietary carbohydrates into ethanol [177]. Various species of *Candida, Saccharomyces, Klebsiella and Enterococcus* are capable of this. These people display symptoms of alcoholic intoxication without consuming any alcohol; their blood tests show the presence of alcohol [177]. In acute cases, antifungal medication can be helpful, but in the long term, a therapeutic carbohydrate restriction (TCR) is required. Clinical experience shows that a large proportion of individuals with abnormal gut flora suffer from this affliction to various degrees.

8.3.2.5 Antinutrients

In clinical practice, individuals with digestive disorders usually cannot handle antinutrients [178]. This is one of the reasons why plant foods present the biggest challenge for this group of patients. Removing the worst offenders out of the diet, such as grains, and preparing vegetables and seeds (beans, pulses, nuts and other) carefully to neutralise antinutrients and make them more digestible, can improve the symptoms and health of those with digestive disorders [178,179]. For more information on antinutrients, refer to Section 2.5.

Diets for gastrointestinal disorders

Tamzyn Murphy

Diets that emphasise real, whole foods and the avoidance of processed food, combined with modification of dietary carbohydrate content, have the best evidence for efficacy for gastrointestinal disorders such as IBD [180,181] and IBS [182]. The specific carbohydrate diet (SCD) and its variation, the antiinflammatory diet, as well as the low-FODMAP diet are perhaps the best evidence-based examples of such diets, though palaeolithic and gluten-free diets have also been used with variable success.

The SCD avoids di- and polysaccharides, which are hypothesised to be poorly absorbed in IBD, resulting in bacterial and yeast overgrowth, mucosal damage and overproduction of mucus. Limited intake of monosaccharides is permitted. The SCD eliminates grains, most legumes, lactose-containing dairy, potatoes and corn, as well as most processed food. It allows unprocessed meat, fruit, most vegetables, lactose-free dairy, butter, wine and honey. The SCD has shown efficacy in IBD, particularly in paediatric populations [183], with an online survey indicating a majority of patients reporting significant clinical improvements on the diet, and 42% reporting clinical remission after six months [184].

The low-FODMAP diet restricts foods high in fermentable and poorly absorbed carbohydrates and polyols (>50 g/day) to improve symptoms of gas, bloating, distension, pain and motility changes in 74% of IBS patients [185]. It is superior to other diets used to treat IBS and has become a first-line treatment for many with the condition. The low-FODMAP diet has been found to be safe and effective for long-term use in IBS patients under dietician supervision [186]. A low-FODMAP diet has also shown efficacy for IBD symptoms (diarrhoea, bloating, pain, nausea, other gut symptoms, but not constipation) [187].

Identifying what the diets that work have in common is key to determining what dietary intervention to recommend for gastrointestinal disorders like IBS and IBD. The key aspects seem to be avoidance of processed foods and restriction of specific (the most fermentable and least absorbable) carbohydrates. The observation that limiting carbohydrates (quantity or type) is common to efficacy is not novel [188]. Logically then, TCR or more specifically, a KD, which limits total carbohydrate to below 50 g/d, will, by definition, also limit problematic carbohydrates (quantity and diversity) to below this level, with a similar efficacy. Unsurprisingly, evidence is emerging indicating that KD may indeed be efficacious for gastrointestinal disorders like IBS and IBD but more research is needed [189,190].

8.3.3 Guiding the patient

The following food lists belong to the *GAPS (Gut and Psychology Syndrome) Diet* [185,191] and incorporate common aspects of the most evidence-based diets for gastrointestinal disorders (e.g. IBS and IBD), namely, SCD, low-FODMAP and palaeolithic diets, together with clinical experience of efficacy.

8.3.3.1 Foods to avoid

Patients with digestive disorders should avoid the following.

- All grains and anything made out of them: wheat, rye, rice, oats, corn, maize, sorghum, barley, buckwheat, millet, spelt, triticale, bulgur, tapioca, quinoa and couscous. Grains contain starch and other complex carbohydrates, proteins (gluten, hordein, secalin and other) and antinutrients, which are very difficult to digest and which can damage the gut lining and other tissues and organs in the human body. These substances have been found to cause harm in healthy individuals, and even more so in individuals with damaged gut flora and a sensitive digestive system. There is no doubt that removing grains is a must for a person with any chronic degenerative illness, physical or mental.
- All starchy vegetables and anything made out of them: potato, yams, sweet potato, parsnip, Jerusalem artichoke, cassava, arrowroot and taro. Apart from starch, potatoes (and other starchy vegetables) contain antinutrients, which can have a damaging effect on many organs in the human body, including the GIT [191].
- Sugar (sucrose) and anything that contains it [185]. Sugar is a perfect food for pathogenic microbes in the gut. There can be no healing in the digestive system or anywhere else in the body without complete avoidance of table sugar.
- Starchy beans; legumes and pulses: soya beans, mung beans, garbanzo beans, bean sprouts, chickpeas, faba beans and many other varieties. Apart from starch, beans, legumes and pulses contain many antinutrients and are generally difficult to digest. When enough healing has happened in the digestive system, properly prepared beans and lentils can be introduced. Proper preparation techniques include soaking, rinsing, sprouting, fermenting and boiling over extended periods [192–194].
- Unfermented dairy products, high in lactose: fluid or dried milk of any type, many commercially produced yoghurts, commercially produced buttermilk and sour cream and processed foods with added lactose. Lactose is a perfect food for pathogenic microbes in the gut and should be avoided by any person with a gastrointestinal disorder [195]. Homemade yoghurt, kefir, sour cream and cheese are lower in lactose (lactose is consumed by lactobacilli during fermentation). They are an important part of the appropriate diet for digestive disorders.
- All processed foods must be avoided, as they contain many damaging ingredients and have low nutritional value. Everything a person with digestive problems eats should ideally be prepared at home from fresh natural ingredients.

8.3.3.2 Recommended foods

- Meats, game, organ meats, poultry, fish and shellfish are excellent sources of nutrition. Contrary to popular belief, it is meats, fish and other animal products that have the highest content of nourishing protein, vitamins, fats, minerals and other nutrients which humans need on a daily basis [141]. Nutrition in meats and fish also comes in the most digestible form for the human digestive system.
- Fresh eggs. Eggs are one the most nourishing and easy-to-digest foods on the planet. Egg yolks provide essential amino acids, vitamins (B1, B2, B6, B7, B12, A, D, E, and K), essential fatty acids, zinc, magnesium and many other nutrients, necessary for healing [196,197].
- Fermented milk products made at home. When fermented, lactose is reduced [179,198], nutrients become more bioavailable and the product is enriched with active enzymes and probiotics. Fermented milk may have therapeutic benefits on the digestive system in the form of kefir, yoghurt, sour cream and cottage cheese [199].
- Nonstarchy vegetables, which include a very wide range of vegetables. Cooked vegetables are easier to digest and are better tolerated than raw. Some fibre will be consumed with vegetables, and an individual has to gauge what amount their gut is ready for. Once grains and starchy vegetables are removed, most people with digestive disorders can tolerate some fibre from nonstarchy vegetables.
- Fermented vegetables, fruit and beverages. Fermentation employs microbes to digest food for us before we consume it. This preserves the food and enriches it with probiotics, enzymes, bioavailable nutrients and healing substances for the gut [199].
- Properly prepared plant seeds, nuts, oily seeds and legumes allow us to bake healthier versions of breads, cakes and deserts. To prepare them, they should be soaked, sprouted or fermented prior to cooking, which will reduce amounts of antinutrients [200]. It is best to avoid all plant seeds initially until enough healing happens in the digestive system and then introduce these foods gradually starting from small amounts.

- Ripe fresh local fruit is introduced, when the digestive system is ready to handle it. Enough healing has to happen in the gut before fruits can be consumed, and it should be introduced gradually starting from small amounts. Once local fresh fruit is tolerated, dried fruit can be used in baking and freshly pressed fruit juices can be consumed in limited amounts.

Individual variation should be accommodated, but based on individual tolerance and the characteristics and severity of the condition being addressed. Clinical experience indicates that more severe conditions or individual sensitivities may require more severe or bespoke restrictions (of carbohydrates or plant foods for example) or even a several day liquid fast.

8.3.4 Dietary approaches to address specific gastrointestinal disorders and motility problems

8.3.4.1 *Irritable bowel syndrome, Inflammatory bowel disease, chronic inflammation and autoimmunity*

Clinical experience indicates that an elimination diet, with components from the SCD, palaeolithic and low-FODMAP diets, including bone broth, muscle and organ meats and seafood, fermented dairy (in those who tolerate it), and in certain cases, well-cooked vegetables, is the best approach to helping patients with IBS, IBD, chronic inflammation and autoimmunity [187,188,190,201]. Clinical experience has shown that in acute stages of Crohn's disease and ulcerative colitis, a liquid fast preceding this elimination diet is often beneficial [105]. Once the inflammatory markers go down to normal and all symptoms are gone, the diet lists above should be followed as a permanent lifestyle.

Apart from the diet, probiotics in the form of fermented foods and commercial supplements help to restore damaged gut flora and have been shown to be useful in many digestive disorders, including IBD [202].

8.3.4.2 *Diarrhoea*

Diarrhoea is a natural cleansing reaction in the body and should not be feared [203]. Many pathogens and toxins are removed from the body through the bowel, and diarrhoea is the natural way for the bowel to flush these toxins out. Short-term diarrhoea, when we have food poisoning or a gastrointestinal infection, is an essential part of healing from these afflictions. However, when diarrhoea becomes chronic, it can be a problem in itself, draining nutrients from the body and making an individual malnourished and weak.

From clinical experience, the most effective treatment for diarrhoea is to drink bone/meat broth, homemade whey, yoghurt or kefir, ginger tea and honey and water and eat well-cooked meat and vegetable soup or stew. In cases of profuse watery diarrhoea, all plant foods should be excluded for a while. Once the stools improve, well-cooked vegetables can be slowly introduced. Fermented dairy products with high-protein content (homemade yoghurt, kefir and whey) are very effective at removing diarrhoea in the majority of cases. Once diarrhoea fully subsides, the patient can consume more of the foods listed above.

In some patients, chronic loose stools and even chronic diarrhoea are the result of faecal impaction with an overspill syndrome [204,205]. This is a situation when the bowel is full of old hard masses 'glued' to the gut wall, so the stool squeezes past these masses and comes out as diarrhoea, an overflow. The stool can also be loose or soft, coming out in strange shapes due to squeezing past the hard masses. Sometimes, the stool can leak out in small amounts and soil underwear [205]. This situation can be seen as a combination of constipation and diarrhoea and has significant associations with many chronic degenerative conditions, from autism [206], antipsychotic-associated constipation in schizophrenia [207] and other psychiatric problems to autoimmune disease [208], neurological illness [209] and fibromyalgia [210]. The compacted old faeces can trigger immune activation [211]. Passing stool typically does not shift the compacted masses and does not empty the bowel. Children and adults with this problem spend a long time on the toilet, feeling that something remains in the bowel and evacuation was not complete. In my clinical experience, following the nutritional protocol outlined above resolves this situation over time.

8.3.4.3 *Constipation*

Constipation is common among people with abnormal gut microbiome and poor bile flow [212,213]. Chronic constipation is associated with many degenerative diseases, such as chronic fatigue syndrome, fibromyalgia, autoimmune illnesses and cancer, including bowel cancer [214]. As an immediate remedy for constipation, there is nothing more effective than an enema or colonic irrigation, used under the advice of your medical practitioner [215,216]. Long-term resolution of constipation takes time and effort.

Management of chronic constipation.

- Impaired bile flow may be a cause of constipation [213]. Clinical experience shows it can respond to an appropriate diet with a gradual increase in fat consumption [217].
- Clinical experience shows that removing dairy from the diet can be helpful, as constipation can rise from cow milk protein allergies presenting as elevated immunoglobulin E (IgE) and β-lactoglobulin proteins [218], where β-lactoglobulins without iron complexes aids in Th2 lymphocyte activation and IgE production, creating an allergic response [219]. For some people, just removing high-protein dairy (yoghurt, kefir, cheese and whey) is sufficient, while continuing to consume high-fat dairy (ghee, butter and sour cream).
- For many people, it is important to reduce lean muscle meats in the diet and replace them with gelatinous meats: soft tissues around joints, bones, feet, skin, bone marrow and organs of animals and birds [220].
- Drinking more water helps in some cases, but homemade fermented beverages (kvass and kombucha) are more effective, providing not only water but probiotics and enzymes to assist digestion and elimination. Kvass can be made from beetroot, cabbage and other vegetables, as well as fruit and berries. These beverages provide magnesium, essential for resolving constipation [221].
- Supplementing magnesium (as citrate, oxide or amino acid chelates) can help [222]. Supplements of spirulina [223], blue-green algae [224] and chlorella [225] also provide magnesium and can be effective laxatives, particularly in children.
- Castor oil can be taken orally as a laxative to provide a quick relief [226].
- For a chronically constipated person, it is important to use a correct position on the toilet (close to the natural position of squatting on the ground); a small foot stool can be used to bring the knees closer to the chest [227].
- While fibre is a ubiquitous prescription for constipation, no studies have sufficiently demonstrated a remedial effect [228] and others have demonstrated benefit from its removal [153].

8.3.5 Nutritional supplements

When it comes to the digestive system, supplements and pharmaceuticals should be prescribed with increased caution, because most of them contain ingredients which can irritate and damage the gut (fillers, binders, preservatives, colourants, sugars, etc.). Since the gut is already damaged in a person with a digestive illness, supplements and pharmaceuticals should be limited to an absolute necessary minimum, with consideration of the ingredient list. Nevertheless, some supplements can be helpful in digestive disorders.

8.3.5.1 Digestive enzymes

8.3.5.1.1 Hypochlorhydria

Hypochlorhydria is pervasive in patients with digestive disorders, particularly in people with stomach problems and reflux [229]. Normal stomach acidity is crucial for proper digestion, so boosting stomach acid production is helpful for many gastrointestinal illnesses [229]. This can be done through the use of nutritional bitters, cabbage juice (natural and fermented) and supplements.

1. Bitter herbs (artichoke, dandelion, gentian, blessed thistle, bitter orange and other) have a good ability to stimulate stomach acid production [230] and have been used for centuries in traditional digestive bitters [230,231]. There are a number of digestive bitters available on the market; a few drops should be taken before meals in some water or meat stock. It is important to experience the bitter taste of the herbs in order for them to work [230], so they cannot be taken in capsules or tablets.
2. Cabbage (fresh and fermented) is a traditional stimulant of stomach acid production. A small helping of fresh cabbage salad, cabbage juice and sauerkraut, consumed at the start of the meals, can be quite effective in preparing the stomach for the arriving food [232].
3. Supplements of stomach acid typically contain *Betaine Hydrochloride* with *pepsin* in different concentrations and should be taken at the beginning of each meal [233]. Improvements in reflux can be expected [234]. Clinically, patients also report improvements in bloating and stool in just a few days from starting Betaine hydrochloride with pepsin. Probiotics should not be taken together with these supplements, as the acid is likely to damage the probiotic microbes [235].

8.3.5.1.2 Digestive enzyme insufficiencies

When stomach acidity is normalised, pancreatic enzymes are produced naturally [236]. However, some people find it helpful [237] to finish their meals with a supplement of pancreatic digestive enzymes, usually containing a mixture of proteases, peptidases, lipases, amylase, lactase and cellulase [237].

Supplements of digestive enzymes do not need to be taken permanently by the majority of people. As the gut starts healing, the person can slowly withdraw the stomach acid supplementation and/or pancreatic enzymes, taking them only with heavy meals, or if something not allowed on the diet has been eaten. Where possible, it is far more natural and practical to use fermented foods, particularly containing fermented cabbage, and digestive bitters to stimulate production of normal amounts of stomach acid [230–232] and digestive enzymes.

For patients with poor fat digestion, which can result in steatorrhea, it is helpful to supplement ox bile with lipase [238].

8.3.5.2 Probiotics

There is a large body of research conducted on the use of probiotics, particularly in the treatment of gastrointestinal disorders:

- Antibiotic-associated diarrhoea [239]
- *Candida Albicans* growth [240]
- Viral infections of the digestive tract [241,242]
- Necrotising enterocolitis in infants [243]
- Acute paediatric diarrhoea (acute gastroenteritis) [244]
- Traveller's diarrhoea [245]
- *Clostridium difficile* enterocolitis [246]
- *Helicobacter* infection [239,240]
- Enteropathogenic *Escherichia coli* infection [247]
- IBD: Crohn's disease [248], ulcerative colitis [249] and chronic pouchitis [250]
- IBS [251]
- Lactose intolerance [252,253]
- Prevention of colonic cancer in laboratory studies [254,255],
- Infantile colic [256]

In clinical practice, adding probiotics to the treatment regimen can improve and, in some cases, even resolve the condition.

Probiotics may also offer benefits in health problems beyond the GIT (often likely through modulation of the gastrointestinal microbiome, such as insulin-resistant conditions (e.g. type 2 diabetes–associated CVD [243,257,258] and obesity [259])); immune conditions (e.g. arthritis [260], allergic rhinitis, eczema and atopy [261–265], some psychiatric conditions [266,267], infections [268–271], and aspects of cancer (specifically improving quality of life in respect of bowel symptoms in colorectal cancer survivors and possibly playing a role in cancer prevention via immune modulation and inflammation pathways [272,273])). Unfortunately, there is high heterogeneity between studies, which are often of low quality. More research is required.

Probiotic supplements and fermented foods can produce a so-called *die-off reaction* (also known as the Herxheimer reaction) [274,275]. As probiotics are introduced into the gut, they start destroying pathogenic bacteria, viruses and fungi [274,275]. When these pathogens die, they release toxins, making the typical symptoms of the patient worse. On top of that, the patient may feel more tired than usual, experience general malaise and develop a headache, a skin rash, or myalgia [276,277]. Die-off is a temporary reaction and usually lasts from a few days to a few weeks in different individuals [277]. To make this reaction milder, the dose of the probiotic (or fermented foods) should be built slowly, starting from a small amount (no larger than half of the recommended dose). Some die-off symptoms may have to be tolerated as part of the treatment, and controlling their intensity is recommended.

Many people do well just with fermented foods (which provide active probiotic microbes), without adding any commercial formulas. For other people, commercial probiotics can be very helpful in combination with fermented foods.

8.3.5.3 *Fibre*

In properly conducted research, no statistically significant differences can be found between supplement groups and controls in fibre supplementation for alleviating constipation [278]. Importantly, some studies indicate that fibre supplementation worsens constipation, and its reduction or elimination instead alleviates symptoms [153].

8.3.5.3.1 Whey for gastritis

Drinking homemade whey, diluted with some warm water, reduces inflammation and initiates healing in the mucosa of the stomach and oesophagus [279]. It is effective for acute gastritis [280]. The gastritis patient should sip it all day between meals and with meals.

8.3.5.3.2 Fat-soluble vitamins for pancreatic problems

The highest concentration of vitamin K2 in the human body has been found in the pancreas, indicating that this organ has particularly high needs for this vital vitamin [281]. Fat-soluble vitamins A, D and K2 work synergistically and are usually globally deficient in patients with acute and chronic pancreatitis [282–285], so vitamins A and D should also be provided and it is best to provide all three vitamins in their bioavailable natural form (i.e. in vitamin-dense animal oils such as fermented cod liver oil [286], quality emu oil [287] and butter oil [286]). Supplementing these vitamins is helpful for people with pancreatic problems [282,283,288,289]. If, initially, no amount of fat is tolerated orally, these oils can be applied as a poultice to provide these vitamins transdermally (rub the oil onto the skin of the abdomen, cover with a towel and a hot-water bottle) [290,291].

8.3.6 Conclusion

Our digestive system holds the roots of our health, and the microbial community inside our gut is the soil around those roots. Clinical experience indicates that patients with diverse systemic illnesses have some form of digestive symptoms as well as abnormal gut microflora. Using the nutritional protocol outlined in this chapter to improve our gastrointestinal microflora and heal the digestive system often results in clinical improvement in other systemic conditions.

8.4 The Microbiome and Therapeutic Carbohydrate Restriction

Sarah M. Rice

8.4.1 Introduction

The role of the microbiome and its contribution to disease and disease management is receiving increasing attention as an area of therapeutic interest across a range of disorders including metabolic [97,292–294], inflammatory [295], neurological [296,297], allergic [298,299], endocrine [300,301] and combinations of these conditions [302].

8.4.2 What does a healthy gut microbiome look like?

The microbiome is influenced by a number of factors and exposures such as diet, toxins, drugs, stress, temperature, age, genetics and pathogens like viruses, bacteria and fungi [292,303–305]. What defines a healthy microbiome has not been clearly determined at a taxonomic level though trends across various metrics have been explored [305–307]. A key driver of an individual's ability to develop a healthy resilient gut flora may be set in infancy with factors such as delivery, maternal microbiome, breastfeeding, weaning and malnutrition being influential [293,295,305,308]. These complex interactions have made the microbiome challenging to categorise. The aspects considered include the ratio of *Firmicutes* to *Bacteroidetes*, alpha species diversity and the relative number of beneficial to harmful or opportunistic flora [308]. In general, an increased number of *Bacteroidetes* and a lower number of *Firmicutes* is associated with positive health markers [97,309], though it is not universal [310].

Trends in microbiome composition with metabolic health and leanness include observations that different bacteria drive differences in SCFA production, which affects metabolic signalling. Emerging as a signal in type 2 diabetes is a shift in the microbiome away from gut bacteria able to produce butyrate (associated with insulin sensitivity) and towards the production of propionate (associated with insulin resistance) [311]. An increase in the SCFA butyrate can stimulate GLP1 and peptide YY via actions on enteroendocrine cells, which help regulate energy homoeostasis, reducing appetite and improving glucose and insulin regulation [305].

Bacteria-derived butyrate also plays a role in intestinal permeability via modulating tight junction protein expression (zonulin and occludin), mucous production and stabilisation of hypoxia-inducible factor, which coordinates intestinal barrier protection [97,312,313].

Lactobacillus reuteri is a gram-positive bacteria from the phylum *Firmicutes*, which has gained interest and is a widely used probiotic. It has an antimicrobial action, which influences the harmful vs commensal bacteria balance, leading to positive remodelling of the microbiome. It may reduce the production of proinflammatory cytokines, support regulatory T cell function and contribute to intestinal barrier function (it can form a biofilm and play a role in reversing leaky gut) [314]. The use of *L. reuteri* has also been explored in decreasing the bacterial load of *H. pylori* [314,315] among other gut, metabolic, immune-related and neurodevelopmental conditions [314,316].

Overall, evidence does not support a clearly defined reference gut microbiota capable of promoting metabolic health due to significant variations across age and environmental exposures [305,306,317], though elements of diversity, homoeostasis and butyrate-producing flora appear to be important [308,311,318].

8.4.3 The Western Diet and the Microbiome

Recent changes in the human diet, moving away from ancestral foods towards agriculture and animal husbandry, may have resulted in shifts in the microbiome, contributing to the increasing prevalence of chronic disease in society [319]. While the many interactions create challenges, comparisons of Western, urbanised populations with traditional, rural populations tend to show a decrease in biodiversity occurring with movement away from ancestral foods and towards a more processed Western diet [320].

Food processing, to different degrees, substantially affects the gut environment [319–321]. It is suggested that more than 70% of the daily energy consumed by the US population come from foods that would have had little prevalence in pre-agricultural society [319]. Over the course of human history, cellular nutrients have been released during digestion and the accessibility of these nutrients is dependent on the food matrix and degree of processing. Acellular nutrients, those not contained in cells, alter absorption kinetics and influence gut flora growth. The production of the most recent ultraprocessed foods uses highly refined starches and oils extracted from seed crops which are highly acellular. In particular, this has the ability to affect the small intestine and may contribute to gut dysbiosis [321]. Likewise, other additives such as preservatives, emulsifiers and artificial sweeteners contribute to altering the gut environment [322]. Taken together, the evidence suggests a trend towards a decrease in the richness and diversity of the microbiome under a Western diet, which may contribute to the development of chronic disease [319–321].

8.4.4 The role of the therapeutic carbohydrate restriction in modulating the microbiome

The negative impact of the Western diet on the microbiome, inflammation and autoimmune disorders is well described [321,323], as is the effect of carbohydrate constituents on the microbiome [324]. Removing processed foods from the diet would be expected to benefit the microbiome.

Sholl et al. [307] considers the metabolic flexibility we evolved with (the ability to burn fat or carbohydrate, as required, with seasonal changes in diet) as the context by which we should evaluate the microbiome in diets that are higher in fat content, such as TCR or KD. Alternate pathways that are influenced by the state of nutritional ketosis and production of beta-hydroxybutyrate are able to support gut function [152,307] and therefore measures of a 'healthy microbiome' may be altered compared to a diet that is glucocentric [325].

8.4.4.1 Short-chain fatty acids

The production of SCFAs, necessary for providing fuel to the gut epithelial cells, is one of the alternate pathways that support gut health in a TCR nutritional approach [307]. Dietary changes modulate SCFA production [326], which is proposed to have a role in health outcomes. A study by David et al. [326], which compared animal-based diet (ABD) with a plant-based diet (PBD), found that the SCFA butyrate production was only slightly elevated on a PBD, but that the ABD produced significantly more isobutyrate, which influences similar receptors to butyrate [307,326]. Four substances are able to be utilised instead of butyrate: acetoacetate, β-HB, isobutyrate, and acylcarnitines. Taken together, these substances are able to support gut function effectively though they have different actions [307].

Preclinical studies have shown that a KD is able to support gut mucosal layer integrity even in the absence of fermentable carbohydrates [325]. In cases of preexisting inflammation, circulating ketones may provide therapeutic benefit as a damaged gut lining impacts butyrate absorption. Ketones can provide fuel, protect gut barrier function and reduce the production of innate lymphoid cells and cytokines [307,327].

8.4.4.2 *Lipopolysaccharide*

With respect to other metabolic pathways which respond to TCR, a higher HDL value increases the ability to manage the bacterial endotoxin LPS. HDL binds and clears LPS, protecting against toxicity [324]. So even in the presence of increased LPS, which has been noted in studies where higher fat diets are consumed [328], other metabolic pathways can compensate. The Western diet, often high in fat and simple carbohydrates, is usually the context where LPS is problematic [329]. Exposure to LPS is largely mediated by gut permeability, so in the setting of robust gut barrier function, which may be supported by a KD, this concern is reduced [307,327].

8.4.4.3 *Trimethylamine N-oxide*

Trimethylamine N-oxide (TMAO) has emerged as a metabolite of interest due to its association with CVD, but in the metabolically healthy, the significance of TMAO is uncertain [330]. Concentrations of TMAO are subject to variations driven by nutrition, microbiome, genetics and liver and kidney function. Two pathways contribute to TMAO levels: diet and microbiome metabolite. Dietary sources for the microbiome pathway are carnitine, choline and phosphatidylcholine, which provide the precursors for trimethylamine converted by the liver to TMAO [330]. These precursors are commonly found in animal products like red meat, eggs, liver, dairy and salt water fish, but also in soybean and sunflower [331]. The microbiome can significantly influence TMAO, increasing it via an excess of *E. coli* [332], or conversely, the activity of *Bilophila* may attenuate TMAO production. *Bilophila* is able to metabolise TMA (derived from ABD) and dietary precursors to dimethylamine instead of TMAO, thereby reducing TMAO [333]. Microbiome composition and metabolic health may be more influential drivers of health than TMAO [330,334].

8.4.4.4 *Bile acids*

Increased bile acids observed with diets higher in fat may support gut barrier integrity by influencing mucous secretion and epithelial cell migration as well as providing an alternative fuel source via acylcarnitines [307,335].

8.4.4.5 *Summary*

Studies reviewed suggest that the pathological or healing potential of the microbiome may be context-dependent, and while it is clear that the microbiome plays an important role, other features of TCR have significant mediating effects on metabolic pathways, which support the therapeutic effect of nutrition on disease [336–338]. These include pathways that influence our mood and relationship with food via the microbiome–gut–brain axis [339,340].

8.4.5 Other lifestyle interventions affecting the microbiome

Other factors that can modulate the microbiome include fasting [341,342], time-restricted eating [343], circadian rhythms [344], exercise [345–347] and stress [348,349].

8.4.6 Conclusion

While dependent on many factors, TCR and lifestyle choices can both modulate the microbiome, showing promise for a range of chronic conditions.

References

[1] Miquel-Kergoat S, Azais-Braesco V, Burton-Freeman B, Hetherington MM. Effects of chewing on appetite, food intake and gut hormones: a systematic review and meta-analysis. Physiol Behav 2015;151:88–96. Available from: https://doi.org/10.1016/j.physbeh.2015.07.017 Epub 2015 Jul 15. PMID: 26188140.

[2] Carpenter GH. The secretion, components, and properties of saliva. Annu Rev Food Sci Technol 2013;4:267–76. Available from: https://doi.org/10.1146/annurev-food-030212-182700 PMID: 23464573.

[3] Keremi B, Beck A, Fabian TK, Fabian G, Szabo G, Nagy A, et al. Stress and salivary glands. Curr Pharm Des 2017;23(27). Available from: https://doi.org/10.2174/1381612823666170215110648.

[4] Dominik N. It's All In Your Mouth. Biological Dentistry and the Surprising Impact of Oral Health on Whole Body Wellness. Chelsea Green Publishing; 2020.
[5] Figdor D, Gulabivala K. Survival against the odds: microbiology of root canals associated with post-treatment disease. Endod Top 2008; 18(1):62–77.
[6] Lasserre JF, Brecx MC, Toma S. Oral microbes, biofilms and their role in periodontal and peri-implant diseases. Materials 2018;11(10):1802.
[7] Bürgers R, Krohn S, Wassmann T. Surface properties of dental materials and biofilm formation. Oral Biofilms and Modern Dental Materials. Cham: Springer; 2021. p. 55–69.
[8] Milhem MM, Al-Hiyasat AS, Darmani H. Toxicity testing of restorative dental materials using brine shrimp larvae (Artemia salina). J Appl Oral Sci 2008;16:297–301.
[9] Schneider JC. Can microparticles contribute to inflammatory bowel disease: innocuous or inflammatory? Exp Biol Med 2007;232(1):1–2.
[10] Deo PN, Deshmukh R. Oral microbiome: unveiling the fundamentals. J Oral Maxillofac Pathol 2019;23(1):122–8.
[11] Docktor MJ, Paster BJ, Abramowicz S, Ingram J, Wang YE, Correll M, et al. Alterations in diversity of the oral microbiome in pediatric inflammatory bowel disease. Inflamm Bowel Dis 2012;18(5):935–42. Available from: https://doi.org/10.1002/ibd.21874.
[12] Wade WG. The oral microbiome in health and disease. Pharmacol Res 2013;69(1):137–43. Available from: https://doi.org/10.1016/j.phrs.2012.11.006.
[13] Ren W, Xun Z, Wang Z, et al. Tongue Coating and the salivary microbial communities vary in children with halitosis. Sci Rep 2016;6:24481. Available from: https://doi.org/10.1038/srep24481.
[14] Kleinstein SE, Nelson KE, Freire M. Inflammatory networks linking oral microbiome with systemic health and disease. J Dental Res 2020; 99(10):1131–9. Available from: https://doi.org/10.1177/0022034520926126.
[15] Casu C, Mosaico G, Natoli V, Scarano A, Lorusso F, Inchingolo F. Microbiota of the tongue and systemic connections: the examination of the tongue as an integrated approach in oral medicine. Hygiene 2021;1(2):56–68. Available from: https://doi.org/10.3390/hygiene1020006.
[16] Okada M, Hisajima T, Ishibashi H, Miyasaka T, Abe S, Satoh T. Pathological analysis of the candida albicans-infected tongue tissues of a murine oral candidiasis model in the early infection stage. Arch Oral Biol 2013;58(4):444–50. Available from: https://doi.org/10.1016/j.archoralbio.2012.09.014.
[17] Panov VE, Krasteva A. Tongue coating in patients with gastrointestinal and liver diseases. J IMAB 2012;18(2):188–90. Available from: https://doi.org/10.5272/jimab.2012182.188.
[18] Femiano F, Lanza A, Buonaiuto C, Gombos F, Nunziata M, Cuccurullo L, et al. Burning mouth syndrome and burning mouth in hypothyroidism: proposal for a diagnostic and therapeutic protocol. Oral Surg Oral Med Oral Pathol Oral Radiol Endod 2008;105(1). Available from: https://doi.org/10.1016/j.tripleo.2007.07.030.
[19] Reamy BV, Derby R, Bunt CW. *Common tongue conditions in primary care*. Am Fam Phys 2010. Retrieved July 7, 2022, Available from: https://www.aafp.org/pubs/afp/issues/2010/0301/p627.html.
[20] Costa MMB. Neural control of swallowing. Arq Gastroenterol 2018;55(Suppl 1):61–75. Available from: https://doi.org/10.1590/S0004-2803.201800000-45. Epub 2018 Aug 23. PMID: 30156597.
[21] Li D, He R, Hou G, Ming W, Fan T, Chen L, et al. Characterization of the esophageal microbiota and prediction of the metabolic pathways involved in esophageal cancer Front Cell Infect Microbiol [Internet] 2020;[cited 2022 Jul 18];10. Available from: https://www.frontiersin.org/articles/10.3389/fcimb.2020.00268.
[22] De Giorgi F, Palmiero M, Esposito I, Mosca F, Cuomo R. Pathophysiology of gastro-oesophageal reflux disease. Acta Otorhinolaryngol Ital 2006;26(5):241–6 PMID: 17345925; PMCID: PMC2639970.
[23] Okereke I, Hamilton C, Wenholz A, Jala V, Giang T, Reynolds S, et al. Associations of the microbiome and esophageal disease. J Thorac Dis 2019;11(Suppl 12):S1588–93. Available from: https://doi.org/10.21037/jtd.2019.05.82 PMID: 31489225; PMCID: PMC6702393.
[24] Mikami DJ, Murayama KM. Physiology and pathogenesis of gastroesophageal reflux disease. Surg Clin North Am 2015;95(3):515–25. Available from: https://doi.org/10.1016/j.suc.2015.02.006 Epub 2015 Mar 24. PMID: 25965127.
[25] Lechien JR, Saussez S, Karkos PD. Laryngopharyngeal reflux disease: clinical presentation, diagnosis and therapeutic challenges in 2018. Curr Opin Otolaryngol Head Neck Surg 2018;26(6):392–402. Available from: https://doi.org/10.1097/MOO.0000000000000486.
[26] Capucilli P, Hill DA. Allergic comorbidity in eosinophilic esophagitis: mechanistic relevance and clinical implications. Clin Rev Allergy Immunol 2019;57(1):111–27. Available from: https://doi.org/10.1007/s12016-019-08733-0 PMID: 30903437; PMCID: PMC6626558.
[27] Vinit C, Dieme A, Courbage S, Dehaine C, Dufeu CM, Jacquemot S, et al. Eosinophilic esophagitis: pathophysiology, diagnosis, and management. Arch De Pédiatrie 2019;26(3):182–90. Available from: https://doi.org/10.1016/j.arcped.2019.02.005.
[28] Eneström S, Hultman P. Does amalgam affect the immune system? A controversial issue (Part 1 of 2). Int Arch allergy immunology 1995; 106(3):180–91.
[29] How does the stomach work? - informedhealth.org - NCBI bookshelf. (2009). Retrieved July 8, 2022, Available from: https://www.ncbi.nlm.nih.gov/books/NBK279304/.
[30] Philpott HL, Nandurkar S, Lubel J, Gibson PR. Drug-induced gastrointestinal disorders. Frontline Gastroenterol 2014;5(1):49–57. Available from: https://doi.org/10.1136/flgastro-2013-100316.
[31] Yuan X, Pan Z, Jin C, Ni Y, Fu Z, Jin Y. Gut microbiota: an underestimated and unintended recipient for pesticide-induced toxicity. Chemosphere 2019;227:425–34. Available from: https://doi.org/10.1016/j.chemosphere.2019.04.088.
[32] Roman S, Pandolfino JE. Environmental—lifestyle related factors. Best Pract Res Clin Gastroenterol 2010;24(6):847–59. Available from: https://doi.org/10.1016/j.bpg.2010.09.010.

[33] Howden CW, Hunt RH. Spontaneous hypochlorhydria in man: possible causes and consequences. Dig Dis 1986;4(1):26–32. Available from: https://doi.org/10.1159/000171134.

[34] Hunt RH, Yaghoobi M. The esophageal and gastric microbiome in health and disease. Gastroenterol Clin North Am 2017;46(1):121–41. Available from: https://doi.org/10.1016/j.gtc.2016.09.009.

[35] Castaño-Rodríguez N, Goh KL, Fock KM, Mitchell HM, Kaakoush NO. Dysbiosis of the microbiome in gastric carcinogenesis. Sci Rep 2017; 7(1):15957. Available from: https://doi.org/10.1038/s41598-017-16289-2 Published 2017 Nov 21.

[36] Cheung KS, Leung WK. Long-term use of proton-pump inhibitors and risk of gastric cancer: a review of the current evidence. Ther Adv Gastroenterol [Internet] 2019;12 [cited 2020 Feb 14].

[37] Lender N, Talley NJ, Enck P, Haag S, Zipfel S, Morrison M, et al. Review article: associations between *Helicobacter pylori* and obesity - an ecological study. Alimentary Pharmacology & Therapeutics 2014;40(1):24–31.

[38] Jeffery PL, McGuckin MA, Linden SK. Endocrine impact of *Helicobacter pylori*: focus on ghrelin and ghrelin o-acyltransferase. World J Gastroenterol 2011;17(10):1249–60.

[39] Sheh A, Fox JG. The role of the gastrointestinal microbiome in *Helicobacter pylori* pathogenesis. Gut Microbes 2013;4(6):505–31. Available from: https://doi.org/10.4161/gmic.26205.

[40] Liu Z, Udenigwe CC. Role of food-derived opioid peptides in the central nervous and gastrointestinal systems. J food Biochem 2019;43(1): e12629.

[41] Cater RE. The clinical importance of Hypochlorhydria (a consequence of chronic helicobacter infection): its possible etiological role in mineral and amino acid malabsorption, depression, and other syndromes. Med Hypotheses 1992;39(4):375–83. Available from: https://doi.org/10.1016/0306-9877(92)90065-k.

[42] Brownie S. Why are elderly individuals at risk of nutritional deficiency. Int J Nurs Pract 2006;12(2):110–18. Available from: https://doi.org/10.1111/j.1440-172x.2006.00557.x.

[43] Kines K, Krupczak T. Nutritional interventions for gastroesophageal reflux, irritable bowel syndrome, and hypochlorhydria: a case report. Integr Med (Encinitas, Calif) 2016;15(4):49–53.

[44] Väkeväinen S, Mentula S, Nuutinen H, Salmela KS, Jousimies-Somer H, Färkkilä M, et al. Ethanol-derived microbial production of carcinogenic acetaldehyde in achlorhydric atrophic gastritis. Scand J Gastroenterol 2002;37(6):648–55.

[45] O'Leary F, Samman S. Vitamin B12 in health and disease. Nutrients 2010;2(3):299–316. Available from: https://doi.org/10.3390/nu2030299.

[46] Pimentel M, Mathur R, Chang C. Gas and the microbiome. Curr Gastroenterol Rep 2013;15(12):356. Available from: https://doi.org/10.1007/s11894-013-0356-y.

[47] Camilleri M, Chedid V, Ford AC, et al. Gastroparesis. Nat Rev Dis Primers 2018;4(1):41. Available from: https://doi.org/10.1038/s41572-018-0038-z Published 2018 Nov 1.

[48] Stein HUBERTJ, Barlow ANTONYP, Demeester TOMR, Hinder RONALDA. Complications of gastroesophageal reflux disease. Ann Surg 1992;216(1):35–43. Available from: https://doi.org/10.1097/00000658-199207000-00006.

[49] Nasser SC, Slim M, Nassif JG, Nasser SM. Influence of proton pump inhibitors on gastritis diagnosis and pathologic gastric changes. World J Gastroenterol 2015;21(15):4599–606.

[50] Wilkinson JM, Cozine EW, Loftus CG. Gas, bloating, and belching: approach to evaluation and management. Am Fam Physician 2019; 99(5):301–9.

[51] Bhandari S, Jha P, Thakur A, Kar A, Gerdes H, Venkatesan T. Cyclic vomiting syndrome: epidemiology, diagnosis, and treatment. Clin Auton Res 2018;28(2):203–9. Available from: https://doi.org/10.1007/s10286-018-0506-2.

[52] Kucik CJ, Martin GL, Sortor BV. Common intestinal parasites. Am Fam Physician 2004;69(5):1161–8 PMID: 15023017.

[53] Wu CY. Initiatives for a healthy stomach. Curr Treat Options Gastro 2019;17:628–35. Available from: https://doi.org/10.1007/s11938-019-00266-x.

[54] Stengel A, Taché Y. Interaction between gastric and upper small intestinal hormones in the regulation of hunger and satiety: ghrelin and cholecystokinin take the central stage. Curr Protein Pept Sci 2011;12(4):293–304. Available from: https://doi.org/10.2174/138920311795906673.

[55] Lynch SV, Pedersen O. The human intestinal microbiome in health and disease. N Engl J Med 2016;375(24):2369–79. Available from: https://doi.org/10.1056/NEJMra1600266 PMID: 27974040.

[56] Pincus IJ, Thomas JE, Rehfuss ME. A study of gastric secretion as influenced by changes in duodenal acidity. Exp Biol Med 1942; 51(3):367–8. Available from: https://doi.org/10.3181/00379727-51-13978p.

[57] Bruno G, Zaccari P, Rocco G, Scalese G, Panetta C, Porowska B, et al. Proton pump inhibitors and dysbiosis: current knowledge and aspects to be clarified. World J Gastroenterol 2019;25(22):2706–19. Available from: https://doi.org/10.3748/wjg.v25.i22.2706.

[58] Filardo S, Scalese G, Virili C, Pontone S, Di Pietro M, Covelli A, et al. The potential role of hypochlorhydria in the development of duodenal dysbiosis: a preliminary report. Front Cell Infect Microbiology 2022;12. Available from: https://doi.org/10.3389/fcimb.2022.854904.

[59] Lauritano EC, Gabrielli M, Scarpellini E, Lupascu A, Novi M, Sottili S, et al. Small intestinal bacterial overgrowth recurrence after antibiotic therapy. Am J Gastroenterol 2008;103(8):2031–5. Available from: https://doi.org/10.1111/j.1572-0241.2008.02030.x PMID: 18802998.

[60] Fasano A. All disease begins in the (leaky) gut: role of zonulin-mediated gut permeability in the pathogenesis of some chronic inflammatory diseases. F1000Res 2020;9:F1000 PMID: 32051759 PMCID: PMC6996528.

[61] Brostoff J, Gamlin L. Food allergies and food intolerance: the complete guide to their identification and treatment. Inner Traditions/Bear & Co; 2000.

[62] Sicherer SH, Sampson HA. Food allergy: epidemiology, pathogenesis, diagnosis, and treatment. J Allergy Clin Immunology 2014; 133(2):291–307.

[63] Nowak-Węgrzyn A, Katz Y, Mehr SS, Koletzko S. Non-IgE-mediated gastrointestinal food allergy. J Allergy Clin Immunol 2015.
[64] Campbell-McBride N. Gut and physiology syndrome. Medinform Publishing; 2020. p. 166–96.
[65] Trefts E, Gannon M, Wasserman DH. The liver. Curr Biol 2017;27(21):R1147–51. Available from: https://doi.org/10.1016/j.cub.2017.09.019 PMID: 29112863; PMCID: PMC5897118.
[66] Dosch AR, Imagawa DK, Jutric Z. Bile metabolism and lithogenesis: an update. Surg Clin North Am 2019;99(2):215–29. Available from: https://doi.org/10.1016/j.suc.2018.12.003 PMID: 30846031.
[67] Kitchen J. Hypochlorhydria: a review, part 1. Townsend Lett Dr Patients 2001;(219) 56-56.
[68] Garrow JS, James WPT, Ralph A. Human nutrition and dietetics. 10th edition Churchill Livingstone; 2000. p. 107–9.
[69] Garrow JS, James WPT, Ralph A. Human nutrition and dietetics. 10th edition Churchill Livingstone; 2000. p. 114–9.
[70] Stokes CS, Gluud LL, Casper M, Lammert F. Ursodeoxycholic acid and diets higher in fat prevent gallbladder stones during weight loss: a meta-analysis of randomized controlled trials. Clin Gastroenterology Hepatology 2014;12(7):1090–100.
[71] Lee JY, Keane MG, Pereira S. Diagnosis and treatment of gallstone disease. Practitioner 2015;259(1783):15–19 2. PMID: 26455113.
[72] Festi D, Colecchia A, Larocca A, Villanova N, Mazzella G, Petroni ML, et al. Review: low caloric intake and gall-bladder motor function. Aliment Pharmacol Ther 2000;14(Suppl 2):51–3. Available from: https://doi.org/10.1046/j.1365-2036.2000.014s2051.x PMID: 10903004.
[73] Wells ML, Venkatesh SK. Congestive hepatopathy. Abdom Radiol (NY) 2018;43(8):2037–51. Available from: https://doi.org/10.1007/s00261-017-1387-x PMID: 29147765.
[74] Gui GP, Cheruvu CV, West N, Sivaniah K, Fiennes AG. Is cholecystectomy effective treatment for symptomatic gallstones? Clinical outcome after long-term follow-up. Ann R Coll Surg Engl 1998;80(1):25.
[75] Palmer RH. Bile acid deficiency and constipation. Clin Gastroenterol Hepatol 2018;16(8):1363–4. Available from: https://doi.org/10.1016/j.cgh.2018.04.018 PMID: 30033178.
[76] Vijayvargiya P, Busciglio I, Burton D, Donato L, Lueke A, Camilleri M. Bile acid deficiency in a subgroup of patients with irritable bowel syndrome with constipation based on biomarkers in serum and fecal samples. Clin Gastroenterology Hepatology 2018;16(4):522–7.
[77] Hosking SW, Smart HL, Johnson AG, Triger DR. Anorectal varices, haemorrhoids, and portal hypertension. Lancet 1989;1(8634):349–52. Available from: https://doi.org/10.1016/s0140-6736(89)91724-8 PMID: 2563507.
[78] Treiber G, Csepregi A, Malfertheiner P. The pathophysiology of portal hypertension. Digestive Dis 2005;23(1):6–10.
[79] Kibret AA, Oumer M, Moges AM. Prevalence and associated factors of hemorrhoids among adult patients visiting the surgical outpatient department in the University of Gondar Comprehensive Specialized Hospital, Northwest Ethiopia. PLoS One 2021;16(4):e0249736.
[80] Lightner AM, Kirkwood KS. Pathophysiology of gallstone pancreatitis. Front Bioscience-Landmark 2001;6(4):66–76.
[81] Lowenfels AB, Sullivan T, Fiorianti J, Maisonneuve P. The epidemiology and impact of pancreatic diseases in the United States. Curr gastroenterology Rep 2005;7(2):90–5.
[82] Fan Y, Hu J, Feng B, Wang W, Yao G, Zhai J, et al. Increased risk of pancreatic cancer related to gallstones and cholecystectomy: a systematic review and meta-analysis. Pancreas 2016;45(4):503–9.
[83] Petrov MS. Diagnosis of endocrine disease: post-pancreatitis diabetes mellitus: prime time for secondary disease. Eur J Endocrinol 2021; 184(4):R137–49.
[84] Leung PS. Physiology of the pancreas. Adv Exp Med Biol 2010;690:13–27. Available from: https://doi.org/10.1007/978-90-481-9060-7_2 PMID: 20700835.
[85] Sugama J, Moritoh Y, Yashiro H, Tsuchimori K, Watanabe M. Enteropeptidase inhibition improves obesity by modulating gut microbiota composition and enterobacterial metabolites in diet-induced obese mice. Pharmacol Res 2021;163:105337.
[86] Del Rosario MA, Fitzgerald JF, Gupta SK, Croffie JM. Direct measurement of pancreatic enzymes after stimulation with secretin versus secretin plus cholecystokinin. J Pediatr Gastroenterol Nutr 2000;31(1):28–32. Available from: https://doi.org/10.1097/00005176-200007000-00008 PMID: 10896067.
[87] Chen YF, Chey WY, Chang TM, Lee KY. Duodenal acidification releases cholecystokinin. Am J Physiol-Gastrointestinal Liver Physiology 1985;249(1):G29–33.
[88] Khan MN, Raza SS, Hussain AK, Nadeem MD, Ullah F. Pancreatic duct stones. J Ayub Med Coll Abbottabad 2017;29(1):154–6. PMID: 28712198.
[89] Marotta F, Labadarios D, Frazer L, Girdwood A, Marks IN. Fat-soluble vitamin concentration in chronic alcohol-induced pancreatitis. Digestive Dis Sci 1994;39(5):993–8.
[90] Tilg H, Adolph TE. Beyond digestion: the pancreas shapes intestinal microbiota and immunity. Cell Metab 2017;25(3):495–6.
[91] Akshintala VS, Talukdar R, Singh VK, Goggins M. The gut microbiome in pancreatic disease. Clin Gastroenterol Hepatol 2019;17(2):290–5. Available from: https://doi.org/10.1016/j.cgh.2018.08.045.
[92] Dominguez-Muñoz JE. Diagnosis and treatment of pancreatic exocrine insufficiency. Curr Opin Gastroenterol 2018;34(5):349–54. Available from: https://doi.org/10.1097/MOG.0000000000000459 PMID: 29889111.
[93] Zhou Q, Melton DA. Pancreas regeneration. Nature 2018;557(7705):351–8. Available from: https://doi.org/10.1038/s41586-018-0088-0 Epub 2018 May 16. Erratum in: Nature. 2018 Aug;560(7720):E34. PMID: 29769672; PMCID: PMC6168194.
[94] Archibugi L, Signoretti M, Capurso G. The microbiome and pancreatic cancer: an evidence-based association? J Clin Gastroenterology 2018;52:S82–5.
[95] Greenwood-Van Meerveld B, Johnson AC, Grundy D. Gastrointestinal physiology and function. Handb Exp Pharmacol 2017;239:1–16. Available from: https://doi.org/10.1007/164_2016_118 PMID: 28176047.
[96] Bik EM. Composition and function of the human-associated microbiota. Nutr Rev 2009;67(suppl_2):S164–71.

[97] Saad MJA, Santos A, Prada PO. Linking gut microbiota and inflammation to obesity and insulin resistance. Physiology 2016;31(4):283–93.
[98] O'Callaghan A, van Sinderen D. Bifidobacteria and their role as members of the human gut microbiota. Front Microbiol 2016;7:925. Available from: https://doi.org/10.3389/fmicb.2016.00925 PMID: 27379055; PMCID: PMC4908950.
[99] Lopetuso LR, Scaldaferri F, Petito V, et al. Commensal Clostridia: leading players in the maintenance of gut homeostasis. Gut Pathog 2013;5:23. Available from: https://doi.org/10.1186/1757-4749-5-23.
[100] Quigley EM. Gut bacteria in health and disease. Gastroenterol Hepatol (N Y) 2013;9(9):560–9 PMID: 24729765; PMCID: PMC3983973.
[101] Holscher HD. Dietary fiber and prebiotics and the gastrointestinal microbiota. Gut Microbes 2017;8(2):172–84. Available from: https://doi.org/10.1080/19490976.2017.1290756.
[102] Simpson HL, Campbell BJ. Review article: dietary fibre-microbiota interactions. Aliment Pharmacol Ther 2015;42(2):158–79. Available from: https://doi.org/10.1111/apt.13248 Epub 2015 May 24. PMID: 26011307; PMCID: PMC4949558.
[103] Martin P, Johansson M, Ek A. A zero carbohydrate, carnivore diet can normalize hydrogen positive small intestinal bacterial overgrowth lactulose breath tests: a case report. Research Square [Internet] 2021; [cited 2022 Jul 18]. https://doi.org/10.21203/rs.3.rs-148500/v1.
[104] Mehrtash F. Sustained Crohn's disease remission with an exclusive elemental and exclusion diet: a case report. Gastrointest Disord 2021; 3(3):129–37.
[105] Arjomand A, Suskind DL. Clinical and histologic remission in an adult Crohn's disease patient following the specific carbohydrate diet and its impact on healthcare costs Cureus [Internet] 2022;14(2)Feb 8 [cited 2022 Feb 13]. Available from: https://www.cureus.com/articles/81257-clinical-and-histologic-remission-in-an-adult-crohns-disease-patient-following-the-specific-carbohydrate-diet-and-its-impact-on-healthcare-costs.
[106] Vighi G, Marcucci F, Sensi L, Di Cara G, Frati F. Allergy and the gastrointestinal system. Clin Exp Immunol 2008;153(Suppl 1):3–6. Available from: https://doi.org/10.1111/j.1365-2249.2008.03713.x.
[107] Wu H-J, Wu E. The role of gut microbiota in immune homeostasis and autoimmunity. Gut Microbes 2012;3(1):4–14.
[108] Jiao Y, Wu L, Huntington ND, Zhang X. Crosstalk between gut microbiota and innate immunity and its implication in autoimmune diseases. Front Immunol 2020;11:282. Available from: https://doi.org/10.3389/fimmu.2020.00282 PMID: 32153586; PMCID: PMC7047319.
[109] Murtaza N, Ó Cuív P, Morrison M. Diet and the microbiome. Gastroenterol Clin North Am 2017;46(1):49–60. Available from: https://doi.org/10.1016/j.gtc.2016.09.005. Epub 2017 Jan 4. PMID: 28164852.
[110] Thompson-Chagoyán OC, Maldonado J, Gil A. Aetiology of inflammatory bowel disease (IBD): role of intestinal microbiota and gut-associated lymphoid tissue immune response. Clin Nutr 2005;24(3):339–52.
[111] Wilkins T, Sequoia J. Probiotics for gastrointestinal conditions: a summary of the evidence. Am Fam Physician 2017;96(3):170–8 PMID: 28762696.
[112] Zhang S, Chen DC. Facing a new challenge: the adverse effects of antibiotics on gut microbiota and host immunity. Chin Med J 2019; 132(10):1135–8.
[113] Gershon MD. The second brain. HarperCollins World; 1999.
[114] Dinan TG, Cryan JF. Brain-gut-microbiota axis and mental health. Psychosom Med 2017;79(8):920–6. Available from: https://doi.org/10.1097/PSY.0000000000000519 PMID: 28806201.
[115] Quigley EMM. Microbiota-brain-gut axis and neurodegenerative diseases. Curr Neurol Neurosci Rep 2017;17(12):94. Available from: https://doi.org/10.1007/s11910-017-0802-6 PMID: 29039142.
[116] Kim DY, Camilleri M. Serotonin: a mediator of the brain-gut connection. Am J gastroenterology 2000;95(10):2698.
[117] Eisenhofer G, Coughtrie MW, Goldstein DS. Dopamine sulphate: an enigma resolved. Clin Exp pharmacology & Physiol 1999;(Supplement, 26):S41–53.
[118] Koopman M, El Aidy S. MIDtrauma consortium. Depressed gut? The microbiota-diet-inflammation trialogue in depression. Curr Opin Psychiatry 2017;30(5):369–77. Available from: https://doi.org/10.1097/YCO.0000000000000350 PMID: 28654462.
[119] Pulikkan J, Mazumder A, Grace T. Role of the gut microbiome in autism spectrum disorders. Adv Exp Med Biol 2019;1118:253–69. Available from: https://doi.org/10.1007/978-3-030-05542-4_13 PMID: 30747427.
[120] Mathee K, Cickovski T, Deoraj A, Stollstorff M, Narasimhan G. The gut microbiome and neuropsychiatric disorders: implications for attention deficit hyperactivity disorder (ADHD). J Med Microbiol 2020;69(1):14–24. Available from: https://doi.org/10.1099/jmm.0.001112 PMID: 31821133; PMCID: PMC7440676.
[121] Caputi V, Giron MC. Microbiome-gut-brain axis and toll-like receptors in Parkinson's disease. Int J Mol Sci 2018;19(6):1689. Available from: https://doi.org/10.3390/ijms19061689 PMID: 29882798; PMCID: PMC6032048.
[122] Lach G, Schellekens H, Dinan TG, Cryan JF. Anxiety, depression, and the microbiome: a role for gut peptides. Neurotherapeutics 2018; 15(1):36–59. Available from: https://doi.org/10.1007/s13311-017-0585-0 PMID: 29134359; PMCID: PMC5794698.
[123] Lin L, Zheng LJ, Zhang LJ. Neuroinflammation, gut microbiome, and Alzheimer's disease Mol Neurobiol. 2018;55(11):8243–50. Available from: https://doi.org/10.1007/s12035-018-0983-2 Epub 2018 Mar 9. Available from: 29524051.
[124] Golofast B, Vales K. The connection between microbiome and schizophrenia. Neurosci Biobehav Rev 2020;108:712–31. Available from: https://doi.org/10.1016/j.neubiorev.2019.12.011 Epub 2019 Dec 9. PMID: 31821833.
[125] Ahlman H. Nilsson. The gut as the largest endocrine organ in the body. Ann Oncol 2001;12(Suppl 2):S63–8. Available from: https://doi.org/10.1093/annonc/12.suppl_2.s63 PMID: 11762354.
[126] Rastelli M, Cani PD, Knauf C. The gut microbiome influences host endocrine functions. Endocr Rev 2019;40(5):1271–84. Available from: https://doi.org/10.1210/er.2018-00280 PMID: 31081896.
[127] Rizzetto L, Fava F, Tuohy KM, Selmi C. Connecting the immune system, systemic chronic inflammation and the gut microbiome: the role of sex. J Autoimmun 2018;92:12–34. Available from: https://doi.org/10.1016/j.jaut.2018.05.008 Epub 2018 Jun 1. PMID: 29861127.

[128] He S, Li H, Yu Z, Zhang F, Liang S, Liu H, et al. The gut microbiome and sex hormone-related diseases Front Microbiol [Internet] 2021;12 [cited 2022 Jul 18]. Available from: https://www.frontiersin.org/articles/10.3389/fmicb.2021.711137.
[129] Baker JM, Al-Nakkash L, Herbst-Kralovetz MM. Estrogen-gut microbiome axis: physiological and clinical implications. Maturitas 2017;103:45–53. Available from: https://doi.org/10.1016/j.maturitas.2017.06.025 Epub 2017 Jun 23. PMID: 28778332.
[130] Francino MP. Antibiotics and the human gut microbiome: dysbioses and accumulation of resistances. Front microbiology 2016;1543.
[131] Alcock J, Maley CC, Aktipis CA. Is eating behaviour manipulated by the gastrointestinal microbiota? Evolutionary pressures and potential mechanisms. Bioessays. 2014;36(10):940–9.
[132] Flint HJ, Scott KP, Duncan SH, Louis P, Forano E. Microbial degradation of complex carbohydrates in the gut. Gut Microbes 2012;3 (4):289–306.
[133] Tomasello G, Mazzola M, Leone A, Sinagra E, Zummo G, Farina F, et al. Nutrition, oxidative stress and intestinal dysbiosis: influence of diet on gut microbiota in inflammatory bowel diseases. Biomed Pap Med Fac Univ Palacky Olomouc Czech Repub 2016;160(4):461–6.
[134] Galland L. The gut microbiome and the brain. J Med Food 2014;17(12):1261–72.
[135] Garrow JS, James WPT, Ralph A. Human Nutrition and Dietetics. 10th edition Churchill Livingstone; 2000.
[136] Malabsorption: Background, Pathophysiology, Etiology. 2021 Apr 3 [cited 2022 Jul 19]; Available from: https://emedicine.medscape.com/article/180785-overview#a5.
[137] Muscogiuri G, Cantone E, Cassarano S, Tuccinardi D, Barrea L, Savastano S, et al. Gut microbiota: a new path to treat obesity. Int J Obes Suppl 2019;9(1):10–19.
[138] Goldstein R, Braverman D, Stankiewicz H. Carbohydrate malabsorption and the effect of dietary restriction on symptoms of irritable bowel syndrome and functional bowel complaints. Isr Med Assoc journal: IMAJ 2000;2(8):583–7.
[139] Nolan JD, Johnston IM, Walters JR. Physiology of malabsorption. Surg (Oxf) 2012;30(6):268–74.
[140] Carbohydrate—an overview | ScienceDirect Topics [Internet]. [cited 2022 Jul 19]. Available from: https://www.sciencedirect.com/topics/psychology/carbohydrate.
[141] Desai MS, Seekatz AM, Koropatkin NM, Kamada N, Hickey CA, Wolter M, et al. A dietary fiber-deprived gut microbiota degrades the colonic mucus barrier and enhances pathogen susceptibility. Cell 2016;167(5):1339–53.
[142] King DE. Dietary fiber, inflammation, and cardiovascular disease. Mol Nutr & food Res 2005;49(6):594–600.
[143] Anderson JW, Gustafson NJ, Bryant CA, Tietyen-Clark J. Dietary fiber and diabetes: a comprehensive review and practical application. J Am Dietetic Assoc 1987;87(9):1189–97.
[144] Reddy BS. Role of dietary fiber in colon cancer: an overview. Am J Med 1999;106(1):16–19.
[145] Brownlee IA, Chater PI, Pearson JP, et al. Dietary fibre and weight loss: where are we now? Food Hydrocoll 2017;68:186–91.
[146] Wu GD, Chen J, Hoffmann C, Bittinger K, Chen YY, Keilbaugh SA, et al. Linking long-term dietary patterns with gut microbial enterotypes. Sci (N York, NY) 2011;334(6052):105–8. Available from: https://doi.org/10.1126/science.1208344.
[147] Nakajima A, Sasaki T, Itoh K, Kitahara T, Takema Y, Hiramatsu K, et al. A soluble fiber diet increases Bacteroides fragilis group abundance and immunoglobulin A production in the gut. Appl Environ microbiology 2020;86(13):e00405–20.
[148] Fung QM, Szilagyi A. Carbohydrate elimination or adaptation diet for symptoms of intestinal discomfort in IBD: rationales for "Gibsons' Conundrum. Int J Inflamm 2012;2012.
[149] Vakil N. Dietary fermentable oligosaccharides, disaccharides, monosaccharides, and polyols (FODMAPs) and gastrointestinal disease. Nutr ClPract 2018;33(4):468–75.
[150] Rivière A, Selak M, Lantin D, Leroy F, De Vuyst L. Bifidobacteria and butyrate-producing colon bacteria: importance and strategies for their stimulation in the human gut. Front microbiology 2016;7:979.
[151] Bach Knudsen KE, Lærke HN, Hedemann MS, Nielsen TS, Ingerslev AK, Gundelund Nielsen DS, et al. Impact of diet-modulated butyrate production on intestinal barrier function and inflammation. Nutrients 2018;10(10):1499.
[152] Mukherjee A, Lordan C, Ross RP, Cotter PD. Gut microbes from the phylogenetically diverse genus *Eubacterium* and their various contributions to gut health. Gut microbes 2020;12(1):1802866. Available from: https://doi.org/10.1080/19490976.2020.1802866.
[153] Ho KS, Tan CY, Mohd Daud MA, Seow-Choen F. Stopping or reducing dietary fiber intake reduces constipation and its associated symptoms. World J gastroenterology 2012;18(33):4593–6. Available from: https://doi.org/10.3748/wjg.v18.i33.4593.
[154] Zoppi G, Cinquetti M, Luciano A, Benini A, Muner A, Minelli EB. The intestinal ecosystem in chronic functional constipation. Acta paediatrica 1998;87(8):836–41.
[155] Youmans BP, Ajami NJ, Jiang ZD, Campbell F, Wadsworth WD, Petrosino JF, et al. Characterization of the human gut microbiome during travelers' diarrhea. Gut microbes 2015;6(2):110–19.
[156] Bellini M, Gambaccini D, Usai-Satta P, De Bortoli N, Bertani L, Marchi S, et al. Irritable bowel syndrome and chronic constipation: fact and fiction. World J Gastroenterology: WJG 2015;21(40):11362.
[157] Barrett JS. How to institute the low-FODMAP diet. J gastroenterology hepatology 2017;32:8–10.
[158] Gibson PR. Use of the low-FODMAP diet in inflammatory bowel disease. J gastroenterology hepatology 2017;32:40–2.
[159] Balakireva AV, Zamyatnin Jr AA. Properties of gluten intolerance: gluten structure, evolution, pathogenicity and detoxification capabilities. Nutrients 2016;8(10):644.
[160] Pal S, Woodford K, Kukuljan S, Ho S. Milk intolerance, beta-casein and lactose. Nutrients 2015;7(9):7285–97.
[161] Arısoy S, Çoban I, Üstün-Aytekin Ö. Food-derived opioids: production and the effects of opioids on human health. From Conventional to Innovative Approaches for Pain Treatment. IntechOpen; 2019.
[162] Ulaş AŞ, Çakır A, Erbaş O. Gluten and casein: their roles in psychiatric disorders. J Exp Basic Med Sci 2022;3(1):13–21.

[163] Sheikh SA, Mishra PS, Bandopadhyay R, Mishra A. Opioid Activity. Bioactive Peptides from Food: Sources, Analysis, and Functions. CRC Press; 2022. p. 427–40.
[164] Lange KW, Hauser J, Reissmann A. Gluten-free and casein-free diets in the therapy of autism. Curr OpClNutr & Metab Care 2015; 18(6):572–5.
[165] Aranburu E, Matias S, Simón E, Larretxi I, Martínez O, Bustamante MÁ, et al. Gluten and FODMAPs relationship with mental disorders: systematic review. Nutrients 2021;13(6):1894.
[166] Van Campen DR, Glahn RP. Micronutrient bioavailability techniques: accuracy, problems and limitations. Field Crop Res 1999;60(1-2):93–113.
[167] Daulatzai MA. Non-celiac gluten sensitivity triggers gut dysbiosis, neuroinflammation, gut-brain axis dysfunction, and vulnerability for dementia. CNS Neurol Disord Drug Targets 2015;14(1):110–31. Available from: https://doi.org/10.2174/1871527314666150202152436 PMID: 25642988.
[168] Sanz Y. Microbiome and Gluten. Ann Nutr Metab 2015;67(Suppl 2):28–41. Available from: https://doi.org/10.1159/000440991.
[169] Molina-Infante J, Santolaria S, Sanders DS, Fernández-Bañares F. Systematic review: noncoeliac gluten sensitivity. Alimentary pharmacology & therapeutics 2015;41(9):807–20.
[170] Hoffman JR, et al. Protein – which is best? J Sprots Sci Med 2004;3(3) Published online 2004 Sep1.
[171] Salter AM. The effects of meat consumption on global health. Rev Sci Tech 2018;37(1):47–55. Available from: https://doi.org/10.20506/rst.37.1.2739 PMID: 30209430.
[172] Yen CLE, Nelson DW, Yen MI. Intestinal triacylglycerol synthesis in fat absorption and systemic energy metabolism. J lipid Res 2015; 56(3):489–501.
[173] Muscogiuri G, Barrea L, Laudisio D, et al. The management of very low-calorie ketogenic diet in obesity outpatient clinic: a practical guide. J Transl Med 2019;17:356. Available from: https://doi.org/10.1186/s12967-019-2104-z.
[174] Dueland AN. Headache and alcohol. Headache: J Head Face Pain 2015;55(7):1045–9.
[175] Dawson D, Reid K. Fatigue, alcohol and performance impairment. Nature 1997;388(6639) 235-235.
[176] Cutter HS, Jones WC, Maloof BA, Kurtz NR. Pain as a joint function of alcohol intake and customary reasons for drinking. Int J Addictions 1979;14(2):173–82.
[177] Malik F, Wickremesinghe P, Saverimuttu J. Case report and literature review of auto-brewery syndrome: probably an underdiagnosed medical condition. BMJ Open Gastroenterology 2019;6(1):e000325.
[178] Hamid R, Masood A. Dietary lectins as disease causing toxicants. Pak J Nutr 2009;8(3):293–303.
[179] Hasan MN, Sultan MZ, Mar-E-Um M. Significance of fermented food in nutrition and food science. J Sci Res 2014;6(2):373–86.
[180] Knight-Sepulveda K, Kais S, Santaolalla R, Abreu MT. Diet and Inflammatory Bowel Disease. Gastroenterol Hepatol (N Y) 2015; 11(8):511–20 PMID: 27118948; PMCID: PMC4843040.
[181] Damas OM, Garces L, Abreu MT. Diet as adjunctive treatment for inflammatory bowel disease: review and update of the latest literature. Curr Treat Options Gastro 2019;17:313–25.
[182] van Lanen AS, de Bree A, Greyling A. Efficacy of a low-FODMAP diet in adult irritable bowel syndrome: a systematic review and meta-analysis. Eur J Nutr 2021;60:3505–22.
[183] Obih C, Wahbeh G, Lee D, Braly K, Giefer M, Shaffer ML, et al. Specific carbohydrate diet for pediatric inflammatory bowel disease in clinical practice within an academic IBD center. Nutrition 2016;32(4):418–25.
[184] Suskind DL, Wahbeh G, Cohen SA, Damman CJ, Klein J, Braly K, et al. Patients perceive clinical benefit with the specific carbohydrate diet for inflammatory bowel disease. Digestive Dis Sci 2016;61(11):3255–60.
[185] Shepherd SJ, Gibson PR. Fructose malabsorption and symptoms of irritable bowel syndrome: guidelines for effective dietary management. J Am dietetic Assoc 2006;106(10):1631–9.
[186] De Palma G, Bercik P. Long-term personalized low FODMAP diet in IBS. Neurogastroenterology & Motil 2022;34(4):e14356.
[187] Zhan YA, Dai SX. Is a low FODMAP diet beneficial for patients with inflammatory bowel disease? A meta-analysis and systematic review. Clin Nutr 2018;37(1):123–9.
[188] Britto S, Kellermayer R. Carbohydrate monotony as protection and treatment for inflammatory bowel disease. J Crohn's Colitis 2019;13 (7):942–8.
[189] Ludwig DS. The ketogenic diet: evidence for optimism but high-quality research needed J Nutr [Internet] 2019;[cited 2019 Dec 13]. Available from: https://academic.oup.com/jn/advance-article/doi/10.1093/jn/nxz308/5673196.
[190] Tóth C, Dabóczi A, Howard M, Miller NJ, Clemens Z. Crohn's disease successfully treated with the paleolithic ketogenic diet. Int J Case Rep Images 2016;7(10):570–8.
[191] Popova A, Mihaylova D. Antinutrients in plant-based foods: a review. Open Biotechnol J 2019;13(1).
[192] Egounlety M, Aworh OC. Effect of soaking, dehulling, cooking and fermentation with Rhizopus oligosporus on the oligosaccharides, trypsin inhibitor, phytic acid and tannins of soybean (Glycine max Merr.), cowpea (Vigna unguiculata L. Walp) and groundbean (Macrotyloma geocarpa Harms). J food Eng 2003;56(2-3):249–54.
[193] Roy M, Imran MZH, Alam M, Rahman M. Effect of boiling and roasting on physicochemical and antioxidant properties of dark red kidney bean (Phaseolus vulgaris). Food Res 2021;5(3):438–45.
[194] Mohammed MA, Mohamed EA, Yagoub AEA, Mohamed AR, Babiker EE. Effect of processing methods on alkaloids, phytate, phenolics, antioxidants activity and minerals of newly developed lupin (Lupinus albus L.) cultivar. J Food Process Preservation 2017;41(1):e12960.
[195] Malik, T.F.; Panuganti, K.K. (2020). "Lactose Intolerance." PMID 30335318.

[196] Geiker NRW, Larsen ML, Dyerberg J, Stender S, Astrup A. [Eggs do not increase the risk of cardiovascular disease and can be safely consumed]. Ugeskr Laeger 2017;179(20) V11160792. Danish. PMID: 28504636.
[197] Réhault-Godbert S, Guyot N, Nys Y. The golden egg: nutritional value, bioactivities, and emerging benefits for human health. Nutrients 2019;11(3):684.
[198] Melse-Boonstra A. Bioavailability of micronutrients from nutrient-dense whole foods: zooming in on dairy, vegetables, and fruits. Front Nutr 2020;7:101.
[199] Sador Ellix K. The art of fermentation: an in-depth exploration of essential concepts and processes from around the world. First Edition Chelsea Green Publishing Co; 2012.
[200] Hassan EG, Alkareem AMA, Mustafa AMI. Effect of fermentation and particle size of wheat bran on the antinutritional factors and bread quality. Pak J Nutr 2008;7(4):521–6.
[201] Krysiak R, Szkróbka W, Okopień B. The effect of gluten-free diet on thyroid autoimmunity in drug-naïve women with Hashimoto's thyroiditis: a pilot study. Exp Clin Endocrinol Diabetes 2019;127(07):417–22.
[202] Dahiya D, Nigam PS. Probiotics, prebiotics, synbiotics, and fermented foods as potential biotics in nutrition improving health via microbiome-gut-brain axis. Fermentation 2022;8(7):303.
[203] Gangarosa EJ. Recent developments in diarrheal diseases. Postgrad Med 1977;62(2):113–17.
[204] Dave D, Ivyanskiy I, Naguib T. S3374 Overflow diarrhea and AKI as a presentation of fecal impaction that led to obstructive uropathy. Am Coll of Gastroenterol 2020;115:S1755.
[205] Kamm MA. Fortnightly review: faecal incontinence. BMJ 1998;316(7130):528.
[206] Marler S, Ferguson BJ, Lee EB, et al. Association of Rigid-Compulsive Behavior with Functional Constipation in Autism Spectrum Disorder. J Autism Dev Disord 2017;47:1673–81. Available from: https://doi.org/10.1007/s10803-017-3084-6.
[207] Sarangi A, Armin S, Vargas A, et al. Management of constipation in patients with schizophrenia—a case study and review of literature. Middle East Curr Psychiatry 2021;28:17. Available from: https://doi.org/10.1186/s43045-021-00097-6.
[208] Sattar B, Chokshi RV. Colonic and anorectal manifestations of systemic sclerosis. Current gastroenterology reports 2019;21(7):1–7.
[209] Grant RL, Drennan VM, Rait G, Petersen I, Iliffe S. First diagnosis and management of incontinence in older people with and without dementia in primary care: a cohort study using The Health Improvement Network primary care database. PLoS medicine 2013;10(8):e1001505.
[210] Slim M, Calandre EP, Rico-Villademoros F. An insight into the gastrointestinal component of fibromyalgia: clinical manifestations and potential underlying mechanisms. Rheumatology international 2015;35(3):433–44.
[211] Khalif IL, Quigley EM, Konovitch EA, Maximova ID. Alterations in the colonic flora and intestinal permeability and evidence of immune activation in chronic constipation. Dig Liver Dis 2005;37(11):838–49. Available from: https://doi.org/10.1016/j.dld.2005.06.008 Epub 2005 Oct 5. PMID: 16169298.
[212] Wang JK, Yao SK. Roles of gut microbiota and metabolites in pathogenesis of functional constipation. Evidence-Based Complementary and Alternative Medicine 2021;2021.
[213] Abrahamsson H, Östlund-Lindqvist AM, Nilsson R, Simrén M, Gillberg PG. Altered bile acid metabolism in patients with constipation-predominant irritable bowel syndrome and functional constipation. Scandinavian journal of gastroenterology 2008;43(12):1483–8.
[214] Triadafilopoulos G, Simms RW, Goldenberg DL. Bowel dysfunction in fibromyalgia syndrome. Digestive diseases and sciences 1991; 36(1):59–64.
[215] Parekh PJ, Burleson D, Lubin C, Johnson DA. Colon irrigation: effective, safe, and well-tolerated alternative to traditional therapy in the management of refractory chronic constipation. J Clin Gastroenterol Hepatol 2018;2(1):5. Available from: https://doi.org/10.21767/2575-7733.100034.
[216] Portalatin M, Winstead N. Medical management of constipation. Clin Colon Rectal Surg. 2012;25(1). Available from: https://doi.org/10.1055/s-0032-1301754 PMID: 23449608; PMCID: PMC3348737.
[217] Al Mushref M, Srinivasan S. Effect of high fat-diet and obesity on gastrointestinal motility. Annals of translational medicine 2013;1(2).
[218] Aslam H, Mohebbi M, Ruusunen A, Dawson SL, Williams LJ, Berk M, et al. Associations between dairy consumption and constipation in adults: a cross-sectional study. Nutrition and Health 2022;28(1):31–9.
[219] Roth-Walter F, Pacios LF, Gomez-Casado C, Hofstetter G, Roth GA, Singer J, et al. The major cow milk allergen bos d 5 manipulates T-helper cells depending on its load with siderophore-bound iron. PLoS One 2014;9(8):e104803. Available from: https://doi.org/10.1371/journal.pone.0104803.
[220] O'Hearn A. Can a carnivore diet provide all essential nutrients? Current Opinion in Endocrinology, Diabetes and Obesity 2020;27(5):312–16.
[221] Kluz MI, Pietrzyk K, Pastuszczak M, Kacaniova M, Kita A, Kapusta I, et al. Microbiological and physicochemical composition of various types of homemade kombucha beverages using alternative kinds of sugars. Foods 2022;11(10):1523.
[222] Schiller LR. The therapy of constipation. Aliment Pharmacol Ther 2001;15(6):749–63.
[223] Ghaeni M, Roomiani L. Review for application and medicine effects of Spirulina, microalgae. J Adv Agric Technol 2016;3(2).
[224] Gupta S, Gupta C, Garg AP, Prakash D. Prebiotic efficiency of blue green algae on probiotics microorganisms. J. Microbiol. Exp 2017;4(4):4–7.
[225] Nishimoto Y, Nomaguchi T, Mori Y, Ito M, Nakamura Y, Fujishima M, et al. The nutritional efficacy of Chlorella supplementation depends on the individual gut environment: a randomised control study. Front Nutr. 2021;31(8):648073. Available from: https://doi.org/10.3389/fnut.2021.648073 PMID: 34136514; PMCID: PMC8200412.
[226] Gaginella TS, Capasso F, Mascolo N, Perilli S. Castor oil: new lessons from an ancient oil. Phytother Res 1998;12(S1):S128–30.
[227] Tanjung Fahrul Azmi, et al. Functional constipation and posture in defecation. Paediatrica Indonesiana 2013;53(2):104–7.
[228] Müller-Lissner SA, Kamm MA, Scarpignato C, Wald A. Myths and misconceptions about chronic constipation. Am Coll Gastroenterol 2005;100(1):232–42.

[229] Wright JV, Lenard L. Why stomach acid is good for you: natural relief from heartburn, indigestion, reflux and GERD. Rowman & Littlefield; 2001.

[230] Capasso F, Gaginella TS, Grandolini G, Izzo AA. Plants and the digestive system. Phytotherapy. Berlin, Heidelberg: Springer; 2003. p. 251–94.

[231] McMullen MK, Whitehouse JM, Towell A. Bitters: time for a new paradigm. Evid Based Complement Alternat Med. 2015;2015:670504. Available from: https://doi.org/10.1155/2015/670504 Epub 2015 May 14. PMID: 26074998; PMCID: PMC4446506.

[232] Brailski H, Galabov T. Influence of juice from fresh or dried cabbage on the secretory and motor functions of the stomach. Voprosy Pitaniya 1957;4:19–26.

[233] Yago MR, Frymoyer AR, Smelick GS, et al. Gastric reacidification with betaine HCl in healthy volunteers with rabeprazole-induced hypochlorhydria. Mol Pharm 2013;10(11):4032–7.

[234] Wald, Honzíková, Lysíková, Masinovský, Murphree II. Systemic Enzyme Support: An Overview [Internet]. 2008. Available from: https://www.oakwayhealthcenter.com/store/DL_Systemic-Enzyme-Support.pdf.

[235] Ouwehand AC, Tölkkö S, Salminen S. The effect of digestive enzymes on the adhesion of probiotic bacteria in vitro. J Food Sci 2001; 66(6):856–9.

[236] Worning H, MÜllertz S. pH and pancreatic enzymes in the human duodenum during digestion of a standard meal. Scand J Gastroenterol 1966;1(4):268–83.

[237] Ianiro G, Pecere S, Giorgio V, Gasbarrini A, Cammarota G. Digestive enzyme supplementation in gastrointestinal diseases. Curr Drug Metab 2016;17(2):187–93. Available from: https://doi.org/10.2174/138920021702160114150137.

[238] Little KH, Schiller LR, Bilhartz LE, Fordtran JS. Treatment of severe steatorrhea with ox bile in an ileectomy patient with residual colon. Digest Dis Sci 1992;37(6):929–33.

[239] Hempel S, Newberry SJ, Maher AR, Wang Z, Miles JN, Shanman R, et al. Probiotics for the prevention and treatment of antibiotic-associated diarrhea: a systematic review and meta-analysis. JAMA 2012;307(18):1959–69.

[240] Matsubara VH, Bandara HMHN, Mayer MP, Samaranayake LP. Probiotics as antifungals in mucosal candidiasis. Clin Infect Dis 2016;62 (9):1143–53.

[241] Liu Y, Tran DQ, Rhoads JM. Probiotics in disease prevention and treatment. J Clin Pharmacol. 2018;58(Suppl 10):S164–79. Available from: https://doi.org/10.1002/jcph.1121.

[242] Reid G. Probiotics: definition, scope and mechanisms of action. Best Pract Res Clin Gastroenterol 2016;30:17–25.

[243] Deshpande G, Rao S, Patole S. Probiotics for prevention of necrotising enterocolitis in preterm neonates with very low birthweight: a systematic review of randomised controlled trials. The Lancet 2007;369(9573):1614–20.

[244] Szajewska H, Mrukowicz JZ. Use of probiotics in children with acute diarrhea. Pediatric drugs 2005;7(2):111–22.

[245] McFarland LV. Meta-analysis of probiotics for the prevention of traveler's diarrhea. Travel medicine and infectious disease 2007;5(2):97–105.

[246] McFarland LV. Meta-analysis of probiotics for the prevention of antibiotic associated diarrhea and the treatment of Clostridium difficile disease. Am J Gastroenterol 2006;101(4):812–22. Available from: https://doi.org/10.1111/j.1572-0241.2006.00465.x PMID: 16635227.

[247] Resta-Lenert S, Barrett KE. Live probiotics protect intestinal epithelial cells from the effects of infection with enteroinvasive *Escherichia coli* (EIEC). Gut 2003;52(7):988–97.

[248] Rolfe VE, Fortun PJ, Hawkey CJ, Bath-Hextall FJ. Probiotics for maintenance of remission in Crohn's disease. Cochrane Database of Systematic Reviews 2006;(4).

[249] Sang LX, Chang B, Zhang WL, Wu XM, Li XH, Jiang M. Remission induction and maintenance effect of probiotics on ulcerative colitis: a meta-analysis. World J Gastroenterol 2010;16(15):1908.

[250] Gionchetti P, Rizzello F, Morselli C, Poggioli G, Tambasco R, Calabrese C, et al. High-dose probiotics for the treatment of active pouchitis. Dis Colon Rectum 2007;50(12):2075–84.

[251] Sandhu BK, Paul SP. Irritable bowel syndrome in children: pathogenesis, diagnosis and evidence-based treatment. World J Gastroenterol 2014;20(20):6013–23.

[252] Oak SJ, Jha R. The effects of probiotics in lactose intolerance: a systematic review. Critical reviews in food science and nutrition 2019; 59(11):1675–83.

[253] Schmid R. The Untold Story of Milk. The History, Politics and Science of Nature's Perfect Food: Raw Milk From Pastured Cows. New Trends Publishing; 2009.

[254] Rafter J, Bennett M, Caderni G, Clune Y, Hughes R, Karlsson PC, et al. Dietary synbiotics reduce cancer risk factors in polypectomized and colon cancer patients. Am J Clin Nutr 2007;85(2):488–96. Available from: https://doi.org/10.1093/ajcn/85.2.488 PMID: 17284748.

[255] Uccello M, Malaguarnera G, Basile F, D'agata V, Malaguarnera M, Bertino G, et al. Potential role of probiotics on colorectal cancer prevention. BMC surgery 2012;12(1):1–8.

[256] Chau K, Lau E, Greenberg S, Jacobson S, Yazdani-Brojeni P, Verma N, et al. Probiotics for infantile colic: a randomized, double-blind, placebo-controlled trial investigating *Lactobacillus reuteri* DSM 17938. J Pediatr 2015;166(1):74–8.

[257] Hendijani F, Akbari V. Probiotic supplementation for management of cardiovascular risk factors in adults with type II diabetes: a systematic review and meta-analysis. Clin Nutr. 2018;37(2):532–41 [PubMed] [Google Scholar].

[258] Wu Y, Zhang Q, Ren Y, Ruan Z. Effect of probiotic Lactobacillus on lipid profile: a systematic review and meta-analysis of randomized, controlled trials. PLoS One 2017;12:e0178868.

[259] Kobyliak N, Conte C, Cammarota G, et al. Probiotics in prevention and treatment of obesity: a critical view. Nutr Metab (Lond) 2016;13:14. Available from: https://doi.org/10.1186/s12986-016-0067-0 Published 2016 Feb 20.

[260] Mohammed AT, Khattab M, et al. The therapeutic effect of probiotics on rheumatoid arthritis: a systematic review and meta-analysis of randomized control trials. Clin. Rheumatol 2017;.

[261] Dang D, Zhou W, Lun ZJ, Mu X, Wang DX, Wu H. Meta-analysis of probiotics and/or prebiotics for the prevention of eczema. J Int Med Res 2013;41:1426–36 [PubMed] [Google Scholar].

[262] Zhang GQ, Hu HJ, Liu CY, Zhang Q, Shakya S, Li ZY. Probiotics for prevention of atopy and food hypersensitivity in early childhood: a PRISMA-compliant systematic review and meta-analysis of randomized controlled trials. Medicine (Baltimore) 2016;95:e2562 [PMC free article] [PubMed] [Google Scholar].

[263] Zuccotti G, Meneghin F, Aceti A, et al. Probiotics for prevention of atopic diseases in infants: systematic review and meta-analysis. Allergy 2015;70:1356–71.

[264] Tang ML, Ponsonby AL, Orsini F, et al. Administration of a probiotic with peanut oral immunotherapy: a randomized trial. J Allergy Clin Immunol 2015;135:737–44 [PubMed] [Google Scholar].

[265] Vliagoftis H, Kouranos VD, Betsi GI, Falagas ME. Probiotics for the treatment of allergic rhinitis and asthma: systematic review of randomized controlled trials. Ann Allergy Asthma Immunol 2008;101:570–9.

[266] Kang Dae-Wook, James BAdams, Gregory Ann C, Borody Thomas, Chittick Lauren, Fasano Alessio, et al. Microbiota transfer therapy alters gut ecosystem and improves gastrointestinal and autism symptoms: an open-label study. Microbiome 2017;5(1):10.

[267] Rudzki Leszek, Szulc Agata. 'Immune Gate' of psychopathology—the role of gut derived immune activation in major psychiatric disorders. Front Psychiatr 2018;9.

[268] Corthesy B, Gaskins HR, Mercenier A. Cross-talk between probiotic bacteria and the host immune system. J Nutr 2007;137:781S–90S.

[269] Wang Y, Li X, Ge T, et al. Probiotics for prevention and treatment of respiratory tract infections in children: a systematic review and meta-analysis of randomized controlled trials. Medicine (Baltimore) 2016;95:e4509.

[270] Gleeson M, Bishop NC, Oliveira M, Tauler P. Daily probiotic's (Lactobacillus casei Shirota) reduction of infection incidence in athletes. Int J Sport Nutr Exerc Metab. 2011;21:55–64.

[271] Liu PC, Yan YK, Ma YJ, et al. Probiotics reduce postoperative infections in patients undergoing colorectal surgery: a systematic review and meta-analysis. Gastroenterol Res Pract 2017;2017:6029075.

[272] Lee JY, Chu SH, Jeon JY, et al. Effects of 12 weeks of probiotic supplementation on quality of life in colorectal cancer survivors: a double-blind, randomized, placebo-controlled trial. Dig Liver Dis 2014;46(12):1126–32. Available from: https://doi.org/10.1016/j.dld.2014.09.004.

[273] Górska A, Przystupski D, Niemczura MJ, Kulbacka J. Probiotic bacteria: a promising tool in cancer prevention and therapy. Curr Microbiol 2019;76(8):939–49. Available from: https://doi.org/10.1007/s00284-019-01679-8.

[274] Karpa KD. Probiotics for Clostridium difficile diarrhea: putting it into perspective. Annals of Pharmacotherapy 2007;41(7–8):1284–7.

[275] White E, Sherlock C. The effect of nutritional therapy for yeast infection (Candidiasis) in cases of chronic fatigue syndrome. J Orthomol Med 2005;20(3):193–209.

[276] Knezevic, S., Lj, D., & Virijevic, S. Jarisch–Herxheimer reaction during therapy of neuroborreliosis.

[277] Butler T. The Jarisch–Herxheimer reaction after antibiotic treatment of spirochetal infections: a review of recent cases and our understanding of pathogenesis. Am J Trop. Med. Hyg. 2017;96(1):46–52.

[278] McRorie JW, Chey WD. Fermented fiber supplements are no better than placebo for a laxative effect. Digest Dis Sci 2016;61(11):3140–6.

[279] Krissansen GW. Emerging health properties of whey proteins and their clinical implications. J Am Coll Nutr 2007;26(6):713S–23S.

[280] Matsumoto H, Shimokawa Y, Ushida Y, ToIDA T, Hayasawa H. New biological function of bovine α-lactalbumin: protective effect against ethanol-and stress-induced gastric mucosal injury in rats. Biosci Biotechnol Biochem 2001;65(5):1104–11.

[281] Ho HJ, Shirakawa H, Hirahara K, Sone H, Kamiyama S, Komai M. Menaquinone-4 amplified glucose-stimulated insulin secretion in isolated mouse pancreatic islets and INS-1 rat insulinoma cells. Int J Mol Sci 2019;20(8):1995. Available from: https://doi.org/10.3390/ijms20081995.

[282] De Waele B, Vierendeels T, Willems G. Vitamin status in patients with acute pancreatitis. Clin Nutr 1992;11(2):83–6. Available from: https://doi.org/10.1016/0261-5614(92)90015-i.

[283] Sikkens EC, Cahen DL, Koch AD, Braat H, Poley JW, Kuipers EJ, et al. The prevalence of fat-soluble vitamin deficiencies and a decreased bone mass in patients with chronic pancreatitis. Pancreatology 2013;13(3):238–42. Available from: https://doi.org/10.1016/j.pan.2013.02.008.

[284] Hoogenboom SA, Lekkerkerker SJ, Fockens P, Boermeester MA, van Hooft JE. Systematic review and meta-analysis on the prevalence of vitamin D deficiency in patients with chronic pancreatitis. Pancreatology 2016;16(5):800–6.

[285] Huh JH, Kim JW, Lee KJ. Vitamin D deficiency predicts severe acute pancreatitis. United European Gastroenterol J 2019;7(1):90–5.

[286] Ravisankar P, Reddy AA, Nagalakshmi B, Koushik OS, Kumar BV, Anvith PS. The comprehensive review on fat soluble vitamins. IOSR J Pharm 2015;5(11):12–28.

[287] Jeengar MK, Shrivastava S, Veeravalli SCM, Naidu VGM, Sistla R. Amelioration of FCA induced arthritis on topical application of curcumin in combination with emu oil. Nutrition 2016;32(9):955–64.

[288] Cai F, Hu C, Chen CJ, Han YP, Lin ZQ, Deng LH, et al. Vitamin D and pancreatitis: a narrative review of current evidence. Nutrients 2022;14(10):2113.

[289] Zhou Y, Wang H, Zhou J, Qiu S, Cai T, Li H, et al. Vitamin A and its multi-effects on pancreas: recent advances and prospects. Front Endocrinol 2021;12:620941.

[290] Mandelbaum J, Schlessinger L. Absorption of vitamin A through human skin. Arch Derm Syphilol 1942;46(3):431–42.

[291] Sadat-Ali M, Bubshait DA, Al-Turki HA, Al-Dakheel DA, Al-Olayani WS. Topical delivery of vitamin d3: a randomized controlled pilot study. Int J Biomed Sci 2014;10(1):21.

[292] Davis CD. The gut microbiome and its role in obesity. Nutr Today 2016;51(4):167–74.

[293] Baothman OA, Zamzami MA, Taher I, Abubaker J, Abu-Farha M. The role of gut microbiota in the development of obesity and diabetes. Lipids Health Dis 2016;15(1):108.

[294] Liébana-García R, Olivares M, Bullich-Vilarrubias C, López-Almela I, Romaní-Pérez M, Sanz Y. The gut microbiota as a versatile immunomodulator in obesity and associated metabolic disorders. Best Pract Res Clin Endocrinol Metab 2021;101542.

[295] Clemente JC, Manasson J, Scher JU. State of the art review: the role of the gut microbiome in systemic inflammatory disease BMJ [Internet] 2018;360[cited 2022 Feb 28]. Available from: https://www.ncbi.nlm.nih.gov/labs/pmc/articles/PMC6889978/.

[296] Fan Y, Wang H, Liu X, Zhang J, Liu G. Crosstalk between the ketogenic diet and epilepsy: from the perspective of gut microbiota Mediat Inflamm [Internet] 2019;2019[cited 2022 Feb 28]. Available from: https://www.ncbi.nlm.nih.gov/labs/pmc/articles/PMC6589192/.

[297] Cryan JF, O'Riordan KJ, Sandhu K, Peterson V, Dinan TG. The gut microbiome in neurological disorders. Lancet Neurol 2020;19(2):179–94.

[298] McKenzie C, Tan J, Macia L, Mackay CR. The nutrition-gut microbiome-physiology axis and allergic diseases. Immunol Rev 2017;278 (1):277–95.

[299] Polkowska-Pruszyńska B, Gerkowicz A, Krasowska D. The gut microbiome alterations in allergic and inflammatory skin diseases - an update. J Eur Acad Dermatol Venereol 2020;34(3):455–64.

[300] Fenneman AC, Rampanelli E, Yin YS, Ames J, Blaser MJ, Fliers E, et al. Gut microbiota and metabolites in the pathogenesis of endocrine disease. Biochem Soc Trans 2020;48(3):915–31.

[301] Zheng P, Li Z, Zhou Z. Gut microbiome in type 1 diabetes: a comprehensive review Diabetes/Metabolism Research and Reviews [Internet] 2018;34(7)[cited 2022 Feb 28]. Available from: https://www.ncbi.nlm.nih.gov/labs/pmc/articles/PMC6220847/.

[302] Ristori MV, Quagliariello A, Reddel S, Ianiro G, Vicari S, Gasbarrini A, et al. Autism, gastrointestinal symptoms and modulation of gut microbiota by nutritional interventions. Nutrients. 2019;11(11):2812.

[303] Luca FD, Shoenfeld Y. The microbiome in autoimmune diseases. Clin Exp Immunol 2019;195(1):74.

[304] Xu F, Fu Y, Sun TY, Jiang Z, Miao Z, Shuai M, et al. The interplay between host genetics and the gut microbiome reveals common and distinct microbiome features for complex human diseases Microbiome [Internet] 2020;8[cited 2022 Feb 28]. Available from: https://www.ncbi.nlm.nih.gov/labs/pmc/articles/PMC7545574/.

[305] Fan Y, Pedersen O. Gut microbiota in human metabolic health and disease. Nat Rev Microbiol 2021;19(1):55–71.

[306] Nagpal R, Yadav H, Marotta F. Gut microbiota: the next-gen frontier in preventive and therapeutic medicine? Front Med 2014;1:15.

[307] Sholl J, Mailing LJ, Wood TR. Reframing nutritional microbiota studies to reflect an inherent metabolic flexibility of the human gut: a narrative review focusing on high-fat diets mBio [Internet] 2021;12(2)[cited 2021 Apr 22]. Available from: https://mbio.asm.org/content/12/2/e00579-21.

[308] Hills RD, Pontefract BA, Mishcon HR, Black CA, Sutton SC, Theberge CR. Gut microbiome: profound implications for diet and disease. Nutrients 2019;11(7):1613.

[309] Yu D, Xie L, Chen W, Qin J, Zhang J, Lei M, et al. Dynamics of the gut bacteria and fungi accompanying low-carbohydrate diet-induced weight loss in overweight and obese adults. Front Nutr 2022;9:846378.

[310] Magne F, Gotteland M, Gauthier L, Zazueta A, Pesoa S, Navarrete P, et al. The Firmicutes/Bacteroidetes ratio: a relevant marker of gut dysbiosis in obese patients? Nutrients 2020;12(5):1474.

[311] Sanna S, van Zuydam NR, Mahajan A, Kurilshikov A, Vich Vila A, Võsa U, et al. Causal relationships among the gut microbiome, short-chain fatty acids and metabolic diseases. Nat Genet 2019;51(4):600–5.

[312] VanHook AM. Butyrate benefits the intestinal barrier Sci Signal [Internet] 2015;[cited 2022 Mar 7]; Available from. Available from: https://www.science.org/doi/abs/10.1126/scisignal.aac6198.

[313] Kelly CJ, Zheng L, Campbell EL, Saeedi B, Scholz CC, Bayless AJ, et al. Crosstalk between microbiota-derived short-chain fatty acids and intestinal epithelial hif augments tissue barrier function. Cell Host Microbe 2015;17(5):662.

[314] Mu Q, Tavella VJ, Luo XM. Role of Lactobacillus reuteri in human health and diseases Front Microbiol [Internet] 2018;9[cited 2022 Mar 29]. Available from: https://www.frontiersin.org/article/10.3389/fmicb.2018.00757.

[315] Francavilla R, Polimeno L, Demichina A, Maurogiovanni G, Principi B, Scaccianoce G, et al. Lactobacillus reuteri strain combination in *Helicobacter pylori* infection: a randomized, double-blind, placebo-controlled study. J Clin Gastroenterol 2014;48(5):407–13.

[316] *Lactobacillus reuteri*—an overview | ScienceDirect Topics [Internet]. [cited 2022 Mar 29]. Available from: https://www.sciencedirect.com/topics/biochemistry-genetics-and-molecular-biology/lactobacillus-reuteri.

[317] Cabrera-Mulero A, Tinahones A, Bandera B, Moreno-Indias I, Macías-González M, Tinahones FJ. Keto microbiota: a powerful contributor to host disease recovery. Rev Endocr Metab Disord 2019;20(4):415–25.

[318] Johnson KVA, Burnet PWJ. Microbiome: should we diversify from diversity? Gut Microbes 2016;7(6):455–8.

[319] González Olmo BM, Butler MJ, Barrientos RM. Evolution of the human diet and its impact on gut microbiota, immune responses, and brain health. Nutrients. 2021;13(1):196.

[320] Barone M, Turroni S, Rampelli S, Soverini M, D'Amico F, Biagi E, et al. Gut microbiome response to a modern Paleolithic diet in a Western lifestyle context. PLoS One 2019;14(8):e0220619.

[321] Zinöcker MK, Lindseth IA. The Western diet–microbiome-host interaction and its role in metabolic disease. Nutrients. 2018;10(3):365.

[322] Seo YS, Lee HB, Kim Y, Park HY. Dietary carbohydrate constituents related to gut dysbiosis and health. Microorganisms. 2020;8(3):427.

[323] Manzel A, Muller DN, Hafler DA, Erdman SE, Linker RA, Kleinewietfeld M. Role of "Western Diet" in inflammatory autoimmune diseases. Curr Allergy Asthma Rep 2013;14(1):404.
[324] German JB, Dillard CJ. Saturated fats: a perspective from lactation and milk composition. Lipids. 2010;45(10):915–23.
[325] Ang QY, Alexander M, Newman JC, Tian Y, Cai J, Upadhyay V, et al. Ketogenic diets alter the gut microbiome resulting in decreased intestinal Th17 cells Cell [Internet] 2020;0(0)[cited 2020 May 24]. Available from: https://www.cell.com/cell/abstract/S0092-8674(20)30490-6.
[326] David LA, Maurice CF, Carmody RN, Gootenberg DB, Button JE, Wolfe BE, et al. Diet rapidly and reproducibly alters the human gut microbiome. Nature. 2014;505(7484):559–63.
[327] Kong C, Yan X, Liu Y, Huang L, Zhu Y, He J, et al. Ketogenic diet alleviates colitis by reduction of colonic group 3 innate lymphoid cells through altering gut microbiome. Signal Transduct Target Ther 2021;6:154.
[328] Moreira APB, Texeira TFS, Ferreira AB, Peluzio M, do CG, Alfenas R, et al. Influence of a high-fat diet on gut microbiota, intestinal permeability and metabolic endotoxaemia. British Journal of Nutrition 2012;108(5):801–9.
[329] Malesza IJ, Malesza M, Walkowiak J, Mussin N, Walkowiak D, Aringazina R, et al. High-fat, western-style diet, systemic inflammation, and gut microbiota: a narrative review. Cells. 2021;10(11):3164.
[330] James KL, Gertz ER, Cervantes E, Bonnel EL, Stephensen CB, Kable ME, et al. Diet, fecal microbiome, and trimethylamine N-oxide in a cohort of metabolically healthy United States adults. Nutrients. 2022;14(7):1376.
[331] Küllenberg D, Taylor LA, Schneider M, Massing U. Health effects of dietary phospholipids. Lipids Health Dis 2012;11(1):3.
[332] Yoo W, Zieba JK, Foegeding NJ, Torres TP, Shelton CD, Shealy NG, et al. High-fat diet–induced colonocyte dysfunction escalates microbiota-derived trimethylamine N-oxide. Science. 2021;373(6556):813–18.
[333] Kivenson V, Giovannoni SJ. An expanded genetic code enables trimethylamine metabolism in human gut bacteria. mSystems. 2020;5(5): e00413–20.
[334] Jia J, Dou P, Gao M, Kong X, Li C, Liu Z, et al. Assessment of causal direction between gut microbiota-dependent metabolites and cardiometabolic health: a bidirectional Mendelian randomization analysis. Diabetes. 2019;68(9):1747–55.
[335] Smith SA, Ogawa SA, Chau L, Whelan KA, Hamilton KE, Chen J, et al. Mitochondrial dysfunction in inflammatory bowel disease alters intestinal epithelial metabolism of hepatic acylcarnitines. J Clin Invest 2021;131(1):e133371.
[336] Murakami M, Tognini P. Molecular mechanisms underlying the bioactive properties of a ketogenic diet. Nutrients. 2022;14(4):782.
[337] Zhu H, Bi D, Zhang Y, Kong C, Du J, Wu X, et al. Ketogenic diet for human diseases: the underlying mechanisms and potential for clinical implementations. Sig Transduct Target Ther 2022;7(1):1–21.
[338] Choi IY, Piccio L, Childress P, Bollman B, Ghosh A, Brandhorst S, et al. A diet mimicking fasting promotes regeneration and reduces autoimmunity and multiple sclerosis symptoms. Cell Rep 2016;15(10):2136–46.
[339] Gupta A, Osadchiy V, Mayer EA. Brain–gut–microbiome interactions in obesity and food addiction. Nature reviews Gastroenterology & hepatology 2020;17(11):655.
[340] Zhu H, Tian P, Zhao J, Zhang H, Wang G, Chen W. A psychobiotic approach to the treatment of depression: a systematic review and meta-analysis. Journal of Functional Foods 2022;91:104999.
[341] Zang BY, He LX, Xue L. Intermittent fasting: potential bridge of obesity and diabetes to health? Nutrients. 2022;14(5):981.
[342] Maifeld A, Bartolomaeus H, Löber U, Avery EG, Steckhan N, Markó L, et al. Fasting alters the gut microbiome reducing blood pressure and body weight in metabolic syndrome patients. Nature Communications 2021;12(1):1970.
[343] Xie Z, Sun Y, Ye Y, Hu D, Zhang H, He Z, et al. Randomized controlled trial for time-restricted eating in healthy volunteers without obesity. Nat Commun 2022;13(1):1003.
[344] Frazier K, Chang EB. Intersection of the gut microbiome and circadian rhythms in metabolism. Trends Endocrinol Metab 2021;20.
[345] Gubert C, Kong G, Renoir T, Hannan AJ. Exercise, diet and stress as modulators of gut microbiota: implications for neurodegenerative diseases. Neurobiol Dis 2020;134:104621.
[346] Suryani D, Subhan Alfaqih M, Gunadi JW, Sylviana N, Goenawan H, Megantara I, et al. Type, intensity, and duration of exercise as regulator of gut microbiome profile. Curr Sports Med Rep 2022;21(3):84–91.
[347] Huang WC, Tung CL, Yang YCSH, Lin IH, Ng XE, Tung YT. Endurance exercise ameliorates Western diet–induced atherosclerosis through modulation of microbiota and its metabolites. Sci Rep 2022;12(1):3612.
[348] Madison A, Kiecolt-Glaser JK. Stress, depression, diet, and the gut microbiota: human–bacteria interactions at the core of psychoneuroimmunology and nutrition. Curr Opin Behav Sci 2019;28:105–10.
[349] Foster JA, Rinaman L, Cryan JF. Stress & the gut-brain axis: regulation by the microbiome. Neurobiology of Stress 2017;7:124–36.

Part 3

Therapeutic carbohydrate restriction for health and fitness

Chapter 9

Exercise and sports performance

Caryn Zinn[1], Cliff Harvey[2], Timothy David Noakes[3,4], James Smith[5], Christopher Webster[5] and Catherine Saenz[6]

[1]Auckland University of Technology, Auckland, New Zealand, [2]Holistic Performance Institute, Auckland, New Zealand, [3]Department of Health and Wellness Sciences, Cape Peninsula University of Technology, Cape Town, South Africa, [4]Nutrition Network, Cape Town, South Africa, [5]Division of Exercise Science and Sports Medicine, University of Cape Town, Cape Town, South Africa, [6]Exercise Science, Ohio State University, Columbus, OH, United States

9.1 Introduction

Caryn Zinn
Cliff Harvey

The in-depth study of human skeletal muscle was made possible by the discovery of the muscle biopsy technique in the 1960s. Since then, scientists have been able to develop an understanding of the storage capacity and fuel utilisation of the working muscle [1]. The limited capacity of the muscle to store carbohydrate (muscle glycogen) and the notion that carbohydrate is the dominant nutrient and fuel source for the exercising muscle have since dominated the direction of nutrition research and practice.

Nutrition guidelines for all types of athletes (endurance, strength, team, recreational, or elite) have historically been centred on a chronic, high carbohydrate-availability model to assure optimal muscle glycogen stores around training and competition. This model presumes that fatigue during most forms of more prolonged exercise is caused by the depletion of glycogen stores in the active muscles. Thus the emphasis is on beginning exercise with muscle glycogen stores that are maximally replete. The problem with the model is that it predicts that muscle fatigue develops when the capacity of the exercising muscles to produce ATP directly from muscle glycogen becomes less than the ATP required for the activity. But this model cannot be correct since muscle ATP depletion would produce muscle rigour which does not happen. Thus more complex mechanisms must be involved [2,3].

Despite the clear logical problems with this model of exercise fatigue [2], generations of athletes and sports dietitians, nutritionists, and sports science professionals have promoted advice on carbohydrate requirements for exercise by matching these requirements with exercise type, intensity, and duration. The principal focus has been on carbohydrate-loading strategies pre-exercise to ensure replete muscle glycogen stores, consumption of carbohydrate during exercise (where appropriate) to minimise or delay depletion of muscle and liver glycogen stores, and postexercise carbohydrate replenishment to restock depleted stores [4]. The most demanding of the carbohydrate fuelling strategies are prescribed for the endurance athlete, for whom much research supports endurance performance benefits when high rates of carbohydrate oxidation are sustained [5]. For the strength and power athlete, despite a lesser demand for carbohydrate compared with endurance athletes, large amounts of carbohydrate are nevertheless recommended.

More recently, low carbohydrate, high (or healthy) fat (LCHF) and very low carbohydrate, or ketogenic diets (KD) have gained the attention of athletes, practitioners, and researchers. This has stemmed largely from anecdotal evidence derived from athlete successes using this dietary approach, and from metabolic health-related literature and clinical outcomes reported in nonathlete populations. Such diets have been shown to be beneficial for the therapeutic management of a wide range of chronic conditions, including those characterised by insulin resistance, that is, obesity, diabetes (pre, type 1 and 2), polycystic ovarian syndrome (PCOS), and neurological conditions, that is, Parkinson's disease, dementia, concussion, brain and other cancers, and medication-resistant epilepsy, for which the KDs have proven highly effective [6–10].

For any athlete (endurance, strength, team, recreational or elite) the idea that the body's metabolic and energy systems could be transformed to preferentially favour fat utilisation over carbohydrate (glycogen) for fuel has appeal, from both the perspectives of performance enhancement and body composition improvements. Research on LCHF and KDs

Ketogenic. DOI: https://doi.org/10.1016/B978-0-12-821617-0.00013-9

and endurance athletes began in the 1980s and since then, interest in these dietary approaches has ebbed and flowed, both in its science and practice. However, there is now a growing interest within the sport and exercise science communities of the importance of athlete metabolic health, alongside the achievement of optimal performance [11]. Athletes with existing metabolic health concerns are seeking dietary approaches that align with both their performance and health goals. In a general sense, metabolically-healthy athletes may have some protection against chronic disease compared to their sedentary counterparts [12]. However, they are far from immune, particularly when their formal athletic career ends. These significant shifts in philosophies towards the importance of athlete health appear to be the driving forces behind the resurgence and maintenance of interest in LCHF and KDs.

The pursuit of individually tailored, optimal dietary formulae that cater for both high performance and optimal health is the future direction of sports nutrition. This chapter provides an account of the evidence and practise of LCHF and KDs in endurance, strength/resistance and team sport, recreational, and elite athlete populations.

9.2 The science of low carbohydrate and ketogenic diets for exercise and sports performance

Caryn Zinn
Cliff Harvey

9.2.1 The endurance athlete

Endurance exercise can be defined as continuous exercise longer than 30 min in duration, with ultraendurance referring to training and events lasting up to and beyond 4–5 h [13]. Any exercise lasting longer than a few minutes is fuelled mainly by carbohydrates and lipids, with protein contributing minute amounts [14], with the longer the duration and the greater the muscle adaptation to endurance exercise, the greater the contribution from fat oxidation [15]. For endurance athletes habitually consuming a diet high in carbohydrates, depletion of the body's limited muscle and liver glycogen stores during training sessions or events lasting longer than 90 min, has been associated with fatigue or suboptimal performance [2,16,17]. Of the two macronutrients fat and carbohydrate, the greater energy contribution of fat compared with carbohydrate, that is, 9 cal/g, versus 4 cal/g, respectively, partnered with the unlimited storage capacity of fat compared with carbohydrate, even in the leanest of athletes, has produced a growing scientific interest into ways to promote fat as a more substantial contributor of fuel for extensive exercise durations. Hence, the interest in LCHF and KDs began with the focus on endurance athletes.

9.2.1.1 Metabolic flexibility and performance

To achieve optimal sports performance, athletes need to effectively metabolise both carbohydrate and fat in a timely manner to support moderate (submaximal) exercise intensities and maximal-intensity efforts that are inherent in endurance and ultraendurance competitions (i.e., surges from breakaways or sprint finishes). This ability to switch between the utilisation of carbohydrate and fat rapidly and efficiently to maximise ATP regeneration has become known in the sporting context as "metabolic flexibility" [18].

The traditional dietary sports nutrition model of high carbohydrate availability has meant a dependence on carbohydrate for fuel, from both endogenous and exogenous sources, and subsequently, an athlete that paradoxically is metabolically inflexible. Whether athletes can access and utilise fat more efficiently during exercise and become metabolically flexible with either the preservation of, or improvement in, their performance compared to the mainstream model is the key question being posed.

The first study to comprehensively investigate the concept of enhanced fat utilisation in the endurance context was conducted by Stephen Phinney and colleagues in 1983. This group demonstrated that after 28 days of consuming a KD, trained cyclists could sustain exercise capacity at submaximal intensities [19]. Subsequent studies have since extensively explored a variety of protocols for enhancing fat utilisation (i.e., becoming more metabolically flexible) and their impact on performance outcomes in trained endurance athletes. Table 9.1 presents relevant studies investigating the impact of an LCHF or KD diet on endurance performance in athletes. Study inclusion (and exclusion) criteria are: (1) dietary interventions that are considered both KDs (defined as dietary carbohydrate <50 g/day) and LCHF (defined as $<$either 130 g/day or $<25\%$ of total energy) in their prescription; (2). fat adaptation strategies of $\geq$ 3 days in duration; (3) studies that report functional performance outcomes and/or body composition measures; (4) controlled and uncontrolled trials, and case studies; (5) English language; (6) human participants; (7) elite, competitive recreational and

TABLE 9.1 Low-carbohydrate high fat diet and ketogenic diet studies on endurance athletes.

Study. Author/ year	Study population	Study design and duration	Prescribed dietary protocols	Anthropometric and performance metrics	Anthropometric outcome	Performance outcome	LCHF or KD outcome Notes/comments
Acute fat- adaptation protocol (≤7 days)							
O'Keeffe et al. [20]	*n* = 7, highly trained female cyclists	RCT, 7 days. All athletes exposed to all three diets	LCHF (CHO 13%; Pro 28%; Fat 59% TE) MCD (CHO 54%; Pro 21%; Fat 25% TE) HCD (CHO 72%; Pro 15%; Fat 12% TE) Isocaloric diets.	n/a TTE	n/a	*Between-group:* TTE: ↓ in LCHF versus MCD and HCD	LCHF detrimental to performance. Time to fatigue increased as dietary carbohydrate content increased.
Burke et al. [21]	*n* = 8 well-trained cyclists	Randomised, double-blind crossover, 5 days	LCHF (Fat >65%; CHO <20% TE) HCD (CHO 70%–75%; fat <15% TE) Both followed by 1-day HCD (10 g/kg BM) Isocaloric diets Water during TT	BM 2 h cycle (70% VO_2 max) followed by 7 kJ/kg BM TT (time and power)	*Between-group:* BM ←→ LCHF versus HCD	*Between-group:* 7 kJ/kg BM TT (time and power) ←→ LCHF versus HCD	No significant benefit in LCHF but no impairment in time trial performance for time or power undertaken after 2 h of submaximal cycling.
Carey et al. [22]	*n* = 7 competitive male cyclists	Randomised cross-over study, 6 days	SCD—1 day (CHO 58%; Fat 27%; Pro 15% TE) followed by 6 days HCD (CHO 70%; Fat 15%) LCHF (Fat 69%; CHO 16% TE) followed by 1-day HCD Isocaloric diets.	n/a 4 h cycle, followed by 1-h TT (distance and power)	n/a	*Between-group:* 1-h TT (distance and power) ←→ LCHF versus HCD.	No significant benefit in LCHF but no impairment in performance in 1-h TT after 4 h of cycling.
Havemann et al. [23]	*n* = 8, well trained cyclists	Randomised single-blind crossover, 6 days	LCHF (Fat 68%; CHO 17%; Pro 15% TE) HCD (CHO 68%; Fat 17%; Pro 15% TE) Both followed by 1 day of CHO loading (CHO: 90% TE) Isocaloric diets	n/a 100 km TT (time) 1 and 4 km sprint (power)	n/a	*Between-groups:* 100 km TT (time) ←→ LCHF versus HCD 1 km sprint (power): ↓ in LCHF versus HCD	No impairment in endurance performance in LCHF, but impairment in high intensity exercise performance.

(Continued)

TABLE 9.1 (Continued)

Study. Author/ year	Study population	Study design and duration	Prescribed dietary protocols	Anthropometric and performance metrics	Anthropometric outcome	Performance outcome	LCHF or KD outcome Notes/comments
Burke et al. [24]	$n = 13$, elite male racewalkers	Parallel groups, 5 days (KD component); 5-day baseline phase (before) and 5-day restoration phase (after). 15-day total study duration.	Baseline phase (5 days): HCD (8.5 g/kg/d; Pro 2–2.2 g/kg/d) Adaptation phase (5 days): HCD (CHO 8.5 g/kg/d; Pro 2–2.2 g/kg/d) KD (CHO <50 g/d; Pro 2.2 g/kg/d; Fat 80% TE) followed by 1 day HCD Isocaloric diets. Restoration phase (5 days): HCD (8.5 g/kg/d; Pro 2–2.2 g/kg/d)	25 km BM (3 walks: baseline, adaptation, restoration) 25 km TT (time). 3 walks: baseline (1), adaptation (2), restoration (3) 10 km TT (time) 2 walks: baseline (1), adaptation (2)	*Between group:* 25 km BM: ←→ KD versus HCD *Within group:* 25 km BM: ↓ in HCD (all walks) 25 km BM ↓ in KD (walks 1 and 3)	*Between group:* 25 km TT (time): ←→ KD versus HCD (all 3 walks) 10 km TT (time): ↓ in HCD versus KD *Within group:* 25 km TT (time): ↑ in KD in walk 2 compared to walk 1 and 3	Impairment in KD performance relative to HCD
McSwiney et al. [25]	$n = 9$ trained males.	Uncontrolled trial, 7 days.	KD (CHO 5%–10%; Pro 15%–20%; Fat 75%–80% TE)	BM BF% FM FFM Wmax (power)	BM, FM, FFM: ↓ BF%: ←→	Wmax (power): ←→	No performance enhancement or impairment in KD; reduction in BM and FFM
Acute fat- adaptation protocol (8–15 days)							
Lambert et al. [26]	$n = 5$ trained cyclists	Crossover trial, 14 days	KD (Fat 70%; CHO 7% TE). HCD (CHO 74%; Fat 12% TE) Isocaloric diets	n/a 30 s Wingate test (power) TTE: HIE-85% PPO, TTE: MIE-50% PPO	n/a	*Between group:* Wingate power: ←→ KD versus HCD TTE-HIE: ←→ KD versus HCD. TTE-MIE: ↑ in KD versus HCD	KD had unimpaired performance in power and high intensity exercise, and improved performance in moderate intensity exercise.
Goedecke et al. [27]	$n = 16$, well trained cyclists.	RCT; 15 days.	LCHF (Fat 69%; CHO 19%; Pro 10% TE) UD (Fat 30%; CHO 53%; Pro 13% TE) Isocaloric diets CHO and MCT solution during TT	n/a 40 km TT (time)	n/a	*Between-groups:* 40 km TT (time): ←→ KD versus UD	No significant benefit for LCHF but no impairment in TT performance.

Lambert et al. [28]	$n = 5$ trained cyclists	RCT; 14 days	LCHF (Fat >65%; CHO <15%; Pro 20% TE) UD (Fat 30%; CHO 53%; Pro 13%; Alc 2% TE) for 10 days Both followed by HCD (CHO >65%; Fat <15%; Pro 20% TE) for 3 days Isocaloric diets MCT solution before trial; 10% glucose + MCT solution during performance test	BM BF 150-min cycle, followed by 20 km TT (time; power)	*Between-group:* BM, BF: ←→ LCHF versus UD.	*Between-group:* 20 kmTT (time): ↓ in LCHF versus UD 20km TT (power): ↑ in LCHF versus UD	Performance benefit of LCHF for 10 days, with 3-day carb replenishment.
Rowlands and Hopkins [29]	$n = 7$, cyclists.	RCT, 14 days.	3 diets, each separated by 2 weeks of SCD HCD (CHO 70%; Pro 14%; Fat 16% TE) LCHF (CHO 15%; Pro 20%; 66% Fat TE) LCHF + 2.5day CHO loading SCD (CHO 49%; Pro 16%; Fat 36% TE)	BM SF 15 min TT (distance; power) 100 km TT (time; power)	*Between group:* BM or SF: ←→ LCHF versus LCHF + CHO-load or HCD.	*Between group:* 15 min TT (distance and power): ←→ LCHF versus LCHF + CHO-load versus HCD 100 km TT (time and power): ←→ LCHF versus LCHF + CHO-load versus HCD 100 km TT (Final 5 km power): ↑ in LCHF + CHO-load versus HCD and SCD *Within group:* 100 km TT (power): ↓ in HCD and SCD Note: Between group metrics are based on the difference in outcomes between treatment diet and SCD	No enhancement or impairment in performance for LCHF. Trends towards enhanced ultra-endurance performance and reduced performance in HIE that can be attenuated with CHO loading.

(*Continued*)

TABLE 9.1 (Continued)

Study. Author/ year	Study population	Study design and duration	Prescribed dietary protocols	Anthropometric and performance metrics	Anthropometric outcome	Performance outcome	LCHF or KD outcome Notes/comments
≥ 15 days							
Zajac et al. [30]	$n = 8$, male endurance-trained off-road cyclists	Crossover trial, 8 weeks (4 weeks each diet)	MD (CHO 50%; Fat 30%; Pro 20% TE) KD (CHO 15%; Fat 70%; Pro 15% TE) Isocaloric diets	BM BMI Fat% Max workload Max workload LT	*Between group:* BM, BMI, fat%: ↓ in KD versus MD	*Between group*: Max workload and max workload LT: ↑ in MD versus KD	The KD showed favourable changes in body mass and body composition. Max workload and the workload at lactate threshold were significantly higher after the mixed diet and compromised in the KD.
Burke et al. [31]	$n = 29$, elite male racewalkers	Nonrandomised parallel group trial, 3 weeks	HCD (CHO 8 g/kg/d; Pro 2.1 g/kg/d; Fat 1.2 g/kg/d) Periodised HCD (CHO 8.3 g/kg/d; Pro 2.2 g/kg/d; Fat 1.2 g/kg/d) KD (CHO <50 g/d; Pro 2.1 g/kg/d; Fat 4.4 g/kg/d) Isocaloric diets	BM 10 km TT walk	*Between group:* BM: ←→ KD versus HDC versus Periodised HCD *Within group:* BM: ↓ in LCD and Periodised HCD	*Between group:* 10 km TT walk (time): ←→ KD versus HDC versus Periodised HCD *Within group:* 10 km walk (time): ↓ in HCD and periodised HCD	No performance enhancement or impairment in race times
Zinn et al. [32]	$n = 5$ competitive multisport athletes	Case study design, 10 weeks	KD (Fat < 50 g/d; Pro 1.5 g/kg/d, ad lib fat)	BM SF TTE Peak power	BM and SF: ↓ (in all athletes)	TTE: ↓ (in all athletes). Peak power: Nonsignificant ↓ (↑ in one athlete; ↓ in 4 athletes)	KD reduced weight and BF; reduced overall mean performance outcomes, but some increases or unchanged outcomes.
Sitko et al. [33]	$n = 11$ trained male road cyclists	Uncontrolled trial, 4 weeks	LCHF (CHO 10%; Pro 25%; Fat 65% TE)	BM BF% AP-5 min RP-5min AP-20 min RP-20min	BM: ↓ (medium-large ES) BF%: ↓ (small-large ES)	AP (5 and 20 min): Nonsignificant ↑ RP-5 min: ↑ (small-medium ES) RP-20 min: ↑ (medium-large ES)	No impact of LCHF on absolute power output, but due to reduced weight and BF%, (increased power: weight ratio) improved relative power.

Prins et al. [34]	*n* = 7, male competitive recreational distance runners	Randomised cross-over trial, 12 weeks (6 weeks per group)	KD (CHO <50 g/; Fat 75%–80%; Pro 15%–20% TE) HCD (CHO 60%–65%, Pro 15%–20%; Fat 20% TE)	BM BF% FM LM TTE (graded exercise test) 5 km TT (time) (performed 4x)	*Between and within group:* BM, BF%, FM, LM: ←→ KD versus HCD	*Between group:* TTE: ←→ KD versus HCD. 5 km TT (time) (in all four tests): ←→ KD versus HCD. *Within group:* TTE: ←→ in KD or HCD 5 km TT (time) (first one only): ↓ in KD	KD did not significantly change body composition relative to HCD. No benefit, but no performance impairment during maximal exercise testing in KD group relative to HCD. Running performance impaired during the initial 5 km TT (performed within the first ~4 days KD exposure) but improved thereafter. No difference in 5 km TT performance on both diets for the remainder of the trial.
Podlogar and Debevec [35]	*n* = 1, recreationally trained male cyclist	Case study, 14 days HCD (in LCHF-adapted athlete)	>6 months KD-adapted (CHO 7%; Pro 18%; Fat 74% TE) HCD (CHO: 64%; Pro 18%; Fat 18% TE)	n/a TTE MICP TTE HICP	n/a	TTE MICP: ↓ TTE HICP: ↑	KD increased ability to perform high-intensity endurance performance while decreased moderate intensity performance.
McSwiney et al. [36]	*n* = 20, male trained athletes	Nonrandomised control trial, 12 weeks	HCD (CHO 65%; Pro 14%; Fat 20% TE) KD (CHO 6%; Pro 17%; Fat 77% TE)	BM BF% 100 km TT (time) 6SS CPT	*Between group:* BM, BF%: ↓ in KD versus HCD.	*Between group:* 100 km TT (time): ←→ KD versus HCD 6SS and CPT: ↑ in KD versus HCD	KD enhanced body composition and performance.
Shaw et al. [37]	*n* = 8; male endurance athletes	Randomised, repeated measures, crossover trial; 31 days	UD (CHO 43%; Pro 19%; Fat 38% TE) KD (CHO 4%; Pro 18%; Fat 78% TE).	n/a TTE (at 70% VO_2max)	n/a	*Between and within group* TTE: ←→ KD versus UD.	No improvement in KD but no impairment in submaximal exercise performance.
Phinney et al. [19]	*n* = 5 elite cyclists.	Crossover trial with order effect (HCD first); 5 weeks (1 week HCD; 4 weeks KD).	HCD (CHO 66% TE; Pro 1.8 g/kg/d; Fat 33% TE) KD (CHO <20 g/d; Pro 1.8 g/kg/d; Fat remaining calories) Isocaloric diets	n/a TTE	n/a	*Between group* TTE: ←→ KD versus HCD	Variable individual effects but no overall improvement or impairment in endurance performance.

(*Continued*)

TABLE 9.1 (Continued)

Study. Author/ year	Study population	Study design and duration	Prescribed dietary protocols	Anthropometric and performance metrics	Anthropometric outcome	Performance outcome	LCHF or KD outcome Notes/comments
Helge et al. [38]	*n* = 20 untrained males	RCT, 8 weeks	7 weeks HCD (CHO 65%; Pro 15%; Fat 20% TE) LCHF (Fat 62%; Pro 17%; CHO 21% TE) followed by 1 week on HCD Isocaloric diets	n/a TTE	n/a	*Between group:* TTE: ↑ in LCHF versus HCD at both 7 and 8 weeks	LCHF was detrimental to performance relative to HCD.
Helge et al. [39]	*n* = 15 untrained males	RCT, 4 weeks	HCD (CHO 65%; Pro 15%; Fat 20% TE) LCHF (Fat 62%; Pro 17%; CHO 21% TE) Isocaloric diets.	n/a TTE	n/a	*Between group:* TTE: ←→ LCHF versus HCD *Within group:* TTE: ↑ in LCHF and HCD	Endurance performance enhanced similarly in LCHF and HCD.
Heatherly et al. [40]	*n* = 8 recreational runners	Crossover trial with order effect (UD first); 4 ½ weeks (7–10 days UD; 3 weeks KD)	KD (CHO 7%; Pro 29%; Fat 64% TE) UD (CHO 43%; Pro 17%; Fat 38% TE)	BM BF% FM FFM 5 km TT (time) (after 10 min test runs in heat) × 2	*Between group:* BM, BF%, FM: ↓ in KD versus UD FFM: ←→ KD versus UD	*Between group:* 5 km TT (time): ←→ KD versus UD	No performance improvement or impairment. Improvement in body composition outcomes.
Fleming et al. [41]	*n* = 20 nonhighly trained male athletes	Two-group trial, 6 weeks	KD (Fat 61% Pro 30%; CHO 8% TE) SCD (Fat 25% Pro 15%; CHO 59% TE)	BM 30 s Wingate (× 2) (peak power) 45 min cycle (work output)	*Between group:* BM: ←→ KD versus SCD *Within group:* BM: ↓ in KD	*Between group:* Wingate power: ←→ KD versus SCD 45 min cycle (work output): ↓ in KD versus SCD *Within group:* Wingate power: (first bout only): ↓ in KD Work output): ↓ in KD	KD showed small impairments in peak power and endurance performance, and reduced body weight.

Webster et al. [42]	$n = 1$, elite endurance athlete	Case study, 7 weeks	4 weeks LCHF + water, followed by 3 weeks LCHF + CHO (60 g/CHO/h) during 8 high intensity training sessions and performance trials.	N/A Power: (30 s, 4 min sprint) 20 km and 100 km TT: (time and power)	N/A	30 s sprint power: ↓ (0.5%) in LCHF + CHO versus LCHF + water. 4-min sprint power: ↑ (1.6%) in LCHF + CHO versus LCHF + water 20 km TT: ↓ time (2.8%); ↑ power (8.1%) in LCHF + CHO versus LCHF + water 100 km TT: ↑ time (1.1%); ↓ power (2.7%) in LCHF + CHO versus LCHF + water	CHO ingestion with LCHF beneficial during high-intensity endurance exercise (4–30 min) but not for short-sprint or prolonged endurance performance.

↓: statistically significant decrease; ←→: no significant difference; min: minute; RCT: randomised controlled trial; CHO: carbohydrate; Pro: protein; Alc: alcohol; TE: total energy; LCHF: Low carbohydrate, high fat; KD: ketogenic diet; MCD: medium carbohydrate diet; HCD: High carbohydrate diet; SCD: standard carbohydrate diet; n/a: not applicable; TTE: Time to exhaustion; Sign: significantly; LCHF: low carbohydrate, high fat diet; TT: time trial; g/d: (grams per day); BM: body mass; BF%: body fat percentage; FM: fat mass; FFM: fat free mass; LM: lean mass; Wmax (maximum power output); HIE: high intensity exercise; MIE: moderate intensity exercise; PPO peak power output; MCT: medium chain triglyceride; UD: usual diet; MD: mixed diet; Max workload LT: Maximum workload at lactate threshold; SF: skinfolds; AP: absolute power; RP: relative power; ES: effect size; MICP: moderate intensity constant power test; HICP: high intensity constant power test; 6SS: 6 s sprint; CPT: critical power test; g/kg/d: grams per kilogram per day.

recreational athletes; (8) studies published in peer reviewed journals, and conference presentations, where adequate information was able to be retrieved. All types of trials have been included, rather than limited to randomised controlled trials, to allow for a broad appreciation of all forms of peer reviewed evidence in this area, based on the context of LCHF or KD application. Only statistically significant outcomes are presented from trials with control or comparison groups and are denoted as follows: ↑ = significant increase; ↓ = significant decrease; ← → = no significant difference. Significant and nonsignificant outcomes are presented from case studies and uncontrolled trials, with nonsignificant outcomes specified where relevant.

9.2.1.2 *Study findings*

When interpreting study findings collectively, it is important to acknowledge the considerable variation across studies in dietary protocol (i.e., the degree of carbohydrate restriction, detail of food quality, carbohydrate refeeding protocols), exercise testing protocols, class of endurance athlete (trained, untrained) and study design. Common to all these studies, both acute and chronic, is the increase in whole-body fat oxidation and decrease in carbohydrate oxidation when athletes consume a LCHF or KD for any length of time (not shown in the study table).

Taken as a whole, the evidence suggests that performance decrements resulting from reductions in acute or chronic carbohydrate intake are most apparent with shorter fat-adaptation times (i.e., less than one week) even when carbohydrate refuelling strategies to restore muscle glycogen stores are applied, and with exercise modalities that involve high volumes of highly glycolytic activity. Time to exhaustion, power, repeated sprint-ability, and muscle tissue gain or retention are improved in the short term on higher-carbohydrate diets compared to lower-carbohydrate diets. However, with sufficient adaptation, these effects appear to be mitigated except for maximum workloads in the glycolytic range.

At extremes of energy provision, that is, for very short (<15 s) or very long bouts of continuous exercise (>4 h) there is unlikely to be any performance decrement resulting from a reduced carbohydrate diet due to the reliance upon creatine phosphate or lipids for fuel provision, respectively. Similarly, performances when undertaking relatively low volumes of activity, even within glycolytic ranges, are unlikely to be affected by a reduced carbohydrate diet.

One of the key physiological limitations proposed to explain the performance decrements seen in some studies in the LCHF or KD arms centres around the downregulation of pyruvate dehydrogenase (PDH). PDH is a key regulatory enzyme involved in the pathways of skeletal muscle fat and carbohydrate metabolism, indicating reduced metabolic flexibility [43]. There is speculation, however, that reduced PDH activity in the context of carbohydrate restriction facilitates the diversion of pyruvate into other metabolites to allow for the continuation of the Citric Acid Cycle for fuel provision as required [44]. These adaptation mechanisms require elucidation with further experimental research over a range of fat-adaption durations. Importantly, the study of [43] failed to show that the apparent reduction in PDH activity was associated with any impairment of exercise performance in the athletes that were studied. Furthermore maximal PDH activity measured during high intensity exercise was not impaired by the high fat diet showing that the "reduced" PDH activity during submaximal exercise following the high-fat diet reflected intact homoeostatic regulation, not an "energy limitation" [2]. The point remains however that if energy supply limits performance (because of downregulation of PDH activity), then the outcome should be skeletal muscle rigour, not fatigue or impaired athletic performance, neither of which were found in this study.

With sufficient fat-adaptation, substrate use will be modified to increase fatty acid utilisation by tissue, preserve both hepatic and muscle glycogen by reducing relative glucose use via glycogenolysis, encourage increased gluconeogenesis (when required), and increase ketogenesis to provide a "crossover" fuel to fill any applied energy shortfall. It has been demonstrated in the FASTER (Fat Adapted Substrate Use in Trained Elite Runners) study that with sufficient time for complete fat adaptation to occur, in this case, up to 20 months, substrate use is markedly altered in athletes following a low-carbohydrate diet. These athletes had a greater capacity to oxidise fat at higher exercise intensities, when compared with athletes habituated to high carbohydrate diets; yet there was no difference in resting muscle glycogen concentrations or rates of glycogen depletion or repletion when compared to athletes eating a standard high-carbohydrate protocol (Fig. 9.1) [45]. This was the first study to demonstrate such an outcome, and while performance outcomes weren't measured in this study, the finding that fat-adapted athletes could maintain normal glycogen concentrations in the context of limited carbohydrate intake is intriguing. The metabolic milieu of highly trained, elite athletes consuming an LCHF or KDs for several months or years is likely vastly different from that after a few days or weeks. It might be that with time additional physiological and biochemical adaptations occur beyond those required for retooling the muscle to adjust to fat burning (such as glycogen restoration); however, further studies are required for this to be substantiated.

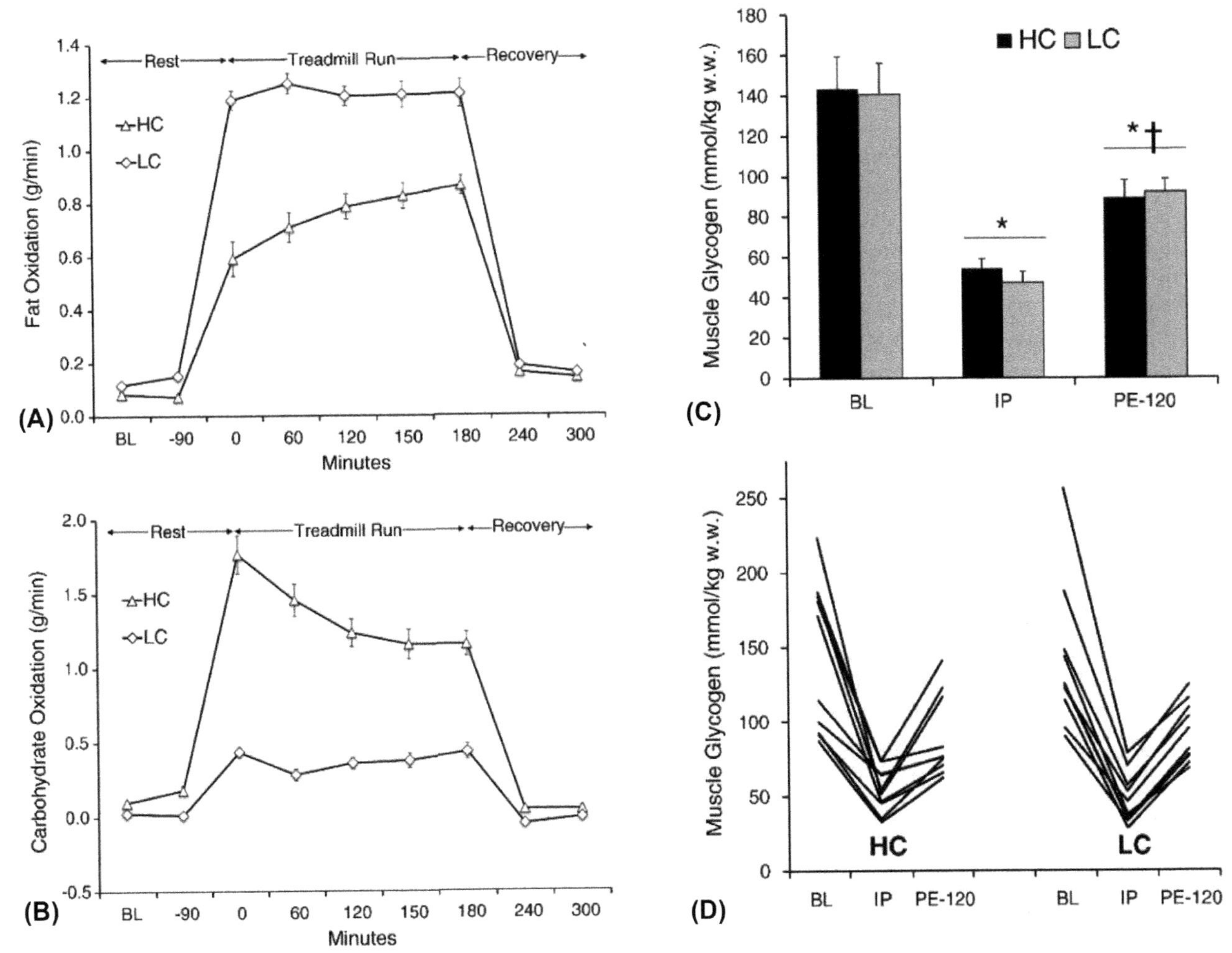

FIGURE 9.1 Fuel oxidation rates and muscle glycogen stores from the FASTER Study. Fat (A) and carbohydrate (B) oxidation rate during 180 min of running at 64% VO_2max and 120 min of recovery. All time points were significantly different between groups. Mean (C) and individual (D) muscle glycogen concentrations at baseline (pre-exercise), immediate postexercise (IP), and 120 postexercise (PE-120). Subjects ran on a treadmill at 64% VO_2max for 180 min. * Indicates significant ($P = 0.000$) difference from baseline. † Indicates significant ($P = 0.000$) difference from IP. No significant differences between groups. *LC*, low-carbohydrate diet group; *HC*, high-carbohydrate diet group. *Reproduced with permission from Volek, J.S., Freidenreich, D.J., Saenz, C., Kunces, L.J., Creighton, B.C., Bartley, J.M., ... et al. (2016). Metabolic characteristics of keto-adapted ultra-endurance runners. Metabolism: Clin Exp, 65(3), 100–110. https://doi.org/10.1016/j.metabol.2015.10.028.*

Another gap in the published literature is the differing effects, if any, of LCHF and KDs on male compared to female athletes. While there are female population groups being studied, the majority of this work has been conducted on males. Considering the stark differences in metabolic make-up between males and females, future studies are needed to determine if any differences in outcomes exist. In the absence of such studies, it may be wise to explain to female athletes that advice on the optimum diet for athletic performance comes largely from studies of male athletes so that self-experimentation might be advisable. Indeed, this advice should apply to all athletes. Whilst scientific studies can determine what may apply to the majority, the possibility is always that the individual may respond quite differently.

In summary, to ensure optimal performance outcomes, endurance athletes should allow sufficient time-to-adaptation before events when embarking on a low-carbohydrate regimen. Equivocal performance results might still be of interest for weight-restricted athletes or those for whom a lighter body weight is advantageous. There are consistent benefits observed for body mass and body fat levels without any performance decrement, leading to improved power-to-weight ratio. In particular, the low-carbohydrate diet specifically enhances loss of visceral fat.

9.2.2 The strength or resistance athlete

The appeal of LCHF and KDs for endurance athletes largely stems from their ability to enhance muscle fat oxidation. However, the physiological rationale partnered with the outcomes borne out in the endurance literature relating to body composition benefits, has renewed interest in this diet among strength- or resistance-trained athletes. Compared to studies conducted on endurance athletes, which began in the 1980s, there is little evidence for the efficacy of LCHF and KDs on strength- or resistance-trained athletes. However, research has been on the rise over the past decade. For this group of athletes, the key metrics of interest are body composition (lean body mass, fat mass and overall body mass) and strength and power performance. Athletes that are typically included in this sporting group include weightlifters, powerlifters, bodybuilders, combat sports, rowing, and CrossFit, but it also includes athletes in sports that involve substantial portions of their training as resistance, such as dancers, gymnasts, and many team sports.

For many of these athletes, body weight reduction strategies particularly for those that have strict weight classes in which they compete are an inherent part of the sporting demands. The practise of rapid weight loss prior to competition has historically used methods such as low calorie or low residue diets, fasting, vomiting, and deliberate dehydration from frequent sauna use, sweat-inducing clothing, and diuretics [46]. Some of these methods can be dangerous and cause lean mass loss and impaired physiological function and health [47]. LCHF and KDs could provide the athletes with a more effective and safer way to reduce weight, both chronically, and more acutely prior to competition.

In many sports, there is a surprising variety in training volumes between (and within) recreational and elite-level athletes and this is no truer than in the strength, power or "crossover" pursuits of CrossFit, bodybuilding, powerlifting, and all-round weightlifting. Athletes who train with low-volumes and maximal loads almost exclusively, are almost completely reliant on the creatine phosphate-ATP energy system and have very low requirements for carbohydrate to fuel their performances. However, increased training volume of any type, but particularly involving high-intensity work bouts $> 10-15$ s will place increasingly greater demands on muscle glycogen reserves and reduce the ability to replete glycogen from available substrates (liver gluconeogenesis from amino acids and glycerol). Thus the relative efficacy of a lower- or higher-carbohydrate diet will be activity- and volume dependent. For example, a powerlifter or all-round lifter performing three 45-min sessions per week focussed mostly on low repetition strength work will require little carbohydrate to fuel the work required. On the other hand, a competitor performing six 90-min sessions per week would likely require a much greater carbohydrate intake, despite being in the same sport, and at the same level of competition. It is therefore difficult to accurately compare diet-sport interactions because of the variability in training loads and volumes between athletes.

Table 9.2 presents relevant studies investigating the impact of an LCHF or a KDs in strength- or resistance-trained athletes. Study inclusion (and exclusion) criteria and presentation of outcomes are the same as selected for Table 9.1 (Endurance) with the difference being the performance metric related to strength or resistance performance outcomes.

9.2.2.1 Study findings

As in the studies of endurance athletes (Table 9.1), these studies also display similar heterogeneities, that is, different dietary protocols, including level of carbohydrate restriction and duration of fat adaptation protocol (4 days to 12 weeks), testing protocols and class of athlete. However, most of these (11/13) employ the KDs rather than the LCHF dietary approach. Taken collectively, the weight of the findings leans towards an improvement in body composition outcomes, specifically body mass, fat mass, body fat %, without negatively impacting performance. The only clear demonstration of a performance impairment was following the application of a 4-day KD, the shortest fat-adaptation duration under study.

In the two studies that reported a detrimental effect of the KDs on fat free mass (or lean mass) loss [56,58] both report nonsignificant reductions in fat free mass, and in both cases no performance impairment. This finding could be explained by a key limitation in LCHF or KDs studies relating to the measurement of body composition, in particular lean mass using DXA, bioelectric impedance, or BODPOD equipment. The evaluation of fat free-mass includes intracellular water, which is stored with muscle glycogen in a $\sim$ 3:1 ratio [61]. In a glycogen- depleted state, intracellular water will be subsequently less, so when fat-free mass is measured in LCHF or KD groups postintervention, losses will likely be exaggerated. Either way, from a practical standpoint, while lean body mass losses are undesirable in general for all athletes, but particularly for strength athletes, this should at least provide some peace of mind for athletes and coaches that LCHF or KDs can be used effectively for more rapid weight loss strategies (i.e., at least two weeks) to qualify for weight classes.

Controlling for dietary equivalency in studies, that is, energy and macronutrient intake, and energy expenditure, is critical when both body composition and performance are the outcome measures of interest. Some of the study

TABLE 9.2 **Low-carbohydrate high fat diet and ketogenic diet studies on strength or resistance athletes.**

Study. Author/ year	Study population	Study design and duration	Prescribed dietary protocols	Anthropometric and performance metrics	Anthropometric outcome	Performance outcome	Benefit of KD: notes/comments
Paoli et al. [48]	*n* = 8; elite artistic male gymnasts	Randomised, crossover trial (3-month washout); 30 days	KD (CHO 4.5%; Pro 40.7%; Fat: 54.8% TE) SCD (CHO 46.8%; Pro 14.7%; Fat: 38.5% TE)	BM FM BF% LM LM% Range of strength tests	*Between groups* None reported. *Within groups*: BM, FM, BF%: ↓ in KD; ←→ in SC LM: ←→ in KD and SCD. LM%: ↑ in KD; ←→ in KD	*Between groups* ←→ KD versus SCD in all strength tests	KD over a short time period (i.e., 30 days) can decrease body weight and body fat without negative effects on strength performance.
Sawyer et al. [49]	*n* = 31; resistance-trained males and females	Repeated measures: 14 days	UD for 7 days (CHO 41%; Pro 22%; Fat 34% TE) Followed by KD for 7 days (CHO 5%; Pro 35%; Fat 54% TE)	BM FFM FM BF% TBW Handgrip dynamometry, vertical jump, 1RM (bench press; back squat), maximum-repetition bench press, 30 s Wingate (peak power).	*Between group* BM, TBW, BF% (females only): ↓ in KD versus UD FFM, FM ←→ KD versus UD	*Between group* Handgrip strength, back squat: ↑ in KD versus UD ←→ KD versus UD in all other variables	KD beneficial for short-term weight loss purposes without compromising strength and power.
Rhyu and Cho [50]	*n* = 20 Taekwondo athletes	RCT, 3 weeks.	Calorie-restricted (75%) KD (CHO 4%; Pro 41%; Fat 55% TE) LCHF (CHO 30%; Pro 40%; Fat 30% TE)	BM BF% FFM BMI 2000m sprint (time) Wingate: Power (peak and mean power), anaerobic fatigue Grip force Back muscle strength Sit-up 100 m sprint Jumps	*Between group* BM, BF%, FFM, BMI: ←→ KD versus LCHF *Within group* BM, BF%, FFM, BMI: ↓ in KD and LCHF	*Between group* 2000m sprint time, Wingate anaerobic fatigue: ↓ in KD versus LCHF All other variables: ←→ KD versus LCHF *Within group* 2000m (time): ↓ in KD and LCHF Back strength, sit-up: ↑ in KD and LCHF	KD can be helpful for weight category athletes by improving aerobic capacity and fatigue resistance.

(Continued)

TABLE 9.2 (Continued)

Study. Author/ year	Study population	Study design and duration	Prescribed dietary protocols	Anthropometric and performance metrics	Anthropometric outcome	Performance outcome	Benefit of KD: notes/comments
Gregory et al. [51]	*n* = 27; nonelite male and female CrossFit athletes	RCT; 6 weeks.	KD (CHO <50 g/d; Pro and fat ad lib) UD (CHO 40%; Pro 22%; Fat 38% TE)	BM BF% FM LM Vertical jump, standing long jump, CrossFit performance test (row, squats, sit-ups, push-ups, pull-ups) (time)	*Between group* BM, BF%, FM: ↓ in KD versus UD LM: ←→ KD versus UD *Within group* ←→ in KD or UD	*Between group* All performance measures: ←→ KD versus UD *Within group* Jumps: ←→ in KD or UD Crossfit performance test (time): ↓ in KD and UD	KD can favourably impact body fat%, fat mass, and weight, while maintaining lean mass and improving performance (but not relative to usual diet).
Chatterton et al. [52]	*n* = 5; subelite weightlifters and powerlifters	Case study; 16 weeks; 4 weeks UD; 8 weeks LCHF; 4 weeks UD	LCHF (1 g/CHO/kg; Pro and fat ad lib) UD (CHO 21.-3.8 g/kg/d; Pro 1.1–2.6 g/kg/d; Fat 0.7–1.7 g/kg/d)	BM BF (skinfolds) 1RM	BM and BF: ↓ in 4 athletes. ←→ in 1 athlete.	1RM: ↑ in 2 athletes; ←→ in 2 athletes; ↓ in one athlete	No impairment in performance in 4 out of 5 athletes. Body composition improvements shown in most athletes.
Wilson et al. [53]	*n* = 25; resistance-trained males	RCT; 11 weeks	KD (wk 1–10) (CHO 5%; Pro 20%; Fat 75% TE), followed by CHO refeed wk 10–11 SCD (wks 1–11) (CHO 55%; Pro 20%; Fat 25% TE)	LM FM 1RM (bench press; back squat); 10 s Wingate (Peak power)	*Between group* LM: ↑ in KD versus SCD (change between wk 1–11 and wk 10–11) FM: ↓ in KD versus SCD (wk 1–10) *Within group* LM: ↑ in KD and SCD (wk 1–10 and wk 1–11). ↑ in KD (wk 10–11) FM: ↓ in KD and SCD (wk 1–10 and wk 1–11). ↑ in KD (wk 10–11)	*Between group* All variables: ←→ KD versus SCD *Within group* 1RM: ↑ in KD and SCD (wk 1–10, wk 10–11). Wingate power: ↑ in KD (wk 1–11); ↑ in SCD (wk 1–10; wk 1–11)	KD can show improvements in body composition relative to SCD, with similar benefits in muscle strength and power.

Miele et al. [54]	HIIT $n = 15$; CrossFit athletes trained for 3 months	RCT; 8 weeks	KD (CHO 5%–10%; Fat 65%–85%; Pro 15%–30% TE) CON (usual diet: not specified)	BM TTE (500 m row) Wingate test (Anaerobic power) 3RM (deadlift)	*Between group* ←→ KD versus CON.	*Between group* All variables: ←→ KD versus CON. *Within group* Wingate power: ↑ in CON.	No impairment in performance for KD.
Vargas et al. [55]	$n = 24$; strength-trained males	RCT; 8 weeks	KD CHO (42 g/d < 10% TE; Pro 2 g/kg/d 20% TE; Fat remaining calories 70% TE) SCD (Pro 2 g/kg/d 20% TE; Fat 25% TE; CHO remaining calories 55% TE) CON: Not stated Hyperenergetic diets across all athletes (39 Cal/kg/d)	BM FM VAT LM	*Between group*: BM, FM, VAT, LM: ←→ KD versus SCD *Within group*: BM: ↑ in SCD. FM and VAT: ↓ in KD LM: ↑ in SCD	N/A	KD may help reduce fat mass and visceral adipose tissue without decreasing lean mass.
Greene et al. [56]	$n = 14$; intermediate to elite level male and female powerlifters and Olympic weightlifters.	Randomised, crossover trial; 3 months (2-week washout)	KD (CHO <50 g/d <10% TE; Fat 70%; Pro 20%; ad lib calories) UD (CHO >250 g/d; ad lib calories)	BM LM FM 1 RM (Self-selection of snatch, clean and jerk, bench press, squat, deadlift)	*Between group*: BM, LM: ↓ in KD versus UD. FM: ←→ KD versus UD *Within group*: BM, LM, FM: ↓ in KD BM, LM, FM: ↑ in UD	*Between group*: 1RM: ←→ KD versus UD *Within group*: 1RM: ↑ in both KD and UD	Impairment in lean body mass for KD, but losses not reflected in lifting performances.
Waldman et al. [57]	$n = 11$; resistance-trained males	Uncontrolled trial; within-subject repeated measures; 15 days	LCHF (CHO <25%; Pro 25%; Fat 50% TE)	BM BF % FFM FM Aerobic only measured. TTE on graduated intensity run protocol.	BM: ↓ BF %, FFM, FM: ←→.	TTE: ←→.	KD showed no impairment in performance.

(*Continued*)

TABLE 9.2 (Continued)

Study. Author/ year	Study population	Study design and duration	Prescribed dietary protocols	Anthropometric and performance metrics	Anthropometric outcome	Performance outcome	Benefit of KD: notes/comments
Kephart et al. [58]	$n = 12$; recreational male and female CrossFit athletes.	Nonrandomised controlled trial; 12 weeks.	KD (CHO 50 g/d; Fat 70% TE). UD (not specified).	BM FM LM (in dual arm, leg, lateralis thickness) 1-RM (back squat; clean); maximum push-ups; 400 m run	*Between group*: BM, FM, LM: ←→ in KD versus UD. *Within group*: BM: ↓ in KD. FM, LM: ←→ in KD and UD.	*Between group*: 1RM: ←→ in KD versus UD. *Within group*: 1RM: ←→ in KD and UD.	Trends towards reductions in whole-body adiposity in KD group; no negative impact on performance. Trends towards reduction in dual-leg muscle mass and vastus lateralis thickness in KD. Needs further investigation.
Wroble et al. [59]	$n = 16$ exercise-trained athletes.	Randomised-sequence, counterbalanced crossover; 4 days on both diets.	KD (CHO <50 g/d <10% TE). HCD (6–10 g/kg/d). Isocaloric diets.	Wingate (power) Yo-yo intermittent recovery run test (distance).	N/A	*Between group* Wingate power, Yo-yo test (distance): ↓ in KD versus HCD.	KD impaired performance.
Vargas-Molina et al. [60]	$n = 21$; strength-trained females.	RCT; 8 weeks.	KD (CHO 30–40 g/d; Pro 1.7 g/kg/d; Fat remaining energy ~120 g/d). SCD (Pro 1.7 g/kg/d; Fat 1 g/kg/d; CHO remaining energy ~280 g/d).	BM FM FFM 1RM (back squat; bench press); CMJ	*Between group*: BM, FM, FFM: ↓ in KD versus SCD. *Within group*: BM, FM: ↓ in KD. FFM: ←→ in KD and SCD.	*Between group* Bench press, squat: ↑ in SCD versus KD. CMJ: ←→ in KD versus SCD. *Within group*: Squat, CMJ: ↑ in KD and SCD. Bench-press: ↑ in SCD; ←→ in KD.	KD helps reduce body mass and fat mass and maintain fat free mass but is suboptimal for increasing fat free mass in females. No performance advantage of KD, but no impairment.

CHO: Carbohydrate; Pro: protein; TE: total energy; KD: ketogenic diet; non-KD: nonketogenic diet; SCD: Standard carbohydrate diet; UD: Usual diet; LCHF: Low carbohydrate, high fat diet; HCD: high carbohydrate diet; CON: control; BM: body mass; BF%: body fat percentage; FM: fat mass; FFM: fat free mass; LM: lean mass; TBW: Total body water; FFM: fat free mass; 1RM: One repetition maximum; RCT: randomised controlled trial; CON: control (usual diet); wk: week; HIIT: high intensity intermittent training; TTE: time to exhaustion; VAT: visceral adipose tissue; CMJ: countermovement jump.

limitations worth mentioning due to their potential to influence outcomes include uncontrolled physical activity outside of structured exercise intervention sessions [51], reduced energy intakes subsequent to diminished appetites in athletes consuming the KDs [55], use of ad lib energy intakes across groups [56], and reported protein variations between groups [49,57]. Finally, a common problem across all dietary studies is the challenge of obtaining dietary records with optimal precision due to measurement error associated with self-reported dietary assessment tools.

In summary, strength and resistance type sports place high importance on the power-to-weight ratio. Considering the efficacy of LCHF and KD diets in reducing body mass and body fat, and maintaining strength performance at high levels, this may be a strong rationale for their application within the strength and power sporting domain. The issue of lean mass loss, irrespective of whether this results in a performance impairment, needs further investigation, alongside further trials on how these diets fare against high-carbohydrate diets in the context of weight- and muscle-gain goals.

9.2.3 The high intensity intermittent training and team athlete

There are very few studies investigating the effects of LCHF or KDs on high-intensity exercise performance. It has long been recognised and accepted that both aerobic and anaerobic exercise performance is highly reliant on carbohydrate availability [62] although this belief has recently been challenged [2]. As a result, dietary carbohydrate availability is believed to be essential for ensuring high intensity exercise performance and high intensity intermittent training (HIIT) exercise in some form is central to the training of many team and individual sports [63]. Consequently, scientists, athletes and their coaches are apprehensive of adopting LCHF or KDs in the anticipation that it impairs the ability to perform high intensity exercise. Table 9.3 summarises the studies to date on low-carbohydrate dietary interventions for athletes involved in high-intensity exercise.

9.2.3.1 Study findings

Despite the relatively few studies of the effects of low-carbohydrate diets for HITT and team athletes, the published studies challenge the common perception that a high carbohydrate diet is necessary to sustain high-intensity exercise performance. In the studies to date, there have been few decrements demonstrated in high-intensity exercise performance, but there have been positive changes in adiposity and weight.

These results are consistent with our emerging understanding of low-carbohydrate diets and performance, namely that larger volumes of glycolytic activity require greater intakes of carbohydrate, especially in the short term, although this may be mitigated by longer-term fat adaptation. For example, in the study by Michalczyk et al. [67] a 4-week low-carbohydrate diet resulted in a significant decrement in the total work performed during the exercise trial, which was likely to have resulted from impaired glycogen stores according to the conventional explanation. Based on our current understanding, this would be expected to improve with sufficient fat-adaptation [45]. In this same study, and indicative of power performance during shorter, higher-intensity bouts, peak power output was unaffected by the LCHF. So, similarly to strength- and resistance-trained athletes, carbohydrate intake should be allocated based on the volume of glycolytic work but within a framework that recognises the value of increased fat-adaptation (and therefore reduced reliance on carbohydrate) over the longer term.

Alternatively, it may be that there is not an obligatory need for muscle glycogen oxidation even during more intense exercise [2].

9.2.4 Low carbohydrate diets and immune and gut health

Two important research areas relating to LCHF and KDs in the athletic population that are gaining interest are the impact of such diets on the immune system and on the microbiome. The few studies that have been undertaken recently on the immune system show mixed outcomes. McKay reported no effect of a 3-week KDs on immune markers in elite racewalkers [69]. In contrast Waldman et al., reported both protective effects on chronic inflammatory markers as well as increases in some proinflammatory markers when the KDs were administered to endurance athletes for 3 weeks [70]. Shaw et al. reported a transient increase in proinflammatory immune markers in trained cyclists consuming KDs for 31 days, but as this did not translate into increased illness outcomes for athletes, the clinical relevance of this finding is unknown [71].

Any analysis of dietary influences on the athlete's immune system is complicated by the multitude of factors contributing to immune compromise, including seasonal (winter) illnesses, physical (prolonged, strenuous exercise) and mental stress, poor sleep, long-haul travel, and micronutrient insufficiencies [72]. Despite this, future research to determine any effects of well-formulated LCHF and KDs on immunity and subsequent illness is warranted.

TABLE 9.3 Low-carbohydrate high fat diet and ketogenic diet studies on athletes involved with HIIT exercise and team sports.

Study. Author/ year	Study population	Study design and duration	Prescribed dietary protocols	Anthropometric and performance metrics	Anthropometric outcome	Performance outcome	Notes/ comments
HIIT							
Dostal et al. [64]	$n = 24$; recreationally trained individuals.	Nonrandomised, parallel-group controlled trial; 12 weeks.	KD (CHO 8%; Pro 29%; Fat 63% TE). UD (CHO 48%; Pro 17%; Fat 35% TE).	BM LM FM TFM TBW GXT-TTE HIIT-TTE (30–15 intermittent fitness test)	*Between groups* Not reported *Within groups* FM, TFM: ↓ in KD.	*Between groups* GXT-TTE and HIIT-TTE: ←→ KD versus UD. *Within groups* GRX-TTE, HIIT-TTE: ↑ in KD and UD.	KD showed no impairment in high intensity continuous or intermittent exercise.
Cipryan et al. [65]	$n = 18$; moderately trained males.	RCT; 4 weeks.	KD (CHO 8%; Pro 29%; Fat 63% TE). UD (CHO 48%; Pro 17%; Fat 35% TE).	BM BF% GXT-TTE	*Between groups* BM, BF%: Likely small differences (reductions in KD and UD). *Note: Analysis conducted by magnitude-based inferences and not statistical significance.*	*Between groups* GRX-TTE: Possibly small-to-trivial differences (increases in KD and UD).	KD showed no evidence of high intensity performance impairment.
Team sport or mix of modalities							
Kysel et al. [66]	$n = 25$ male recreational resistance and aerobic training athletes.	RCT, 8 weeks.	CKD Weekly cycles of 5 days: KD (CHO < 30 g; Pro: 1.6 g/kg; Fat remaining calories), followed by 2 days HCD (CHO 70%; Pro 15%; Fat 15% TE). RD (CHO 55%; Fat 30%; Pro 15% TE). Both diets calorie reduced (500 Cal).	BM BF% LM FM Peak workload 1RM for 3 lifts (Wmax) Work capacity (W170max/kg)	*Between group* BM, BF%, LM, FM: ←→ CKD versus RD. *Within group:* BM, BF% LM, FM: ↓ in KD and RD.	*Between group* 1RM, work capacity: ←→ CKD versus RD. *Within group:* 1RM, work capacity: ↑ in RD.	No improvement or impairment in body composition or performance in a cyclical KD relative to RD.

Michalczyk et al. [67]	$n = 15$ competitive basketball athletes.	Crossover trial with order effect (HCD first), 9 weeks.	HCD for 4 weeks (CHO 55%; Pro 25%; Fat 31% TE). Followed by LCHF for 4 weeks (CHO 10%; Pro 31%; Fat 59% TE). Followed by Carbo-L for 1 week (CHO 75%; Pro 16%; Fat 9% TE).	BM FM% FFM TW PP TPP	*Between group* BM, FM%: ↓ in LCHF versus HCD. FFM: ↑ in Carbo-L versus LCHF.	*Between group* TW: ↓ in LCHF versus HCD; ↑ in Carbo-L versus LCD. PP, TPP: ←→ in HCD versus LCF versus Carbo-L.	LCHF improved body composition and impaired total work output, but performance was restored after carbohydrate replenishment.
[a][68]	$n = 12$ recreational endurance and strength athletes.	Pilot case study, 35–50 days: median 38 days.	KD (CHO < 20 g/d; fat 75% TE).	BM FM FFM TTE PP (Graded treadmill running)	BM (10/12 athletes), FM (11/12 athletes): ↓FFM: ←→	TTE, PP: ←→	KD improved body composition, with no improvement or impairment in performance.

RCT: randomised controlled trial; TE: total energy; BM: body mass; BF%: body fat percentage; FM: fat mass; FFM: fat free mass; LM: lean mass; TFM: trunk fat mass; TBW: total body water; GXT: graded exercise tests; TTE: time to exhaustion; HCD: high carbohydrate diet; CKD: cyclical ketogenic diet; RD: calorie-reduction diet; W170max.kg: maximum working capacity at 170m heart rate 170bpm; DC Conventional diet; TW: total work; PP: peak power; TPP: Time to peak power; Carbo-L: carbohydrate loaded diet.

[a]*This study has not been conducted on team or HIIT athletes, but rather on a combination of athletes with pooled statistical outcomes. The performance test was <15 m and therefore classed as high intensity exercise modality.*

Current understanding of the human microbiome indicates that the microbial environment can be altered by diet in as little as 48 h [73], and that a richness in microbial diversity and the presence of beneficial bacterial strains have been associated with good health [74].

Evidence on the impact of LCHF or KDs on the microbiome in the general population is limited, and to date there have been no studies conducted in athletes [75]. Nonathlete human and animal KD studies show mixed outcomes on the microbiome and include reports of positive effects on reshaping bacterial composition and biological gut functions, and negative effects such as reduced microbial diversity and increased proinflammatory bacteria [76]. Further research is needed to elucidate the impact of LCHF and KDs on the gut flora of athletes to determine whether changes in flora have a positive, negative, or neutral effect on athlete health or performance, or both.

9.3 Practical application of low-carbohydrate high fat diet and ketogenic diets in athletes

Caryn Zinn
Cliff Harvey

To date, evidence has provided important insights into carbohydrate-restricted diets for a range of athletes, including contexts where fat-adaptation protocols show a beneficial, neutral, or harmful effect on performance and body composition. Of further interest to the practitioner across all sports are two important areas that are not always well-explored in the research.

1. Individual variability
2. Individual prescription (and periodisation) of macronutrient intakes

Within any dietary paradigm, there are responders and nonresponders, and those that need more or less of a particular macronutrient or micronutrient based on their metabolic make-up. Within the research summarised in this chapter, there are examples of participants who responded more, or less favourably to either of the prescribed interventions. In a real-life situation, a dietary prescription will also be individualised, and this could encompass a large range of carbohydrate intakes not constrained by common definitions of "low carbohydrate" or "ketogenic" diets in the literature. This individualisation of diet might consist of greater amounts of carbohydrate in a diet that remains functionally low carbohydrate due to a large overall energy requirement, or could involve periodisation of carbohydrate, or the use of relatively large amounts of exogenous carbohydrate during training or events as suggested by Maunder, Kilding, and Plews in *Substrate Metabolism During Ironman Triathlon: Different Horses on the Same Courses* [77]. It is also important to state that there is no evidence to date to suggest that different dietary requirements are needed for male and female athletes or for female athletes of reproductive versus nonreproductive age. However, considering the physical and hormonal differences between males and females, and across female life-stages, it is wise to assume a more cautious approach when applying any dietary regime in females that results in extreme energy and/or macronutrient manipulations. It is also prudent to apply close monitoring to assure that outcomes are beneficial for both sports performance and health.

9.3.1 How to apply low-carbohydrate diets for athletes

Nutrition for the athlete should always be tailored to their overall goals in the short and longer term, whether it be performance, body composition, health, or a combination of these. Elements to consider with a dietary prescription include the timing of the competition or event, the physiology of the athlete, fuel requirements of the sport and current training volumes, lifestyle preferences, and metabolic health (level of carbohydrate tolerance).

The purpose of the training phase is to integrate the training stimuli and the nutrition strategies to facilitate muscle mitochondrial and other system adaptations. During this period, fuelling strategies should be periodised, based on training demands of varying intensities and durations, body composition goals should be targeted, and competition strategies should be practised. Irrespective of the protocols, the dietary foundations of the training phase should be prioritised, including ensuring sufficient micronutrients and fibre, and consolidating food and meal planning and preparation habits. The purpose of the competition phase is to execute the event strategy, both from an exercise and nutrition perspective, that has been planned in the lead-up training phase.

9.3.2 The training diet

9.3.2.1 *Prescribing nutrition for the endurance athlete*

1. Decide on the pathway to fat-adaptation

   that is, rapid fat-adaptation (KD) or gradual time to fat-adaptation (LCHF) and a suitable time frame for this. The initial fat adaptation phase should take place in the training season, where competition is months away, to allow time for individual adjustments and optimal adaptation without compromising competition performance.

   a. For the endurance athlete, while there is no consensus on the exact time for complete fat adaptation, allow for at least 12 weeks.
   b. For the strength athlete, shorter fat adaptation timeframes (>2 weeks) could be useful to achieve body composition goals, without compromising performance.

2. Training reduction

   Due to potential reductions, or perceptions of reductions in exercise capacity while the metabolic adaptations of switching substrates (from carbohydrate to fat) are taking place, exercise intensity and duration of training should be decreased for the first 1–3 weeks.

3. Set macronutrient targets

   Carbohydrate

   a. For a KD, total carbohydrate $<10\%$ total energy (TE) or <50 g total carbohydrate (<30 g net or glycaemic carbohydrate).
   b. For LCHF, total carbohydrate $<25\%$ TE or (<130 g per day).
   Note: total carbohydrate includes fibre; net or glycaemic carbohydrate excludes fibre.

   Protein

   a. For endurance athletes, aim for approximately 1.4–2 g of protein per kilogram of ideal body weight per day [78]. For strength athletes, protein requirements should be adjusted up if dieting or actively attempting to lose weight or body fat for competition. Research suggests a range up to 2.5 g protein per kilogram of bodyweight per day to preserve muscle when dieting [79].

   Fat

   a. Remaining calories.
   b. For LCHF, aim for $\geq 50\%$ of total energy.
   c. For KD, aim for $\geq 75\%$ of total energy. As ketogenic adaptation is not reliant on thresholds for fat, but rather limiting carbohydrates, the fat recommendation may vary between individuals.

4. Supplementation

   The following supplements can be considered under certain contexts.

   a. Medium Chain Triglycerides (MCT) can be used to enhance ketonaemia and ketogenesis, while ketone salts or esters can increase ketonaemia and potentially improve fuelling without increasing endogenous ketone production. Thus nutritional ketosis can be obtained with lower levels of dietary fat and higher levels of dietary carbohydrate with supplementation [80].
   b. Multivitamin/mineral preparations could be considered in certain contexts to prevent or correct any chronic subthreshold micronutrient deficiencies. For example, (1) for athletes with a restricted overall energy intake (i.e., for body composition goals or other reasons); (2) in travelling situations to countries with an uncertain supply of usual or familiar foods; (3) to correct any diagnosed deficiency state.
   c. Protein powders could be necessary for vegetarian or vegan athletes and for any other athlete for convenience. Whole food from high-quality sources and reputable brands are recommended.

5. Energy (calories)

   Total energy intake will need to be carefully considered in athletes who have strict body composition goals. The appropriate level of energy reduction needs to be considered in the context of minimising the risk of low energy availability, driven by undereating and/or overtraining, especially in, but not limited to, female athletes. Reductions in total energy intake during the fat-adaptation period may also be associated with "keto flu" symptoms [81]. For strength athletes aiming to gain lean mass, an energy surplus is recommended. In this case, an LCHF rather than KDs may be preferred due to the specific goal of facilitating insulin-driven amino acid uptake into muscle.

6. Look out for and address any problems commonly associated with fat-adaptation (see Table 9.4).

TABLE 9.4 A guide to trouble-shooting fat-adaptation.

First phase of fat-adaptation (3–4 days)
Cautions: Ketu-flu: Light-headedness, headache, irritability, lack of concentration, dizziness, feeling "off".
Solutions: Keep well hydrated; consume sufficient additional sodium (i.e., 1–2 grams per day; ½-1 tsp salt); consume sufficient food sources of potassium (i.e., leafy greens, avocado, mushrooms, salmon, meat); ensure energy intake is sufficient (i.e., not in a substantial deficit).
First phase of fat-adaptation (first 1–3 weeks).
Cautions: Possible reductions in exercise capacity/increased perceptions of effort.
Solutions: Reduce exercise intensity and duration during this time.
First phase of fat-adaptation (hydration).
Cautions: Possible increased thirst at the start of endurance exercise due to normal plasma volume expansion [83].
Solutions: Consume 1–2 cups (250–500 mL) water prior to exercise.
Micronutrient deficiencies
Cautions: Micronutrients might be compromised under the following circumstances:
1. Low energy diet
2. Regular intermittent fasting
3. Vegetarian/vegan diet
4. Food allergies/intolerances without suitable nutrient-rich food alternatives
5. KD

Solutions: Consume a well-formulated LCHF or KD diet, that is, sufficient good quality meats, fish, poultry, eggs, full-fat dairy or alternatives, nuts and seeds, and plenty of vegetables with a range of different colours (nonstarchy focus for KD). Consult with a Registered Dietitian or nutrition professional specialising in sports nutrition to assess whether supplementation is required.
Muscle cramps
Cautions: cramps during, after exercise, or at night, could be signs that your body is low in magnesium.
Solution: Take a magnesium supplement (400 mg of elemental magnesium; select the most bioavailable preparation, that is, magnesium glycinate, citrate or malate).
Bowel habits
Cautions: You may experience a change in bowel habits in the early stages of fat adaptation. This should resolve after a short period of time; if not, seek help from a nutrition professional specialising in low-carb nutrition and with gut health expertise.
Solutions: For constipation: Increase or restrict fibre, water, and fat intake. If unchanged, supplement with magnesium. For diarrhoea, remove aggravating foods and assess.
Other side effects (e.g., hair loss/menstrual dysfunction/altered sleep/mental health disturbances/body rash/heat rate irregularities).
Cautions: These are unlikely to be part of your experience; however, some people can be more sensitive to extreme dietary changes than others, especially females.
Solutions: Gradually increase the total carbohydrate content of your diet (add good quality whole food sources) and/or total energy, ensure optimal hydration, and assess symptoms. It is recommended that you seek help from a nutrition professional specialising in low carbohydrate nutrition, and a supportive medical professional.

7. Monitoring
   a. Macronutrients and energy. This practice is highly recommended, particularly for serious/elite athletes. Use a smartphone app that provides a tally for each macronutrient. This allows for easy application and establishes good food composition knowledge.
   b. General well-being. It is also highly recommended to regularly monitor how the athlete feels overall. If any untoward side effects are experienced, such as hair loss, sleep irregularities, anxiety, heart rate irregularities, or menstrual dysfunction, it is recommended to apply a less extreme dietary manipulation (i.e., not too low in carbohydrate or total energy) and to seek help.
8. Nutritional ketosis
   a. Symptoms: In the first few days (days 3–5) athletes might experience a reduction in overall well-being (termed "keto flu"); this typically includes symptoms such as light-headedness, headache, irritability, lack of concentration, and dizziness [82,83]. This is likely a result of the initial renal response to carbohydrate-restriction, that is, a reduction in insulin causing sodium, potassium, and water excretion [84].
   b. Measurement: Measure ketones to establish level of ketosis. For consistency, ketones should be measured fasted in the morning upon rising.
      i. Urine ketones (acetoacetate) can be measured with urine test strips, which change colour with higher levels of urine ketones. However, this may not be a very accurate measure of mild ketosis, and the presence of urinary ketones may diminish over time as fat adaptation occurs [85].
      ii. Blood ketones (beta hydroxybutyrate—BOHB) can be measured with a ketone metre. Values ≥ 0.5 mmol/L (3 mg/dL) indicate mild ketosis; and between 1 and 4 mmol/l (6–23 mg/dL) indicate deep ketosis.

iii. Breath ketones (acetone) can be measured using a breath metre/analyser; there are many already on the market with more being added, regularly.

Note: The science around nutritional ketosis in athletes is still emerging. There is no consensus on which is the optimal diagnostic device to use to measure ketones; however blood ketones are the most frequently reported in the athlete literature. Variations in ketone readings are shown across the time course of a day and after different exercise durations and intensities, the meaning of which has yet to be established.

9. Micronutrients

Ensure a range of nutrient-dense foods are selected to ensure a good dietary foundation of micronutrients and fibre.

a. Nutrient-dense protein-based foods: Select high quality meats, fish, poultry, eggs, organ meats, full fat dairy produce, nuts, seeds, and if vegetarian or vegan, minimally processed soya-based foods (tofu, tempeh). Avoid foods with commercially made batters or marinades.

b. Nutrient-dense carbohydrate-based foods: Select vegetables with a wide range of colours (plenty of non- or low- starch vegetables, some higher-starchy varieties, some fruit (low sugar ones preferred, i.e., berries), full cream dairy produce. Avoid commercial grains (unless they are bespoke low-carbohydrate products). Note: A broader selection of foods can be consumed with LCHF (i.e., some higher-starch vegetables and fruit than for KDs due to the moderate level of carbohydrate restriction). Entering foods into a food tracking app will allow for immediate feedback and help guide food selection in relation to carbohydrate thresholds. To preserve gut health, include fermented food and beverages and natural foods containing natural prebiotics and probiotics (yoghurt, water and milk kefir, kimchi, and fermented vegetables).

c. Nutrient-dense fat-based foods: To obtain an optimal balance of essential fats, omega 3 and 6, focus on increasing omega 3 fats from food (fatty fish, eggs, hemp, walnuts, and chia seeds) and avoid processed seed oils that provide high amounts of omega 6 fats (soybean, sunflower, canola, safflower, rice bran oil, and margarine). Choose other oils or foods rich in monounsaturated fat and saturated fat (olive, avocado, coconut, hemp oil, nut, lard, butter, and full-fat dairy produce).

Note: Concern has been raised of the micronutrient status of individuals eating an LCHF or KDs on a chronic basis. There are no athlete-specific daily micronutrient recommendations, apart from iron for endurance athletes, but considering the physical demands of athletes, one could only speculate that their needs would be greater than those of the nonathletic population. A hypothetical case study reported that a well-formulated LCHF diet for moderately active adults could exceed nutrient requirements for all micronutrients apart from iron (which was marginally below the recommended intake) and dietary fibre [86]. *To date, only one study has been conducted on micronutrient status in athletes. McSwiney* et al. *reported several nutrients below the national threshold for daily requirements in male endurance athletes consuming KDs for 12 weeks, including iron, zinc, copper, manganese, folic acid and Vitamin C.* [87]. *Despite subthreshold intakes of iron, serum ferritin levels were reported as uncompromised. The question of whether other subthreshold nutrient values translate into compromised nutrient stores or future deficiencies remains unanswered.*

For athletes with a restricted overall energy intake (i.e., body composition goals or other reasons), subthreshold intakes of some nutrients could be expected for LCHF, KD, or any other dietary approach; in this case, a general multivitamin/mineral supplement could be considered. Further investigation into both the development of athlete-specific micronutrient recommendations, and the assessment of dietary and micronutrient adequacy in athletes undertaking an LCHF or KD diet is warranted.

10. Fluid requirements

These do not differ substantially across different dietary approaches, with the emphasis being on the establishment of individualised drinking plans. In general, guidelines are to begin exercise in an euhydrated state and to drink according to the dictates of thirst during exercise. This will prevent the dual risk of drinking either too little or too much [88] during exercise. Athletes are advised to utilise practical measurement strategies (i.e., body weight differences before and after exercise; sweat rates) to determine optimal fluid consumption strategies to complement this "drink to thirst" advice. In the case of the LCHF or KD approach, consuming water and/or other beverages that are low in total carbohydrate is recommended.

During the first 1–4 days of beginning KDs (and possibly other low-carbohydrate diets), reduced insulin levels can result in increased urinary sodium, potassium, and water losses; it is therefore prudent to increase water intake along with electrolytes (below) by approximately 500–1000 mL per day over habitual intakes [84,89–91].

11. Electrolytes

Sodium (i.e., salt) requirements are increased during the first 2 weeks of starting the LCHF or KD, with some individuals requiring the continuation of this level of sodium intake for a longer duration. An amount between 1 and 3 teaspoons of salt should be consumed (in food/beverages) per day; with more required if symptoms of light-headedness or dizziness persist. During exercise, additional sodium should be consumed when large sweat losses occur. Some athletes might need a potassium or magnesium supplement (in the case of cramping) if dietary sources do not adequately cover their needs [83].

Note: Fluid and electrolyte requirements during training and competition will likely be greater for the endurance athlete compared with the strength athlete.

It is advisable that if an athlete wishes to adopt an LCHF or KD, he or she should seek the expertise of an experienced nutrition professional (Registered Dietitian, nutritionist or other health professional that has undergone training in this area).

9.3.2.1.1 Adjusting nutrition for the endurance athlete

After an initial period of consistently consuming an LCHF or KDs to achieve fat adaptation, more or less carbohydrate can be introduced based on the phase or type of training the athlete is undertaking. This can be adjusted to meet the changing demands of the athlete. There is no peer-reviewed evidence addressing optimal carbohydrate periodisation strategies, but rather this is based on the findings from the consistent clinical experience of practitioners who regularly apply LCHF and KD nutrition interventions with endurance athletes [92].

9.3.2.1.2 When to consider *increasing* carbohydrate

1. If after the initial fat adaptation phase, with increased volumes of glycolytic activity (i.e., added sessions of conditioning-style workouts), especially if the athlete is unable to achieve optimal performance.
2. If sleep quality decreases, menstrual irregularities appear, anxiety levels increase or unwanted symptoms appear (e.g., hair loss, keto-rash). Note: This may be more prevalent in females purely due to a higher hormonal sensitivity than males to sudden changes in diet or overall energy availability.
3. If the athlete prefers (and is more adherent to) dietary strategies with a greater carbohydrate intake.
4. If the athlete is consistently undereating
5. Specific to the strength athlete:
   a. when trying to gain large amounts of mass or muscle
6. Specific to the endurance athlete:
   a. during longer sessions that include >60 min of higher intensity glycolytic work (i.e., intervals, hill climbs, sprints).
   b. during competition periods
   c. If not gaining muscle during a hypertrophy phase of training (assuming sufficient protein and energy intake)

In any of the above conditions, small amounts of carbohydrate (i.e., 10–20 g increments from whole food sources) are to be titrated into the athlete's diet at a suitable time (often before or after exercise sessions) until the desired effect is achieved (i.e., top-end performance is improved, symptoms or side-effects disappear).

9.3.2.1.3 When to consider *reducing* carbohydrate

1. During the initial fat-adaptation phase
2. If the athlete is consistently overeating (also consider if protein intake is adequate)
3. If excess and unwanted body fat needs reducing, or overall body mass need reducing
4. If the volume of total activity and especially highly glycolytic activity is decreasing
5. If the athlete does not like or adhere well to higher-carbohydrate intakes
6. If a lower carbohydrate approach is preferred for the management of coexisting metabolic (i.e., type 1 or 2 diabetes) or neurological conditions.
7. Specific for the strength athlete:
   a. When losing body fat or "cutting" for competition

9.3.3 The competition diet

As with the training diet protocols, there is no direct peer-reviewed evidence for optimal competition nutrition strategies, but rather protocols are derived from the experience of LCHF/KDs successful athletes and experienced practitioners.

1. For the endurance athlete:
   a. Consider including carbohydrate supplementation during events and pre-event training
   b. Titrate dose of carbohydrate to gut tolerance and to perceived performance benefit starting at ~15 g carbohydrate per hour

c. Type of supplementation: Pre-event carbohydrate supplement should ideally be in the form of whole food wherever possible. During events, select sources based on convenience, taste and texture preference.
d. High molecular weight starch products (known as super-starch) can be used for athletes who wish to decrease the digestion and absorption rate of carbohydrate during exercise.
e. Note: There may be times when refined sugar sources, that is, regular consumption of sports drink and/or gels throughout an event is required. While such practise is not recommended for optimal health, it might be necessary in the context of achieving optimal performance (e.g., during an event), particularly for elite and highly competitive athletes.
f. Fluid replacement during competition will be guided by strategies identified during training. Goals include preventing excessive dehydration ($>2\%$ BW loss from water deficit) and excessive changes in electrolyte balance, to avoid compromised exercise performance [93]. Overconsuming fluid is discouraged to prevent hyponatraemia [94].

2. For the strength athlete:
   a. There is little requirement for carbohydrate during strength events (such as in powerlifting, all-round, and Olympic weightlifting); carbohydrate should therefore be consumed at a level appropriate to the athlete's health conditions, comfort, behavioural tendencies, and psychosocial milieu.
   b. Pre-event carbohydrate intake should be consistent with the athlete's overall plan and should include whole, unrefined carbohydrate foods.
   c. If cutting weight for competition, attention should be paid to water repletion after the weigh-in and then the athlete should eat unrefined foods ad libitum for comfort and satiety.
   d. Where extreme fat and water cutting is carried out, and the athlete is not highly fat-adapted, supplementation with fast digesting carbohydrate in addition to water and electrolytes should be considered on a case-by-case basis.
   e. During competition, food should be eaten ad libitum and according to the athlete's overall plan.
   f. Hydration is a key concern as in indoor events, insidious water loss can be appreciable. Athletes should aim for ~500–1000 mL of water per hour of events with 500–1000 mg of sodium per litre.

9.3.4 The recreational athlete

The foundation dietary principles of LCHF or KDs are applicable across the athlete spectrum. In general, recreational athletes tend to have a lower training volume, and LCHF and KDs are typically able to be used without extensive modifications. Recreational athletes may require less dietary stringency than the more serious, elite athlete as there is less at stake. As such, the level of adherence to and the acceptability of the diet are primary considerations.

Table 9.5 is a summary of carbohydrate requirements for the mainstream and LCHF and KD approaches for training and competition.

9.3.5 Conclusion

For athletes to be appropriately lean for their sport, high performing and healthy, they need to be metabolically flexible, that is, able to utilise carbohydrate and fat as fuel interchangeably with ease and efficiency. Research has progressed over the last 40 years and led us to a more comprehensive understanding of the area of fat-adaptation and metabolic flexibility in athletes. There is clear evidence that both acute and chronic adaptation to an LCHF or KDs creates substantial cellular changes in favour of enhanced fat oxidation during exercise, that has likely occurred to its maximum capacity by 3–4 weeks.

However, there are still several unknowns and gaps in the literature about how to get the best of LCHF or KD applications for optimal performance. To enhance our understanding of this field, we need further research on carbohydrate periodisation and performance outcomes, and the differences between males and females, the impact of such diets on the microbiome and the immune system, the independent impact of ketone utilisation by the muscle, and the real-world meaning of a reduction in exercise economy as seen in some studies. The most provocative unknown is the extreme variability in responsiveness between athletes on the LCHF or KD diet. Based on the scientific evidence that we have to date, there is insufficient evidence to conclusively recommend LCHF or KDs over high carbohydrate diets for endurance athletes *based on performance outcomes alone*. What is important to consider is that in the context of no impairment in performance outcomes, athletes can assess whether any further benefit in metabolic health and wellness, and body composition benefits they might experience on an LCHF or KD, make it a viable option.

TABLE 9.5 Carbohydrate requirements for training and competition.

	Conventional nutrition guidelines (training and competition)	LCHF/KD guidelines (training)	LCHF/KD guidelines (competition)
General training recommendations	5–12 g carbohydrate/ kg body weight	LCHF: <130 g/day Keto: <50 g total carbohydrate (or 20–30 net carbohydrate)	
Prior to exercise	1–4 g carbohydrate /kg body weight: 1–4 h before	Highly individualised Nothing (fasted training) to a little or portion of your daily LCHF or KD carbohydrate allowance. Amount based on sport and periodised to programme and acceptability. Never a lot.	Highly individualised Small amounts based on comfort and acceptability, possibly more than training, especially in endurance events. Never a lot. All strategies and foods consumed practised in training sessions.
During exercise			
<45 m	None	None	None
45–75 m	Small amounts (carbohydrate mouth rinse)	None	Small amounts
1–2.5 h	30–60 g/h	None	15–60 g/h
>2.5 h	Up to 90 g/h	None or a little (15–30 g)	15–90 g/h
Recovery	1–1.2 g/kg body weight	Small amounts based on sport and periodised to programme and acceptability. Never a lot.	Small amounts based on comfort and acceptability. More leeway for greater amounts in LCHF than KD.

9.4 Evidence that the oxidation of liver- (or gut-) derived glucose, but not muscle glycogen, is obligatory for sustained exercise performance in humans

Timothy David Noakes

9.4.1 Introduction

By allowing the direct measurement of muscle and liver glycogen content for the first time, the introduction of the needle muscle (and liver) biopsy technique after 1967 [95] revolutionised the sports and nutrition sciences.

Early studies found that a high-carbohydrate diet prior to exercise increased muscle glycogen content, allowing exercise at 75% VO_{2max} to be sustained for substantially longer than when a low-carbohydrate diet was eaten [96] (Fig. 9.2). A subsequent study reported that a pre-exercise high-carbohydrate diet allowed some to finish a 30 km running race up to 15 min faster [97] than when they ate their normal diet.

The conclusion was that muscle glycogen provides the obligatory source of energy during exercise. This became known as the Anaplerotic Theory (TAT) [98–100].

But TAT is not supported by the evidence [2]:

9.4.1.1 TAT is biologically implausible and has been disproven by 5 different studies

TAT predicts that muscle ATP concentrations reach very low levels at exhaustion, especially during prolonged exercise. But four published studies have disproved this [101–104]. Another study [43] found that a high-fat diet homeostatically

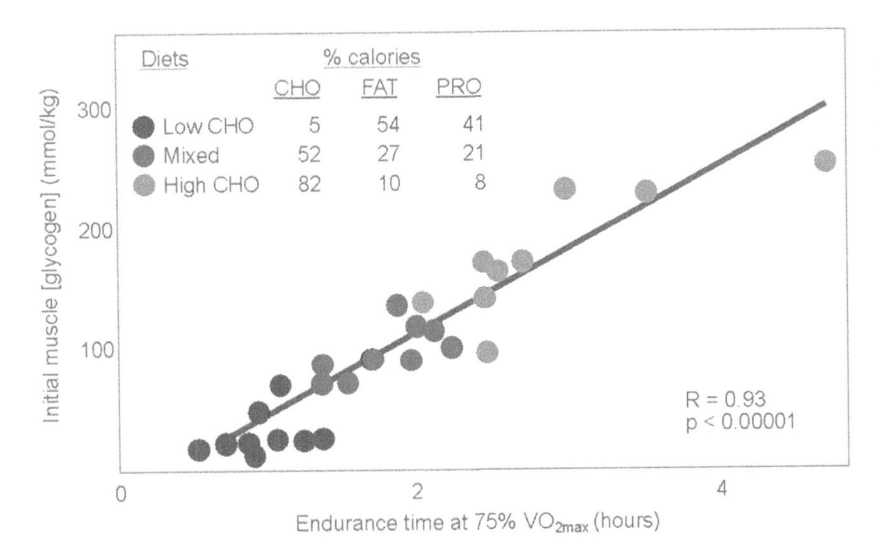

FIGURE 9.2 A linear (associational) relationship between initial muscle glycogen concentrations and endurance time at 75%VO_{2max}. *Redrawn using data from Bergström, J.; Hermansen, L.; Hultman, E.; Saltin, B. Diet, muscle glycogen and physical performance. Acta Physiol Scand. 1967, 71, 140–150.*

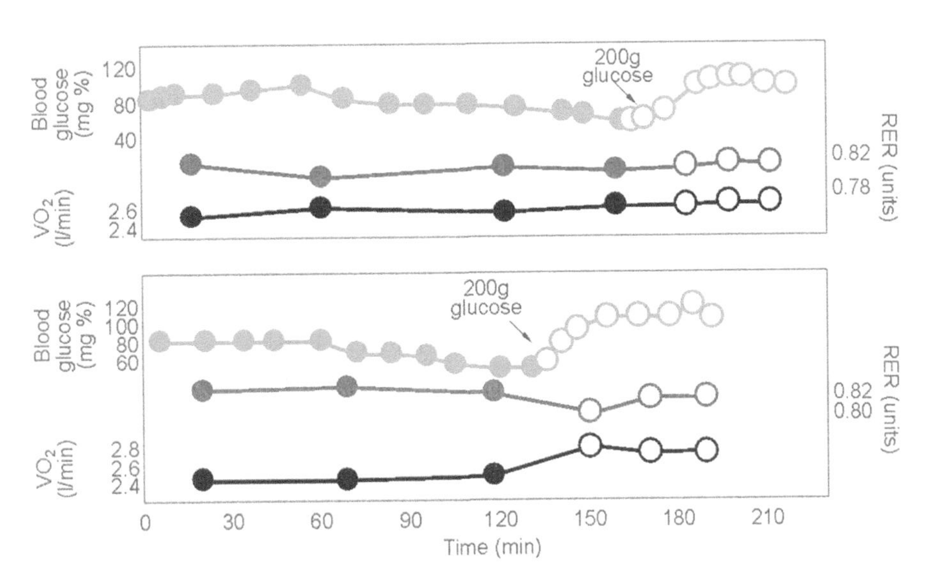

FIGURE 9.3 Changes in blood glucose concentrations, oxygen consumption (VO_2) and respiratory exchange ratio in two athletes during prolonged exercise before and after they ingested 200 g glucose (arrows). *Redrawn from [107] Christensen, E.H., and Hansen, O. Hypoglykame, arbeitsfähigkeit und ermudung. Skand Arch Physiol 1939, 81, 172–179.*

reduces skeletal muscle pyruvate dehydrogenase (PDH) activity during submaximal exercise without altering exercise performance [2].

Muscle ATP depletion must produce skeletal muscle rigour [105], not fatigue [2,17]. No case of exercise-induced muscle rigour has ever been reported in the scientific literature, ultimately disproving TAT.

9.4.1.2 Carbohydrate ingestion acutely reverses fatigue associated with exercise-induced hypoglycaemia. This effect cannot be due to the immediate reversal of muscle glycogen depletion

In 1939 Christiansen and Hansen [106] showed that subjects eating a low-carbohydrate diet developed EIH and terminated submaximal exercise prematurely. A second study [107] showed that glucose ingestion at the point of fatigue, rapidly reversed both (Fig. 9.3).

An exquisite series of modern studies [108–111] have extended these findings (Fig. 9.4)

Crucially, carbohydrate ingestion increased endurance by preventing the development of EIH (arrow 1), not by influencing muscle glycogen use (arrows 2 and 3) (Fig. 9.4.).

In a subsequent study the authors concluded [111]:

Interestingly, the extent to which fatigue was delayed in the present study (i.e., by 30–60 min) by carbohydrate ingestion late in exercise is similar to that observed in previous studies in which carbohydrate was ingested throughout the duration of exercise bout. This suggests that ***there may be no practical benefit to be gained by the ingestion of carbohydrate supplements***

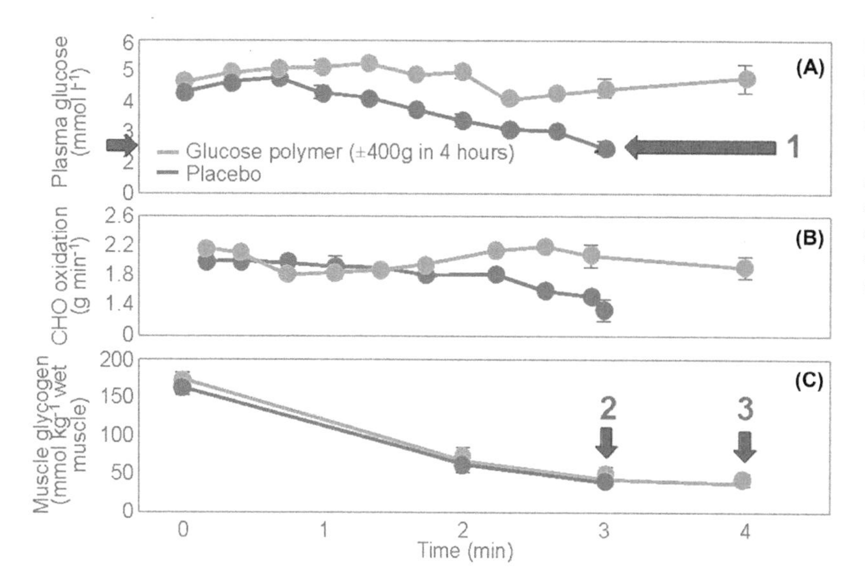

FIGURE 9.4 Changes in plasma glucose and muscle glycogen concentrations, and rates of carbohydrate (CHO) oxidation during prolonged exercise in athletes when they ingested either 100 g glucose/h or placebo during exercise. Athletes did not eat for 12 h before exercise. *Reproduced from [109] Coyle, E.F.; Coggan, A.R. Muscle glycogen utilization during prolonged strenuous exercise when fed carbohydrate. J Appl Physiol 1986, 61, 165–172.*

> ***throughout exercise***. *Rather, what appears to be critical is the ability of such carbohydrate supplements to supply glucose into the blood at sufficiently high rates late in exercise* ***to prevent a decline in the plasma glucose concentration and R [respiratory exchange ratio]*** *(emphasis added).*

Within a short time, however, these authors became certain that their main conclusion was incorrect. Instead, they began to promote the dictum that when muscle glycogen depletion occurs during exercise, high rates of carbohydrate ingestion are essential to maintain optimum rates of muscle carbohydrate oxidation. Accordingly, athletes were advised to ingest glucose at rates of 1.0 g/min [112] to 2.4 g/min [113] during more prolonged exercise. It is difficult to reconcile this 1992 advice [112] with the 1989 conclusion that high rates of carbohydrate ingestion during exercise "may be of no practical benefit" [111,114].

But ultimately the TAT-friendly interpretation became the established doctrine [109,115,116]:

> *lowering of blood glucose during the latter stages of prolonged strenuous exercise plays a major role in the development of [muscular] fatigue* ***by not allowing leg glucose uptake to increase sufficiently in order to offset reduced [muscle] glycogen availability*** *(added emphasis).*

Yet Coggan and Coyle nevertheless noted that "plasma glucose is the predominant carbohydrate energy source in the latter stages of prolonged exercise at ~70%VO_{2max}" [110] at the precise time when "the rate of [glucose] entry into the blood was unable to match its rate of removal" [110]. This is the perfect physiological recipe for the development of EIH [117–120].

9.4.1.3 In studies finding that carbohydrate improves exercise performance (in the carbohydrate-intervention group), EIH always develops in the nonintervention control group

A key finding, hidden for 55 years, was that subjects who followed the low- or mixed-carbohydrate diets in the original study (Fig. 9.2; [96]) developed a progressive EIH (Fig. 9.5).

Since EIH is a known cause of premature exercise termination (Figs. 9.3 and 9.4), these authors could not possibly conclude with absolute certainty that a difference in pre-exercise muscle glycogen concentrations was the exclusive cause of these variances in exercise performance (Fig. 9.2). Pre-exercise liver glycogen concentrations would also have varied, depending on the pre-exercise diet, being highest after the high-carbohydrate diet. Starting exercise with higher liver glycogen concentrations would delay the onset of EIH, increasing exercise performance unrelated to any dietary effect on muscle glycogen concentrations.

Coyle et al. [108] also observed that carbohydrate ingestion does not improve performance in those who maintain normal blood glucose concentrations when they exercise either with or without carbohydrate supplementation. Which should indicate that it is a falling blood glucose concentration [2], not muscle glycogen depletion, that impairs this type of exercise performance.

Indeed the evidence is highly suggestive that when pre-exercise carbohydrate loading or carbohydrate ingestion improved performance during prolonged exercise (>1.5 h), then the subjects in the control (noncarbohydrate comparison condition) will have developed a progressive EIH. Whereas carbohydrate loading before or carbohydrate ingestion

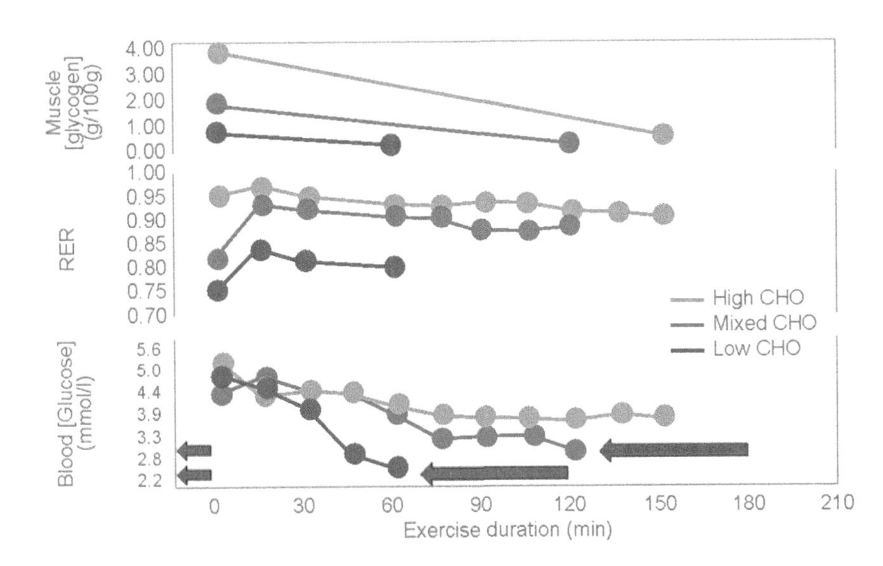

FIGURE 9.5 Changes in muscle glycogen concentrations, Respiratory Exchange Ratio (RER) and blood glucose concentrations during prolonged exercise in subjects who ate either high-, mixed- or low-carbohydrate diets before exercise. *Reproduced from [96] Bergström, J.; Hermansen, L.; Hultman, E.; Saltin, B. Diet, muscle glycogen and physical performance. Acta Physiol Scand. 1967, 71, 140–150.*

during exercise then prevented or reversed EIH in the carbohydrate intervention group. This is so clearly established by 40 studies [96,107–111,120–154] that it appears to be a biological certainty. In contrast, if blood glucose concentrations remain in the normal range in the control condition during more prolonged exercise then, with one exception [155], carbohydrate ingestion [156–162] or pre-exercise carbohydrate loading [163] or continuous glucose infusion producing hyperglycaemia [164] does not improve performance in the carbohydrate intervention group.

Carbohydrate ingestion (135 g) 4 h before exercise or continuous ingestion (approximately 40 g/h) prevented the development of EIH during 2 h of high effort exercise [165], showing that relatively little carbohydrate is required to prevent EIH. This is best explained if the main effect of the ingested carbohydrate is to preserve those "precious few grams of glucose" present in the human bloodstream [166].

During exercise of shorter duration and higher intensity (<1.5–2 h), carbohydrate ingestion can clearly improve performance [167] without the need to prevent EIH [168–179]. This is likely the result of a cerebral motor cortex reflex response to the presence of carbohydrate in the mouth [180].

Flynn et al. [156] explained why carbohydrate ingestion does not always enhance endurance performance: "when experienced cyclists elevate muscle glycogen stores, the dependence on exogenous sources of carbohydrate during 2 h of high intensity exercise is greatly reduced". Or: "From these studies it would appear that as long as muscle glycogen is available, carbohydrate feeding will not elicit a performance-enhancing effect" [160]. A more plausible explanation would be that the same high-carbohydrate pre-exercise diet that raises muscle glycogen concentrations also raises liver glycogen concentrations. This will delay the inevitable EIH that must develop during prolonged exercise in subjects who do not ingest any carbohydrate during exercise [166].

Not to be ignored is the evidence that EIH can develop during short duration exercise of high- intensity [181] and may impair exercise performance [182].

Another critical piece of information is that mice that overexpress the protein targeting to glycogen (PTG) specifically to the liver (PTG^{OE} mice) that increases liver glycogen content at rest, during exercise and in response to fasting, maintain higher blood glucose concentrations and have superior endurance without alterations in muscle glycogen use during prolonged exercise [183]. The authors conclude:

> *these results identify hepatic glycogen as a key regulator of endurance capacity in mice, an effect that may be exerted through the maintenance of blood glucose levels. Thus in endurance sports such as marathon running and long-distance cycling, increasing liver glycogen stores should maintain blood glucose and delay the onset of hypoglycaemia or "hitting the wall".*

9.4.1.4 Muscle glycogen use is not spared during exercise. Rather its use is determined almost exclusively by the starting muscle and liver glycogen concentrations

If the oxidation of carbohydrate (muscle glycogen early in exercise followed by blood glucose later in exercise) is obligatory for sustained exercise performance, then logically the body would attempt to spare especially muscle glycogen use immediately as exercise begins. Indeed scientists routinely advise athletes to train their bodies to burn fats and "spare glycogen" during exercise [184]. Yet attempts to develop nutritional interventions including pre-exercise carbohydrate-loading [185] or carbohydrate ingestion during exercise [109,120,128–130,133,143,151,152,186–191] to "spare" muscle glycogen use during exercise have proved largely fruitless (Fig. 9.4) except early in exercise [192] or when muscle glycogen concentrations fall below 70 mmol/kg wet weight during exercise lasting more than 2 h [193].

Even glucose infused intravenously at rates sufficient to produce profound hyperglycaemia and high rates of carbohydrate oxidation, fails to influence muscle glycogen use (Fig. 9.6) [194].

So the unresolved paradoxes remain: If glycogen is supposedly the one obligatory fuel for muscle metabolism, why are fasting [195] or intralipid and heparin infusions [181,196–198], the sole interventions that can "spare" muscle glycogen use during exercise (other than beginning exercise with low muscle glycogen concentrations)? If muscle glycogen provides the obligatory carbohydrate for oxidation during exercise, why is it not "spared" by exogenous glucose delivered at high rates either intravenously or via the gastrointestinal tract? Indeed, why is an "obligatory" fuel seemingly always burned in excess especially when present in abundance?

9.4.1.5 *In contrast, liver glycogenolysis and blood glucose oxidation may be subject to "sparing" during prolonged exercise*

Studies of changes in liver glycogen concentrations during exercise are limited by the invasive nature of the liver biopsy technique, specifically the risk of uncontrolled bleeding. But it requires no experimental evidence to "prove" that liver glycogen/blood glucose oxidation must be tightly regulated, especially during intense or prolonged exercise.

Brooks [166] describes the biological dilemma:

> *...relative to the meagre 4–5 g blood glucose pool size in a postabsorptive individual ... [exercise-induced] hypoglycemia would occur in less than a minute during hard exercise because blood glucose disposal rate (Rd) could easily exceed glucose production (Ra) from hepatic glycogenolysis and gluconeogenesis.*

Whereas higher starting muscle glycogen concentrations increase muscle glycogen use during exercise [185,199–208], carbohydrate ingestion or infusion during exercise spares the use of liver [117,144,151,152,189,209–213] but not muscle glycogen [109,120,128–130,133,143,151,152,186–191,194].

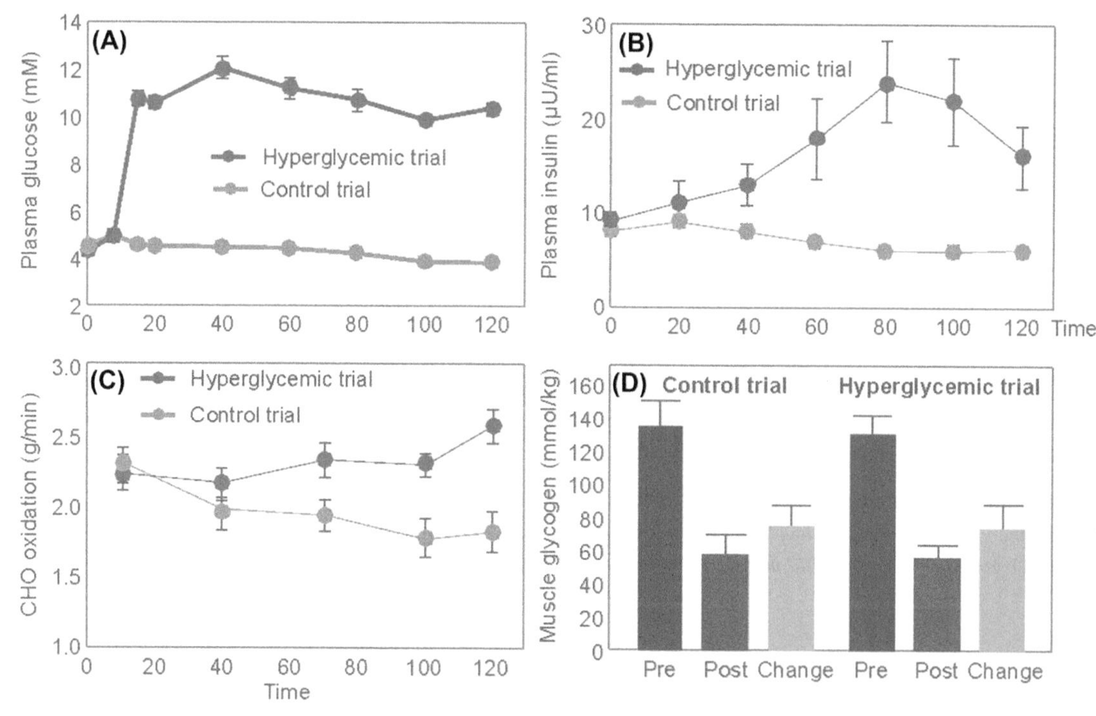

FIGURE 9.6 Glucose infused at rates sufficient to produce profound hyperglycaemia (panel A), increased plasma insulin concentrations (panel B), and which increased rates of carbohydrate (CHO) oxidation (panel C), failed to influence the rate of muscle glycogen use during prolonged exercise (panel D). *Reproduced from [194] Coyle, E.F.; Hamilton, M.T.; Alonso, J.G.; Montain, S.J.; Ivy, J.L. Carbohydrate metabolism during intense exercise when hyperglycemic. J Appl Physiol 1991, 70, 834–840.*

Paradoxically and yet to be explained, increasing circulating free fatty acid (FFA) (and glycerol) concentrations in rats had a much greater glycogen-sparing effect in the liver [196,197] than in skeletal muscle associated with a greater than twofold increase in blood glycerol concentrations for the final 2 h of a 3-h exercise bout [197]. Exercise time to exhaustion was increased by 1 h, associated with a delayed fall in blood glucose concentrations [197]. Heparin infusions that increased plasma FFA concentration in humans spared muscle glycogen use [198] also increased plasma glycerol concentrations more than 10-fold and elevated blood glucose concentrations during exercise.

Conversely, blood glucose oxidation during exercise is not altered by higher starting muscle glycogen concentrations [185,205]. Glucose infusion during exercise also inhibits hepatic glucose production in proportion to the elevation of the blood glucose concentration [211,212]. This effect may be caused by a direct inhibitory action of the elevated blood glucose concentration on hepatic glucose production [214] through allosteric regulation of glycogen phosphorylase activity [215]. Thus Hawley et al. [213] suggest that "glucose oxidation by skeletal muscle is precisely regulated by the prevailing plasma glucose concentration which, in turn, regulates hepatic glucose uptake and release".

Importantly, at very high rates of glucose infusion, approximately 40% of the infused glucose could not be accounted for by oxidative removal [213]. Therefore the fate of this excess glucose disappearance is currently unknown. The most likely fate is conversion to triglyceride in the liver [216,217].

The conclusion must be that the mechanism by which carbohydrate interventions improve athletic performance, cannot be by "sparing" muscle glycogen. This has been known since at least 1985 [190] but has been largely ignored. Rather carbohydrate interventions that enhance exercise performance, most likely act by delaying the onset of EIH (Figs. 9.3–9.5; [96,107–111,120–154], probably by reducing liver glycogen use [218] and perhaps by stimulating hepatic gluconeogenesis [196,197].

Liver glycogen concentrations in turn directly influence muscle lipid (and hence muscle glycogen) oxidation via a specific liver → brain → adipose tissue reflex that increases adipose tissue lipolysis [219,220] and, as a result, increases fat oxidation by muscle (Fig. 9.7), whenever liver glycogen content falls. A similar mechanism by which muscle glycogen content might regulate liver glycogen/blood glucose oxidation has, to this author's knowledge, not yet been described [166,221].

The functional importance of this liver → brain → adipose tissue reflex for the prevention of EIH has been established by Weltan et al. [204]. As they explain:

> *...glucose oxidation is not increased by reduced muscle glycogen content in subjects with similar blood glucose concentrations; instead, a switch takes place towards lipid oxidation even when plasma glucose concentrations are hyperglycemic. This strengthens the argument in our previous study [203] that this may be a teleological mechanism to compensate for a reduced availability of intramuscular carbohydrate without predisposing to hypoglycaemia.*

Indeed the finding that blood glucose oxidation is not increased by hyperglycaemia in those who begin exercise with low muscle glycogen concentrations [204] is perhaps the strongest currently available evidence disproving the dictum that there is an obligatory role for muscle carbohydrate oxidation during exercise.

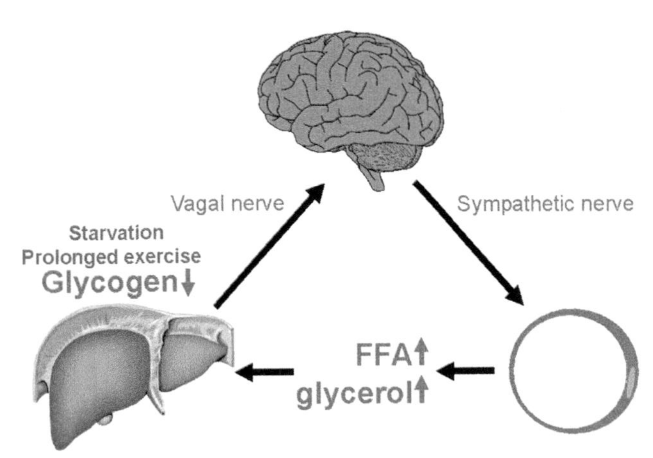

FIGURE 9.7 A liver → brain → adipose tissue reflex that increases adipose tissue lipolysis in response to falling liver glycogen concentrations has been described by Izumida et al. [219] and Yahagi [220]. Unrecognised until now is that whereas increasing blood free fatty acid (FFA) and glycerol concentrations spares muscle glycogen use during exercise [181,196–198], the effect on liver glycogen use and the prevention of EIH is, at least in rats, much greater [196,197]. The mechanism for this effect is currently unknown but could be the result of glycerol-induced stimulation of hepatic gluconeogenesis. *Redrawn from [220] Yahagi, N. Hepatic control of energy metabolism via the autonomic nervous system. J Atheroscler Thromb 2017, 24, 14–18.*

Instead, the metabolic response to prolonged exercise in humans appears to be designed to delay the onset of EIH for as long as possible; in part by increasing skeletal muscle fat oxidation to prevent excessive and uncontrolled blood glucose oxidation as liver glycogen content falls and perhaps by as yet to be described direct effects on liver glycogenolysis and gluconeogenesis. The following section explains why this is so important, especially during more prolonged exercise.

9.4.1.6 Whereas whole body carbohydrate oxidation reduces during prolonged exercise; blood glucose oxidation increases progressively, regardless of exercise intensity

The respiratory exchange ratio (RER) falls progressively during prolonged exercise (Fig. 9.5) indicating a gradual shift from carbohydrate to fat metabolism [210,222]. In contrast, blood glucose (as opposed to whole body carbohydrate) oxidation increases progressively [109,117,143,150,152,154,185,186,191–193,203–210,223,224]. This effect and its consequences are best illustrated by data from Hargreaves et al. [205] (Fig. 9.8).

Fig. 9.8 shows that blood glucose concentration (Panel A) begins to fall early in exercise after a low-carbohydrate (CHO) diet when starting liver glycogen concentrations will be low. Glucose Rd initially increases equally and progressively regardless of starting liver (and muscle) glycogen concentrations (Panel B) but reaches higher rates in the CHO-replete state (arrow 1 in Panel B). In contrast, glucose Ra (Panel C) in the CHO-depleted state lags glucose Rd in the CHO-replete state throughout exercise. The result is that whereas glucose Ra matches glucose Rd in the CHO-replete state (arrow 3 in Panel C; arrow 1 in Panel B), glucose Ra is substantially less than glucose Rd at the termination of exercise in the CHO-depleted state (arrow 4 in Panel C; arrow 2 in Panel B). This explains why EIH develops in the CHO-depleted state [117–120]. Note that glucose Rd is also higher in the carbohydrate-replete state (compare arrows 1 and 2 in Panel B) indicating a smaller contribution from fat oxidation in specific tissues.

Panel D shows that unlike blood glucose Rd (Panel C), which is clearly independent of starting liver glycogen concentrations, rates of muscle glycogen disappearance (use) are determined by starting muscle glycogen concentrations as repeatedly established [185,199–208].

The fact that blood glucose Rd increases progressively even when the exercise begins in a carbohydrate-depleted state, makes no immediate sense since it must lead to EIH [117–120,166,221] if carbohydrate is not ingested during exercise.

But this acceleration of blood glucose Rd makes perfect sense if it serves an obligatory role supporting an increasing need for glucose oxidation by the brain as brain glycogen concentrations begin to fall during prolonged exercise [226,227].

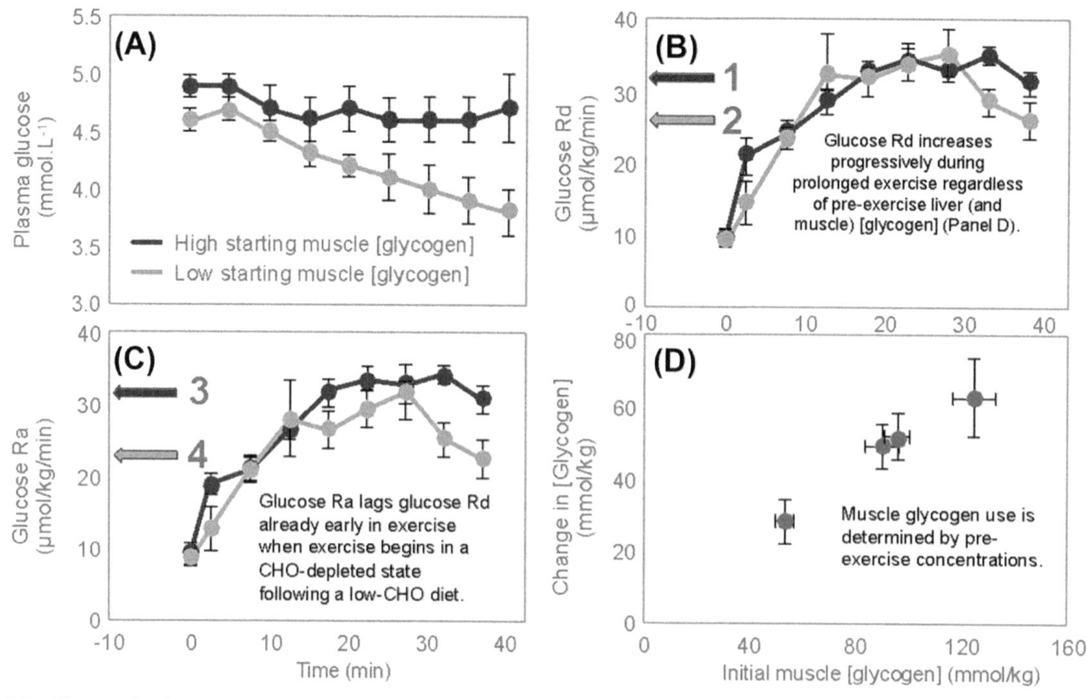

FIGURE 9.8 Changes in plasma glucose concentrations (Panel A), rates of glucose disappearance (Rd) (Panel B) and glucose appearance (Ra) (Panel C), and muscle glycogen use (Panel D) during exercise that began with either high or low muscle glycogen concentrations. Redrawn from [205]. Note that the maximum glucose Rd is 24 g/h (0.4 g/min) (for a 70 kg subject). Similar values were reported by Trimmer et al. [223]. Brain glucose Rd at rest is ~0.1 g/min [225].

Chronic adaptation to a low-carbohydrate diet reduces total carbohydrate oxidation during exercise by 55% with some reduction in glucose Rd [228]. This would provide additional protection against the development of EIH. Part of this effect might be due to the substitution of blood ketones [225,229] or lactate [166] or both, for this "obligatory" glucose use by the brain.

9.4.1.7 Blood glucose concentrations during exercise must be homeostatically regulated in part by a hypothalamus → motor cortex reflex that regulates the extent of skeletal muscle recruitment that it will allow

The Central Governor Model of Exercise [230] predicts that exercise performance is regulated "in anticipation" by a brain mechanism that protects the body from harm. Hypoglycaemic brain damage is one such major threat [231]. A model describing brain (hypothalamic) mechanisms for the homoeostatic regulation of blood glucose concentrations [232] under resting condition, does not include a mechanism to regulate the major source of blood glucose Rd during exercise – the extent of skeletal muscle recruitment.

Fig. 9.9 advances that model to include a hypothalamus → motor cortex reflex that would regulate the extent of skeletal muscle recruitment during exercise. Once the hypothalamus detects a falling blood glucose concentration, it

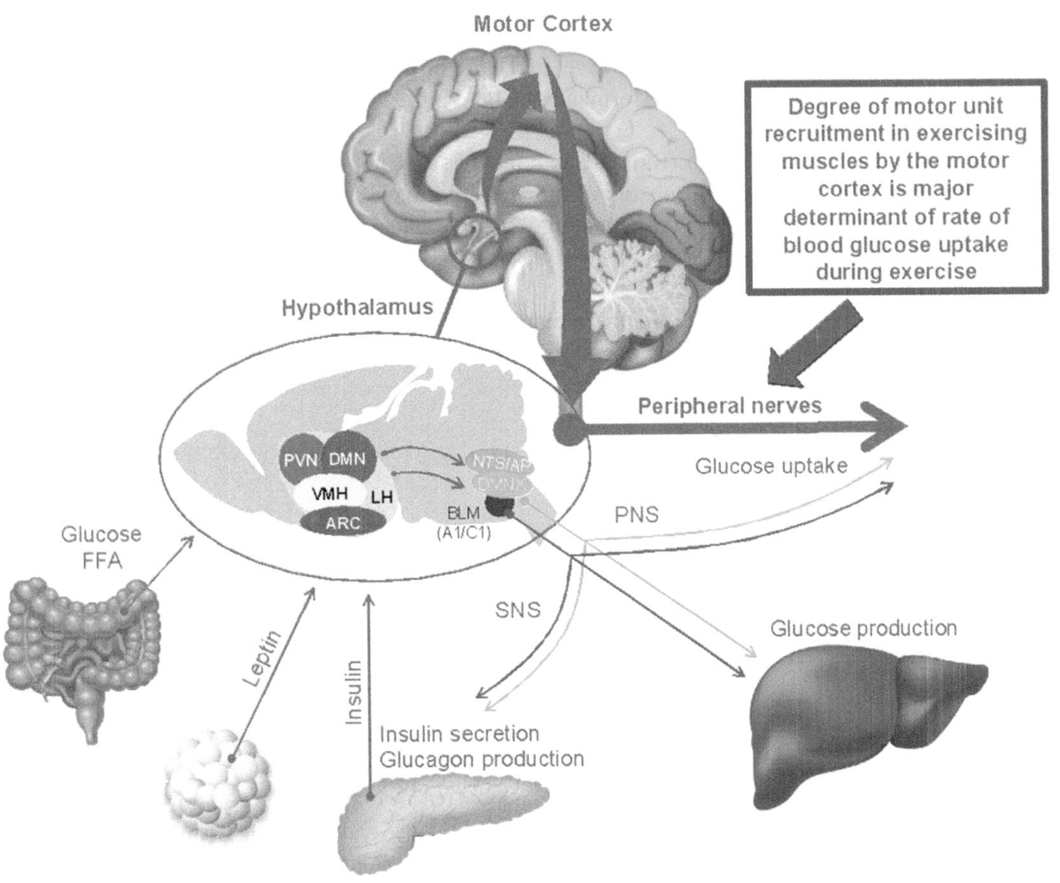

FIGURE 9.9 Specialised brain areas in the hypothalamus and brainstem (AP, area postrema; ARC, arcuate nucleus; BLM, basolateral medulla; DMN, dorsomedial nucleus; DMNX, dorsal motor nucleus of the vagus; LH, lateral hypothalamus; NTS, nucleus of the solitary tract; PNS, parasympathetic nervous system; PVN, paraventricular nucleus; SNS, sympathetic nervous system; VMH, ventromedial hypothalamus) sense peripheral metabolic signals through hormones and nutrients to regulate glucose metabolism. The autonomic nervous system contributes by modulating pancreatic insulin/glucagon secretion, hepatic glucose production, and skeletal muscle glucose uptake. Text adapted from reference [232]. Missing from this diagram is a necessary link between these hypothalamic and brain stem centres and the motor cortex specifically to prevent excessive skeletal muscle recruitment during prolonged exercise when liver glycogen depletion develops causing a progressive EIH. Without this added control, all forms of prolonged exercise would ultimately cause EIH [117–120,166,221] and hypoglycaemic brain damage [231]. Also missing is the effect of the blood glucose concentration in directly regulating hepatic glucose production [214,215]. *Redrawn from [232] Roh, E.; Song, D.K.; Kim, M.-S. Emerging role of the brain in the homeostatic regulation of energy and glucose metabolism. Exp Mol Med 2016, 48, e216. with additions.*

must reduce the central motor drive to the exercising muscles in order to protect itself from hypoglycaemic brain damage [231]. This would explain why exercise performance begins to fall progressively "in anticipation" as blood glucose concentrations drop during prolonged exercise [96,107–111,120–154] in those who do not ingest carbohydrate during exercise [2].

The studies of Nybo and colleagues [233,234] clearly establish that EIH impairs cerebral uptake of glucose and oxygen and impairs the ability of the motor cortex to activate skeletal muscle, exactly as predicted by this model.

9.4.2 Conclusion

There is no convincing evidence that muscle glycogen is an obligatory fuel for use during exercise [2]. It has been known since 1967 [96] (Fig. 9.2) that muscle glycogen use is increased if exercise begins with higher muscle glycogen concentrations. It's also been known from at least 1985 [190] that carbohydrate ingestion during exercise does not "spare" muscle glycogen use during exercise. Thus muscle glycogen "sparing" cannot explain how carbohydrate interventions enhance exercise performance.

Rather the evidence shows that blood glucose disappearance (Rd), mainly through oxidation, increases during exercise regardless of the state of carbohydrate stores in the liver or muscle. This suggests that blood glucose is serving an obligatory metabolic role during exercise. That obligatory carbohydrate role could be the provision of glucose (and lactate) to sustain brain metabolism. In the absence of a supply of ingested (exogenous) glucose during more prolonged exercise, the rate of liver glucose appearance (Ra) must inevitably become less than glucose Rd, leading to EIH [117–120,166,221]. The development of a progressive EIH will provoke an anticipatory brain-directed reduction in skeletal muscle recruitment causing exercise performance to fall (Fig. 9.9) and ultimately to terminate, specifically to prevent hypoglycaemic brain damage [231].

Thus the rate of liver glucose production (Ra) and its removal (Rd), not the rate of muscle glycogen oxidation, are likely to be the more important metabolic regulators of human performance during prolonged exercise. The rate of glucose Rd during prolonged exercise is not inconsequential, reaching values as high as 0.4 g/min (Fig. 9.8) [205,223] in athletes adapted to high-carbohydrate diets. But this can easily be matched by similar rates of carbohydrate ingestion during exercise in places of rates of 1.0–2.4 g/min [112,113] as currently prescribed.

Chronic adaptation to a low-carbohydrate, high-fat diet reduces total carbohydrate oxidation during exercise with some reduction in rates of glucose Rd during prolonged exercise [228], perhaps by increasing the "metabolic flexibility" of the brain, thereby allowing blood-borne ketones [225,229] and lactate [166] to substitute for this "obligatory" role of cerebral blood glucose oxidation during exercise.

Conventional exercise training has a similar effect [234–237] suggesting that this effect is likely to be fundamental to improving performance during prolonged exercise in humans.

9.5 Nutritional supplementation for athletic performance

Smith J
Webster C
Catherine Saenz

9.5.1 Introduction

Dietary supplements are defined as "a food, food component, nutrient, or nonfood compound that is purposefully ingested in addition to the habitually consumed diet with the aim of achieving a specific health and/or performance benefit" [238]. The commercial market is flooded with dietary supplements and their use by athletes is widespread, however only a handful of supplements are supported by consistent evidence and even this evidence has important limitations. For example, most studies test supplements in isolation or in combination with one or two other supplements, yet commercial products may contain many ingredients [239]. Women and elite athletes are generally underrepresented in supplement research and studies in keto-adapted athletes are virtually nonexistent. Additionally, the performance outcomes are often very specific and laboratory-based, which can limit their application to real performance scenarios. This is particularly the case when exercise *capacity* is tested using time to exhaustion trials at fixed workloads. *Performance* trials, where a fixed distance or workload must be completed in the fastest time, are more reflective of actual events but it can be difficult to detect small but meaningful changes in performance. While supplements can be a convenient way to meet unique nutrient requirements, athletes and clinicians should weigh the potential benefits against the added expense of supplements, the risk of other untested ingredients, the risk of accidental doping (if the supplement contains unknown or hidden banned substances) and the risk of becoming too reliant on supplements (potentially leading to other nutrient deficiencies).

With these caveats in mind, there are a few dietary supplements that have reasonably strong evidence to support a performance advantage for certain scenarios. These include macronutrients such carbohydrate and protein, as well as dietary supplements like creatine, caffeine, nitrate, sodium bicarbonate and beta alanine. Two additional supplements with equivocal evidence may also be attractive to keto-adapted athletes because they support nutritional ketosis, namely MCT and exogenous ketones. Table 9.6 summarises this body of research by describing these supplements and the dosing protocols used most often in studies. The physiological effects that may affect performance are described, as well as a summary of actual performance outcomes. It is important to note that almost all of these studies were conducted on athletes eating more traditional, moderate-to-high carbohydrate diet. Since keto-adapted athletes have different metabolic environments and nutrient needs than those eating a high carbohydrate diet, it is unclear whether they would benefit more, less, or the same from using these supplements or whether different dosing protocols are required. The final column discusses some of the theoretical implications of using these supplements in the context of keto-adaptation. In summary, the supplements in Table 9.6 may offer a potential, but untested, performance advantage for keto-adapted athletes. If they are to be used, athletes and their coaches would need to experiment with them out of competition, while monitoring performance, health, and potential side effects.

9.5.2 Medium chain triglycerides

Medium chain triglycerides (MCTs) have been relatively well researched for their potential to improve endurance performance in athletes habitually eating a conventional high-carbohydrate diet. The premise of MCTs as a supplement is that they would "spare" endogenous carbohydrate stores by stimulating fat oxidation. Ultimately, this research has failed to demonstrate a clear performance-enhancing or glycogen-sparing effect of acute MCT ingestion. Moderate doses of MCTs (25–30 g) are well tolerated and increase plasma ketone bodies but do not affect endogenous substrate metabolism [270]. Ingesting larger doses of pure MCTs (~86 g) is generally associated with a decrease in performance which was attributed to GI symptoms [246,271]. Coingesting MCTs with carbohydrate increases the proportion of ingested MCTs that are oxidised during exercise [272] but does not appear to reduce the severity of GI symptoms [271]. While one study showed a positive effect on endurance performance by adding a high dose of MCT to a carbohydrate supplement [271], most studies showed no effect [145,246,273] and one study showed a detrimental effect on ultra-endurance performance which was attributed to GI symptoms [145]. In a recent nonrandomised study in recreationally active individuals, exercise time to exhaustion was extended by daily supplementation with low doses of MCTs (6 g) with carbohydrate for 2 weeks, compared to carbohydrate alone [272]. However, this finding should be interpreted with caution until repeated in a randomised trial with trained individuals. The effect of MCT supplementation on performance, metabolism and GI symptoms has not been researched in athletes who are well adapted to an LCHF diet, however, it is generally accepted that MCTs are not a viable performance supplement for nonfat adapted athletes.

9.5.3 Exogenous ketones

Nutritional ketosis can also be achieved acutely without dietary carbohydrate restriction, via the ingestion of exogenous ketone supplements, such as ketone salts, ketone esters, or ketone precursors [274]. Because ketone bodies theoretically offer a more economical source of energy than carbohydrate and they can be readily oxidised by the brain for energy, ketone supplements have received considerable scientific interest over the past 5 years for their potential to improve exercise performance and recovery [249,275]. It is important to consider that the vast majority of studies have been conducted in athletes who were not habitually consuming a low carbohydrate diet, so their relevance for keto-adapted athletes is unclear. While ketone supplements are considered safe for human consumption [276], they have been associated with gastrointestinal (GI) symptoms that ranged from negligible or mild [277,278] to moderate [279] and even severe [280,281]. Overall, it appears as though exogenous ketones are unlikely to offer an exercise performance advantage with two studies showing a positive effect [277,282], two showing a negative effect [280,283] and nine showing no effect [279,281,284–290] of a ketone supplement compared to a control. Interestingly, the only study which included keto-adapted athletes found a positive effect of a ketone salt supplement on subsequent high intensity endurance performance [277], however the supplement also contained caffeine and amino acids, and there may have been a placebo effect as the participants were not blinded

TABLE 9.6 Summary of supplement recommendations with regards to the ketogenic athlete.

Supplement, reference and examples	Common/effective dosing protocols in studies	Metabolic effects related to performance	Performance effect	Potential implications for the keto-adapted athlete
Carbohydrate [62,240–245] Rapidly absorbed sugars and starches, for example, glucose, glucose polymers, fructose, sucrose, galactose. Supplement products often contain combinations that target different gut transport proteins (multiple transportable carbohydrates). Slow-release starch, for example, hydrothermally modified starch (HMS). Blunts glucose and insulin spikes and attenuates decline in fat oxidation, compared to rapidly absorbed carbohydrate.	*Fast release CHO:* 1–4 g/kg, 1–4 h before exercise plus 30–60 g/h during exercise lasting 1–2.5 h or 60–90 g/h of multiple transportable carbohydrates during exercise lasting > 2.5 h. *Slow release CHO:* ~1 g/kg BM ingested either as a single dose 30 min before exercise or as split doses (before and during exercise) OR Mouth rinsing with 6% carbohydrate solution during high intensity endurance exercise	Provides exogenous fuel during exercise, particularly for skeletal muscle and the brain. Maintains high rates of carbohydrate oxidation and prevents low plasma glucose concentrations (but suppresses fat oxidation). Reduces muscle glycogen use in some but not most studies. Stimulatory effect on the central nervous system. May cause GI distress at higher doses.	Improves endurance performance and capacity in events lasting more than 1 h. Improves capacity for high intensity intermittent-type exercise (~ team sports). Reduces perceived effort and decline in motor skills during intermittent exercise. Mouth rinse may slightly improve higher intensity endurance performance lasting 25–60 min.	No well controlled studies in keto-adapted athletes, however there are anecdotal reports of its use for endurance and ultra-endurance competition. Some of the potential ergogenic mechanisms listed here may be less applicable to keto-adapted athletes as they are less reliant on carbohydrate for energy production (i.e. fat adapted). Will likely reduce nutritional ketosis and fat oxidation during exercise.
MCT [145,246,247] Triglycerides with fatty acid chain length between 6 and 10 carbons (absorbed and oxidised more rapidly than long chain triglycerides)	30–86 g MCT ingested as single or split doses within 60 min before and/or during endurance exercise. Often co-ingested with ~60 g/h carbohydrate (e.g., glucose), which increases MCT absorption and oxidation rates.	Provides exogenous fuel for skeletal muscle. Results in acute nutritional ketosis (elevated plasma ketone bodies). Most (but not all) studies suggest that MCT ingestion does not reduce rates of carbohydrate oxidation nor muscle glycogen utilisation during exercise. May cause GI symptoms at higher doses, particularly if ingested alone.	MCT ingestion alone may have no effect or a possible negative effect on endurance performance compared to placebo or carbohydrate ingestion. In one study, MCT co-ingested with carbohydrate improved endurance performance compared to carbohydrate alone but most studies showed no performance effect of adding MCT to carbohydrate.	No studies in keto-adapted athletes. Compatible with nutritional ketosis and keto-adaption. Keto adapted athletes may tolerate MCTs better than mixed macronutrient diet athletes.
Protein [248] Good quality protein supplements should be rich in leucine and essential amino acids. Whey is the most common protein supplement in studies. Others include casein, milk, milk protein, soy protein, egg protein, or whole food (beef, yoghurt).	Supplements can be useful to increase daily protein intake to 1.6 g/kg BW/d (ergogenic effects are limited if habitual protein intake is above this) 20–44 g protein, ingested pre and/or post resistance exercise session. Additional smaller doses are sometimes consumed during the recovery period.	Enhances amino acid pool to increase muscle protein synthesis and anabolic signalling.	Acute effects after resistance exercise: • Improves recovery (muscle function), markers of repair and regrowth of lean tissue. • Reduces delayed onset muscle soreness. Chronic effects with training: • Increases lean mass (skeletal muscle, bone, and connective tissues). • Improves body composition and power to weight ratio. Increases maximal strength and endurance performance.	No studies investigating the effect of post exercise protein supplementation in keto-adapted athletes. High bolus of glucogenic amino acids and higher protein diets may reduce ability to sustain nutritional ketosis.

Exogenous ketones [37,249–251] Ketone esters (KE), for example, R-BD D-βHB monoester Ketone salts (KS), for example, KB + sodium, potassium, calcium, magnesium. Ketone precursors, for example, R,S-1,3-butanaediol (BD)	Either ingested in 1 dose 0–30 min before exercise or split doses before and during exercise. KE: 250 to 750 mg/kg BW. Increases blood D-βHB to 0.3–3.5 mM. KS: 300–380 mg/kg BW. Dose limited by high salt load. Increases blood D-βHB to 0.3–1 mM. BD: 2 × 350 mg/kg BW. Increases blood D-βHB to ~1 mM.	Results in acute nutritional ketosis lasting several hours (Note that this shares some properties with, but is a distinct metabolic state to, keto adaptation). Provide an alternative fuel for the brain, skeletal muscle and the heart. Influence a variety of cellular and gene signals. In some studies (but not all) they reduce rates of carbohydrate oxidation and muscle glycogenolysis and increase intramuscular triglyceride oxidation during exercise. Preliminary but inconclusive evidence that they reduce muscle protein degradation during fasting/starving and augment markers of protein synthesis after exercise. Inconclusive effect on post exercise muscle glycogen synthesis. Higher doses are associated with GI distress ranging from mild to severe.	Performance research is limited. Most studies show no effect of acute ingestion on endurance or high intensity performance, with only one study showing a positive effect (improved endurance performance with R-BD D-βHB monoester). R-BD D-βHB monoester may attenuate decline in cognitive function during high intensity exercise. Chronic use of a R-BD D-βHB monoester after high intensity exercise sessions may reduce symptoms of overreaching and improve training effect on performance.	No exogenous ketone specific studies in keto-adapted athletes. One study used a combination supplement of KS, caffeine and amino acids and found a positive effect on high intensity endurance performance, which was irrespective of keto-adaptation, but there may have been a placebo effect (not blinded) and the specific effect of the KS is difficult to interpret. Compatible with nutritional ketosis and keto-adaption.
Creatine [252,253] Creatine monohydrate.	Daily supplementation during a loading phase to "saturate" muscles with creatine, which may then be followed by a maintenance phase. Rapid loading: ~20 g/d split over 4 doses for 5–7 d. Slow loading: 3 g/d for 28 d. Maintenance: 3–10 g/d depending on athlete size. Ingestion with carbohydrate or carbohydrate and protein can aid in muscle creatine retention.	Increases the capacity of the phosphocreatine (PCr) system, allowing greater rates of ATP resynthesis during very high-intensity exercise. Helps maintain glycolytic flux in the mitochondria, which reduces markers of oxidative stress. Increases anaerobic threshold. Increases anabolic signalling after exercise. Reduces muscle damage and increases glycogen resynthesis after high intensity exercise. Increases BW and lean mass which may be advantageous or disadvantageous depending on event.	Increases performance in single and repeated bouts of high intensity exercise lasting <150 s with greatest benefit seen in bouts lasting <30 s. Enhances training effect on high intensity performance, muscle mass and maximal strength. Possibly protects against neurodegenerative complications related to traumatic head injuries. Inconclusive evidence suggests that supplementation may be particularly ergogenic for vegetarians who have less plasma and muscle creatine stores.	No studies in keto-adapted athletes.

(Continued)

TABLE 9.6 (Continued)

Supplement, reference and examples	Common/effective dosing protocols in studies	Metabolic effects related to performance	Performance effect	Potential implications for the keto-adapted athlete
Caffeine [254–259] Anhydrous caffeine in pill or powder form. Research using caffeinated foods and drinks is limited because less able to control dose.	The most common dose used in studies is 3–6 mg/kg BW, ingested either as a single dose 60–90 min pre-exercise, or split, with additional doses during exercise. Lower doses (2–3 mg/kg BW) are also common and appear to elicit most but not all ergogenic effects. Higher doses may be associated with negative side effects.	Adenosine receptor antagonist which stimulates CNS function. Stimulates catecholamine release. Enhances arousal, vigilance, and concentration. Decreases perception of pain, effort, and fatigue during exercise. Enhances skeletal muscle calcium dynamics and muscle contraction. Inhibits muscle glycogenolysis and increases fatty acid metabolism. Side effects may include nausea, anxiousness, insomnia, and restlessness.	Variable individual response that is at least partly genetic. Improves endurance performance (> 60 min) and sustained high intensity performance (1–60 min) in most but not all studies (cycling, running, rowing, swimming). May improve intermittent high-intensity exercise performance (e.g., individual and team sports) Equivocal effect on maximal strength and power events.	No specific research in keto-adapted athletes but the performance effect is unlikely to be affected by keto-adaption.
Sodium bicarbonate [257,260–262]	0.2–0.4 g/kg BW ingested as a single dose (or in multiple smaller doses over 60 min), 60–120 min prior to high intensity exercise. The time to achieve peak blood Bicarbonate ($HCO3^-$) concentrations has been inconsistent between studies and individuals, ranging from 60 to 180 min.	Raises blood HCO_3^- concentrations, which increases extracellular pH, creating a H^+ gradient and allowing greater efflux of H^+ from muscle cells. This increases the acid buffering capacity during high-intensity exercise. Influences multiple metabolic pathways and intermediates, which may also be ergogenic. Proposed to have a central ergogenic effect. May cause GI distress which could negate ergogenic effects. Coingestion with small amounts of carbohydrate or spreading ingestion over 60 min may minimise GI distress.	High individual and day to day variation with greater ergogenic effect seen with trained individuals. Likely improves single bout supramaximal (all out) performance (<4 min). Likely improves performance in intermittent very high intensity exercise e.g., repeated sprints (however studies with sport simulations failed to show a positive effect). Equivocal effect on performance in endurance events lasting > 4 min. Likely improves skill-based performance during fatiguing exercise.	No studies in keto-adapted athletes. Inconclusive whether keto-adaptation affects buffering capabilities during high-intensity exercise so it is unclear whether it will alter the performance effects of sodium bicarbonate.

Beta alanine [30,255,260,263–265]	Dosing protocols involve chronic ingestion with daily intake of 3.2–6.4 g for 4–12 weeks. Daily doses were often split into 0.8–1.6 g doses every 3–4 h.	2–4 weeks of supplementation increases skeletal muscle carnosine concentrations by up to ~65%, which increases muscle buffering capacity (beta alanine is a precursor to carnosine, which is a buffer that protects against the accumulation of H^+ in muscle during high intensity exercise). May cause side effects such as flushing, skin rashes or transient paraesthesia, which may be reduced by using multiple smaller doses throughout the day.	Improves high intensity performance and particularly capacity for continuous and intermittent exercise sessions lasting 30 s -10 min. Improvements are likely to be greater in less trained individuals but still evident in trained individuals. Ergogenic effect may be further improved with sodium bicarbonate. Does not appear to affect performance for exercise lasting < 30 s and possibly not for exercise longer than 10 min.	No studies in keto-adapted athletes.
Nitrate (NO_3^-) [257,260,266–269] Leafy green and root vegetables with most studies using beetroot juice	A variety of acute and chronic dosing protocols have been studied. Ingesting beetroot juice with a NO_3^- dose of 5–20 mmol, 2–3 h before the onset of exercise appears to be most ergogenic. This effect does not appear to be significantly enhanced by chronic supplementation (daily for 2–15 d).	Increases nitric oxide bioavailability in the circulation, which increases blood flow to working muscle, particularly type II fibres. Improves oxygen uptake during submaximal exercise. Increases mitochondrial respiration efficiency and reduces oxygen cost of submaximal exercise (improved exercise economy). Proposed to help maintain PCr concentrations during repeated high intensity bouts. Improves the release and reuptake of calcium from the sarcoplasmic reticulum (which may improve muscle power production) Minimal side effects reported.	Promising but variable effect, with 32% out of 80 studies showing an ergogenic effect. Ergogenic effect appears to be blunted in women (albeit limited evidence) and absent in highly trained athletes. Ergogenic effect seen across numerous exercise types (e.g., cycling, rowing, running, weight lifting/ resistance) but may be particularly effective for small muscle group exercises (e.g., handgrip) Likely improves endurance capacity, particularly in events lasting <40 min (absent or blunted effect when TT performance was assessed). Possibly improves performance and capacity in very high intensity intermittent exercise with short recovery intervals (e.g., repeated sprints, weightlifting, resistance training)	No studies in keto-adapted athletes. Carbohydrate in beetroot juice may reduce nutritional ketosis and rates of fat oxidation before and during exercise. Nitric oxide pathway may be enhanced with keto-adaption so unclear whether effects of nitrate supplementation will be additive.

CHO, carbohydrate; GI, gastro intestinal; BW, body weight; TT, time trial; d, day; h, hour; min, minutes; s, seconds.

to which trial they were taking part in. The effects of exogenous ketone supplements on substrate metabolism have also been inconsistent with some studies suggesting a glucose sparing effect during exercise (reduced muscle glycogen use, reduced blood lactate accumulation and increase intramuscular triglyceride use) but others reporting no change in substrate metabolism [275].

Performance studies have varied considerably in the type of ketone supplement used, dose and timing of supplement ingestion, degree of ketosis achieved, nutritional status (fasting vs fed), other nutrients coingested with the supplement or control drink (e.g., MCT, carbohydrate, caffeine, electrolytes or amino acids), training status, severity of GI symptoms and the duration and intensity of the performance test [249,275]. Because of this heterogeneity in study design and inconsistent findings, the specific conditions required for a ketone supplement to be potentially ergogenic without causing GI symptoms have been difficult to pinpoint. As such, there is not currently sufficient evidence to recommend ketone as supplements for exercise performance, but is a growing area of research to help provide more insight into if/how they may fit into the performance paradigm.

9.6 Case study

Webster C
Smith J

This case study documents the habitual diet and performance history of a 34-year-old male athlete who competed in elite endurance events while following a strict LCHF diet. It then monitored his performance in a laboratory setting as he started supplementing his exercise sessions with carbohydrate [42]. His habitual diet contained ~8% of calories as carbohydrate, ~ 75% as fat, and 17% as protein, which he said reflected how he had eaten for the previous 2 years. He also predominantly ingested only water during training and racing. During this time, he won several national-level triathlon and Ironman competitions and consistently placed in the top 20 in elite international competitions, often winning his age group category. This case study demonstrates that it is possible, at least for this individual, to be highly competitive at elite ultra-endurance events while following a strict LCHF diet and without carbohydrate supplementation. This is noteworthy given that many exercise scientists consider carbohydrate-rich diets and carbohydrate supplementation as essential for elite level endurance performance [291].

The performance-enhancing benefits of carbohydrate ingestion during exercise have been well established in athletes who follow conventional high-carbohydrate diets. Carbohydrate ingestion helps these athletes, who only have a moderate capacity for fat oxidation, to maintain high rates of carbohydrate oxidation while sparing their limited endogenous carbohydrate stores. The presence of carbohydrate in the mouth can also have a stimulatory effect on performance, which is likely to be centrally regulated as it occurs even when the supplement is not swallowed. LCHF-adapted athletes are much less dependent on carbohydrate oxidation during exercise, and have much higher rates of fat oxidation so it is not immediately clear whether supplying additional carbohydrate during exercise would be beneficial. This case study therefore examined the athlete's performance before and after he started ingesting carbohydrate during exercise. After a 3-week baseline control period of standardised habitual training and habitual LCHF diet, he completed a 30 s sprint, a 4-min sprint, a 20 km time trial, and a 100 km time trial while ingesting only water. He then completed another 3 weeks of identical training and similar habitual LCHF diet with the exception that he ingested carbohydrate (at an average rate of 1 g/min) during training sessions to become accustomed to the supplement. The follow-up performance tests were then repeated with carbohydrate supplementation.

An interesting result was that his 100 km time trial was similar or even slightly slower (1%) when he ingested carbohydrate compared to water. By contrast his 20 km time trial was slightly faster (~2%) with carbohydrate ingestion than with water. His 30 s and 4 min sprints were identical between conditions. During the 100 km time trial, his rate of carbohydrate oxidation increased throughout the trial with carbohydrate ingestion, whereas it decreased with water ingestion (Fig. 9.10). However, his rate of fat oxidation decreased during the trial with carbohydrate ingestion such that his overall energy expenditure was largely similar between trials. This may explain the lack of an ergogenic effect of carbohydrate ingestion. The mechanism by which his performance improved in the 20 km time trial is not clear, however it is possible that both metabolic and/or central effects were involved.

In summary, this particular LCHF elite athlete does not appear to benefit from carbohydrate supplementation before very short (up to 4 min) or during prolonged endurance events (~3 h) but may benefit during shorter high- intensity endurance events lasting ~30 min. Whether this is a general trend for other fat-adapted athletes is not currently known, as no published studies have investigated the metabolic and performance enhancing effects of carbohydrate supplementation during exercise in this population.

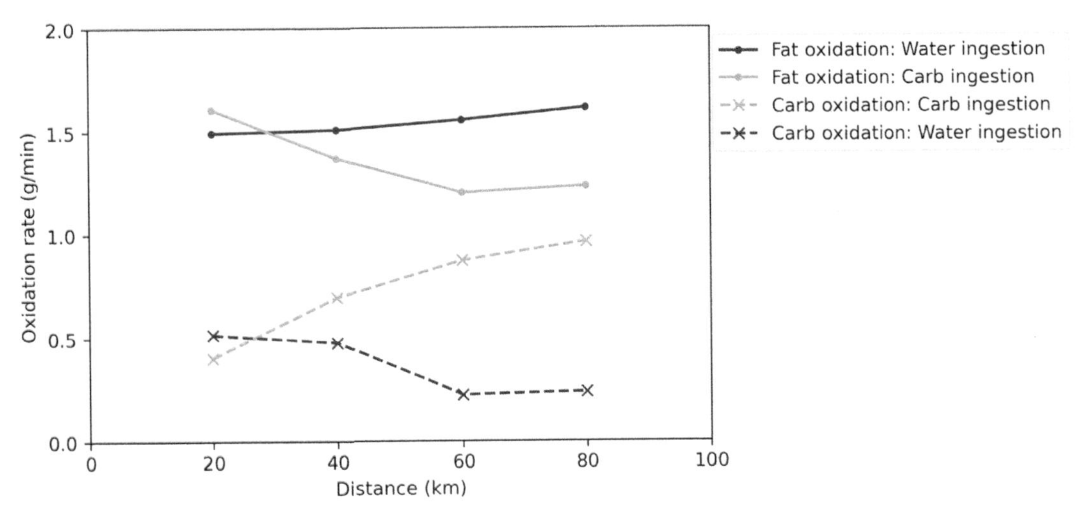

FIGURE 9.10 Fat and carbohydrate oxidation rates during two 100 km time trials where either water or carbohydrate (at an average rate of 1 g/min) were ingested.

References

[1] Greene J, Louis J, Korostynska O, Mason A. State-of-the-art methods for skeletal muscle glycogen analysis in athletes-the need for novel non-invasive techniques. Biosensors 2017;7(1). Available from: https://doi.org/10.3390/bios7010011.

[2] Noakes TD. What is the evidence that dietary macronutrient composition influences exercise performance? A narrative review. Nutrients. 2022;14(4):862.

[3] Noakes TD, St Clair Gibson A. Logical limitations to the "catastrophe" models of fatigue during exercise in humans. Br J Sports Med 2004;38 (5):648–9. Available from: https://doi.org/10.1136/bjsm.2003.009761.

[4] Burke LM, Hawley JA, Wong SH, Jeukendrup AE. Carbohydrates for training and competition. J Sports Sci 2011;29(Suppl 1):S17–27. Available from: https://doi.org/10.1080/02640414.2011.585473.

[5] Burke LM. Ketogenic low-CHO, high-fat diet: the future of elite endurance sport? J Physiol 2020. Available from: https://doi.org/10.1113/JP278928.

[6] Choi YJ, Jeon SM, Shin S. Impact of a ketogenic diet on metabolic parameters in patients with obesity or overweight and with or without type 2 diabetes: A meta-analysis of randomized controlled trials. Nutrients 2020;12(7). Available from: https://doi.org/10.3390/nu12072005.

[7] Davis JJ, Fournakis N, Ellison J. Ketogenic diet for the treatment and prevention of dementia: a review. J Geriatric Psychiatry Neurol 2020. Available from: https://doi.org/10.1177/0891988720901785 891988720901785.

[8] Paoli A, Rubini A, Volek JS, Grimaldi KA. Beyond weight loss: a review of the therapeutic uses of very-low-carbohydrate (ketogenic) diets. Eur J Clin Nutr 2013;67(8):789–96. Available from: https://doi.org/10.1038/ejcn.2013.116.

[9] Sourbron J, Klinkenberg S, van Kuijk SMJ, Lagae L, Lambrechts D, Braakman HMH, et al. Ketogenic diet for the treatment of pediatric epilepsy: review and meta-analysis. Child's Nerv Syst 2020;36(6):1099–109. Available from: https://doi.org/10.1007/s00381-020-04578-7.

[10] Zhang X, Zheng Y, Guo Y, Lai Z. The effect of low carbohydrate diet on polycystic ovary syndrome: a meta-analysis of randomized controlled trials. Int J Endocrinol 2019;2019:4386401. Available from: https://doi.org/10.1155/2019/4386401.

[11] Maffetone PB, Laursen PB. Athletes: fit but unhealthy? Sports Med - Open 2016;2:24. Available from: https://doi.org/10.1186/s40798-016-0048-x.

[12] Kujala UM, Marti P, Kaprio J, Hernelahti M, Tikkanen H, Sarna S. Occurrence of chronic disease in former top-level athletes. Predominance of benefits, risks or selection effects? Sports Med 2003;33(8):553–61. Available from: https://doi.org/10.2165/00007256-200333080-00001.

[13] Saris WH, Antoine JM, Brouns F, Fogelholm M, Gleeson M, Hespel P, et al. PASSCLAIM - physical performance and fitness. Eur J Nutr 2003;42(Suppl 1):I50–95. Available from: https://doi.org/10.1007/s00394-003-1104-0.

[14] Egan B, Zierath JR. Exercise metabolism and the molecular regulation of skeletal muscle adaptation. Cell Metab 2013;17(2):162–84. Available from: https://doi.org/10.1016/j.cmet.2012.12.012.

[15] Spriet LL. New insights into the interaction of carbohydrate and fat metabolism during exercise. Sports Med 2014;44(Suppl 1):S87–96. Available from: https://doi.org/10.1007/s40279-014-0154-1.

[16] Jeukendrup AE. Nutrition for endurance sports: marathon, triathlon, and road cycling. J Sports Sci 2011;29(Suppl 1):S91–9. Available from: https://doi.org/10.1080/02640414.2011.610348.

[17] Noakes T. Physiological models to understand exercise fatigue and the adaptations that predict or enhance athletic performance. ScJ Med Sci Sports 2000;10(3):123–45. Available from: https://doi.org/10.1034/j.1600-0838.2000.010003123.x.

[18] Goodpaster BH, Sparks LM. Metabolic flexibility in health and disease. Cell Metab 2017;25(2):1027–36.

[19] Phinney SD, Bistrian BR, Evans WJ, Gervino E, Blackburn GL. The human metabolic response to chronic ketosis without caloric restriction: preservation of submaximal exercise capability with reduced carbohydrate oxidation. Metabolism: Clin Exp 1983;32(8):769–76. Available from: https://doi.org/10.1016/0026-0495(83)90106-3.

[20] O'Keeffe KA, Keith RE, Wilson GD, Blessing DL. Dietary carbohydrate intake and endurance exercise performance of trained female cyclists. Nutr Res 1989;9(8):819–30. Available from: https://doi.org/10.1016/S0271-5317(89)80027-2.

[21] Burke LM, Angus DJ, Cox GR, Cummings NK, Febbraio MA, Gawthorn K, et al. Effect of fat adaptation and carbohydrate restoration on metabolism and performance during prolonged cycling. J Appl Physiol 2000;89(6):2413–21.

[22] Carey AL, Staudacher HM, Cummings NK, Stepto NK, Nikolopoulos V, Burke LM, et al. Effects of fat adaptation and carbohydrate restoration on prolonged endurance exercise. J Appl Physiol 2001;91(1):115–22.

[23] Havemann L, West SJ, Goedecke JH, Macdonald IA, St Clair Gibson A, Noakes TD, et al. Fat adaptation followed by carbohydrate loading compromises high-intensity sprint performance. J Appl Physiol 2006;100(1):194–202. Available from: https://doi.org/10.1152/japplphysiol.00813.2005.

[24] Burke LM, Whitfield J, Heikura IA, Ross MLR, Tee N, Forbes SF, et al. Adaptation to a low carbohydrate high fat diet is rapid but impairs endurance exercise metabolism and performance despite enhanced glycogen availability. J Physiol 2020. Available from: https://doi.org/10.1113/JP280221.

[25] McSwiney FT, Fusco B, McCabe L, Lombard A, Crowley P, Walsh J, et al. Changes in body composition and substrate utilization after a short-term ketogenic diet in endurance-trained males. Biol Sport 2020;38(1):145–52.

[26] Lambert EV, Speechly DP, Dennis SC, Noakes TD. Enhanced endurance in trained cyclists during moderate intensity exercise following 2 weeks adaptation to a high fat diet. Eur J Appl Physiol Occup Physiol 1994;69(4):287–93.

[27] Goedecke JH, Christie C, Wilson G, Dennis SC, Noakes TD, Hopkins WG, et al. Metabolic adaptations to a high-fat diet in endurance cyclists. Metabolism: Clin Exp 1999;48(12):1509–17. Available from: https://doi.org/10.1016/s0026-0495(99)90238-x.

[28] Lambert EV, Goedecke JH, van Zyl C, Murphy K, Hawley JA, Dennis SC, et al. High-fat diet versus habitual diet prior to carbohydrate loading: Effects on exercise metabolism and cycling performance. Int J Sports Nutr Exerc Metab 2001;11(2):209–25.

[29] Rowlands DS, Hopkins WG. Effects of high-fat and high-carbohydrate diets on metabolism and performance in cycling. Metabolism: Clin Exp 2002;51(6):678–90. Available from: https://doi.org/10.1053/meta.2002.32723.

[30] Zajac A, Poprzecki S, Maszczyk A, Czuba M, Michalczyk M, Zydek G. The effects of a ketogenic diet on exercise metabolism and physical performance in off-road cyclists. Nutrients 2014;6(7):2493–508. Available from: https://doi.org/10.3390/nu6072493.

[31] Burke LM, Ross ML, Garvican-Lewis LA, Welvaert M, Heikura IA, Forbes SG, et al. Low carbohydrate, high fat diet impairs exercise economy and negates the performance benefit from intensified training in elite race walkers. J Physiol 2017;595(9):2785–807. Available from: https://doi.org/10.1113/JP273230.

[32] Zinn C, Wood M, Williden M, Chatterton S, Maunder E. Ketogenic diet benefits body composition and well-being but not performance in a pilot case study of New Zealand endurance athletes. J Int Soc Sports Nutr 2017;14:22. Available from: https://doi.org/10.1186/s12970-017-0180-0.

[33] Sitko S, Cirer-Sastre R, Lopez Laval I. Effects of a low-carbohydrate diet on performance and body composition in trained cyclists. Nutricion Hospitalaria 2019;36(6):1384–8. Available from: https://doi.org/10.20960/nh.02762.

[34] Prins PJ, Noakes TD, Welton GL, Haley SJ, Esbenshade NJ, Atwell AD, et al. High rates of fat oxidation induced by a low-carbohydrate, high-fat diet, do not impair 5-km running performance in competitive recreational athletes. J Sports Sci Med 2019;18(4):738–50.

[35] Podlogar T, Debevec T. Effects of a 14-day high-carbohydrate diet on exercise performance of a low-carbohydrate adapted athlete – case study. Kinesiol Slovenica 2016;22(1):37–46.

[36] McSwiney FT, Wardrop B, Hyde PN, Lafountain RA, Volek JS, Doyle L. Keto-adaptation enhances exercise performance and body composition responses to training in endurance athletes. Metabolism: Clin Exp 2018;83:e1–2. Available from: https://doi.org/10.1016/j.metabol.2017.11.016.

[37] Shaw DM, Merien F, Braakhuis A, Maunder ED, Dulson DK. Effect of a ketogenic diet on submaximal exercise capacity and efficiency in runners. Med Sci Sports Exerc 2019;51(10):2135–46. Available from: https://doi.org/10.1249/MSS0.0000000000002008.

[38] Helge JW, Richter EA, Kiens B. Interaction of training and diet on metabolism and endurance during exercise in man. J Physiol 1996;492(Pt 1):293–306. Available from: https://doi.org/10.1113/jphysiol.1996.sp021309.

[39] Helge JW, Wulff B, Kiens B. Impact of a fat-rich diet on endurance in man: role of the dietary period. Med Sci Sports Exerc 1998; 30(3):456–61.

[40] Heatherly AJ, Killen LG, Smith AF, Waldman HS, Seltmann CL, Hollingsworth A, et al. Effects of ad libitum low-carbohydrate high-fat dieting in middle-age male runners. Med Sci Sports Exerc 2018;50(3):570–9. Available from: https://doi.org/10.1249/MSS.0000000000001477.

[41] Fleming J, Sharman MJ, Avery NG, Love DM, Gomez AL, Scheett TP, et al. Endurance capacity and high-intensity exercise performance responses to a high fat diet. Int J Sport Nutr Exerc Metab 2003;13(4):466–78. Available from: https://doi.org/10.1123/ijsnem.13.4.466.

[42] Webster CC, Swart J, Noakes TD, Smith JA. A carbohydrate ingestion intervention in an elite athlete who follows a low-carbohydrate high-fat diet. Int J Sports Physiol Perform 2018;13(7):957–60. Available from: https://doi.org/10.1123/ijspp.2017-0392.

[43] Stellingwerff T, Spriet LL, Watt MJ, Kimber NE, Hargreaves M, Hawley JA, et al. Decreased PDH activation and glycogenolysis during exercise following fat adaptation with carbohydrate restoration. Am J Physiol Endocrinol Metab 2006;290(2):E380–8. Available from: https://doi.org/10.1152/ajpendo.00268.2005.

[44] Wood T. Lost metabolic machinery during ketosis? Depends where you are looking. Strenth Conditioning J 2017;39(5):94.

[45] Volek JS, Freidenreich DJ, Saenz C, Kunces LJ, Creighton BC, Bartley JM, et al. Metabolic characteristics of keto-adapted ultra-endurance runners. Metabolism: Clin Exp 2016;65(3):100–10. Available from: https://doi.org/10.1016/j.metabol.2015.10.028.
[46] Oppliger RA, Steen SA, Scott JR. Weight loss practices of college wrestlers. Int J Sport Nutr Exerc Metab 2003;13(1):29–46. Available from: https://doi.org/10.1123/ijsnem.13.1.29.
[47] Cadwallader AB, de la Torre X, Tieri A, Botre F. The abuse of diuretics as performance-enhancing drugs and masking agents in sport doping: pharmacology, toxicology and analysis. Br J Pharmacol 2010;161(1):1–16. Available from: https://doi.org/10.1111/j.1476-5381.2010.00789.x.
[48] Paoli A, Grimaldi K, D'Agostino D, Cenci L, Moro T, Bianco A, et al. Ketogenic diet does not affect strength performance in elite artistic gymnasts. J Int Soc Sports Nutr 2012;9(1):34.
[49] Sawyer JC, Wood RJ, Davidson PW, Collins SM, Matthews TD, Gregory SM, et al. Effects of a short-term carbohydrate-restricted diet on strength and power performance. J Strength Conditioning Res 2013;27(8):2255–62. Available from: https://doi.org/10.1519/JSC.0b013e31827da314.
[50] Rhyu HS, Cho SY. The effect of weight loss by ketogenic diet on the body composition, performance-related physical fitness factors and cytokines of Taekwondo athletes. J Exerc Rehabilitation 2014;10(5):326–31. Available from: https://doi.org/10.12965/jer.140160.
[51] Gregory RM, Hamdan H, Torisky DM, Akers JD. A low-carbohydrate ketogenic diet combined with 6-weeks of crossfit training improves body composition and performance. Int J Sports Exerc Med 2017;3(2). Available from: https://doi.org/10.23937/2469-5718/1510054.
[52] Chatterton S, Zinn C, Helms E, Storey A. The effect of an 8-week low carbohydrate high fat (LCHF) diet in sub-elite Olympic weightlifters and powerlifters on strength, body composition, mental state and adherence: a pilot case-study. J Australian Strength Conditioning 2017;25(2):6–13.
[53] Wilson JM, Lowery RP, Roberts MD, Sharp MH, Joy JM, Shields KA, et al. The effects of ketogenic dieting on body composition, strength, power, and hormonal profiles in resistance training males. J Strength Conditioning Res 2017. Available from: https://doi.org/10.1519/JSC.0000000000001935.
[54] Miele E, Vitti S, Christoph L, O'Neill E, Matthews T, Wood R. The effects of a six-week ketogenic diet on the performance of short-duration, high-intensity exercise: a pilot study. Med Sci Sports Exerc 2018;50(5S Suppl 1):792.
[55] Vargas S, Romance R, Petro JL, Bonilla DA, Galancho I, Espinar S, et al. Efficacy of ketogenic diet on body composition during resistance training in trained men: a randomized controlled trial. J Int Soc Sports Nutr 2018;15(1):31. Available from: https://doi.org/10.1186/s12970-018-0236-9.
[56] Greene DA, Varler BJ, Hartwig TB, Chapman P, Rugney M. A low-carbohydrate ketogenic diet reduces body mass without compromising performance in powerlifting and olympic weightlifting athletes. Strength Conditioning Res 2018;32(12):3373–82. Available from: https://doi.org/10.1519/JSC.0000000000002904.
[57] Waldman HS, Krings BM, Basham SA, Smith JEW, Fountain BJ, McAllister MJ. Effects of a 15-day low carbohydrate, high-fat diet in resistance-trained men. J Strength Conditioning Res 2018;32(11):3103–11. Available from: https://doi.org/10.1519/JSC.0000000000002282.
[58] Kephart WC, Pledge CD, Roberson PA, Mumford PW, Romero MA, Mobley CB, et al. The three-month effects of a ketogenic diet on body composition, blood parameters, and performance metrics in crossfit trainees: a pilot study. Sports 2018;6(1). Available from: https://doi.org/10.3390/sports6010001.
[59] Wroble KA, Trott MN, Schweitzer GG, Rahman RS, Kelly PV, Weiss EP. Low-carbohydrate, ketogenic diet impairs anaerobic exercise performance in exercise-trained women and men: a randomized-sequence crossover trial. J Sports Med Phys Finess 2019;59(4):600–7. Available from: https://doi.org/10.23736/S0022-4707.18.08318-4.
[60] Vargas-Molina S, Petro JL, Romance R, Kreider RB, Schoenfeld BJ, Bonilla DA, et al. Effects of a ketogenic diet on body composition and strength in trained women. J Int Soc Sports Nutr 2020;17(1):19. Available from: https://doi.org/10.1186/s12970-020-00348-7.
[61] Bergstrom J, Furst P, Holmstrom BU, Vinnars E, Askanasi J, Elwyn DH, et al. Influence of injury and nutrition on muscle water electrolytes: effect of elective operation. Ann Surg 1981;193(6):810–16. Available from: https://doi.org/10.1097/00000658-198106000-00017.
[62] Cermak NM, van Loon LJ. The use of carbohydrates during exercise as an ergogenic aid. Sports Med 2013;43(11):1139–55. Available from: https://doi.org/10.1007/s40279-013-0079-0.
[63] Buchheit M, Laursen PB. High-intensity interval training, solutions to the programming puzzle. Part II: anaerobic energy, neuromuscular load and practical applications. Sports Med 2013;43(10):927–54. Available from: https://doi.org/10.1007/s40279-013-0066-5.
[64] Dostal T, Plews DJ, Hofmann P, Laursen PB, Cipryan L. Effects of a 12-week very-low carbohydrate high-fat diet on maximal aerobic capacity, high-intensity intermittent exercise, and cardiac autonomic regulation: Non-randomized parallel-group study. Front Physiol 2019;10:912. Available from: https://doi.org/10.3389/fphys.2019.00912.
[65] Cipryan L, Plews DJ, Ferretti A, Maffetone PB, Laursen PB. Effects of a 4-week very low-carbohydrate diet on high-intensity interval training responses. J Sports Sci Med 2018;17(2):259–68.
[66] Kysel P, Haluzikova D, Dolezalova RP, Lankova I, Lacinova Z, Kasperova BJ, et al. The influence of cyclical ketogenic reduction diet vs. Nutritionally balanced reduction diet on body composition, strength, and endurance performance in healthy young males: a randomized controlled trial. Nutrients 2020;12(9). Available from: https://doi.org/10.3390/nu12092832.
[67] Michalczyk MM, Chycki J, Zajac A, Maszczyk A, Zydek G, Langfort J. Anaerobic performance after a low-carbohydrate diet (lcd) followed by 7 days of carbohydrate loading in male basketball players. Nutrients 2019;11(4). Available from: https://doi.org/10.3390/nu11040778.
[68] Klement R, Frobel T, Albers T, Fikenzer S, Prinzhausen J, Ulrike K. A pilot case study on the impact of a self-prescribed ketogenic diet on biochemical parameters and running performance in healthy and physically active individuals. Nutr Med 2013;1(1):10–37.
[69] McKay AKA, Pyne DB, Peeling P, Sharma AP, Ross MLR, Burke LM. The impact of chronic carbohydrate manipulation on mucosal immunity in elite endurance athletes. J Sports Sci 2019;37(5):553–9. Available from: https://doi.org/10.1080/02640414.2018.1521712.

[70] Waldman HS, Heatherly AJ, Killen LG, Hollingsworth A, Koh Y, O'Neal EK. A 3-week, low-carbohydrate, high-fat diet improves multiple serum inflammatory markers in endurance-trained males. J Strength Conditioning Res 2020. Available from: https://doi.org/10.1519/JSC.0000000000003761.

[71] Shaw DM, Merien F, Braakhuis A, Keaney L, Dulson DK. Adaptation to a ketogenic diet modulates adaptive and mucosal immune markers in trained male endurance athletes. ScJ Med Sci Sports 2020. Available from: https://doi.org/10.1111/sms.13833.

[72] Walsh NP. Nutrition and athlete immune health: new perspectives on an old paradigm. Sports Med 2019;49(Suppl 2):153–68. Available from: https://doi.org/10.1007/s40279-019-01160-3.

[73] David LA, Maurice CF, Carmody RN, Gootenberg DB, Button JE, Wolfe BE, et al. Diet rapidly and reproducibly alters the human gut microbiome. Nature 2014;505(7484):559–63. Available from: https://doi.org/10.1038/nature12820.

[74] Ellerbroek A. The effect of ketogenic diets on the gut microbiota. J Exerc Nutr 2018;1(5).

[75] Hughes RL. A review of the role of the gut microbiome in personalized sports nutrition. Front Nutr 2019;6:191. Available from: https://doi.org/10.3389/fnut.2019.00191.

[76] Paoli A, Mancin L, Bianco A, Thomas E, Mota JF, Piccini F. Ketogenic diet and microbiota: friends or enemies? Genes 2019;10(7). Available from: https://doi.org/10.3390/genes10070534.

[77] Maunder E, Kilding A, Plews D. Substrate metabolism during ironman triathlon: different horses on the same courses. Sports Med 2018;48(10):2219–26.

[78] Campbell B, Kreider RB, Ziegenfuss T, La Bounty P, Roberts M, Burke D, et al. International Society of Sports Nutrition position stand: protein and exercise. J Int Soc Sports Nutr 2007;4:8. Available from: https://doi.org/10.1186/1550-2783-4-8.

[79] Helms ER, Zinn C, Rowlands DS, Brown SR. A systematic review of dietary protein during caloric restriction in resistance trained lean athletes: a case for higher intakes. Int J sport Nutr Exerc Metab 2014;24(2):127–38. Available from: https://doi.org/10.1123/ijsnem.2013-0054.

[80] Harvey CJd C, Schofield GM, Williden M. The use of nutritional supplements to induce ketosis and reduce symptoms associated with keto-induction: a narrative review. PeerJ 2018;6:e4488. Available from: https://doi.org/10.7717/peerj.4488.

[81] Harvey CJd C, Schofield G, Zinn C, Thornley SJ. Effects of differing levels of carbohydrate restriction on the achievement of nutritional ketosis, mood, and symptoms of carbohydrate withdrawal in healthy adults: a randomized clinical trial. Nutrition: X 2019;2(100005).

[82] Volek J, Phinney S. The art and science of low carbohydrate living: an expert guide to making the life-saving benefits of carbohydrate restriction sustainable and enjoyable. Beyond Obesity Llc; 2011.

[83] Volek JS, Phinney SD. The art and science of low carbohydrate performance; beyond obesity. Miami, FL: LLC; 2012.

[84] Tiwari S, Riazi S, Ecelbarger CA. Insulin's impact on renal sodium transport and blood pressure in health, obesity, and diabetes. Am J Physiol: Ren Physiol 2007;293(4):F974–84. Available from: https://doi.org/10.1152/ajprenal.00149.2007.

[85] Gibson AA, Eroglu EI, Rooney K, Harper C, McClintock S, Franklin J, et al. Urine dipsticks are not accurate for detecting mild ketosis during a severely energy restricted diet. Obes Sci Pract 2020;6(5):544–51. Available from: https://doi.org/10.1002/osp4.432.

[86] Zinn C, Rush A, Johnson R. Assessing the nutrient intake of a low-carbohydrate, high-fat (LCHF) diet: a hypothetical case study design. BMJ Open 2018;8:e018846. Available from: https://doi.org/10.1136/bmjopen-2017-018846.

[87] McSwiney FT, Doyle L. Low-carbohydrate ketogenic diets in male endurance athletes demonstrate different micronutrient contents and changes in corpuscular haemoglobin over 12 weeks. Sports 2019;7(9). Available from: https://doi.org/10.3390/sports7090201.

[88] Noakes T, Immda. Fluid replacement during marathon running. Clin J Sport Med 2003;13(5):309–18. Available from: https://doi.org/10.1097/00042752-200309000-00007.

[89] DeFronzo RA. The effect of insulin on renal sodium metabolism. A review with clinical implications. Diabetologia 1981;21(3):165–71. Available from: https://doi.org/10.1007/BF00252649.

[90] DeFronzo RA, Goldberg M, Agus ZS. The effects of glucose and insulin on renal electrolyte transport. J Clin Investig 1976;58(1):83–90. Available from: https://doi.org/10.1172/JCI108463.

[91] Hamwi GJ, Mitchell MC, Wieland RG, Kruger FA, Schachner SS. Sodium and potassium metabolism during starvation. Am J Clin Nutr 1967;20(8):897–902. Available from: https://doi.org/10.1093/ajcn/20.8.897.

[92] Schofield G, Zinn C, Rodger C. What the fat? Sports performance: leaner, fitter, faster on low-carb healthy fat. Auckland, New Zealand: The Real Food Publishing Company; 2016.

[93] American College of Sports M, Sawka MN, Burke LM, Eichner ER, Maughan RJ, Montain SJ, et al. American College of Sports Medicine position stand. Exercise and fluid replacement. Med Sci Sports Exerc 2007;39(2):377–90. Available from: https://doi.org/10.1249/mss.0b013e31802ca597.

[94] Noakes T. Waterlogged: serious Probl overhydration endurance sports. Human Kinetics; 2012.

[95] Bergstrom J. Percutaneous needle biopsy of skeletal muscle in physiological and clinical research. Scan J Clin Lab Invest 1975;35:609–16.

[96] Bergström J, Hermansen L, Hultman E, Saltin B. Diet, muscle glycogen and physical performance. Acta Physiol Scand 1967;71:140–50.

[97] Karlsson J, Saltin B. Diet, muscle glycogen, and endurance performance. J Appl Physiol 1971;31:203–6.

[98] Gollnick PD. Metabolism of substrates: energy substrate metabolism during exercise and as modified by training. Fed Proc 1985;44:353–7.

[99] Conlee RK. Muscle glycogen and exercise endurance: a twenty-year perspective. Exerc Sport Sci Rev 1987;15:1–28.

[100] Fitts RH. Cellular mechanisms of muscle fatigue. Physiol Rev 1994;74:49–93.

[101] Febbraio MA, Dancey J. Skeletal muscle energy metabolism during prolonged, fatiguing exercise. J Appl Physiol 2003;87:2341–7.

[102] Parkin JM, Carey MF, Zhao S, Febbraio MA. Effect of ambient temperature on human skeletal muscle metabolism during fatiguing submaximal exercise. J Appl Physiol 1999;86:902–8.

[103] Baldwin J, Snow RF, Carey MF, Febbraio MA. Muscle IMP accumulation during fatiguing submaximal exercise in endurance trained and untrained men. Am J Physiol (Regulatory Integr Comp Physiol 1999;277:R295–300 46).
[104] Baldwin J, Snow RJ, Gibala MJ, Garnham A, Howarth K, Febbraio MA. Glycogen availability does not affect the TCA cycle or TAN pools during prolonged, fatiguing exercise. J Appl Physiol 2003;94:2181–7.
[105] Lorand L. 'Adenosine triphosphate-creatine transphosphorylase' as relaxing factor of muscle. Nature 1953;172:1181–3.
[106] Christensen EH, Hansen O. Arbeitsfähigkeit und ernährung. Skand Arch Physiol 1939;81:160–71.
[107] Christensen EH, Hansen O. Hypoglykame, arbeitsfähigkeit und ermudung. Skand Arch Physiol 1939;81:172–9.
[108] Coyle EF, Hagberg JM, Hurley BF, Martin WH, Ehsani AA, Holloszy JG. Carbohydrate feeding during prolonged strenuous exercise can delay fatigue. J Appl Physiol 1983;55:230–5.
[109] Coyle EF, Coggan AR. Muscle glycogen utilization during prolonged strenuous exercise when fed carbohydrate. J Appl Physiol 1986;61:165–72.
[110] Coggan AR, Coyle EF. Reversal of fatigue during prolonged exercise by carbohydrate infusion or ingestion. J Appl Physiol 1987;63:2388–95.
[111] Coggan AR, Coyle EF. Metabolism and performance following carbohydrate ingestion late in exercise. Med Sci Sports Exerc 1989;21:59–65.
[112] Coyle EF. Carbohydrate feeding during exercise. Int J Sports Med 1992;13:S126–8.
[113] Jeukendrup AE. Carbohydrate feeding during exercise. Eur J Sport Sci 2008;8:77–86.
[114] Jeukendrup AE, Jentjens R. Oxidation of carbohydrate feedings during prolonged exercise: current thoughts, guidelines and directions for future research. Sports Med 2000;29(6):407–24. Available from: https://doi.org/10.2165/00007256-200029060-00004. PMID 10870867.
[115] Costill DL, Hargreaves M. Carbohydrate nutrition and fatigue. Sports Med 1992;13:86–92. Available from: https://doi.org/10.2165/00007256-199213020-00003.
[116] Bourdas DL, Souglis A, Zacharakis ED, Geladas ND, Travlos AK. Meta-analysis of carbohydrate solution intake during prolonged exercise in adults: from the last 45 + years' perspective. Nutrients 2021;13:4223.
[117] Rauch LHG, Bosch AN, Noakes TD, Dennis SC, Hawley JA. Fuel utilization during prolonged low-to-moderate intensity exercise when ingesting water or carbohydrate. Pflug Arch 1995;430:971–7.
[118] Wahren J, Felig G, Ahlborg G, Jorfeldt L. Glucose metabolism during leg exercise in man. J Clin Invest 1971;50:2715–25.
[119] Wahren J. Glucose turnover during exercise in man. Ann N Y Acad Sci 1977;301:45–55.
[120] Smith JEW, Zachwieja JJ, Peronnet F, Passe DH, Massicotte D, Lavoie C, et al. Fuel selection and cycling endurance performance with ingestion of [^{13}C]glucose: evidence for a carbohydrate dose response: evidence for a carbohydrate dose response. J Appl Physiol 2010;108:1520–9.
[121] Green LF, Bagley R. Ingestion of a glucose syrup drink during long distance canoeing. Brit J Sports Med 1972;6:125–8.
[122] Ivy JL, Costill DL, Fink WJ, Lower RW. Influence of caffeine and carbohydrate feedings on endurance performance. Med Sci Sports Exerc 1979;11:6–11.
[123] Ivy JL, Miller W, Dover V, Goodyear LG, Sherman WM, Farrell S, et al. Endurance improved by ingestion of a glucose polymer supplement. Med Sci Sports Exerc 1983;15:466–71.
[124] Bjorkman O, Sahlin K, Hagenfeldt L, Wahren J. Influence of glucose and fructose ingestion on the capacity for long-term exercise in well-trained men. Clin Physiol 1984;4:483–94.
[125] Hargreaves M, Costill DL, Coggan A, Fink WJ, Nishibata I. Effect of carbohydrate feedings on muscle glycogen utilization and exercise performance. Med Sci Sports Exerc 1984;16:219–22.
[126] Neufer PD, Costill DL, Flynn MG, Kirwan JP, Mitchell JB, Houmard J. Improvements in exercise performance: effects of carbohydrate feedings and diet. J Appl Physiol 1987;62:983–8.
[127] Murray R, Eddy DE, Murray TW, Seifert JG, Paul GL, Halaby GA. The effect of fluid and carbohydrate feedings during intermittent cycling exercise. Med Sci Sports Exerc 1987;19:597–604.
[128] Mitchell JB, Costill DL, Houmard JA, Flynn MG, Fink WJ, Beltz JD. Effects of carbohydrate ingestion on gastric emptying and exercise performance. Med Sci Sports Exerc 1988;20:110–15.
[129] Mitchell, J.B.. The effect of carbohydrate ingestion on gastric emptying, glycogen metabolism, and exercise performance. (Ph.D. thesis). Ball State University, 1988.
[130] Hargreaves M, Briggs GA. Effect of carbohydrate ingestion on exercise metabolism. J Appl Physiol 1988;65:1553–5.
[131] Riley ML, Israel RG, Holbert D, Tapscott EB, Dohm GL. Effect of carbohydrate ingestion on exercise endurance and metabolism after a 1-day fast. Int J Sports Med 1988;9:320–4.
[132] Davis JM, Lamb DR, Pate RR, Slentz CA, Burgess WA, Bartoli WP. Carbohydrate-electrolyte drinks: effects on endurance cycling in the heat. Am J Clin Nutr 1988;48:1023–30.
[133] Mitchell JB, Costill DB, Houmard JA, Fink WJ, Pascoe DD, Pearson DR. Influence of carbohydrate dosage on exercise performance and glycogen metabolism. J Appl Physiol 1989;67:1843–9.
[134] Williams C, Nute MG, Broadbank L, Vinall S. Influence of fluid intake on endurance running performance. A comparison between water, glucose and fructose solutions. Eur J Appl Physiol 1990;60:112–19.
[135] Wright DA, Sherman WM, Dernbach AR. Carbohydrate feedings before, during, or in combination improve cycling endurance performance. J Appl Physiol 1991;71:1082–8.
[136] Williams C, Brewer J, Walker M. The effect of a high carbohydrate diet on running performance during a 30-km treadmill time trial. Eur J Appl Physiol 1992;65:18–24.
[137] Murray R, Paul GL, Seifert JG, Eddy DE. Responses to varying rates of carbohydrate ingestion during exercise. Med Sci Sports Exerc 1991;23:713–18.

[138] Tsintzas K, Liu R, Williams C, Campbell I, Gaitanos G. The effect of carbohydrate ingestion on performance during a 30-km race. Int J Sport Nutr 1993;3:127–39.

[139] Widrick JJ, Costill DL, Fink WJ, Hickey MS, McConell GK, Tanaka H. Carbohydrate feedings and exercise performance: effects of initial muscle glycogen concentrations. J Appl Physiol 1993;74:2998–3005.

[140] Kang J, Robertson RJ, Denys BG, DaSilva SG, Visich P, Suminski RR, et al. Effect of carbohydrate ingestion subsequent to carbohydrate supercompensation on endurance performance. Int J Sport Nutr 1995;5:329–43.

[141] Anantaraman R, Carmines AA, Gaesser GA, Weltman A. Effects of carbohydrate supplementation on performance during 1 hour of high-intensity exercise. Int J Sports Med 1995;16:461–5.

[142] McConell G, Kloot K, Hargreaves M. Effect of timing of carbohydrate ingestion on endurance exercise performance. Med Sci Sports Exerc 1996;28:1300–4.

[143] McConell G, Snow RJ, Proietto J, Hargreaves M. Muscle metabolism during prolonged exercise in humans: influence of carbohydrate availability. J Appl Physiol 1999;87:1083–6.

[144] McConell G, Canny BJ, Daddo MC, Nance MJ, Snow RJ. Effect of carbohydrate ingestion on glucose kinetics and muscle metabolism during intense endurance exercise. J Appl Physiol 2000;89:1690–8.

[145] Angus DJ, Hargreaves M, Dancey J, Febbraio MA. Effect of carbohydrate or carbohydrate plus medium-chain triglyceride ingestion on cycling time trial performance. J Appl Physiol 2000;88(1):113–19.

[146] Febbraio MA, Chiu A, Angus DJ, Arkinstall MJ, Hawley JA. Effects of carbohydrate ingestion before and during exercise on glucose kinetics and performance. J Appl Physiol 2000;89:2220–6.

[147] Ivy JL, Res PT, Sprague RC, Widzer MO. Effect of a carbohydrate-protein supplement on endurance performance during exercise of varying intensity. Int J Sport Nutr Exerc Metab 2003;13:382–95.

[148] Currell K, Jeukendrup AE. Superior endurance performance with ingestion of multiple transportable carbohydrates. Med Sci Sports Exerc 2008;40:275–81.

[149] Newell ML, Hunter AM, Lawrence C, Tipton KD, Galloway SDR. The ingestion of 39 or 64 g.hr^{-1} of carbohydrate is equally effective at improving endurance exercise performance in cyclists. Int J Sport Nutr Exerc Metabl 2015;25:285–92.

[150] Newell ML, Wallis GA, Hunter AM, Tipton KD, Galloway SDR. Metabolic responses to carbohydrate ingestion during exercise: association between carbohydrate dose and endurance performance. Nutrients 2018;10:37.

[151] King AJ, O'Hara JP, Morrison DJ, Preston T, King RFGJ. Carbohydrate dose influences liver and muscle glycogen oxidation and performance during prolonged exercise. Physiol Rep 2018;6:e13555.

[152] King AJ, O'Hara JP, Arjomandkhah NC, Rowe J, Morrison DJ, Preston T, et al. Liver and muscle glycogen oxidation and performance with dose variation of glucose-fructose ingestion during prolonged (3 h) exercise. Eur J Appl Physiol 2019;119:1157–69.

[153] Fell JM, Hearris MA, Ellis DG, Moran JEP, Jevons EFP, Owens DJ, et al. Carbohydrate improves exercise capacity but does not affect subcellular lipid droplet morphology, AMPK and p53 signalling in human skeletal muscle. J Physiol 2021;599:2823–49.

[154] Rowe J, King RFGJ, King AJ, Morrison DJ, Preston T, Wilson OJ, et al. Glucose and fructose hydrogel enhances running performance, exogenous carbohydrate oxidation and gastrointestinal tolerance. Med Sci Sports Exerc 2022;54:129–40.

[155] Tsintzas OK, Williams C, Singh R, Wilson W, Burrin J. Influence of carbohydrate-electrolyte drinks on marathon running performance. EurJ Appl Physiol 1995;70:154–60.

[156] Flynn MG, Costill DG, Hawley JA, Fink WJ, Neufer PD, Fielding RA, et al. Influence of selected carbohydrate drinks on cycling performance and glycogen use. Med Sci Sports Exerc 1987;16:37–40.

[157] Sasaki H, Takaoka I, Ishiko T. Effects of sucrose or caffeine ingestion on running performance and biochemical responses to endurance running. Int J Sports Med 1987;8:203–7.

[158] Davis JM, Burgess WA, Slentz CA, Bartoli WP, Pate RR. Effects of ingesting 6% and 12% glucose/electrolyte beverages during prolonged intermittent cycling in the heat. Eur J Appl Physiol 1988;57:563–9.

[159] Noakes TD, Lambert EV, Lambert MI, McArthur PS, Myburgh KH, Benade AJS. Carbohydrate ingestion and muscle glycogen depletion during marathon and ultramarathon racing. Eur J Appl Physiol 1988;57:482–9.

[160] Zachwieja JJ, Costill DL, Beard GC, Robergs RA, Pascoe DD, Anderson DE. The effects of a carbonated carbohydrate drink on gastric emptying, gastrointestinal distress, and exercise performance. Int J Sport Nutr 1992;2:239–50.

[161] Madsen K, MacLean DA, Kiens B, Christensen D. Effects of glucose, glucose plus branched-chain amino acids, or placebo on bike performance over 100 km. J Appl Physiol 1996;81:2644–50.

[162] Pettersson S, Edin F, Bakkman L, McGawley K. Effects of supplementing with an 18% carbohydrate-hydrogel drink versus a placebo during whole-body exercise in -5°C with elite cross-country ski athletes: a crossover study. J Int Soc Sports Nutr 2019;16:46.

[163] Burke LM, Hawley JA, Schabort EJ, St Clair Gibson A, Mujika I, Noakes TD. Carbohydrate loading failed to improve 100-km cycling performance in a placebo-controlled trial. J Appl Physiol 2000;88:1284–90.

[164] Bosch AN, Kirkman M. Maintenance of hyperglycaemia does not improve performance in a 100 km cycling time trial. S Afr J Sports Med 2007;19(3):94–8.

[165] Chryssanthopoulos C, Williams C, Wilson W, Asher L, Hearne L. Comparison between carbohydrate feedings before and during exercise on running performance during a 30-km treadmill time trial. Int J Sport Nutr 1994;4:374–84.

[166] Brooks GA. The precious few grams of glucose during exercise. Int J Molec Sci 2020;21:5733.

[167] Jeukendrup A, Brouns F, Wagenmakers AJM, Saris WHM. Carbohydrate-electrolyte feedings improve 1 h time trial cycling performance. Int J Sports Med 1997;18:125–9.

[168] Murray R, Paul GL, Seifert JG, Eddy DE, Halaby GA. The effect of glucose, fructose, and sucrose ingestion during exercise. Med Sci Sports Exerc 1989;21:275–82.

[169] Maughan RJ, Fenn CE, Leiper JB. Effects of fluid, electrolyte and substrate ingestion on endurance capacity. Eur J Appl Physiol 1989;58:481–6.

[170] Murray RS, Seifert JG, Eddy DE, Paul GA, Halaby GA. Carbohydrate feeding and exercise: effect of beverage carbohydrate content. Eur J Appl Physiol 1989;59:152–8.

[171] Wilber RL, Moffatt RJ. Influence of carbohydrate ingestion on blood glucose and performance in runners. Int J Sport Nutr 1992;2:317–27.

[172] El-Sayed MS, Rattu AJM, Roberts I. Effects of carbohydrate feeding before and during prolonged exercise on subsequent maximal exercise performance capacity. Int J Sport Nutr 1995;5:215–24.

[173] Below PR, Rodriguez R, Gonzalez-Alonso J, Coyle EF. Fluid and carbohydrate ingestion independently improve performance during 1 hr of intense exercise. Med Sci Sports Exerc 1995;27:200–10.

[174] Maughan RJ, Bethell LR, Leiper JB. Effects of ingested fluids on exercise capacity and on cardiovascular and metabolic responses to prolonged exercise in man. Exp Physiol 1996;81:847–59.

[175] Tsintsaz OK, Williams C, Wilson W, Burrin J. Influence of carbohydrate supplementation early in exercise on endurance running capacity. Med Sci Sports Exerc 1996;28:1373–9.

[176] El-Sayed MS, Balmer J, Rattu AJM. Carbohydrate ingestion improves endurance performance during a 1 h simulated cycling time trial. J Sports Sci 1997;15:223–30.

[177] Millard-Stafford M, Rosskopf LB, Snow TK, Hinson BT. Water versus carbohydrate-electrolyte ingestion before and during a 15-km run in the heat. Int J Sport Nutr 1997;7:26–38.

[178] Rollo I, Williams C. Influence of ingesting a carbohydrate-electrolyte solution before and during a 1-hr running performance test. Int J Sport Nutr Exerc Metab 2009;19:645–58.

[179] Flood TR, Montanari S, Wicks M, Blanchard J, Sharp H, Taylor L, et al. Addition of pectin-alginate to a carbohydrate beverage does not maintain gastrointestinal barrier function during exercise in hot-humid conditions better than carbohydrate ingestion alone. Appl Physiol Nutr Metab 2020;45:1145–55.

[180] Burke LM, Maughan RJ. The Governor has a sweet tooth – mouth sensing of nutrients to enhance sports performance. Eur J Sport Sci 2014;15:29–40.

[181] Costill DL, Coyle E, Dalsky G, Evans W, Fink W, Hoopes D. Effects of elevated plasma FFA and insulin on muscle glycogen usage during exercise. J Appl Physiol 1977;43:695–9.

[182] Foster C, Costill DL, Fink WJ. Effects of preexercise feedings on endurance performance. Med Sci Sports 1979;11:1–5.

[183] Lopez-Soldado I, Guinovart JJ, Duran J. Increased liver glycogen levels enhance exercise capacity in mice. J Biol Chem 2021;297:100976.

[184] Yeo WK, Carey AL, Burke L, Spriet L, Hawley JA. Fat adaptation in well-trained athletes: effects on cell metabolism. Appl Physiol Nutr Metab 2011;36:12–22.

[185] Bosch AN, Dennis SC, Noakes TD. Influence of carbohydrate loading on fuel substrate turnover and oxidation during prolonged exercise. J Appl Physiol 1993;74:1923–7.

[186] Bosch AN, Dennis SC, Noakes TD. Influence of carbohydrate ingestion on fuel substrate turnover and oxidation during prolonged exercise. J Appl Physiol 1994;76:2364–72.

[187] Jeukendrup AE, Raben A, Gijsen A, Stegen JHCH, Brouns F, Saris WHM, et al. Glucose kinetics during prolonged exercise in highly trained human subjects: effect of glucose ingestion. J Physiol 1999;515:579–89.

[188] Gonzalez JT, Fuchs CJ, Smith FE, Thelwall PE, Taylor R, Stevenson EJ, et al. Ingestion of glucose or sucrose prevents liver but not muscle glycogen depletion during prolonged endurance-type exercise in trained cyclists. Am J Physiol Endocrinol Metab 2015;309:E1031–9.

[189] Jeukendrup AE, Wagenmakers AJM, Stegen JHCH, Gijsen AP, Brouns F, Saris WHM. Carbohydrate ingestion can completely suppress endogenous glucose production during exercise. Am J Physiol Endocrinol Metab 1999;39:E672–83.

[190] Fielding RA, Costill DL, Fink WJ, King DS, Hargreaves M, Kovaleski JE. Effect of carbohydrate feeding frequencies and dosage on muscle glycogen use during exercise. Med Sci Sports Exerc 1985;17:472–6.

[191] Wallis GA, Dawson R, Achten J, Webber J, Jeukendrup AE. Metabolic response to carbohydrate ingestion during exercise in males and females. Am J Physiol Endocrinol Metab 2006;290:E708–15.

[192] Stellingwerff T, Boon H, Gijsen AP, Stegen J,HCH, Kuipers H, van Loon LJC. Carbohydrate supplementation during prolonged cycling exercise spares muscle glycogen but does not affect intramuscular lipid use. Pflug Arch 2007;454:635–47.

[193] Bosch AN, Weltan SM, Dennis SC, Noakes TD. Fuel substrate turnover and oxidation and glycogen sparing with carbohydrate ingestion in non-carbohydrate-loaded cyclists. Pflug Arch 1996;432:1003–10.

[194] Coyle EF, Hamilton MT, Alonso JG, Montain SJ, Ivy JL. Carbohydrate metabolism during intense exercise when hyperglycemic. J Appl Physiol 1991;70:834–40.

[195] Horowitz JF, Mora-Rodriguez R, Byerley LO, Coyle EF. Lipolytic suppression following carbohydrate ingestion limits fat oxidation during exercise. Am J Physiol Endocrinol Metab 1997;36:E768–75.

[196] Rennie MJ, Winder WW, Holloszy JO. A sparing effect of increased plasma free fatty acids on muscle and liver glycogen content in the exercising rat. Biochem J 1976;156:647–55.

[197] Hickson RC, Rennie MJ, Conlee RK, Winder WW, Holloszy JO. Effects of increased plasma free fatty acids on glycogen utilization and endurance. J Appl Physiol 1977;43:829–33.

[198] Odland LM, Heigenhauser GJF, Wong D, Hollidge-Horvat MG, Spriet LJ. Effects of increased fat availability on fat-carbohydrate interaction during prolonged exercise in men. Am J Physiol Regulatory Integr Comp Physiol 1998;43:R894–902.

[199] Gollnick PD, Piehl K, Saubert CW, Armstrong RB, Saltin B. Diet, exercise, and glycogen changes in human muscle fibers. J Appl Physiol 1972;33:421–5.

[200] Gollnick PD, Pernow B, Essen B, Jansson E, Saltin B. Availability of glycogen and plasma FFA for substrate utilization in leg muscle of man during exercise. Clin Physiol 1981;1:27–42.

[201] Shearer J, Marchand I, Tarnopolsky MA, Dyck DJ, Graham TE. Pro- and macroglycogenolysis during repeated exercise: roles of glycogen content and phosphorylase activation. J Appl Physiol 2001;90:880–8.

[202] Wojtaszewski JFP, MacDonald C, Nielsen JN, Hellsten Y, Hardie DG, Kemp BE, et al. Regulation of 5'AMP-activated protein kinase activity and substrate utilization in exercising human skeletal muscle. Am J Physiol Endocrinol Metab 2003;284:E813–22.

[203] Weltan SM, Bosch AN, Dennis SC, Noakes TD. Influence of muscle glycogen content on metabolic regulation. Am J Physiol Endocrinol Metab 1998;274:E72–82.

[204] Weltan SM, Bosch AN, Dennis SC, Noakes TD. Preexercise muscle glycogen content affects metabolism during exercise despite maintenance of hyperglycemia. Am J Physiol Endocrinol Metab 1998;274:E83–8.

[205] Hargreaves M, McConell G, Proietto J. Influence of muscle glycogen on glycogenolysis and glucose uptake during exercise in humans. J Appl Physiol 1995;78:288–92.

[206] Arkinstall MJ, Bruce CR, Clark SA, Rickards CA, Burke LM, Hawley JA. Regulation of fuel metabolism by preexercise muscle glycogen content and exercise intensity. J Appl Physiol 2004;97:2275–83.

[207] Spencer, M.K.; Yan, Z.; Katz, A.. Effect of low glycogen on carbohydrate and energy metabolism in human muscle during exercise. *Am. J. Physiol. Cell Physiol*. 31, 1992, C975-C979.

[208] Margolis LM, Wilson MA, Whitney CC, Carrigan CT, Murphy NE, Hatch AM, et al. Exercising with low muscle glycogen content increases fat oxidation and decreases endogenous, but not exogenous carbohydrate oxidation. Metab Clin Exp 2019;97:1–8.

[209] McConell G, Fabris S, Proietto J, Hargreaves M. Effects of carbohydrate ingestion on glucose kinetics during exercise. J Appl Physiol 1994;77:1537–41.

[210] Rauch HGL, Hawley JA, Noakes TD, Dennis SC. Fuel metabolism during ultra-endurance exercise. Pflug Arch 1998;436:211–19.

[211] Bosch AN, Weltan SM, Dennis SC, Noakes TD. Fuel substrate kinetics of carbohydrate loading differs from that of carbohydrate ingestion during prolonged exercise. Metabolism 1996;45:415–23.

[212] Hawley JH, Bosch AN, Weltan SM, Dennis SC, Noakes TD. Effect of glucose ingestion or glucose infusion on fuel substrate kinetics during prolonged exercise. Eur J Appl Physiol 1994;68:381–9.

[213] Hawley JH, Bosch AN, Weltan SM, Dennis SC, Noakes TD. Glucose kinetics during prolonged exercise in euglycaemic and hyperglycaemic subjects. Pflug Arch 1994;426:378–86.

[214] Jenkins AB, Chrisholm DJ, Ho JKY, Kraegen EW. Exercise-induced hepatic glucose output is precisely sensitive to the rate of systemic glucose supply. Metabolism 1985;34:431–6.

[215] Newsholme E, Leech T. Chapter 6. Carbohydrate metabolism. In: Newsholme E, Leech T, editors. Functional biochemistry in health and disease. West Sussex, UK: Wiley-Blackwell; 2009.

[216] Acheson KJ, Schutz Y, Bessard T, Anantharaman K, Flatt J-P, Jequier E. Glycogen storage capacity and de novo lipogenesis during massive carbohydrate overfeeding in man. Am J Clin Nutr 1988;48:240–7.

[217] Parks EJ. Effect of dietary carbohydrate on triglyceride metabolism in humans. J Nutr 2001;131:2772S–4S.

[218] Gonzalez JT, Fuchs CJ, Betts JA, van Loon LJC. Liver glycogen metabolism during and after prolonged endurance-type exercise. Am J Physiol Endocrinol Metab 2016;311:E543–53.

[219] Izumida Y, Yahagi N, Takeuchi Y, Nishi M, Shikama A, Takarada A, et al. Glycogen shortage during fasting triggers liver–brain–adipose neurocircuitry to facilitate fat utilization. Nat Comm 2013;4:2930.

[220] Yahagi N. Hepatic control of energy metabolism via the autonomic nervous system. J Atheroscler Thromb 2017;24:14–18.

[221] Wasserman DH. Four grams of glucose. Am J Physiol Endocrinol Metab 2009;296:E11–21.

[222] Romijn JA, Coyle EF, Sidossis LS, Gastaldelli A, Horowitz JF, Endert E, et al. Regulation of endogenous fat and carbohydrate metabolism in relation to exercise intensity and duration. Am J Physiol Endocrinol Metab 1993;28:E380–91.

[223] Trimmer JK, Schwarz J-M, Casazza GA, Horning MA, Rodriguez N, Brooks GA. Measurement of gluconeogenesis in exercising men by mass isotopomer distribution analysis. J Appl Physiol 2002;93:233–41.

[224] Jeukendrup A, Moseley L, Mainwaring GL, Samuels S, Perry S, Mann CH. Exogenous carbohydrate oxidation during ultraendurance exercise. J Appl Physiol 2006;100:1134–41.

[225] Owen OE, Morgan AP, Kemp HG, Sullivan JM, Herrera MG, Cahill GF. Brain metabolism during fasting. J Clin Invest 1967;46:1589–95.

[226] Matsui T, Ishikawa T, Ito H, Okamoto M, Inoue K, Lee M-C, et al. Brain glycogen supercompensation following exhaustive exercise. J Physiol 2012;590:607–16.

[227] Matsui T, Omuro H, Liu Y-F, Soya M, Shima T, McEwan BS, et al. Astrocytic glycogen-derived lactate fuels the brain during exhaustive exercise to maintain endurance capacity. Proc Nat Acad Sci 2017;114:6358–63.

[228] Webster CC, Noakes TD, Chacko SK, Smith JA. Gluconeogenesis during endurance exercise in cyclists habituated to a long-term low-carbohydrate high-fat diet. J Physiol 2016;594:4389–405.

[229] Owen OE. Ketone bodies as a fuel for the brain during starvation. Biochem Mol Biol Edu 2005;33:246–51.

[230] Noakes TD. Fatigue is a brain-derived emotion that regulates the exercise behavior to ensure the protection of whole body homeostasis. Front Physiol 2012;3:82.

[231] Auer RN. Hypoglycemic brain damage. Metab Brain Dis 2004;19:169–75.

[232] Roh E, Song DK, Kim M-S. Emerging role of the brain in the homeostatic regulation of energy and glucose metabolism. Exp Mol Med 2016;48:e216.

[233] Nybo L, Moller K, Pedersen BK, Nielsen B, Secher NH. Association between fatigue and failure to preserve cerebral energy turnover during prolonged exercise. Acta Physiol Scand 2003;179:67–74.

[234] Nybo L. CNS fatigue and prolonged exercise: effect of glucose supplementation. Med Sci Sports Exerc 2003;35:589–94.

[235] Coggan AR, Kohrt WM, Spina RJ, Bier DM, Holloszy JO. Endurance training decreases plasma glucose turnover and oxidation during moderate-intensity exercise in men. J Appl Physiol 1990;68:990–6.

[236] Coggan AR. Plasma glucose metabolism during exercise: effect of endurance training in humans. Sports Med 1997;29:620–7.

[237] Fitts RH, Booth FW, Winder WW, Holloszy JO. Skeletal muscle respiratory capacity, endurance, and glycogen utilization. Am J Physiol 1975;228:1029–33.

[238] Maughan RJ, Burke LM, Dvorak J, Larson-Meyer DE, Peeling P, Phillips SM, et al. IOC consensus statement: dietary supplements and the high-performance athlete. Br J Sports Med 2018;52(7):439–55. Available from: https://doi.org/10.1136/bjsports-2018-099027.

[239] Peeling P, Castell LM, Derave W, de Hon O, Burke LM. Sports foods and dietary supplements for optimal function and performance enhancement in track-and-field athletes. Int J Sport Nutr Exerc Metab 2019;29(2):198–209. Available from: https://doi.org/10.1123/ijsnem.2018-0271.

[240] Baur DA, Vargas F, de CS, Bach CW, Garvey JA, Ormsbee MJ. Slow-absorbing modified starch before and during prolonged cycling increases fat oxidation and gastrointestinal distress without changing performance. Nutrients 2016. Available from: https://doi.org/10.3390/nu8070392.

[241] Burke LM, Hawley JA, Wong SHS, Jeukendrup AE. Carbohydrates for training and competition. J Sports Sci 2011. Available from: https://doi.org/10.1080/02640414.2011.585473.

[242] de Oliveira EP, Burini RC. Carbohydrate-dependent, exercise-induced gastrointestinal distress. Nutrients 2014. Available from: https://doi.org/10.3390/nu6104191.

[243] Pöchmüller M, Schwingshackl L, Colombani PC, Hoffmann G. A systematic review and meta-analysis of carbohydrate benefits associated with randomized controlled competition-based performance trials. J Int Soc Sports Nutr 2016. Available from: https://doi.org/10.1186/s12970-016-0139-6.

[244] Quinones MD, Lemon PWR. Hydrothermally modified corn starch ingestion attenuates soccer skill performance decrements in the second half of a simulated soccer match. Int J Sport Nutr Exerc Metab 2019. Available from: https://doi.org/10.1123/ijsnem.2018-0217.

[245] Peart DJ. Quantifying the effect of carbohydrate mouth rinsing on exercise performance. J Strength Cond Res 2017. Available from: https://doi.org/10.1519/JSC.0000000000001741.

[246] Jeukendrup AE, Thielen JJ, Wagenmakers AJ, Brouns F, Saris WH. Effect of medium-chain triacylglycerol and carbohydrate ingestion during exercise on substrate utilization and subsequent cycling performance. Am J Clin Nutr 1998;67(3):397–404.

[247] Clegg ME. Medium-chain triglycerides are advantageous in promoting weight loss although not beneficial to exercise performance. Int J Food Sci Nutr 2010. Available from: https://doi.org/10.3109/09637481003702114.

[248] Jäger R, Kerksick CM, Campbell BI, et al. International society of sports nutrition position stand: protein and exercise. J Int Soc Sports Nutr 2017. Available from: https://doi.org/10.1186/s12970-017-0177-8.

[249] Valenzuela PL, Morales JS, Castillo-García A, Lucia A. Acute ketone supplementation and exercise performance: a systematic review and meta-analysis of randomized controlled trials. Int J Sports Physiol Perform 2020;15(3):298–308.

[250] Margolis LM, O'Fallon KS. Utility of ketone supplementation to enhance physical performance: a systematic review. Adv Nutr 2020. Available from: https://doi.org/10.1093/advances/nmz104.

[251] Poffé C, Ramaekers M, Van Thienen R, Hespel P. Ketone ester supplementation blunts overreaching symptoms during endurance training overload. J Physiol 2019. Available from: https://doi.org/10.1113/JP277831.

[252] Kreider RB, Kalman DS, Antonio J, et al. International Society of Sports Nutrition position stand: safety and efficacy of creatine supplementation in exercise, sport, and medicine. J Int Soc Sports Nutr 2017. Available from: https://doi.org/10.1186/s12970-017-0173-z.

[253] Kaviani M, Shaw K, Chilibeck PD. Benefits of creatine supplementation for vegetarians compared to omnivorous athletes: a systematic review. Int J Env Res Public Health 2020. Available from: https://doi.org/10.3390/ijerph17093041.

[254] Grgic J, Grgic I, Pickering C, et al. Infographic. Wake up and smell the coffee: caffeine supplementation and exercise performance. Br J Sports Med 2020. Available from: https://doi.org/10.1136/bjsports-2019-101097.

[255] Stecker RA, Harty PS, Jagim AR, Candow DG, Kerksick CM. Timing of ergogenic aids and micronutrients on muscle and exercise performance. J Int Soc Sports Nutr 2019. Available from: https://doi.org/10.1186/s12970-019-0304-9.

[256] Salinero JJ, Lara B, Del Coso J. Effects of acute ingestion of caffeine on team sports performance: a systematic review and meta-analysis. Res Sport Med 2019. Available from: https://doi.org/10.1080/15438627.2018.1552146.

[257] Burke LM. Practical issues in evidence-based use of performance supplements: supplement interactions, repeated use and individual responses. Sport Med 2017. Available from: https://doi.org/10.1007/s40279-017-0687-1.

[258] Spriet LL. Exercise and sport performance with low doses of caffeine. Sport Med 2014. Available from: https://doi.org/10.1007/s40279-014-0257-8.

[259] Burke LM. Caffeine and sports performance. Appl Physiol Nutr Metab 2008;33:1319–34. Available from: https://doi.org/10.1139/H08-130.

[260] Peeling P, Binnie MJ, Goods PSR, Sim M, Burke LM. Evidence-based supplements for the enhancement of athletic performance. Int J Sport Nutr Exerc Metab 2018. Available from: https://doi.org/10.1123/ijsnem.2017-0343.

[261] McNaughton LR, Gough L, Deb S, Bentley D, Sparks SA. Recent developments in the use of sodium bicarbonate as an ergogenic aid. Curr Sports Med Rep 2016. Available from: https://doi.org/10.1249/JSR.0000000000000283.

[262] Hadzic M, Eckstein ML, Schugardt M. The impact of sodium bicarbonate on performance in response to exercise duration in athletes: a systematic review. J Sport Sci Med 2019. Available from: https://doi.org/10.25932/publishup-42807.

[263] Carr AJ, Sharma AP, Ross ML, Welvaert M, Slater GJ, Burke LM. Chronic ketogenic low carbohydrate high fat diet has minimal effects on acid–base status in elite athletes. Nutrients 2018. Available from: https://doi.org/10.3390/nu10020236.

[264] Trexler ET, Smith-Ryan AE, Stout JR, et al. International society of sports nutrition position stand: beta-alanine. J Int Soc Sports Nutr 2015. Available from: https://doi.org/10.1186/s12970-015-0090-y.

[265] Saunders B, Elliott-Sale K, Artioli GG, et al. β-Alanine supplementation to improve exercise capacity and performance: a systematic review and meta-analysis. Br J Sports Med 2017. Available from: https://doi.org/10.1136/bjsports-2016-096396.

[266] Rojas-Valverde D, Montoya-Rodríguez J, Azofeifa-Mora C, Sanchez-Urena B. Effectiveness of beetroot juice derived nitrates supplementation on fatigue resistance during repeated-sprints: a systematic review. Crit Rev Food Sci Nutr 2020. Available from: https://doi.org/10.1080/10408398.2020.1798351.

[267] San Juan AF, Dominguez R, Lago-Rodríguez Á, Montoya JJ, Tan R, Bailey SJ. Effects of dietary nitrate supplementation on weightlifting exercise performance in healthy adults: a systematic review. Nutrients 2020. Available from: https://doi.org/10.3390/nu12082227.

[268] Greco T, Glenn TC, Hovda DA, Prins ML. Ketogenic diet decreases oxidative stress and improves mitochondrial respiratory complex activity. J Cereb Blood Flow Metab 2016. Available from: https://doi.org/10.1177/0271678X15610584.

[269] Senefeld JW, Wiggins CC, Regimbal RJ, Dominelli PB, Baker SE, Joyner MJ. Ergogenic effect of nitrate supplementation: a systematic review and meta-analysis. Med Sci Sports Exerc 2020. Available from: https://doi.org/10.1249/MSS.0000000000002363.

[270] Décombaz J, Arnaud MJ, Milon H, et al. Energy metabolism of medium-chain triglycerides versus carbohydrates during exercise. Eur J Appl Physiol Occup Physiol 1983;52(1):9–14.

[271] Van Zyl CG, Lambert EV, Hawley JA, Noakes TD, Dennis SC. Effects of medium-chain triglyceride ingestion on fuel metabolism and cycling performance. J Appl Physiol 1996;80(6):2217–25.

[272] Jeukendrup AE, Saris WH, Schrauwen P, Brouns F, Wagenmakers AJ. Metabolic availability of medium-chain triglycerides coingested with carbohydrates during prolonged exercise. J Appl Physiol 1995;79(3):756–62.

[273] Goedecke JH, Elmer-English R, Dennis SC, Schloss I, Noakes TD, Lambert EV. Effects of medium-chain triaclyglycerol ingested with carbohydrate on metabolism and exercise performance. Int J Sport Nutr 1999;9(1):35–47.

[274] Shaw DM, Merien F, Braakhuis A, Maunder E, Dulson DK. Exogenous ketone supplementation and keto-adaptation for endurance performance: disentangling the effects of two distinct metabolic states. Sports Med 2019;50(4):641–56.

[275] Margolis LM, O'Fallon KS. Utility of ketone supplementation to enhance physical performance: a systematic review. Adv Nutr 2019;31 (6):834–8.

[276] Soto-Mota A, Vansant H, Evans RD, Clarke K. Safety and tolerability of sustained exogenous ketosis using ketone monoester drinks for 28 days in healthy adults. Regulatory Toxicol Pharmacol 2019. Available from: https://doi.org/10.1016/j.yrtph.2019.104506.

[277] L KM, A SJ, N HP, et al. A pre-workout supplement of ketone salts, caffeine, and amino acids improves high-intensity exercise performance in keto-naïve and keto- adapted individuals. J Am Coll Nutr 2020;0(0):1–11.

[278] Stubbs BJ, Cox PJ, Kirk T, Evans RD, Clarke K. Gastrointestinal effects of exogenous ketone drinks are infrequent, mild, and vary according to ketone compound and dose. Int J Sport Nutr Exerc Metab 2019;29(6):596–603.

[279] Evans M, Egan B. Intermittent running and cognitive performance after ketone ester ingestion. Med Sci Sports Exerc 2018;50(11):2330–8.

[280] Leckey JJ, Ross ML, Quod M, Hawley JA, Burke LM. Ketone diester ingestion impairs time-trial performance in professional cyclists. Front Physiol 2017;8: 41–10.

[281] Shaw DM, Merien F, Braakhuis A, Plews D, Laursen P, Dulson DK. The effect of 1,3-butanediol on cycling time-trial performance. Int J Sport Nutr Exerc Metab 2019;29(5):466–73.

[282] Cox PJ, Kirk T, Ashmore T, et al. Nutritional ketosis alters fuel preference and thereby endurance performance in athletes. Cell Metab 2016;24(2):256–68.

[283] O'Malley T, Myette-Côté É, Durrer C, Little JP. Nutritional ketone salts increase fat oxidation but impair high-intensity exercise performance in healthy adult males. Appl Physiol Nutr Metab 2017;42(10):1031–5.

[284] Dearlove DJ. Nutritional ketoacidosis during incremental exercise in healthy athletes. *fphys-10-00290tex*, 2019; 1–6.

[285] Evans M, McSwiney FT, Brady AJ, Egan B. No benefit of ingestion of a ketone monoester supplement on 10-km running performance. Med Sci Sports Exerc 2019;51(12):2506–15.

[286] Faull OK. Beyond RPE: the perception of exercise under normal and ketotic conditions. *fphys-10-00229tex*, 2019; 1–10.

[287] Prins PJ, Koutnik AP, D'Agostino DP, et al. Effects of an exogenous ketone supplement on five-kilometer running performance. J Hum Kinetics 2020;72(1):115–27.

[288] Rodger S, Plews D, Laursen P, Driller MW. Oral β-hydroxybutyrate salt fails to improve 4-minute cycling performance following submaximal exercise. 2017; 6(1):26–31.

[289] Scott BE, Laursen PB, James LJ, et al. The effect of 1,3-butanediol and carbohydrate supplementation on running performance. J Sci Med Sport 20181–5.

[290] Waldman HS, Shepherd BD, Egan B, McAllister MJ. Exogenous ketone salts do not improve cognitive performance during a dual-stress challenge. Int J Sport Nutr Exerc Metab 2020;30(2):120–7.

[291] Hargreaves M, Spriet LL. Skeletal muscle energy metabolism during exercise. Nat Metab 2020. Available from: https://doi.org/10.1038/s42255-020-0251-4.

Chapter 10

Therapeutic fasting

Jason Fung[1], Connor Ostoich[1], Mateja Stephanovic[1], Nadia Pataguana[2] and Nasha Winters[3]

[1]*Scarborough Hospital Network, Scarborough, Ontario, Canada,* [2]*Public Health Collaboration, United Kingdom,* [3]*Metabolic Terrain Institute of Health, Wilmington, DE, United States*

10.1 Introduction

Fasting can be defined as the voluntary abstinence from food for religious, spiritual, health, political or any other reasons. Essentially, if one is not eating, one is fasting. It differs substantially from starvation because of the element of control. Starvation is involuntary, whereas fasting is entirely voluntary. A person who is starving wants to eat, but cannot, for various reasons such as poverty, war, civil unrest, or famine. A person who is fasting chooses not to eat food that is readily available. There is no standard duration, and one may begin or break a fast at any time.

Fasting has been practiced throughout human history. The ancient Greeks noted that most animals naturally avoid eating when sick, and deduced that fasting was a natural remedy for many types of illness, a sort of "fasting instinct." Fasting also significantly improves mental cognition. The legendary mathematician Pythagoras is said to have fasted for 40 days before exams. Later, he would also require that his own students fast prior to class to maximise learning [1]. Fasting for spiritual reasons remains part of almost every major religion in the world. Fasting is often prescribed on certain days of the year, commonly referred to as a "cleansing" or "purification" ritual.

Fasting is considered a part of the normal eating cycle—alternating feeding and fasting. If you eat your morning meal at 8am and your evening meal at 8 pm, there exists a 12-hour period of feeding and a 12-hour period of fasting. In the English language, the first meal is termed "break-fast," or the meal that breaks your fast, for this reason.

In the United States, daily fasting duration has significantly decreased. In 1977, the average American ate three times each day. A typical eating window lasted from 8 am to 6 pm (10 hours), balanced with 14 hours of fasting. Notably, obesity and type 2 diabetes were not nearly as large a problem as they are today. By the mid 2000s, the average American had increased the number of daily eating opportunities from three to almost six [2]. Snacking, which had previously been rare, had become an everyday event, significantly decreasing the daily fasting period (Fig. 10.1).

10.2 Physiology

10.2.1 Energy storage and retrieval

Food energy (calories) can be stored in two forms:

- Glycogen
- Body fat

The liver has limited capacity for glycogen so high insulin concentrations stimulate de novo *lipogenesis*, which converts any excess glucose into fatty acids. These fatty acids are then esterified with glycerol into triglycerides [3]. This newly created fat can be stored in the liver or exported through the bloodstream to fat deposits in other organs and adipocytes [3]. The major advantage of storing food energy as triglycerides is that there is effectively no upper limit.

Fasting represents the transition from the fed (high-insulin, storing energy) state to the fasted (low-insulin, using stored energy) state [4]. During fasting, the process of storing food energy (calories) is reversed. Falling insulin concentrations signal retrieval of previously stored energy. Hepatic glycogenolysis first provides glucose which, if storage is full, lasts approximately 24 hours. Afterwards, gluconeogenesis begins before lipolysis takes over. The transition from the fed to fasted state occurs classically in five stages, as described by Dr. George Cahill (Table 10.1) [5].

Ketogenic. DOI: https://doi.org/10.1016/B978-0-12-821617-0.00003-6

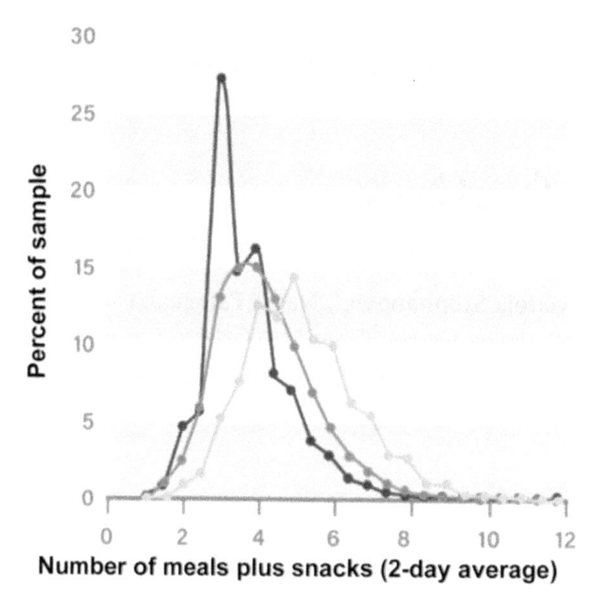

FIGURE 10.1 The average number of meals and snacks consumed by adults increased from three per day in 1977–78 to almost six per day in 2003–06 [2].

TABLE 10.1 The five stages of metabolism.

Phase	Events
Feeding	• Serum glucose and insulin concentrations rise • Excess glucose stored as glycogen (*glycogenesis*) or converted to fat (*de novo lipogenesis*)
Post-absorptive phase 6–24 h after beginning fasting	• Serum glucose and insulin concentrations fall • Breakdown of glycogen (*glycogenolysis*)
Gluconeogenesis 24 h to 2 days after beginning fasting	• Breakdown of amino acids for conversion to glucose (*gluconeogenesis*)
Ketosis 2–3 days after beginning fasting	• Breakdown of triglycerides (*lipolysis*) • Most tissues, except for brain, switch to triglyceride metabolism • Glycerol backbone is metabolised for gluconeogenesis • Fatty acids are metabolised into ketone bodies, capable of crossing the blood-brain-barrier ◦ Ketones, including beta-hydroxybutyrate and acetoacetate, can increase over seventy-fold
Protein conservation phase 5 days after beginning fasting	• Growth hormone maintains lean mass [6] • Blood glucose is maintained by glycerol metabolism and gluconeogenesis

During fasting, blood glucose concentrations are maintained by breaking down stored glycogen and producing new glucose through gluconeogenesis [5].

Fasting is simply the natural process of switching fuel sources from food energy to stored sources of energy (predominantly glycogen and body fat) [7]. Periods of low food availability have always been a natural part of human history and our bodies have evolved these mechanisms to help us survive [8].

10.2.2 Water and electrolyte balance

Fasting, due to lower insulin concentrations, reduces sodium reabsorption in the proximal tubule of the nephron [9]. This diuretic effect has the potential to lower blood pressure [9].

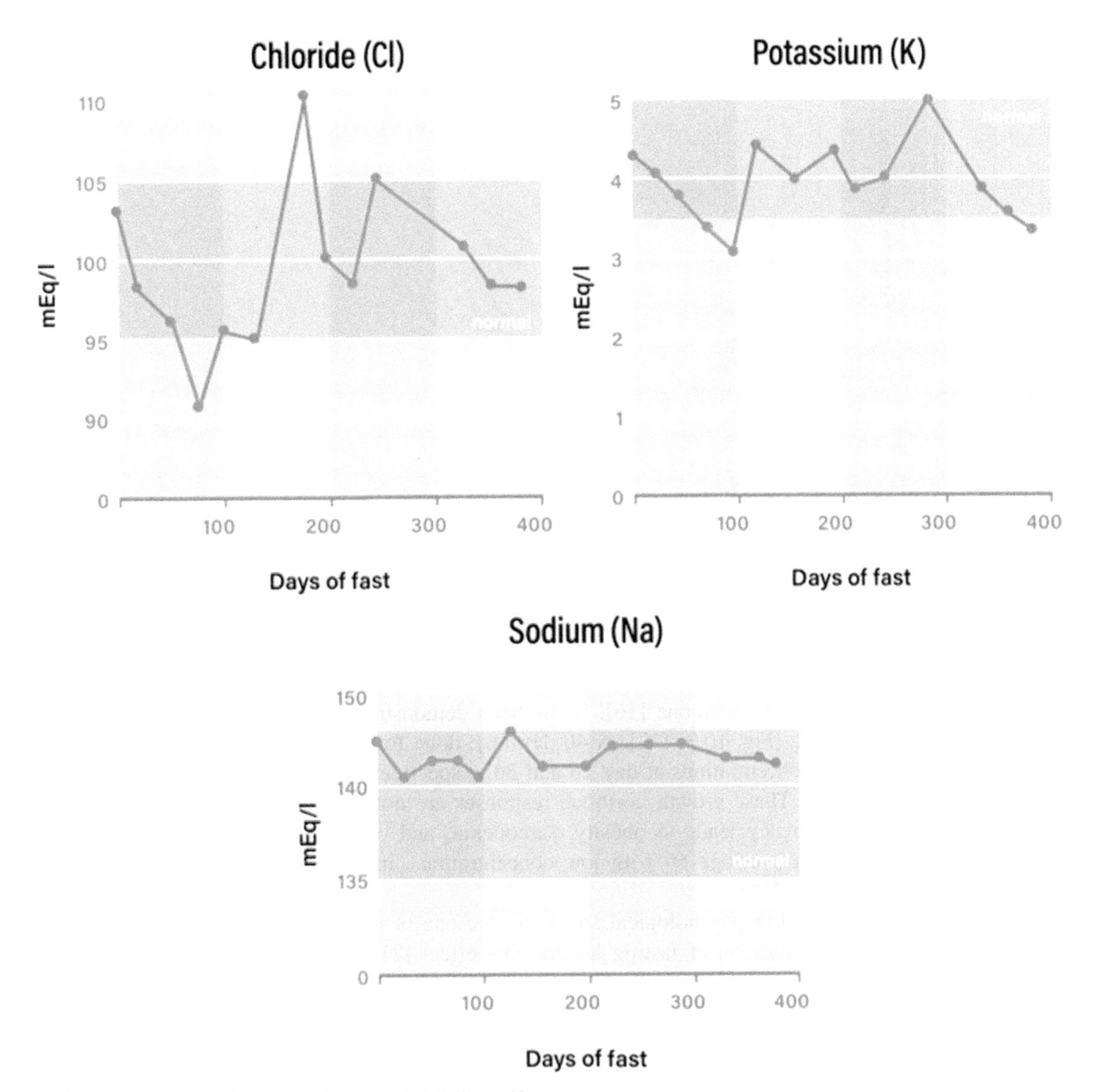

FIGURE 10.2 Electrolytes remain stable during extended fasting [12].

On the other hand, serum electrolyte concentrations, including sodium, potassium, and chloride, are tightly controlled and vary little during fasting, even for extended periods [10]. During prolonged fasting, the kidneys reabsorb and retain virtually all of the electrolytes that are filtered at the glomerulus [10]. Accordingly, extended studies of fasting have found no evidence of electrolyte imbalances, and salt supplementation is rarely required [11].

Serum potassium, magnesium, calcium, and phosphorus concentrations may decrease slightly during fasting, but they generally remain in the normal range (Fig. 10.2) [11]. If necessary, a general multivitamin supplement can provide the recommended daily amount of micronutrients. A case report of a supervised 117-day fast, maintained only on water and vitamins, demonstrated no change in serum electrolytes, lipids, proteins, or amino acid concentrations [11]. Another case report of a 382-day therapeutic fast, demonstrates that maintenance with only a multivitamin caused no ill effects on that individual's health [12].

10.2.3 Counterregulatory hormones

Fasting decreases serum insulin concentrations, while increasing the concentrations of other hormones, including glucagon, adrenalin, noradrenalin, growth hormone, and cortisol [13]. Collectively, these so-called counterregulatory hormones activate the sympathetic nervous system [14].

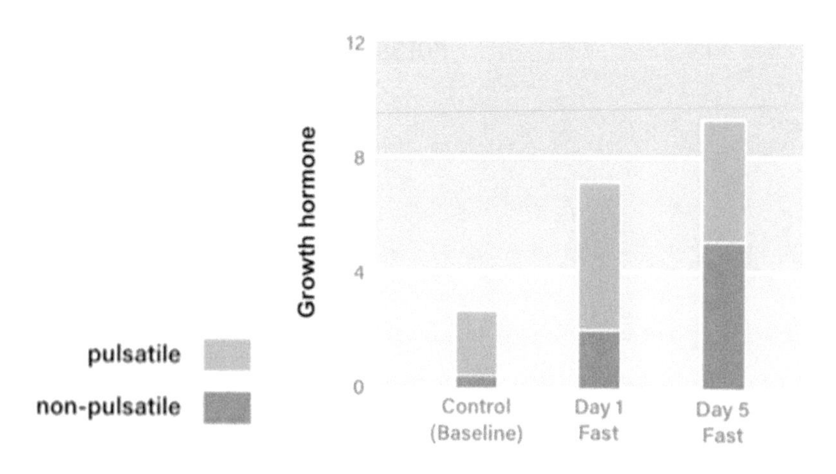

FIGURE 10.3 Fasting significantly increases growth hormone [17].

Increased adrenaline (epinephrine) and noradrenalin (norepinephrine) concentrations facilitate glycogenolysis and lipolysis. They can boost resting energy expenditure by up to 12% during a 4-day fast [1].

Growth hormone increases lipolysis by stimulating key enzymes, such as lipoprotein lipase and hepatic lipase [1]. This reduces the need for glucose and helps maintain stable blood glucose concentrations during fasting [15]. Overeating suppresses growth hormone concentrations by as much as 80% [1]. Whereas fasting is the most potent stimulus for the natural secretion of growth hormone [16]. It has been demonstrated that growth hormone secretion more than doubled over 5 days of fasting (Fig. 10.3) [17]. A 40-day fast, done for religious reasons, resulted in 1250% and 518% increased growth hormone concentrations at day 26 and 36, respectively [8]. A 2-day fast increased growth hormone concentrations fivefold [18]. These growth hormone responses are not reproducible with very low-calorie diets [18]. Adult growth hormone deficiency leads to obesity, sarcopenia, and osteopenia in both men and women [19]. Replacing growth hormone in men over age 60 with low concentrations, increased lean mass by 3.7 kg (8.2 lb) and decreased fat mass by 2.4 kg (5.2 lb) [19].

Cortisol, released during physical or psychological stress, is also one of the counter-regulatory hormones [20], and rises during acute fasting. Longer duration of fasting lessens this effect [21], and even a 72-hour fast failed to raise concentrations significantly [22].

10.2.4 Basal metabolic rate

Daily energy (caloric) reduction is known to reduce the basal metabolic rate (BMR) by 25%–30% [23], which limits weight loss efforts. Conversely, fasting does not significantly reduce BMR, due to the protective effect of increased counterregulatory hormones [14]. Increased sympathetic tone and noradrenalin concentrations allow glycogenolysis, gluconeogenesis, and lipolysis to proceed, ensuring adequate provision of energy from body stores [14]. Since body stores provide adequate energy, there is no need to reduce metabolic rate. This is the precise reason why humans carry glycogen and body fat, to be used for energy when none is available. When sufficient stores of body fat are available, there is no need to reduce BMR.

During a 4-day fast, average resting energy expenditure increased from 3.97 to 4.43 kJ/min and VO_2 increased from 199 to 229 mL/min; likely in part driven by the 117% increase in serum noradrenaline concentrations (Fig. 10.4) [14]. Another study found that a 72-hour fast increased resting energy expenditure from 1684 to 1729 kcal over 24 hours, largely due to increased noradrenaline [24] and adrenaline [25,26] spillover from adipose tissue. In longer-term studies, a 22-alternate-day fast resulted in no measurable decrease in BMR, although fat oxidation increased by 58% and carbohydrate oxidation decreased by 53%. Serum fatty acids concentrations also increased over 370% as the body switched over from burning glucose to burning stored fats [27].

10.2.5 Lean body mass

Fasting appears to have little effect on lean body mass as the body switches to lipolysis for energy, sparing protein in the process (Fig. 10.5). Adipocytes store triglycerides as a potential source of energy in the body [28], and proteins and

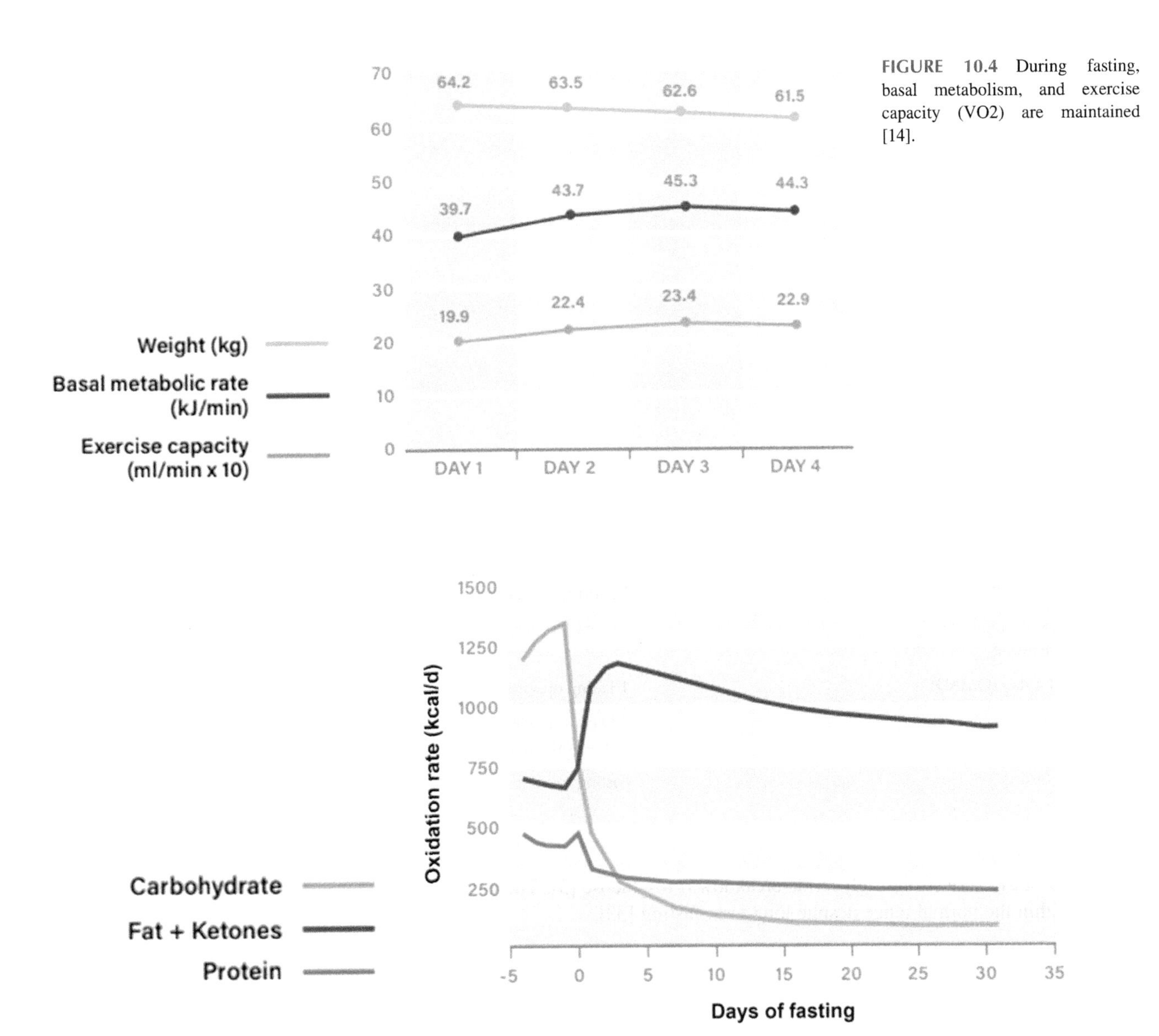

FIGURE 10.4 During fasting, basal metabolism, and exercise capacity (VO2) are maintained [14].

FIGURE 10.5 During fasting, the body switches from burning carbohydrates to fat for energy. Protein is spared [23].

lean mass are generally preserved unless body fat is unavailable. The increased adrenaline and growth hormone concentrations during fasting lead to the preservation of fat-free mass (lean muscles and bones) [14,29]. In a study of alternate-day fasting over 70 days, a 5.8% decrease in weight was demonstrated, with an 11.4% fat mass reduction, yet lean mass (muscle and bone) was unchanged (Fig. 10.6) [30]. Furthermore, a 32-week study of alternate daily fasting found no significant decrease in lean mass [31].

10.2.6 Blood glucose concentrations

Multiple physiological mechanisms maintain blood glucose concentrations within the normal range during fasting. Hepatic glycogenolysis may provide sufficient glucose for 24 hours, after which gluconeogenesis begins [14]. In conjunction, most tissues, other than the brain, convert to triglyceride metabolism to conserve glucose [32]. Ketone bodies are produced, which may cross the blood-brain-barrier to provide energy for the brain, further reducing glucose requirements [14]. After 4 days of fasting, approximately 75% of the energy used by the brain is provided by ketone metabolism [5]. One does not need to ingest glucose in order for the brain to function and for blood glucose concentrations to remain normal. During longer fasts, the body enters the protein conservation phase with a combination of lowered glucose requirements and

	Baseline	Alternate-Day Fasting
	Day 1	Day 70
Body weight (kg)	96.4 ± 5.3	90.8 ± 4.8*
BMI (kg/m²)	33.7 ± 1.0	31.4 ± 0.9*
Fat mass (kg)	43.0 ± 2.2	38.1 ± 1.8*
Fat-free mass (kg)	52.0 ± 3.6	51.9 ± 3.7
Waist circumference (cm)	109 ± 2	105 ± 3

FIGURE 10.6 There was no loss of fat-free mass during 70 days of alternate-day fasting [30].

TABLE 10.2 Fasting regimens.

Fasting regimen	Feeding pattern
Intermittent fasting/time restricted feeding	12–23 h of fasting/1- to 12-h eating period
One meal a day (OMAD)	1 Eating opportunity in a 24-h period
5:2 Fasting	5 Days eating regularly with 2 days of very low-calorie consumption (500–700 calories)
Extended fasting	Fasting more than 24 h

conversion of glycerol (from triglyceride breakdown) to glucose [5]. These mechanisms all maintain serum glucose concentrations within the normal range despite long-term fasting [33].

10.3 Therapeutic fasting

10.3.1 Fasting regimens

There is no standard definition or period of fasting. Fasting regimens generally differ with respect to two variables:

1. What may be consumed
2. The duration of the fasting period.

Classically, fasts only allow the consumption of water, but many variations exist. Dry fasting prohibits food or drinks and thus, also produces dehydration. More lenient fasting variations allow non-caloric beverages like teas and herbal teas, a limited number of calories, or certain foods. The duration of fasts also vary and include time restricted feeding [34,35], the 5:2 diet [36], alternate-day fasting [37,38], and extended multi-day fasting [39] (Table 10.2).

Therapeutic fasting regimens offer many advantages compared to other diets including:

- Simplicity
- Convenience
- Time-saving
- Effectiveness
- Unlimited power
- Flexibility
- Works with any diet

10.3.2 Benefits of fasting

Calorie restriction of 15% in animal and human studies reduces many risk factors for age-related diseases including type 2 diabetes mellitus, cancer, and cardiovascular disease [40]. Animal studies also suggest a reduction in inflammation [41,42]. Protein restriction alone may confer some of these benefits [43], however, it can also lead to increased frailty and sarcopenia [44]. The benefits of calorie restriction are generally believed to be mediated by changes in cellular substrates like NAD^+ and AMP, with subsequent downstream changes in nutrient sensing pathways like sirtuins (SIRT1) [45], AMP-activated protein kinase (AMPK) [46], insulin/insulin-like growth factor (IGF-1) [47], mammalian target of rapamycin (mTOR) and phosphoinositide 3-kinase (PI3K) [48]. While beneficial, chronic calorie restriction is difficult or impossible to sustain for most people [49]. This reveals the need for alternative dietary interventions, such as IF, that may optimise healthspan, while increasing compliance and minimising side effects [50]. Of note, fasting involves both a restrictive and a refeeding phase, which may be accompanied by regenerative processes such as autophagy, and which may not be activated during chronic calorie restriction [51].

Fasting is indicated in the treatment of obesity and type 2 diabetes mellitus [52]. A recent literature review listed 27 trials of IF which produced weight loss of 0.8%–13%, with no serious adverse effects [53]. However, several more recent randomised controlled trials suggest that fasting may not be more effective than chronic calorie restriction [38,54]. Given the known poor results of calorie restricted diets in the treatment of obesity though, fasting remains a viable and interesting alternative.

In humans, the liver is the main reservoir of glucose in the form of glycogen. Fasting depletes hepatic glycogen stores and it typically decreases serum glucose concentrations (from 4.9 to 3.5 mmol/L over 4 days) and insulin concentrations (from 71 to 59 pmol/L over 4 days) [14], accompanied by a switch in metabolic mode toward fat burning. This combination has great potential for the treatment and prevention of type 2 diabetes; [55,56] although larger studies are still required. Fasting may represent a promising therapeutic and preventative avenue for many other chronic conditions also associated with insulin resistance/hyperinsulinemia [57]. Several studies have shown more metabolic benefits using fasting when compared to chronic caloric restriction [58,59]. Furthermore, fasting has exhibited potential therapeutic effects in fatty liver disease [60].

10.3.2.1 Aging and longevity

Fasting extends longevity in multiple animal models [61,62]. It activates many molecular mechanisms with varied anti-aging benefits, potentially accomplished through reduced activity of nutrient sensing pathways including insulin, mTOR, and AMPK [63]. The pharmacologic inhibition of mTOR extends lifespan in animals [64].

Fasting may improve brain function, aging, and memory [65]. A higher body mass is associated with decreased blood flow to brain regions involved in attention, focus, reasoning and more complex, abstract thought [66]. Hence through the mechanism of weight loss, fasting represents a promising intervention. Additionally, animal studies suggest that IF slows the age-related deterioration of neurons and the symptoms of Alzheimer's disease, Parkinson's disease, and Huntington's disease [67].

Aging rats markedly improved motor coordination, cognition, learning and memory with fasting, displaying increased brain connectivity and new neuron growth from stem cells [63]. Brain-derived neurotrophic factor (BDNF), which supports neuron growth and memory, is significantly increased in fasting mice [63]. In rat studies, a 40% reduction in calories consumed increased the synaptic and electrical activity in the brain, and significantly improves memory [67]. Concerns that fasting may reduce cognitive performance are not substantiated. Human studies of fasting find no impairment in attentional focus, reaction time, memory, activity, sleep, or mood [68,69].

10.3.2.2 Autophagy

The mTOR pathway is the key regulator of autophagy, the natural process that removes damaged, old or unnecessary cellular components [70]. Increased nutrient availability, as detected by increased concentrations of glucose, insulin and dietary amino acids, increase mTOR and suppress autophagy [70]. Low mTOR activity during periods of very low nutrient availability, such as fasting, stimulates autophagy, an effect not always seen in chronic caloric restriction [63]. The presence of hepatic glycogen and body fat is irrelevant for mTOR and autophagy, as mTOR dormancy is predominantly related to short-term nutrient availability [71].

Certain diseases, like Alzheimer's disease [72] and cancer [73,74], are known to be associated with disordered autophagy. Accordingly, the role of fasting in the inhibition of mTOR and the stimulation of autophagy provides an interesting prospect for cancer prevention; [75] in fact, multiple mTOR inhibitors have already been approved by the Food and Drug Administration (FDA) for cancer treatment, with many more currently in clinical trials [76]. Moreover,

TABLE 10.3 Fasting cautions and contraindications.

Absolute contraindications	Caution
• Children under 18 years of age • Severely malnourished or underweight individuals • Pregnant women • Breastfeeding women	• Gout [78] • Taking medications or supplements (e.g., metformin, iron, magnesium) • Type 1 or type 2 diabetes • GERD • Gallstones [79] • History of anorexia nervosa

fasting demonstrates potential to protect normal cells against damage from chemotherapy, while sensitising the cancer cells (see Chapter 7) [77].

10.3.3 Risks of fasting

10.3.3.1 Contraindications to extended fasting

Fasting restricts calories, but it also restricts the intake of vitamins, minerals, and other essential micronutrients. Consequently, specific populations at risk of under-nourishment should avoid extended fasts longer than 24 hours. Medical supervision is additionally recommended for those with certain medical conditions (see Table 10.3).

10.3.3.2 Refeeding syndrome

Refeeding syndrome is a potentially fatal condition, caused by rapid refeeding following a period of malnutrition [80]. Hypophosphatemia is the hallmark electrolyte imbalance, although hypokalemia, hyponatremia, and hypomagnesemia may also be problematic [80].

Refeeding syndrome is caused by sudden metabolic and hormonal changes that occur with rapid refeeding after a period of prolonged undernutrition; intracellular minerals become depleted while blood concentrations are still normal [80]. During refeeding, increased blood glucose concentrations lead to increased insulin and decreased glucagon secretion, stimulating fat and protein synthesis. This requires minerals like phosphate and magnesium, as well as cofactors like thiamine [80]. The intracellular shift may result in severe and occasionally fatal hypophosphatemia, as well as, less commonly, hypokalemia or hypomagnesemia [80]. The higher insulin concentrations during refeeding can also cause renal retention of salt and water, which may appear as swelling of the feet and ankles, termed "refeeding edema" [81].

The incidence of severe hypophosphatemia, however, is generally low, at an estimated 0.43% of hospitalised patients [82]. However, malnutrition and diabetic ketoacidosis are amongst the most important risk factors, with 10.4% and 14.6% respectively experiencing refeeding syndrome after a period of extended fasting [82]. Additional individuals at high risk include those with anorexia nervosa, chronic alcoholism, postoperative patients, oncology patients, and the elderly [83].

10.4 Conclusion

In conclusion, fasting is the voluntary abstinence from food that has been practiced throughout human history. It has become less common with today's increased prevalence of eating opportunities. However, it presents an intriguing option for combating aging and various medical diseases.

The transition from the fed, high-insulin state to the fasted, low-insulin state is classically described in five stages. As insulin level falls, counter-regulatory hormones including the concentrations of glucagon, adrenalin, noradrenalin, growth hormone and cortisol, all rise. The body maintains the ability to regulate electrolyte and glucose concentrations, even during prolonged fasts.

Fasting studies in both animals and humans have presented numerous potential physiologic and cognitive benefits. Fasting offers an opportunity to increase basal metabolic rate, while maintaining lean body mass. It may also improve brain function, counter aging, and extend lifespan. Furthermore, fasting may be indicated in the treatment and prevention of various diseases such as type 2 diabetes, obesity, fatty liver disease, and metabolic syndrome. Many fasting regimens can be incorporated into a daily eating routine, although certain populations with specific medical conditions should seek medical supervision before initiating a period of fasting.

Myth 1: Eating more often is healthy and helps control body weight.

Nadia Pataguana, ND

TheFastingMethod.com

Prior to 1977, not only did we eat more dietary fat and fewer refined grains, we also ate less often. The National Health and Nutrition Examination Survey (NHANES) study in 1977 found that most people ate three times per day: breakfast, lunch, and dinner [84]. Snacking was considered neither necessary nor healthy. Yet, many nutrition authorities now recommend eating more frequently to aid weight loss. This is likely due to heavy advertising by food companies. As no scientific study has ever proved that snacking causes weight loss or is even healthy. In fact, to the contrary, The Adventist Health Study [85] looked at the dietary habits of over 50,000 adults and found that the more often you eat, the heavier you are likely to be. The study also noted that the longer your nightly fast, the less you weigh. By 2004, most people were eating almost six times per day. Snacking has become the norm and likely plays a significant role in the current obesity crisis.

There really is no such thing as a healthy snack. Recent studies [86] show that fewer than 10% of people eat three times per day or less. The top 10% of people ate an astounding 10 times per day. Essentially, many people start eating as soon as they get up and don't stop until they go to bed. The median time during which people eat is 14.75 hours per day. For example, if they break their fast at 8 am, they don't, on average, put the last bite of food in their mouth until 10:45 pm. Practically the only time people stopped eating was while sleeping. This contrasts with a 1970s-era style of eating breakfast at 8 am and dinner at 6 pm, an eating duration of only 10 hours.

By reducing snacks, we allow our body the time it needs to digest the food and metabolise it, before putting more food into our mouths. One further problem with snacks is that they need to be relatively easy to carry (portable) and convenient, requiring little cooking. Snack foods are often highly processed and pre-packaged, containing refined grains and sugar, which do not require refrigeration. After all, very few people will grill a small piece of salmon for a mid-morning snack.

Myth 2: Food cravings develop in the absence of food.

Nadia Pataguana, ND

TheFastingMethod.com

One of the persistent myths about fasting is that it promotes hunger resulting in uncontrolled binging on processed food. Thus recommendations to eat six or seven times a day, to stave off those cravings. The research shows exactly the opposite. Constant eating feeds cravings. Conversely, eating less often reduces cravings and hunger. Research shows that severe caloric restriction is significantly more effective at reducing cravings than a higher-calorie (1200 kcal/day) diet [87,88]. Experience and literature on fasting, indicates that fasting, when done consistently, decreases hunger and helps control cravings [88]. Eating a moderately restricted diet may not reduce hunger or cravings [89]. People who reduce their sugar intake very close to zero, for example, find that their sweet tooth goes away [90]. In contrast, if you eat more sugar, cravings don't get better. They get worse.

Myth 3: Breakfast is the most important meal of the day.

Nadia Pataguana, ND

TheFastingMethod.com

The exact same food will elicit different insulin responses at different times of the day. A study showed that the same meal taken at dinner, compared to breakfast, produced 25%–50% more insulin [91]. Food is more fattening when you eat it later at night because more of the food energy is directed towards storage rather than usage.

The body's circadian rhythm also affects our appetite. Hunger is lowest in the morning and greatest in the evening, around 8:00 pm or so [92]. Other studies show that eating later at night results in a lower metabolic rate [93]. When metabolism is burning fewer calories, weight loss is harder.

So eating the largest meal late in the day is problematic for three reasons:

1. Eat more (due to increase appetite)
2. The food eaten is more fattening (due to double the rise in insulin)
3. Less energy expenditure (and more adipogenesis).

We tend to eat later only because of our work-life schedules, not because it is healthy. Since many people work or go to school during the day, we leave our main meal, which we eat as a family, until the evening. And this dinner often gets pushed later and later into the evening because of longer commuting times and more families in which both parents work outside the home.

Fasting fortifies the mind.

Nasha Winters, ND, F

Metabolic Terrain Institute of Health

The modern Western relationship with food is troubling, and it takes only a brief look at human evolution to understand why. Before modern luxuries, the nomadic lifestyle required humans to hunt and gather their food, which took time, effort, energy, and some luck. Like other wild species, early humans were at the mercy of the migratory patterns of animals and natural weather events. Bouts of feast and famine marked much of early nomadic life, and the species was built not only to withstand those conditions but also to thrive in them.

Our ancestors were alert during times of famine; they had to be in order to track, hunt, and secure their next meal. Unsurprisingly then, modern humans often report feeling invigorated, alive, and keenly in touch with the world around them when they practice intermittent fasting (de Cabo and Mattson) [62].

During the fasting process, glycogen stores are depleted and ketones are produced from adipose-cell-derived fatty acids. This metabolic switch is accompanied by cellular adaptation of neural networks in the brain. Intermittent fasting has been shown to increase the production of brain-derived neurotrophic factor (BDNF), which helps the brain to build more neurons and work more efficiently. Fasting also promotes neuroplasticity and makes the brain more resistant to injury and disease Mattson et al. [94].

If fasting sharpens our cognitive ability and mental acuity, then the opposite must also be true. In 2013, a population-based study examined the association of high energy intake on cognitive function. The study found an association between high energy intake and mild cognitive impairment Geda et al. [95]. The American colloquial expression, a "food coma" describes the sleepy, groggy, and lethargic feeling caused by overeating.

Interestingly, fasting is just now emerging as a possible preventative treatment for neurodegenerative diseases like Alzheimer's. In 2018, Shin et al., reported that fasting improved glucose tolerance and prevented memory loss in rats. They determined that intermittent fasting may prevent some of the metabolic pathologies associated with age-related memory decline.

References

[1] Hippocrates, Chadwick J, Lloyd GER, Mann WN. Hippocratic writings. Harmondswerth: Penguin Books; 1983.

[2] Popkin BM, Duffey KJ. Does hunger and satiety drive eating anymore? Increasing eating occasions and decreasing time between eating occasions in the United States. Am J Clin Nutr 2010;91(5):1342–7. Available from: https://doi.org/10.3945/ajcn.2009.28962.

[3] Ameer F, Scandiuzzi L, Hasnain S, Kalbacher H, Zaidi N. De novo lipogenesis in health and disease. Metabolism 2014;63(7):895–902. Available from: https://doi.org/10.1016/j.metabol.2014.04.003.

[4] Cohen P, Spiegelman BM. Cell biology of fat storage. Mol Biol Cell 2016;27(16):2523–7. Available from: https://doi.org/10.1091/mbc.e15-10-0749.

[5] Cahill GF. Fuel metabolism in starvation. Annu Rev Nutr 2006;26(1):1–22. Available from: https://doi.org/10.1146/annurev.nutr.26.061505.111258.

[6] Møller N, Jørgensen JOL. Effects of growth hormone on glucose, lipid, and protein metabolism in human subjects. Endocr Rev 2009;30(2):152–77. Available from: https://doi.org/10.1210/er.2008-0027.

[7] Izumida Y, Yahagi N, Takeuchi Y, et al. Erratum: corrigendum: glycogen shortage during fasting triggers liver–brain–adipose neurocircuitry to facilitate fat utilization. Nat Commun 2013;4(1). Available from: https://doi.org/10.1038/ncomms3930.

[8] Kerndt PR, Naughton JL, Driscoll CE, Loxterkamp DA. Fasting: the history, pathophysiology and complications. West J Med 1982;137(5):379–99.

[9] Heyman SN, Bursztyn M, Szalat A, Muszkat M, Abassi Z. Fasting-induced natriuresis and SGLT: a new hypothesis for an old enigma. Front Endocrinol 2020;11(1):217. Available from: https://doi.org/10.3389/fendo.2020.00217.

[10] Weinsier RL. Fasting—a review with emphasis on the electrolytes. Am J Med 1971;50(2):233–40. Available from: https://doi.org/10.1016/0002-9343(71)90152-5.

[11] Drenick EJ, Swendseid ME, Blahd WH, Tuttle SG. Prolonged starvation as treatment for severe obesity. JAMA. 1964;187(2). Available from: https://doi.org/10.1001/jama.1964.03060150024006.

[12] Stewart WK, Fleming LW. Features of a successful therapeutic fast of 382 days' duration. Postgrad Med J 1973;49(569):203–9. Available from: https://doi.org/10.1136/pgmj.49.569.203.

[13] Lager I. The insulin-antagonistic effect of the counterregulatory hormones. J Gen Intern Med 1991;735:41–7.

[14] Zauner C, Schneeweiss B, Kranz A, et al. Resting energy expenditure in short-term starvation is increased as a result of an increase in serum norepinephrine. Am J Clin Nutr 2000;71(6):1511–15. Available from: https://doi.org/10.1093/ajcn/71.6.1511.

[15] Oscarsson J, Ottosson M, Edén S. Effects of growth hormone on lipoprotein lipase and hepatic lipase. J Endocrinol Investigation 1999;22(5 Suppl):2–9.

[16] Roth J, Glick SM, Yalow RS, Berson SA. Hypoglycemia: a potent stimulus to secretion of growth hormone. Science 1963;140(3570):987–8. Available from: https://doi.org/10.1126/science.140.3570.987.

[17] Ho KY, Veldhuis JD, Johnson ML, et al. Fasting enhances growth hormone secretion and amplifies the complex rhythms of growth hormone secretion in man. J Clin Investigation 1988;81(4):968–75. Available from: https://doi.org/10.1172/jci113450.

[18] Hartman ML, Thorner MO, Samojlik E, et al. Augmented growth hormone (GH) secretory burst frequency and amplitude mediate enhanced GH secretion during a two-day fast in normal men. J Clin Endocrinol Metab 1992;74(4):757–65. Available from: https://doi.org/10.1210/jcem.74.4.1548337.

[19] Rudman D, Feller AG, Nagraj HS, et al. Effects of human growth hormone in men over 60 years old. N Engl J Med 1990;323(22):1561–3. Available from: https://doi.org/10.1056/nejm199011293232212.

[20] Verberne AJM, Sabetghadam A, Korim WS. Neural pathways that control the glucose counterregulatory response. Front Neurosci 2014;8(1). Available from: https://doi.org/10.3389/fnins.2014.00038.

[21] Nakamura Y, Walker BR, Ikuta T. Systematic review and meta-analysis reveals acutely elevated plasma cortisol following fasting but not less severe calorie restriction. Stress 2016;19(2):151–7. Available from: https://doi.org/10.3109/10253890.2015.1121984 Epub 2016 Jan 7.

[22] Steekumaran Nair K, Woolf PD, Welle SL, Mathews DE. Leucine, glucose and energy metabolism after 3 days of fasting in healthy subjects. Am J Clin Nutr 1987;46(4):557–62. Available from: https://doi.org/10.1093/ajcn/46.4.557.

[23] McCue MD. Comparative physiology of fasting, starvation, and food limitation. Berlin: Springer Berlin; 2014.

[24] Patel JN, Coppack SW, Goldstein DS, Miles JM, Eisenhofer G. Norepinephrine spillover from human adipose tissue before and after a 72-hour fast. J Clin Endocrinol Metab 2002;87(7):3373–7. Available from: https://doi.org/10.1210/jcem.87.7.8695.

[25] Webber J, Macdonald IA. The cardiovascular, metabolic and hormonal changes accompanying acute starvation in men and women. Br J Nutr 1994;71(3):437–47. Available from: https://doi.org/10.1079/bjn19940150.

[26] Mansell PI, Fellows IW, Macdonald IA. Enhanced thermogenic response to epinephrine after 48-h starvation in humans. Am J Physiol-Regulat Integr Comp Physiol 1990;258(1). Available from: https://doi.org/10.1152/ajpregu.1990.258.1.r87.

[27] Heilbronn LK, Smith SR, Martin CK, Anton SD, Ravussin E. Alternate-day fasting in nonobese subjects: effects on body weight, body composition, and energy metabolism. Am J Clin Nutr 2005;81(1):69–73. Available from: https://doi.org/10.1093/ajcn/81.1.69.

[28] Keys AB, Drummonds JC. The biology of human starvation. Minneapolis: The Univ. of Minnesota Pr; 1950.

[29] Norrelund H, Nair KS, Jorgensen JO, Christiansen JS, Moller N. The protein-retaining effects of growth hormone during fasting involve inhibition of muscle-protein breakdown. Diabetes. 2001;50(1):96–104. Available from: https://doi.org/10.2337/diabetes.50.1.96.

[30] Bhutani S, Klempel MC, Berger RA, Varady KA. Improvements in coronary heart disease risk indicators by alternate-day fasting involve adipose tissue modulations. Obesity. 2010;18(11):2152–9. Available from: https://doi.org/10.1038/oby.2010.54.

[31] Catenacci VA, Pan Z, Ostendorf D, et al. A randomized pilot study comparing zero-calorie alternate-day fasting to daily caloric restriction in adults with obesity. Obesity. 2016;24(9):1874–83. Available from: https://doi.org/10.1002/oby.21581.

[32] Jensen MD, Ekberg K, Landau BR. Lipid metabolism during fasting. Am J Physiol Endocrinol Metab 2001;281(4). Available from: https://doi.org/10.1152/ajpendo.2001.281.4.e789.

[33] Secor SM, Carey HV. Integrative physiology of fasting. Compr Physiol 2016;6(2):773–825. Available from: https://doi.org/10.1002/cphy.c150013.

[34] Che T, Yan C, Tian D, Zhang X, Liu X, Wu Z. Time-restricted feeding improves blood glucose and insulin sensitivity in overweight patients with type 2 diabetes: a randomised controlled trial. Nutr Metab (Lond) 2021;18(1):88.

[35] Chow LS, Manoogian ENC, Alvear A, Fleischer JG, Thor H, Dietsche K, et al. Time-restricted eating effects on body composition and metabolic measures in humans with overweight: a feasibility study. Obes (Silver Spring) 2020; Apr 9.

[36] Harvie MN, Pegington M, Mattson MP, et al. The effects of intermittent or continuous energy restriction on weight loss and metabolic disease risk markers: a randomized trial in young overweight women. Int J Obes 2010;35(5):714–27. Available from: https://doi.org/10.1038/ijo.2010.171.

[37] Varady KA, Dam VT, Klempel MC, et al. Erratum: corrigendum: effects of weight loss via high fat vs. low fat alternate day fasting diets on free fatty acid profiles. Sci Rep. 2015;5(1). Available from: https://doi.org/10.1038/srep08806.

[38] Trepanowski JF, Kroeger CM, Barnosky A, et al. Effect of alternate-day fasting on weight loss, weight maintenance, and cardioprotection among metabolically healthy obese adults. JAMA Intern Med 2017;177(7):930. Available from: https://doi.org/10.1001/jamainternmed.2017.0936.

[39] Wilhelmi de Toledo F, Grundler F, Bergouignan A, Drinda S, Michalsen A. Safety, health improvement and well-being during a 4 to 21-day fasting period in an observational study including 1422 subjects. PLoS One 2019;14(1). Available from: https://doi.org/10.1371/journal.pone.0209353.

[40] Fontana L, Partridge L, Longo VD. Extending healthy life span—from yeast to humans. Science. 2010;328(5976):321–6. Available from: https://doi.org/10.1126/science.1172539.

[41] Abe T. Suppression of experimental autoimmune uveoretinitis by dietary calorie restriction. Japanese J Ophthalmol 2001;45(1):46–52. Available from: https://doi.org/10.1016/s0021-5155(00)00303-8.

[42] Jolly CA, Fernandes G. Diet modulates Th-1 and Th-2 cytokine production in the peripheral blood of lupus-prone mice. J Clin Immunol 1999;19(3):172–8. Available from: https://doi.org/10.1023/a:1020503727157.

[43] Solon-Biet SM, Mitchell SJ, Coogan SCP, et al. Dietary protein to carbohydrate ratio and caloric restriction: comparing metabolic outcomes in mice. Cell Rep 2015;11(10):1529–34. Available from: https://doi.org/10.1016/j.celrep.2015.05.007.

[44] Paddon-Jones D, Rasmussen BB. Dietary protein recommendations and the prevention of sarcopenia. Curr OpClNutr Metab Care 2009;12 (1):86–90. Available from: https://doi.org/10.1097/mco.0b013e32831cef8b.

[45] D'Onofrio N, Servillo L, Balestrieri ML. SIRT1 and SIRT6 signaling pathways in cardiovascular disease protection. Antioxid Redox Signal 2018;28(8):711–32. Available from: https://doi.org/10.1089/ars.2017.7178.

[46] Schwalm C, Jamart C, Benoit N, et al. Activation of autophagy in human skeletal muscle is dependent on exercise intensity and AMPK activation. FASEB J 2015;29(8):3515–26. Available from: https://doi.org/10.1096/fj.14-267187.

[47] Cheng C-W, Adams GB, Perin L, et al. Prolonged fasting reduces IGF-1/PKA to promote hematopoietic-stem-cell-based regeneration and reverse immunosuppression. Cell Stem Cell 2014;14(6):810–23. Available from: https://doi.org/10.1016/j.stem.2014.04.014.

[48] Ersahin T, Tuncbag N, Cetin-Atalay R. The PI3K/AKT/mTOR interactive pathway. Mol Biosyst 2015;11(7):1946–54. Available from: https://doi.org/10.1039/c5mb00101c.

[49] Fontana L, Partridge L. Promoting health and longevity through diet: from model organisms to humans. Cell. 2015;161(1):106–18. Available from: https://doi.org/10.1016/j.cell.2015.02.020.

[50] Anton S, Leeuwenburgh C. Fasting or caloric restriction for Healthy Aging. Exp Gerontol 2013;48(10):1003–5. Available from: https://doi.org/10.1016/j.exger.2013.04.011.

[51] Mattson MP, Longo VD, Harvie M. Impact of intermittent fasting on health and disease processes. Ageing Res Rev 2017;39:46–58. Available from: https://doi.org/10.1016/j.arr.2016.10.005.

[52] Zubrzycki A, Cierpka-Kmiec K, Kmiec Z, Wronska A. The role of low-calorie diets and intermittent fasting in the treatment of obesity and type-2 diabetes. J Physiol Pharmacol 2018;69(5). Available from: https://doi.org/10.26402/jpp.2018.5.02.

[53] Welton S, Minty R, O'Driscoll T, et al. Intermittent fasting and weight loss: systematic review. Can Family Phys 2020;66(2):117–25.

[54] Lowe DA, Wu N, Rohdin-Bibby L, et al. Effects of time-restricted eating on weight loss and other metabolic parameters in women and men with overweight and obesity. JAMA Intern Med 2020;180(11):1491. Available from: https://doi.org/10.1001/jamainternmed.2020.4153.

[55] Arnason TG, Bowen MW, Mansell KD. Effects of intermittent fasting on health markers in those with type 2 diabetes: a pilot study. World J Diabetes 2017;8(4):154. Available from: https://doi.org/10.4239/wjd.v8.i4.154.

[56] Furmli S, Elmasry R, Ramos M, Fung J. Therapeutic use of intermittent fasting for people with type 2 diabetes as an alternative to insulin. BMJ Case Rep 2018;. Available from: https://doi.org/10.1136/bcr-2017-221854.

[57] Stange R, Pflugbeil C, Michalsen A, Uehleke B. Therapeutic fasting in patients with metabolic syndrome and impaired insulin resistance. Forschende Komplementärmedizin/Res Complem Med 2013;20(6):421–6. Available from: https://doi.org/10.1159/000357875.

[58] Gabel K, Kroeger CM, Trepanowski JF, et al. Differential effects of alternate-day fasting versus daily calorie restriction on insulin resistance. Obesity. 2019;27(9):1443–50. Available from: https://doi.org/10.1002/oby.22564.

[59] Stekovic S, Hofer SJ, Tripolt N, et al. Alternate day fasting improves physiological and molecular markers of aging in healthy, non-obese humans. Cell Metab 2020;31(4):878–81. Available from: https://doi.org/10.1016/j.cmet.2020.02.011.

[60] Drinda S, Grundler F, Neumann T, et al. Effects of periodic fasting on fatty liver index—a prospective observational study. Nutrients. 2019;11 (11):2601. Available from: https://doi.org/10.3390/nu11112601.

[61] Weir HJ, Yao P, Huynh FK, et al. Dietary restriction and AMPK increase lifespan via mitochondrial network and peroxisome remodeling. Cell Metab 2017;26(6):884–96. Available from: https://doi.org/10.1016/j.cmet.2017.09.024.

[62] de Cabo R, Mattson MP. Effects of intermittent fasting on health, aging, and disease. N Engl J Med 2019;381(26):2541–51. Available from: https://doi.org/10.1056/NEJMra1905136.61.

[63] Longo VD, Mattson MP. Fasting: molecular mechanisms and clinical applications. Cell Metabolism. 2014;19(2):181–92. Available from: https://doi.org/10.1016/j.cmet.2013.12.008.

[64] Harrison DE, Strong R, Sharp ZD, et al. Rapamycin fed late in life extends lifespan in genetically heterogeneous mice. Nature 2009;460 (7253):392–5. Available from: https://doi.org/10.1038/nature08221.

[65] Witte AV, Fobker M, Gellner R, Knecht S, Floel A. Caloric restriction improves memory in elderly humans. Proc Natl Acad Sci 2009;106 (4):1255–60. Available from: https://doi.org/10.1073/pnas.0808587106.

[66] Willeumier KC, Taylor DV, Amen DG. Elevated BMI is associated with decreased blood flow in the prefrontal cortex using SPECT imaging in healthy adults. Obesity. 2011;19(5):1095–7. Available from: https://doi.org/10.1038/oby.2011.16.

[67] Halagappa VK, Guo Z, Pearson M, et al. Intermittent fasting and caloric restriction ameliorate age-related behavioral deficits in the triple-transgenic mouse model of Alzheimer's disease. Neurobiol Dis 2007;26(1):212–20. Available from: https://doi.org/10.1016/j.nbd.2006.12.019.

[68] Mattson MP. Energy intake and exercise as determinants of brain health and vulnerability to injury and disease. Cell Metab 2012;16 (6):706–22. Available from: https://doi.org/10.1016/j.cmet.2012.08.012.

[69] Lieberman HR, Caruso CM, Niro PJ, et al. A double-blind, placebo-controlled test of 2 d of calorie deprivation: effects on cognition, activity, sleep, and interstitial glucose concentrations. Am J Clin Nutr 2008;88(3):667–76. Available from: https://doi.org/10.1093/ajcn/88.3.667.

[70] Mizushima N. Autophagy: process and function. Genes Dev 2007;21(22):2861–73. Available from: https://doi.org/10.1101/gad.1599207.

[71] Glick D, Barth S, Macleod KF. Autophagy: cellular and molecular mechanisms. J Pathol 2010;221(1):3–12. Available from: https://doi.org/10.1002/path.2697.

[72] Cataldo AM, Peterhoff CM, Troncoso JC, Gomez-Isla T, Hyman BT, Nixon RA. Endocytic pathway abnormalities precede amyloid β deposition in sporadic Alzheimer's disease and down syndrome. Am J Pathol 2000;157(1):277–86. Available from: https://doi.org/10.1016/s0002-9440(10)64538-5.

[73] Hanahan D, Weinberg RA. Hallmarks of cancer: the next generation. Cell 2011;144(5):646–74. https://doi.org/10.1016j.cell/2011.02.013.

[74] Sato T, Nakashima A, Guo L, Coffman K, Tamanoi F. Single amino-acid changes that confer constitutive activation of mTOR are discovered in human cancer. Oncogene. 2010;29(18):2746–52. Available from: https://doi.org/10.1038/onc.2010.28.

[75] Nencioni A, Caffa I, Cortellino S, Longo VD. Fasting and cancer: molecular mechanisms and clinical application. Nat Rev Cancer 2018;18 (11):707–19. Available from: https://doi.org/10.1038/s41568-018-0061-0.

[76] Tian T, Li X, Zhang J. mTOR signaling in cancer and mTOR inhibitors in solid tumor targeting therapy. Intern J Mol Sci 2019;20(3):755. Available from: https://doi.org/10.3390/ijms20030755.

[77] Raffaghello L, Lee C, Safdie FM, et al. Starvation-dependent differential stress resistance protects normal but not cancer cells against high-dose chemotherapy. Proc Natl Acad Sci 2008;105(24):8215–20. Available from: https://doi.org/10.1073/pnas.0708100105.

[78] Rajpal A, Ismail-Beigi F. Intermittent fasting and "metabolic switch": effects on metabolic syndrome, pre-diabetes and type 2 diabetes mellitus. Diabetes Obes Metab 2020;22(9):1496–510. Available from: https://doi.org/10.1111/dom.1408077.

[79] Sichieri R, Everhart JE, Roth H. A prospective study of hospitalization with gallstone disease among women: role of dietary factors, fasting period, and dieting. Am J Public Health 1991;81(7):880–4. Available from: https://doi.org/10.2105/ajph.81.7.880.

[80] Crook MA, Hally V, Panteli JV. The importance of the refeeding syndrome. Nutrition. 2001;17(7–8):632–7. Available from: https://doi.org/10.1016/s0899-9007(01)00542-1.

[81] Drenick EJ, Hunt IF, Swendseid ME. Influence of fasting and refeeding on body composition. Am J Public Health Nations Health 1968;58 (3):477–84. Available from: https://doi.org/10.2105/ajph.58.3.477.

[82] Camp MA, Allon M. Severe hypophosphatemia in hospitalized patients. Miner Electrolyte Metab 1990;16(6):365 268.

[83] Mehanna HM, Moledina J, Travis J. Refeeding syndrome: what it is, and how to prevent and treat it. Br Med J 2008;336(7659):1495–8. Available from: https://doi.org/10.1136/bmj.a301.

[84] Piernas C, Popkin BM. Snacking increased among U.S. adults between 1977 and 2006. J Nutr 2010;140(2):325–32. Available from: https://doi.org/10.3945/jn.109.112763.

[85] Kahleova H, et al. Meal frequency and timing are associated with changes in body mass index in adventist health study 2. J Nutr 2017;147 (9):1722–8.

[86] Gill S, Panda S. A smartphone app reveals erratic diurnal eating patterns in humans that can be modulated for health benefits. Clin Transl Rep 2015;22(5):P789–98.

[87] Martin CK, et al. Changes in food cravings during low-calorie and very-low-calorie diets. Obesity 2006;14(1):115–21.

[88] Ravussin E, Beyl RA, Poggiogalle E, Hsia DS, Peterson CM. Early time-restricted feeding reduces appetite and increases fat oxidation but does not affect energy expenditure in humans. Obesity 2019;27(8):1244–54.

[89] Johnstone AM, Horgan GW, Murison SD, Bremner DM, Lobley GE. Effects of a high-protein ketogenic diet on hunger, appetite, and weight loss in obese men feeding ad libitum. Am J Clin Nutr 2008;87(1):44–55.

[90] Castro AI, Gomez-Arbelaez D, Crujeiras AB, Granero R, Aguera Z, Jimenez-Murcia S, et al. Effect of a very low-calorie ketogenic diet on food and alcohol cravings, physical and sexual activity, sleep disturbances, and quality of life in obese patients Nutrients [Internet] 2018;10(10) Sep 21 [cited 2019 Jul 11]. Available from: https://www.ncbi.nlm.nih.gov/pmc/articles/PMC6213862/.

[91] Van Cauter E, et al. Circadian modulation of glucose and insulin responses to meals: relationship to cortisol rhythm. Am J Physiol 1992;262 (4 Pt 1):E467–76.

[92] Scheer FA, et al. The internal circadian clock increases hunger and appetite in the evening independent of food intake and other behaviors. Obesity 2013;21(3):431–3.

[93] Bo S, et al. Is the timing of caloric intake associated with variation in diet-induced thermogenesis and in the metabolic pattern? A randomized cross-over study. Int J Obes (Lond) 2015;39(12):1689–95. Available from: https://doi.org/10.1038/ijo.2015.138.

[94] Mattson MP, Moehl K, Ghena N, Schmaedick M, Cheng A. Intermittent metabolic switching, neuroplasticity and brain health. Nature reviews. Neuroscience 2018;19(2):63–80. Available from: https://doi.org/10.1038/nrn.2017.156.

[95] Geda YE, Ragossnig M, Roberts LA, Roberts RO, Pankratz VS, Christianson TJ, et al. Caloric intake, aging, and mild cognitive impairment: a population-based study. J Alzheimer's Dis JAD 2013;34(2):501–7. Available from: https://doi.org/10.3233/JAD-121270.

Further reading

Cornford AS, Barkan AL, Horowitz JF. Rapid suppression of growth hormone concentration by overeating: potential mediation by hyperinsulinemia. J Clin Endocrinol Metab 2011;96(3):824–30. Available from: https://doi.org/10.1210/jc.2010-1895.

Overview: Nutrition support for adults: oral nutrition support, enteral tube feeding and parenteral nutrition. National Institute for Health and Care Excellence. https://www.nice.org.uk/guidance/cg32. [accessed 20.03.21].

Shin BK, Kang S, Kim DS, Park S. Intermittent fasting protects against the deterioration of cognitive function, energy metabolism and dyslipidemia in Alzheimer's disease-induced estrogen deficient rats. Exp Biol Med (Maywood, NJ) 2018;243(4):334–43. Available from: https://doi.org/10.1177/1535370217751610.

Part 4

Managing the patient

Chapter 11

Psychological, behavioural, and ethical considerations

Joan Adams[1], David Unwin[2], Jen Unwin[2], Trudi Deakin[3], Joan Ifland[4] and Mark I. Friedman[5]
[1]HPCSA Professional Conduct Commitee, Arcadia, Pretoria, South Africa, [2]Norwood Surgery, Southport, United Kingdom, [3]X-PERT Health, Hebden Bridge, West Yorkshire, United Kingdom, [4]Food Addiction Reset LLC, Vashon, WA, United States, [5]Nutrition Science Initiative, San Diego, CA, United States

11.1 Introduction

A dietary intervention is only effective in the long term if it is sustainable. Sustainable health improvements require persistent changes in thoughts and behaviour, as well as control over eating. There are techniques healthcare practitioners can employ to guide patients towards behaviour change, while encouraging them to take responsibility for their own health and achieve lasting improvements. Therapeutic carbohydrate restriction (TCR) gives patients a physiological advantage by controlling hunger (despite reduced caloric intake and weight loss); offering a sustainable alternative to conventional hypocaloric weight loss interventions, which usually result in hunger and rebound weight gains. Evidence indicates that ultra-processed food (UPF) may also play a role in cravings and eating control, promoting addictive eating behaviours that thwart health and weight loss efforts. TCR, eliminates UPF and thus, as an adjunct to other behavioural and psychological interventions, may offer a treatment modality to address addictive eating. While TCR is a relatively novel nutritional evidence-based modality that challenges current dietary guidelines, healthcare practitioners have an ethical responsibility to fulfil the Hippocratic values that underlie western medical ethics to first do no harm. In the light of evidence indicating the harmful effects of conventional high-carbohydrate diets on metabolic health, TCR public health advocacy is one of the most crucial ethical duties of healthcare professionals in modern times.

11.2 Behaviour change

11.2.1 Motivating for change

Trudi Deakin

Introducing Dr Trudi Deakin, a registered dietitian and founder/chief executive of the registered charity 'X-PERT Health' that has provided self-management education and support to over half million people with metabolic syndrome, obesity, prediabetes, Type 1 and Type 2 diabetes.

11.2.1.1 Introduction

> In nature there are neither rewards nor punishments—there are consequences.
>
> Robert G.

The cornerstone to motivating patients to change their diet and lifestyle is recognising that the person is completely responsible for managing his or her illness [1]. This is non-negotiable and inescapable and rests on three characteristics:

11.2.1.1.1 Choices

Each day patients make choices about eating, physical activity, stress, and sleep management that have a far greater impact on their overall health and well-being than the care provided to them by healthcare professionals (HCPs).

Ketogenic. DOI: https://doi.org/10.1016/B978-0-12-821617-0.00014-0

11.2.1.1.2 Control

The patient is in control. HCPs may plead, beg, cajole, threaten, advise, prescribe, or order patients to change their behaviour, but when they leave the consultation, they can ignore any recommendation, no matter how important or relevant it is deemed to be.

11.2.1.1.3 Consequences

The consequences happen to the patient, not to the HCP. Therefore, the patient needs to take responsibility and weigh up the pros and cons, the benefits and risks for each lifestyle decision they make (Fig. 11.1). HCP can help by making sure that the decisions are based on correct and up-to-date information.

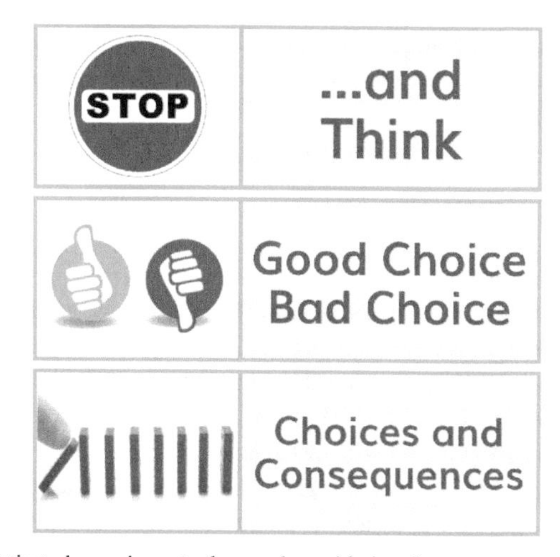

FIGURE 11.1 **Motivations for change.** Patient change is centred around considering the consequences of their actions. *Source: X-PERT Health © Dr Trudi Deakin 2003.*

Motivating consultations start with supporting patients in recognising that they often do things due to habits and providing an opportunity for them to *Stop and think*. Once patients take responsibility for their diet and lifestyle, they will recognise that they have *choices* and those choices have *Consequences*. *Good choices* are more likely to lead to better consequences, whereas *bad choices* more commonly lead to poorer consequences.

HCPs may have strongly held beliefs about what patients should do. After seeing the devastation caused by poor diets and lifestyles, they may believe that patients owe it to themselves and their families to work hard to prevent the potential complications of poor metabolic health. Many HCPs think that it is *their* responsibility to *get* patients to change their health behaviour. However compliance and adherence are dysfunctional concepts in behaviour change [2]. Non-compliance can be described as two people working towards two different goals [3]. Shifting from a compliance paradigm to an empowering collaborative goal-setting approach based on informed decision-making requires new defined roles for patients and HCPs. The empowerment philosophy frees HCPs from the responsibility of attempting to solve patients' problems. Instead, it allows them to enter into a dialogue with patients during which solutions to problems emerge naturally from an exploration of issues in a relationship based on trust and respect.

11.2.1.2 The five essential steps to the empowerment approach

Working through the five-step empowerment approach supports patients in making informed decisions and setting meaningful goals to change their diet and lifestyle. A climate for change begins with a discussion about who is responsible for what in the management of their health. HCPs cannot relieve patients of their responsibility, but they can help them develop the skills and supply them with resources to help them carry out informed decision-making. Focusing on goal setting can only happen after the patient has identified their concern and viewed their feelings about it and have a desire to solve the problem or concern. Sometimes patients want to set goals that the HCP believes are not appropriate, are too ambitious or are not compatible with established guidelines. However, it is the patient's prerogative to set their own goals, and the HCP's job to be sure that they understand the costs and benefits of their decisions.

5 Essential Steps to Goal Setting

1 What is my biggest concern about my health?

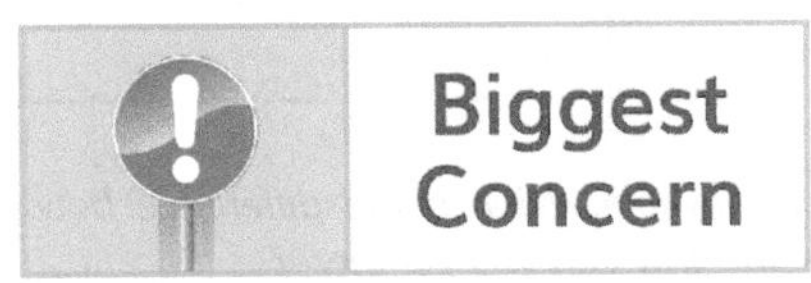

2 How do I feel about the concern?

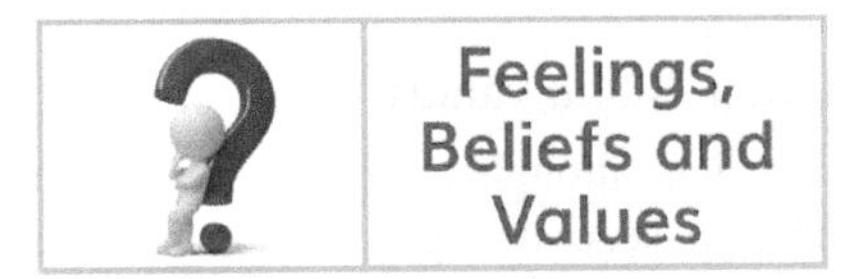

3 What steps could I take to tackle the concern?

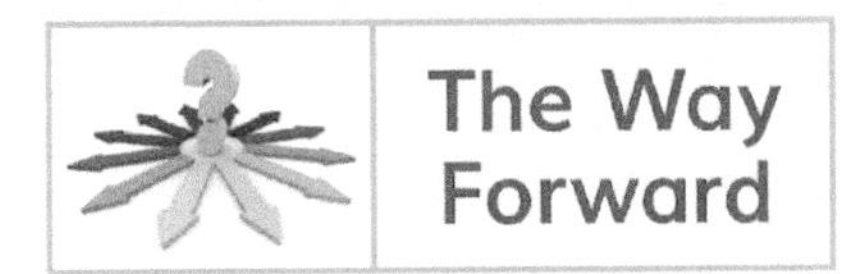

4 What is the first step I'm going to take?

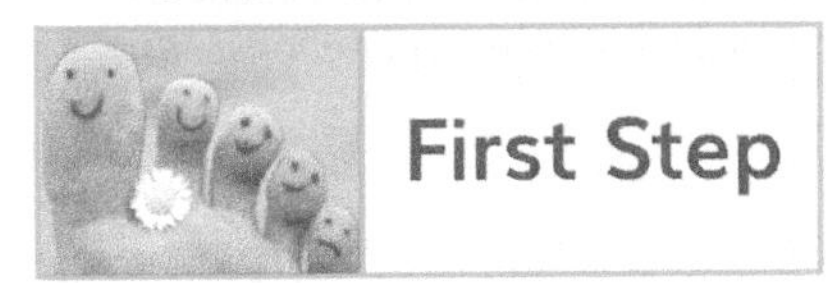

5 What happened? Did it work?

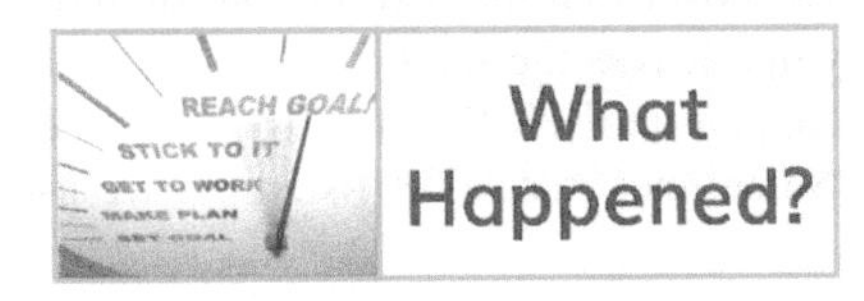

FIGURE 11.2 **Steps of goal setting.** Goal setting is centred around the patient's feelings about their health empowering them to take action. *Source: X-PERT Health © Dr Trudi Deakin 2003.*

One criticism of the empowerment approach to goal setting is that it requires time. However, once the HCP sets aside their need to feel in control and stops setting goals *for* the patient, it can be carried out in a 10-min consultation (Fig. 11.2).

If you do what you've always done, you'll get what you've always gotten.

Peter Bender.

11.2.1.2.1 Step 1: Identifying the biggest concern

This entails exploring how patients currently feel about their health. Many patients expect to continue living their lives in the same way that they did when they were younger. If they become unwell, they assume healthcare will intervene in order for their lives to continue unchanged. However, when health improvement is reliant on dietary or lifestyle change, this is not possible. Changing habits is not easy but having a degree of control over the process of change is fundamental to reducing levels of distress. Assisting patients in managing and accepting change in their lives is a core skill for HCPs.

Questions to ask

- *Do you feel healthy at the moment?*
- *Consider a 'desired future self' that is achievable. What is the difference between the expected future self (if behaviour doesn't change) and the desired future self? How can you get there?*
- *What is the hardest thing about caring for your health? Tell me more about that*
- *What would you have to do to improve your health? Are there some specific examples you can give me?*

11.2.1.2.2 Step 2: Discussing feelings, beliefs and values

Behaviour is usually an expression of our beliefs, thoughts, emotions, attitudes, and values. These underpin and influence the visible behaviour seen by all. Thus, the second step is to help patients identify how they feel about the behaviour (or concern) that they are hoping to change.

Patients can write down their thoughts then review them to try and identify any unhelpful ones. These can then be challenged to promote self-efficacy and contemplation of change.

Questions to ask

- *How do you feel about....?*
- *What are your thoughts about....?*
- *How will you feel if things don't change?*
- *How will you feel if you achieve your goal?*
- *Are you feeling (insert feelings) because of (insert biggest concern)?*
- *Have you tried to tackle this concern before? If so, what was your experience?*
- *How do you feel when your results do not appear to reflect your efforts?*

11.2.1.2.3 Step 3: The way forward

One approach for developing a plan is to ask patients to generate a list of options that might be effective in helping them achieve their goal. It is important for patients to come up with as many of their own strategies as possible before offering suggestions, as this helps them to discover that they are in control and can solve their own problems. If you are required to offer strategies, do so in a way that leaves the final decision up to the patient.

Learning to listen attentively cannot happen until HCPs let go of the expectation that they must come up with an answer. This can be very difficult to do. Sometimes instead of listening, we use the time the patient is talking to think about what we will say next.

> Knowledge speaks, but wisdom listens.
>
> Jimi Hendrix

Have you ever had the experience of working with someone and realised that you had different goals? How did you feel? Frustrated? Angry? Did you feel that no matter how hard you were trying to reach your goals, your efforts were being criticised and thwarted? That interaction is often repeated in healthcare with both patients and health professionals stating, 'We don't seem to be getting anywhere'.

Whenever a patient makes significant changes in their lives, they give up some things (costs) and gain other things (benefits). Changes are made when the benefits of solving a problem outweigh the costs of changing. The decision that a goal is worthwhile can only be made by the patient with the problem.

Cost-benefit analysis This technique allows patients to list the costs and benefits and score them on a scale of 0 to 10 based on how important they are to evaluate if a specific change is right for them.

The example presented in Table 11.1 shows a cost-benefit analysis for adopting a therapeutic carbohydrate-restricted (TCR) diet. In this example, the benefits outweigh the costs and the change seems to make sense based on the individuals' own belief system. It may also be possible to maximise some of the benefits and minimise or remove some of the costs.

TABLE 11.1 Example of a cost-benefit analysis for adopting a therapeutic carbohydrate restricted (TCR) diet.

Costs	Score	Benefits	Score
Will need to do more food prep	3	Feel fitter – less breathless	8
Will miss bread and potatoes	8	Help to control blood glucose concentrations	8
It'll be more difficult to eat out	3	Help to lose weight	8
Will have to explain to friends/family	5	Feel good factor and reduce stress	8
Total	19	Total	32

Questions to ask

- *How would this situation have to change for you to feel better about it?*
- *What will you gain if you change?*
- *Are you willing to take action to improve the situation?*
- *What needs to happen for you to get to where you want to be?*
- *What are your options?*
- *What are the costs and benefits?*
- *Who could help you?*
- *What could happen if you didn't do anything?*
- *How important is it that you do something about it?*
- *How important is it, on a scale of 1 to 10, for you to do something about this?*

11.2.1.2.4 Step 4: The first real step – facilitating goal setting

Advice is like castor oil, easy enough to give but dreadful uneasy to take.

Josh Billings

The fourth step is for patients to develop a plan of action. The experiments and subsequent discussions also help patients discover and enhance their abilities to solve problems and adjust their behaviour to meet their needs. It is often easy to set long-term goals, but it can be hard to achieve them without identifying a series of concrete steps that lead to the goal.

Making a commitment: Encourage patients to write out their goals and plan, and make a written or verbal commitment to it. This helps to move the individual from preparation to action. It may also be helpful for patients to add a reward or reinforcement to their plan.

Diaries: By keeping a record of the concern can enable the true severity of the problem to be established and identify patterns so far unnoticed. This can be therapeutic. Diaries can be as simple or as complex as the patient is happy to keep and can include thoughts, images, emotions as well as avoidance behaviour.

Encourage goals to be SMART: i.e. specific, measurable, attainable, relevant and time-bound [4].

Paraphrasing and summarising: Picking up the meaning of the patient's words and putting it back to them to check that you understand what is being conveyed can be used to help focus on the main thoughts and feelings.

Assessing self-efficacy: Patients need to believe they can do it. Ask them to score on a scale of 1–10 how likely they think they are to achieve this goal. If they score seven or higher, it is likely to be attainable. However, if the score is below seven, ask what aspects of the plan they do not feel able to complete (reinforcing the positive aspects). It may be that the first step is too ambitious and a more realistic goal needs to be set.

> What lies behind us and what lies before us are tiny matters compared to what lies within us.
>
> Ralph Waldo Emerson

Questions to ask

- *Are you willing to do what you need to do to solve this problem?*
- *What are some steps you could take?*
- *What are you going to do and when?*
- *How will you know if you have succeeded?*
- *What is one thing you will do when you leave here today?*
- *Does this sound like something you can do and are you committed?*
- *What will you do to reward yourself for making this change?*
- *On a scale of 1–10, how confident are you that you can achieve this goal?*

11.2.1.2.5 Step 5: What happened? Enabling evaluation

Evaluation is both the beginning and the end of the behaviour change process. At the beginning patients evaluate their lifestyle and/or health status to identify the concern or problem. Once we have assisted patients in identifying a goal and a plan, we have an important role in helping them monitor and evaluate the effectiveness of the strategies they have chosen. The feedback allows them to discover and keep those behaviours that are effective and revise those that are not.

> Nothing is a waste of time if you use the experience wisely.
>
> Auguste Rodin

Encourage patients to think of their goal-setting plan as a series of experiments. Experiments that do not appear to work are as valuable as those that do for setting future goals.

Questions to ask

- *How will you know if you have succeeded?*
- *Did it help you reach your short-term goals?*
- *What did you learn about yourself from this experience?*
- *What would you do differently next time? What would you do the same?*
- *What barriers did you encounter? What ideas do you have for strategies to overcome those barriers?*
- *How do you feel about what you accomplished?*
- *Were you able to do more or less than you thought you would be able to do? Why?*
- *Is this still an area on which you want to work?*
- *Did you learn things about the type of support you have, want, or need?*
- *What did you learn about how you feel about this problem or area of change?*

11.2.1.3 Interactive learning strategies

The following are interactive learning strategies that can be used to promote behaviour change:

- **Open-ended questions**: These are the most effective techniques for promoting patients to think critically about their health.
- **Wait for answers**: It takes most people three to five seconds to formulate an answer.
- **Use appropriate voice tone and body language**: These are often greater contributors to communication than the spoken word.
- **Role-playing**: This is an excellent method for practising behavioural skills for a situation that may have a high degree of emotional intensity. For example, patients may practise asking their HCP questions or practise responding to social pressure to eat or drink when they do not wish to do so.

11.2.1.4 *Assess your facilitation skills*

A highly effective way to improve your facilitation skills is to record interactions with patients and then to watch/listen and reflect on our practice. Rate each of your responses using the scoring system below. Add the scores for each response and divide by the number of responses. This gives you an overall numerical score for your interaction. Using a numerical rating system provides you with a way to quantify your progress in using the empowerment approach.

+2 Focusing on feelings or goals e.g., *'how do you feel about that?', 'What are you willing to do?'*
+1 Problem exploration e.g., *'Tell me more about that?', 'Why is that a problem for you?'*
0 Miscellaneous e.g., collection of factual data and technical questions
−1 Solving problems for the patient e.g., *'Why don't you try...?,' 'A better way to handle that is...'*
−2 Judging the patient e.g., *'Don't worry everyone finds it hard', 'I'm sure you can do better'*

Behaviour change skills are not adopted overnight and HCP are strongly encouraged to reflect on their experiences so that they can continuously improve their skills.

REFLECTION QUESTIONS

- What barriers make it difficult for you to listen to your patients? How can you overcome them?
- How comfortable are you sitting in silence for a few moments whilst the patient considers the question?
- What would you do differently if you repeated the consultation?
- How do you feel about setting goals *with* rather than *for* patients?
- How do you know when you have succeeded in establishing a partnership with a patient?
- What do you do when you are unable to establish a partnership with a patient?
- How do you know when you have succeeded or failed with a patient?
- How do you respond to patients who are 'successful'?
- How do you respond to patients who are 'unsuccessful'?
- How do you communicate that the person is responsible for, and in control of, their healthcare behaviour?

11.2.1.5 *Conclusion*

The patient is responsible for both their decision to undertake TCR and their adherence to it following acceptance of the protocol. Practitioners should be careful not to judge the patient or assume control in goal setting and management, and make an effort to take a patient, question-centred approach. Ultimately, the patient is behind their own success, and practitioners are the facilitators.

11.2.2 Promoting sustainable dietary changes and improving adherence: the psychology of positive change

David and Jen Unwin

> He is the best physician who is the most ingenious inspirer of hope.
>
> Samuel Taylor Coleridge, 1833

Introducing Dr Jen Unwin, a consultant clinical health psychologist interested in the difference hope makes to chronic disease and how best to help motivate people and change behaviour.
Introducing Dr David Unwin, works at the Norwood Surgery in Southport near Liverpool, United Kingdom, where he has cared for the same population since 1986 as a family doctor.

Together we have run a low carb service for our 9800-patient practice, achieving T2D drug-free remission for 51% of those who choose our approach (128 individuals to date) and substantial drug-budget savings of about £68,000 a year. We have published ten peer reviewed papers on our work. In 2016, David was awarded 'NHS Innovator of the year' for his low carb approach to T2D which has been covered by national TV, The Times, and New Scientist magazine.

How often is improving outcomes in chronic disease actually about changing behaviour? As clinicians we are full of good advice about diet, exercise, or sleep but so often patients say 'yes, but I just couldn't live without bread, potatoes' etc. and fail to change. Changing behaviour is a psychological challenge, requiring a psychological approach. In this section, we look at motivation and the initiation of change, then in the next section we focus on monitoring, how to deal with failure and effective longer-term support.

Firstly, as with any relationship, picking the best time to make a suggestion or enquiry is key. When are we most likely to be listened to? We suggest it's when there is a sudden change in the course of someone's case. David calls these 'golden opportunities' and actively seeks them out. The moment we inform a patient about abnormal blood tests, alarm bells ring and far more attention will be paid to any relevant information we supply. For our purposes, this means any results relevant to the metabolic syndrome and so may include not only blood tests like worsening HbA1c, triglyceride or liver function tests but also blood pressure problems, increasing weight or even waist circumference. It is at this point we like to offer our patients alternatives to lifelong medication, which is so often the reflex response of most doctors. In clinical practice, we find offering the choice of lifestyle modification or initiation of drugs results in 99% choosing the lifestyle option. So the first consideration is a matter of timing.

Secondly, we would like to share our simple model for consultations with patients that not only inspires hope for a better future but also helps people notice what works for them, thus promoting positive lifestyle behaviour changes. The model derives from positive psychology and solution-focused therapy and can be easily applied in brief appointments. The approach focuses on four steps: establishing patients' own goals, personal resources, self-chosen next steps and shared noticing of success and progress. In the following sections, ideas will be explored for trying out the model in practice, illustrated by an example of a clinical success story. Our ideas can also be applied to group work in relation to dietary and other lifestyle changes. Adopting this approach encourages both clinicians and patients to remain focused on sustainable change to achieve and maintain desired health outcomes.

Psychological theory and practice can seem complex and time consuming to translate into busy clinical settings. However, a large proportion of all consultations are for chronic physical and mental health conditions exacerbated by behavioural/lifestyle factors such as smoking, alcohol consumption, inactivity, and poor nutrition. Health professionals often lack the confidence and competence to address these issues in clinic, assuming a lack of patient motivation or fearing opening a 'can of worms' in an all too short consultation. Even when professionals understand the science of low-carbohydrate lifestyles, they can struggle with engaging patients in long-term behaviour change. The result can be worsening well-being, repeat consulting, poly-pharmacy and increasing healthcare costs. We have devised a simple four-step plan that we have been using in 10-min GP appointments for over 15 years. Our plan enhances the hope that people have for achieving their personal goals and hence their ability to make significant and lasting positive changes in their well-being and health. Specifically, it is part of an approach that has helped us achieve drug-free remission for 128 people with T2D to date, along with significant practice drug budget savings [5].

11.2.2.1 The importance of hope

Hope has been defined as the belief that pathways exist towards our desired goals and that we have the motivation and skill to pursue those pathways. Hope is the belief in a preferred future. A positive psychology researcher, Charles Snyder [6] summarised the research in this area. Hope is a major component of well-being and adjustment to adversity. High-hope individuals have greater self-reported well-being and health. This group is less likely to get ill and they cope better if they do [7,8]. They visit doctors less. They even live longer. Hopeful people are happier and happy people do better on a whole range of metrics related to health, well-being, and longevity [9,10].

Perhaps that is not too surprising. However, what is surprising is that these powerful effects of hope on well-being and health status are so rarely harnessed or even considered in healthcare settings. In fact, often the exact opposite happens in practice. Consultations focus for the most part on what is *wrong* with people (symptoms) and possible risks to health, with a reliance on passive acceptance of medication. This negative emphasis can result in greater patient anxiety, unnecessary prescriptions and tests that do not lead enhance patient self-efficacy but instead increase learned helplessness and passivity.

Another way to understand the importance of hope is to look at research into the power of the ubiquitous placebo effect. The placebo effect is hope in action. Studies have to be designed to eliminate the placebo effect by having a control arm with a treatment that contains none of the active substance. It is well known that placebo treatments are effective in many conditions, even when the patient knows they are taking a placebo. 'Doctors should seek fervently to harness the power of hope in their consultations, by enhancing belief in an achievable preferred future' [11]. The result of focusing on hopeful consultations is patients who are seen as competent rather than problematic and clinicians who are uplifted and sustained by hearing stories of success on a daily basis [12].

11.2.2.2 *A simple model to enhance hope: G.R.I.N. (Goals. Resources. Increments. Noticing.)*

Goals. Resources. Increments. Noticing.

Our simple conversational model is based on enhancing hope by using questions from a solution-focused approach [13]. Solution-focused therapy started as a form of brief family therapy in the United States but is now widely used in health, education, and business settings. This approach assumes that people already have the knowledge and skills to move towards their goals or preferred future and that the helper's role is to uncover that existing confidence, competence, and motivation by asking useful questions. Clinicians must learn to hold back their advice until they have established these essential factors.

The approach we have developed has four stages that can be pursued in any order but always requires an initial understanding of the person's goals (hopes) or preferred future (Fig. 11.3). We have used the techniques described, in direct patient work, groups, and even remote digital interventions to help people with T2DM achieve significant improvements in glycaemic control [14,15,16].

11.2.2.2.1 Step 1: Goals

The first and most important step is establishing what 'better' would look like to the patient. What is their preferred future? Here are some example questions to try.

> 'What are your best hopes for our consultation today?'
> 'If in 6 months' time, things were how you wanted them to be-what would that look like?'
> 'Are there any particular ways you would like your health to improve?'
> 'If a miracle happened and your problems had resolved, what would be better?'

Usually, people will come up with concrete goals such as 'I want to breathe better', 'I want to lose ten kilos', or 'I want to have no pain in my knees'.

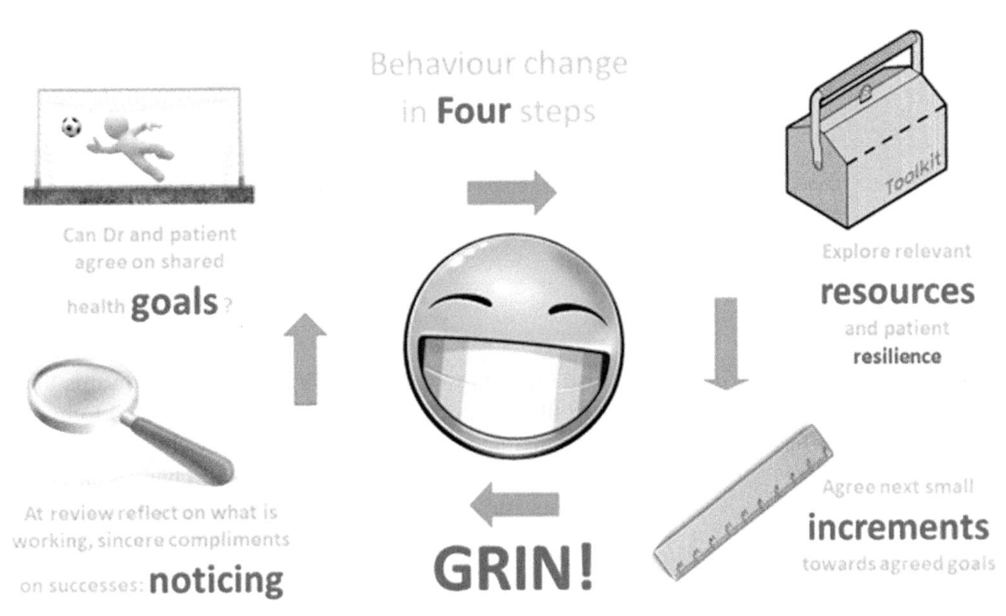

FIGURE 11.3 The GRIN model.

The clinician can then find a rich source of information and insight into the person by following up with this key question to uncover a person's motivation and values.

'What difference would that make to your life?'

Patients then respond with something of central importance to them. For example, someone might say 'then I can help with my grandchildren more' or 'I could keep walking the dog'.

This then allows the clinician to feedback to the patient what they have now learned. For example, 'It sounds like family is really important to you'. This kind of questioning, listening and feedback is a very powerful way of engaging people and uncovering what matters to them.

Another very useful question in this approach is 'what else?' This can be used to deepen and expand on what people say, allowing more rich information to emerge.

'You would be able to keep walking the dog. What else?'

11.2.2.2.2 Step 2: Resources

The second stage is to explore what is already working in the patient's life that is going to help them make progress. This enhances the person's belief in their abilities to make changes. An alternative is to ask for an example from the past. For example, 'Have you ever managed to lose weight in the past? What seemed to work then? When people come for help they are often demoralised and have lost hope in their ability to effect change. This stage is about uncovering resources but also resilience and past success.

Who is supporting/helping you right now or might do so?
What helps your (symptom) now? When are things even slightly better?
What has helped you in the past?
What personal strengths do you have that could help?
What else?

Sometimes the strength question is difficult for people to answer. A different slant can be to give the person a sincere compliment from what you already know of them or to ask what a loved one would say.

'I know you are a very determined/organised/positive/caring person and that this will help you to make good progress'
'What would your wife/best friend say are your best qualities?'
'What else?'

11.2.2.2.3 Step 3: Increments

So many people have goals they never realise because they fail to take those first small steps towards their goal. So the third stage of the conversation is either about what would be happening if the person first started to make progress and what they might notice when they do, or committing to some specific small steps they think would be helpful. This stage is about encouraging people into a future focused mindset and encouraging small changes in behaviour that are determined by the patient. It's important that the clinician isn't giving advice or suggesting what needs to be done. This can be quite a challenge when most of us are trained to give copious advice and to believe in our expertise. In this case, think of the patient as the expert in themselves.

What will be the next small sign that you are making progress towards (goal)?
What will your wife/best friend notice that will tell them you are making progress?
What will tell us you are making progress?
Bearing in mind your goal, can you think of a small change you can easily make before we meet again?*
What else?

This last question can lead to permission for regular measurements and tests such as waist circumference, weight, BP, or HbA1c for example.

11.2.2.2.4 Step 4: Noticing

So often the medical paradigm is about noticing negative things like pain or depression and asking how bad things are. In this model we are trying to shift the focus to positive experiences by asking what is working and what a person has noticed about any improvement. These questions are very useful at follow-up appointments to keep the conversation progress focused. These questions are novel to most practitioners but also to most patients, so take time to practice them and to give people time to think. We have noticed that people often start a consultation with what is worse but can easily generate a list of what is better if the clinician is persistent.

What is better since we last met?
I'm interested to hear about any improvements you have noticed since the last appointment
What difference has that made to you? Who else in the family noticed?
What seems to be working well for you right now?
What else?

The healthcare professional should also be highly attuned to noticing progress and giving positive feedback. The power of this cannot be underestimated.

I have noticed that you are smiling more/came without your stick/are breathing better this week
Your (test) tells me that you have been successful in making important changes...
Wow! You have lost (measurement) off your waist. How did you do that? (Get details).

We have found that patients respond really positively to graphs of progress printed from the GP computer system (an example is given below) and like to show family and friends how much progress they have made. In a nutshell, noticing supplies feedback and feedback is an important part of motivation and maintenance of behaviour change.

11.2.2.3 An example of a G.R.I.N. case study (based closely on a consented patient)

A 63-year-old lady, Carol, went through the practice's diabetes screening program and was found to have a raised HbA1c of 46 mmol/mol (6.4%) (normal range <42 mmol/mol (6%)). The practice nurse made her an appointment to discuss this with a GP in 2018 when she weighed 110 kg (Fig. 11.4).

She had a background of low mood, severe brittle asthma and bronchiectasis and so was a frequent attender.

On 24 May 2018 Carol weighed 110 kg. Over the next 10 months she lost 11.5 kg with the help of the GRIN approach and therapeutic carbohydrate restriction (TCR). The two acute spikes in body weight seen between 30 September 2018 and 31 March 2019 were due to steroid courses for asthma.

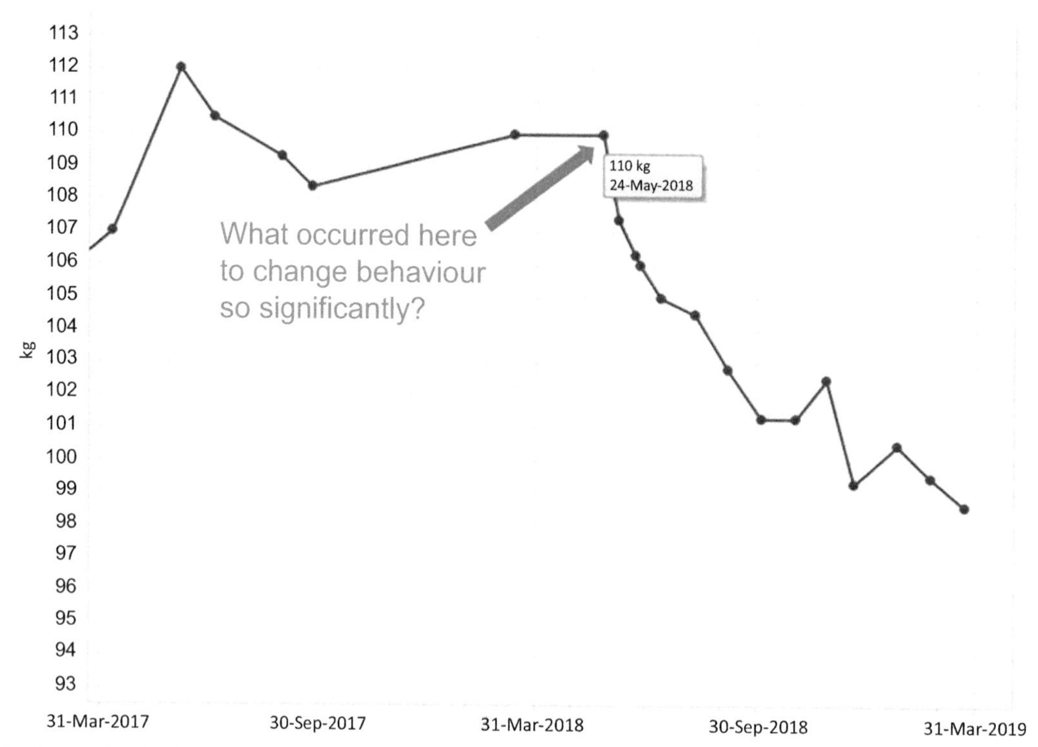

FIGURE 11.4 Case study: Carol's weight change over 2 years.

11.2.2.3.1 Patient's individual health goals

Doctor: '*Carol, in general what would you most like to see improve in your health?*'
Patient: 'To be able to breathe better – I get really scared at times.'

Note that she was not really interested in her raised HbA1c. That just made her even more worried. Instead it was better to pursue a positive, more solution-focused line.

Doctor: '*If you could breathe better what difference would that make to your life?*'
Patient: 'Well, it would be so great to worry less about my breathing –sometimes I wonder where this will all end…'

The next question employs the useful 'what else?' aspect to get more details.
Doctor: 'What else would be better if you could breathe more easily?'
Patient: 'I help look after my three-year-old grandson and I would love to be able to be more active with him, he's so lively!'

The tone of the consultation improves as we move from fears to hopes. Also, the more someone adds detail to a preferred future, the more likely they are to believe in it and want it. My next question would be around what activities breathing better might allow her to share with her little grandson. The more she imagines and inhabits a preferred future the more likely she is to make the necessary changes to achieve her goals.

Doctor: 'In your experience what might help you breathe better? Or when has your breathing been even a little better?'

Note we are still not talking about my goal around the HbA1c because it's not hers. But with patience we will get there. I am trying to find a shared goal.

Patient: 'Well it's obvious I need to lose weight; stairs are a nightmare for me!'

11.2.2.3.2 Exploring resources and resilience

It's important to resist the urge to give advice before further exploring the strengths and wisdom your patient already has.
Doctor: 'If you have ever lost weight successfully before, what has helped you succeed in the past?
Patient: 'Being organised seems to help me, getting the fridge "sin free" for a start.'
Doctor: 'What else?'

Patient: 'Also, I'm quite a fan of social media, so I found some good advice last time and Facebook can be a support too. My neighbour and I used to go walking together which I enjoyed.'

11.2.2.3.3 Increments

So many of us have a grand scheme but those first steps towards a goal are the most important.
Doctor: 'Carol, can you think of something you can commit to right now, today, to help you lose weight?'
Patient: 'Really, I suppose in view of the diabetes thing the nurse mentioned, the biscuits and cake should be the first to go.'

At this point some strong reinforcement can help. Perhaps discuss exactly how this is to be achieved, what difference that action would make and agree on a next appointment to re-weigh and monitor progress.

Doctor: 'What a great idea! What do you hope to be telling me in two weeks time? How will you/I/your family know this is working well?'

11.2.2.3.4 Noticing

Noticing may be the most powerful part of positive psychology. Noticing both what works and crucially, what feels better, seems to be central to further success and sustainability. The classical medical paradigm is the opposite of this, focusing as it does on symptoms of disease, like pain or depression. The patient gets the doctor's attention by citing her maladies, and the doctor focuses on those accordingly. A negative effect results, for patient and doctor alike. In this case, Carol agreed to be reweighed after 3 weeks. Looking at the graph, you can see she had lost an impressive 2.8 kg.

Doctor: 'Carol that is amazing! Well done! I'm really interested, what other improvements have you noticed?'
Patient: 'Yes! My family says that I'm more cheerful. It feels good to be more in control and I didn't miss the biscuits as much as I expected.'
Doctor: 'What else?'
Patient: 'I've started walking again with my neighbour too and have enjoyed chatting to her.'

We see noticing as closely related to feedback, an important part of motivation. In Carol's case, printing off her weight graph supplied more positive feedback, as I could point out she was the lightest she had been for over a year.

That completed this GRIN cycle. So now the process can be repeated at future appointments to build on her success.

Doctor: 'Right Carol, that's biscuits and cakes beaten, what's your next step?'
Patient: 'I was wondering if perhaps I eat too much toast –I know it's fattening...'
Doctor: 'You're right! How will you know when you've beaten toast? What will you be eating instead?'

Over a year, Carol lost more weight than ever before in her life. The two transient blips on her graph are due to courses of steroids for her asthma, but she didn't end up in the hospital once in the winter. She is pleased to notice that it's not just that she breathes better but she also feels healthy.

Doctor: 'What else is better?'
Patient: 'My family are so proud of me! Oh and I buy smaller clothes now. And you know I don't miss bread a bit, and yes I can bend over to play with my grandson easily these days. The best bit is to feel less scared and more in control of my own health!'

Her HbA1c reduced to 41 mmol/mol (5.9%) (in the normal range). This shows how holistic a hope-based, patient-centred approach can be. Carol's blood pressure improved too.

This process affected David, her doctor, as well. Having looked after Carol for over 30 years, he only recently noticed what a resourceful, determined person she is. It seems wrong that she is so grateful, because it has been her efforts that have made such a difference. These days we look forward to hearing how she is getting on. Cases like this give hope and energy back to the doctor and can improve healthcare professional resilience as well as patient health and happiness.

11.2.2.4 Applying GRIN

The approach can be used in brief appointments. We called it GRIN to help you remember the four components but in pressurised clinical practice it is fine to use any one or two of the four in a consultation. For instance, in a case with multiple morbidities, if all you manage is to explore your patient's health goals or relevant resources, your time is very well spent. Practitioners who are new to this might have the goal of using a minimum of one of the elements in each case. A useful training exercise is to see how many times in a morning clinic you are able to give out a sincere compliment or comment on some improvement, then notice how that affects your patient interactions.

Using a solution-focused approach challenges the traditional model that any problem must be understood and analysed in detail before progress can be made. It gets away from diagnosing the problem to envisioning the solution. Most clinicians believe that taking a history detailing the causal events that led up to illness is always important in finding the remedy. In fact, though this may help understanding, sometimes it can hamper progress. For example take obesity, a detailed history of a lifelong weight problem can sometimes lead to people feeling worse. In a case like this, particularly if time is short, an alternative could be to notice resilience with a sincere enquiry about *toughness* by asking, 'that sounds so hard, I'm interested to understand how you managed to get through those difficult times?' This may be an excellent prelude to exploring goals, and a much more productive and cheerful use of time than taking your patient through a very painful, detailed examination of past difficulties. In this way, progress can be fast and sometimes surprisingly so. Practitioners must be ready to give up advice and rather have sincere faith in the patient's expertise and strengths. The practitioner's knowledge and experience is then used to support the patient's efforts and progress.

We have found this approach to be easily incorporated into a wide range of clinical scenarios. It is positive, patient-centred and less burdensome on staff. Surely, this is much needed in helping both patients and staff remain happy, resilient, and well.

11.2.2.5 Resources

https://www.dietdoctor.com/motivating-people-change-lives
https://youtu.be/3WTY74j3DAg
http://www.ukasfp.org

11.2.3 Monitoring, how to deal with failure and effective longer-term support

David & Jen Unwin

In clinical practice, all sorts of things work at the beginning but what counts is longer term results. It is vital to think about how your service will monitor clients, deal with problems and support maintenance. In this way, our National Health Service T2D remission rates (defined as HbA1c <48 mmol/mol (6.5%) and being drug-free) have actually improved over the years from 31% in 2017 to 51% in March 2023. Let us help you to achieve similar results.

11.2.3.1 The psychological aspects of maintenance

Applying our GRIN model, discussed earlier, at review, always be on the lookout for the opportunity for sincere compliments (Noticing). The first things we notice in our patients are often:

- Improving skin quality
- Eyes look larger as periorbital fat is lost very early in the diet
- Reduced belly size

Next, actively look for the benefits of their lifestyle changes. Ask if they have noticed any improvements before moving on to the problems or challenges they may be facing. Common early observations are:

- Surprise at not being hungry [17]
- More energy
- Loss of brain fog

If they have done well, it is possible to take them round the GRIN cycle again. 'In view of these improvements I'm wondering what your next steps will be? . . .' And so on.

At review don't forget to revisit baseline measurements and use these metrics to give feedback. Feedback is the bedrock of behaviour change. This is how we notice what works and do more of it. In our practice, the computer system generates graphs, which is one good way to do this. In addition, perhaps encourage your patients to weigh themselves or do serial waist or blood pressure measurements. This is great if the metrics improve, but what to do if your client regresses?

11.2.3.2 Reframing failure

What can you do if your patient encounters problems, such as gaining weight or their health condition regressing?

It may help to prepare patients for challenges at the start, and explore how they might handle them or organise their lives to reduce temptation.

A common scenario is weight gain after Christmas or a holiday. Give them hope for future success by saying something like, 'As we grow older, we learn from our mistakes.' 'We all make mistakes',; 'wise people only make the same mistake once (or twice!)'. Instead of seeing the mistake as a failure, reframe by asking, '*what would you do differently next time*?'. Encourage clear and concise, actionable answers. Explore planning in advance for the next time to make success easier. In this case you may suggest replanning foods or drinks they could enjoy at Christmas. Also examine exactly what went wrong: 'who really eats those biscuits you have for the Grandchildren?', 'how could this be better handled?'

11.2.3.2.1 Willpower or habits

Many people blame a lack of willpower for mistakes or lack of success. Perhaps their goals aren't clear or actionable enough. Firstly, with respect to patient goals, ask yourself: are they clear and actionable? Many people would like to lose weight in a vague way. Clarify by revising the difference that losing weight would make to their lives.

Willpower may be overrated. It doesn't withstand stress, poor health, and all sorts of other things. Getting into good habits is far more useful [18]. Think about it, we do all sorts of things on a daily basis that don't require willpower. Many of them are habits that require little thought or energy, such as brushing teeth, hanging up the car keys or locking the door. It's possible to develop healthy dietary habits too. Many of our patients get into the habit of not eating breakfast, which becomes an established habit after a few weeks, requiring no willpower at all.

11.2.3.3 Repeated failure: What is really going on?

Again, sometimes the patient may benefit from revisiting their goals, are they valid?

Sometimes external factors, such as problems with relationships, housing, and finances, may play a role in failure. Weight loss may not be a priority right now. It's important to allow people to step back and to signal they are welcome back in the future. Some of our patients have returned years later saying, 'Now I'm ready to sort this.'

A common pattern is yo-yo dieting prior to working with us. There are people whose weight goes up and down all their lives. Note the oscillatory nature of the weight in Fig. 11.5 – we see this pattern often.

Other people just become steadily heavier. For years we wondered why advice around moderation and cutting back to help some people with weight loss seemed so ineffective, even after pointing out the serious risk to patient health that obesity and Type 2 diabetes brings. Then one day we realised some of our very obese patients were exhibiting similar behaviours to other people who struggle with moderation: those addicted to drugs or alcohol. What if they really could not easily just cut back any more than a person with an alcohol problem can stop at a small whiskey. It could make far more sense if obesity for some, rather than being a result of dietary choice or greed, was part of a compulsion to eat certain foods even while knowing the dangers involved. A similar scenario exists for most cigarette smokers. Bear in mind the actual problem for people who are yo-yo dieters and also those who gain weight steadily could be food addiction.

11.2.3.4 Food addiction

Once we accepted food addiction as a possible explanation for the behaviour of many of our patients with significant weight problems, we came to find more and more clinical cases to support it as a theory. This was particularly true for those with a BMI over 35. There are people for whom the very idea of life without bread, mashed potato or chips is quite unthinkable. Some panic and eat more just at the thought of restricting carbohydrate. But for others the suggestion of food addiction will be the first time they have understood a lifetime of overeating. Moderation in dietary terms has all sorts of problems such as how to measure it, but one of its greatest setbacks is revealed if there is an underlying compulsion to eat certain foods. Just a single biscuit or half a chocolate bar can be just as impossible as half a cigarette. Once we are clear which foods are involved two possible strategies are possible; cold turkey and abstinence, or transitioning. An example of the latter was David's approach to biscuits. Over nearly a year he transitioned from chocolate biscuits to oat biscuits to almonds to no snacks at all, and has maintained this as a good habit for nearly 7 years now.

We all live in an obesogenic environment that makes maintaining a low carbohydrate diet difficult (Fig. 11.6). Most patients find maintenance difficult at some point. The graph above illustrates this for one of our patients. In 2014, he

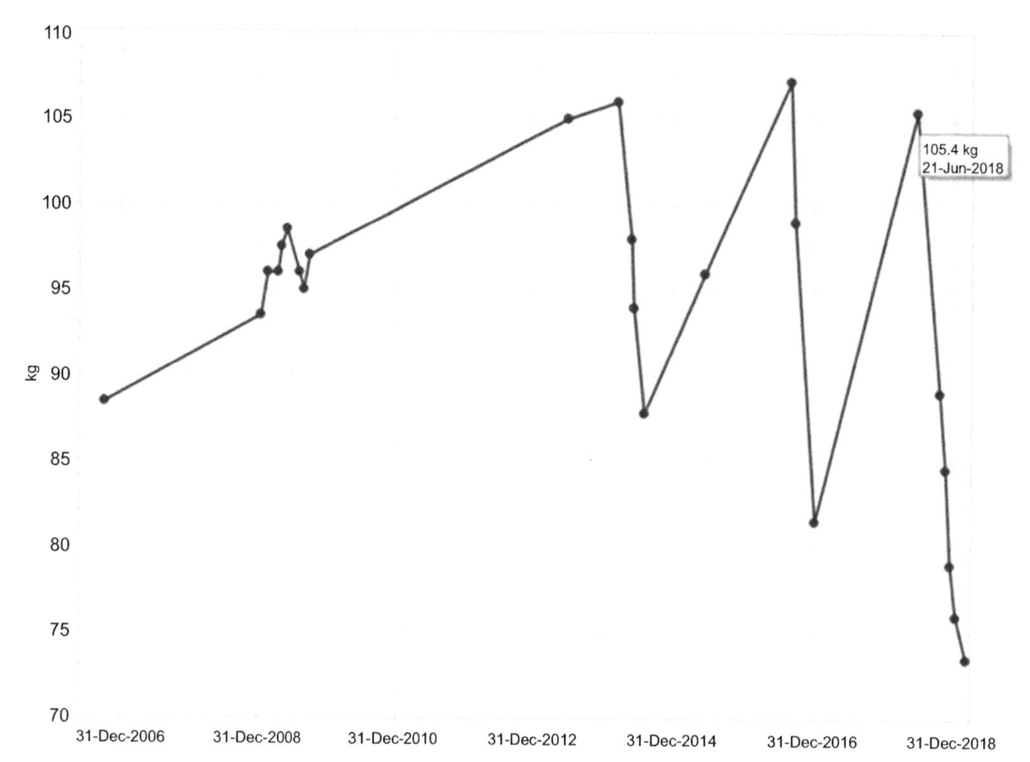

FIGURE 11.5 Body weight (kg) over 12 years as a result of Yo-yo dieting. Body weight oscillates as the patient endures the vicious cycle of relapse.

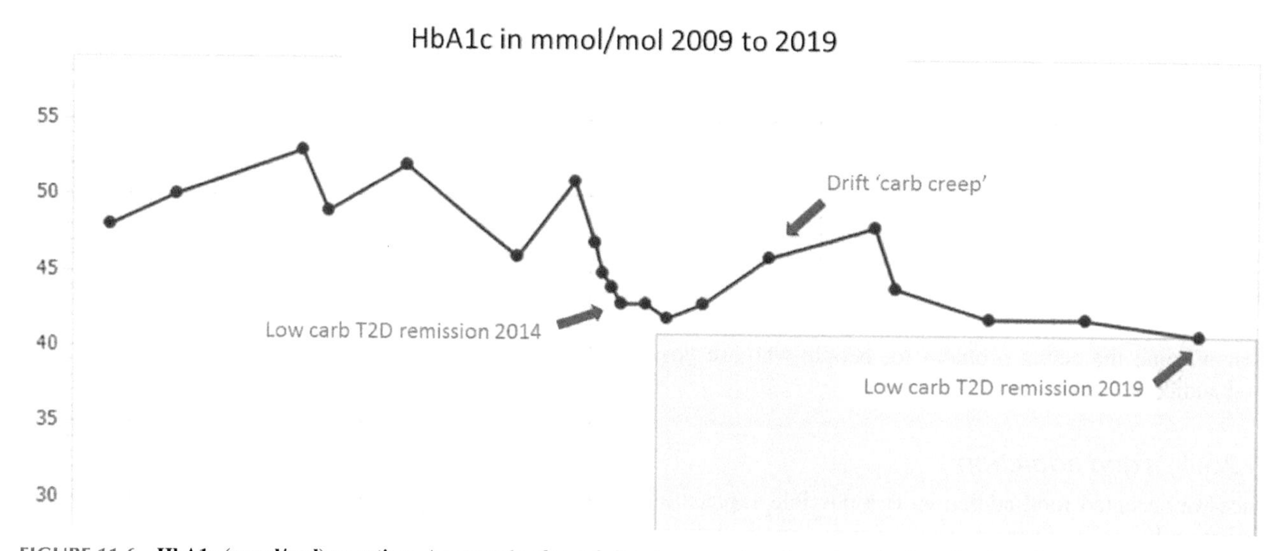

FIGURE 11.6 **HbA1c (mmol/mol) over time.** An example of type 2 diabetes regressing after reintroduction of carbohydrates.

achieved drug free T2D remission but after 18 months his diabetic control deteriorated and his HbA1c started to climb. It is important that clinicians don't necessarily start medication at this point, assuming that diet has failed, as in reality slow reintroduction of carbohydrate rich foods may mean that the patient isn't truly on the diet any more. When we asked if sugar was creeping back, the patient acknowledged that it was, and he knew exactly how. He was then keen to rectify matters rather than go back on the medication. It is so important to train all members of your team in the approach and to review patients' results on a regular basis over the years to ensure dietary compliance, effective patient support and sustainable health changes.

11.2.3.5 Making maintenance both economical and effective

We work in the cash-strapped British National Health Service (NHS) and have been forced to become innovative in the absence of any funding for our service. We started running our group consultations in 2013, holding the meetings approximately once a month. Just as in the one-on-one work we encourage participants to consider their individual health goals, the resources available to them, setting realistic steps and enabling the individual to notice what works for them using the GRIN approach. Patient relatives and carers are welcome to attend as some patients rely on others for food shopping or cooking. Group sessions also provide a forum for patients to offer practical support to their peers and for the training of new staff. On average, 30 patients attend each session, which lasts 90 minutes. They are held in the evening so working people can attend. Over time some patients become happy to act as mentors to help newcomers. A practical point is that we find two staff members are needed to run these meetings, also they are an ideal environment to train new staff as they see first-hand what can be achieved. Post-COVID these sessions are easily morphed into virtual meetings via Zoom.

11.2.3.6 Clinical patterns to look out for

Firstly, rarely there is weight loss and yet a worsening of HbA1c. We have recently seen this twice, watch out for it. In one case, the patient had in fact developed type 1 diabetes and needed insulin. Further investigation into the other case led to the diagnosis of a hidden malignancy.

Another worrying pattern is where a low HbA1c does not fit with the clinical picture, a very low HbA1c makes it easier to guess what is going on here. Many of us forget that anaemia gives a low HbA1c too.

11.3 Eating control

11.3.1 Hunger

Mark I. Friedman

11.3.1.1 Introduction

Considering that increased hunger can undermine dietary treatments for weight loss [19,20], losing weight with less hunger would be a significant benefit for overweight and obese individuals who are dieting. Physicians have long observed that their patients experience little hunger despite substantial weight reduction when they eat a diet that is severely restricted in carbohydrate, high in fat, and containing adequate protein [21]. Results of controlled clinical trials using self-reporting methodologies to assess hunger in patients eating such KDs are consistent with these clinical observations.

11.3.1.2 Measurement of hunger

Subjective hunger feelings and sensations are most commonly measured using either visual analogue scales (VAS) or questionnaires. VAS pose a question (e.g., 'How hungry do you feel?') and the study subject makes a hash mark on a 100 mm line that is anchored on either end by extreme answers (e.g., 'Not at all' to 'As hungry as I've ever been'). The distance in millimetres from the zero or minimal response ('Not at all') to the hash mark is the quantitative equivalent of the intensity of their subjective feeling or sensation. Another instrument, the Eating Inventory/Three-Factor Eating Questionnaire [22], consists of a series of true/false questions and predetermined numerical rating (Likert) scales that tap into various aspects of eating behaviour, appetite and weight control. 'Hunger' is one of the three dimensions of eating behaviour derived by factor analysis of responses to the Eating Inventory and the score on this factor is used to assess the experience of hunger.

As with any measure of subjective experience, such assessments of hunger have limitations. The instruments described above appear to measure different aspects of hunger, making interpretation and comparisons across studies difficult. For example, the Eating Inventory was originally thought to measure a trait reflecting long-term or overall experience of hunger cues, but it appears that it may at least in part reflect the immediate experience or state of hunger depending on when the questionnaire is completed relative to mealtime [23]. Another limitation of these commonly used measurements of hunger is that they do not reflect individual differences in the physical sensation of hunger [24]. A more granular assessment of the physical locus and extent of hunger sensations not only offers a qualitative picture of the subjective experience of hunger not captured by VAS, but may provide a more sensitive measure because it varies over a larger range of hunger intensities [24,25]. Importantly, it may more adequately reflect the experience of hunger in obese than in normal weight individuals [25].

11.3.1.3 Clinical studies

Inpatient studies provide rigorous control over diet consumption and composition, although they can be less relevant to 'real world' conditions than are trials with free-living participants. One inpatient study found no increase in hunger ratings despite lower energy intake and weight loss in obese participants eating a KD *ad libitum* when compared with baseline measures taken when participants ate their usual high-carbohydrate diet [26]. Another inpatient trial using a counterbalanced crossover design found that whereas obese subjects consumed fewer calories, they lost more weight and experienced less hunger eating a KD as compared with a high-carbohydrate diet [27]. In both studies, elevated blood ketone body concentrations validated the intended effect of the KD.

Studies of free-living patients who are overweight or obese have typically compared the effects of a KD with a high-carbohydrate diet that either served as a baseline diet or was one of the two diets to which participants were randomly assigned. When a KD was compared with a high-carbohydrate/low-fat diet, the latter was restricted in calories in an attempt to control for the reduction in energy intake typically seen with ad libitum consumption of KDs. Adherence to the KD was validated by measurement of blood or urinary ketone bodies except in one study [28] in which ketosis may have been likely given that subjects eating the KD consumed on average only 43 g per day of carbohydrate [29].

Free-living patients who were switched from their usual baseline high-carbohydrate diet to a KD reported reduced hunger despite significant weight loss [30,31] and lower energy intakes [31]. In studies comparing diets using a between-subjects design, those assigned to a KD reported less hunger than those eating a high-carbohydrate diet despite greater [28,32] or equivalent [33] weight loss. Hunger was assessed once weekly or at the beginning and end of the trials, which lasted from 1 month to 2 years. The reduction of hunger associated with eating a KD apparently persisted for up to 6 months [32,33]. After this time, hunger returned to levels seen in subjects eating a high-carbohydrate diet possibly due to a liberalisation of carbohydrate intake over time [33,34].

Very low carbohydrate KDs may contain relatively high amounts of protein as well as fat. However, whereas high protein diets may suppress hunger relative to diets with normal amounts of protein [35], this effect appears independent of the reduction of hunger associated with consumption of a KD. Veldhorst et al. [36] found that hunger ratings in normal weight subjects were lower on high-protein diets regardless of carbohydrate content, but were even lower when they ate a carbohydrate-free diet that was high in both protein and fat. Studies in obese patients also suggest that the effect of KDs on hunger is not solely related to the protein content of the diet. Protein intakes were similar in inpatient studies of obese participants who reported reduced hunger eating a KD [26,27]. Trials in free-living patients have found a relative absence or suppression of hunger with KDs whether dietary protein content was higher or lower than that in high-carbohydrate/low-fat diets [28,32].

11.3.1.4 Mechanisms

Elevated blood ketone body concentrations acting in the brain are often thought to be the cause of the attenuated hunger associated with consumption of a KD, but there is no direct evidence for this assumption. Certainly, circulating ketone body concentrations increased in each of the studies reviewed above in which it was measured. Similarly, very low energy diets that restrict intake to less than 800 kcal/day (3347 kJ/day) also produce ketosis, presumably by restricting carbohydrates along with calories, and prevent an increase in hunger despite weight loss [37,38]. However, although suggestive, these correlational data do not permit a causal inference regarding the effects of ketone bodies on hunger.

Stubbs et al. concluded that increased circulating concentrations of ketone bodies directly suppress hunger based on their observation that ketosis induced by the ingestion of a ketone monoester beverage after an overnight fast reduced hunger compared to the ingestion of a similar isocaloric glucose drink [39]. It is difficult to interpret the significance of this result given the unusual and unphysiological route of delivery and metabolism required for the conversion of the monoester into ketone bodies and the acute increase in ketones to 3.0 mM, which is the limit of what may be considered nutritional ketosis [40]. The effects on hunger of intravenous infusion of β-hydroxybutyrate that mimic the degree of ketosis associated with ingestion of a KD would be a more informative test of the hypothesis that blood ketone bodies *per se* suppress hunger.

The circulating concentration of the gut hormone, ghrelin, is elevated during fasting and after weight loss, and infusion of ghrelin elicits sensations of hunger in humans [41]. As with its effect on subjective hunger ratings, consumption of a KD [31] or a very low energy diet that results in ketosis [37,38] prevents the expected increase in blood ghrelin concentrations after reduced energy intake and weight loss. Similarly, ingestion of a ketone monoester beverage caused ketosis and suppressed hunger, and decreased ghrelin concentrations in fasted subjects [39]. Whereas these observations may suggest that suppression of ghrelin secretion provides a mechanism for the reduced hunger associated with eating KDs, its role appears complex given that ghrelin deficiency has no significant effect on food intake or eating behaviour in mice [41]. Ghrelin infusion may affect hunger indirectly through its other effects on gastrointestinal function and fuel metabolism in mice [41]. Even though changes in circulating ghrelin concentrations may not be the mechanism by which KDs affect hunger, they may serve as an objective marker for hunger that complements and helps validate subjective hunger ratings.

Studies in human subjects suggest that susceptibility to obesity is associated with a decreased capacity to oxidise fat [42,43]. Results from experiments in laboratory rodents are consistent with these observations and suggest that the predisposition to obesity and any accompanying excessive hunger or food intake is tied specifically to lower rates of fatty acid oxidation in the liver [44,45]. Given that ketone bodies are generated primarily by the hepatic oxidation of fatty acids, it is possible that an increase in fatty acid oxidation, not circulating ketone bodies *per se*, provides a signal that works to prevent or restrain hunger when one eats a KD.

11.3.1.5 Conclusions

Clinical observations and measurements of subjective hunger in clinical trials indicate that KDs attenuate hunger despite weight loss, although the mechanism for this dietary effect on appetite is unknown. Because persistent hunger may undermine weight loss efforts, the attenuation of hunger should benefit patients by improving adherence to their KD.

Acknowledgements

The author thanks David Ludwig and Gary Taubes for their helpful comments.

11.3.2 Processed Food Addiction

Joan Ifland

11.3.2.1 Introduction

Diet-related diseases are the leading cause of preventable death worldwide. Health practitioners would like to recommend real food-based Low Carbohydrate High Fat (LCHF) food plans to put diet-related diseases into remission, but they may find that their patients and clients are not able to adhere to them. Research shows that in spite of significant, even life-saving benefits of ketogenic diets (KD) [46] patients continue to consume high carbohydrate processed foods. This is a source of frustration to practitioner and patient alike.

This section offers a novel explanation for why some patients may not be able to adhere to an LCHF food plan. There is evidence that processed foods have addictive properties. Thus individuals who cannot adhere to an LCHF food plan may be suffering from addictive cravings that are severe enough to overwhelm the desire to improve health [47]. There is evidence for addictive properties in sugars [48,49], flours [50], gluten [51], excessive salt [52], processed fats [53], dairy [54], caffeine [55], and food additives [56].

The epidemic of diet-related diseases coincides with the entry of the tobacco industry into processed foods in the 1980s. The tobacco industry developed the Addiction Business Model consisting of five components: (1) addictive ingredients in the product, (2) advertising, (3) availability, (4) affordability, and (5) young age of onset [57]. When this model was applied to processed foods, the obesity epidemic and accompanying metabolic syndrome ensued.

Practitioners can overcome hidden barriers to successful implementation of LCHF diets by understanding the business and cultural pressure on neurological processes that drive food addiction. Understanding how processed food addiction is fostered by the Addiction Business Model could give practitioners the tools they need to help patients implement and adhere to an LCHF diet.

11.3.2.2 Evidence

Due to widespread research into obesity, eating disorders, and drug addiction, extensive evidence for processed food addiction exists [58,59]. Existing research illuminates aspects of addictive use of processed foods. Addictions in general exhibit extensive constellations of consequences and processed food addiction is no exception. The evidence is organised into four categories. (1) Addictions alter neurofunctioning which impairs the individual's capabilities. (2) This dysfunction in the individual radiates out into family systems. (3) There are addictive properties in the substances being abused, that is specific processed foods. (4) In order for an epidemic of addiction to flourish as tobacco once did and processed foods do now, there must be macro factors in place. The following describes this evidence.

11.3.2.2.1 The individual

1. Neurofunctioning. The brains of drug-addicted people and overeaters exhibit altered function in similar ways. Reward centres are hyperactivated as are stress pathways. Blood flow to the frontal lobe is impaired [60].
2. Cue Reactivity. Reward centres in the brain react easily and strongly to cues for substances of abuse for drug-addicted people and to processed foods for overeaters [61].
3. Cognitive Impairment. As blood flow is diverted from the frontal lobe to the addicted neurons, cognitive impairments develop. These include attention span, learning, decision-making, memory, and impulse control [62].
4. Pavlovian Conditioning of Neurons. In both drug addiction and addictive eating, research shows that reward neurons become hyperactive through a process of repeat exposure to addictive substances and cues for the substances [63].
5. Genetics and Epigenetics. In both drug and food addiction, similar genetic anomalies are found [64]. Further, environment plays a role in activating addictive genes [65]
6. Manifestations of the DSM 5 Substance Use Disorder Criteria. Manifestations of the 11 diagnostic criteria for alcoholism also appear in overeaters. These include unintended use, failure to cut back, time spent, cravings, failure to fulfil roles, relationship problems, activities given up, hazardous use, use in spite of consequences, increased use over time, and use to avoid withdrawal [66].
7. Behaviours. Behavioural dysfunction includes poor impulse control, numbing, blaming, shame, denial, minimising, normalising, and emotional avoidance. These behaviours are found in both drug-addicted people and overeaters [67].
8. Sense of taste. Both tobacco and sodas are associated with loss of taste. This is important for recovering food-addicted people because it impairs enjoyment of unprocessed real foods and creates a barrier to acceptance of low carbohydrate foods [68,69].
9. Comorbidities. Both drug and food addiction generate a constellation of consequences. In both syndromes, the consequences can be measured by the same instrument, The Addiction Severity Index [70,71].

11.3.2.2.2 Family systems

10. Inherited Patterns of Use. In both addictive use of drugs and of food, the syndromes are inherited through family systems [72,73].
11. Adverse Childhood Experiences (ACE). Both drug addiction and overeating correlate with ACE [74,75].
12. Foetal Syndrome. Children born to women who abuse substances and women who abuse processed foods during pregnancy have congenital defects [76,77].

11.3.2.2.3 Addictive Substances

13. Psychoactive Characteristics of Substances. Both processed foods and addictive drugs elicit similar neuro-adaptations [78,79].
14. Drugs and Processed Foods are Interchangeable. Drug-addicted people substitute food for the drug in withdrawal and recovery. Overeaters may turn to drugs such as diet-pills or nicotine to stop the use of processed foods [60].
15. Patterns of Polysubstance Use. Drug addiction and food abuse are both characterised by the simultaneous use of several substances. Combining alcohol and nicotine is an example of polysubstance use. Fast food typically contains sweetener, flour, gluten, excessive salt, dairy, processed fats, and caffeine [80,81].
16. Abstinence in Treatment. In both drug/alcohol recovery and food addiction recovery, abstinence from the substances leads to control [82,83].

11.3.2.2.4 Macro factors

17. Epidemiological Patterns. Tobacco addiction and overweight both reached about 65% of the US population [84,85]. This is evidence for the reach of corporations using the Addiction Business Model.
18. Business Practices. Businesses selling addictive products such as alcohol and tobacco use the same business model as those selling processed foods. This includes enhancing addictive properties of the products, heavy advertising, cheap prices, widespread availability, and targeting the youngest possible user [57].
19. Cost to Society. Overeating, drug abuse, alcoholism, and tobacco create a significant cost to society [86,87].
20. Government Subsidies. Subsidies make substances cheap enough to be bought often enough to addict reward neurons [88,89].

The evidence that people are experiencing overeating in the same way as drug addiction is strong and consistent. It is also temporal in that the epidemic of diet-related diseases followed the entry of the tobacco industry's Addictive Model into processed food, just as tobacco related diseases followed the worldwide spread of smoking.

Advising on the possibility that patients and clients have developed an addiction to processed foods will lead to tremendous relief. Patients and clients have been blamed for being failures at weight loss and compulsive eating. Finding out that overeating is the result of the same business practices that led to smoking as the leading cause of preventable death will relieve patients of guilt and even self-stigmatisation.

The findings of addiction to processed foods also stop ineffectual approaches that can and often do make food addiction worse. These approaches include insufficient calories, addictive diet products, transference of food addiction to drug and alcohol addiction in bariatric surgery, weight regain, the side-effects of pharmaceuticals, and failed residential stays. These are all painful conditions that food-addicted people have commonly endured. The finding of addiction to processed food brings hope to the defeated patient because treatment for food addiction recovery is radically different than it is for weight-loss or eating disorders.

11.3.2.3 Treatment

Treatment of addictions is difficult at best. Research shows that in recovery, relapse is normal [90] and can persist for an average of 8 years in the case of drug and alcohol addiction [91]. Both the addicted person and the people around the addicted person suffer the roller coaster of ups and downs as the addiction slowly goes into remission. About 50%–60% of addicted people attain permanent remission from drug and alcohol addiction but less than 1% of overweight people recover from processed food addiction as evidenced by research showing that most people who lose weight regain it [92].

It may be harder to put processed food addiction into remission than drug and alcohol addiction. Research shows certain factors correlate with longer periods of relapse before remission. These include early age of onset [93], use of multiple substances [80], cuing inside the household [94], cuing in social circles [95], and a history of weight cycling [96]. It is common for food-addicted people to experience many of these complicating factors.

Nonetheless, the approach to recovery from addiction to processed foods responds to the same approaches as recovery from drug/alcohol addiction. Primary protocols include motivational interviewing, abstinence, cue avoidance, and lifetime support.

11.3.2.3.1 Motivational interviewing

Stages of motivational interviewing include learning about reasons for change, recognising problems and benefits of resolving problems, gaining optimism and confidence about changing, and committing to change through development of options [97]. Redefining the problem from one of needing to just eat less to lose weight, all the way to needing years to retrain severely addiction reward neurons, is a significant leap. It can be accomplished by asking about the 11 DSM 5 substance use disorders Criteria as well as the presence of complicating factors [98].

11.3.2.3.2 Abstinence

Abstinence from processed foods can be attained by eliminating the full range of addictive substances that manufacturers have added to our food [99,100]. Dividing food into addictive versus non-addictive follows the structure of dividing drinks into alcoholic and non-alcoholic. It can take months, even years for food-addicted people to eliminate all addictive processed foods.

11.3.2.3.3 Cue avoidance

Classic addiction recovery calls for avoiding people, places, and things associated with substance use. Research shows that cue avoidance is just as important in recovery from addiction to processed foods [47]. Cue avoidance in food addiction recovery is much more difficult due to the sheer volume of processed food cues that pervade environments [101] and the vast quantity of processed foods that people consume [102].

11.3.2.3.4 Lifelong support

Although evidence shows less than a 15% chance that alcohol- and drug-addicted people will relapse after attaining 5 years of abstinence, the risk remains. Alcoholics Anonymous for example, may have members with over 50 years of abstinence. They continue to attend meetings and socialise with friends in recovery. They avoid extensive socialising with drinkers to avoid activating the drive to conform to them.

Lifelong support for people in recovery from processed food addiction is even more essential because of the intense proliferation of food cues and the common use of processed foods in all walks of life. Food-addicted people will endure more stimulation of addicted reward centres than drug- and alcohol-addicted people. More stimulation combined with neurons that have been increasingly sensitised since birth means that food-addicted people will be more vulnerable to cravings and relapse for life.

11.3.2.3.5 Special issues in treatment of processed food addiction

Early onset, intense cuing and polysubstance use all mean that processed food addiction will be characterised by more deeply conditioned neurons, more persistent cravings, and more lapsing. In addition to these challenges, competing theories about the cause of overeating are always there to pull food-addicted people off their recovery path and back into harmful weight-loss schemes. Because addictive substances are presented as food, or hidden in food, it is hard for observers to define overeating as a pure substance use disorder. Consumption looks like it must have something to do with eating even though at its core, it is like alcoholism or nicotine addiction.

11.3.2.4 Conclusion

Making the shift to seeing overeating as a severe addiction ends the frustration of practitioners and the suffering of patients and clients. The severity of food addiction is a match for an intensive outpatient program. Practitioners do well to never waiver from the focus on addictive substances posing as processed foods.

11.4 Legal and ethical aspects to therapeutic carbohydrate restriction

11.4.1 Legal and ethical aspects of prescribing therapeutic carbohydrate restriction

Joan Adams

Senior Legal Counsel (RSA) with a special interest in ethics. Chairperson of the HPCSA Professional Conduct Committee who acquitted Noakes in 2017.

> *In most diseases, there is a tendency to natural cure and, if the patient's constitution is supported by simple means (food and fluids), recovery will follow.*
>
> Hippocrates [103]

Around 400 BC Hippocrates gave birth to the Westernised European concept of medical ethics with the formulation of its central tenet, which still persists to this day: 'do no harm'. During the intellectual revolution of the 18th century (Renaissance), Thomas Percival published the 'Code of Medical Ethics' in 1803. Further codes of ethics and conduct followed as a result of, inter alia, outrage due to the medical and scientific atrocities committed by the Nazi regime, as exposed in the Nuremberg trials, and the 40-year Study of Untreated Syphilis at Tuskegee, in the United States (1932–72). A well-researched historical perspective of these developments, which also places them in an international context, is provided and tabulated concisely in the article *Ups and downs in the history of medical ethics* [104].

The current concept of Western medical ethics has been well developed, based mainly on core ethical principles and standards of good practice: beneficence, non-maleficence, autonomy and justice, aptly described as follows:

'The four principles plus scope approach provides a simple, accessible, and culturally neutral approach to thinking about ethical issues in healthcare. The approach, developed in the United States, is based on four common, basic *prima facie* moral commitments – respect for autonomy, beneficence, non-maleficence, and justice – plus concern for their scope of application' [105].

These four principles in turn have been further expanded, with various theories of their application on a philosophical level, inter alia that of 'reflective equilibrium' as expounded by J Summers, namely a weighing-up of the interaction and respective merits of each of the four principles for each ad hoc decision, based on an intimate and thorough knowledge of such principles by the professional considering the case [106].

On a global more practical level, various governing and regulatory bodies of the medical and healthcare professions in every state, consisting of members of the profession, have developed similar ethical rules of conduct and standards of good practice, for application in various branches of the profession. Some form of professional accountability and regulation of the healthcare professions would indeed appear to be imperative in the interest of public safety.

Codes of practice and codes of good conduct as tabulated by various regulatory bodies are not, however, ethics themselves, but guidelines as to how to achieve and arrive at ethical decision-making. Ethics is a branch of moral philosophy entailing a critical and objective assessment of what should and should not be done, of what is good and what is not good [107]. It must be borne in mind that ethics, as with medical advancement and science, is not static and is constantly evolving with the times, in a highly dynamic environment. Social media ethics, which include virtual consultations and e-health, are examples of modern day digital ethics, unheard of a few years ago.

Due regard being given to the centuries of existence and development of medical ethics, one would imagine that a trained physician and healthcare provider prescribing a healthy wholesome natural diet, and healthy dietary lifestyle choices in general, would be commonplace. In fact, it should at least be as commonplace as prescribing other healthy lifestyle strategies, including a good night's sleep, relaxation and stress reduction techniques, sufficient hydration, limited alcohol intake, no smoking, healthy weight management, and moderate exercise and physical activity. Diet and nutrition indeed go hand-in-hand with a robust immune system and general health and wellbeing, not to mention disease prevention and management. It has oft been said: 'Let food be thy medicine', the origin of which is uncertain but it is often, erroneously it would seem, attributed to Hippocrates.

The doctor/healthcare [103] professional provider–patient relationship is an autonomous one. A healthcare practitioner has a duty to conduct a thorough clinical examination, which may include diagnostic investigations and tests. The doctor is also enjoined to record a proper and comprehensive medical history, provide an independent professional opinion and impart objective practical advice, dietary or otherwise, in the best interests of the patient (beneficence). It is the health practitioner who is in the best position to treat a patient and clinically prescribe what is best on an individual patient-specific basis. In applying her or his mind professionally, impartially, and ethically, the healthcare practitioner must treat patients fairly and justly, without fear or favour (justice), with due regard to anecdotal clinical evidence, robust scientific evidence and best practice. The healthcare practitioner is expected to place the medical interests, health and well-being of the patients even above her or his own personal self-interest (bias; financial and/or pecuniary interests) and/or professional interests (vested food production, business, corporate and pharmaceutical interests, and other perverse incentives; sponsorships; peer, political and/or institutional pressure, etc.). This is, indeed, the essence of non-maleficence and doing no harm. The patient has the right to self-determination (and autonomy) and the freedom to make healthy lifestyle and dietary choices, and informed decisions, based on objective, unbiased and transparent professional advice. This is the essence of informed consent and the cornerstone of a democracy.

It would appear obvious that healthcare practitioners should be treating patients holistically with and by all natural healthy means possible, with due regard to the importance of adequate daily nutrition and a healthy natural diet, with the least invasive medical, surgical, pharmaceutical, chemical and diagnostic means. There was, however, unprecedented regulatory furore, well-publicised globally, relating to at least two relatively recent professional conduct disciplinary hearings, concerning relatively benign dietary advice pertaining to a low carbohydrate and high (healthy) fat (LCHF) diet by members of the medical profession: that of Professor Tim Noakes in South Africa, by the Health Professions Council of South Africa (HPCSA) [108], during the period 2015–18, and that of Dr Gary Fettke of Tasmania, by the Australian Health Practitioner Regulation Agency (AHPRA), during the period 2016–18. In both instances complaints had been lodged with the respective regulators by dieticians, in what the evidence seemed to suggest were professional 'turf wars', with alleged food production, pharmaceutical and/or other vested interests. Hence the Noakes hearing was aptly dubbed by the media as 'The Nutrition Hearing of The Century' as it was a first of its kind in modern day medicine. If dispensing natural healthy dietary advice and healthy lifestyle choices is, and should be, commonplace for a healthcare practitioner, the disciplinary proceedings launched against the two mentioned professionals, highlighted an ethical dilemma not witnessed before in modern medicine, and neither on such a global scale.

In neither of the above hearings were the merits of the LCHF diet, as such, adjudicated on. Both hearings did, however, provide a platform to lead vast expert, professional and/or scientific evidence, in order to refute the charges. The complaint by the HPCSA against Noakes, resulted in an acquittal, which was upheld on appeal, and the conviction of Fettke was repealed by the AHPRA. Fettke was, unlike Noakes, issued a formal written apology by the AHPRA.

In complying with his ethical and professional duty, a healthcare practitioner is enjoined to be well-informed, and keep abreast of scientific advancement (including natural healthy dietary and nutrition strategies) pertaining to the profession and/or speciality, including clinical best practices and evidence-based protocols. A healthcare practitioner, indeed, has a duty to attain the necessary professional skills to do so properly. This should ideally not be confined to the bare minimum regulatory requirements, annually or bi-annually, relating to continuing professional development (CPD) points, but should be on an ongoing permanent basis. That said, practitioners are duty bound to perform professional acts only in the field of medicine and healthcare in which they **are** educated and trained, and in which they have gained experience, and to act within their scope of practice (a global pandemic and an international 'medical emergency' created, for example, by the Covid-19 coronavirus, is a rare exception to the duty to act within the confines of scope of practice - based on the defence of necessity due to an emergency).

As indicated, ethics is evolving with the (modern) times. What may in the past have been regarded as unconventional, and thus unethical and unprofessional, may be regarded as conventional, best practice, and thus be entirely ethical and professional today. Likewise, what was once regarded as conventional wisdom, evidence-based science and best practice, may now simply be rejected due to being proven to be bad science. Science is advanced only by challenging it. Medical dogma, ideologies, and egos have no place in science. The same goes for ethics.

Indeed, on a broader scale, the tragic and well-known travails of Dr Ignaz Semmelweis, in the mid-1800s clearly indicate that, at times, prevailing institutional wisdom may be inherently unscientific and blatantly incorrect, and even contribute significantly to high mortality rates. Semmelweis persisted, in the face of ridicule, in advocating basic hygiene and hand disinfection in obstetrical clinics, to combat puerperal fever in patients. History has since determined this to be correct procedure (rigorous hand washing was, for example, inter alia, also notably followed during the Covid-19 coronavirus pandemic). He lost his job, was ostracised and his life ended most tragically and prematurely in an asylum. Today Semmelweis is duly recognised as an early pioneer of antiseptic procedures.

Considering the considerable opprobrium, subsequently shown to be unjustified, heaped upon the proponents of the LCHF diet, as evidenced in the Noakes and Fettke professional conduct disciplinary hearings, the necessary question must be asked whether there is any safe way for a healthcare practitioner to negotiate the ethical minefield relating to dietary advice. This is especially so as current (the United States) dietary guidelines (followed in many countries and states) predominantly focus on HCLF (high carbohydrate low fat) diets, cereals, and maize, despite growing scientific evidence to the contrary.

The ethical conundrum faced by a medical practitioner, whose professional dietary convictions conflict with the prescripts of a regulating body, or official dietary guidelines, and a suggested ethical resolution of this dilemma, is concisely dealt with by Dr S.J. Genuis in a paper entitled *Dismembering the ethical physician* [109]. Certain passages warrant quotation in full:

> *Many times throughout history, existing medical dogma has been proved utterly wrong with the passage of time; accordingly, it should be permissible for practitioners to pursue truth, scientific fact, and moral behaviour as ultimate authority, rather than simply accepting authority or experts as the ultimate source of ethics, morality, or truth.*

Attempts to suppress this behaviour in medical practitioners, according to Dr Genuis, consists of an infringement on the medical practitioner's autonomy. One could go further and argue that the same would also amount to an infringement on the healthcare professional's constitutional right to self-determination.

He concludes the paper with the following:

> *... history has repeatedly shown that doctrinaire wisdom may ultimately be wrong and efforts to thwart independent thinking can stifle progress. Aristotle suggested that virtue lies as a mean between extremes. To facilitate advancement in ethical medicine and to avoid dismembering the ethical integrity of principled physicians, it is vital that the medical community, healthcare institutions, and governing organisations actively pursue a healthy and judicious tension between administrative regulation and support for personal autonomy in medical practice.*

Insofar as a medical practitioner's considered independent professional dietary advice may run contrary to institutional wisdom, ethics place a duty on such a practitioner to act according to his considered convictions. Referral to another practitioner who would not give advice in line with what the referring practitioner considers beneficial, and in the best interests of the patient, would conflict with the principle of 'do no harm' and not be in accordance with correct ethics. In the event of such non-alignment with institutional wisdom, it would be incumbent, however, on such a practitioner to inform the patient of such non-alignment, and of the right to seek other professional advice, and consult another healthcare practitioner. The healthcare practitioner has an ethical duty to ensure that the patient is fully informed of natural healthy dietary interventions and healthy lifestyle choices, and the various available health, treatment and management options and alternatives. It remains the patient's ultimate decision as to whether or not, and to what extent, to implement such professional advice, based on informed (consensual) decision-making.

In this modern day and age, with severe lifestyle disease and obesity, diet and nutrition have an important role to play in the management and prevention of disease, particularly chronic and non-communicable disease [110]. The medical health benefits of a robust immune system, accomplished, inter alia, by means of the utilisation of healthy natural dietary strategies and interventions, cannot be denied.

11.4.2 Public health: advocating for change

Joan Adams
Senior Legal Counsel (RSA) with a special interest in ethics. Chairperson of the HPCSA Professional Conduct Committee who acquitted Noakes in 2017.

Continued research, based on technological development in methodologies, as part of the advancement of science, often produces new knowledge that will and must ultimately change medical dogma, dietary guidelines and nutrition recommendations. Science is, after all, not static and is continually evolving. Science is only advanced by challenging it (legally and ethically). Most literature concerning the methods and ethical considerations relating to advocating for change, relate to political lobbying, which may be read *mutatis mutandis* in relation to advocating a medical interest, healthy natural wholesome diet and healthy lifestyle.

In an essay relating to the impact of expenditure by the pharmaceutical industry on lobbying in the United States [111] suggest that physicians have a responsibility to indulge in lobbying as well, as they should play an important role in shaping and policing the national healthcare system. This also applies to the matter under discussion, pertaining to dietary recommendations imposed carte blanche on a population as a whole. They suggest that physicians become educated and organised about creating political change. This challenge of medical and scientific dogma, established mindset and institutional 'wisdom' will bring about much needed change to international and national dietary guidelines.

It is trite that any form of lobbying must, however, be honest, transparent and done with integrity.

The appropriate approach would appear to be that espoused by Fernandez [112] who postulates that 'the most effective way to advocate any public policy is to be equipped with credible policy-analytic information.' The benefits of TCR are not only expounded by anecdotal clinical evidence, but also by multiple evidence-based scientific studies by reputable bodies, both completed and in the process of recruiting, much of which is freely available – it only requires objectivity and the absence of bias and vested interests. Reference to this credible evidence-based analytic information, properly circumscribed as not being a blanket panacea for all persons and all malaises, is both an available and persuasive tool.

Lobbying and advocating for change must, however, be performed in terms of core ethical rules and standards of practice relating to the medical and healthcare professions. Some form of professional accountability and regulation of the healthcare industry would indeed appear to be imperative in the interest of public safety and wellbeing. The attacks on proponents of TCR and the LCHF diet may, however, not come through rational and logical scientific evidence-based opposition, but disingenuously from governing or regulatory professional ethical rules (and even more so, the practical application and interpretation of those rules) relating to scope of practice and/or the doctor-patient relationship (as in the Fettke and Noakes [108] professional conduct disciplinary hearings in Australia and the RSA, respectively).

There are various forms of media available for the purpose of lobbying, especially social media platforms, where there is the potential for exponential and influential reach to patients, professionals, institutions, local communities, principalities, governments, and the general public alike. It is commonplace in this day and age for presidents, politicians, celebrities, so-called 'influencers', institutions and regulatory bodies to tweet and use other social media platforms to further their cause, and reach their followers, supporters, subscribers, registered members and the general public. Media and social media should, however, be used with circumspection and regulatory guidelines adhered to whenever available. Subsequent to the finalisation of the disciplinary and appeal hearing of Noakes during 2018, wherein Twitter took centre stage, the Health Professions Council of South Africa (HPCSA) was prompted to publish social media ethical guidelines [113]. Prior thereto regulatory HPCSA social media ethical guidelines were non-existent. The advice of Kushel and Bindman (*supra)* should be followed in this respect and proponents of TCR should be educated in respect of both the strengths and pitfalls of public media lobbying.

Current official dietary guidelines are somewhat inflexible, heavily in favour of cereals, maize, and carbohydrates, with the concomitant limitation of fatty foods – namely high carbohydrate, low fat (HCLF) diets [114]. There is, however, growing support globally for TCR and a good recent example is the United States. Every 5 years, the US Dietary Guidelines should be [112] updated to reflect the current body of scientific evidence on nutrition, food, and health. In July 2019, a coalition of doctors, academics, and American consumers, called the Low-Carb Action Network (LCAN), made compelling arguments before US nutrition leaders, to include a low carbohydrate diet, as part of the 2020 Dietary Guidelines for Americans (DGA) [115]. The exclusion in June 2020, by the Dietary Guidelines Advisory Committee, of all low-carbohydrate clinical studies, all clinical trials on weight-loss and other health benefits, and the failure to address numerous process and methodological concerns in its final report [116], is a strong sign that this battle is, unfortunately, far from over.

Advocating for change, and health and wellbeing of the general public, is a constitutional imperative in every democracy, with the concomitant freedom of expression (which includes freedom of opinion and freedom of scientific opinion); freedom of conscience; freedom of association and freedom to pursue legitimate interests and careers. Healthcare practitioners should indeed be encouraged to publish peer-reviewed articles and participate in scientific evidence-based clinical studies, become actively involved utilising diverse forms of advertising and marketing, inter alia, radio, television, documentaries and social media. To constructively influence national government it is necessary to work from the 'bottom-up' and to start at grass roots level, in educating the healthcare profession as a whole [108], the general public and communities, and local municipalities and principalities. By so doing institutional mindset, policy makers, national governments and states may ultimately be constructively persuaded and encouraged, by means of a growing support base of TCR proponents, including professionals, experts and scientists of high esteem, armed with robust, credible, and irrefutable scientific evidence. Formal evidence-based written submissions should be made, wherever possible, and certainly in response to draft legislation and policies. Endeavours should be made to testify before panels, and parliamentary and/or dietary advisory bodies, in order to refute medical and dietary dogma and ideologies. Healthcare professionals have a duty to become health activists in the interest of public health and safety.

References

[1] De Silva D. Helping People Help Themselves: A Review of the Evidence Considering Whether it is Worthwhile to Support Self-management. London: Health Foundation; 2011.

[2] Anderson RM, Funnell MM. Compliance and adherence are dysfunctional concepts in diabetes care. Diabetes Educ 2000;26(4):597–604.

[3] Anderson R, Funnell M. The Art of Empowerment: Stories and Strategies for Diabetes Educators. Virginia: American Diabetes Association; 2000.

[4] Mehrabian A. Silent Messages. Belmont, California: Wadsworth Publishing Company; 1971.

[5] Unwin D, Delon C, Unwin J, Tobin S, Taylor R. What predicts drug-free type 2 diabetes remission? Insights from an 8-year general practice service evaluation of a lower carbohydrate diet with weight loss. BMJ Nutr Prev Health 2023:e000544.

[6] Snyder C. Hope theory: rainbows in the mind. Psychological Inq 2002;13(4):249–75.

[7] Unwin J, Kacperek L, Clark C. A prospective study of positive adjustment to lower limb amputation. Clin Rehabil 2009;23:1044–50.

[8] Billington E, Simpson J, Unwin J, Bray D, Giles D. Does hope predict adjustment to end stage renal failure? Br J Health Psychol 2008;13 (4):683–700.

[9] Diener E, Chan M. Happy people live longer. Appl Psychol 2011;3(1):1–43.

[10] Unwin J, Dickson J. Goal focused hope, spiritual hope and well-being. Soc Sci Study Religion 2010;21:161–74.

[11] Frank J, Frank J. Persuasion and Healing. John Hopkins University press; 1993.

[12] Unwin D. SFGP! Why a solution-focused approach is brilliant in. Prim care Solut N 2005;1(4):10–12.

[13] O'Connell B. Solution-focused Therapy. Sage Publications Ltd.; 2012.

[14] Unwin D, Tobin S. A patient request for some 'deprescribing'. BMJ 2015;351:h4023.

[15] Unwin D, Khalid AA, Unwin J, Crocombe D, Delon C, Martyn K, et al. Insights from a general practice service evaluation supporting a lower carbohydrate diet in patients with type 2 diabetes mellitus and prediabetes: a secondary analysis of routine clinic data including HbA1c, weight and prescribing over 6 years. BMJ BMJ Nutr Prev Health 2020:bmjnph-2020-000072.

[16] Saslow L, Summers C, Aikens J, Unwin D. Outcomes of a digitally delivered low-carbohydrate type 2 diabetes self-management program. JMIR Diabetes 2018;3(3):e12.

[17] Hu T, Yao L, Reynolds K, Niu T, Li S, Whelton P, et al. The effects of a low-carbohydrate diet on appetite: a randomized controlled trial. Nutr Metab Cardiovasc Dis 2016;26(6):476–88.

[18] Neal DT, Wood W, Drolet A. How do people adhere to goals when willpower is low? The profits (and pitfalls) of strong habits. J Personality Soc Psychol 2013;104(6):959–75.

[19] Elfhag K, Rossner S. Who succeeds in maintaining weight loss? A conceptual review of factors associated with weight loss maintenance and weight regain. Obes Rev 2005;6(1):67–85. Available from: https://doi.org/10.1111/j.1467-789X.2005.00170.x.

[20] Pasman WJ, Saris WHM, Westerterp-Plantenga MS. Predictors of weight maintenance. Obes Res 1999;7(1):43–50. Available from: https://doi.org/10.1002/j.1550-8528.1999.tb00389.x.

[21] Taubes G. Good Calories Bad Calories. Knopf; 2007. p. 336–7.

[22] Stunkard AJ, Messick S. The three-factor eating questionnaire to measure dietary restraint, disinhibition and hunger. J Psychosom Res 1985;29 (1):71–83. Available from: https://doi.org/10.1016/0022-3999(85)90010-8.

[23] Yeomans MR, McCrickerd K. Acute hunger modifies responses on the three factor eating questionnaire hunger and disinhibition, but not restraint, scales. Appetite 2017;110:1–5. Available from: https://doi.org/10.1016/j.appet.2016.12.008.

[24] Friedman MI, Ulrich P, Mattes RD. A figurative measure of subjective hunger sensations. Appetite 1999;32(3):395–404. Available from: https://doi.org/10.1006/appe.1999.0230.

[25] Lowe MR, Friedman MI, Mattes R, Kopyt D, Gayda C. Comparison of verbal and pictorial measures of hunger during fasting in normal weight and obese subjects. Obes Res 2000;8(8):566–74. Available from: https://doi.org/10.1038/oby.2000.73.

[26] Boden G, Sargrad K, Homko C, Mozzoli M, Stein TP. Effect of a low-carbohydrate diet on appetite, blood glucose levels, and insulin resistance in obese patients with yype 2 diabetes. Ann Intern Med 2005;142(6):403–11. Available from: https://doi.org/10.7326/0003-4819-142-6-200503150-00006.

[27] Johnstone AM, Horgan GW, Murison SD, Bremner DM, Lobley GE. Effects of a high-protein ketogenic diet on hunger, appetite, and weight loss in obese men feeding ad libitum. Am J Clin Nutr 2008;87(1):44–55. Available from: https://doi.org/10.1093/ajcn/87.1.44.

[28] Nickols-Richardson SM, Coleman MD, Volpe JJ, Hosig KW. Perceived hunger is lower and weight loss is greater in overweight premenopausal women consuming a low-carbohydrate/high-protein vs high-carbohydrate/low-Fat diet. J Am Dietetic Assoc 2005;105(9):1433–7. Available from: https://doi.org/10.1016/j.jada.2005.06.025.

[29] Feinman RD, Pogozelski WK, Astrup A, Bernstein RK, Fine EJ, Westman EC, et al. Dietary carbohydrate restriction as the first approach in diabetes management: Critical review and evidence base. Nutrition 2015;31(1):1–13. Available from: https://doi.org/10.1016/j.nut.2014.06.011.

[30] Anguah KO-B, Syed-Abdul MM, Hu Q, Jacome-Sosa M, Heimowitz C, Cox V, et al. Changes in food cravings and eating behavior after a dietary carbohydrate restriction intervention trial. Nutrients 2019;12(1):52. Available from: https://doi.org/10.3390/nu12010052.

[31] Ratliff J, Mutungi G, Puglisi MJ, Volek JS, Fernandez ML. Carbohydrate restriction (with or without additional dietary cholesterol provided by eggs) reduces insulin resistance and plasma leptin without modifying appetite hormones in adult men. Nutr Res 2009;29(4):262–8. Available from: https://doi.org/10.1016/j.nutres.2009.03.007.

[32] McClernon FJ, Yancy WS, Eberstein JA, Atkins RC, Westman EC. The effects of a low-carbohydrate ketogenic diet and a low-fat diet on mood, hunger, and other self-reported symptoms. Obesity 2007;15(1):182. Available from: https://doi.org/10.1038/oby.2007.516.

[33] Martin CK, Rosenbaum D, Han H, Geiselman PJ, Wyatt HR, Hill JO, et al. Change in food cravings, food preferences, and appetite during a low-carbohydrate and low-fat diet. Obesity 2011;19(10):1963–70. Available from: https://doi.org/10.1038/oby.2011.62.

[34] Foster GD, Wyatt HR, Hill JO, Makris AP, Rosenbaum DL, Brill C, et al. Weight and metabolic outcomes after 2 years on a low-carbohydrate versus low-fat diet. Ann Intern Med 2010;153(3):147–57. Available from: https://doi.org/10.7326/0003-4819-153-3-201008030-00005.

[35] Johnston CS, Tjonn SL, Swan PD. High-protein, low-fat diets are effective for weight loss and favorably alter biomarkers in healthy adults. J Nutr 2004;134(3):586–91. Available from: https://doi.org/10.1093/jn/134.3.586.

[36] Veldhorst MAB, Westerterp KR, van Vught AJAH, Westerterp-Plantenga MS. Presence or absence of carbohydrates and the proportion of fat in a high-protein diet affect appetite suppression but not energy expenditure in normal-weight human subjects fed in energy balance. Br J Nutr 2010;104(9):1395–405. Available from: https://doi.org/10.1017/S0007114510002060.

[37] Deemer SE, Plaisance EP, Martins C. Impact of ketosis on appetite regulation—A review. Nutr Res 2020;77:1–11. Available from: https://doi.org/10.1016/j.nutres.2020.02.010.

[38] Gibson AA, Seimon RV, Lee CMY, Ayre J, Franklin J, Markovic TP, et al. Do ketogenic diets really suppress appetite? A systematic review and meta-analysis: Do ketogenic diets really suppress appetite? Obes Rev 2015;16(1):64–76. Available from: https://doi.org/10.1111/obr.12230.

[39] Stubbs BJ, Cox PJ, Evans RD, Cyranka M, Clarke K, de Wet H. A ketone ester drink lowers human ghrelin and appetite. Obesity 2018;26(2):269–73. Available from: https://doi.org/10.1002/oby.22051.

[40] Volek J, Phinney SD. The Art and Science of Low Carbohydrate Performance: A Revolutionary Program to Extend Your Physical and Mental Performance Envelope. Beyond Obesity LLC; 2012. p. 89–90.

[41] Müller TD, Nogueiras R, Andermann ML, Andrews ZB, Anker SD, Argente J, et al. Ghrelin. Mol Metab 2015;4(6):437–60. Available from: https://doi.org/10.1016/j.molmet.2015.03.005.

[42] Begaye B, Vinales KL, Hollstein T, Ando T, Walter M, Bogardus C, et al. Impaired metabolic flexibility to high-fat overfeeding predicts future weight gain in healthy adults. Diabetes 2020;69(2):181–92. Available from: https://doi.org/10.2337/db19-0719.

[43] Giacco R, Clemente G, Busiello L, Lasorella G, Rivieccio AM, Rivellese AA, et al. Insulin sensitivity is increased and fat oxidation after a high-fat meal is reduced in normal-weight healthy men with strong familial predisposition to overweight. Int J Obes 2003;27(7):790–6. Available from: https://doi.org/10.1038/sj.ijo.0802306.

[44] Ji H, Friedman MI. Reduced capacity for fatty acid oxidation in rats with inherited susceptibility to diet-induced obesity. Metabolism 2007;56(8):1124–30. Available from: https://doi.org/10.1016/j.metabol.2007.04.006.

[45] Ji H, Friedman MI. Reduced hepatocyte fatty acid oxidation in outbred rats prescreened for susceptibility to diet-induced obesity. Int J Obes 2008;32(8):1331–4. Available from: https://doi.org/10.1038/ijo.2008.71.

[46] Paoli A, Rubini A, Volek JS, Grimaldi KA. Beyond weight loss: a review of the therapeutic uses of very-low-carbohydrate (ketogenic) diets. Eur J Clin Nutr 2013;67(8):789–96.

[47] Boswell RG, Kober H. Food cue reactivity and craving predict eating and weight gain: a meta-analytic review. Obes Rev 2016;17(2):159–77.

[48] Avena NM, Bocarsly ME, Hoebel BG. Animal models of sugar and fat bingeing: relationship to food addiction and increased body weight. Methods Mol Biol 2012;829:351–65.

[49] Tukey DS, Ferreira JM, Antoine SO, D'Amour J A, Ninan I, Cabeza de Vaca S, et al. Sucrose ingestion induces rapid AMPA receptor trafficking. J Neurosci 2013;33(14):6123–32.

[50] Spreadbury I. Comparison with ancestral diets suggests dense acellular carbohydrates promote an inflammatory microbiota, and may be the primary dietary cause of leptin resistance and obesity. Diabetes Metab Syndr Obes 2012;5:175–89.

[51] Takahashi M, Fukunaga H, Kaneto H, Fukudome S, Yoshikawa M. Behavioral and pharmacological studies on gluten exorphin A5, a newly isolated bioactive food protein fragment, in mice. Jpn J Pharmacol 2000;84(3):259–65.

[52] Cocores JA, Gold MS. The salted food addiction hypothesis may explain overeating and the obesity epidemic. Med Hypotheses 2009;73 (6):892–9.

[53] Ziauddeen H, Alonso-Alonso M, Hill JO, Kelley M, Khan NA. Obesity and the neurocognitive basis of food reward and the control of intake. Adv Nutr 2015;6(4):474–86.

[54] Teschemacher H, Koch G, Brantl V. Milk protein-derived opioid receptor ligands. Biopolymers 1997;43(2):99–117.

[55] Ferré S. Mechanisms of the psychostimulant effects of caffeine: implications for substance use disorders. Psychopharmacol (Berl) 2016;233 (10):1963–79.

[56] Onaolapo AY, Onaolapo OJ. Food additives, food and the concept of 'food addiction': Is stimulation of the brain reward circuit by food sufficient to trigger addiction? Pathophysiology 2018;25(4):263–76.

[57] Ifland JR, Preuss HG. Focusing the fight against food addiction. In: Preuss HG, Bagchi D, editors. Dietary Fat, Salt, and Sugar in Dietary Health. New York: Elsevier; 2020.

[58] Gordon EL, Ariel-Donges AH, Bauman V, Merlo LJ. What is the evidence for "food addiction?" A systematic review. Nutrients [Internet] 2018;10(4). Available from: https://www.ncbi.nlm.nih.gov/pmc/articles/PMC5946262/.

[59] Pedram P, Wadden D, Amini P, Gulliver W, Randell E, Cahill F, et al. Food addiction: its prevalence and significant association with obesity in the general population. PLoS One 2013;8(9):e74832.

[60] Volkow ND, Wang GJ, Fowler JS, Tomasi D, Baler R. Food and drug reward: overlapping circuits in human obesity and addiction. Curr Top Behav Neurosci 2012;11:1–24.

[61] Noori HR, Cosa Linan A, Spanagel R. Largely overlapping neuronal substrates of reactivity to drug, gambling, food and sexual cues: A comprehensive meta-analysis. Eur Neuropsychopharmacol 2016;26(9):1419–30.

[62] Esch T, Stefano GB. The neurobiology of pleasure, reward processes, addiction and their health implications. Neuro Endocrinol Lett 2004;25 (4):235–51.

[63] Kelley AE, Schiltz CA, Landry CF. Neural systems recruited by drug- and food-related cues: studies of gene activation in corticolimbic regions. Physiol Behav 2005;86(1-2):11–14.

[64] Stice E, Dagher A. Genetic variation in dopaminergic reward in humans. Forum Nutr 2010;63:176–85.

[65] Blum K, Thanos PK, Badgaiyan RD, Febo M, Oscar-Berman M, Fratantonio J, et al. Neurogenetics and gene therapy for reward deficiency syndrome: are we going to the Promised Land? Expert Opin Biol Ther 2015;15(7):973–85.

[66] Ifland JR, Marcus MT, Preuss HG, editors. Processed Food Addiction: Foundations, Assessment, and Recovery. Boca Ratan, FL: CRC Press; 2018.

[67] Mole TB, Irvine MA, Worbe Y, Collins P, Mitchell SP, Bolton S, et al. Impulsivity in disorders of food and drug misuse. Psychol Med 2015;45 (4):771–82.

[68] Suliburska J, Duda G, Pupek-Musialik D. Effect of tobacco smoking on taste sensitivity in adults. Przegl Lek 2004;61(10):1174–6.

[69] Sartor F, Donaldson LF, Markland DA, Loveday H, Jackson MJ, Kubis HP. Taste perception and implicit attitude toward sweet related to body mass index and soft drink supplementation. Appetite 2011;57(1):237–46.

[70] McLellan AT, Cacciola JC, Alterman AI, Rikoon SH, Carise D. The addiction severity index at 25: origins, contributions and transitions. Am J Addict 2006;15(2):113–24.

[71] Ifland J, Sheppard KK, Wright HT. The Addiction severity index in the assessment of processed food addiction. In: Ifland J, Marcus MT, Preuss HG, editors. Processed Food Addiction: Foundations, Assessment, and Recovery. Boca Ratan, FL: CRC Press; 2017. p. 289–306.

[72] Raimo EB, Smith TL, Danko GP, Bucholz KK, Schuckit MA. Clinical characteristics and family histories of alcoholics with stimulant dependence. J Stud Alcohol 2000;61(5):728–35.

[73] Krahnstoever Davison K, Francis LA, Birch LL. Reexamining obesigenic families: parents' obesity-related behaviors predict girls' change in BMI. Obes Res 2005;13(11):1980–90.

[74] Dube SR, Anda RF, Felitti VJ, Croft JB, Edwards VJ, Giles WH. Growing up with parental alcohol abuse: exposure to childhood abuse, neglect, and household dysfunction. Child Abuse Negl 2001;25(12):1627–40.

[75] Mason SM, Flint AJ, Field AE, Austin SB, Rich-Edwards JW. Abuse victimization in childhood or adolescence and risk of food addiction in adult women. Obes (Silver Spring) 2013;21(12):E775–81.

[76] Mattson SN, Roesch SC, Fagerlund A, Autti-Ramo I, Jones KL, May PA, et al. Toward a neurobehavioral profile of fetal alcohol spectrum disorders. Alcohol Clin Exp Res 2010;34(9):1640–50.

[77] Goran MI, Plows JF, Ventura EE. Effects of consuming sugars and alternative sweeteners during pregnancy on maternal and child health: evidence for a secondhand sugar effect. Proc Nutr Soc 2019;78(3):262–71.

[78] Swedberg MD. Drug discrimination: A versatile tool for characterization of CNS safety pharmacology and potential for drug abuse. J Pharmacol Toxicol Methods 2016;81:295–305.

[79] Moore CF, Sabino V, Koob GF, Cottone P. Pathological overeating: emerging evidence for a compulsivity construct. Neuropsychopharmacol. 2017;42:1375–89.

[80] Connor JP, Gullo MJ, White A, Kelly AB. Polysubstance use: diagnostic challenges, patterns of use and health. Curr Opin Psychiatry 2014;27 (4):269–75.

[81] Schulte EM, Avena NM, Gearhardt AN. Which foods may be addictive? The roles of processing, fat content, and glycemic load. PLoS One 2015;10(2):e0117959.

[82] Food Addicts Anonymous (2010). Port St. Lucie, FL.

[83] Reis RK, Fiellin DA, editors. The ASAM Principles of Addiction Medicine. Wolters Kluwer Health; 2014.

[84] Giovino GA, Henningfield JE, Tomar SL, Escobedo LG, Slade J. Epidemiology of tobacco use and dependence. Epidemiol Rev 1995;17 (1):48–65.

[85] Ogden CL, Yanovski SZ, Carroll MD, Flegal KM. The epidemiology of obesity. Gastroenterology 2007;132(6):2087–102.

[86] Finkelstein EA, Trogdon JG, Cohen JW, Dietz W. Annual medical spending attributable to obesity: payer-and service-specific estimates. Health Aff (Millwood) 2009;28(5):w822–31.

[87] National Institute of Drug Abuse. (2015). Costs of Substance Abuse. Retrieved March 10, 2017, from https://www.drugabuse.gov/related-topics/trends-statistics.

[88] Tillotson JE. America's obesity: conflicting public policies, industrial economic development, and unintended human consequences. Annu Rev Nutr 2004;24:617–43.

[89] Glynn T, Seffrin JR, Brawley OW, Grey N, Ross H. The globalization of tobacco use: 21 challenges for the 21st century. CA Cancer J Clin 2010;60(1):50–61.

[90] Volkow ND, Koob GF, McLellan AT. Neurobiologic advances from the brain disease model of addiction. N Engl J Med 2016;374 (4):363–71.

[91] Kelly JF, Greene MC, Bergman BG, White WL, Hoeppner BB. How many recovery attempts does it take to successfully resolve an alcohol or drug problem? estimates and correlates from a national study of recovering U.S. adults. Alcohol Clin Exp Res 2019;43(7):1533–44.

[92] Turk MW, Yang K, Hravnak M, Sereika SM, Ewing LJ, Burke LE. Randomized clinical trials of weight loss maintenance: a review. J Cardiovasc Nurs 2009;24(1):58–80.

[93] Johnson BA, Cloninger CR, Roache JD, Bordnick PS, Ruiz P. Age of onset as a discriminator between alcoholic subtypes in a treatment-seeking outpatient population. Am J Addict 2000;9(1):17–27.

[94] Schuz B, Bower J, Ferguson SG. Stimulus control and affect in dietary behaviours. An intensive longitudinal study. Appetite 2015;87C:310–17.

[95] Powell K, Wilcox J, Clonan A, Bissell P, Preston L, Peacock M, et al. The role of social networks in the development of overweight and obesity among adults: a scoping review. BMC Public Health 2015;15:996.

[96] Martire SI, Westbrook RF, Morris MJ. Effects of long-term cycling between palatable cafeteria diet and regular chow on intake, eating patterns, and response to saccharin and sucrose. Physiol Behav 2015;139:80–8.

[97] Donovan. Evidence-based assessment: strategies and measures in addictive behaviors. In: McCrady B, Epstein E, editors. Addictions: A Comprehensive Guidebook. Oxford: Oxford University Press; 2013.

[98] Donovan DM, Ifland J. Diagnosing and assessing processed food addiction. In: Ifland J, Marcus MT, Preuss HG, editors. Processed Food Addiction: Foundations, Assessment, and Recovery. Boca Ratan, FL: CRC Press; 2017. p. 121–36.

[99] Khan TA, Sievenpiper JL. Controversies about sugars: results from systematic reviews and meta-analyses on obesity, cardiometabolic disease and diabetes. Eur J Nutr 2016;55(Suppl 2):25–43.

[100] Ifland J, Preuss HG, Marcus MT, Wright HT, Taylor WC, Sheppard K, et al. Abstinent food plans for processed food addiction. In: Ifland J, Marcus MT, Preuss HG, editors. Processed Food Addiction: Foundations, Assessment, and Recovery. Boca Ratan, FL: CRC Press; 2017. p. 462.

[101] Lifshitz F, Lifshitz JZ. Globesity: the root causes of the obesity epidemic in the USA and now worldwide. Pediatr Endocrinol Rev 2014;12 (1):17–34.

[102] Ifland JR, Preuss HG, Marcus MT, Rourke KM, Taylor WC, Burau K, et al. Refined food addiction: a classic substance use disorder. Med Hypotheses 2009;72(5):518–26.

[103] Allison S. Basics in clinical nutrition: Ethical and legal aspects. E-spen, Eur E-journal Clin Nutr Metab 2008;3. Available from: https://doi.org/10.1016/j.eclnm.2008.07.004.

[104] Chandramohan P. Ups and downs in the history of medical ethics. Arch Med Health Sci 2013;1(Issue 2):191–4.

[105] Gillon R. Medical ethics: four principles plus attention to scope. BMJ 1994;309(6948):184–8. Available from: https://doi.org/10.1136/bmj.309.6948.184.

[106] Summers J. Health Care Ethics: Critical Issues for the 21st Century. 2nd edition Sudbury, MA: Jones and Bartlett Publishers; 2009. p. 41–58.

[107] De Villiers F. Ethical decision-making in clinical nutritional practice. Food Nutr Sci 2011;2:641–6. Available from: https://doi.org/10.4236/fns.2011.26089.

[108] Noakes T. Lore of Nutrition: Challenging conventional dietary beliefs. Penguin Random House South Africa; 2017 Nov 1.

[109] Genuis SJ. Dismembering the ethical physician. Postgrad Med J 2006;82(966):233–8. Available from: https://doi.org/10.1136/pgmj.2005.037754.

[110] Kris-Etherton P, Akabas S, Douglas P. Nutrition competencies in health professionals' education and training: a new paradigm. Adv Nutr 2015;6(Issue 1):83–7. Available from: https://doi.org/10.3945/an.114.006734.

[111] Kushel M, Bindman AB. Health care lobbying: time make patients spec interest. Am J Med 2004;116(Issue 7):496–7. Available from: https://doi.org/10.1016/j.amjmed.2004.02.011.

[112] A.N. Fernandes, Ethical Considerations of the Public Sector Lobbyist, 41 McGeorge L. Rev. (2009). https://scholarlycommons.pacific.edu/mlr/vol41/iss1/6.

[113] Health Professions Council of South Africa (HPCSA) Ethical Guidelines. Booklet 16: Ethical Guidelines on Social Media (2019). https://www.hpcsa.co.za/Uploads/Professional_Practice/Ethics_Booklet.pdf.

[114] Dietary Guidelines for Americans (2020–2025). 164. https://www.dietaryguidelines.gov/sites/default/files/2020-12/Dietary_Guidelines_for_Americans_2020-2025.pdf.
[115] https://www.foodnavigator-usa.com/Article/2019/12/20/Coalition-pushes-for-low-carb-diet-to-be-added-to-2020-Dietary-Guidelines.
[116] https://lowcarbaction.org/science-excluded-from-dga-advisory-committee-report/.

Further reading

Malpass T. The Hope That I Have: To Remission and Beyond. Print2Demand; 2018.
Unwin D, Unwin J. A simple model to find patient hope for positive lifestyle changes: GRIN. J Holist Healthc 2019;16(2).
Wortley KE, Anderson KD, Garcia K, Murray JD, Malinova L, Liu R, et al. Genetic deletion of ghrelin does not decrease food intake but influences metabolic fuel preference. Proc Natl Acad Sci USA 2004;101(21):8227–32. Available from: https://doi.org/10.1073/pnas.0402763101 PMID:15148384 PMCID: PMC419585.

Acronyms

PD	Parkinson's disease
HCPs	Healthcare professionals
BBB	Blood–brain barrier
CNS	Central nervous system
T2D	Type 2 diabetes
TZD	Thiazolidinediones
T1D	Type 1 diabetes
KD	Ketogenic diet
MetS	Metabolic syndrome
GNG	Gluconeogenesis
BOHB	Beta-hydroxybutyrate
AcAc	Acetoacetate
DHA	Docosahexaenoic acid
LCHF	Low-carbohydrate high-fat
CAD	Coronary artery disease
IR	Insulin resistance
IS	Insulin secretion
ATP	Adenosine triphosphate
NS	Nitrogen species
ROS	Reactive oxygen species
AGE	Advanced glycation end products
IRS	Insulin receptor substrate
TCR	Therapeutic carbohydrate restriction
MMT	Mitochondrial metabolic theory of cancer
SMT	Somatic mutation theory of cancer
OxPhos	Oxidative phosphorylation
mSLP	Mitochondrial substrate-level phosphorylation
FG	Fasting glucose
OGTT	Oral glucose tolerance test
LDL	Low-density lipoproteins
PV	Portal vein
ARR	Absolute risk reduction
EEG	Electroencephalogram
LCT	Long-chain triglycerides
MAD	Modified Atkins diet
MCT	Medium-chain triglycerides
LGIT	Low-glycemic index treatment
AD	Alzheimer's disease
MCI	Mild cognitive impairment
MoCA	Montreal cognitive assessment
MDD	Major depressive disorders
GI	Glycemic index
MPTP	1-methyl-4-phenyl-1,2,3,6-propionoxypiperidine
ASD	Autism spectrum disorder
SGLT	Sodium-coupled glucose transporters
ALS	Amyotrophic lateral sclerosis
TBI	Traumatic brain injury

GCS	Glasgow coma scale
ATLS	Advanced trauma life skills
CT	Computerised tomography
SIBO	Small intestinal bacterial overgrowth
PFA	Processed food addiction
KD-R	Restricted ketogenic diet
TCA	Tricarboxylic acid
SLP	Substrate-level phosphorylation
FAD	Flavin adenine dinucleotide
NAD	Nicotinamide adenine dinucleotide
DON	6-diazo-5-oxo-L-norleucine
CR	Calorie restriction
GKI	Glucose ketone index
2-DG	2-deoxyglucose
GBM	Glioblastoma multiforme
HBOT	Hyperbaric oxygen therapy
FFA	Free fatty acids
NAD +	Nicotinamide adenine dinucleotide
Nrf2	NF-E2-related factor 2
AMP	Adenosine monophosphate
AMPK	AMP-activated protein kinase
BDNF	Brain-derived neurotrophic factor
BMI	Body mass index
DM	Diabetes mellitus
GERD	Gastroesophageal reflux disease
GH	Growth hormone
IF	Intermittent fasting IF
IGF-1	Insulin-like growth factor
FDA	Food and Drug Administration
mTOR	Mammalian target of rapamycin
NHANES	National Health and Nutrition Examination Survey
NICE	National Institute for Health and Clinical Excellence
PI3K	Phosphoinositide 3-kinase
SIRT1	Sirtuin 1

Index

Note: Page numbers followed by "*f*," "*t*," and "*b*" refer to figures, tables, and boxes, respectively.

A

B

F

I

K

M

O

P

Q

R

U

V

9780128216170